P9-CRS-879

ACUTE MYOCARDIAL INFARCTION

Second Edition

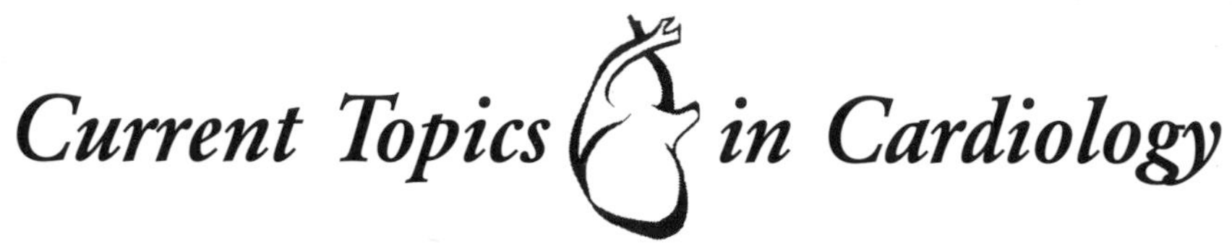

Series Editor

Shahbudin H. Rahimtoola, MB, FRCP
George C. Griffith Professor of Cardiology
Chief, Division of Cardiology
University of Southern California School of Medicine
Los Angeles, California

Acute Myocardial Infarction Second Edition
Bernard J. Gersh, MB, ChB, DPhil, FRCP
Shahbudin H. Rahimtoola, MB, FRCP

Heart Failure
David McCall, MD, PhD
Shahbudin H. Rahimtoola, MB, FRCP

A Primer of Molecular Biology
Robert Roberts, MD
Jeffrey Towbin, MD
Thomas Parker, MD, PhD
Roger D. Bies, MD

ACUTE MYOCARDIAL INFARCTION

Second Edition

edited by

Bernard J. Gersh, MB, ChB, DPhil, FRCP

W. Proctor Harvey Teaching Professor in Cardiology
Chief, Division of Cardiology
Georgetown University Medical Center

Shahbudin H. Rahimtoola, MB, FRCP, MACP

Distinguished Professor, George C. Griffith Professor of Cardiology,
Professor of Medicine, University of Southern California

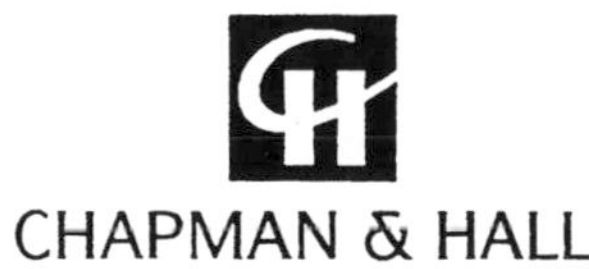

CHAPMAN & HALL

ITP® International Thomson Publishing

New York • Albany • Bonn • Boston • Cincinnati • Detroit • London • Madrid • Melbourne
Mexico City • Pacific Grove • Paris • San Francisco • Singapore • Tokyo • Toronto • Washington

No responsibility is assumed by the Publisher for any injury and/or damage to persons or property as a matter of products liability, negligence or otherwise, or from any use or operation of any methods, products, instructions or ideas contained in the material herein. No suggested test or procedure should be carried out unless, in the reader's judgement, its risk is justified. Because of rapid advances in the medical sciences, we recommend that independent verification of diagnoses and drug dosages should be made. Discussion, views and recommendations as to medical procedures, choice of drugs, and drug dosages are the responsibility of the authors.

Cover Design: Andrea Meyer, emDASH inc.

Printed in the United States of America

For more information, contact:

Chapman & Hall
115 Fifth Avenue
New York, NY 10003

Chapman & Hall
2-6 Boundary Row
London SE1 8HN
England

Thomas Nelson Australia
102 Dodds Street
South Melbourne, 3205
Victoria, Australia

Chapman & Hall GmbH
Postfach 100 263
D-69442 Weinheim
Germany

International Thomson Editores
Campos Eliseos 385, Piso 7
Col. Polanco
11560 Mexico D.F.
Mexico

International Thomson Publishing-Japan
Hirakawacho-cho Kyowa Building, 3F
1-2-1 Hirakawacho-cho
Chiyoda-ku, 102 Tokyo
Japan

International Thomson Publishing Asia
221 Henderson Road #05-10
Henderson Building
Singapore 0315

1 2 3 4 5 6 7 8 9 10 XXX 01 00 99 97

Library of Congress Cataloging-in-Publication Data

Acute myocardial infarction / [edited by] Bernard J. Gersh, Shahbudin H. Rahimtoola,—2nd ed.
p. cm. — (Current topics in cardiology)
Includes bibliographical references and index.
ISBN 0-412-07341-2 (alk. paper)
1. Myocardial infarction. I. Gersh, Bernard J. II. Rahimtoola, Shahbudin H. III. Series.
[DNLM: 1. Myocardial Infarction—diagnosis.
2. Myocardial Infarction—pathology. 3. Myocardial Infarction—therapy. WG 300 A189 1996]
RC685.I6A2372 1996
616.1'237—dc20
DNLM/DLC
for Library of Congress
96-16761
CIP

British Library Cataloguing in Publication Data available

To order this or any other Chapman & Hall book, please contact **International Thomson Publishing, 7625 Empire Drive, Florence, KY 41042.** Phone: (606) 525-6600 or 1-800-842-3636.
Fax: (606) 525-7778, e-mail: order@chaphall.com.

For a complete listing of Chapman & Hall's titles, send your requests to
Chapman & Hall, Dept. BC, 115 Fifth Avenue, New York, NY 10003.

This book is dedicated to our families and colleagues.

Contents

Foreword to the Series

My career in Cardiology extends over four decades and has spanned a period of great excitement. This period has witnessed the development of better and more sophisticated diagnostic methods and therapeutic approaches; the excitement continues at an accelerated pace. The Series, CURRENT TOPICS IN CARDIOLOGY, is intended to collate, in a comprehensive manner, the important aspects of the rapidly expanding knowledge in a variety of topics in cardiovascular medicine. It is hoped that the series will be of value to practicing physicians and specialists, investigators, and academicians.

I am grateful to Chapman & Hall for their generous support, encouragement, and above all patience; this has provided me with the excitement and thrill of putting this series together. The editors of each book deserve the credit for the volume they put together; I am grateful to them for their hard work and willingness to undertake an important task.

I would like to dedicate this Series to those who have made all of this excitement possible for me. They include: (1) patients who have willingly consented to partake in clinical research, (2) close collaboration between basic and clinical scientists, (3) investigators, in particular, the clinician-clinical investigators who have created a milieu of great excitement and have also been responsible for the rapid transfer of research findings to clinical care, (4) several teachers and colleagues who have influenced me greatly, (5) colleagues and friends throughout the world for exchange of thoughts and ideas and collaboration in research endeavors, and (5) my family, my wife Shameem, and our children, Aly, Nadia, and Yasmin.

Shahbudin H. Rahimtoola, MB, FRCP, MACP

Foreword

At the beginning of this century, coronary occlusion was generally considered to be immediately and invariably fatal. In the second decade it became appreciated that survival could occur, and soon thereafter the clinical features of the syndrome, the principal clinical-pathologic correlations, and characteristic diagnostic electrocardiographic changes of acute myocardial infarction were described. Acute myocardial infarction and death therefrom were observed with increasing frequency. By mid-century acute myocardial infarction was recognized as the most common cause of death in industrialized nations. One-third of all afflicted patients died before even reaching the hospital and an equal fraction then succumbed prior to hospital discharge; the mortality rate of survivors following discharge was also high. To make matters worse, many patients were struck down in the prime of life. The physician was little more that a helpless bystander who was able to offer little more than pain relief and to order bed rest and anticoagulants.

Then, at first slowly and subsequently more rapidly, the tide began to turn. The diagnosis and successful treatment of cardiac arrhythmias coupled with the development of the coronary care unit made the first large dent in mortality. The recognition that myocardial infarction is a dynamic process that can be modified *after* coronary occlusion, followed by the development of thrombolytic therapy and other techniques of reperfusion led to further decisive reductions in mortality. As we approach the end of the century, the in-hospital mortality has now declined to about 5%, and the one-year mortality for patients discharged from the hospital is just 2%. Thus, mortality is now reduced to about one sixth of what it was just three decades ago. Even the *incidence* of acute myocardial infarction is declining.

What is responsible for this success story? Certainly not a single discovery, such as the development of a vaccine or antibiotic. Rather, it has involved a chipping away at numerous aspects of the problem. *Acute Myocardial Infarction,* well written by recognized experts in every aspect of the condition and superbly edited by Drs. Gersh and Rahimtoola, two leaders of contemporary cardiology, provides a comprehensive survey of every up-to-date development that has been responsible for these notable improvements in outcome; These include diagnosis, prehospital treatment, emergency management, the prevention, early recognition and prompt treatment of complications, risk stratification, and post-hospital management based on this stratification.

Several aspects of this book are particularly notable. First, it achieves the often elusive but important blend of the practical and the theoretical. While it provides much useful down-to-earth information on the management of the patient with acute myocardial infarction, this book is *much* more than an excellent manual of coronary care. It provides the scientific underpinnings of pathogenesis, pathophysiology and pharmacology necessary for the understanding of the disease process and the many subtle aspects of its management. Second, due to the skill of the editors, it maintains a clear objective, and keeps the scope, content and length all within reasonable bounds. Third, this book is as current as this month's journals, a difficult editorial task in a field that is changing so swiftly.

While we have come a long way in the care of the patients with acute myocardial infarction, there is still much to accomplish and *Acute Myocardial Infarction* points the way to the future by identifying problems which must now be addressed. The next challenge is to prevent the development of acute coronary events. If this challenge is met successfully (and there are many provocative ideas in this book as to how this might be achieved), then we will have come full circle and should be able to enter the next century with coronary artery disease low on the list of mankind's fatal, disabling illnesses.

Although the first edition of *Acute Myocardial Infarction* was superb, as happens so often with outstanding textbooks, the second edition is superior. Important new material has been added and an even higher standard of excellence has been achieved. I look forward to the third edition.

Eugene Braunwald, MD
Vice President for Academic Programs
Partners HealthCare System
Distinguished Hersey Professor of Medicine,
Harvard Medical School
Boston, MA

Preface

Acute myocardial infarction is one of the most important CURRENT TOPICS IN CARDIOLOGY today. Many factors—including changing epidemiology of coronary artery disease, earlier diagnosis, and more effective treatment—have radically altered the management of patients with this disorder. The emergence of therapy aimed at acute reperfusion has heralded an era of profound change: a therapeutic revolution. There has been a virtual explosion of data about diagnosis, pathophysiology, characterization of clinical subgroups, and treatment of patients with acute myocardial infarction. The first edition was received with great enthusiasm which has led to this edition, the second one. In this edition, a couple of chapters have been deleted, all the remaining chapters have been revised and updated. In addition, several new chapters are included. This monograph is designed to provide a comprehensive, detailed overview of acute myocardial infarction in the current era; we hope this will lead to better care of patients.

Bernard J. Gersh, MB, ChB, DPhil, FRCP
Shahbudin H. Rahimtoola, MB, FRCP, MACP

Contributors

JOSEPH S. ALPERT, MD
Robert S. and Irene P. Flinn Chair of Medicine
Professor of Medicine
University of Arizona College of Medicine
Tucson, Arizona

JOHN A. AMBROSE, MD
Professor of Medicine
Mount Sinai Medical Center
New York, New York

GEORGE A. BELLER, MD, FACC
Ruth C. Heede Professor Cardiology and Professor of Internal Medicine
Chief, Cardiovascular Division, Department of Internal Medicine
University of Virginia Health Sciences Center
Charlottesville, Virginia

ANIL K. BHANDARI, MBBS
Director, Electrophysiology Laboratory
Good Samaritan Hospital
Clinical Associate Professor of Medicine
University of Southern California School of Medicine
Los Angeles, California

ROBERT M. CALIFF, MD, FACC
Professor of Medicine
Duke University Medical Center
Director, Duke Clinical Research Institute
Durham, North Carolina

JAMES H. CHESEBRO, MD
Professor of Medicine
Director of Clinical Research
Cardiovascular Institute
Mount Sinai Medical Center
New York, New York

MYLAN C. COHEN, MD, MPH
Cardiovascular Division
Deaconess Hospital
Harvard Medical School
Boston, Massachusetts

LAURA J. COLLINS, MD
Instructor in Medicine
Department of Medicine
Cardiology Division
University of Texas Health Science Center
San Antonio, Texas

LOUIS J. DELL'ITALIA, MD
Associate Professor, Clinical Director
Cardiology Fellowship Training Program
The University of Alabama at Birmingham
School of Medicine
Birmingham, Alabama

PAMELA S. DOUGLAS, MD
Associate Professor of Medicine
Harvard Medical School
Director, Noninvasive Cardiology
Beth Israel Hospital
Boston, Massachusetts

WILLIAM D. EDWARDS, MD
Consultant, Division of Anatomic Pathology
Professor of Pathology, Mayo Medical School
Mayo Graduate School of Medicine
Rochester, Minnesota

PAUL R. EISENBERG, MD, MPH
Associate Professor of Medicine
Washington University School of Medicine
Medical Director, Cardiac Care Unit
Barnes-Jewish Hospital
St. Louis, Missouri

GERALD F. FLETCHER, MD
Professor of Medicine
Mayo Medical School
Senior Associate Consultant
Cardiovascular Diseases
Mayo Clinic Jacksonville
Jacksonville, Florida

MERVYN B. FORMAN, MD Bch, PhD, FRCP (Ed)
Clinical Professor of Medicine
Department of Medicine
Emory University
Atlanta, Georgia

WILLIAM H. FRISHMAN, MD
Professor and Associate Chairman
Department of Medicine
Albert Einstein College of Medicine
Bronx, New York

VALENTIN FUSTER, MD, PhD
Arthur M. and Hilda E. Master Professor of Medicine
Director, Cardiovascular Institute
Mount Sinai School of Medicine
New York, New York

W. BRUCE FYE, MD, MA
Chair, Cardiology Department, Marshfield Clinic
Clinical Professor of Medicine and Adjunct Professor of the History of Medicine
University of Wisconsin, Madison
Madison, Wisconsin

RICHARD GALLO, MD, FRCPC
Associate Professor of Medicine
University of Montreal Faculty of Medicine
Montreal, Quebec Canada

BERNARD J. GERSH, MB, ChB, DPhil, FRCP
Dr. Proctor Harvey Teaching Professor of Cardiology
Chief, Division of Cardiology
Georgetown University Medial Center
Washington, DC

LEONARD S. GETTES, MD
Professor of Medicine
Division of Cardiology
University of North Carolina
Chapel Hill, North Carolina

ROBERT S. GIBSON, MD
Professor and Vice-Chairman
Department of Medicine
University of Virginia School of Medicine
Charlottesville, Virginia

J. ANTHONY GOMES, MD
Professor of Medicine
Mount Sinai School of Medicine of CUNY
Director, Section of Electrophysiology and Electrocardiography
Mount Sinai Medical Center
New York, New York

JUDITH S. HOCHMAN, MD
Associate Professor of Medicine
College of Physicians & Surgeons of Columbia University
Director, Cardiac Care Unit & Cardiac Step Down Unit
St. Luke's / Roosevelt Hospital Center
New York, New York

DAVID R. HOLMES, JR., MD
Professor of Medicine
Mayo Medical School
Director of Adult Cardiac Catheterization Laboratory
Mayo Clinic
Rochester, Minnesota

ALLAN S. JAFFE, MD
Professor and Chief of the Division of Cardiovascular Medicine
Department of Medicine
State University of New York Health Science Center at Syracuse
Syracuse, New York

DALANE W. KITZMAN, MD
Assistant Professor of Internal Medicine
Director of Echocardiography
Bowman Gray School of Medicine of Wake Forest University
Winston-Salem, North Carolina

HARLAN M. KRUMHOLZ, MD
Assistant Professor of Medicine and Epidemiology
Section of Cardiology
Yale School of Medicine
New Haven, Connecticut

KEVIN R. KRUSE, MD
Fellow, Division of Cardiology, Department of Medicine
Duke University Medical Center
Durham, North Carolina

FREDERICK E. KUHN, MD
Clinical Assistant Professor of Medicine
Georgetown University Medical Center
Washington, DC

DANIEL L. KULICK, MD
Interventional Cardiologist
Mission Hospital Regional Medical Center
Clinical Assistant Professor of Medicine
University of Southern California
Los Angeles, California

CRAIG HJEMDAHL-MONSEN, MD
Associate Professor of Clinical Medicine
New York Medical College
Valhalla, New York

JAMES E. MULLER, MD
Professor of Internal Medicine
Chief, Division of Cardiology
University of Kentucky College of Medicine
Lexington, Kentucky

JOHN J. MURRAY, MD, PhD
Associate Professor of Medicine
Departments of Medicine and Pharmacology
Vanderbilt University
Nashville, Tennessee

RICK A. NISHIMURA, MD
Professor of Internal Medicine
Consultant, Cardiovascular Diseases
Mayo Clinic
Rochester, Minnesota

ROBIN M. NORRIS, MD, FRCP, FRACP
Honorary Consultant Cardiologist
Senior Visiting Fellow
Royal Sussex County Hospital
Brighton, England

CHRISTOPHER M. O'CONNOR, MD, FACP, FACC
Director, Clinical Trials
DUCCS (Duke University Cooperative Cardiovascular Studies) Organization
Assistant Professor of Medicine
Duke University School of Medicine
Durham, North Carolina

ROBERT A. O'ROURKE, MD
Charles Conrad Brown Professor in Cardiovascular Disease
The University of Texas Health Science Center at San Antonio
San Antonio, Texas

JAE K. OH, MD
Associate Professor of Internal Medicine
Consultant, Division of Cardiovascular Diseases
Mayo Clinic
Rochester, Minnesota

E. MAGNUS OHMAN, MD, FACC, FRCP
Assistant Professor of Medicine
Duke University Medical Center
Director, Clinical Trials—Interventional Cardiology
Duke Clinical Research Institute
Durham, North Carolina

LIONEL H. OPIE, MD, DPhil, FRCP
Director, Heart Research Unit of the Medical Research Council
University of Capetown Medical School
Capetown, South Africa

ASHISH PARIKH, MD
Clinical Fellow
Division of Cardiology
Cedars-Sinai Medical Center and UCLA School of Medicine
Los Angeles, California

MARC A. PFEFFER, MD, PhD
Director, Heart Failure/Transplant Center
Brigham and Women's Hospital
Associate Professor of Medicine
Harvard Medical School
Boston, Massachusetts

CHARLES E. RACKLEY, MD
Professor
Division of Cardiology
Department of Medicine
Director, Lipid Disorder Clinic
Georgetown University Medical Center
Washington, DC

SHAHBUDIN H. RAHIMTOOLA, MB, FRCP, MACP
Distinguished Professor
George C. Griffith Professor of Cardiology
Chairman, Griffith Center
Professor of Medicine
University of Southern California
Los Angeles, California

HARTZELL V. SCHAFF, MD
Stuart W. Harrington Professor of Surgery
Mayo Clinic and Mayo Foundation
Rochester, Minnesota

PREDIMAN K. SHAH, MD, FACC
Director, Division of Cardiology and Atherosclerosis Research Center
Cedars-Sinai Medical Center
Shapell and Webb Chair in Cardiology and Professor of Medicine
UCLA School of Medicine
Los Angeles, California

SCOTT D. SOLOMON, MD
Assistant Professor of Medicine
Harvard Medical School
Associate Director of Noninvasive Cardiology
Brigham & Women's Hospital
Boston, Massachusetts

CAROLE A. WARNES, MD, MRCP, FACC
Consultant in Cardiovascular Diseases, Internal Medicine and Pediatric Cardiology
Mayo Clinic
Associate Professor
Mayo Medical School
Rochester, Minnesota

J. WAYNE WARNICA, MD, FRCPC
Professor of Medicine
University of Calgary
Director of Coronary Care
Foothills Hospital
Calgary, Alberta Canada

JOHN G. WEBB, MD
Clinical Associate Professor of Medicine
University of British Columbia

Director, Coronary Care Unit
St. Paul's Hospital
Vancouver, British Columbia Canada

MARK W. I. WEBSTER, MD, ChB, FRACP
Consultant Cardiologist
Green Land Hospital
Auckland, New Zealand

JEANNE Y. WEI, MD, PhD
Associate Professor of Medicine
Director, Division on Aging
Harvard Medical School
Chief, Gerontology Division
Beth Israel Hospital
Boston, Massachusetts

ALAN WOELFEL, MD
Director of Electrophysiology
Butterworth Hospital
Grand Rapids, Michigan

PART I

Historical Perspective, Pathology, Pathophysiology and Natural History

1

Acute Myocardial Infarction: A Historical Summary

W. Bruce Fye, MD, MA

INTRODUCTION

The clinical syndrome of acute myocardial infarction was first described just before World War I (1). This seems remarkable when it is recalled that angina pectoris was reported in 1772 (2). While patients had heart attacks before the twentieth century, doctors did not view their symptoms and signs as part of a discrete syndrome. Their complaints and findings were classified as severe angina, so-called *status anginosus*. Many factors contributed to the nearly 140-year delay between the first published descriptions of angina and acute myocardial infarction.

There are various ways to interpret the process that led eventually to the delineation of acute myocardial infarction as a distinct clinical syndrome. In a recent essay, British historian Christopher Lawrence argued that myocardial infarction came to be viewed as a specific disease after a dynamic "restructuring" of "clinical and pathological experience" took place early in the twentieth century. While this is true, Lawrence's interpretation of the social dynamics that led to this restructuring is more provocative. He thinks that the characteristic clinical and electrocardiographic features of myocardial infarction were defined through a "process of negotiation and persuasion over a period of time" and that the outcome was determined mainly by the "social interests of cardiologists and academic physicians"(3). My view is more traditional: a series of isolated and sometimes interconnected experiments and clinical observations led gradually to the recognition (and ultimately the acceptance) of a new disease entity, acute myocardial infarction (4).

William Osler, the English-speaking world's most acclaimed physician, explained in 1910 that "diseases have their destiny." Doctors and patients label signs and symptoms to communicate with each other, and their lexicon changes over time to reflect the definition or recognition of "new cohorts of disease" as well as the "disappearance of familiar enemies." Osler suggested that Heberden, if he could return a century after his death, would enjoy writing "new commentaries upon old diseases with new names"(5). As experimental evidence accumulated and clinical experience grew, a few physicians began sketching a new boundary—one that distinguished acute myocardial infarction from angina pectoris and other noncardiac conditions.

Several factors contributed to the delay in the recognition of acute myocardial infarction as a distinct clinical entity until the early twentieth century: (i) the belief that sudden coronary occlusion was invariably fatal; (ii) the variable relationship between symptoms and pathological findings in ischemic heart disease; (iii) the dependence on auscultation as an indicator of cardiac disease; (iv) the failure to examine the coronary arteries and myocardium routinely at autopsy; (v) the slow incorporation of new pathological and physiological knowledge into clinical practice; (vi) the preoccupation of physicians and medical scientists with the new field of bacteriology; (vii) the lack of any diagnostic tests to identify coronary artery obstruction or its consequences during life; and (viii) satisfaction with the standard classification scheme, which lumped what came to be called acute myocardial infarction with angina pectoris (4).

PATHOLOGICAL OBSERVATIONS ON CORONARY ARTERY DISEASE

During the second half of the nineteenth century, a series of observations and discoveries led to a clearer understanding of the pathological sequelae of coronary occlusion. In the 1840s a few British doctors began to study the coronary circulation experimentally. John Erichsen investigated the relationship of experimental coronary occlusion and cardiac arrest. Richard Quain distinguished simple epicardial fat from "fatty degeneration" of the myocardium, which he attributed to a fundamental chemical or physical change in the muscle fibers. Quain argued that fatty degeneration had been overlooked previously because doctors rarely used the microscope to examine the heart at autopsy. He concluded in 1850 that there was a significant association between coronary artery disease and fatty degeneration: "I have seen the coronary artery extremely ossified, going directly to the only part of the heart affected"(6).

A few of Quain's contemporaries recognized that coronary occlusion could result in fatty degeneration and cardiac rupture; Swedish physicians J. P. Malmsten and G. W. Düben reported this in 1859 (7). Seven years later, French physician Edme Vulpian reported the case of a 75-year-old woman who died shortly after a stroke. Autopsy revealed that a thrombus obliterated her severely atherosclerotic left anterior descending coronary artery. Vulpian thought the atheromatous changes in the artery had predisposed to clot formation. The muscle supplied by this obstructed vessel was thin and soft and had eventually ruptured—the fatal event in this case (8). Although Vulpian's interpretation of the pathophysiology of coronary occlusion was advanced, he did not address the clinical aspects of coronary thrombosis or suggest how practitioners might recognize such an event, however.

While some pathologists proposed a causal relationship between thrombotic coronary occlusion and myocardial degeneration, clinicians were unaware of (or unimpressed by) their conclusions. In 1872 German pathologist Georg Rindfleisch attributed fatty degeneration to "atheromatous degeneration of the coronary arteries with plugging of one of their larger branches by a thrombus . . . in every instance"(9). Austin Flint, sometimes called the "American Laennec" for his voluminous writings on auscultation, claimed in 1859 that it was possible to diagnose fatty degeneration during life if poor exercise tolerance, dyspnea on exertion, palpitations, and precordial distress were present (10). But these symptoms were nonspecific. Their presence reflected myocardial dysfunction, but they did not help physicians identify the cause of the disorder. Neither Flint nor any one else had yet diagnosed coronary thrombosis during life.

St. Louis physician Adam Hammer is usually credited with first recognizing coronary thrombosis during life (11,12). But it is apparent from his 1878 case report that Hammer's case was not atherosclerotic coronary artery disease. At autopsy, the patient's coronary artery was obstructed by a thrombus attached to an aortic valve vegetation. In his discussion, Hammer exhibits no true insight into the relationship between acute coronary occlusion and myocardial necrosis.

Researchers in Julius Cohnheim's pathological laboratory at the University of Leipzig made important observations on ischemic heart disease during the final quarter of the nineteenth century. In an 1880 article, Carl Weigert discussed the pathological appearance of "infarcts" in the heart and several other organs. He concluded that atherosclerotic coronary arteries were predisposed to thrombotic or embolic occlusion. If a vessel became obstructed slowly and adequate collaterals had developed, the muscle it supplied would be gradually replaced by fibrous tissue. On the other hand, if abrupt occlusion occurred, large areas of scar developed. Weigert's paper is a milestone in our evolving understanding of the pathophysiology of myocardial infarction (13).

Two years later, Weigert's clinical colleague Carl Huber published the histories of several patients found at autopsy to have pathological evidence of myocardial infarction. Based on his own clinical observations and Weigert's pathological studies, Huber proposed that the clinical syndrome of angina pectoris and the pathological findings of myocardial infarction were both manifestations of coronary artery disease. Cohnheim agreed, writing, "It is now known that the very great majority of the myocarditic indurations . . . are due to an advanced sclerosis . . . of the coronary arteries supplying the affected part." Most pathologists now agreed that fatty degeneration was caused by coronary artery disease. Cohnheim thought that "the degeneration usually affects first the papillary muscles, next the subendocardial layer of muscle fibres, and finally, in extreme cases, the whole thickness of the muscular wall." While Cohnheim thought that sudden coronary occlusion was often fatal, he acknowledged that death was not inevitable (14).

The Leipzig group's important observations had no apparent impact on contemporary medical practice, however. In retrospect, the clinical event we denote acute myocardial infarction was occasionally described, but it was not distinguished from angina. Contemporary practitioners termed prolonged anginal attacks—some of which surely represented acute myocardial infarction—status anginosus. While the pathological features of myocardial infarction were sometimes discovered at autopsy and were found to be associated with coronary occlusion, the relationship of symptoms to pathological findings remained obscure.

The inconstant relationship of symptoms and pathological findings was one factor that made it difficult for physicians to distinguish the various ischemic heart disease syndromes we now recognize. British physician Samuel West, who had studied the coronary circulation using postmortem injection techniques, wrote in 1884, "It is very remarkable how large an amount of obstruction there may be to both coronary arteries without any cardiac symptoms during life, or any gross pathological change recognizable in the muscle of the heart after death"(15). Cohnheim also emphasized the poor correlation of coronary anatomy with symptoms.

In 1882 Swiss pathologist Ernst Ziegler proposed the term "myomalacia cordis" for the pathological changes of the myocardium that accompanied coronary occlusion. He agreed that coronary occlusion was not always fatal and described the evolution of histological changes as the age of the infarction increased. British physician Donald MacAlister (who translated Ziegler's pathology text) viewed myomalacia cordis as "anaemic necrosis" and concluded that it was "not a rare affection." When the process was "at all extensive it brings about death by failure or rupture of the heart"(16).

Practitioners were frustrated that they could not diagnose myocardial disease with certainly. While British pathologist and practitioner Charles Fagge was impressed with how often myocardial scars were detected at autopsy, he complained in 1886 that, "Clinically, fibroid disease and aneurism of the heart can very seldom, if ever, be diagnosed"(17). Still, the fact that doctors did not recognize acute myocardial infarction a century ago does not mean the syndrome did not exist. British pathologist A. D. Morgan explained in 1968: "Although ischaemic heart disease may have masqueraded in the nineteenth century as angina pectoris, fatty degeneration, rupture of the heart, cardiac aneurysm, fibroid degeneration or chronic myocarditis, there would seem to have been . . . quite a lot of it about"(18).

Gradually, the pathological concept of coronary occlusion and myocardial infarction began to appear in the clinical literature. In 1889, William Osler, who had studied with Cohnheim and Weigert, suggested the possibility of short-term survival following coronary occlusion: "The local disturbances of nutrition caused by the blocking of a terminal branch of a coronary artery produce the condition known as infarct of the heart." Osler explained, "The danger is not alone at the period of preliminary softening, but time gradually effects a transformation of the softened areas into fibrous tissue, which yield and lead in many cases to aneurism of the cardiac wall and rupture. . . . In a number of cases death occurs suddenly, without any premonition; in other cases, precordial distress, pain in the left side, and signs of cardiac trouble have preceded the fatal illness for days or even weeks"(19,20).

Confusion about the pathophysiology of ischemic heart disease syndromes persisted, however. In 1889 Osler's Johns Hopkins colleague William Welch, a pathologist who had also studied with Cohnheim and Weigert, presented a specimen "in which a thrombus had formed in the apex of the left ventricle, a portion breaking off obstructed the anterior coronary artery completely, thus causing anaemia of the wall, coagulation necrosis, and a white infarction." Although these pathological observations were undoubtedly accurate, Welch's interpretation of the sequence of events reveals his lack of understanding of the pathophysiology of myocardial infarction and its sequelae (21).

Meanwhile, Harvard physiologist William Porter had begun a series of innovative experiments on the effects of coronary artery occlusion in animals (22). He found that experimental coronary ligation or embolization caused a decline in peak intraventricular pressure, often triggered fatal cardiac arrhythmias, and led to characteristic gross and microscopic pathologic changes (23,24). Walter Baumgarten, a graduate student working with Porter, published the most comprehensive and insightful article on myocardial infarction written by an American in the nineteenth century. Addressing the relationship between ischemia and myocardial contractility, Baumgarten reported that "portions of the mammalian ventricle will resume their contractions if fed with defibrinated blood" up to 11 hours following experimental coronary occlusion. He also concluded that contractility was most impaired in the central zone of the ischemic area and least impaired at the periphery (25).

There was growing awareness that coronary occlusion was not invariably fatal. American internist George Dock reported one of the first antemortem diagnoses of myocardial infarction in 1896. Dock had studied in Germany with Weigert, Huber, and Ernst von Leyden after graduating from the University of Pennsylvania School of Medicine in 1884. He attributed the renewed interest in the coronary arteries to the growing awareness of their significance in cases of sudden death (26). William Welch declared in 1899, "Thrombosis of the coronary arteries is an affection of great clinical importance." While he thought that "the symptoms associated with coronary thrombosis are those of the angiosclerotic heart, so that it is hardly possible to make a positive diagnosis of thrombotic occlusion of the coronary arteries," Welch proclaimed, "cardiac infarction is more common than would appear from the meager attention usually given to the subject in text-books, and is of much anatomical and clinical interest"(27).

Ludolf Krehl, a German physician and proponent of pathologic physiology—a disease paradigm in which symptoms were viewed as manifestations of disordered function rather than abnormal structure—discussed the clinical aspects of acute coronary thrombosis in 1901 (28). Denying that sudden coronary occlusion was invariably fatal, Krehl proposed that a severe attack of angina or a "temporary attack of cardiac failure" might in fact be a manifestation of this event. In some instances, the patient "lives on and never suspects what an abyss he has escaped." Krehl thought that abrupt coronary obstruction might lead to "marked subjective symptoms, especially pressure on the chest, pain, and a sensation of fear—in short, all the symptoms described under stenocardia." Troubled by the broad spectrum of responses to experimental occlusion of the coronary arteries, Krehl thought "there is some intermediate link of which we are still ignorant between occlusion of a coronary artery and the occurrence of heart failure"(29).

Some researchers speculated that coronary anastomoses might be this missing link—they might explain the variable consequences of experimental and clinical coronary occlusion. British physician Richard Lower had first demonstrated anastomoses in the coronary circulation by injection techniques in 1669, but generations of researchers thought these collateral vessels had little or no functional significance. The x-ray, a powerful new technology invented in 1895, helped to settle the question. In 1907 Friedrich Jamin and Hermann Merkel of Germany published the first atlas of x-ray images of the human coronary arteries. In their postmortem study, they injected a radio-opaque solution into the coronary system of excised human hearts and then x-rayed the organ (30). Their images revealed a rich anastomotic network in the human coronary circulation.

THE CLINICAL SYNDROME OF ACUTE MYOCARDIAL INFARCTION

Russian physicians W. P. Obrastzow and N. D. Straschesko published the first paper describing the typical clinical features of acute myocardial infarction in 1910. Speculating that certain signs and symptoms accompanied acute coronary thrombosis, they emphasized two main findings: prolonged chest discomfort (status anginosus) and persistent dyspnea (status dyspnoeticus). After presenting case summaries with autopsy correlations, Obrastzow and Straschesko concluded that "the differential diagnosis of coronary thrombosis from angina pectoris is made by the presence of status anginosus with coronary thrombosis and its absence with isolated attacks of angina pectoris." They also stressed that the signs and symptoms of cardiac failure resolved promptly following a simple anginal attack, but they persisted if coronary thrombosis had occurred (31,32). Their paper, published in a German journal of clinical medicine, attracted little attention.

Chicago physician James Herrick was familiar with Obrastzow and Straschesko's report. Herrick deserves credit for convincing the English-speaking medical community that coronary thrombosis was not invariably fatal and could be recognized during life. His 1912 paper "Certain clinical features of sudden obstruction of the coronary arteries" is a milestone in our understanding of the pathophysiology of coronary artery disease, angina pectoris, and myocardial infarction. Based on his own experience as well as a wide variety of experimental, clinical, and pathological reports, Herrick concluded that acute coronary thrombosis was not invariably fatal—some patients even recovered completely.

Herrick provided a detailed explanation for the spectrum of symptoms he attributed to acute coronary thrombosis: "The clinical manifestations of coronary obstruction will evidently vary greatly, depending on the size, location and number of vessels occluded. The symptoms and end-results must also be influenced by blood-pressure, by the condition of the myocardium not immediately affected by the obstruction, and by the ability of the remaining vessels properly to carry on their work, as determined by their health or disease. No simple picture of the condition can, therefore, be drawn." Herrick advocated absolute bed rest following acute coronary thrombosis and emphasized the role of collateral vessels: "The hope for the damaged myocardium lies in the direction of securing a supply of blood through friendly neighboring vessels so as to restore so far as possible its functional integrity"(33).

The initial response to Herrick's masterful synthesis of the pathophysiology and clinical manifestations of acute myocardial infarction was negligible. Practitioners were used to classifying patients with sustained chest pain as suffering from a severe attack of angina. Many years later, Herrick recalled that his presentation on coronary thrombosis before the leading internists of the day "fell like a dud" and the publication of his manuscript "aroused no more comment than it did when it had been read six months before"(34). His observations attracted little attention until physicians had some objective way to prove that a patient's chest discomfort and associated symptoms were unequivocally cardiac in origin.

In 1916 Victor Vaughan, dean of the University of Michigan School of Medicine, told a Colorado doctor that "the diagnosis of disease depends now largely upon laboratory tests"(35). During the 1920s, physicians came to rely on the electrocardiograph to help them recognize acute myocardial infarction. Willem Einthoven, a Dutch physiologist, invented a string galvanometer to record the heart's electrical activity in 1901 and published the first electrocardiograph the following year (36).

Initially, the electrocardiograph was used almost exclusively to investigate cardiac arrhythmias (37). New York physician Bernard Oppenheimer was one of the first clinical investigators to extend electrocardiographic studies beyond disturbances of impulse formation and conduction to include abnormalities of the wave forms. He reported his results at the annual meeting of the American Medical Association in 1917. During the discussion, New York internist Emanuel Libman emphasized how difficult it was to recognize coronary thrombosis clinically and speculated that "an electrocardiograph examination might be of value in confirming the diagnosis"(38).

Herrick, also present for Oppenheimer's presentation, told the audience that he was studying the electrocardiographic features of experimental coronary occlusion in dogs. Herrick noted a similarity between the electrocardiogram recorded from one of Oppenheimer's patients found at autopsy to have coronary thrombosis and those he had recorded from dogs following ligation of the left coronary artery (39). Herrick's assistant Fred Smith published the results of their electrocardiographic study of experimental coronary occlusion in 1918 (40). Herrick argued that characteristic electrocardiographic changes accompanied coronary occlusion and that these might help physicians recognize the clinical event of acute coronary thrombosis (41). Thus he provided clinicians with both an intellectual framework for conceptualizing survival after coronary thrombosis and a new diagnostic approach to help them recognize the event in individual patients.

During the 1920s and 1930s, clinical investigators in Great Britain and America (including Evan Bedford, Harold Pardee, John Parkinson, Frank Wilson, Charles Wolferth, and Francis Wood) made important observations on the value of electrocardiography in myocardial infarction. Pardee published a paper in 1920 in which he described dramatic ST segment elevation in leads 2 and 3 in a patient who had a clinical event consistent with an acute myocardial infarction. Electrocardiograms recorded over the next few weeks revealed progressive T wave inversions in those leads and the return of isoelectric ST segments. Pardee concluded that these serial changes were due to "muscle degeneration" following acute coronary occlusion (42). Precordial leads were introduced in 1932 by Wolferth and Wood of Philadelphia, who emphasized their value in the electrocardiographic diagnosis of myocardial infarction (43).

In a comprehensive 1923 review on coronary thrombosis and myocardial infarction, Joseph Wearn of Boston claimed that this clinical problem was more common than was generally believed: "When one reads almost daily of sudden death from 'heart failure,' 'acute indigestion,' or 'cerebral hemorrhage,' one questions if he is not reading of the result of a thrombus in a coronary artery." For treatment, Wearn emphasized the importance of "absolute rest," noting that the patient should avoid "any bodily exertion." If signs of cardiac failure appeared, fluid restriction was ordered and digitalis was administered. Nitrates and morphine were prescribed for pain, and caffeine and camphor were used to treat hypotension (44).

American physicians and clinical investigators John McNee, Emanuel Libman, Warfield Longcope, Canby Robinson, Henry Christian, and William Thayer published significant papers on the pathophysiology and clinical features of coronary thrombosis in this period. In a classic 1928 review British physicians John Parkinson and Evan Bedford proposed that coronary thrombosis was analogous to cerebral thrombosis "both pathologically and in its clinical manifestations." Their comprehensive summary of the clinical manifestations, electrocardiographic features, complications, treatment, and prognosis of acute myocardial infarction stimulated widespread interest among British and American physicians in coronary thrombosis (45).

The following year, Samuel Levine of Boston published the first book in English on coronary thrombosis. Based on the published experiences of others and his own series of 145 patients, Levine provided a detailed summary of the complications of myocardial infarction including cardiac arrhythmias, cardiac rupture, and embolic events. The pharmacological treatment of life-threatening arrhythmias dates to this era when Levine and others advocated quinidine for the treatment of ventricular tachycardia. The nonpharmacological aspects of care that Levine and his contemporaries advocated became standard practice for a generation. Levine advocated 6 to 8 weeks of "absolute bed rest"(46).

Oxygen was routinely administered to patients following myocardial infarction, especially after Barach demonstrated in 1931 that this intervention reduced mortality (47). Boston physicians Kenneth Mallory, Paul Dudley White and Jorge Salcedo-Salgar published an article in 1939 that supported the practice of prolonged bed rest following acute myocardial infarction. Their clinico-pathological study of 72 cases led them to conclude that it took up to two months for an infarct to heal completely (48). By the late forties, some physicians had begun to question the need for prolonged bed rest, however, citing the complications that accompanied immobilization (49,50). Gradually, earlier ambulation gained in popularity and hospitalizations became shorter.

THE CORONARY CARE UNIT: A NEW HEART CARE PARADIGM

Acute myocardial infarction with its associated risk of sudden death is the most feared complication of coronary artery disease. The coronary care unit (CCU) was an innovation designed to improve survival following acute myocardial infarction. Advances in the detection and treatment of cardiac arrhythmias introduced during the 1950s set the stage for the invention of the coronary care unit concept in the early sixties. Two new technologies gave doctors the power to treat some life-threatening arrhythmias. The electric defibrillator was useful for treating ventricular tachycardia and ventricular fibrillation, while electronic pacemakers were useful for treating symptomatic bradycardia (51,52).

During the middle of the twentieth century, several teams of researchers (that often included electrical engineers, cardiologists, physiologists, and surgeons) made discoveries and invented devices that led to the introduction of the defibrillator and pacemaker into clinical medicine. Claude Beck, a heart surgeon at Western Reserve University, reported the first successful human resuscitation using a defibrillator in 1947. He delivered the electric shock directly to the heart after opening his patient's chest to compress the organ, so-called direct cardiac massage. Beck's report stimulated great interest in defibrillation as an adjunct to the drug treatment of cardiac arrest (53).

During the fifties, surgeons and cardiologists viewed cardiac arrest differently. Surgeons saw it as a surgical problem because 85 percent of cardiac arrests in hospitalized patients occurred in the operating room and treatment required an operative procedure (immediate thoracotomy to expose the heart so it could be manually compressed). Meanwhile, cardiologists and other nonsurgeons saw cardiac arrest as a catastrophe that might occur anywhere and at any time in patients with heart disease. Even if they were present when the arrest occurred (and they rarely were), few doctors were trained to open a patient's chest in order to perform direct cardiac massage.

In 1956 Boston cardiologist Paul Zoll reported that ventricular fibrillation could be terminated by a shock delivered through the chest wall. His transthoracic defibrillator was a major advance in the treatment of this life-threatening arrhythmia (54,55). Because irreversible brain damage occurred within 5 minutes following cardiac arrest, immediate treatment was necessary. Zoll knew this and advocated using a "practical monitoring device" in patients thought to be at risk for cardiac arrest "to signal immediately the cessation of circulation" so resuscitation attempts could begin at once (56).

Electrical engineer William Kouwenhoven and his colleagues at Johns Hopkins reported their nonoperative method for treating cardiac arrest in 1960. It consisted of closed chest cardiac massage, mouth-to-mouth artificial respiration, and transthoracic defibrillation (57–59). This widely publicized innovation changed the way doctors treated patients with cardiac arrest. It quickly replaced open cardiac massage and demystified the technique of cardiopulmonary resuscitation (CPR). No longer would cardiac resuscitation be limited to surgeons and a few nonsurgeons bold enough to wield a scalpel when a patient suffered a cardiac arrest.

Meanwhile, other groups had developed practical methods for accelerating the heartbeat. Physiologists began using electricity to stimulate the heartbeat in the nineteenth century. New York practitioner cardiologist Albert Hyman invented an "artificial cardiac pacemaker" for clinical use in the early 1930s, but it was impractical because its power supply lasted only a few minutes (60,52). In 1950, Canadian surgeons Wilfred Bigelow and John Callaghan reported their research on the electrical stimulation of the heartbeat. Two years later, Zoll described how he had used a transthoracic pacemaker to stimulate the heart of a patient who had developed asystole (61). Later in the decade, other researchers—most notably Walton Lillehei's group in Minneapolis and Seymour Furman and his colleagues in New York City—developed reliable cardiac pacemakers for clinical use.

These inventions led a few doctors to devise new strategies for delivering care to heart attack patients. The cathode ray oscilloscope made continuous electrocardiographic monitoring practical, and doctors now had tools (defibrillators, pacemakers, and antiarrhythmic drugs) to treat the arrhythmias the machine detected. In 1961 Desmond Julian of Edinburgh, Scotland, and Hughes Day of Kansas City, Kansas, independently developed a team approach for promptly resuscitating patients who had a cardiac arrest while hospitalized with a myocardial infarction (62–64). The innovation was to group vulnerable patients in a specific hospital setting—the coronary care unit, or CCU—equipped with medicine's new electronic tools and staffed with nurses trained to use them (along with mouth-to-mouth respiration and closed chest cardiac massage) to resuscitate patients. Their creation of the CCU concept heralded a new era in cardiology—one in which increasing attention was focused on coronary artery disease (65,66).

Day published the first comprehensive description of the cardiac arrest team concept in 1962. Impressed with Kouwenhoven's CPR technique, he formed a "code blue emergency" team of trained staff who responded immediately to any cardiac arrest in his hospital. Day created a "crash cart," a large mobile cabinet that included a defibrillator, thoracotomy instruments, intubation and tracheostomy equipment, a temporary pacemaker, and several cardiac drugs (epinephrine, calcium chloride, quinidine gluconate, procaine amide, digitoxin, levophed, and other vasopressors). His hospital was creating an "intensive coronary care area" where patients with acute cardiac conditions would be continuously monitored with an "Electrodyne scope-pacemaker." Day closed his article claiming that recent advances made it "imperative that all hospitals should establish programs of cardiac resuscitation"(67).

In 1963 Day reported that his CCU staff treated 32 heart attack patients during the first five months the unit was open. All 7 patients who had cardiac arrests (during 8,567 hours of monitoring) survived. Day was convinced that the *staff* rather than the *structure* of the facility was what mattered. Nurses were taught CPR and empowered to initiate resuscitation. Day thought the "greatest impact in an acute coronary care area comes from its constant nursing attention." His detailed description of the facility, equipment, staff, procedures, and philosophy provided a model for other institutions seeking to establish a CCU (68).

The CCU concept was a new heart care paradigm that united high-risk heart patients, technology, and specialized staff—nurses and doctors—in a specific hospital environment. This innovation had implications for both doctors and patients. It was no longer possible simply to put a person with a heart attack in a quiet room, prescribe sedatives, and leave them unattended. Once they were admitted to a CCU, heart attack patients found themselves connected to a monitor in a bright, noisy room with little if any privacy. Now, physicians had effective approaches to treat many of the arrhythmias that complicated acute myocardial infarction—if only they could be used before hypoperfusion and hypoxemia led to irreversible ischemia of the heart or brain and death.

The CCU was an innovation that spread quickly because it worked. Early reports showed that admission to a CCU instead of a regular room conferred a significant survival advantage. The rapid diffusion of CCUs into community hospitals expanded the cardiology job market during the sixties and seventies (69,70). Continuous cardiac monitoring of heart attack patients also helped to clarify how they died. While cardiac arrhythmias were shown to cause almost one-half of in-hospital heart attack deaths, an equal number of patients died from shock and congestive heart failure due to muscle loss and resulting pump failure. Despite aggressive management of the cardiac arrhythmias that complicated heart attacks, the death rate remained around 20 percent (71). These findings led to new treatment strategies and stimulated research into ways to limit the size of heart attacks (72).

It was recognized that the extent of myocardial necrosis was related to survival. Various techniques to quantitate infarct size were developed to aid physicians in establishing a prognosis and to help clinical scientists evaluate new approaches to myocardial preservation. Tests to identify and quantitate myocardial necrosis using serum enzyme assays, electrocardiographic mapping, radioisotopes, ultrasound, and angiocardiography were introduced and refined during the past quarter century. Physiology came to the bedside in 1970 with the invention of a balloon-tipped flow-directed cardiac catheter that could be used to continuously monitor intracardiac pressures. The Swan–Ganz catheter gave clinicians a powerful new tool to help them manage the sickest heart attack patients (73). Interventions could now be selected to address specific hemodynamic abnormalities (74).

ANTICOAGULANT AND THROMBOLYTIC THERAPY FOR CORONARY THROMBOSIS

By 1920 it was generally accepted that sudden thrombotic occlusion of a diseased coronary artery triggered acute myocardial infarction. Shortly after the anticoagulants heparin and bishydroxycoumarin (dicumarol) were developed half a century ago, some clinical investigators thought they might be useful in the treatment of heart attack patients. In 1938 Canadian physiologists Donald Solandt and Charles Best reported that heparin (first administered to humans one year earlier) prevented intracoronary thrombus formation in an animal model (75). The following year, they reported that heparin inhibited the development of mural thrombi after experimental myocardial infarction (76). Because heparin was impractical for long term use, attention soon shifted to the oral anticoagulant dicumerol (first administered to humans in 1941).

By 1946 anecdotal experience had convinced several investigators and clinicians that dicumerol significantly reduced mortality and embolic events following myocardial infarction (77–79). Based on a multi-institutional study of 800 patients with acute myocardial infarction, New York internist Irving Wright and his colleagues concluded in 1948 that those treated with anticoagulants had a lower incidence of death and thromboembolic events during the first 6 weeks following the index event than those who did not receive these agents. As a result, they advocated anticoagulants for "all cases of coronary thrombosis with myocardial infarction unless a definite contraindication exists"(80). Enthusiasm for anticoagulant therapy following myocardial infarction gradually diminished, however, as criticisms of the design of Wright's and other studies were voiced and the risks of chronic anticoagulation were recognized (81). One reviewer explained that by the 1970s "the anticoagulant era, which had begun with such high hopes, ended with a whimper"(82).

Meanwhile, there was growing interest in the role of thrombolytic agents in the treatment of acute myocardial infarction. In 1933 New York bacteriologist William Tillett discovered that β-hemolytic streptococci produced a fibrinolytic substance which he termed fibrinolysin (later named streptokinase—the term used throughout this essay for the sake of consistency) (83). Streptokinase was first administered to humans in 1947 in an attempt to dissolve chronic empyemas. Five years later, Tillett's group reported that an intravenous infusion of streptokinase lysed blood clots that had been induced experimentally in the ear veins of rabbits. They concluded that intravenous streptokinase created "an active lytic system"(84). In 1955 Tillett reported the results of a clinical trial in which streptokinase was administered intravenously to 11 patients to assess its side effects. The "most noteworthy toxic effects" were a pyrogenic response and hypotension (85).

Anthony Fletcher, Sol Sherry (who had worked with Tillett), and their associates reported the results of a trial of "massive and prolonged" administration of intravenous streptokinase in 24 patients with acute myocardial infarction in 1958. Impressed with the results, they speculated: "The rapid dissolution of a coronary thrombus by enzymatic means could result in reduction of the final area of muscle infarction, reduction of the degree of electrical instability present during the early critical phase of infarction and prevent the appearance of or lyse mural thrombi"(86). The following year, they concluded that streptokinase was "a highly effective activator of human plasminogen"(87).

In 1960 Paul Boyles and his associates in Coral Gables and Miami, Florida, reported their observations on the intra-arterial administration of streptokinase. They concluded that the "segmental injection" of the agent near the clot was necessary to obtain "effective *in vivo* lysis of arterial thrombi"(88). The same year, Robert Boucek and his colleagues at the University of Miami administered streptokinase to eight myocardial infarction patients 4 to 12 hours after the onset of pain. In an attempt to obtain "segmental perfusion," they delivered it through a cardiac catheter placed in one of the sinuses of Valsalva (89). The authors concluded that coronary thrombolysis probably occurred in six of their patients, but they could not be sure because they did not perform coronary angiography before or after the administration of streptokinase (89). This reflected the fact that Mason Sones had not yet reported his invention of selective coronary angiography, and available nonselective methods did not predictably provide adequate visualization of the vessels (90).

The clinical application of streptokinase for thromboembolic disorders was retarded because of concerns regarding the pyrogenicity and antigenicity of the substance. These concerns led some investigators to study urokinase, a plasminogen activator of human origin extracted from urine (91). Debate about the pathophysiology of acute myocardial infarction also retarded the diffusion of thrombolytic therapy. For a quarter of a century after Herrick's classic 1912 paper on "sudden obstruction of the coronary arteries," it was accepted that myocardial infarction was caused by an acute thrombotic occlusion of the vessel. In 1939 Charles Friedberg reported an autopsy study of 1,000 patients with myocardial infarction. Because 31 percent did not have evidence of recent coronary thrombosis at autopsy, he concluded that myocardial infarction was not invariably the result of coronary thrombosis, but might "also be due solely to progressive coronary narrowing of extreme degree"(92).

During the next quarter century debate intensified as to whether coronary thrombosis might *result from* rather than *cause* acute myocardial infarction. San Francisco cardiologist Meyer Friedman acknowledged in 1966 that there was "considerable argument" regarding the relationship of thrombus formation and underlying atherosclerosis and "even between thrombosis and infarction." His findings supported the view held by some (but not all) pathologists that "the thrombus lay in direct communication with a pre-existing intramural atheromatous process"(93). Pathologist William Roberts of the National Institutes of Health wrote several papers on the subject in the seventies. In 1972 he explained that several postmortem findings "suggest that coronary thrombi are consequences rather than causes of acute myocardial infarction"(94). Four years later, British pathologist Michael Davies protested that it was "hardly credible that there should be continuing debate about what is ostensibly so simple a morphological problem, the relation of coronary thrombosis to acute myocardial infarction"(95).

While pathologists debated the role of coronary thrombosis in causing acute myocardial infarction, investigators in Europe and America continued to explore the therapeutic value of anticoagulants and thrombolytic therapy. The European Working Party reported the results of their multicenter controlled trial of streptokinase in acute myocardial infarction in 1971. After reviewing the results of this trial in which 764 patients were randomized prospectively to treatment with intravenous streptokinase or heparin, they concluded that streptokinase was superior to heparin in reducing early mortality and reinfarction in the first 6 weeks following infarction. But their study revealed only a "limited reduction in mortality," and they advocated "further extensive trials of streptokinase in acute myocardial infarction"(96).

In 1976 E. I. Chazov and colleagues from Russia reported their experience with two patients who underwent coronary angiography before and after the intracoronary administration of streptokinase and heparin during acute myocardial infarction. Reperfusion was successful in the patient who received thrombolytic therapy 4 hours after the onset of symptoms; it was unsuccessful in the patient who was treated 10 hours after the onset of symptoms (97). This paper, published in Russian with a brief English summary, was unknown to most Europeans and Americans working in the area of thrombolytic therapy (98).

The modern era of thrombolytic therapy for acute myocardial infarction began in 1979 when Peter Rentrop and his associates from Göttingen, Germany published a report on the intracoronary administration of streptokinase in five patients. Rentrop accepted the "classical pathologic theory" that acute myocardial infarction was typically caused by "coronary thrombosis superimposed upon high-degree atherosclerotic lesions." He used selective coronary angiography before and after the infusion of streptokinase to document that in four cases the obstruction was reduced by this therapeutic intervention (99). Simultaneously, the European Cooperative Study Group for Streptokinase Treatment in Acute Myocardial Infarction reported the results of their randomized controlled trial of a 24-hour intravenous infusion of streptokinase. The mortality rate of patients treated with streptokinase was significantly lower at 6 months than those who received an infusion of glucose (100).

The debate regarding the role of thrombus in acute myocardial infarction was resolved in 1980 when Spokane cardiologist Marcus DeWood and his colleagues published a paper on the angiographic prevalence of total coronary occlusion during the early hours of myocardial infarction. Of 126 patients who underwent coronary angiography within 4 hours of the onset of symptoms, 87% were found to have total coronary occlusion. Based on their study, they concluded that "total coronary occlusion is frequent during the early hours of transmural infarction and decreases in frequency during the initial 24 hours"(101). The papers by Rentrop and DeWood led to widespread introduction of intracoronary thrombolytic therapy with streptokinase. Soon, several European and American groups published studies demonstrating the efficacy of intravenous streptokinase (102,103). This was relevant because most patients with acute myocardial infarction did not present to hospitals with cardiac catheterization laboratories.

Meanwhile, other European groups were interested in another thrombolytic agent. Danish biologists Tage Astrup and Per Permin had discovered an activator of plasminogen in tissue in 1947 (104). A third of a century later, W. Weimar, Désiré Collen, and their associates in Belgium and the Netherlands reported the successful intravenous administration of tissue plasminogen activator (t-PA) in an attempt to lyse a renal and iliofemoral thrombus in a renal transplant recipient. They were optimistic about the therapeutic potential of t-PA because animal studies had shown that "thrombolysis was obtained without systemic fibrinolytic activation." Although t-PA was very scarce because it could only be obtained from a melanoma cell line, the authors speculated that it could be produced by genetic engineering techniques (105).

Several investigators were enthusiastic about t-PA because it appeared to be clot-specific and had a short half-life. This led them to conclude that it would cause less systemic lytic activity than streptokinase or urokinase, the agents then available for clinical use. Shortly after Collen began collaborating with Steven Bergmann, Burton Sobel, and other investigators at Washington University in St. Louis, Missouri, they reported successful coronary thrombolysis when t-PA was administered to dogs in whom an intracoronary thrombus had been induced experimentally. These authors claimed that once t-PA was available in greater quantities using recombinant DNA technology it offered "particular promise for widely applicable, prompt, safe dissolution of coronary thrombi accompanied by restitution of metabolism in jeopardized myocardium in patients"(106).

In 1983 Collen and several scientists at Genentech, Inc. (a biotechnology company formed in San Francisco seven years earlier) reported a method for producing human t-PA using recombinant DNA technology. The successful cloning and expression of the human t-PA gene meant that sufficient quantities of the substance could be produced for clinical research and (eventually) commercial marketing (107). With Collen and his group in Belgium, a group of investigators at Washington University reported the first clinical trial of intravenous and intracoronary t-PA for acute myocardial infarction in 1984 (108). Later that year, these groups collaborated with researchers at the Johns Hopkins Hospital and Massachusetts General Hospital in a prospective, placebo-controlled trial sponsored by Genentech. They concluded that intravenous or intracoronary t-PA "induced coronary thrombolysis without eliciting clinically significant fibrinolysis in patients with evolving myocardial infarction due to thrombotic coronary occlusion"(109).

The many clinical trials of thrombolytic therapy during the 1980s and 1990s are beyond the scope of this historical review. The cardiological community was inundated with clever acronyms like GISSI, ISIS, GUSTO, and LATE, to name but a few. It soon became clear that thrombolytic therapy using either streptokinase or t-PA saved lives (110). Mechanical—as opposed to pharmacological—intervention for acute myocardial infarction is a recent extension of percutaneous transluminal coronary angioplasty (PTCA). This innovative catheter-based approach for dilating stenotic coronary arteries was introduced in 1977 by Andreas Grüntzig for the treatment of angina pectoris (111). Recent clinical trials have shown that direct (or immediate) PTCA is an effective way to achieve reperfusion early after the onset of acute myocardial infarction.

It was necessary to exclude from this brief historical review certain topics relating to acute myocardial infarction. I have attempted to show how basic and clinical research were combined with experience at the bedside and in the clinic to achieve our current understanding of the pathophysiology, diagnosis, and treatment of acute myocardial infarction. The rest of this book will describe the current status and future prospects of a wide range of topics as they relate to acute myocardial infarction. As you read it I urge you to reflect on the provocative question, "Where does a review of the literature end and history begin?"

REFERENCES

1. Leibowitz JO: *The History of Coronary Heart Disease.* London, Wellcome Institute of the History of Medicine, 1970.
2. Heberden W: Some account of a disorder of the breast. *Medical Transactions, Published by the College of Physicians of London* 1772;2:59–67.
3. Lawrence C: "Definite and material": Coronary thrombosis and cardiologists in the 1920s, in Rosenberg CE, Golden J (eds): *Framing Disease.* New Brunswick, NJ, Rutgers University Press, 1992, pp 50–82.
4. Fye WB: The delayed diagnosis of acute myocardial infarction: It took half a century. *Circulation* 1985;72:262–271.
5. Osler W: The Lumleian lectures on angina pectoris. *Lancet* 1910;1:697–702, 839–844, 973–977.
6. Quain R: On fatty diseases of the heart. *Med Chir Trans* 1850;33:121–196.
7. Johansson BW, Nicol P: A Swedish report on acute myocardial infarction in 1859. *Br Med J* 1982;284:888.
8. Vulpian EFA: Ramollissement cérébral . . . Caillot ancien dans l'auricle gauche. Infarctus de la paroi du ventricule gauch du coeur coincidant avec l'existence d'un caillot ancien dans l'une des arterès coronaires etc. *Un Méd (Paris)* 1866;n.s. 29:417–419. Translated in Leibowitz, JO: *The History of Coronary Heart Disease,* 1970, pp 184–186.
9. Rindfleisch E: *A Manual of Pathological History to serve as an Introduction to the Study of Morbid Anatomy.* Baxter EB (trans). London, New Sydenham Society, 1872.
10. Flint A: *A Practical Treatise on the Diagnosis, Pathology, and Treatment of Diseases of the Heart.* Philadelphia, Blanchard & Lea, 1859.
11. Hammer A: Ein Fall von thrombotischem Verchlusse einer der kranzarterien des Herzens. *Wiener Med Wochesnchr* 1878;28:97–102.
12. Lie JT: Centenary of the first correct antemortem diagnosis of coronary thrombosis by Adam Hammer (1818–1878); English translation of the original report. *Am J Cardiol* 1978;42:848–852.
13. Weigert C: Ueber die pathologische Gerinnungs-Vorgänge. *Arch Pathol Anat* 1880;79:87–123.
14. Cohnheim J: *Lectures on General Pathology.* McKee AB (trans). London, New Sydenham Society, 1889.
15. West S: Cases of complete obliteration of one coronary artery, with remarks upon the coronary circulation. *Trans Pathol Soc London* 1884;35: 110–114.
16. Ziegler E: *A Text-book of Pathological Anatomy and Pathogenesis.* MacAlister D (trans, ed). New York, William Wood & Co., 1887.
17. Fagge CH: *The Principles and Practice of Medicine.* Philadelphia, P. Blakiston, Son & Co., 1886.
18. Morgan AD: Some forms of undiagnosed coronary disease in nineteenth-century England. *Med Hist* 1968;12:344–358.
19. [Osler W]: Rupture of the heart. *Med News* 1889;54:129–130.
20. Dock G: Historical notes on coronary occlusion: From Heberden to Osler. *JAMA* 1939;113: 563–568.
21. Welch W: Diseases of the coronary arteries and alterations in the muscular walls of the heart. *Proc Trans Pathol Soc Toronto* 1889;1:8–9.
22. Fye WB: Acute coronary occlusion always results in death, or does it? The observations of William T. Porter. *Circulation* 1985;71:4–10.

23. Porter WT: On the results of ligation of the coronary arteries. *J Physiol* 1893;15:121–138.
24. Porter WT: Further researches on the closure of the coronary arteries. *J Exp Med* 1896;1:46–70.
25. Baumgarten W: Infarction in the heart. *Am J Physiol* 1899;2:243–265.
26. Dock G: *Notes on the Coronary Arteries.* Ann Arbor, MI Inland Press, 1896.
27. Welch WH: Thrombosis and embolism, in Allbutt C (ed): *A System of Medicine.* London, MacMillan & Co. 1899, pp 155–285.
28. Krehl L: *Die Erkrankungen des Herzmuskels und die nervösen Herzkrankheiten.* Vienna, Alfred Hölder, 1901.
29. Krehl L: Diseases of the myocardium and nervous diseases of the heart, in Dock G (ed): *Diseases of the Heart.* Philadelphia, W.B. Saunders & Co. 1908, pp 421–763.
30. Jamin F, Merkel H: *Die Koronararterien des menschlichen Herzens unter normalen und pathologischen Verhältnissen.* Jena, Gustav Fischer, 1907.
31. Obrastzow WP, Straschesko ND: Zur Kenntnis der Thrombose der Koronararterien des Herzens. *Z Klin Med* 1910;71:116–132.
32. Muller JE: Diagnosis of myocardial infarction: Historical notes from the Soviet Union and the United States. *Am J Cardiol* 1977;40:269–271.
33. Herrick JB: Certain clinical features of sudden obstruction of the coronary arteries. *JAMA* 1912;59:2015–2020.
34. Herrick JB: An intimate account of my early experience with coronary thrombosis. *Am Heart J* 1944;27:1–18.
35. Vaughan VC to Corwin RW, 24 April 1916, in Michigan University, Medical School, miscellaneous correspondence, box 32, July 1916, A N. Bentley Library, University of Michigan, Ann Arbor.
36. Fye WB: A history of the origin, evolution, and impact of electrocardiography. *Am J Cardiol* 1994;73:937–949.
37. Howell JD: Early perceptions of the electrocardiogram: From arrhythmia to infarction. *Bull Hist Med* 1984;58:83–98.
38. Libman E: Discussion of B. S. Oppenheimer and M. A. Rothschild, Electrocardiographic changes associated with myocardial involvement. *JAMA* 1917;69:429–431.
39. Herrick JB: Discussion of B. S. Oppenheimer and M. A. Rothschild, Electrocardiographic changes associated with myocardial involvement. *JAMA* 1917;69:429–431.
40. Smith FM: The ligation of coronary arteries with electrocardiographic study. *Arch Int Med* 1918; 22:8–27.
41. Herrick JB: Thrombosis of the coronary arteries. *JAMA* 1919;72:387–390.
42. Pardee HEB: An electrocardiographic sign of coronary artery obstruction. *Arch Int Med* 1920;26: 244–257.
43. Wolferth CC, Wood FC: The electrocardiographic diagnosis of coronary occlusion by the use of chest leads. *Am J Med Sci* 1932;183: 30–35.
44. Wearn JT: Thrombosis of the coronary arteries, with infarction of the heart. *Am J Med Sci* 1923; 165:250–276.
45. Parkinson J, Bedford E: Cardiac infarction and coronary thrombosis. *Lancet* 1928;1:4–11.
46. Levine SA: *Coronary Thrombosis: Its Various Clinical Features.* Baltimore, Williams & Wilkins, 1929.
47. Barach A: The therapeutic use of oxygen in heart disease. *Ann Int Med* 1931;5:428–440.
48. Mallory GK, White PD, Salcedo-Salgar J: The speed of healing of myocardial infarction. *Am Heart J* 1939;18:647–671.
49. Irvin CW Jr, Burgess AM Jr: The abuse of bed rest in the treatment of myocardial infarction. *N Engl J Med* 1950;243:486–489.
50. Levine SA, Lown B: Armchair treatment of acute coronary thrombosis. *JAMA* 1952;148:1365–1369.
51. Fye WB: Ventricular fibrillation and defibrillation: Historical perspectives with emphasis on the contributions of John MacWilliam, Carl Wiggers, and William Kouwenhoven. *Circulation* 1985;71: 858–865.
52. Schechter DC: *Exploring the Origins of Electrical Cardiac Stimulation: Selected Works of David Charles Schechter, M.D., F.A.C.S., on the History of Electrotherapy.* Minneapolis, Medtronic, Inc., 1983.
53. Beck CS: Reminiscences of cardiac resuscitation. *Rev Surg* 1970;27:77–86.
54. Zoll PM, Linenthal AJ, Gibson W, Paul MH, Norman LR: Termination of ventricular fibrillation in man by externally applied electric countershock. *N Engl J Med* 1956;254:727–732.
55. Kouwenhoven WB: The development of the defibrillator. *Ann Int Med* 1969;71:449–458.
56. Zoll PM, Linenthal AJ, Norman LR, Paul MH, Gibson W: External electric stimulation of the heart in cardiac arrest. *Arch Int Med* 1955; 96:639–653.

57. Kouwenhoven WB, Jude JR, Knickerbocker GG: Closed-chest cardiac massage. *JAMA* 1960;173: 94–97.
58. Kouwenhoven WB, Jude JR, Knickerbocker GG: Heart activation in cardiac arrest. *Mod Concepts Cardiovasc Dis* 1961;30:639–643.
59. Kouwenhoven WB, Langworthy OR: Cardiopulmonary resuscitation: An account of forty-five years. *Johns Hopkins Med J* 1973;132:186–193.
60. Hyman AS: Resuscitation of the stopped heart by intracardial therapy. II. Experimental use of an artificial pacemaker. *Arch Int Med* 1932;50: 283–305.
61. Zoll PM: Resuscitation of the heart in ventricular standstill by external electric stimulation. *N Engl J Med* 1952;247:768–771.
62. Julian DG: The history of coronary care units. *Br Heart J* 1987;57:497–502.
63. Day HW: History of coronary care units. *Am J Cardiol* 1972;30:405–407.
64. Julian D to Fye WB. 22 March 1994.
65. Russell LB: *Technology in Hospitals: Medical Advances and Their Diffusion.* Washington, The Brookings Institution, 1979.
66. Julian DG: Treatment of cardiac arrest in acute myocardial ischaemia and infarction. *Lancet* 1961; 2:840–844.
67. Day HW: A cardiac resuscitation program. *Journal-Lancet* 1962;82:153–156.
68. Day HW: Preliminary studies of an acute coronary care area. *Journal-Lancet* 1963;83:53–55.
69. Bloom BS, Peterson OL: Patient needs and medical-care planning: The coronary-care unit as a model. *N Engl J Med* 1974;290:1171–1177.
70. Bloom BS, Peterson OL: End results, cost and productivity of coronary-care units. *N Engl J Med* 1973;288:72–78.
71. Meltzer LE, Kitchell JR: The development and current status of coronary care, in Meltzer LE (ed): *Textbook of Coronary Care.* Philadelphia, Charles Press Publishers, 1972, pp 3–25.
72. Braunwald E: Efforts to limit myocardial infarct size: Historical considerations. *Eur Heart J* 1985;6: E1–E4.
73. Swan HJC, Ganz W, Forrester JS: Catheterization of the heart in man with the use of a flow-directed balloon-tipped catheter. *N Engl J Med* 1970;283:447–451.
74. Gunnar R, Loeb H: Shock in acute myocardial infarction: Evolution of physiologic therapy. *J Am Coll Cardiol* 1983;1:154–163.
75. Solandt DY, Best CH: Heparin and coronary thrombosis in experimental animals. *Lancet* 1938; 2:130–132.
76. Solandt DY, Nassim R, Best CH: Production and prevention of cardiac mural thrombosis in dogs. *Lancet* 1939; 2:592–595.
77. Peters HR, Guyther JR, Brambel CE: Dicumarol in acute coronary thrombosis. *JAMA* 1946;130:398–403.
78. Wright IS: The discovery and early development of anticoagulants: A historical symposium. *Circulation* 1959;19:73–134.
79. Mueller RL, Scheidt S: History of drugs for thrombotic disease: Discovery, development, and directions for the future. *Circulation* 1994;89: 432–449.
80. Wright IS, Marple CD, Beck DF: Report of the committee for the evaluation of anticoagulants in the treatment of coronary thrombosis with myocardial infarction. *Am Heart J* 1948;36: 801–815.
81. Gifford RH, Feinstein AR: A critique of methodology in studies of anticoagulant therapy for acute myocardial infarction. *N Engl J Med* 1969;280: 351–357.
82. Mitchell JRA: Anticoagulants in coronary heart disease—retrospect and prospect. *Lancet* 1981;1: 257–262.
83. Tillett WS, Garner RL: The fibrinolytic activity of hemolytic streptococci. *J Exp Med* 1933; 58:485–502.
84. Johnson AJ, Tillett WS: The lysis in rabbits of intravascular blood clots by the streptococcal fibrinolytic system (streptokinase). *J Exp Med* 1952;95:449–463.
85. Tillett WS, Johnson AJ, McCarty WR: The intravenous infusion of the streptococcal fibrinolytic principles (streptokinase) into patients. *J Clin Invest* 1955;34:169–185.
86. Fletcher AP, Alkjaersig N, Smyrniotis F, Sherry S: The treatment of patients suffering from early myocardial infarction with massive and prolonged streptokinase therapy. *Trans Assoc Am Physicians* 1958;71:287–296.
87. Fletcher AP, Alkjaersig N, Sherry S: The maintenance of a sustained thrombolytic state in man. I.

Induction and effects. *J Clin Invest* 1959;38: 1096–1110.

88. Boyles PW, Meyer WH, Graff J, Ashley CC, Ripic RG: Comparative effectiveness of intravenous and intra-arterial fibrinolysin therapy. *Am J Cardiol* 1960;6:439–444.
89. Boucek RJ, Murphy WPJ: Segmental perfusion of the coronary arteries with fibrinolysin in man following a myocardial infarction. *Am J Cardiol* 1960;6:525–533.
90. Sones FM Jr, Shirey EK: Cine coronary arteriography. *Mod Concepts Cardiovasc Dis* 1962;31: 735–738.
91. Fletcher AP, Alkjaersig N, Sherry S, Genton E, Hirsh J, Bachmann F: The development of urokinase as a thrombolytic agent. Maintenance of a sustained thrombolytic state in man by its intra venous infusion. *J Lab Clin Med* 1965;65:713–731.
92. Friedberg CK, Horn H: Acute myocardial infarction not due to coronary artery occlusion. *JAMA* 1939;112:1675–1679.
93. Friedman M, Van den Bovenkamp GJ: The pathogenesis of a coronary thrombus. *Am J Path* 1966;48:19–44.
94. Roberts WC, Buja LM: The frequency and significance of coronary arterial thrombi and other observations in fatal acute myocardial infarction: A study of 107 necropsy patients. *Am J Med* 1972; 52:425–443.
95. Davies MJ, Woolf N, Robertson WB: Pathology of acute myocardial infarction with particular reference to occlusive coronary thrombi. *Br Heart J* 1976;38:659–664.
96. European Working Party: Streptokinase in recent myocardial infarction: A controlled multicentre trial. *Br Med J* 1971;3:325–331
97. Chazov EI, Matveeva LS, Mazaev AV, Sargin KE, Sadovskaya GV, Ruda MY: Intracoronary administration of fibrinolysin in acute myocardial infarction. *Terapevticheskii Arkhiv* 1976;48:8–19.
98. Braunwald E: The path to myocardial salvage by thrombolytic therapy. *Circulation* 1987;76 (Suppl II):II-3–II-7.
99. Rentrop KP, Blanke H, Karsch KR, et al: Acute myocardial infarction: Intracoronary application of nitroglycerin and streptokinase. *Clin Cardiol* 1979;2:354–363.
100. European Cooperative Study Group for streptokinase treatment in acute myocardial infarction: Streptokinase in acute myocardial infarction. *N Engl J Med* 1979;301:797–802.
101. DeWood MA, Spores J, Notske R, et al: Prevalence of total coronary occlusion during the early hours of transmural myocardial infarction. *N Engl J Med* 1980;303:897–902.
102. Schröder R, Biamino G, Leitner E, et al: Intravenous short-term infusion of streptokinase in acute myocardial infarction. *Circulation* 1983;67: 536–548.
103. Taylor GJ, Mikell FL, Moses HW, et al: Intravenous versus intracoronary streptokinase therapy for acute myocardial infarction in community hospitals. *Am J Cardiol* 1984;54:256–260.
104. Astrup T, Permin PM: Fibrinolysis in the animal organism. *Nature* 1947;159:681–682.
105. Weimar W, Stibbe J, Van Seyen AJ, Billiau A, De Somer P, Collen D: Specific lysis of an iliofemoral thrombus by administration of extrinsic (tissue-type) plasminogen activator. *Lancet* 1981;2: 1018–1020.
106. Bergmann SR, Fox KA, Ter-Pogossian MM, Sobel BE: Clot-selective coronary thrombolysis with tissue-type plasminogen activator. *Science* 1983;220:1181–1183.
107. Pennica D, Holmes WE, Kohr WJ, et al: Cloning and expression of human tissue-type plasminogen activator cDNA in *E. coli*. *Nature* 1983;301: 214–221.
108. Van de Werf F, Ludbrook PA, Bergmann SR, et al: Coronary thrombolysis with tissue-type plasminogen activator in patients with evolving myocardial infarction. *N Engl J Med* 1984;310: 609–613.
109. Collen D, Topol EJ, Tiefenbrunn AJ, et al: Coronary thrombolysis with recombinant human tissue-type plasminogen activator: A prospective, randomized, placebo-controlled trial. *Circulation* 1984;70:1012–1017.
110. Yusuf S, Colins R, Peto R, et al: Intravenous and intracoronary fibrinolytic therapy in acute myocardial infarction: Overview of results of mortality, reinfarction and side-effects from 33 randomized controlled trials. *Eur Heart J* 1985;6:556–585.
111. Grüntzig A: Transluminal dilatation of coronary artery stenosis. *Lancet* 1978;1:263.

2

Pathology of Myocardial Infarction and Reperfusion

William D. Edwards, MD

CORONARY ARTERY DISEASE

Obstructive coronary artery disease may be chronic and stable in nature, or it may be acute and unstable. Chronic stenosis is generally related to atherosclerosis, and acute obstruction is usually the result of thrombosis, spasm, or both. Critical to an understanding of the pathophysiology of the acute coronary syndromes is the realization that nearly all cases of acute myocardial infarction occur in patients with preexisting coronary atherosclerosis.

Chronic Coronary Obstruction

Among patients with chronic obstructive coronary artery disease, atherosclerosis is the most prevalent cause and accounts for at least 90% of the cases (1).

Chronic Atherosclerotic Disease

Coronary atherosclerosis is limited to the epicardial vessels and tends to be most severely obstructive in the proximal half of the left anterior descending and circumflex arteries (and their proximal branches) and anywhere in the right coronary artery (2,3). Severe distal stenosis tends to occur only in hearts with severe proximal disease and to produce shorter and more discrete lesions than observed proximally. High-grade obstruction of the left main coronary artery is usually associated with severe disease in the other three major epicardial vessels.

Atherosclerosis is a chronic, progressive, multifocal *intimal* disease. Its basic lesion, the atheroma, represents a raised plaque with a necrotic core and a fibrous outer coat. The core generally contains foam cells, degenerating blood elements, necrotic debris, cholesterol crystals, loose granulation tissue, smooth muscle cells, mononuclear leukocytes, and occasional giant cells or iron pigment. The fibrous coat varies appreciably in thickness, and the overlying endothelium often exhibits small areas of denudation with focal adherence of monocytes and platelets (4). Plaque calcification is also commonly observed and appears to be related to the severity of stenosis and the age of the patient (5).

The relative composition of atheromas varies considerably, not only between individuals but also in the same heart and within the same artery. As a result, the compliance of plaques is quite variable. Some are soft and moldable; others are firm and rigid (Fig. 2–1). In general, lipid-rich cores are observed most frequently in younger patients, in younger plaques, and in the setting of appreciable hyperlipidemia (6). After the age of 50, atheromas tend to become more fibrotic or fibrocalcific, especially if shallow thrombus has played a role. Clini-

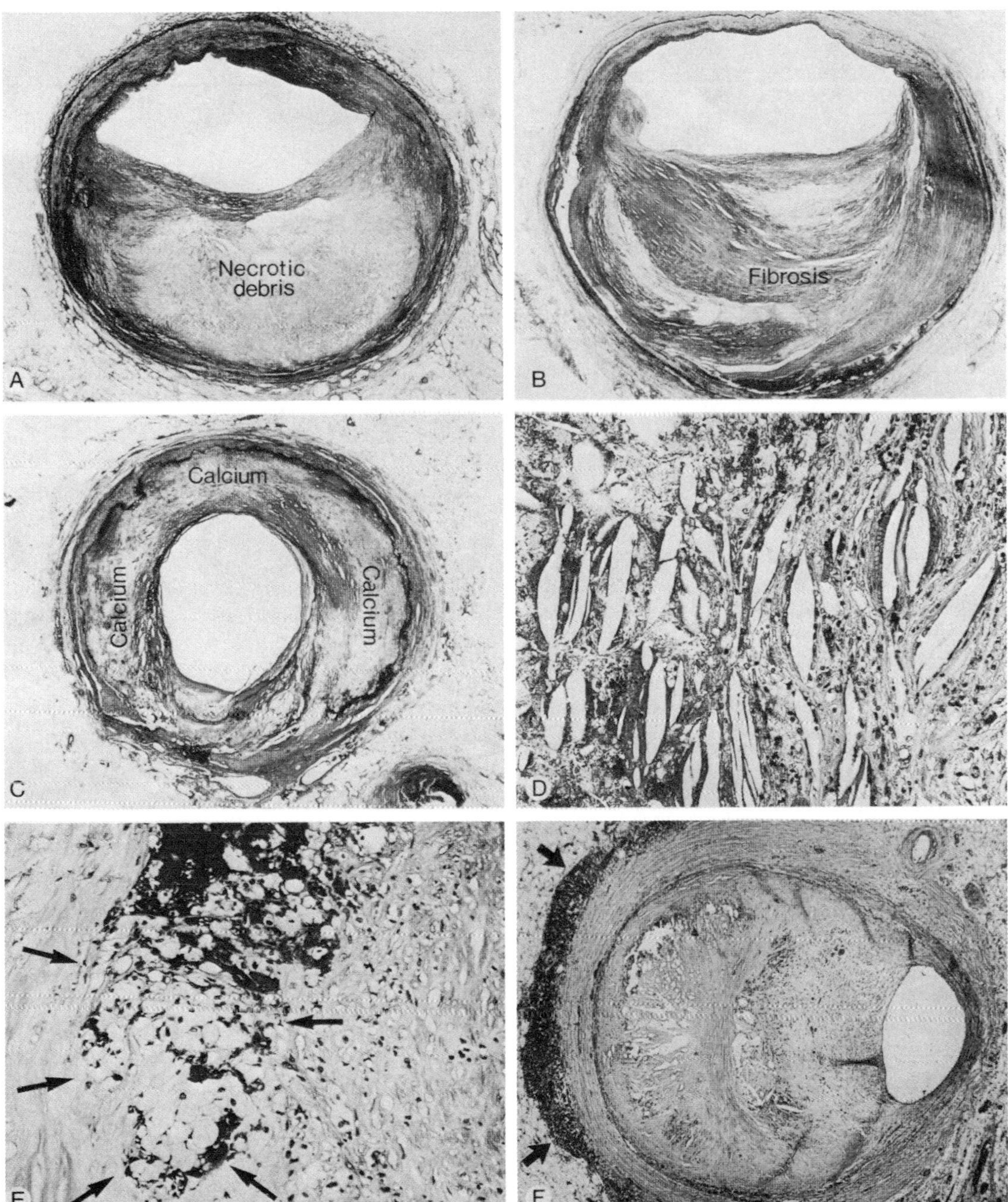

Figure 2–1. Variation in plaque composition. **A.** Eccentric soft plaque. **B.** Eccentric firm plaque. **C.** Concentric calcified atheroma. **D.** Necrotic atheromatous debris with needle-like cholesterol crystals. **E.** Collection of foam cells within plaque (arrows). **F.** Extensive adventitial lymphocytes (arrows).

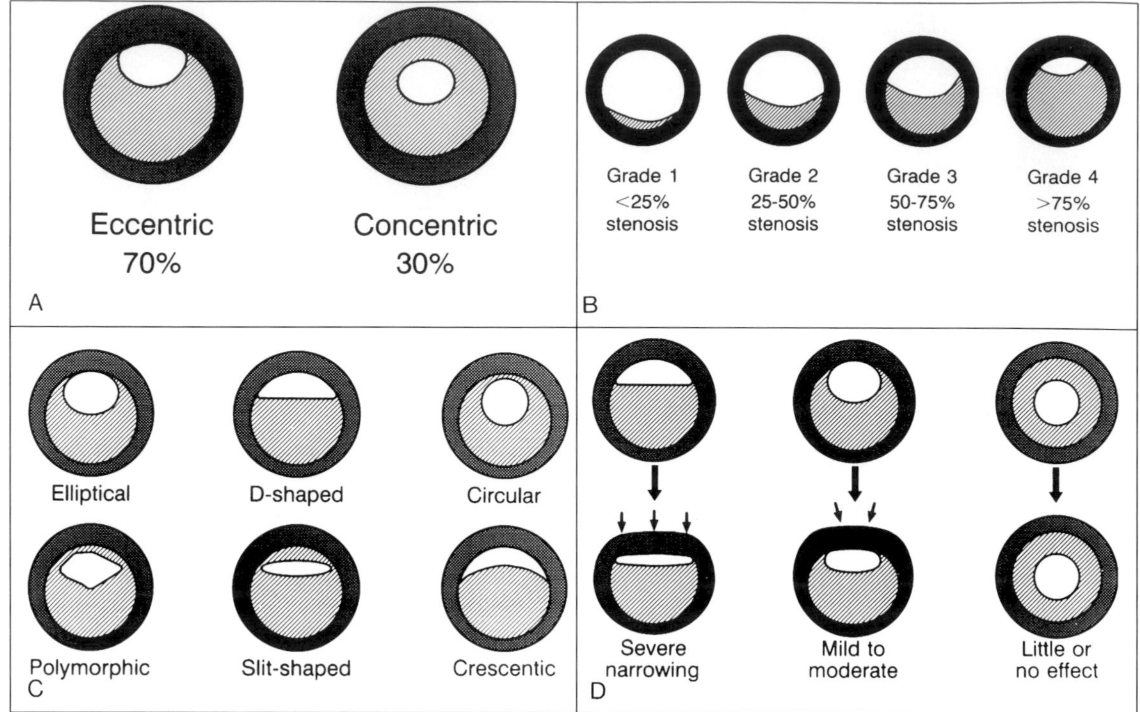

Figure 2–2. Variations in plaque and luminal shapes (schematic). **A.** Comparison of eccentric and concentric plaques. **B.** Four grades of coronary atherosclerosis. **C.** Commonly encountred luminal shapes. **D.** Effect of coronary artery spasm on lumens of varying size, shape, and location.

cally, the distinction between soft and firm plaques can be achieved using invasive intravascular ultrasound. Moreover, the presence of calcium, indicative of a firm plaque, can be detected noninvasively by ultrafast computed tomography (7).

About 70% of atherosclerotic plaques are eccentric in location. Consequently, residual lumens also tend to be eccentric, such that their borders are formed partly by atheroma and partly by a disease-free portion of arterial wall (Fig. 2–2) (8,9). Concentric plaques that form the entire luminal border account for only about 30% of lesions. For high-grade stenoses, of either eccentric or concentric type, the residual lumens are often noncircular and attain shapes that are elliptical, D-shaped, or rarely, polymorphic, crescentic, or slitlike.

Although atherosclerosis is an intimal disease, the subjacent media may become thinned as a result of stretching or atrophy. As atherosclerosis develops, the artery dilates so that luminal size remains constant and the plaque is nonstenotic. This process continues until the atheroma achieves a cross-sectional area similar to that of the lumen. Angiographically there would be no obstruction, whereas microscopically the artery would harbor up to a 50% lesion. At this point, dilation is complete, and further plaque progression produces luminal narrowing. The extent of focal coronary dilation varies appreciably both between individuals and within the same heart (10–12). Expansion beyond twice the expected arterial diameter is considered aneurysmal.

The media opposite an atheroma may also exhibit secondary alterations. In vessels with eccentric plaques, the disease-free wall is often involved by compensatory medial hypertrophy.

The adventitia beneath a plaque occasionally contains dense lymphoplasmacytic infiltrates, with a propensity for perineural involvement. Inflammation may also be observed in the media and the intimal atheroma. Although this process does not represent vasculitis, it does indicate an unstable plaque.

Chronic Nonatherosclerotic Disease

Among nonatherosclerotic causes of chronic coronary artery obstruction, ostial stenosis is the most common. Calcification of the aortic sinotubular junction is the usual cause, and it favors the right ostium (13). Other causes of chronic ostial stenosis include aortitis and congenital malformations.

Acute Coronary Obstruction

Dynamic changes in the coronary circulation that cause acute myocardial infarction are complex and multifaceted. Most transmural infarctions are associated with acute thrombotic coronary occlusion. In contrast, subendocardial infarctions either may exhibit acute obstruction as a result of thrombosis or spasm or may be associated only with chronic coronary disease acting in concert with hypotension or hypoxemia.

Acute Coronary Thrombosis

Thrombosis represents the most common cause of acute coronary obstruction, and it is usually the result of plaque erosion, fissures, or rupture. The cause of atheromatous rupture is unknown, but it is probably related to hemodynamic stresses, unstable aspects of plaque structure, and altered molecular mechanisms at the endothelial and subendothelial levels (14) (see Ch. 4). Morphologic features associated with plaque disruption include a soft atheroma with a large necrotic core, a thin overlying fibrous cap, collections of foam cells within the cap, giant cells engaged in atherophagocytosis, intimal clusters of leukocytes, and adventitial bands of mononuclear leukocytes (1,15–17). Thus, soft plaques are more likely to rupture than firm ones.

Plaque disruption causes exposure of thrombogenic collagen and atheromatous debris to the luminal blood (see Chs. 4 and 20). The resulting thrombus may be composed primarily of platelets, red blood cells, or a layered mixture of the two, and it may cause partial or complete obstruction. It is, however, important to emphasize that even partial obstruction may produce acute ischemic myocardial injury.

The opposing effects of thrombosis and intrinsic thrombolysis, coupled with the hemodynamic effects of pulsatile luminal blood flow, lead to rapid alterations in thrombus size. This dynamic process has been directly observed by coronary angioscopy (18). With time, as the fibrin content increases, the thrombus begins to stabilize such that microembolization ceases.

The consequences of plaque rupture and secondary thrombosis are variable (Figs. 2–3 to 2–5). In most instances, chronic progression of atherosclerosis occurs as a result of plaque hemorrhage or organization of nonocclusive thrombus. In others, shallow platelet–fibrin thrombi are associated with distal microfocal embolization. And in still others, expansion of the thrombus by fibrin entrapment of red blood cells causes sufficient obstruction to produce myocardial ischemia. With time, some restitution of coronary blood flow may occur because of partial thrombolysis and organization with recanalization.

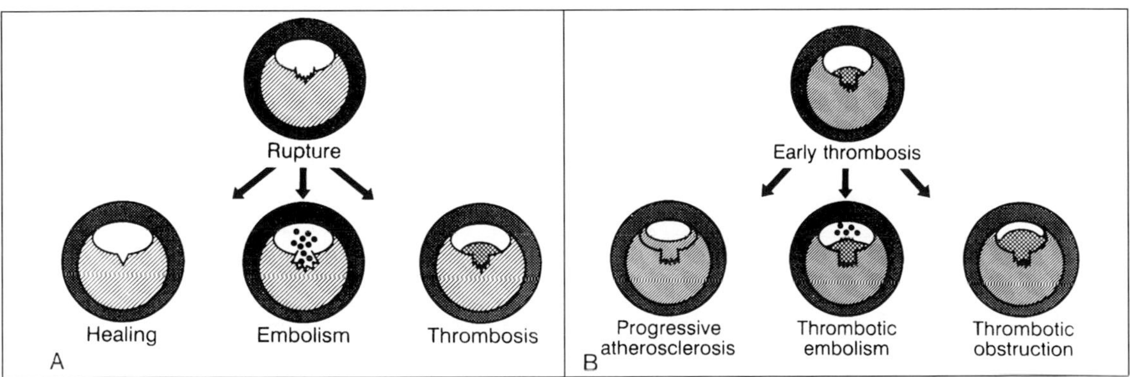

Figure 2–3. Consequences of acute plaque lesions (schematic). **A.** Plaque rupture. **B.** Coronary thrombosis.

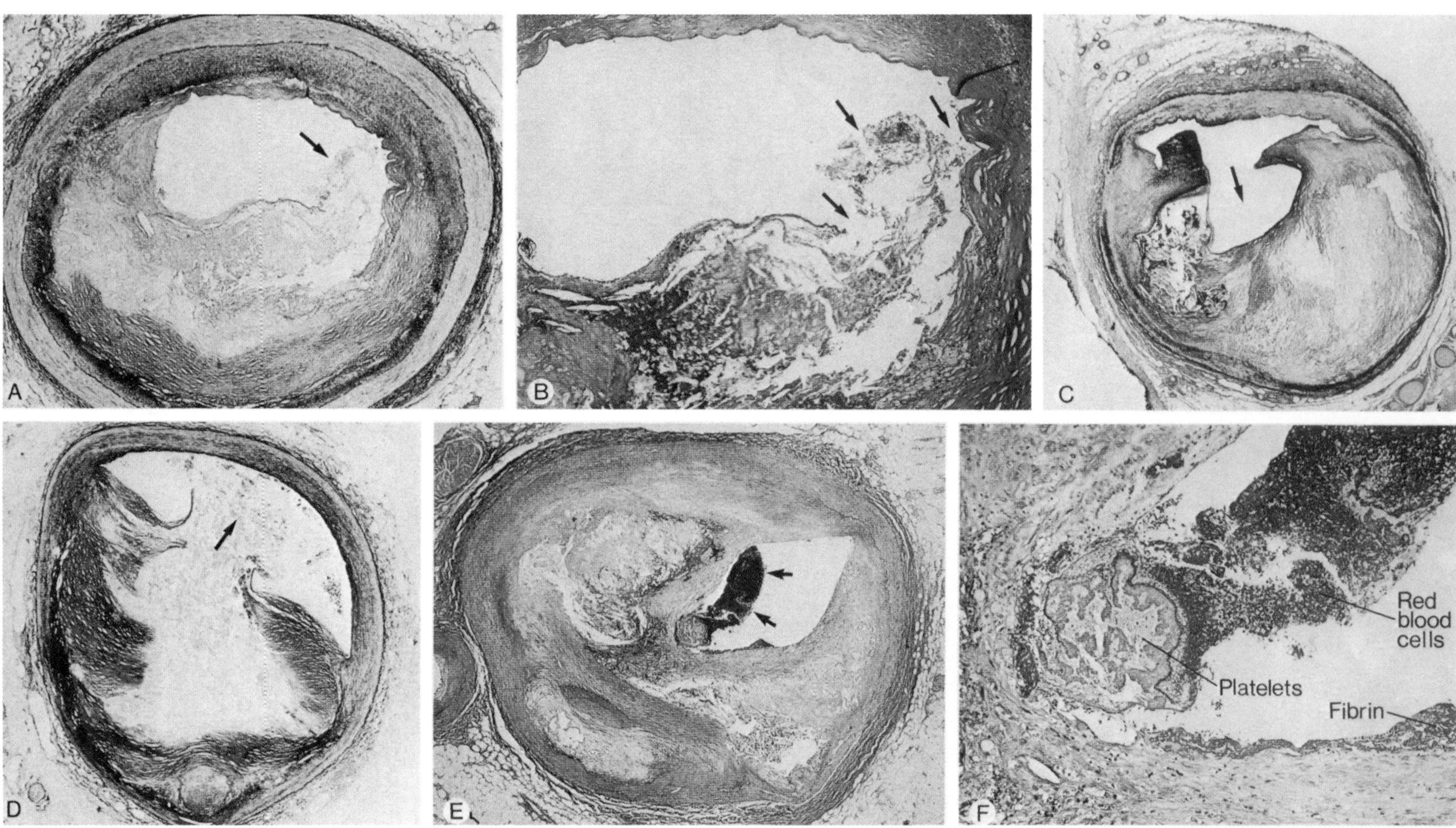

Figure 2–4. Plaque rupture and its consequences. **A,B.** Focal surface disruption (arrows) at low power (**A**) and high power (**B**). **C.** Healed rupture site (arrow), without thrombus. **D.** Plaque rupture with embolization of atheromatous debris (arrow). **E,F.** Acute nonocclusive thrombosis (arrows) at low power (**E**) and high power (**F**).

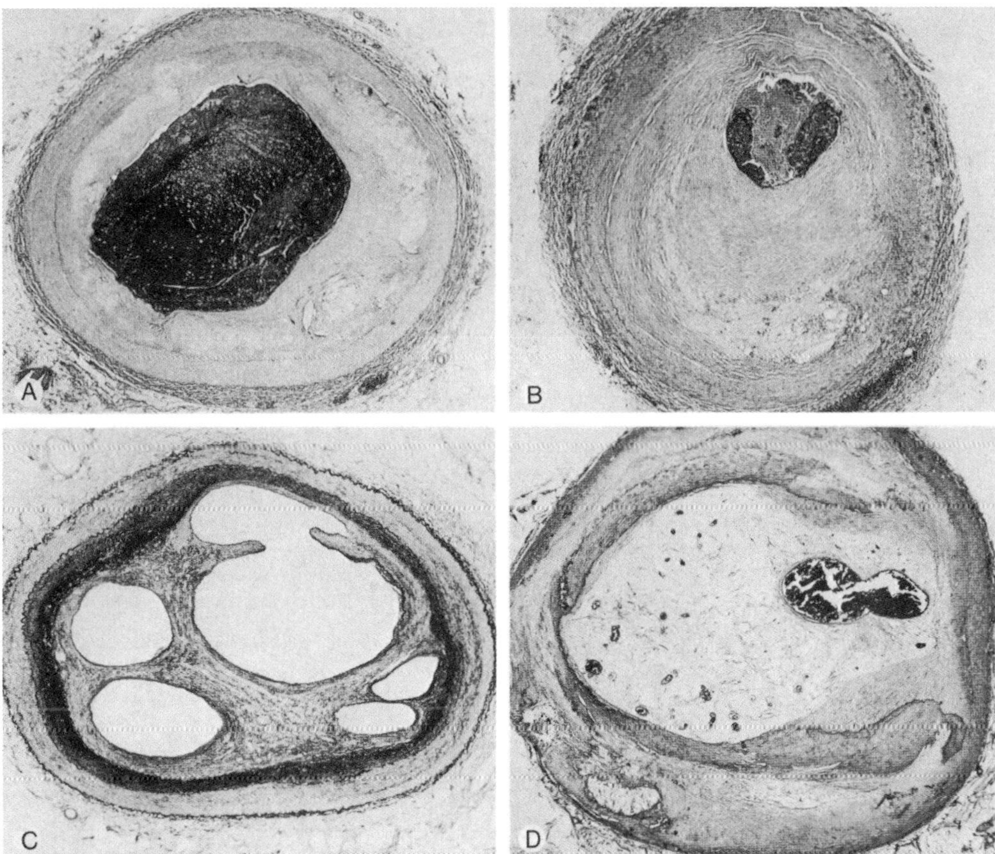

Figure 2–5. Thrombosis and its consequences. **A,B.** Occlusive thrombi involving grade 2 (**A**) and grade 4 (**B**) plaques. **C,D.** Organization and fibrosis of thrombus, with (**C**) and without (**D**) appreciable lysis and recanalization.

Numerous studies support the concept that plaque rupture and secondary thrombosis are important in the pathogenesis of unstable angina, acute myocardial infarction, and sudden coronary death (Tables 2–1 and 2–2) (1,19,20). Thrombi tend to be occlusive in transmural infarctions and nonocclusive in unstable angina, subendocardial infarctions, and sudden coronary death. Moreover, microembolization may play a role in the induction of ventricular arrhythmias (21). In contrast, acute coronary thrombosis is rarely associated with stable angina or chronic heart failure (ischemic cardiomyopathy). For subendocardial infarctions, particularly circumferential ones, hypotension and hypoxemia may be more prevalent causes than thrombosis.

Thrombotic coronary occlusions that lead to acute myocardial infarction are as likely to involve noncritical atherosclerotic plaques as critical ones (22,23). Clinically, the only two coronary features routinely evaluated are the severity of luminal nar-

Table 2–1. Chronic and Acute Forms of Ischemic Myocardial Disease

Chronic Disease	Acute Disease[a]
Silent myocardial ischemia	Unstable angina pectoris
Stable angina pectoris	Subendocardial infarction
Variant angina pectoris	Transmural infarction
Chronic heart failure	Sudden coronary death

[a]Acute forms of ischemic myocardial disease are usually the result of acute coronary obstruction caused by plaque rupture and secondary thrombosis. Obstruction tends to be complete with transmural infarction and to be incomplete with the others.

Table 2–2. Correlation Between Clinical Manifestation of Coronary Artery Disease and Pathologic Features of Atherosclerotic Plaques*

Clinical State	Microscopic Features of Coronary Atherosclerosis
Asymptomatic	Stable noncritical plaques; occasionally, critical stable plaques (generally one-vessel disease)
Angina pectoris	
Chronic stable (exertional)	Stable critical plaques (usually two-vessel or three-vessel disease)
Variant (Prinzmetal's)	Stable noncritical or critical plaques; evidence of plaque progression; occasionally an unstable atheroma
Microvascular (syndrome X)	No significant disease of epicardial coronary arteries; medial and intimal thickening of intramural arteries; swollen capillary endothelial cells
Unstable (preinfarction)	Unstable plaque, either critical or noncritical, with rupture and acute nonocclusive platelet-rich thrombus; also stable critical plaques (usually three-vessel disease)
Myocardial infarction (MI)	
Acute myocardial ischemia⁺	Unstable plaque, either critical or noncritical, with rupture and acute thrombus, either nonocclusive or occlusive; often associated with other stable critical plaques
Acute subendocardial MI	Same as for unstable angina
Acute transmural MI	Unstable plaque, either critical or noncritical, with rupture and acute occlusive fibrin-rich thrombus; also stable critical plaques (usually two-vessel or three-vessel disease)
Chronic myocardial ischemia‡	Stable critical plaques (usually two-vessel or three-vessel disease)
Old healed MI (scars > 1 cm)	Stable critical plaques (usually two-vessel or three-vessel disease); old organized thrombus, especially with old transmural infarcts
Chronic heart failure	Stable critical plaques (usually two-vessel or three-vessel disease); old organized thrombus; evidence of plaque progression
Sudden death	Unstable plaque, either critical or noncritical, with rupture and acute thrombus, either nonocclusive or occlusive; associated with other stable critical plaques (two-vessel or three-vessel disease in 80%, one-vessel disease in 15%, and four-vessel disease in 5%)

*Represents autopsied cases only (a source of bias). See text for detailed descriptions.

⁺Characterized microscopically by contraction band necrosis or by nuclear pyknosis and intense sarcoplasmic staining with eosin, occurring in the *absence* of an infiltrate of neutrophils or, with reperfusion, macrophages. These features generally represent preinfarction changes in which the patient died before leukocytic infiltration occurred.

‡Characterized microscopically by patchy subendocardial collections of vacuolated myocytes or by small (<1 cm) subendocardial patches of fibrosis or granulation tissue.

From Edwards (15), with permission.

rowing and the extent of calcification. Neither of these, however, is a risk factor for plaque rupture and subsequent thrombosis. Consequently, disease progression in individual patients represents a highly unpredictable process (24,25).

Acute Coronary Spasm

Medial spasm generally involves sites with eccentric plaques and produces contraction along the hypertrophied disease-free wall. Acute stenosis may be severe, depending on luminal size, shape, and eccentricity (see Fig. 2–2). Spasm may also induce distortions along the endothelial surface of adjacent plaques and thereby play a role in plaque fissuring. Subsequent platelet thrombosis can promote further spasm by release of thromboxane A_2, resulting in a cycle of spasm and thrombosis until luminal narrowing is sufficient to cause acute myocardial ischemia (1,19,20,26). This cycle may also be responsible for microembolization of platelet-fibrin thrombi.

Other Acute Obstructions

Acute coronary obstruction, unassociated with underlying thrombosis or spasm, may occur in acute aortic dissection and in the setting of embolization from infective or noninfective left-sided valvular vegetations or from left-sided mural thrombi. Many other rare causes have also been described (27).

Clinicopathologic Correlations

Angiographic and pathologic evaluations of chronically obstructed coronary arteries generally provide comparable results (1). However, the two methods of evaluation differ appreciably. Angiographers interpret luminograms that exhibit vessels longitudinally, and they express stenosis as the percentage of reduction in diameter. Pathologists, in contrast, interpret vessels cut in cross section and record the percentage of reduction in cross-sectional luminal area. Mathematically, the two methods are comparable only if circular lumens exist. For high-grade lesions, residual lumens are often noncircular, and results of the two methods are therefore only approximately equivalent.

Nomenclature

Pathologists grade the severity of coronary atherosclerosis by comparing the actual luminal area with the expected normal luminal area (that is, the area bounded by the internal elastic membrane.) Four grades are described on the basis of 25% increments (see Fig. 2–2). Cross-sectional area must be reduced by at least 75% to interfere with hyperemic coronary blood flow during exertion, and it must be narrowed by at least 90% to reduce flow at rest (1). Grade 4 lesions (that is, obstructions >75%) are considered to represent critical stenoses.

Angiographically, lesions are considered to be critically obstructive if the luminal diameter is diminished by 70% or more. For circular lumens, 75% and 90% reductions in cross-sectional area correspond to 50% and 70% reductions in diameter, respectively. Thus critical lesions differ between pathologists and clinicians. Perhaps this could be remedied by defining the reduction in cross-sectional area as 76% to 90% for grade 4 lesions, 91% to 99% for grade 5, and 100% for grade 6. Lesions could then be described as "severe" for grade 4, "critical" for grade 5, and "occluded" for grade 6.

Coronary Calcification

In general, radiographically visible calcium in the epicardial coronary arteries heralds the presence of atherosclerotic disease (28). Furthermore, coronary calcification tends to be a good prognostic indicator of future myocardial ischemic events. In living patients the amount of coronary calcium can be quantitated by electron beam computed tomography (7). Although in older patients there is a positive correlation between the amount of calcium and the degree of obstruction, the correlation fails in patients younger than 50 years, in whom calcification is relatively uncommon.

Angiographic Misinterpretation

The use of two orthogonal (biplane) x-ray cameras to evaluate coronary angiograms has appreciably reduced errors of interpretation related to noncircular lumens. There persists, however, a tendency to underestimate the extent of coronary artery stenosis, particularly in the left main artery. This is related to several factors, including the fact that with a luminogram, the severity of obstruction is evaluated by comparison with an adjacent segment that is assumed to be free of atherosclerosis (1,29,30). This is often a false assumption, and the extent of adjacent disease that is actually present then determines the degree of underestimation (Fig. 2–6).

It is important to recognize that the percentage of stenosis alone is not the only factor that determines the adequacy of myocardial perfusion. Other variables include the size of the vessel, length of the lesion, shape of the lumen, presence of multiple stenoses, extent of collateral flow, coronary perfusion pressure, and the presence of myocardial hypertrophy.

Pathologic Misinterpretation

High-grade lesions may remain undetected if pathologists step-section coronary arteries at such wide intervals that stenotic lesions lie between cuts. Moreover, slides do not necessarily contain the most narrowed region of the arterial segment submitted for microscopy. These two potential sources for underestimation of the severity of stenosis are easily remedied by decalcifying vessels, step-sectioning at 3-mm intervals, cutting vessels in cross section, and embedding sections properly for microscopy.

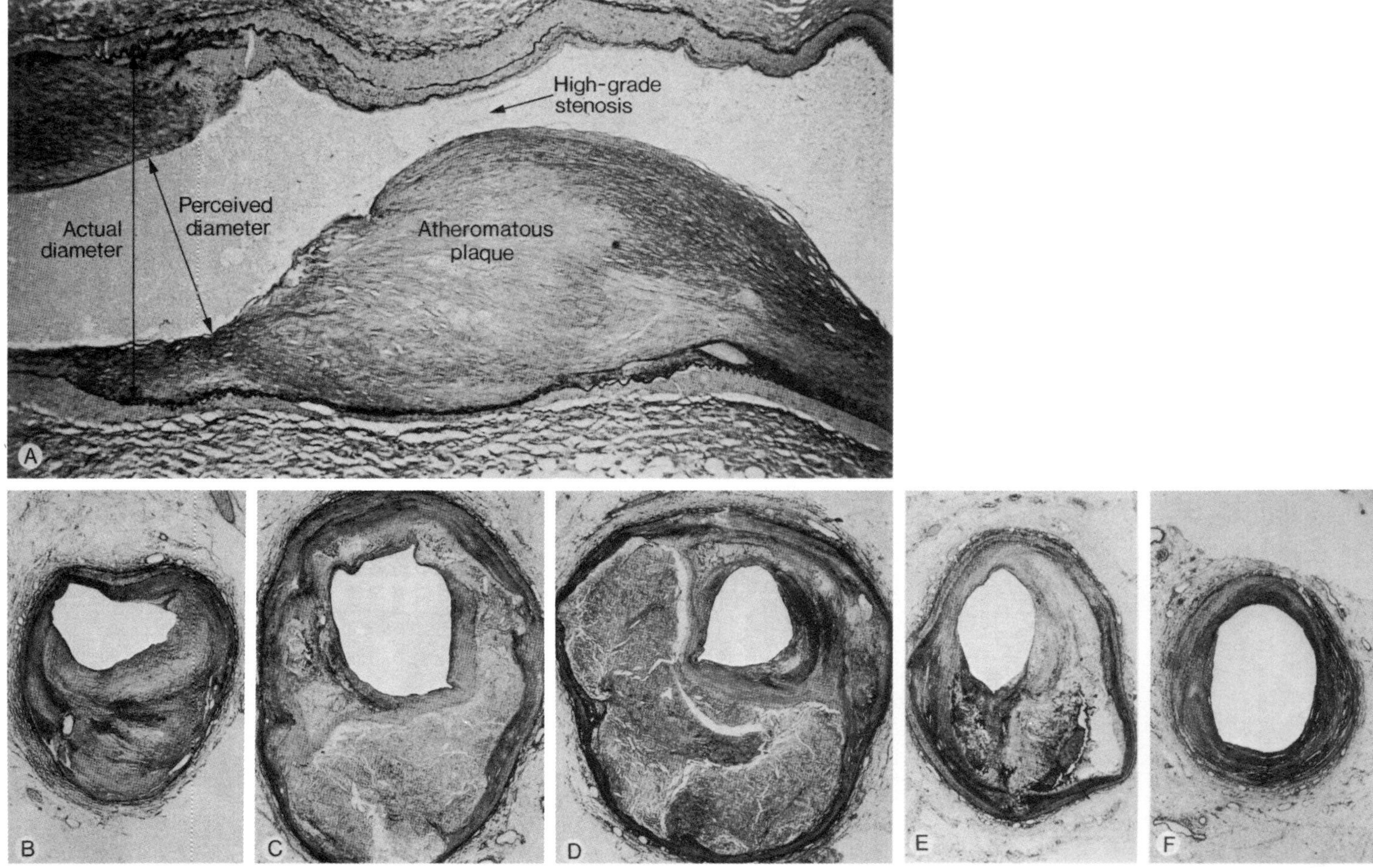

Figure 2–6. Pathologic-angiographic correlations. **A.** Coronary artery is cut in longitudinal section to simulate luminogram obtained angiographically. If segment of artery adjacent to high-grade plaque is considered disease-free angiographically, then calculated degree of obstruction will be underestimated. **B–F.** Five consecutive cross sections show effect of dilation on luminal narrowing. Although **C** and **D** exhibit critical grade 4 lesions, their absolute luminal sizes do not differ appreciably from those in the other three nondilated segments.

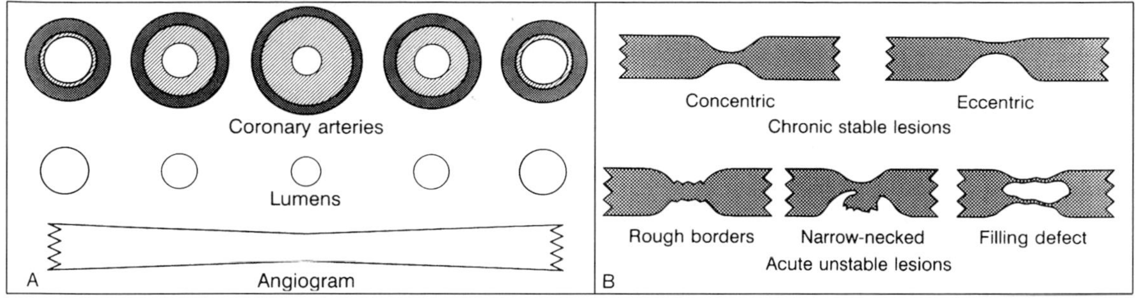

Figure 2–7. Pathologic–angiographic correlations (schematic). **A.** Effect of dilation (remodeling) on absolute luminal narrowing and on pathologist's estimate of grade of stenosis (compare with Fig. 2–6). **B.** Angiographic appearance of stable and unstable coronary atherosclerotic lesions.

If coronary arteries are not perfusion fixed, collapse of the disease-free portion of a vessel with an eccentric lesion will result in overestimation of the degree of stenosis. Other artifacts of tissue processing may also limit the accuracy of determining luminal stenosis microscopically (31).

Another cause of overestimation is inadequate assessment of coronary dilation. In a dilated segment even with grade 4 stenosis, the absolute size of the residual lumen may not vary appreciably from that in an adjacent nondilated segment without a critical lesion (12). In this setting, coronary angiography would more accurately reflect the luminal patency and the adequacy of coronary blood flow than would the use of microscopic grades (Fig. 2–7; also see Fig. 2–6). The effect of dilation, however, is greater for low-grade than high-grade obstructions (11).

Stable and Unstable Lesions

Angiographically, chronic stable atheromatous lesions in the coronary arteries are characterized by smooth borders (see Ch. 4). Concentric lesions produce an hourglass appearance, and eccentric processes result in wide-mouthed defects along one side of the vessel. Acute unstable lesions, in contrast, are associated with a more complex appearance, including rough borders with scalloped or irregular surfaces, narrow-necked defects with jagged or overhanging borders, luminal filling defects that are outlined by contrast material, and haziness of contrast material (see Fig. 2–7) (32,33). Microscopically, this angiographic morphology corresponds to plaque rupture and secondary thrombosis.

ACUTE MYOCARDIAL INFARCTION

General Features

For pathologists, transmural infarctions involve more than 50% of the ventricular wall thickness, and subendocardial (or nontransmural) infarctions occupy less than 50% (Fig. 2–8) (see Ch. 18). Some infarctions exhibit mixed patterns of transmural and subendocardial necrosis. Most infarctions occur in the distribution of a single coronary artery or at the border zone between two vessels. Among acute lesions, about 30% are nontransmural, and many are clinically silent, especially in women and older men. Regardless of the type of infarction, however, a thin (1- to 2-mm) rim of subendocardium usually survives, as a result of diffusion of nutrients from the ventricular blood, unless hindered by overlying mural thrombus.

In general, transmural infarctions are associated clinically with ST segment elevation and the development of abnormal Q waves. By comparison, subendocardial infarctions are usually characterized by ST and T wave changes without abnormal Q waves. Clinical enzymatic estimations of infarct size, which correlate well with pathologic determinations, indicate that Q wave infarctions are generally larger than non-Q wave lesions (34,35). Q wave processes are usually caused by acute coronary occlusion, whereas non-Q wave infarctions are associated either with incomplete obstruction (about 75% of cases) or with complete occlusion and ample collateral circulation. Although the short-term prognosis is better for non-Q wave than

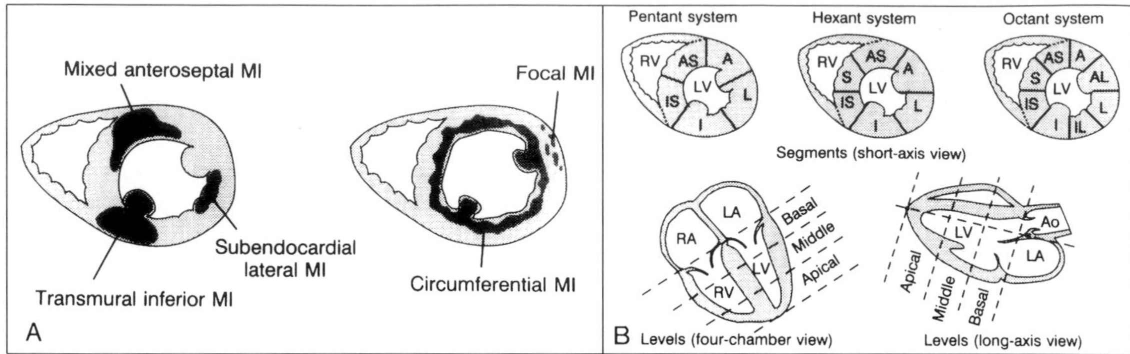

Figure 2–8. General features of myocardial infarctions (schematic). **A.** Types and locations of infarcts. **B.** Various systems for evaluation of infarct location by cardiac regions. A = anterior, AL = anterolateral, Ao = aorta, AS = anteroseptal, I = inferior, IL = inferolateral, IS = inferoseptal, L = lateral, LA = left atrium, LV = left ventricle, MI = myocardial infarction, RA = right atrium, RV = right ventricle, S = septal.

Q wave infarctions, the long-term mortality is similar for both types.

In contrast to these two patterns are circumferential and focal myocardial infarctions. Circumferential subendocardial necrosis is generally associated with global myocardial ischemia resulting from hypotension or hypoxemia. Focal small infarctions, not limited to the subendocardium, are often the result of coronary embolization, most commonly caused by valvular vegetations.

The location of an infarct is designated in terms of the wall thickness involved (transmural or subendocardial), the segment involved (such as anteroseptal), and the level involved (apical, midventricular, or basal) (see Fig. 2–8). With knowledge of the percentage of left ventricular muscle mass that normally constitutes each region (Table 2–3), the relative size of an infarction may be estimated and expressed as a percentage of total left ventricular mass (36). Subendocardial necrosis generally involves about 30% of the wall thickness, and transmural disease usually accounts for 75% to 90%.

Although most myocardial infarctions involve the left ventricle, it is recognized that atrial and right ventricular lesions also occur (37). Right ventricular infarctions generally occur as an extension of an inferoseptal left ventricular process, although isolated lesions and those associated with anteroseptal infarctions may also develop (38) (see Ch. 17). They tend to affect right ventricles that are hypertrophied and dilated as a result of pulmonary hypertension caused by left ventricular hypertrophy or failure or by chronic pulmonary disease.

Table 2–3. Percentage of Regional Left Ventricular Mass

	LV Mass per Region (%)			
LV Level	Pentant	Hexant	Octant	Total
Basal	8.5	7.1	5.3	42.5
Middle	7.2	6.0	4.5	36.0
Apical	4.3	3.6	2.7	21.5
Total	20.0	16.7	12.5	100.0

LV = left ventricular.

Modified from Edwards (36).

Inflammation and Repair

The evolution of acute myocardial infarction represents a clinicopathologic spectrum that begins with unstable angina and extends through subendocardial and then transmural infarction. In experimental animals, necrosis begins subendocardially and progresses transmurally as a wavefront phenomenon. Within the first hour of cessation of regional blood flow, confluent patches of irreversibly injured myocytes are observed in the subendocardial one-third. By 3 hours, fingers of necrosis extend into the middle third, and by 12 to 24 hours, the entire wall thickness is involved.

By transmission electron microscopy, the earliest changes of reversible ischemic injury include glycogen depletion, cellular and mitochondrial swelling, myofibrillar relaxation, and margination of nuclear chromatin (39). With prolonged ischemia, the development of amorphous mitochondrial densities and sarcolemmal disruptions heralds the onset of irreversible myocyte injury. As dying cells undergo further disruption, features of necrosis become visible by light microscopy, as described in the next paragraph. Capillary injury may also occur, with endothelial swelling and, eventually, necrosis.

By light microscopy, clusters of ischemic myocardial cells form peninsulas within areas of viable myocardium and initially exhibit intense sarcoplasmic eosin staining, nuclear pyknosis and, occasionally, stretched and wavy myocytes. As the infarction becomes established, contraction band necrosis is prominent in cases with reperfusion, and coagulation necrosis prevails in those without (39,40). Thus, in general, contraction bands are a feature of subendocardial infarctions, and coagulation necrosis is characteristic of transmural infarctions, although some overlap occurs. Degeneration of dead myocytes elicits a typical inflammatory response that sets the stage for healing by fibrosis (Fig. 2–9 and Table 2–4).

Neutrophils begin to accumulate in the region of infarction by the end of the first day and achieve maximum intensity by 3 to 4 days (see Ch. 21). They release enzymes and thereby prepare the necrotic tissue for phagocytosis by macrophages. Paradoxically, neutrophils may actually cause further myocyte injury, either by releasing enzymes or by plugging capillaries (41). Neutrophils survive only a few days in the hostile acidic and hypoxic environment of infarcted myocardium. By 5 to 7 days, necrotic and partially dissolved myocytes are surrounded by basophilic interstitial debris that contains fragments of necrotic neutrophils (so-called nuclear dust). Eosinophils are occasionally observed, usually in small numbers, but giant cells are not.

Whereas the first week after infarction is characterized by a neutrophilic infiltrate, the second week is marked by the appearance of macrophages, and their numbers peak between days 8 and 10. Lymphokines control the activation of blood monocytes into tissue macrophages. These resilient cells phagocytose not only necrotic myocytes but also necrotic interstitial cells and neutrophils. They often become filled with lipofuscin pigment of myocyte origin. The remaining interstitium, with its collapsed extracellular skeleton of collagen and reticulin, forms the scaffolding on which repair takes place. At the infarct border, ischemic but viable myocytes may exhibit large nucleoli that resemble viral inclusions.

By day 12, fibrovascular granulation tissue forms along the outer border of large infarcts and spreads toward the center, led by a band of macrophages. By the beginning of the third week, plump and active fibroblasts begin to deposit extracellular collagen, as scar formation commences. During the course of the next several weeks, the scar becomes less cellular and vascular and generally becomes more dense and collagenous. A few small clusters of chronic inflammatory cells usually persist. Some degree of scar retraction takes place and contributes to wall thinning, as do stretching (expansion) of the area of infarction and compensatory hypertrophy of noninfarcted regions of the left ventricle. Some scars contain elastin or abundant adipose tissue. Calcification is rare except in some thin-walled aneurysms.

The intensity of the inflammatory infiltrate depends on many factors, including the size of the infarction, the presence of other inflammatory disorders (such as pneumonia), and the age and nutritional state of the patient. Similarly, the rate of healing is influenced by infarct size, the presence of reperfusion, and the patient's age and nutritional state. Coexistent hematologic or immunologic disorders may also interfere with the extent or rate of inflammation and repair.

COMPLICATIONS OF MYOCARDIAL INFARCTION

Among patients with a diagnosis of acute myocardial infarction, approximately one-half will experience one or more complications. The type of complication is often related to the patient's age and gender and to the size and location of the infarction

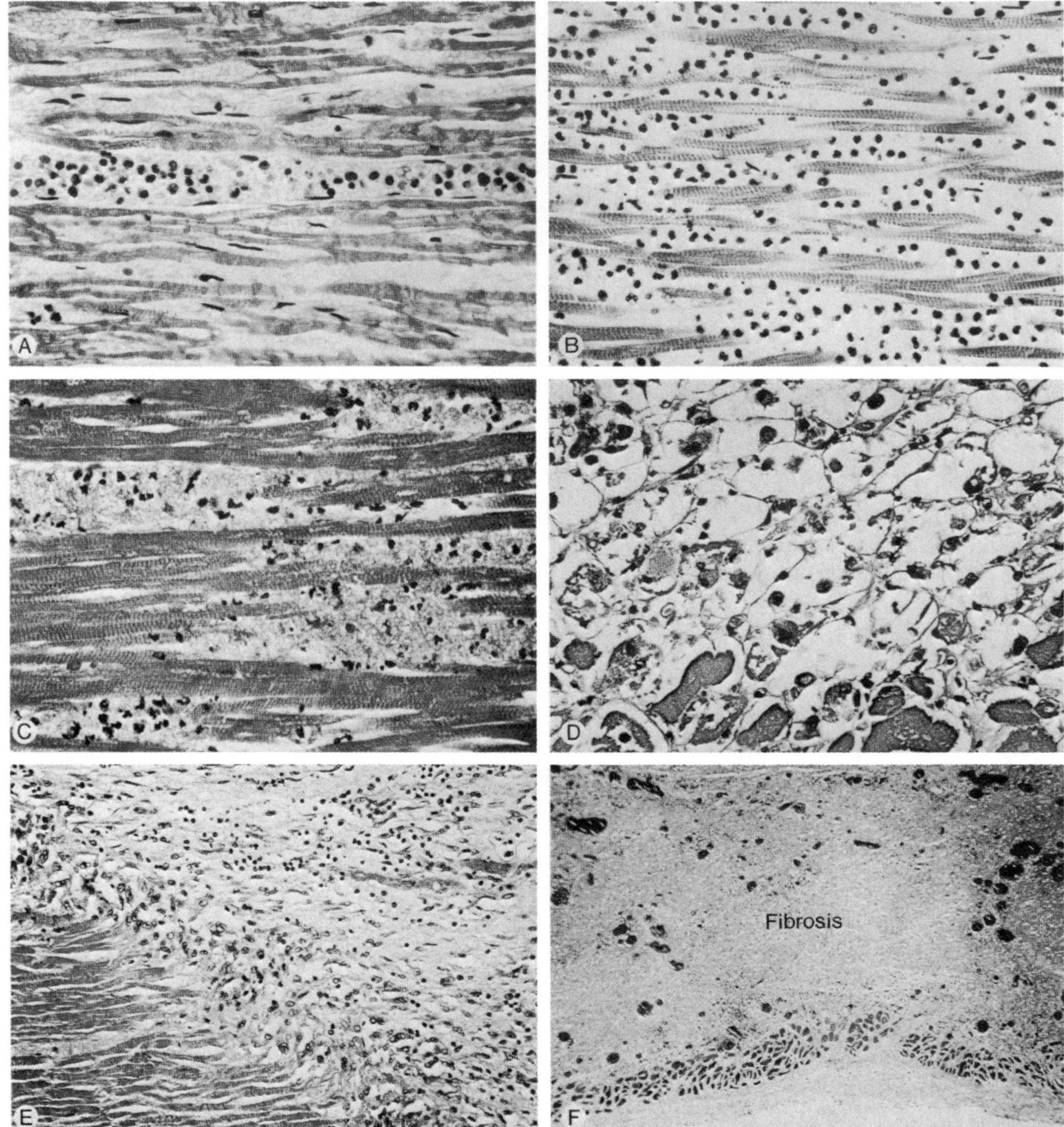

Figure 2–9. Histopathology of myocardial infarction. **A.** Acute myocyte ischemic injury, insterstitial edema, and early neutrophilic infiltration (1 day old). **B.** Necrotic myocytes and extensive neutrophilic infiltrate (2 to 4 days). **C.** Necrotic myocytes and basophilic interstitial debris (5 to 7 days). **D.** Extensive accumulation of macrophages within infarcted myocardium (8 to 11 days). **E.** Fibrovascular granulation tissue at border of infarct (12 to 16 days). **F.** Dense fibrosis, at low power (older than 16 days).

(see Chs. 10, 13, and 16). Some complications, for example, occur only in the setting of transmural necrosis (Fig. 2–10). Heart failure is more likely to complicate transmural disease, whereas angina and recurrent infarction occur more often with subendocardial disease. Mechanical complications are more common with anteroseptal infarctions, and conduction disturbances are more frequent with inferior ones. Large or anterior infarctions have a worse prognosis than others.

Table 2–4. Age-Related Features of Myocardial Infarction

Age	Gross Features	Light Microscopy
< 4 hours	No change	No change
4–12 hours	Slight mottling, with areas of dark discoloration	Intense sacroplasmic eosinophilia and nuclear pyknosis; contraction bands, with reperfusion
12–24 hours	Mottled and mildly edematous, with bulging cut surface	As above, with early interstitial edema and neutrophilic infiltrates
2–4 days	Soft yellow-tan core with mottled border	Maximum neutrophilic infiltrate; nuclear loss and sarcoplasmic coagulation
5–7 days	Yellow-tan core and irregular hyperemic red-brown border	Basophilic interstitial debris; early macrophage infiltration; dilated capillaries at border
8–10 days	Yellow-gray core and red-brown border; depressed cut surface	Numerous macrophages, with active phagocytosis; pigmented macrophages filled with lipofuscin
11–14 days	Yellow-gray core and red-gray border; depressed cut surface	Granulation tissue along border; ongoing phagocytosis at core
2–4 weeks	Core becoming smaller; border becoming larger, grayer, firmer, and less gelatinous; less depressed cut surface	Ongoing scar formation, dense at outer border; chronic inflammation; dilated peripheral small vessels; central core of necrotic tissue
>1 month	Firm gray-white or red-gray scar, with scar retraction and variable wall thinning	Mature scar (dense collagen, focal elastin, and hypocellularity); focal lymphocytes

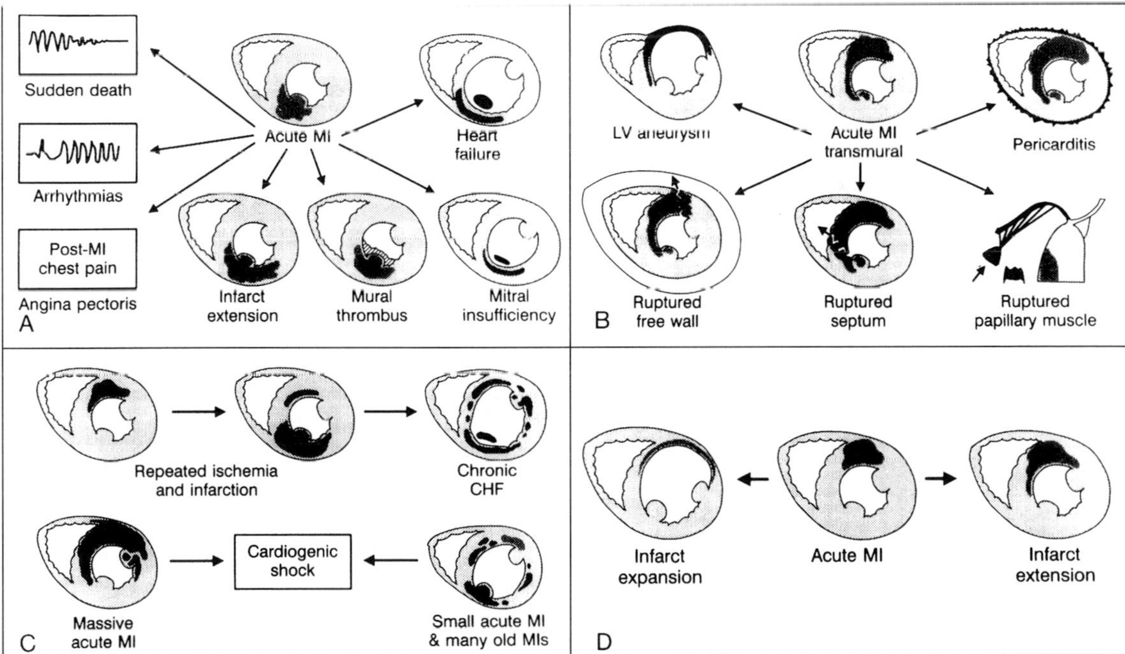

Figure 2–10. Complications of myocardial infarction (schematic). **A.** General complications. **B.** Complications of transmural infarctions. **C.** Cardiogenic shock, as a result of either a massive acute infarction or a small acute process in a heart already involved by multiple old infarctions. **D.** Comparison of infarct expansion (aneurysm formation) and infarct extension (reinfarction). CHF = congestive heart failure, LV = left ventricle, MI = myocardial infarction.

Acute Events

During the course of myocardial infarction certain complications can occur and lead to the acute onset of symptoms. These are related primarily to arrhythmias, cardiogenic shock, infarct extension, various forms of cardiac rupture, and embolization.

Arrhythmias

The primary function of the cardiac conduction system is impulse conduction rather than contraction. Consequently, the modified myocytes in this sytem are far less susceptible to ischemic injury than contracting myocytes. Moreover, the subendocardial position of the left bundle branch favors its nourishment by ventricular blood, and the atrioventricular (His) bundle has a dual blood supply. These factors serve to protect the atrioventricular conduction tissues from acute ischemic injury (see Ch. 15).

Thus, although arrhythmias associated with acute myocardial infarction may originate in the conduction tissues, they more commonly arise in the ventricular myocardium. They appear to be related to electrically unstable ischemic myocardium at the border of the infarction, to arrhythmogenic metabolites released by the infarcted tissues, or to microembolization from a thrombosed coronary artery. Metabolites may produce arrhythmias locally or through their distant effect on the atrioventricular node, as a result of the numerous coronary venous and lymphatic channels that drain through or adjacent to the node. Arrhythmias that develop late after infarction may originate in ischemic myocardium at the border or within the infarct scar.

Cardiogenic Shock

Shock occurs when ventricular function is insufficient to sustain the viability of vital organs. It is associated with loss of at least 40% of the left ventricular mass, although not all infarcts of this size are associated with cardiogenic shock (Figs. 2–10 and 2–11) (see Ch. 13). Shock may be related either to massive acute infarction or to a smaller area of necrosis in a ventricle already ravaged by previous infarctions. In one autopsy study, cardiogenic shock was the most common cause of death among pa-

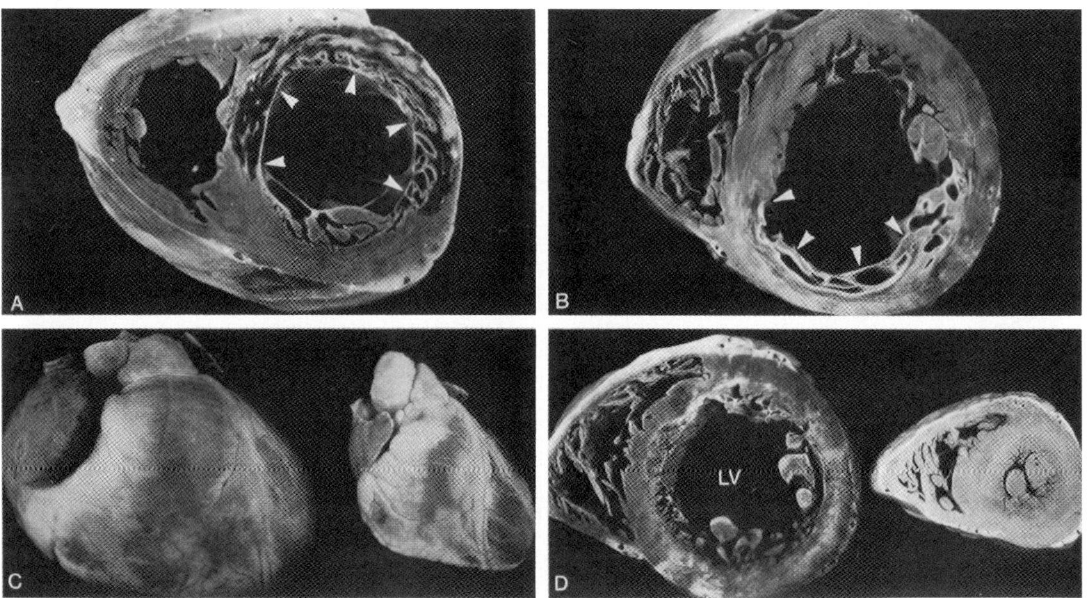

Figure 2–11. Impaired left ventricular function. **A.** Massive acute anteroseptal myocardial infarction (arrowheads) associated with cardiogenic shock. **B.** Old inferior (posterior) myocardial infarction (arrowheads) associated with left ventricular dilation and chronic congestive heart failure. **C,D.** So-called ischemic cardiomyopathy, viewed anteriorly (**C**) and in short-axis cross section (**D**), with normal hearts at right for comparison. LV = left ventricle.

tients with myocardial infarction, accounting for 44% of the deaths; ventricular rupture and arrhythmias accounted for 27% and 16%, respectively (42).

Microscopically, the shock state is associated not only with an acute infarction but also with infarct extension and with small areas of acute subendocardial necrosis elsewhere in the ventricles. Thus cardiogenic shock is characterized by a vicious cycle of ongoing myocardial injury and progressive left ventricular dysfunction.

Infarct Extension

Extension represents a specific form of reinfarction that develops within the context of a recent myocardial infarction. It is associated with an increase in the absolute amount of necrotic myocardium and may involve either ventricle (see Fig. 2–10). Risk factors for infarct extension include subendocardial infarction, female gender, previous infarctions, and a large infarction associated with cardiogenic shock (43,44).

Extension most often occurs between 2 and 10 days after the initial infarction and tends to form along its lateral and subepicardial borders. Microscopically, necrotic myocardium in an area of extension appears younger than the original infarction and occurs outside its peripheral border of macrophages or granulation tissue.

Ruptured Ventricular Free Wall

Among patients with fatal transmural myocardial infarctions who come to autopsy, the cause of death is rupture of the left ventricular free wall in 8% to 9% (44) (see Chs. 10 and 16). Once rupture occurs, death is relatively rapid because of hemopericardium and cardiac tamponade (Fig. 2–12).

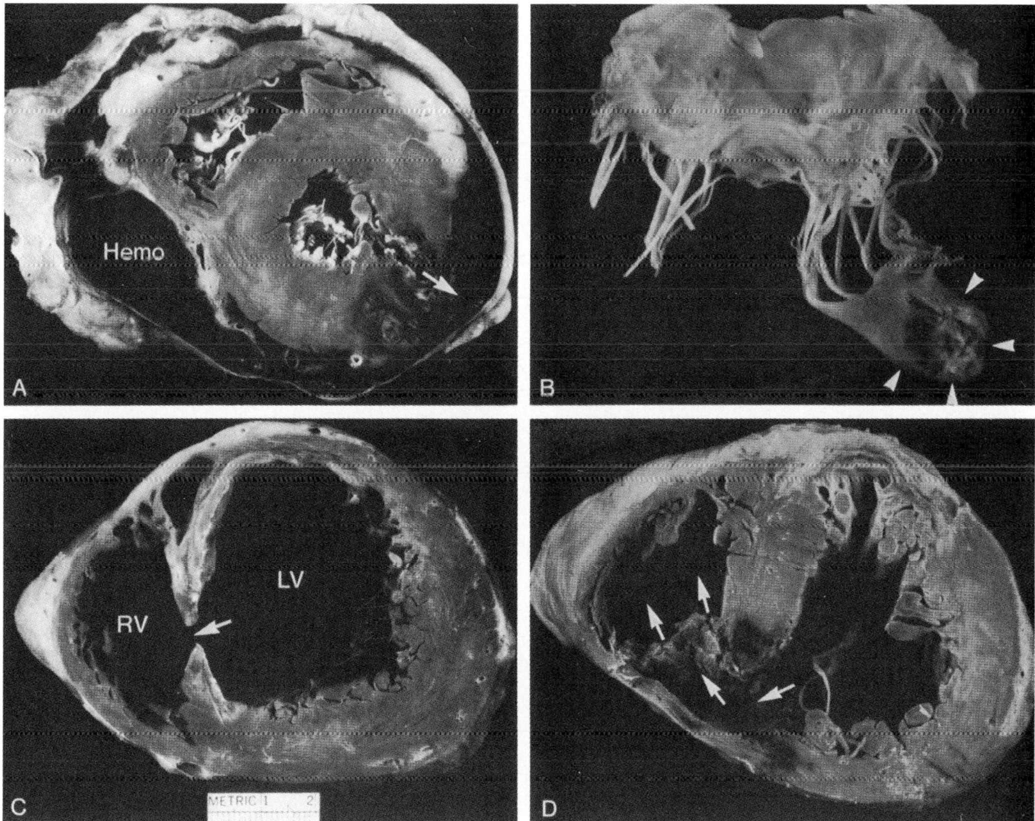

Figure 2–12. Postinfarction cardiac ruptures. **A.** Free wall rupture (arrow), with hemopericardium (Hemo). **B.** Rupture of infarcted mitral papillary muscle (arrowheads) (from surgically excised specimen). **C,D.** Septal ruptures of simple (**C**) and complex (**D**) types. LV = left ventricle, RV = right ventricle.

Most patients have severe multivessel coronary atherosclerosis.

Ruptures affect the lateral wall more frequently than the anterior or inferior walls, and the midventricular level more often than the apical or basal levels (45,46). This may be related to the excess stress placed on the lateral midventricular region by contraction of mitral papillary muscles. Moreover, rupture tends to occur at the edge of a transmural infarction rather than its midportion. This probably relates to shear forces that exist at the interface between viable contracting myocardium and necrotic muscle that is akinetic or dyskinetic (see Color Plate 1).

Rupture tends to occur during the first week, when coagulative necrosis and neutrophilic infiltration have appreciably weakened the infarcted myocardium. Interstitial eosinophils may also play a role (47). However, 13% to 28% of ruptures occur within 24 hours, before necrosis and inflammation are well established (45). In this regard, rapid or age-related changes in the structural integrity of extracellular connective tissue may favor cardiac rupture.

The reported risk factors for free wall rupture include age greater than 60 years, female gender, preexisting hypertension, absence of left ventricular hypertrophy, first myocardial infarction, and midventricular or lateral transmural infarctions (45,46, 48). Although ventricular aneurysms may rupture during the early phase of their development, they almost never rupture after healing by fibrosis occurs.

Certain ECG changes, occuring during the evolution of a transmural infarction, may allow the identification of patients with a particularly high likelihood of myocardial rupture (49). However, in a recent review of 100 cases of postinfarction rupture of the left ventricular free wall, half represented out-of-hospital sudden deaths and were therefore under the jurisdiction of a medical examiner or coroner (45).

Ruptured Ventricular Septum

Postinfarction rupture of the ventricular septum occurs much less frequently than that of the free wall (see Chs. 10 and 16). It is a complication of transmural infarction, and two types have been described pathologically and echocardiographically (Fig. 2–12; see Color Plate 2) (50,51). Simple ruptures tend to be relatively linear and to involve the anteroapical aspect of the septum. In contrast, complex ruptures generally occur inferobasally and follow a serpiginous course through the septum, occasionally extending into the adjacent ventricular free walls.

Septal rupture most commonly occurs during the first week, when the infarcted myocardium is weakest, and it results in an acquired ventricular septal defect of variable size. A left-to-right shunt and acute heart failure or shock are the most common manifestations. The ragged edge of the rupture tract may be a source for embolization of thrombus or necrotic myocardium. Risk factors for rupture of a large transmural septal infarction include first infarction and an occluded coronary artery with little collateral circulation (52). Mortality is higher with inferoseptal than anteroseptal infarctions as a result of the greater likelihood of right ventricular involvement and shock (53).

Ruptured Papillary Muscle

In contrast to postinfarction ruptures of the free wall or septum, those involving the mitral papillary muscles are less frequent and occur with subendocardial as well as transmural necrosis (see Chs. 10 and 16). The underlying infarction may be small and represent the first ischemic event, and the observation of contraction band necrosis and hemorrhage suggests that reperfusion occurs in many (54,55). Coronary atherosclerosis, therefore, is generally less extensive than for other patients with myocardial infarction. Papillary muscle rupture tends to occur during the first week, as do the other forms of postinfarction rupture.

Although mitral regurgitation is sudden in onset, its severity is variable and determined primarily by the extent of papillary muscle involvement (see Fig. 2–12 and Color Plate 3). Rupture near the tip, with only partial involvement of a papillary muscle group, causes less severe regurgitation than disruption of the entire muscle.

The posteromedial muscle is the site of rupture in about 85% of the cases. This is probably related to the fact that its blood supply is usually from only one source, the dominant coronary artery, whereas the anterolateral muscle is nourished by arterial branches from both the left anterior descending artery and the left circumflex coronary arteries. Rarely, right ventricular infarction may be associated with rupture of a tricuspid papillary muscle.

Mural Thrombus and Embolization

The development of mural thrombus in the left ventricular chamber is favored by hemodynamic stasis and endocardial inflammation and is thereby related to infarct size and location (see Chs. 10 and 20). Thrombus is observed in about 50% of patients with large apical anteroseptal infarctions or postinfarction aneurysms (Fig. 2–13) (56). Although small thrombi usually become organized and incorporated into the thickened endocardium, large thrombi tend to organize slowly and incompletely, and they may exhibit liquid cores or calcified borders. Chronic left ventricular dysfunction and dilation are often associated with the progressive development of laminated mural thrombi.

Systemic thromboembolism represents yet another potential acute complication of myocardial infarction. Dislodgement may occur along unstable and friable surfaces of recent thrombi or from surface erosions along old partially organized thrombi. The latter liberates necrotic debris from the core of the thrombus and may result not only in embolization but also in fever. In patients with ischemic heart disease and atrial fibrillation, the left atrium is another potential site for mural thrombus and a source of systemic embolization.

Although the release of small particles from mural thrombi may be asymptomatic, embolization of larger fragments often leads to symptomatic ischemia or infarction and may affect the brain, eyes, kidneys, spleen, bowel, legs, or heart. Thromboemboli are observed microscopically at autopsy in about one-third of cases but are apparent clinically in only 5% to 6%. Even so, it is estimated that 15,000 to 25,000 strokes occur each year in the United States as a result of embolization from postinfarction left ventricular mural thrombus (57). The risk for embolization is greatest in the first few weeks after infarction.

Chronic Events

The chronic effects of myocardial infarction are related primarily to heart failure, left ventricular aneurysm, mitral regurgitation, angina pectoris, and pericarditis.

Chronic Heart Failure

The severity of postinfarction heart failure depends on the extent of cumulative muscle loss by infarction and ischemia, both acutely and chronically. Persistent chronic heart failure has a poor prognosis and represents end-stage ischemic heart disease, or

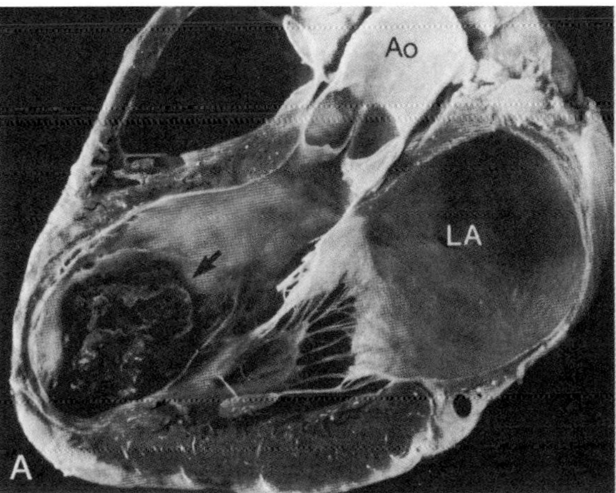

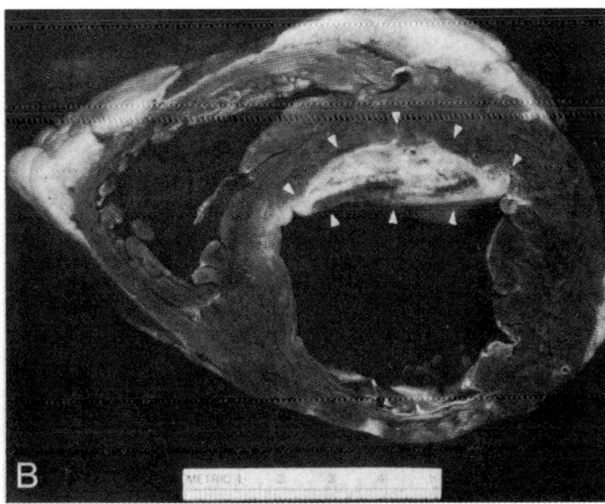

Figure 2–13. Postinfarction left ventricular mural thrombus. **A.** Recent thrombus (arrow), with central ulceration and systemic embolization, in long-axis view. **B.** Old organized thrombus (arrowheads), in short-axis view. Ao = aorta, LA = left atrium.

so-called ischemic cardiomyopathy. Some patients, especially diabetics, with no past history of angina pectoris or myocardial infarction, may be misdiagnosed clinically as having idiopathic dilated cardiomyopathy.

Among patients who die of chronic postinfarction heart failure, the coronary arteries at autopsy are generally the site of critical two-vessel or three-vessel atherosclerosis, although collaterals are generally well developed. It is uncommon, however, to encounter either plaque rupture and luminal thrombosis or critical left main coronary disease.

Hearts show gross cardiomegaly, with moderate biventricular hypertrophy and moderate to marked four-chamber dilation (see Fig. 2–11). The left ventricular myocardium is usually the site of one or more healed myocardial infarctions, some of which may have been clinically silent. Some patients have no gross evidence of myocardial infarction, though (58,59). Microscopically, however, all show evidence of chronic subendocardial ischemia, with sarcoplasmic vacuolization of myocytes and patchy areas of interstitial fibrosis. Mural thrombus may be present in any cardiac chamber, and microscopic evidence of embolization is commonly observed in other organs.

Elsewhere, the effects of chronic biventricular failure are evident. The lungs exhibit typical changes of chronic pulmonary venous hypertension, and the abdominal viscera are enlarged by chronic congestion. Peripheral edema and pleural or pericardial effusions are also commonly encountered. Terminally, shock may ensue, as manifested by hemorrhagic centrilobular hepatic necrosis and acute renal tubular necrosis.

True Aneurysm (Infarct Expansion)

Within a few hours to a few days after transmural myocardial infarction, the pulsatile force of left ventricular contractions acting on a necrotic and weakened wall commonly results in stretching and thinning of the infarcted region (see Ch. 10). This remodeling of left ventricular shape, without an increase in the absolute size of infarction, represents infarct expansion (in contrast to infarct extension) and is the precursor of aneurysm formation (see Fig. 2–10) (60). It occurs most often in hearts with large infarctions and little hypertrophy (61). Early infarct expansion may be more apparent clinically than at autopsy.

As transmural infarctions evolve and later heal by fibrosis, a spectrum exists from those with relatively normal wall thickness, to those with thinned walls and a uniformly dilated left ventricle, to those with a thinned wall that bulges beyond the expected contour of the left ventricle. Only the last are considered to represent postinfarction true aneurysms.

Among patients with left ventricular aneurysms, the coronary arteries are generally involved by critical two-vessel or three-vessel disease (62). Although coronary thrombotic occlusion usually causes the underlying transmural infarction, most hearts that develop aneurysms also have little collateral blood flow (63). This suggests that once transmural infarction is already established, adequate collateral blood flow may be necessary during the healing phase to prevent aneurysm formation.

More than 80% of left ventricular aneurysms involve the apical anteroseptal region (Fig. 2–14). They affect men more often than women and have a poor prognosis if associated with heart failure or arrhythmias (64). As healing occurs, the aneurysmal walls, though thinned, become densely fibrotic and may even calcify. Microscopically, they exhibit features of all three cardiac layers (endocardium, myocardium, epicardium), although myocytes are often sparse and focal disruption of myocardial continuity may be observed.

Heart failure and arrhythmias are responsible for most of the deaths related to postinfarction aneurysms. A thick fibroelastic endocardial rind forms the lining of most aneurysms associated with ventricular tachycardia (65). Although laminated mural thrombus forms within about 50% of aneurysms, it is associated with systemic embolization in fewer than 5% (66). Despite their thinness (only 1 mm in some cases), left ventricular aneurysms have tough fibrous or fibrocalcific walls that are not prone to rupture, unless acute infarctions involve their borders.

False Aneurysm (Contained Rupture)

Rarely, postinfarction rupture of the left ventricular free wall is incomplete because the structural integrity of the overlying epicardium is maintained (see Chs. 10 and 16). Subsequent epicardial dilation results in a flask-shaped pseudoaneurysm, whose neck is formed by the myocardial dissection tract and whose body is formed by epicardial expansion (see Fig. 2–14) (67). Parietal pericardial adhesions may form and reinforce the aneurysmal wall. Microscopically, the false aneurysm consists of fibroadipose connective tissue, without myocardial elements, and a lining of laminated thrombus.

Although the distinction between true and false aneurysms is made microscopically, certain gross features may serve to differentiate the two in most cases. True aneurysms tend to have wide necks and involve the apical anteroseptal wall, whereas false aneurysms generally have narrow necks and commonly occur along the inferior or lateral walls (see Color Plate 4). It should, however, be noted that narrow-necked true aneurysms and wide-necked false aneurysms occur and that distinction between true and false types by clinical imaging techniques is not always accurate, particularly for inferolateral aneurysms.

Because pseudoaneurysms represent contained left ventricular ruptures, their associated coronary artery and myocardial lesions are the same as those for patients with acute transmural infarction and rupture of the left ventricular free wall. Unlike true aneurysms, false aneurysms have a propensity to rupture and to cause death by hemopericardium and cardiac tamponade. This is prevented, however, if fibrous adhesions obliterate the pericardial space.

Mitral Regurgitation

Mitral regurgitation can develop suddenly as a consequence of papillary muscle rupture, as previously discussed. However, it may also develop as a chronic complication (Fig. 2–15).

In some cases, it is related to ischemia or infarc-

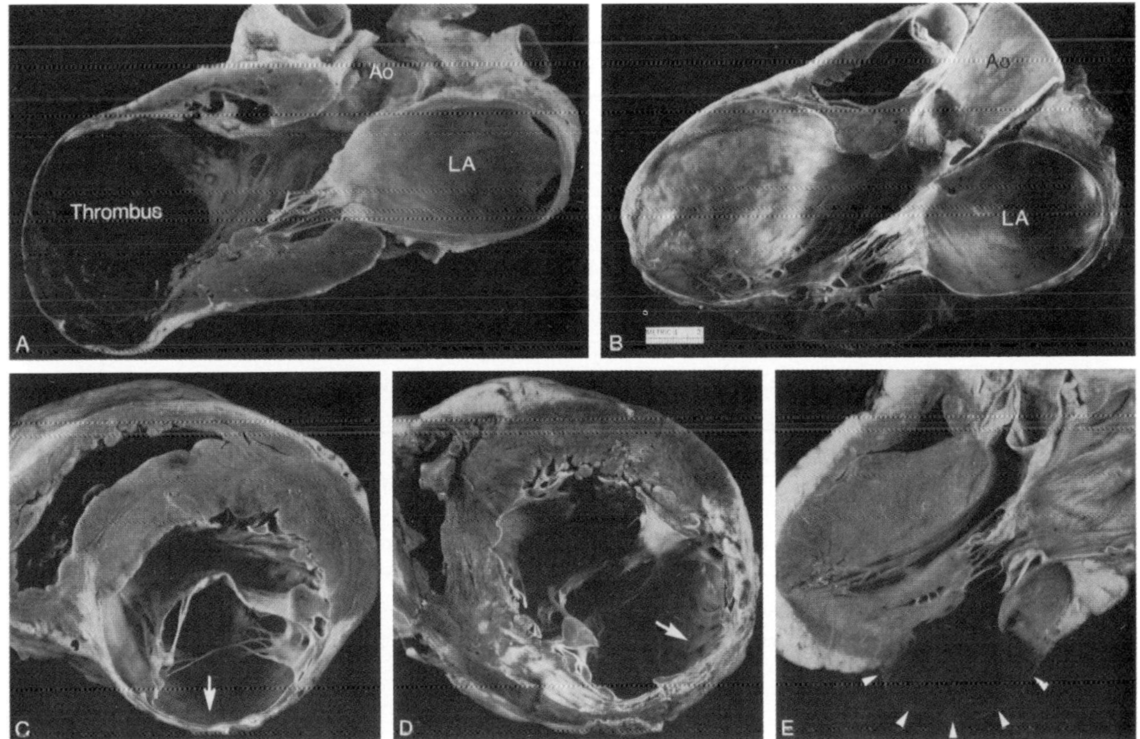

Figure 2–14. Postinfarction left ventricular aneurysms. **A,B.** Apical anteroseptal aneurysms, with (**A**) and without (**B**) mural thrombus, in long-axis views. **C,D.** Inferior (**C**) and lateral (**D**) aneurysms (arrows), in short-axis views. **E.** Thrombus-filled false aneurysm (arrowheads), involving inferolateral wall, in long-axis view. Ao = aorta, LA = left atrium.

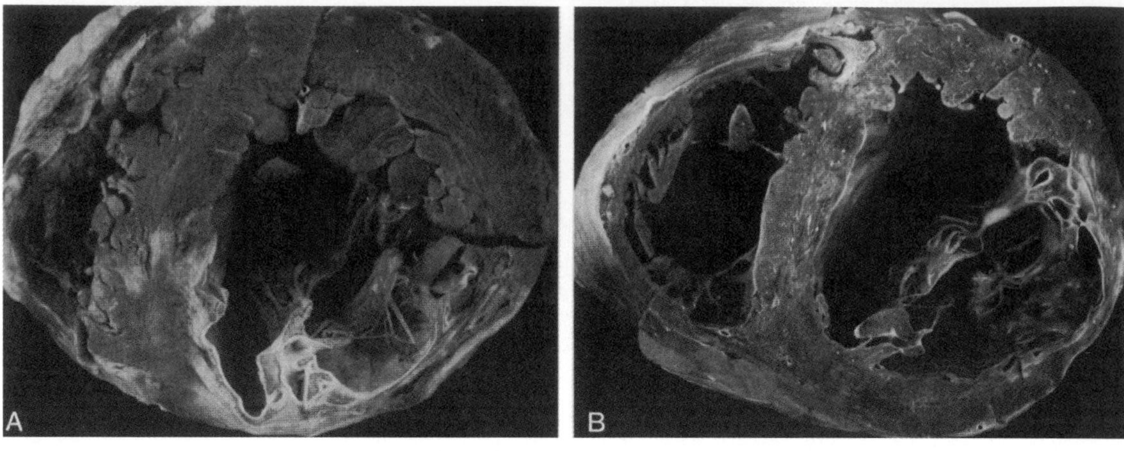

Figure 2–15. Chronic postinfarction mitral regurgitation. **A.** Old infarction involving mitral papillary muscles, in short-axis view. **B.** Mitral insufficiency resulting from left ventricular dilation and chronic heart failure, in short-axis view.

tion, with subsequent fibrosis of one or both papillary muscle groups. This constitutes the syndrome of papillary muscle dysfunction. The ischemic area usually involves both a papillary muscle and its subjacent free wall.

In other cases, mitral regurgitation is related to chronic heart failure with left ventricular dilation. In this setting, valvular incompetence is associated with geometric displacement of the papillary muscles and mild annular dilation (68).

Postinfarction Angina

Angina pectoris develops in some patients *after* myocardial infarction and occurs more commonly with subendocardial than transmural necrosis. Chest pain is due to ischemia either in the distribution of the infarct-related coronary artery, or paradoxically, in the distribution of a second critically narrowed artery, perhaps as a result of interrupted collateral blood flow. During episodes of angina, most cells in the ischemic area sustain only reversible injury, although a few are lethally damaged. Acute and chronic changes occur in the myocardium that reflect the altered homeostasis resulting from ischemia (Fig. 2–16).

Microscopically, acute ischemic changes include sarcoplasmic eosinophilia, pyknotic nuclei, and early formation of contraction bands. No inflammatory infiltrates are observed. In contrast, chronic ischemic changes are characterized by sarcoplasmic vacuolization (so-called myocytolysis) and microfocal patches of interstitial granulation tissue or fibrosis. Granulation tissue often is loose and contains pigmented macrophages. Although the aforementioned myocyte lesions are considered reversible, patchy areas of granulation tissue and fibrosis are not.

Postinfarction Pericarditis

Fibrinous pericarditis is a potential complication of acute transmural myocardial infarctions and usually occurs during the first week. It is associated not only with infarcts of large size but also those with arrhythmias and heart failure (69). In some cases pericarditis is localized to the area overlying the infarction, whereas in others it involves the pericardial sac diffusely. The inflammatory exudate is rich in fibrin and produces a shaggy coat both along the epicardial surface and along areas of contact with the opposing surface of parietal pericardium. Clinically, this results in chest pain and a pericardial friction rub. Organization of the exudate can result in localized or diffuse fibrous pericardial adhesions.

Postmyocardial infarction syndrome (Dressler's syndrome) occurs weeks to months after myocardial infarction and is prone to recurrence. It is characterized clinically by low-grade fever, pleuropericardial chest pain, a pericardial friction rub, and pericardial and pleural effusions that may be hemorrhagic.

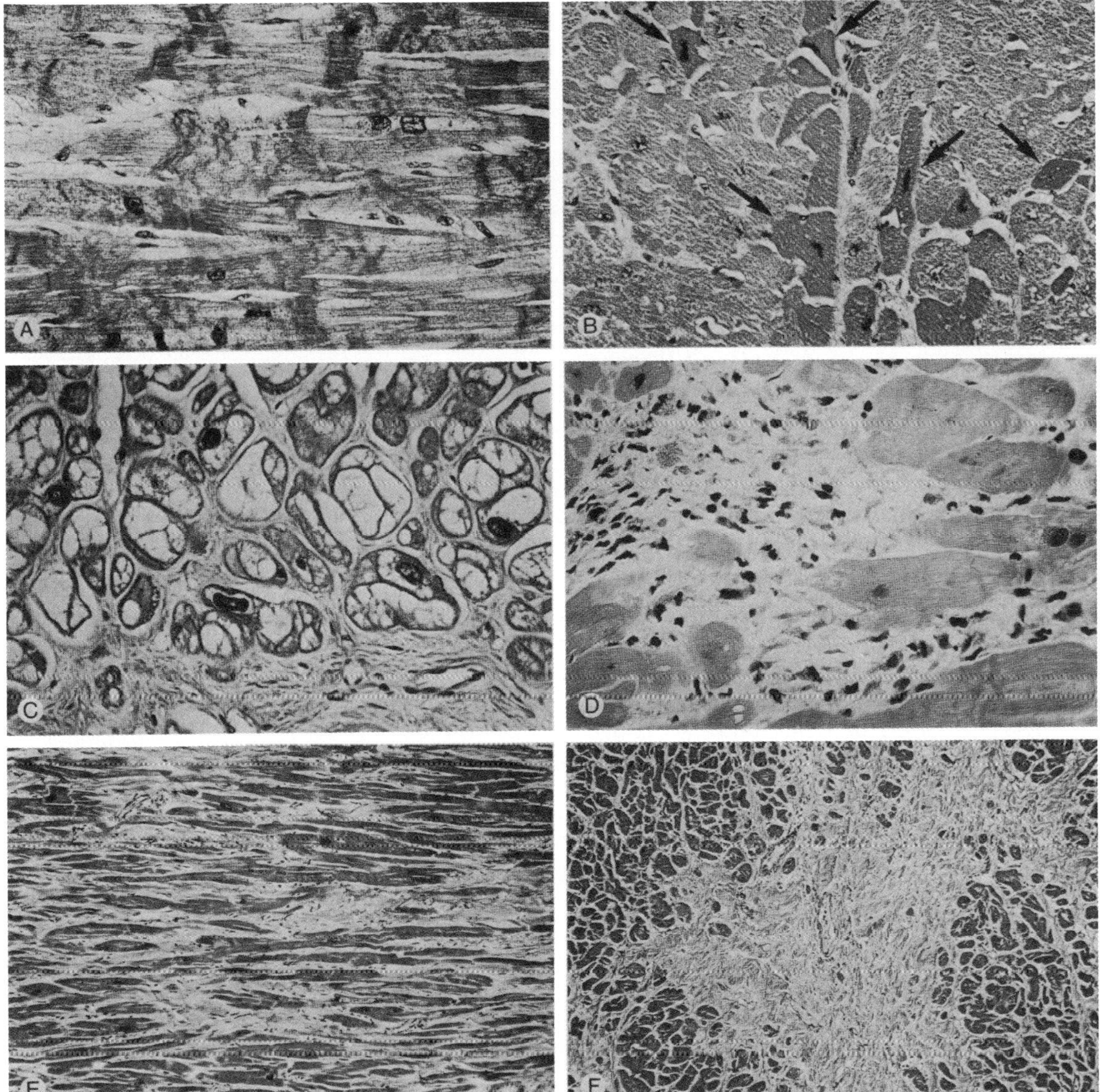

Figure 2–16. Histopathology of acute and chronic myocardial ischemia. **A.** Contraction bands. **B.** Sarcoplasmic eosinophilia and pyknotic nuclei (arrows). **C.** Myocytolysis with sarcoplasmic vacuolization. **D.** Patchy microfocal granulation tissue. **E.** Pericellular fibrosis. **F.** Microfocal replacement fibrosis.

Nonspecific diffuse pericarditis and occasional myocarditis are the histopathologic correlates.

The cause of this syndrome is unknown, but it is currently thought to be related to an autoimmune mechanism or anticoagulant therapy (70). In this regard, acute fibrinous pericarditis and the postmyocardial infarction syndrome may be related disorders. Recent studies, however, indicate that the incidence of the syndrome is decreasing. Although serious complications are rare, cardiac tamponade and constrictive pericarditis have been described.

Other Complications

Rarely, in patients with an acute myocardial infarction, secondary infections occur either within the necrotic myocardium or in an overlying mural thrombus (71). Calcification occurs relatively frequently in the walls of postinfarction aneurysms but only rarely in nonaneurysmal infarctions (72).

Fatal pulmonary thromboembolism occasionally occurs in the setting of acute myocardial infarction and may originate in the leg veins or within the right atrium or right ventricle (73).

MYOCARDIAL REPERFUSION

Myocardial ischemia and infarction are the consequences of critical obstructive coronary artery disease, and they may represent acute or chronic lesions. In contrast to infarction, which denotes irreversible damage, ischemia indicates injured but viable myocytes that are potentially salvageable if an adequate blood supply can be reestablished. With these considerations in mind, the goals of reperfusion therapy are to limit infarct size, improve myocardial function, prevent future infarctions, and improve survival (74). For all currently available surgical and nonsurgical procedures, however, restenosis represents the most prevalent complication, and it is generally the result of thrombosis or intimal hyperplasia.

Surgical Interventions

Operative revascularization procedures include bypass of critical stenoses with autogenous vascular grafts, usually saphenous veins or internal mammary (thoracic) arteries, and removal of plaque by endarterectomy.

Aortocoronary Saphenous Vein Bypass Grafts

The hospital mortality rate for coronary bypass operations is less than 1%; perioperative myocardial infarctions occur in fewer than 3%; and the 5-year survival rate is about 90% (75). The role of coronary bypass surgery in acute myocardial infarction is discussed in Chapter 23. Obstruction is the primary complication of bypass grafts and may occur at the aortic anastomosis site, within the body of the graft, or at the distal coronary artery anastomosis site.

The approximate rates of graft occlusion are 10% at 1 month, 20% at 1 year, 30% at 5 years, and 40% at 10 years (76). Antiplatelet therapy has resulted in improved patency rates (77). Risk factors for graft occlusion include preexisting phlebosclerosis, operative injury to the vein graft, low blood flow in the graft, small luminal size of the grafted artery, atheromatous plaques or arterial branching at the coronary anastomosis site, mechanical factors (such as graft compression or kinking), and postoperative hyperlipidemia or continued smoking.

In general, obstruction is the result of thrombosis, intimal hyperplasia, or atherosclerosis, and these may occur either alone or in various combinations (Fig. 2–17) (76). The hemodynamic stress of high-pressure pulsatile blood flow within venous grafts favors endothelial injury, platelet aggregation, and development of these obstructive lesions. Moreover, preexisting phlebosclerosis can cause significant stenosis at the time of graft insertion. Spasm of vein grafts is also occasionally responsible for postoperative obstruction (78).

Within the first postoperative month, thrombosis accounts for virtually all cases of graft occlusion. This generally occurs when distal coronary perfusion is poor, because of either small arterial size or the presence of critical atherosclerotic narrowing beyond the distal anastomosis site. Plaque disruption at the coronary anastomosis may also result in thrombotic occlusion.

Between 1 month and 1 year postoperatively, intimal hyperplasia is the most frequent cause of graft stenosis. Although intimal thickening develops in all vein grafts, it is excessive in some and consists of an exuberant proliferation of smooth muscle cells, with a few fibroblasts, and deposition of variable amounts of extracellular glycosaminoglycans and collagen. Thus its microscopic appearance is similar to that observed with postangioplasty restenosis. Platelets and their release of smooth muscle growth factor are considered important in the pathogenesis of intimal hyperplasia.

After the first year, and particularly after the third, atherosclerosis of vein grafts becomes more important than intimal proliferation as a cause of stenosis. Plaques tend to involve aneurysmally dilated segments of saphenous vein grafts and are usually soft and friable, with extensive necrotic debris, cholesterol crystals, foam cells, blood elements,

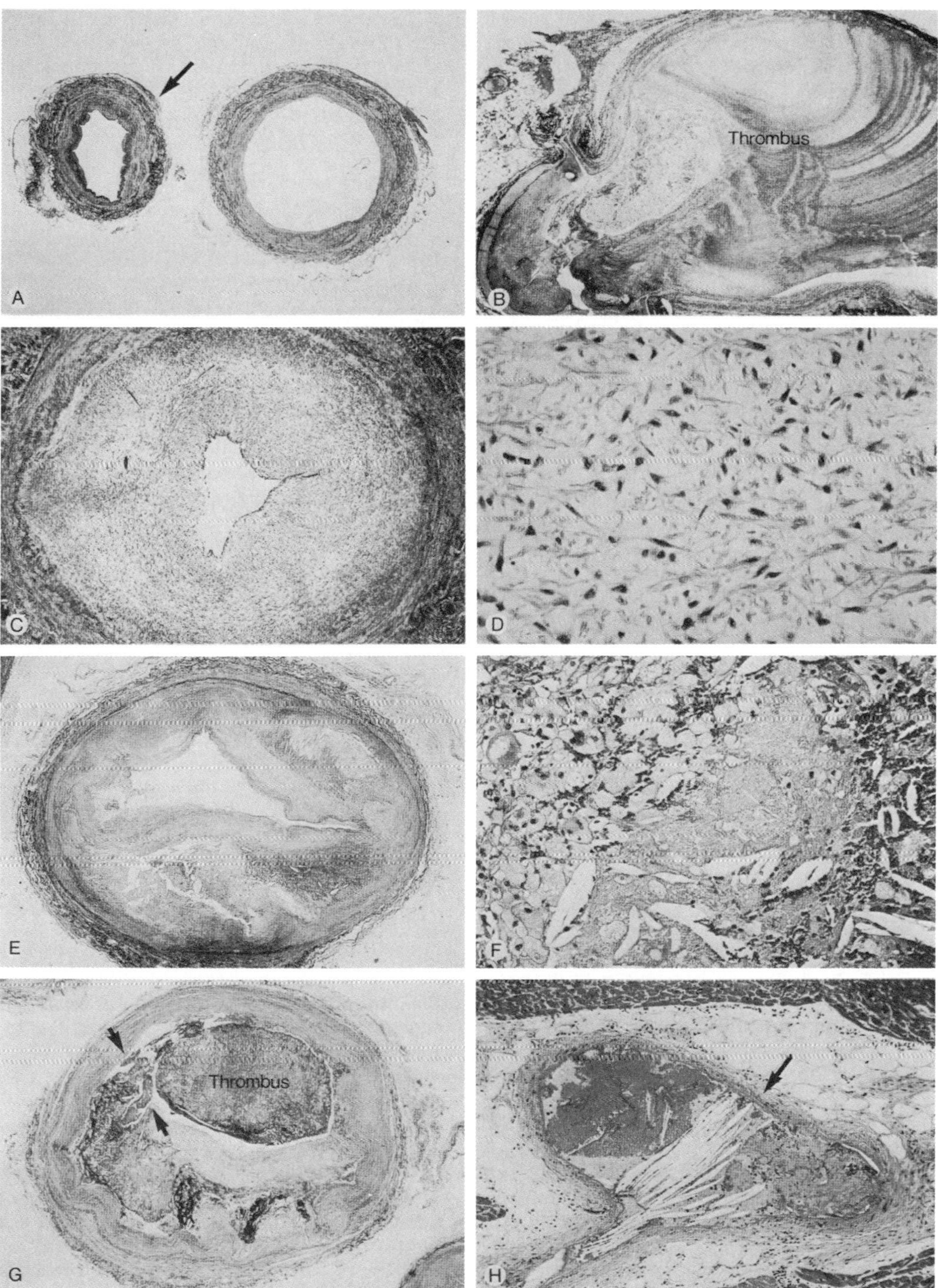

Figure 2–17. Complications of saphenous vein grafts. **A.** Phlebosclerotic narrowing (arrow), with adjacent normal segment for comparison. **B.** Acute thrombotic occlusion, involving distal anastomosis site. **C,D.** Intimal fibroplasia, at low power (**C**) and high power (**D**). **E,F.** Vein graft atherosclerosis, at low power (**E**) and high power (**F**). Compare with Fig. 2–1. **G.** Vein graft atherosclerosis, with spontaneous plaque rupture (between arrows) and secondary thrombotic occlusion. **H.** Atheroembolization to myocardium (arrow) after manipulation of graft at reoperation.

giant cells, and inflammation. Atheromas in vein grafts, as in the coronary arteries, are subject to plaque rupture and secondary embolization or thrombosis. Manipulation of such grafts, during later operative or angioplastic procedures, may result in appreciable embolization of atheromatous debris and subsequent angina pectoris, myocardial infarction, acute left ventricular dysfunction, or ventricular arrhythmias.

Internal Mammary Artery Grafts

Although coronary and internal mammary (thoracic) arteries are similar in size, they differ appreciably in structure. Coronary arteries are muscular and prone to atherosclerosis, whereas internal mammary arteries are elastic and rarely develop plaques (79). Furthermore, when blood flow is low, internal mammary arteries are resistant to the development of thrombotic occlusion. As a result of these features, their patency rate when used as bypass grafts is about 90% at 10 years, greatly exceeding the rate of 60% for saphenous vein grafts (76). Late graft obstruction may occur, however, and is usually the result of intimal hyperplasia (80). Rarely, occlusion occurs on the basis of graft spasm, thrombosis, or medial dissection of the graft at the anastomosis site (81).

Coronary Endarterectomy

Surgical endarterectomy of the coronary arteries has been performed as an isolated procedure or at the anastomosis site of a bypass graft. The procedure results in removal of not only the intimal plaque but also variable amounts of media. Consequently, a thrombogenic surface remains that is prone to acute postoperative thrombosis or late restenosis by neointimal proliferation, similar to that observed after angioplasty (76). Platelets and growth factor are thought to play a role in this process. Creation of an obstructive intimal flap is another potential complication of endarterectomy.

Nonsurgical Interventions

Because acute myocardial infarction is generally associated with acute coronary thrombosis, it is reasonable to direct therapy toward dissolution, disruption, or dislodgement of the thrombotic material (see Chs. 19-21). To this end, thrombolytic or angioplastic treatments, or the two in combination, are applicable (76,82). For chronic coronary disease, angioplasty and other newer procedures, including atherectomy and stents, are available. Currently, restenosis is a prevalent complication.

Thrombolytic Agents

Streptokinase, urokinase, and tissue-type plasminogen activator are the three most commonly used thrombolytic agents (see Chs. 19–22). They reestablish coronary blood flow by dissolution of freshly formed thrombus. If their action is incomplete, residual shallow mural thrombus or thin strands of luminal thrombus are observed. Moreover, the nidus that caused thrombosis (such as plaque rupture) still remains and represents an unstable lesion until reendothelialization takes place.

Most complications of thrombolytic therapy are related to hemorrhage, reperfusion arrhythmias, coronary rethrombosis, and thrombolytic failure (76). Hemorrhage may involve the acutely infarcted myocardium or distant sites such as the brain. Reocclusion occurs in 15% to 35% of patients and appears to be related to incomplete thrombolysis and the unstable nature of the underlying atherosclerotic plaque. Failure of therapy to effect thrombolysis occurs in 20% to 30% of patients and is related to the presence of critical plaques, plaque rupture with luminal obstruction by thromboatheromatous debris, and old organizing thrombus. Other complications include coronary embolism and hemopericardium.

Percutaneous Transluminal Coronary Angioplasty

Percutaneous transluminal coronary angioplasty (PTCA) is applicable to the treatment of both chronic and acute obstructions (see Ch. 22). It is successful in 85% to 95% of cases and is associated with a mortality rate of 1% (76). The procedure entails dilation of a stenotic lesion by multiple inflations of an intraluminal balloon catheter under relatively high pressure (usually 8 to 12 atm). The mechanism for relief of stenoses by PTCA is variable, owing to the complex nature of coronary atheromas, plaque ruptures, and luminal thrombi.

In general, a successful procedure is more likely for eccentric than concentric plaques.

For chronic stable lesions, the most common alteration observed after PTCA is intimal laceration at the junction between an eccentric plaque and the disease-free wall (Fig. 2–18) (76,82,83). This results in partial separation of the plaque from its internal elastic membrane and the formation of a small intimal flap. Extension of the fracture into the subjacent media commonly occurs and produces a localized shallow dissection. In other cases, disruption begins along the thin intima opposite an eccentric atheroma and extends back toward the plaque.

For either eccentric or concentric plaques, shallow erosions or deep lacerations can involve the thin fibrous cap over an atheroma and lead to disruption and hemorrhage into the soft necrotic core. Stretching of the disease-free media opposite an eccentric plaque, with or without intimal tears, may also result in a successful procedure. Thus the mechanisms by which PTCA produces adequate luminal expansion are numerous. Some apply only to eccentric plaques, and some, such as medial stretching, are reversible processes. In most cases, the procedure causes actual tissue injury and the production of a thrombogenic surface that requires healing and reendothelialization.

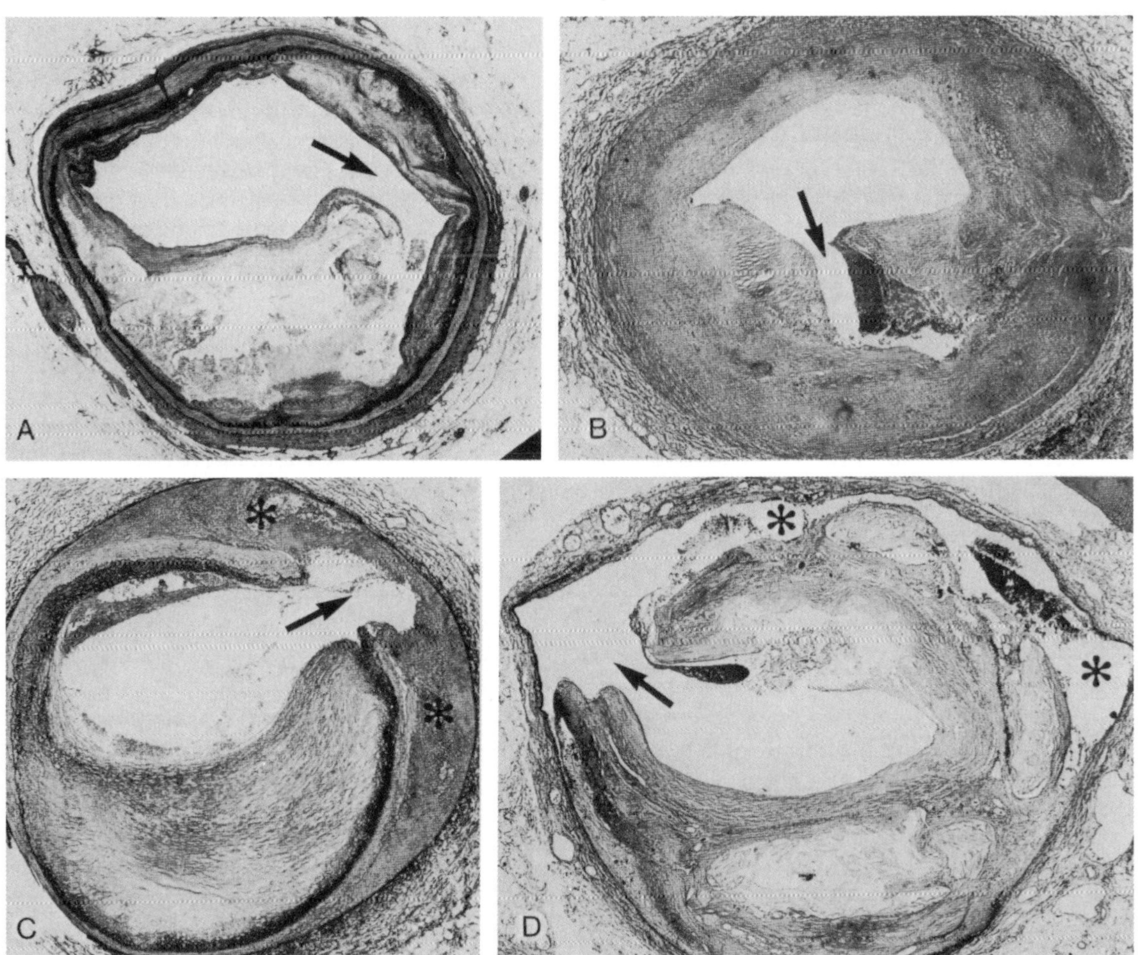

Figure 2–18. Mechanisms of successful percutaneous transluminal coronary angioplasty. **A.** Fracture near junction of plaque with disease-free wall (arrow). **B.** Disruption along midportion of plaque (arrow). **C.** Fracture near plaque junction (arrow), associated with medial dissection (*). **D.** Fracture of concentric plaque at most narrow region (arrow), associated with extensive medial dissection (*).

Acute or unstable coronary lesions (such as plaque erosions, fissures, and ruptures) may be indistinguishable microscopically from certain patterns of disruption produced by PTCA. Moreover, balloon dilation often causes further extension of these spontaneous lesions. Fresh thrombus is also mechanically disrupted and dislodged by the angioplasty procedure. Thus PTCA of unstable lesions may produce not only luminal expansion but also large thrombogenic surfaces.

Microscopically, distinction must be made between lesions that occur spontaneously or are caused by angioplasty and clefts that represent artifacts of tissue processing. Although artifactual clefts superficially resemble plaque ruptures, the absence of red blood cells, platelets, or a reparative response along artifactual rupture tracts allows their identification to be made readily.

Angioplasty has numerous potential complications. The procedure may be unsuccessful or, rarely, balloon dilation may cause embolization or arterial rupture. Early complications occur in 5% to 10% of patients and are usually the result of acute coronary occlusion or femoral hematoma (76,82). Occlusion may be related to acute thrombosis, an obstructive intimal flap or medial dissection, or arterial spasm. Acute thrombosis more commonly occurs on unstable plaques than chronic stable ones. Early coronary complications may be associated with angina pectoris, acute myocardial infarction, arrhythmias, or sudden death. Emergency coronary bypass surgery is necessary in some patients.

The most commonly observed late complication of PTCA is restenosis, and it affects at least 30% to 40% of vessels (76,82). Most restenotic lesions develop between 2 and 6 months after the angioplasty procedure. They are usually treated adequately by repeated PTCA procedures, although some patients have bypass surgery.

Microscopically, most restenotic lesions are characterized by an exuberant healing response in which a proliferation of intimal smooth muscle cells (presumably of medial origin) not only fills in erosions, fissures, and dissection channels but also progresses and causes luminal obstruction (Fig. 2–19). Endothelial disruption, deep vascular injury, platelet aggregation, release of growth factors, and turbulent blood flow are each thought to play a role in this process (83,84).

Numerous risk factors for restenosis resulting from excessive intimal hyperplasia have been identified. They are related primarily to procedural aspects (balloon size and inflation pressure and times), vascular aspects (plaque rupture, luminal thrombosis, lesions at arterial bend points), and patient aspects (diabetes mellitus, hypertension, continued smoking).

For vessels in which stretching of the disease-free wall opposite an atheroma is the primary mechanism for relief of obstruction, subsequent restitution of medial tone represents a cause of early restenosis (82). Progressive coronary atherosclerosis is another potential cause of late restenosis.

Angioplasty has also been applied to obstructions in saphenous vein grafts, internal mammary artery grafts, and coronary arteries in transplanted hearts. The success rate is about 90% for vein grafts and 95% for internal mammary arteries. For vein grafts less than 1 year old, intimal tears and wall stretching represent the primary alterations, and for older grafts, plaque rupture is the most common lesion observed. Angioplasty of old saphenous vein grafts that are involved by atherosclerosis and by aneurysmal dilation pose a particular risk for significant atheromatous embolization and myocardial infarction (85). Restenosis occurs in about 40% and involves the same mechanisms described for coronary arteries.

Other Nonsurgical Interventions

Although the techniques discussed in this section are usually employed in patients with stable lesions, some are applicable to patients with acute myocardial infarction as well. *Coronary laser angioplasty* is intended to ablate plaque material, rather than simply produce fractures, and may be used independently or as an adjunct to balloon angioplasty (76,82). It is applicable to stenoses in coronary arteries and has even been used in saphenous vein grafts. Currently, four different lasers are effective: argon, carbon dioxide, excimer (xenon chloride), and Nd–YAG (neodymium–yttrium aluminum garnet). Selective absorption of laser light energy by an atheroma results in focal rapid heating to high tem-

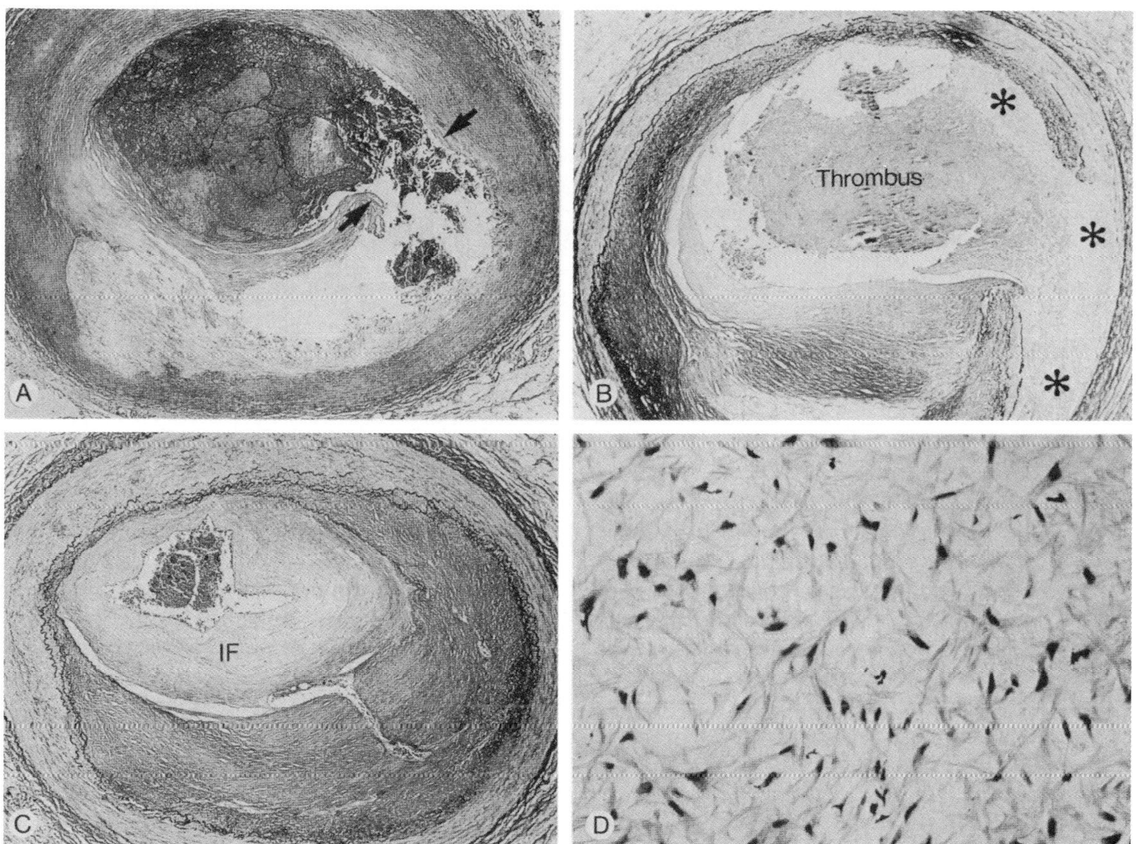

Figure 2–19. Mechanisms of restenosis after percutaneous transluminal coronary angioplasty. **A.** Acute thrombotic occlusion after plaque rupture (between arrows). **B.** Thrombosis of lumen and early fibroplasia along intima and medial dissection channel (*). **C,D.** Intimal fibroplasia (IF), at low power (**C**) and high power (**D**). Compare with Fig. 2–17**D.**

peratures and subsequent vaporization of the affected lesion. The composition of an atheromatous plaque determines the extent to which laser light is absorbed.

With the use of percutaneous catheters, laser energy may be delivered as a continuous wave or as a pulse. Continuous-wave lasers produce not only a crater lesion, through tissue vaporization, but also peripheral charring with coagulation necrosis and tissue vacuolization, through thermal injury (76). Pulsed lasers, in contrast, produce clean incisions and vaporization craters, with little thermal damage to adjacent tissues. Thus laser angioplasty produces focal arterial injury that undergoes healing by organization and reendothelialization. Potential complications of the procedure include thrombosis, dissection, spasm, intimal hyperplasia, aneurysmal dilation, and arterial perforation.

Coronary atherectomy of primary or restenosis lesions is achieved percutaneously with a catheter that contains a circular blade that rotates at high speed, mechanically resecting lesions from arterial walls and then trapping the resected tissue fragments in its metal housing (86,87). It thus creates a type of injury different from that associated with balloon dilation. Resected tissue can be used for cell culture studies (88). Deep arterial resection, including medial and even adventitial elements, occurs frequently but has not been associated with acute symptomatic complications. The procedure does produce thrombogenic surfaces, however, and initial results indicate that restenosis by intimal hyperplasia is as common with atherectomy as with PTCA.

Coronary stents represent expandable tubes of metallic mesh that are inserted percutaneously to preserve luminal patency, particularly at sites of balloon angioplasty (89,90). The procedure has been applied not only to coronary arteries but also to saphenous vein grafts. Restenosis may occur as a result of thrombosis or intimal hyperplasia, but its rate of development is currently unknown. It is possible that impregnation of coated stents with various drugs may decrease the rate of postprocedural restenosis (91).

Other procedures are being developed and include the use of radiofrequency energy to remodel plaques or to fuse intimal tears, and the use of ultrasonic energy to ablate atheromas by a mechanism similar to lithotripsy.

Effects of Reperfusion on the Myocardium

After interventions for acute coronary obstruction, certain alterations may be observed in the myocardium that are related to the effects of reperfusion (92) (see Ch. 21). In most patients, the effects are beneficial and include limitation of infarct size and accelerated healing. Other patients, however, experience various types of reperfusion injury, including hemorrhagic infarction, injury by oxygen free radicals, the no reflow phenomenon, and arrhythmias. Acute myocardial infarction is thus a complex process, and the success of clinical interventions cannot always be predicted accurately.

Limitation of Infarct Size

On the basis of results of animal studies, successful reperfusion within the first few hours after the onset of an acute myocardial infarction should be associated with the limitation of necrosis to a subendocardial process. With no interventional therapy, any limitation of infarct size will depend primarily on the extent of collateral vessels and on intrinsic coronary thrombolysis.

With early intervention, the results of clinical trials indicate that the benefits of reperfusion therapy occur but that they cannot be explained by modest limitations of infarct size alone. Effects on remodeling of the left ventricle, including prevention of dilation, and other factors, such as fewer postinfarction arrhythmias, are also important. Thus the lowered mortality in patients with reperfusion therapy appears to be related to factors other than only limiting infarct size and improving left ventricular function (76).

Accelerated Healing

For acute myocardial infarctions, the typical sequence of inflammatory and reparative responses is well established and relatively predictable (see Table 2–4). However, when blood flow is reestablished to an area of necrosis, the rate of healing tends to be accelerated in nonhemorrhagic infarctions (93). In general, the neutrophilic response is blunted or absent, and macrophages are the most prevalent inflammatory cells. The proliferation of interstitial fibroblasts (a reparative process that usually occurs only after day 12) can be observed at the infarct border within several days of reperfusion. Thus, even young infarctions are characterized by an admixture of necrotic myocytes, plump macrophages (often rich in lipofuscin pigment), and active fibroblasts (Fig. 2–20). As a result, the ability of pathologists to determine infarct age accurately is hampered.

Hemorrhagic Infarction

During acute myocardial infarction, small intramural vessels may be damaged by ischemia to such an extent that vascular disruption occurs (see Ch. 21). If subsequent reperfusion is successful, hemorrhage into the area of infarction can occur (see Fig. 2–20). Hemorrhage tends to be more extensive in patients treated with thrombolytic agents or with bypass surgery than in those treated with angioplasty. Complications of appreciable myocardial hemorrhages are related to infarct expansion and delayed healing. The results of some studies indicate that the late administration of thrombolytic therapy increases the likelihood of ventricular rupture, whereas other studies do not support this conclusion (94,95).

Injury by Oxygen Free Radicals

Although restitution of coronary blood flow is beneficial in most patients with an acute myocardial infarction, it may be associated with further myocar-

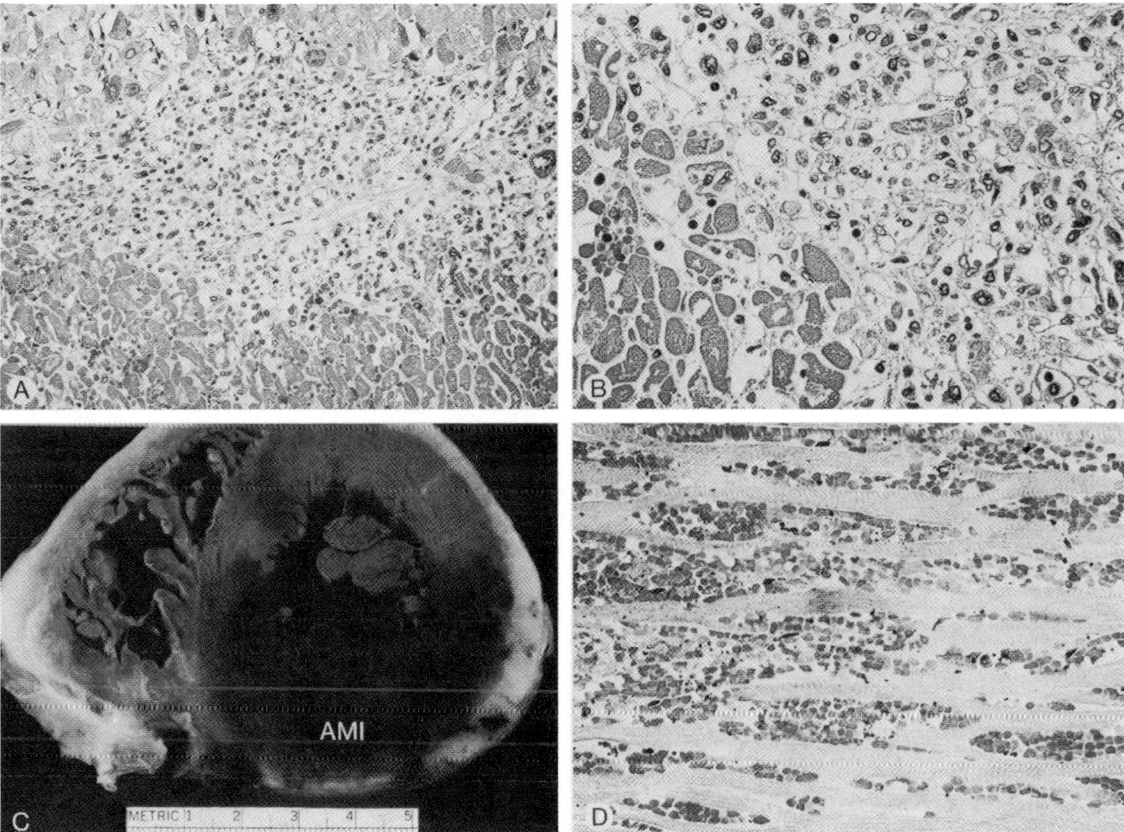

Figure 2–20. Myocardial effects of reperfusion. **A,B.** Accelerated healing, at low power (**A**) and high power (**B**), with mixture of macrophages and fibroblasts in 5-day-old infarct. **C,D.** Hemorrhagic acute myocardial infarction (AMI) of inferior wall, shown grossly (**C**) and microscopically (**D**).

dial injury in others (see Ch. 21). This appears to be related to the production of oxygen free radicals by endothelial cells or neutrophils after reperfusion. Damage caused by these chemical mediators include stunned myocardium and reperfusion-induced arrhythmias (96,97). Whether oxygen-derived free radicals can cause lethal reperfusion injury, with actual myocyte necrosis, is currently an unsettled issue. Studies in animals that receive free radical scavengers before reperfusion have shown conflicting results (92). Hibernating myocardium represents a chronic sublethal form of injury that appears to be unrelated to oxygen free radicals (98).

No Reflow Phenomenon

In some patients, alleviation of an acute coronary occlusion is not associated with restitution of blood flow to the infarcted region. This is known as the no reflow phenomenon and appears to be related to several factors, including interstitial and endothelial edema, ischemic contracture of myocytes with compression of adjacent capillary channels, and plugging of the local microcirculation with neutrophils and platelets (41,92). When the no reflow phenomenon occurs, limitation of infarct size is not achieved by reperfusion.

Reperfusion Arrhythmias

The occurrence of arrhythmias after reperfusion therapy appears to be related to myocyte injury caused by oxygen free radicals, calcium, or postprocedural microembolization (99,100) (see Ch. 14). Risk factors include the extent of myocardial ischemia, the extent of reperfusion, and heart rate.

Patients with adequate collateral blood flow have a lower incidence of reperfusion arrhythmias. It is of interest that reperfusion injury may also play a role in the production of ventricular tachycardia and fibrillation in patients with coronary artery spasm or sudden coronary death.

REFERENCES

1. Buja LM, Willerson JT: The role of coronary artery lesions in ischemic heart disease: Insights from recent clinicopathologic, coronary arteriographic, and experimental studies. *Major Probl Pathol* 1991;23:42–60.
2. Jost S, Deckers JW, Nikutta P, et al: Progression of coronary artery disease is dependent on anatomic location and diameter. *J Am Coll Cardiol* 1993;21:1339–1346.
3. Hochman JS, Phillips WJ, Ruggieri D, Ryan SF: The distribution of atherosclerotic lesions in the coronary arterial tree: Relation to cardiac risk factors. *Am Heart J* 1988;116:1217–1222.
4. Davies MJ, Woolf N, Rowles PM, Pepper J: Morphology of the endothelium over atherosclerotic plaques in human coronary arteries. *Br Heart J* 1988;60:459–464.
5. Kragel AH, Reddy SG, Wittes JT, Roberts WC: Morphometric analysis of the composition of atherosclerotic plaques in the four major epicardial coronary arteries in acute myocardial infarction and in sudden coronary death. *Circulation* 1989;80:1747–1756.
6. Stary HC: The sequence of cell and matrix changes in atherosclerotic lesions of coronary arteries in the first forty years of life. *Eur Heart J* 1990;11(Suppl E):3–19.
7. Rumberger JA, Schwartz RS, Simons DB, et al: Relation of coronary calcium determined by electron beam computed tomography and lumen narrowing determined at autopsy. *Am J Cardiol* 1994;74:1169–1173.
8. Waller BF: The eccentric coronary atherosclerotic plaque: Morphologic observations and clinical relevance. *Clin Cardiol* 1989;12:14–20.
9. Saner HE, Gobel FL, Salomonowitz E, et al: The disease-free wall in coronary atherosclerosis: Its relation to degree of obstruction. *J Am Coll Cardiol* 1985;6:1096–1099.
10. Clarkson TB, Prichard RW, Morgan TM, et al: Remodeling of coronary arteries in human and nonhuman primates. *JAMA* 1994;271:289–294.
11. Stiel GM, Stiel LSG, Schofer J, et al: Impact of compensatory enlargement of atherosclerotic coronary arteries on angiographic assessment of coronary artery diseases. *Circulation* 1989;80:1603–1609.
12. Glagov S, Weisenberg E, Zarins CK, et al: Compensatory enlargement of human atherosclerotic coronary arteries. *N Engl J Med* 1987;316:1371–1375.
13. Tveter KJ, Edwards JE: Calcified aortic sinotubular ridge: A source of coronary ostial stenosis or embolism. *J Am Coll Cardiol* 1988;12:1510–1514.
14. Ross R: The pathogenesis of atherosclerosis: A perspective for the 1990s. *Nature* 1993;362:801–809.
15. Edwards WD: Atherosclerotic plaques: Natural and unnatural history, in Schoen FJ, Gimbrone MA Jr (eds): *Cardiovascular Pathology: Clinicopathologic Correlations and Pathogenetic Mechanisms,* USCAP Monograph No. 37. Baltimore, Williams & Wilkins, 1995, pp 12–46.
16. van der Wal AC, Becker AE, van der Loos CM, Das PK: Site of intimal rupture or erosion of thrombosed coronary atherosclerotic plaques is characterized by an inflammatory process irrespective of the dominant plaque morphology. *Circulation* 1994;89:36–44.
17. Baroldi G, Silver MD, Mariani F, Giuliano G: Correlation of morphological variables in the coronary atherosclerotic plaque with clinical patterns of ischemic heart disease. *Am J Cardiovasc Pathol* 1988;2:159–172.
18. Mizuno K, Satomura K, Miyamoto A, et al: Angioscopic evaluation of coronary artery thrombi in acute coronary syndromes. *N Engl J Med* 1992;326:287–291.
19. Fuster V, Badimon L, Badimon JJ, Chesebro JH: The pathogenesis of coronary artery disease and the acute coronary syndromes. *N Engl J Med* 1992;326:242–250.
20. Davies MJ: A macro and micro view of coronary vascular insult in ischemic heart disease. *Circulation* 1990;82 (Suppl II):II-38–II-46.
21. Frink RJ, Rooney PA Jr, Trowbridge JO, Rose JP: Coronary thrombosis and platelet/fibrin microemboli in death associated with acute myocardial infarction. *Br Heart J* 1988;59:196–200.

22. Qiao J-H, Fishbein MC: The severity of coronary atherosclerosis at sites of plaque rupture with occlusive thrombosis. *J Am Coll Cardiol* 1991;17: 1138–1142.
23. Ambrose JA, Tannenbaum MA, Alexopoulos D, et al: Angiographic progression of coronary artery disease and the development of myocardial infarction. *J Am Coll Cardiol* 1988;12:56–62.
24. Bruschke AVG, Kramer JR Jr, Bal ET, et al: The dynamics of progression of coronary atherosclerosis studied in 168 medically treated patients who underwent coronary arteriography three times. *Am Heart J* 1989;117:296–305.
25. Haft JI, Haik BJ, Goldstein JE, Brodyn NE: Development of significant coronary artery lesions in areas of minimal disease: A common mechanism for coronary disease progression. *Chest* 1988; 94:731 736.
26. Lambert CR Jr, Pepine CJ: Coronary artery spasm and acute myocardial infarction. *Cardiovasc Clin* 1989;20(1):131–140.
27. Waller BF: Atherosclerotic and nonatherosclerotic coronary artery factors in acute myocardial infarction. *Cardiovasc Clin* 1989;20(1):29–104.
28. Loecker TH, Schwartz RS, Cotta CW, Hickman JR Jr: Fluoroscopic coronary artery calcification and associated coronary disease in asymptomatic young men. *J Am Coll Cardiol* 1992;19:1167–1172.
29. Mintz GS, Painter JA, Richard AD, et al: Atherosclerosis in angiographically "normal" coronary artery reference segments: An intravascular ultrasound study with clinical correlations. *J Am Coll Cardiol* 1995;25:1479–1495.
30. Stone PH, Gibson M, Pasternak RC, et al: Natural history of coronary atherosclerosis using quantitative angiography in men, and implications for clinical trials of coronary regression. *Am J Cardiol* 1993;71:766–772.
31. Siegel RJ, Swan K, Edwalds G, Fishbein MC: Limitations of postmortem assessment of human coronary artery size and luminal narrowing: Differential effects of tissue fixation and processing on vessels with different degrees of atherosclerosis. *J Am Coll Cardiol* 1985;5:342–346.
32. Haft JI, Goldstein JE, Niemiera ML: Coronary arteriographic lesion of unstable angina. *Chest* 1987;92:609–612.
33. Ambrose JA, Winters SL, Arora RR, et al: Angiographic evolution of coronary artery morphologic in unstable angina. *J Am Coll Cardiol* 1986;7: 472–478.
34. van der Laarse A, van Leeuwen FT, Krul R, et al: The size of infarction as judged enzymatically in 1974 patients with acute myocardial infarction: Relation with symptomatology, infarct localization and type of infarction. *Int J Cardiol* 1988;19: 191–207.
35. Hackel DB, Reimer KA, Ideker RE, et al: Comparison of enzymatic and anatomic estimates of myocardial infarct size in man. *Circulation* 1984; 70:824–835.
36. Edwards WD: Anatomic basis for tomographic analysis of the heart at autopsy. *Cardiol Clin* 1984; 2(4):485–506.
37. Isner JM: Right ventricular myocardial infarction. *JAMA* 1988;259:712–718.
38. Andersen HR, Falk E, Nielsen D: Right ventricular infarction: Frequency, size and topography in coronary heart disease: A prospective study comparing 107 consecutive autopsies from a coronary care unit. *J Am Coll Cardiol* 1987;10:1223–1232.
39. Reimer KA, Ideker RE: Myocardial ischemia and infarction: Anatomic and biochemical substrates for ischemic cell death and ventricular arrhythmias. *Hum Pathol* 1987;18:462–475.
40. Miyazaki S, Fujiwara H, Onodera T, et al: Quantitative analysis of contraction band and coagulation necrosis after ischemia and reperfusion in the porcine heart. *Circulation* 1987;75:1074–1082.
41. Mehta J, Dinerman J, Mehta P, et al: Neutrophil function in ischemic heart disease. *Circulation* 1989;79:549–556.
42. Stevenson WG, Linssen GCM, Havenith MG, et al: The spectrum of death after myocardial infarction: A necropsy study. *Am Heart J* 1989;118: 1182–1188.
43. Muller JE, Rude RE, Braunwald E, et al: Myocardial infarct extension: Occurrence, outcome, and risk factors in the multicenter investigation of limitation of infarct size. *Ann Intern Med* 1988;108: 1–6.
44. Weisman HF, Healy B: Myocardial infarct expansion, infarct extension, and reinfarction: Pathophysiologic concepts. *Prog Cardiovasc Dis* 1987;30: 73–110.
45. Batts KP, Ackermann DM, Edwards WD: Postinfarction rupture of the left ventricular free wall: Clinicopathologic correlates in 100 consecutive autopsy cases. *Hum Pathol* 1990;21:530–535.

46. Mann JM, Roberts WC: Rupture of the left ventricular free wall during acute myocardial infarction: Analysis of 138 necropsy patients and comparison with 50 necropsy patients with acute myocardial infarction without rupture. *Am J Cardiol* 1988;62:847–859.
47. Atkinson JB, Robinowitz M, McAllister HA, Virmani R: Association of eosinophils with cardiac rupture. *Hum Pathol* 1985;16:562–568.
48. Pohjola-Sintonen S, Muller JE, Stone PH, et al: Ventricular septal and free wall rupture complicating acute myocardial infarction: Experience in the Multicenter Investigation of Limitation of Infarct Size. *Am Heart J* 1989;117:809–818.
49. Oliva PB, Hammill SC, Edwards WD: Cardiac rupture, a clinically predictable complication of acute myocardial infarction: Report of 70 cases with clinicopathologic correlation. *J Am Coll Cardiol* 1993;22:720–726.
50. Edwards BS, Edwards WD, Edwards JE: Ventricular septal rupture complicating acute myocardial infarction: Identification of simple and complex types in 53 autopsied hearts. *Am J Cardiol* 1984;54:1201–1205.
51. Topaz O, Mallon SM, Chahine RA, et al: Acute ventricular septal rupture: Angiographic–morphologic features and clinical assessment. *Chest* 1989;95:292–298.
52. Skehan JD, Carey C, Norrell MS, et al: Patterns of coronary artery disease in post-infarction ventricular septal rupture. *Br Heart J* 1989;62:268–272.
53. Cummings RG, Califf R, Jones RN, et al: Correlates of survival in patients with postinfarction ventricular septal defect. *Ann Thorac Surg* 1989;47:824–830.
54. Barbour DJ, Roberts WC: Rupture of a left ventricular papillary muscle during acute myocardial infarction: Analysis of 22 necropsy patients. *J Am Coll Cardiol* 1986;8:558–565.
55. Nishimura RA, Schaff HV, Shub C, et al: Papillary muscle rupture complicating acute myocardial infarction: Analysis of 17 patients. *Am J Cardiol* 1983;51:373–377.
56. Küpper AJF, Verheugt FWA, Peels CH, et al: Left ventricular thrombus incidence and behavior studied by serial two-dimensional echocardiography in acute anterior myocardial infarction: Left ventricular wall motion, systemic embolism and oral anticoagulation. *J Am Coll Cardiol* 1989;13:1514–1520.
57. Halperin JL, Fuster V: Left ventricular thrombus and stroke after myocardial infarction: Toward prevention or perplexity? (editorial). *J Am Coll Cardiol* 1989;14:912–914.
58. Atkinson JB, Virmani R: Congestive heart failure due to coronary artery disease without myocardial infarction: Clinicopathologic description of an unusual cardiomyopathy. *Hum Pathol* 1989;20:1155–1162.
59. Ross EM, Roberts WC: Severe atherosclerotic coronary arterial narrowing and chronic congestive heart failure without myocardial infarction: Analysis of 18 patients studied at necropsy. *Am J Cardiol* 1986;57:51–56.
60. McKay RG, Pfeffer MA, Pasternak RC, et al: Left ventricular remodeling after myocardial infarction: A corollary to infarct expansion. *Circulation* 1986;74:693–702.
61. Pirolo JS, Hutchins GM, Moore GW: Infarct expansion: Pathologic analysis of 204 patients with a single myocardial infarct. *J Am Coll Cardiol* 1986;7:349–354.
62. Cabin HS, Roberts WC: True left ventricular aneurysm and healed myocardial infarction: Clinical and necropsy observations including quantification of degrees of coronary arterial narrowing. *Am J Cardiol* 1980;46:754–763.
63. Hirai T, Fujita M, Nakajima H, et al: Importance of collateral circulation for prevention of left ventricular aneurysm formation in acute myocardial infarction. *Circulation* 1989;79:791–796.
64. Meizlish JL, Berger HJ, Plankey M, et al: Functional left ventricular aneurysm formation after acute anterior transmural myocardial infarction: Incidence, natural history, and prognostic implications. *N Engl J Med* 1984;311:1001–1006.
65. Hochman JS, Platia EB, Bulkley BH: Endocardial abnormalities in left ventricular aneurysms: A clinicopathologic study. *Ann Intern Med* 1984;100:29–35.
66. Lapeyre AC III, Steele PM, Kazmier FJ, et al: Systemic embolism in chronic left ventricular aneurysm: Incidence and the role of anticoagulation. *J Am Coll Cardiol* 1985;6:534–538.
67. March KL, Sawada SG, Tarver RD, et al: Current concepts of left ventricular pseudoaneurysm: Pathophysiology, therapy, and diagnostic imaging methods. *Clin Cardiol* 1989:12:531–540.

68. Kono T, Sabbah HN, Rosman H, et al: Left ventricular shape is the primary determinant of functional mitral regurgitation in heart failure. *J Am Coll Cardiol* 1992;20:1594–1598.

69. Tofler GH, Muller JE, Stone PH, et al: Pericarditis in acute myocardial infarction: Characterization and clinical significance. *Am Heart J* 1989; 117:86–92.

70. Khan AH: The postcardiac injury syndromes. *Clin Cardiol* 1992;15:67–72.

71. Venezio FR, Thompson JE, Sullivan H, et al: Infection of a ventricular aneurysm and cardiac mural thrombus: Survival after surgical resection. *Am J Med* 1984;77:551–554.

72. Roberts WC, Kaufman RJ: Calcification of healed myocardial infarcts. *Am J Cardiol* 1987;60: 28–32.

73. Ahdout DJ, Damani PM, Ultan LB: Recurrent acute pulmonary emboli in association with acute myocardial infarction. *Chest* 1989;96:682–684.

74. Califf RM, Topol EJ, Gersh BJ: From myocardial salvage to patient salvage in acute myocardial infarction: The role of reperfusion therapy (editorial). *J Am Coll Cardiol* 1989;14:1382–1388.

75. Daily PO: Early and five-year results for coronary artery bypass grafting: A benchmark for percutaneous transluminal coronary angioplasty. *J Thorac Cardiovasc Surg* 1989;97:67–77.

76. Schoen FJ: *Interventional and Surgical Cardiovascular Pathology: Clinical Correlations and Basic Principles.* Philadelphia, WB Saunders, 1989, pp 59–107.

77. Goldman S, Copeland J, Moritz T, et al: Saphenous vein graft patency 1 year after coronary artery bypass surgery and effects of antiplatelet therapy: Results of a Veterans Administration cooperative study. *Circulation* 1989;80:1190–1197.

78. Maleki M, Manley JC: Venospastic phenomena of saphenous vein bypass grafts: Possible causes for unexplained postoperative recurrence of angina or early or late occlusion of vein bypass grafts. *Br Heart J* 1989;62:57–60.

79. Sisto T, Isola J: Incidence of atherosclerosis in the internal mammary artery. *Ann Thorac Surg* 1989; 47:884–886.

80. Shelton ME, Forman MB, Virmani R, et al: A comparison of morphologic and angiographic findings in long-term internal mammary artery and saphenous vein bypass grafts. *J Am Coll Cardiol* 1988;11:297–307.

81. Stone GW, Hartzler GO: Spontaneous reversible spasm in an internal mammary artery graft causing acute myocardial infarction. *Am J Cardiol* 1989;64:822–823.

82. Waller BF: "Crackers, breakers, stretchers, drillers, scrapers, shavers, burners, welders and melters"—the future treatment of atherosclerotic coronary artery disease? A clinical–morphologic assessment. *J Am Coll Cardiol* 1989;13:969–987.

83. Virmani R, Farb A, Burke AP: Coronary angioplasty from the perspective of atherosclerotic plaque: Morphologic predictors of immediate success and restenosis. *Am Heart J* 1994;127: 163–179.

84. Casscells W, Enger D, Willerson JT: Mechanisms of restenosis. *Texas Heart Inst J* 1994;21:68–77.

85. Saber RS, Edwards WD, Holmes DR Jr, et al: Balloon angioplasty of aortocoronary saphenous vein bypass grafts: A histopathologic study of six grafts from five patients, with emphasis on restenosis and embolic complications. *J Am Coll Cardiol* 1988;12:1501–1509.

86. Miller MJ, Kuntz RE, Friedrich SP, et al: Frequency and consequences of intimal hyperplasia in specimens retrieved by directional atherectomy of native primary coronary artery stenosis and subsequent restenoses. *Am J Cardiol* 1993;71: 652–658.

87. Garratt KN, Edwards WD, Kaufmann UP, et al: Differential histopathology of primary atherosclerotic and restenotic lesions in coronary arteries and saphenous vein bypass grafts: Analysis of tissue obtained from 73 patients by directional atherectomy. *J Am Coll Cardiol* 1991;17:442–448.

88. MacLeod DC, Strauss BH, de Jong M, et al: Proliferation and extracellular matrix synthesis of smooth muscle cells cultured from human coronary atherosclerotic and restenotic lesions. *J Am Coll Cardiol* 1994;23:59–65.

89. Serruys PW, de Jaegere P, Kiemeneij F, et al: A comparison of balloon-expandable-stent implantation with balloon angioplasty in patients with coronary artery disease. *N Engl J Med* 1994; 331: 489–495.

90. Fischman DL, Leon MB, Baim DS, et al: A randomized comparison of coronary-stent placement and balloon angioplasty in the treatment of coronary artery disease. *N Engl J Med* 1994;331. 496–501.

91. Holmes DR Jr, Camrud AR, Jorgenson MA, et al: Polymeric stenting in the porcine coronary artery model: Differential outcome of exogenous fibrin

sleeves versus polyurethane-coated stents. *J Am Coll Cardiol* 1994;24:525–531.

92. Jennings RB, Steenberger C Jr, Reimer KA: Myocardial ischemia and reperfusion, in Schoen FJ, Gimbrone MA Jr (eds): *Cardiovascular Pathology: Clinicopathologic Correlations and Pathogenetic Mechanisms,* USCAP Monograph No. 37. Baltimore, Williams & Wilkins, 1995, pp 47–80.
93. Reichenbach D, Cowan MJ: Healing of myocardial infarction with and without reperfusion. *Major Probl Pathol* 1991;23:86–99.
94. Honan MB, Harrall FE Jr, Reimer KA, et al: Cardiac rupture, mortality and the timing of thrombolytic therapy: A meta-analysis. *J Am Coll Cardiol* 1990;16:359–367.
95. Becker RC, Charlesworth A, Wilcox RG, et al: Cardiac rupture associated with thrombolytic therapy: Impact of time to treatment in the late assessment of thrombolytic efficacy (LATE) study. *J Am Coll Cardiol* 1995;25:1063–1068.
96. Mangano DT: Myocardial stunning: An overview. *J Card Surg* 1993;8(Suppl):204–213.
97. Bolli R: Mechanism of myocardial "stunning." *Circulation* 1990;82:723–738.
98. Rahimtoola SH: The hibernating myocardium (editorial). *Am Heart J* 1989;117:211–221.
99. Reimer KA, Richard VJ, Murry CA, Ideker RE: Myocardial ischemia and infarction: Anatomic and biochemical substrates for ischemic cell death and ventricular arrhythmias. *Major Probl Pathol* 1991;23:61–85.
100. Saber RS, Edwards WD, Bailey KR, et al: Coronary embolization after balloon angioplasty or thrombolytic therapy: An autopsy study of 32 cases. *J Am Coll Cardiol* 1993;22:1283–1288.

3

Pathophysiology and Biochemistry of Ischemia, Necrosis, and Reperfusion

Lionel H. Opie, MD, DPhil, FRCP

ISCHEMIA

By ischemia is meant a reduction of the blood supply to the myocardium. The Greek *ischo* means "to hold back," and *haima* means "blood." Ischemia is recognized when it is sufficiently severe to cause characteristic metabolic and electrocardiographic (ECG) changes that are reversible when the ischemia ceases. Ischemia is therefore, by definition, a reversible deficiency of the myocardial blood supply. As ischemia progresses, ultimately a state of infarction develops. Infarction (meaning "stuffed in") is a pathological term indicating that the cell is so damaged that the changes can be recognized by a pathologist using light microscopy. A closely related term is necrosis, the state of death (*necro* = "death").

In clinical terminology, however, the term *acute myocardial infarction* has come to mean the whole spectrum of events starting with initial chest pain and characteristic ECG changes of ischemia and evolving into a large-scale enzyme loss from the cell and the formation of Q waves. In reality, therefore, the initial stages of this process cannot be called "infarction." This seemingly small semantic difference between ischemia and infarction is of crucial importance in the present era of thrombolytic therapy, where thrombolysis can be expected to benefit cells reversibly damaged by ischemia but not those cells irreversibly damaged and necrotic. This chapter concentrates on early metabolic changes and their ionic consequences. The "point of no return" is discussed, and factors leading to necrosis are evaluated. The problem of reperfusion injury is also assessed.

Metabolic Pathways in Ischemia

High-Energy Phosphates

Important consequences of ischemia follow from the impaired oxygen supply. One of the earliest and most rapid changes is breakdown of creatine phosphate and formation of inorganic phosphate (Fig. 3 1). Creatine phosphate breakdown buffers the level of adenosine triphosphate (ATP), maintaining it relatively constant until later. The increase of inorganic phosphate (P_i) is of fundamental importance in stimulating the activity of an important enzyme that controls glycolysis, namely phosphofructokinase [for details, see Opie (1)]. Enhanced glycolytic flux results in increased production of glycolytic ATP. Although the rate of this compensatory increase of anaerobic ATP is insufficient to remedy the consequences of oxygen imbalance on ATP, nonetheless enhanced glycolysis may have benefits. For example, glycolysis may provide ATP that is crucially located to protect the ischemic cell membrane by helping to close the ATP-depen-

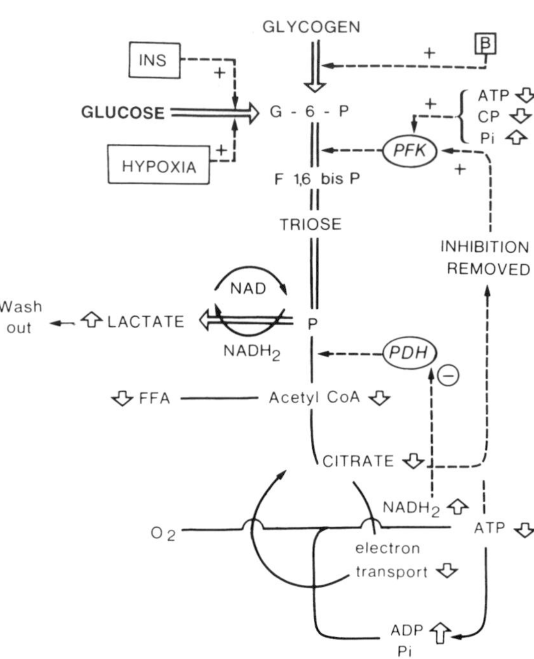

Figure 3–1. Simplified schematic of glycolysis and effect of mild ischemia. Mechanisms whereby mild ischemia enhances glycolytic flux are shown in outline. The major factors stimulating glycolysis are at the level of input (factors concerned: increased uptake of glucose and increased breakdown of glycogen) and at the level of phosphofructokinase (factors concerned: decreased energy status of cell and decreased citrate level). G = glucose, G-6-P = glucose 6-phosphate, F 1,6 bis P = fructose 1,6-biphosphate, P = pyruvate, FFA = free fatty acids, PFK = phosphofructokinase, INS = insulin, β = beta-adrenergic receptor stimulation, CP = creatine phosphate, P_i = inorganic phosphate, PDH = pyruvate dehydrogenase. *Figure copyright by LH Opie.*

dent potassium channel (2) and also assisting in the control of ion pumps concerned with calcium homeostasis (see later).

Although the rate of ATP breakdown is buffered by the creatine phosphate reserves, ATP does break down, to form adenosine diphosphate (ADP), adenosine monophosphate (AMP), inorganic phosphate (P_i), and adenosine [for details, see De Jong (3)]. The fall in the ratios ATP/AMP and creatine phosphate/inorganic phosphate are powerful signals for the stimulation of glycolysis at the level of phosphofructokinase.

Adenosine

Adenosine has a complex function in ischemia: it is a vasodilator stimulating distal arteriolar dilation in response to ischemia, so that the coronary blood supply can be closely matched to the metabolic demands of the tissue, provided that the coronary artery is free of disease. In addition, recently its capacity to inhibit the atrioventricular node by hyperpolarization has been used in the therapy of atrioventricular reentry arrhythmias. The proposal is that adenosine formed during states of myocardial oxygen imbalance can inhibit the atrioventricular node, acting as a negative feedback signal to slow down the ventricular rate and thereby helping to restore the oxygen balance (4). This property of adenosine may explain why in developing inferior infarcts there is a tendency toward atrioventricular block.

Adenosine has two other proposed effects. It may be involved in the production of ischemia and chest pain (5). Also, adenosine may stimulate the activity of protein kinase C and play a role in preconditioning.

Anaerobic Glycolysis: Does It Produce Protons?

Glycolysis is by definition the conversion of glucose 6-phosphate at the "top" of the glycolytic flux pathway to pyruvate at the "bottom" of the pathway (see Fig. 3–1). Operation of this pathway does not, contrary to common opinion, result in the production of protons as examination of the following equation shows:

$$\text{glucose} + 2\text{NAD}^+ \rightarrow 2\text{ pyruvate} + 2\text{NADH} + 2\text{H}+$$

Then, during anaerobic glycolysis,

$$2\text{ pyruvate} + 2\text{NADH} + 2\text{H}^+ \rightarrow 2\text{ lactate} + 2\text{NAD}^+$$

net

$$\text{glucose} \rightarrow 2\text{ lactate}$$

allowing for ATP synthesis:

$$\text{glucose} + 2\text{MgADP}^- + 2\text{ P}^{2-} \rightarrow 2\text{ lactate}^- + 2\text{MgATP}^{2-}$$

Because of the overall energy deficit:

$$2MgATP^{2-} \rightarrow 2MgADP^{-} + 2\ Pi^{2-} + 2H^{+}$$

If all the preceding factors are considered, and if there is net breakdown of ATP, then and only then

$$\text{glucose} \rightarrow 2\ \text{lactate}^{-} + 2H^{+}$$

Thus, in mild ischemia and when the ATP demand is decreased by contractile arrest, glycolysis can proceed without ATP breakdown and therefore without proton production. In severe ischemia, proton production proceeds by several different mechanisms (Table 3–1).

Glycolytic Inhibition: End-products or Glucose Delivery

When lactate accumulates (as in "supply" ischemia with inadequate washout of metabolites), the equilibrium between lactate and pyruvate is altered so that in addition to lactate, some $NADH_2$ builds up as the equilibrium struggles to return to normal. An increase of $NADH_2$ has several harmful consequences, including inhibition of pyruvate dehydrogenase, preventing any residual oxygen available for mitochondrial metabolism from using pyruvate as a substrate; and inhibition of the glycolytic enzyme glyceraldehyde-3-phosphate dehydrogenase, which leads to inhibition of the glycolytic pathway (Fig. 3–2). Furthermore, the continued breakdown of ATP and the formation of protons therefrom result in an intracellular acidosis, which inhibits another glycolytic enzyme, phosphofructokinase, thereby creating an additional site for glycolytic inhibition (Fig. 3–2). Thus, during severe ischemia the buildup of lactate, $NADH_2$, and protons may inhibit glycolytic flux. In addition, the more important factor inhibiting glycolysis in severe ischemia is reduced delivery of glucose (6), hypothetically lessening the ATP available for control of cellular membrane events and potentially impairing control of such ions as potassium and calcium. Thus, for the benefits of provision of glucose to become available to the ischemic myocardium, requires an adequate blood flow as in reperfusion.

Ischemic Potassium Loss

Very soon after the onset of coronary occlusion, within less than a minute, there is a loss of potassium from the ischemic cells with an increase in the potassium concentration of the extracellular space (Fig. 3–3). Among the simultaneous changes in

Table 3–1. Sources of Production of Protons in Anoxia or Ischemia

Process	Mechanism of generation	Comment
Inhibition of mitochondrial oxidation of $NADH_2$	Inhibition of mitochondrial metabolism	$NADH_2$ formed by anaerobic glycolysis is regenerated to NAD by conversion of pyruvate to lactate; other processes must be responsible for increased cytosolic $NADH_2$/NAD ratio in ischemia.
Anaerobic glycolysis	ATP breakdown	Anaerobic glycolysis results in no proton production; protons form during breakdown of ATP.
Increased tissue CO_2	Continued residual respiration Poor washout	Only in ischemia.
Triglyceride–free fatty acid cycle	Continued breakdown and resynthesis of triglyceride; ATP lost with proton production	3 ATP used per cycle, 6–7 protons produced per cycle.
Glycogen turnover	Excess recycling uses ATP and produces protons	1 ATP, 1 UTP, and 1 proton per cycle.
Mitochondrial uptake of calcium	Countertransport of protons with calcium ATP breakdown	Uptake of calcium by mitochondria utilizes ATP and therefore produces protons.

Reproduced from Opie LH: Myocardial metabolism in ischemia, in Heusch G, (ed): Pathophysiology and Rational Therapy of Myocardial Ischemia. New York, Springer, 1990, with permission.

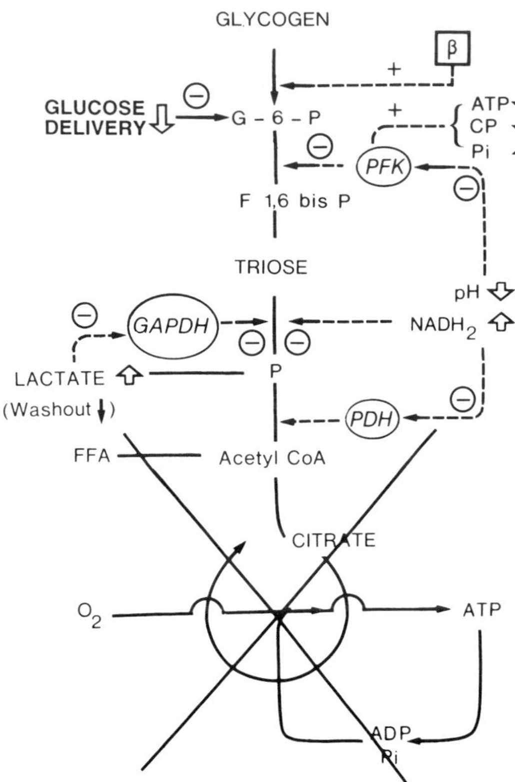

Figure 3–2. Proposed mechanisms whereby glycolysis is decreased by severe ischemia. The major mechanism is by impaired glucose delivery (6). In severe ischemia, there is also an intracellular accumulation of lactate and of protons that inhibit, respectively, glyceraldehyde phosphate dehydrogenase (GAPDH) and phosphofructokinase. The inhibition by protons at phosphofructokinase exceeds the stimulation by the decreased energy status of the cell. NADH accumulation inhibits both pyruvate dehydrogenase and glyceraldehyde phosphate dehydrogenase. Therefore, in severe ischemia, the stimulatory mechanisms shown in Fig. 3–1 are overcome by the inhibitory mechanisms shown in this figure. For abbreviations, see Fig. 3–1. *Figure copyright by LH Opie.*

coronary venous blood are increases in the concentrations of hydrogen ion, lactate, and inorganic phosphate (7). It is the potassium loss that is detected as changes in the degree of membrane polarization and, hence, in ST segment changes on the surface ECG. Harris et al (8) associated early ischemic potassium loss with simultaneously occurring ventricular arrhythmias.

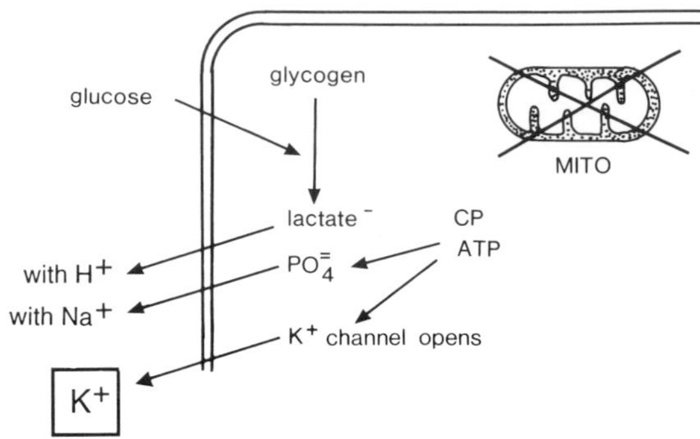

Figure 3–3. Schematic of early potassium loss, depending on opening of the potassium channel rather than on cotransport of potassium with negatively charged ions such as lactate and phosphate. *Figure copyright by LH Opie.*

Three major theories account for early potassium loss, and these are dealt with in historical sequence.

Sodium–Potassium Pump

It seemed logical that inhibition of the sodium–potassium pump (Na^+/K^+ ATPase) could result from the reduction in energy that occurs during myocardial ischemia. As a consequence, the cell would be unable to pump the potassium ion inward against the concentration gradient and to expel the sodium ion outward against its concentration gradient. Although inhibition of this pump may well explain late-phase potassium loss and sodium gain, this theory is currently less favored because there is a large discrepancy between the ATP concentration required for the activity of the pump (very low) and the ATP content of the ischemic cell at the start of potassium loss, and potassium loss can be detected before the increase in intracellular sodium when nuclear magnetic resonance techniques are used to measure the latter (9).

Covalent Ionic Loss

Hypothetically, covalent ionic loss of potassium can occur together with a loss of negatively charged phosphate and lactate ions, thereby maintaining ionic balance (10). Yet a fixed ratio of ionic loss has not been found (11), and so the subject must be regarded as open. The transport of both lactate and phosphate ions is electroneutral, therefore unlikely to account for potassium egress (12).

Potassium Channel Opening

Potassium channel opening is the most recent hypothesis. The ATP-dependent potassium channel has been described by Noma and Shibasaki (13), who propose that as cellular ATP falls, the channel opens. Thus a major problem is understanding why the ATP-dependent potassium channel "opens" when the overall ATP level of the ischemic cell is still relatively high. One possible explanation is compartmentation of ATP, as is strongly suggested by the data of Weiss and Venkatesh (2). They studied isolated myocytes subject to a model of ischemia in which there were both glycolysis and residual mitochondrial metabolism. Energy from glycolytic metabolism was better able to keep the potassium channel closed than was energy from mitochondrial metabolism. According to another explanation, as cellular energy decreases, other metabolic changes occur—for example, an increase in cellular ADP or GDP—that seem to sensitize the channel to small falls in ATP, so that activation of the potassium-losing channel can more readily be explained (14).

Sulfonylureas have a very specific effect in closing the channel (15). Glibenclamide (glyburide) lessens potassium loss and decreases early ventricular arrhythmias in ischemic rat hearts (16). Conversely, cromakalim, which activates the potassium channel, tends to increase potassium loss (17) and may aggravate early arrhythmias (18).

A recent hypothesis is that opening of this channel, by allowing an accumulation of K^+ on the external surface of the ischemic myocyte, can induce "local cardioplegia," thereby helping to protect against ischemic damage [for review, see Ref. (19)].

Cytosolic Calcium in Ischemia

Ischemic Contracture

Energy in the form of ATP is required for calcium homeostasis, when one bears in mind the vast range of concentrations in which calcium is found from the cytosol to the sarcoplasmic reticulum and, especially, across the sarcolemma to the extracellular space. An important phenomenon is the development of ischemic contracture, which theoretically could have as its basis one of two events—either a loss of ATP sufficiently severe to cause rigor bond formation, or a rise in intracellular calcium. The former is likely on the basis of isolated myocyte experiments (20). In the globally underperfused rat heart, ischemic contracture develops when the rate of supply of ATP from glucose falls below 2 μmol/g wet weight per minute (21). It is proposed that sufficient glycolytic flux from glucose can provide the ATP required to maintain ATP-dependent ion pumps, such as the sodium-potassium pump (21A). Hypothetically, when this pump fails, cytosolic Ca^{2+} rises as a result of sodium-calcium exchange (21A).

Glycogen Breakdown

Owen et al (22) suggest that glycogen may not be as good a source of protective glycolytic flux as glucose, for obscure reasons. Possibly the location of glycogen near the sarcoplasmic reticulum, and not close to the sarcolemma, may provide a structural basis for the compartmentation. Inability of glycogen to protect against ischemia was also reported by Neely and Grotyohann (23), but not by Lagerstrom et al (24). The answer to this controversy appears to lie in the severity and duration of ischemia (24A). When ischemia is brief, there is enough glycogen to be protective. But when ischemia is severe and prolonged, glycogen is depleted and increased acidosis promotes myocardial injury (24A).

Measurement

In isolated ferret muscle superfused with nitrogen, there is a rise in cytosolic calcium (as measured by aequorin) together with the development of contracture (25). Also, in the aequorin-injected isolated heart, there is a rise in cytosolic calcium during the ischemic period (26). These data support the earlier finding of Lee et al (27) made with Indo-I in the perfused rabbit heart: that internal calcium rises rapidly and substantially with the onset of severe ischemia. This rise in cytosolic calcium may have important electrophysiologic consequences such as the development of delayed after depolarizations (28) and electrical alternans (29), both of which predispose to early ventricular arrhythmias. Nonetheless, it should be emphasized that the techniques for the measurement of cytosolic calcium remain controversial, and the problem is not settled.

"Supply" Versus "Demand" Ischemia

There is an important difference between "supply" ischemia and "demand" ischemia (Fig. 3–4). In supply ischemia, the basic problem is occlusion of the coronary artery, as in the initial stages of development of acute myocardial infarction. The consequences of supply ischemia are the simultaneous development of a lack of cellular oxygen and impaired washout of metabolites (Table 3–2). In demand ischemia, the oxygen demand rises as a consequence of exercise, while coronary artery disease restricts potential coronary dilation. In demand ischemia, there is still washout of metabolites despite the relative lack of coronary blood flow. Demand ischemia

Table 3–2. Causes of Impaired Contractility in "Supply" Ischemia (with Flaccid Myocardium)[a]

Accumulation of metabolites
Intracellular acidosis with displacement of Ca^{2+} from intracellular binding sites
Accumulation of inorganic phosphate and ADP with inhibition of actin–myosin interaction
Accumulation of neutral lactate
Changes in ATP level or availability
Decreased turnover of ATP
Decreased level of ATP in a "contractile" subcompartment
Decreased free energy change of ATP hydrolysis
Mechanical effects of decreased coronary flow
Reversed "garden hose" or "erectile" effect

[a]Note contrast with increased myocardial stiffness in "demand" ischemia; see Table 3–3.

For references, see Opie (1).

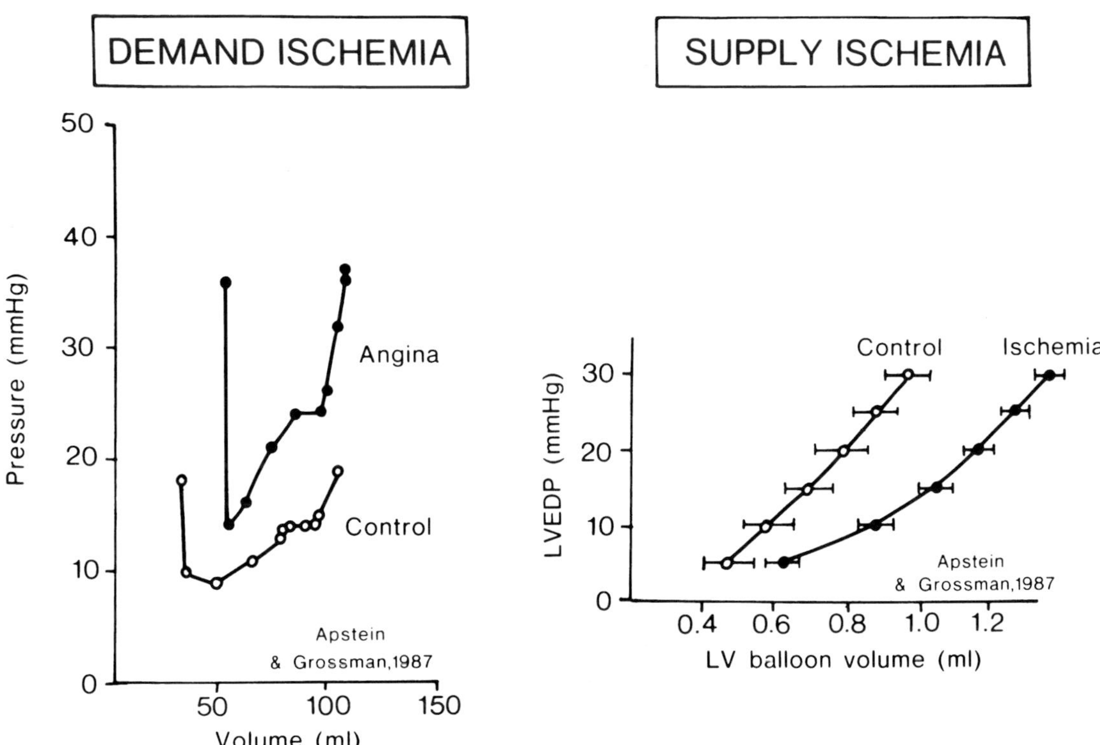

Figure 3–4. Examples of "demand" and "supply" ischemia. **A.** During demand ischemia caused by pacing a patient with angina pectoris, the left ventricular diastolic pressure–volume curve is moved upward, so that the myocardium is stiffer. **B.** In contrast, supply ischemia caused by total reduction of coronary flow in a perfused rabbit heart shows that for any given left ventricular end-diastolic pressure (LVEDP) the left ventricular volume (LV balloon volume) is greater. *Reproduced from Apstein CS, Grossman W: Opposite initial effects of supply and demand ischemia on left ventricular diastolic compliance: The ischemia-diastolic paradox. J Mol Cell Cardio 1987;19:119–128, with permission.*

is typical of effort angina and is seldom so severe and so sustained that it progresses to infarction. This chapter therefore concentrates on supply ischemia, which ultimately may lead to cell necrosis.

Different metabolic and mechanical changes occur in the two different types of ischemia, in contrast to the situation in severe hypoxia (Table 3–3). In supply ischemia, the ischemic tissue becomes flaccid. There is both decreased delivery of oxygen and impaired washout of metabolites, so that the rise of internal calcium is "balanced" by the rise in inorganic phosphate and protons. Protons can prevent the effect of an increase in cytosolic calcium and the interaction with the contractile elements (25). The overall result is that despite the measured rise in cytosolic calcium, contractile activity in the ischemic zone falls (Fig. 3–5).

On the other hand, in demand ischemia, where there still is a relatively high rate of washout of metabolites, there is less of an increase of protons and inorganic phosphate in the cytosol, so that the metabolically induced rise of calcium is not "buffered." The effect of the increased cytosolic calcium is myocardial stiffening and a loss of compliance, typical of early angina pectoris in humans

Table 3–3. Metabolic and Mechanical Differences Between Anoxia (or Severe Hypoxia) and Ischemia, Comparing Mild with Severe Ischemia

	Anoxia/ hypoxia	Mild ischemia	Severe ischemia
Glucose uptake	++	+	–
Tissue acidosis	+/–	+	++
Tissue lactate	+/–	+	++
Tissue inorganic phosphate	+/–	+	++
Residue oxidative metabolism	I	I /	I
Mechanical compliance	––	–	+
Diastolic tension	++	+	I
Systolic pressure development	–	–	––

\+ = increased compared with control; ++ = considerably increased compared with control; – = decreased compared with control; –– = markedly decreased compared with control; I = inhibition compared with control.

Reproduced from Opie LH: Myocardial metabolism in ischemia, in Heusch G (ed): Pathophysiology and Rational Therapy of Myocardial Ischemia. New York, Springer, 1990, with permission.

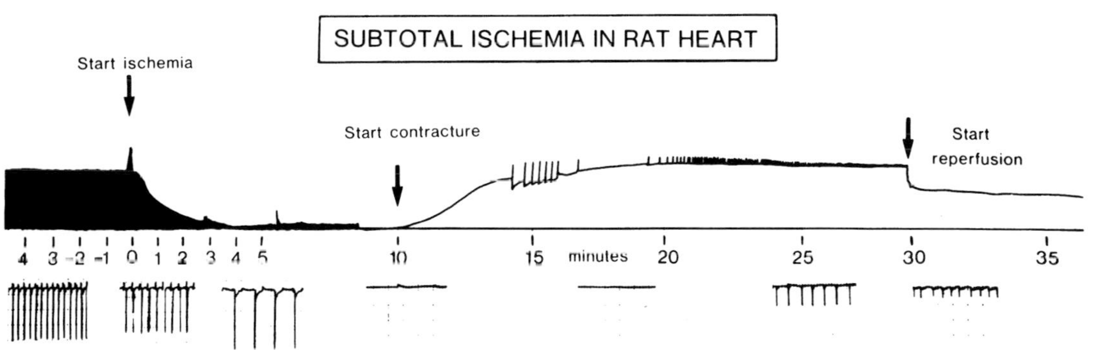

Figure 3–5. Example of supply ischemia with ischemic contracture and induction of irreversibility. On the left is shown cardiac contraction during normal perfusion of an isolated rat heart (Langendorff mode). At the left arrow, the perfusion pressure is abruptly reduced to about 5% to 10% of normal. Note the fall in systolic contraction and the unchanged diastolic tension. This is typical of supply ischemia. Later, after about 10 minutes (middle arrow), note the increase in diastolic tension, probably caused by an increase in internal calcium [see Allen et al (25)]. The diastolic tension eventually rises to equal the previous systolic level. On reperfusion (right arrow), the diastolic tension falls somewhat but does not return to normal, even with prolonged reperfusion of 30 minutes (unpublished observations). Supply ischemia has therefore become irreversible. The ECG traces in the lower panel show first, during supply ischemia, a slowing of sinus node activity (5 minutes) and then extreme slowing with loss of contraction (10 minutes). Note that the loss of sinus node activity is completely dissociated from the latter rise of diastolic tension, as these are caused by different events. Later, during reperfusion, there is sinus node recovery, even in the presence of irreversible left ventricular contracture.

(30). In reality, these distinctions between supply and demand ischemia are not absolute. The real differences may lie more in the severity of ischemia than in the mode of its production. Thus, balloon occlusion during angioplasty is more likely to produce severe ischemia and an increased distensibility than is pacing ischemia in the same patient (30A, 30B).

Cytosolic Magnesium in Ischemia

It has been supposed that a cytosolic magnesium deficiency could develop in acute myocardial ischemia; this would constitute an argument for the therapeutic administration of magnesium salts. Studies in a rat model of global ischemia, in which cytosolic calcium was measured by nuclear magnetic resonance, have shown for the first time a dramatic increase in cytosolic magnesium during severe ischemia (31). The initial value of cytosolic magnesium was about 0.60 mM, not far from that found by others [0.72 mM, (32)]. This value rose to more than 6.5 mM over 15 minutes of severe ischemia (31). The increase could be accounted for by liberation of magnesium from the concurrent fall in ATP. There was very little or no leakage of magnesium into the extracellular space.

DEVELOPMENT OF NECROSIS: THE POINT OF NO RETURN

Jennings and colleagues used the posterior papillary muscle of the dog to define a period of 40 to 60 minutes as the point of irreversible damage in response to severe ischemia. Severe cell damage was coupled with an overall loss of ATP (33). As elegant as these experiments were, they may not be directly relevant to the situation in humans with coronary artery disease, in whom there are usually extensive collaterals. Schaper et al (34) have clearly defined factors influencing the rate of irreversibility.

Collateral Circulation

The more extensive the collaterals, the longer it takes to develop irreversible cell damage. For example, the dog has a better collateral supply than the pig and, correspondingly, takes longer to develop irreversibility. The guinea pig has such a good collateral supply that coronary occlusion appears to have no consequences at all, whereas the rat has a very limited collateral supply and coronary occlusion results in rapid infarction. As Schaper so elegantly stated (35): "How guinea pigs win the rat race."

Myocardial Oxygen Uptake

The other major determinant of the rate of development of necrosis is myocardial oxygen uptake, as stressed by Braunwald and his group (36). The higher the oxygen uptake, the more rapid the development of necrosis. These concepts fit in well with the standard oxygen supply-and-demand concept. An increased supply is obtained by prior collaterals; a decreased demand by low myocardial oxygen uptake. In pigs with poor collateral flow, substantial necrosis can develop in 40 to 60 minutes; whereas in dogs with many collaterals and low myocardial oxygen uptake, even after 3 hours irreversibility is not complete. In patients with coronary artery disease, the progression to irreversibility seems to correspond more closely to the situation in the dog than to that in the pig.

Biochemical Marker of Irreversibility

There is no problem in diagnosing irreversibility when the sarcolemma is extensively damaged, the mitochondrial architecture lost, and the myofibrils pulled apart by contracture; however, these are clearly late events (see Ch. 21). There is considerable and continuing controversy regarding the precise biochemical event that is the early sign of irreversibility and, therefore, of cell necrosis. Increased sarcolemmal permeability can be detected by structural changes at electron microscopy (33), with the development of pores in the sarcolemma, and is an important step along the road to irreversibility. Such increased sarcolemmal permeability corresponds closely to the understanding of clinicians who know that modest increases in cardiac enzymes in the circulation indicate marginal necrosis, whereas major increases in release of intracardiac enzymes, such as the MB isoenzyme creatine kinase, indicate definite infarction. The other major electron microscopic contender for the sign of irreversibility is the development of mitochondrial dense bodies, thought to be calcium phosphate precipitates. These are specific to the ischemic process (37).

Excess of Cytosolic Calcium

Currently, among the markers linked to the development of cell necrosis is an excess of cytosolic calcium. The excess calcium may (i) activate membrane phospholipases, leading to production of membrane active fatty acids and destruction of cell membranes, particularly the sarcolemma, with release of intracardiac enzymes; (ii) induce ischemic contracture (22); and (iii) increase uptake of calcium by mitochondria, leading to impairment of mitochondrial metabolism and decreased ATP production, which is the explanation proposed for intramitochondrial flocculent dense bodies (37).

Membrane Damage

Besides activation of phospholipases, numerous other biochemical factors act simultaneously to cause cell membrane damage (Fig. 3–6). An important event preceding overt membrane damage is the loss of regulation of cell volume (33), suggesting that osmotic pressure may "pop open" the ischemic cell to rupture the sarcolemma. Such a role for the osmolar load in the genesis of irreversible cell injury has been proposed by Jennings et al (38), which may explain why a rise in the cellular ratio of sodium to potassium (Na^+/K^+ ratio) correlates well with histologic evidence of cell necrosis (39). A novel suggestion is that ischemia also depresses the synthesis of membrane phospholipids (40).

Lysophospholipids and Fatty Acids

Lysophospholipids, formed by the action of phospholipases, have an unexpected effect in "un-

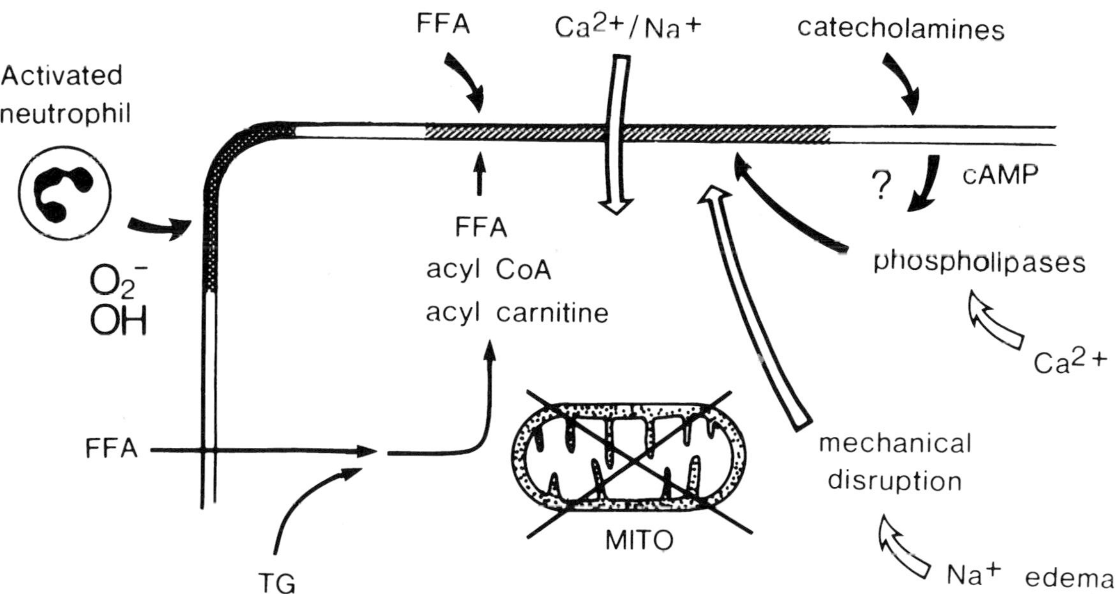

Figure 3–6. Schematic of role of neutrophils and fatty acid metabolites in causing membrane damage. FFA = free fatty acids, cAMP = cyclic AMP, CoA = coenzyme A, MITO = mitochondria, TG = triglyceride. *Figure copyright by LH Opie.*

covering" α_1 receptors (41), thereby bringing such receptors into play, an additional factor likely to increase intracellular cytosolic calcium. Free fatty acids begin to accumulate in the ischemic cell about 30 to 60 minutes after the onset of ischemia and can be expected to be highly damaging to the membranes (42).

Free Radicals

Free radicals form not only during the reperfusion period but also during ischemia (43). Free radicals are highly membrane active and can be expected to contribute to membrane destruction.

Glycolysis, Lipolysis, and Cell Viability

A hypothesis favored by the author of this chapter is that glycolysis helps to protect the cell membranes against ischemia (44). In a variety of circumstances, agents promoting glycolytic flux decrease myocardial ischemic damage, whereas agents promoting lipolysis (fatty acid metabolism) increase damage. Addition of glycolytic flux to a partially ischemic cell decreases the fatty acid–mediated damage (45), "protects" the sarcolemma (46), and improves synthesis of membrane phospholipids (40). When glycolysis ceases or becomes severely inhibited, then, it is hypothesized, the risk of cell necrosis increases (Fig. 3–7).

In trying to ascertain whether lack of glycolysis or accumulation of fatty acid intermediates is of fundamental importance in causing ischemic damage, Lopaschuk et al (47) used the agent etoximor, which decreased fatty acid oxidation and increased glucose oxidation. Both a decreased rate of glycolysis and increased accumulation of lipid intermediates contribute to ischemic contracture (47a). Clearly these two factors (glycolytic flux and lipolysis) have an opposing, seesaw quality, so that promotion of one leads to inhibition of the other. This could be called an intracellular "Randle cycle"(48).

REPERFUSION INJURY

When a coronary artery is occluded, reperfusion is undoubtedly the most effective measure in relieving ischemia (see Chs. 2 and 21). Nonetheless, reperfusion is not an unmixed blessing, and numerous animal experiments attest to the development of reper-

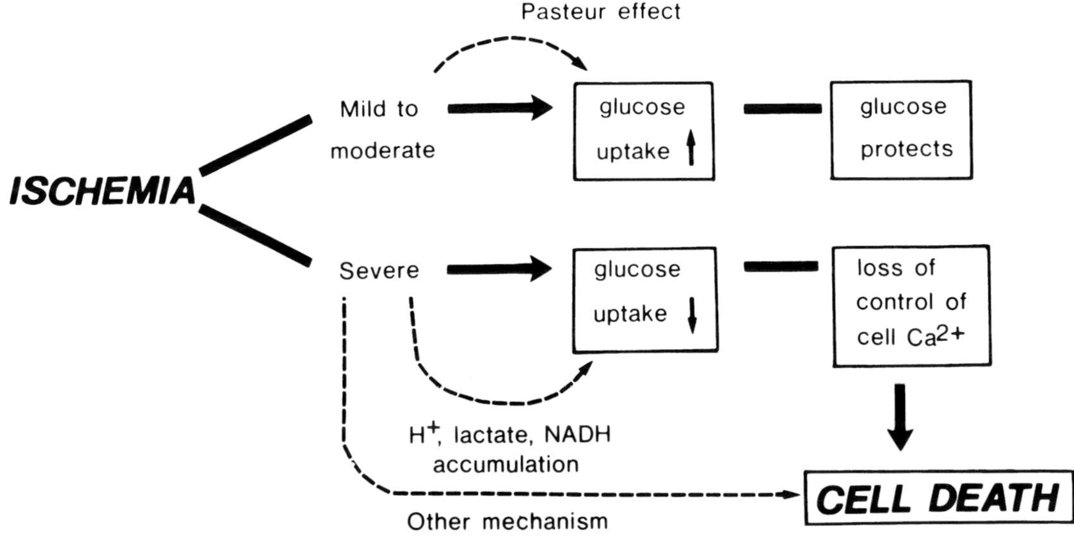

Figure 3–7. Hypothesis relating the rate of glycolysis to cell death. During mild to moderate ischemia, glucose uptake is increased, providing the benefit of increased glycolytic ATP. During severe ischemia, the rate of glucose delivery becomes limiting (6). In addition, the accumulation of protons, lactate, and NADH inhibits glycolysis and glucose uptake. Consequently, there is a loss of control of intracellular calcium with the formation of ischemic contracture. *Figure copyright by LH Opie.*

fusion injury (49–51). The whole issue of reperfusion injury has been clouded by complex definitions. For Jennings and his group (38), true reperfusion injury specifically means only an absolute increase in cell necrosis after reperfusion, that is, more necrosis than there would have been with continued ischemia. Because irreversibility is judged as the failure to respond to reperfusion, and because reperfusion injury is a potential hazard, it becomes extremely difficult to determine whether in any given preparation reperfusion has been achieved without the development of further necrosis. The experimental use of free radical scavengers before reperfusion (52) suggests that there is an additional element in reperfusion causing more extensive cell necrosis, and that this element is countered by the addition of free radical scavengers. In other experiments, the effect of the addition of free radical scavengers on the extent of necrosis has not been so clear-cut [see review by Opie (53)]. Leaving aside the controversial question of the possibility of increased cell necrosis on reperfusion, there are three other aspects of reperfusion injury: (i) reperfusion ventricular arrhythmias; (ii) reperfusion stunning; and (iii) microvascular injury.

Arrhythmias

Although reperfusion arrhythmias do not appear to be of major clinical importance in the use of intravenous thrombolytics, they draw attention to reversible cellular abnormalities occurring during the reperfusion period, expressing themselves as temporary arrhythmias (see Chs. 14 and 21). The peak period of risk for such arrhythmias occurs soon after reperfusion and is over within 10 to 15 minutes. During that period there does, however, exist the risk of fatal reperfusion ventricular fibrillation. Why such severe arrhythmias, frequently found in animal models, are not of major clinical importance during thrombolytic reperfusion remains unknown. It may be relevant that the rate of reperfusion in humans is probably measured in many minutes rather than in seconds, in contrast to abrupt reperfusion after release of the coronary artery occlusion in animal experiments.

The two major mechanisms proposed for reperfusion arrhythmias are an increase in cytosolic calcium and free radical formation.

Excess Cytosolic Calcium

Calcium-mediated injury is thought to play a role as follows. Initially, a high cytosolic concentration of calcium is established as a result of the excessive rhythmical uptake and release of calcium into and out of the sarcoplasmic reticulum, as ATP returns to the previously ischemic cell [see the model for hypoxia and reoxygenation of Allshire et al (54)]. It has already been proposed that cytosolic calcium rises during ischemia, but that the normal oscillations may be dampened by the lack of energy. Then, on the return of high-energy phosphates with reperfusion, the cytosolic calcium starts to undergo large oscillations, with the production of a calcium-dependent transient inward current (55) and early ventricular arrhythmias (28,56). As energy is restored, the electrophysiologic effects of excess calcium cycling become apparent. In energy-depleted preparations, such calcium-dependent electrophysiologic changes cannot occur (57). Evidence for a role of the sarcoplasmic reticulum in recycling of calcium is the abolition of such arrhythmias by internal calcium inhibition using the agent ryanodine (58), or by inhibitors of the calcium uptake pump (59).

Free Radical Formation

Formation of free radicals is the second major theory for reperfusion arrhythmias (see Ch. 21). Such formation undoubtedly occurs in animal preparations with sudden reperfusion. The relationship of free radical formation to ventricular reperfusion arrhythmias remains controversial (60). Excessively rapid formation of free radicals can cause the rapid onset of arrhythmias, but the real questions concern rates of formation of free radicals during ordinary reperfusion and the significance of these presumably lower rates. A useful concept is that the effects of free radicals and calcium ions can be interactive and synergistic (53,61).

Stunning

Stunning is the development of impaired mechanical function despite complete restoration of blood flow; the impairment is of a temporary nature, and so there is spontaneous recovery. It is useful to distinguish between early stunning, as often studied experimentally and lasting hours, and long-term stunning over days and weeks. One of the early theories of early stunning involved ATP depletion and slow rates of resynthesis of ATP after the loss of adenine nucleotides; however, recent data have shown that there is no real defect in the capacity to produce energy (62). Furthermore, there is no relation between overall levels of ATP and reperfusion recovery. At present the two main theories used to explain early reperfusion stunning are based on formation of free radicals and/or calcium overload (Fig. 3–8).

Cytosolic Calcium and Stunning

Excess cytosolic calcium is an attractive theory to explain early stunning in view of the strong evidence for such excess cycling as the basis of reperfusion arrhythmias. On the other hand, it is difficult to relate an excess of calcium to mechanical impairment. One proposal is that the early excess of calcium damages such organelles as the sarcoplasmic reticulum and the myofibers, leading to their later relative insensitivity to even a normal internal calcium (63). Thus, in the late stages of reperfusion injury, according to the calcium theory, there is a failure to respond to calcium, which would explain the benefit of calcium infusions and of catecholamines (64). Further evidence favoring the calcium hypothesis is that specific inhibition of the Na^+/H^+ exchanger during reperfusion lessens stunning (65). The proposal is that there is indirect inhibition of the Na^+/Ca^{2+} exchanger (see also section in this chapter on Sodium–Calcium Exchange).

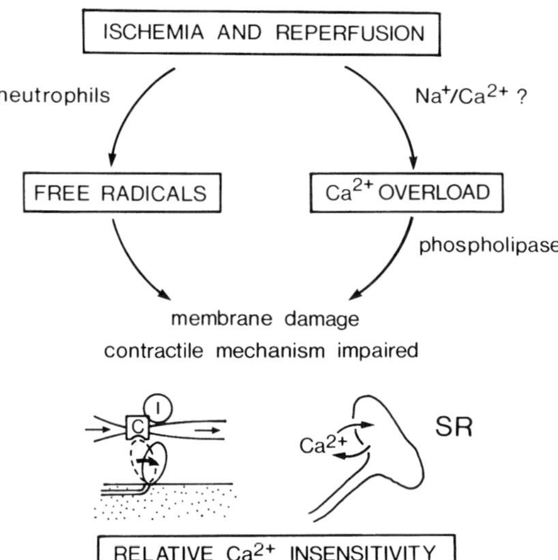

Figure 3–8. Illustration of the two major mechanisms for reperfusion injury: free radical formation and cytosolic calcium overload. This schematic reconciles these apparently conflicting hypotheses, showing the proposed combined role of free radicals and calcium overload in causing membrane damage and relative calcium insensitivity of the contractile mechanism [actin–myosin interaction on left and sarcoplasmic reticulum (SR) on right]. *Reproduced from Opie (53), with the permission of Circulation and the American Heart Association.*

Free Radicals and Stunning

Many more studies have tried to relate reperfusion stunning to formation of free radicals. A review of this hypothesis (53) shows that in the majority of cases, free radical scavengers have been added during the ischemic process, and the benefits in decreasing stunning could have resulted from inhibition of free radical formation during ischemia, not during reperfusion. Nonetheless, Bolli et al (66) showed very convincingly that there is a sudden burst of free radicals in the first minute of abrupt reperfusion, because scavengers were effective in preventing stunning when added just before reperfusion but not when added 1 minute after reperfusion. Further support for this hypothesis lies in the direct measurement of the burst of free radicals in the early reperfusion period (67).

The major cause of the free radical formation may be the return of circulation with the interaction between neutrophils and endothelium, as a number of experiments have shown the benefits of neutrophil depletion, provided that ischemia is sufficiently long (68).

The major defect of the free radical theory is that with the radicals formed during the first minute of abrupt reperfusion, the situation would appear to be different from the more gradual reperfusion attained in patients undergoing thrombolysis. Thus far no free radical scavengers have been shown to diminish reperfusion stunning in humans.

Long-Term Stunning

Whereas short-term stunning typically follows periods of severe or total ischemia lasting 15 to 20 minutes and is never accompanied by cell necrosis, longer periods may be associated with cell necrosis and hence inability to achieve full recovery on reperfusion. Although this condition is not, by definition, true stunning, nonetheless in animal models of prolonged coronary occlusion, reperfusion is followed by a graded recovery of mechanical function, albeit not to preocclusion levels. Similarly, in patients after thrombolysis, left ventricular function may only gradually improve. The mechanism of these changes is almost certainly different from that of short-term calcium-dependent stunning, and it may involve a host of alterations in protein synthesis, including production of protective proteins such as the heat shock proteins (69).

Sodium–Calcium Exchange in Reperfusion: A Mechanism for Calcium Overload

During the ischemic period, an accumulation of intracellular protons is followed by a washout of such protons with reperfusion. The hypothesis is that the washout and transfer of protons to the extracellular space promote proton–sodium exchange in such a direction that intracellular sodium accumulates, to be followed later by accumulation of calcium according to the sodium–calcium exchange. Indirect evidence has been obtained for such a sequence, both as a contribution to ventricular arrhythmias (70) and in the case of mechanical stunning by Tani and Neely (71) and du Toit and Opie (65). Inhibition of sodium–calcium exchange may be a profitable way to lessen reperfusion stunning. Experimentally, a recently synthesized direct inhibitor of this system is now available (72).

Microvascular Damage

Increasing evidence suggests that in addition to the myocardium, the vascular endothelium can also be damaged. Such damage can be diminished by the use of certain fluorocarbons or adenosine (73). Although maintenance of endothelial integrity is poorly understood, the increasing emphasis on a major role for the endothelium in regulating coronary flow as well as in preventing platelet aggregation merits attention. It can safely be prophesied that the role of microvascular injury will be increasingly emphasized in the overall spectrum of reperfusion injury. Massive degrees of microvascular injury can lead to the no reflow phenomenon, a feared complication of cardiac surgery; however, part of the no reflow phenomenon may result from massive calcium overload and the development of ischemic contracture.

NEW ISCHEMIC SYNDROMES

This term refers to a variety of newly described entities, including stunning, hibernation, preconditioning, and ischemic left ventricular dysfunction. Hibernation is the term to describe the condition in patients with coronary artery disease in whom left ventricular function is chronically reduced and in which the function of myocytes improves on reperfusion (74). Preconditioning is the state in which a period of temporary severe ischemia followed by reperfusion protects the myocardium against subsequent ischemia. The mechanism is metabolic in origin, hypothetically the result of stimulation of protein kinase C by adenosine (75). Again, it is useful to distinguish between such short-term preconditioning and long-term preconditioning, the latter lasting for 24 to 48 hours and possibly the result of synthesis of heat shock proteins (76). Ischemic left ventricular dysfunction is a spectrum of clinical conditions, including stunning, hibernation, and preconditioning, but also referring to postinfarct left ventricular diastolic dysfunction of the type that responds to calcium antagonist therapy (77).

CONCLUSIONS

Cellular biochemical events explain the phenomena of early ischemia, necrosis, and reperfusion injury. Emphasis is shifting from the fundamental role of a deficiency of energy to a better understanding of the consequences of the energy deficit, including primarily abnormalities of ion control. In the very early phases of ischemia, the newly described ATP-dependent potassium channel very probably plays a role in the early potassium loss, which can have severe and grave electrophysiologic consequences, such as fatal ventricular fibrillation. At the same time, "local cardioplegia" by the high extracellular potassium protects the ischemic myocyte. Loss of control of calcium leads to an increase in cytosolic calcium, with further implications for arrhythmia development and impaired mechanical function.

Prolonged ischemia leads to necrosis. One proposal is that the critical metabolic event in this change is the decreased glycolytic flux by the low rate of delivery of glucose, which in turn results in loss of control of cytosolic calcium and rigor formation. Also, as a result of impaired control of membrane ionic pumps after depletion of glycolytic energy, a late rise in cell sodium predisposes to edema with rupture of the sarcolemma and release of enzymes. Membrane damage is also promoted by the combined effects of an accumulation of free fatty acids, calcium-activated phospholipase activity, circulating catecholamines, and free radical formation.

In considering the time scale leading to the point of no return, the classical oxygen supply-and-demand equation is a useful framework. An increase in the oxygen supply can be achieved through the preexisting collaterals or by thrombolysis. A decrease in the oxygen demand can be achieved by early beta-blockade. In the presence of preexisting collaterals and a low oxygen demand, the time to necrosis may be several hours; in the absence of such factors, cell death occurs within 1 hour.

Reperfusion injury encompasses a wide range of events, including arrhythmias, stunning, microvascular injury, and accelerated cell death. Of these, evidence for reperfusion-induced arrhythmias and stunning is excellent, that for microvascular injury is good, and that for accelerated cell death is controversial. Excess cytosolic calcium at the time of reperfusion is thought to predispose to enhanced calcium recycling occurring at the time of restoration of energy. According to this concept, such excess calcium can explain both early reperfusion arrhythmias and later stunning, the latter following internal organelle damage as a result of the calcium excess. The other major mechanism proposed for reperfusion injury is the formation of free radicals. The free radical hypothesis does not exclude the calcium hypothesis, and in fact, the two mechanisms appear to act synergistically.

Attention is now shifting from the well-known effects of ischemia (angina versus infarction versus reperfusion) to the new ischemic syndromes, including preconditioning, stunning, hibernation, and ischemic LV dysfunction. The biochemical basis for these syndromes is perhaps best understood in the case of mechanical stunning, but new concepts are required to explain hibernation. These complex entities highlight the heterogeneous reactions to ischemia, made all the more difficult to simplify by the infinitely variable anatomy of coronary artery disease.

ACKNOWLEDGMENTS

The author thanks the South African Medical Research Council, the Chris Barnard Fund, and the University of Cape Town for ongoing support.

REFERENCES

1. Opie LH: Myocardial ischemia—metabolic pathways and implications of increased glycolysis. *Cardiovasc Drugs Ther* 1990;4:777–790.
2. Weiss JN, Venkatesh N: Metabolic regulation of cardiac ATP-sensitive K^+ channels. *Cardiovasc Drugs Ther* 1993;7:499–505.
3. De Jong JW (ed): *Myocardial Energy Metabolism*. Dordrecht, Martinus Nijhoff, 1988.
4. Jenkins JR, Belardinelli L: Atrioventricular nodal accommodation in isolated guinea pig hearts: Physiological significance and role of adenosine. *Circ Res* 1988;63:97–116.
5. Sylven C: Mechanisms of pain in angina pectoris—a critical review of the adenosine hypothesis. *Cardiovasc Drugs Ther* 1993;7:745–759.
6. King LM, Boucher F, Opie LH: Coronary flow rate and glucose delivery as determinants of contracture in the ischaemic myocardium. *J Mol Cell Cardiol* 1995;27:701–720.
7. Opie LH, Owen P, Thomas M, Samson R: Coronary sinus lactate measurements in the assessment of myocardial ischemia. Comparison with changes in the ratios lactate/pyruvate and beta-hydroxybutyrate/acetoacetate and with release of hydrogen, phosphate and potassium ions from the heart. *Am J Cardiol* 1973;32:295–305.
8. Harris AS, Bisteni A, Russell RA, et al: Excitatory factors in ventricular tachycardia resulting from

myocardial ischemia: Potassium a major excitant. *Science* 1954;119:200–203.

9. Bittl JA, Balschi JA, Ingwall JS: Contractile failure and high-energy phosphate turnover during hypoxia: ^{31}P-NMR surface coil studies in living rat. *Circ Res* 1987;60:871–878.

10. Kleber AG: Extracellular potassium accumulation in acute myocardial ischemia. *J Mol Cell Cardiol* 1984;16:389–394.

11. Opie LH, Owen P, Riemersma RA: Relative rates of oxidation of glucose and free fatty acids by ischemic and non-ischemic myocardium after coronary artery ligation in the dog. *Eur J Clin Invest* 1973;3:419–435.

12. Wilde AAM, Aksnes G: Myocardial potassium loss and cell depolarisation in ischaemia and hypoxia. *Cardiovasc Res* 1995,29.1–15.

13. Noma A, Shibasaki T: Membrane current through adenosine-triphosphate-regulated potassium channels in guinea-pig ventricular cells. *J Physiol* 1985;363:463–480.

14. Dunne MJ, Petersen OH: GTP and GDP activation of K^+ channels that can be inhibited by ATP. *Pflugers Arch* 1986;407:561 565.

15. Fosset M, De Weille JR, Green RD, et al: Antidiabetic sulfonylureas control action potential properties in heart cells via high affinity receptors that are linked to ATP-dependent K^+ channels. *J Biol Chem* 1988;263:7933–7936.

16. Kantor PF, Coetzee WA, Carmeliet EE, et al: Reduction in ischemic K^+ loss and arrhythmias: The effect of the sulfonylurea, glibenclamide. *Circ Res* 1990;66:478–485.

17. Sanguinetti MC, Scott AL, Zingaro GJ, Siegl PKS: BRL 34915 (cromakalim) activates ATP-sensitive K^+ current in cardiac muscle. *Proc Natl Acad Sci USA* 1988;85:8360–8364.

18. Wolleben CD, Sanguinetti MC, Siegl PKS: Influence of ATP-sensitive potassium channel modulators on ischemia-induced fibrillation in isolated rat hearts. *J Mol Cell Cardiol* 1989;21:783–788.

19. Opie LH: Modulation of ischemia by regulation of the ATP-sensitive potassium channel. *Cardiovasc Drugs Ther* 1993;7:507–513.

20. Bowers KC, Allshire AP, Cobbold PH: Bioluminescent measurement in single cardiomyocytes of sudden cystolic ATP depletion coincident with rigor. *J Mol Cell Cardiol* 1992;24:213–218.

21. Owen P, Thomas M, Young V, Opie LH: Comparison between metabolic changes in local venous and coronary sinus blood after acute experimental coronary arterial occlusion. *Am J Cardiol* 1970;25: 562–570.

21A. Cross HR, Radda GK, Clarke K: The role of Na^+/K^+ ATPase activity during low flow ischemia in preventing myocardial injury: a ^{31}P, ^{23}Na and ^{87}Rb NMR spectroscopic study. *Magn Reson Med* 1995;34:673–685.

22. Owen P, Dennis S, Opie LH: Glucose flux rate regulates onset of ischemic contracture in globally underperfused rat hearts. *Circ Res* 1990;66:344–354.

23. Neely JR, Grotyohann LW: Role of glycolytic products in damage to ischemic myocardium. Dissociation of adenosine triphosphate levels and recovery of function of reperfused ischemic hearts. *Circ Res* 1984;55:816–824.

24. Lagerstrom CF, Walker WE, Taegtmeyer H: Failure of glycogen depletion to improve left ventricular function of the rabbit heart after hypothermic ischemic arrest. *Circ Res* 1988;63:81–86.

24A. Cross HR, Opie LH, Radda GK, Clarke K: Is a high glycogen content beneficial or detrimental to the ischemic rat heart? A controversy resolved. *Circ Res* 1996;78:482–491.

25. Allen DG, Lee JA, Smith GL: The effects of simulated ischemia on intracellular calcium and tension in isolated ferret ventricular muscle. *J Physiol (Lond)* 1988;401:81P.

26. Meissner A, Morgan JP: Contractile dysfunction and abnormal Ca^{2+} modulation during postischemic reperfusion in rat heart. *Am J Physiol* 1995; 268:H100–H111.

27. Lee H-C, Smith N, Mohabir R, Clusin WT: Cytosolic calcium transients from the beating mammalian heart. *Proc Natl Acad Sci USA* 1987;84: 7793–7797.

28. Opie LH, Coetzee WA, Dennis SC, Thandroyen FT: A potential role of calcium ions in early ischemic and reperfusion arrhythmias. *Ann NY Acad Sci* 1988;522:464–477.

29. Lee H-C, Mohabir R, Smith N, et al: Effect of ischemia on calcium-dependent fluorescence transients in rabbit hearts containing Indo-I. Correlation with monophasic action potentials and contraction. *Circulation* 1988;78:1047–1059.

30. Isoyama S, Apstein CS, Wexler LF, et al: Acute decrease in left ventricular diastolic chamber distensibility during simulated angina in isolated hearts. *Circ Res* 1987;61:925–933.

30A. De Bruyne B, Bronzwaer JGF, Heyndrickx GR, Paulus WJ: Comparative effects of ischemia and hypoxemia on left ventricular systolic and diastolic function in humans. *Circulation* 1993;88:461–471.

30B. Takano H, Glantz SA: Left ventricular contractility predicts how the end-diastolic pressure-volume relation shifts during pacing-induced ischemia in dogs. *Circulation* 1995;91:2423–2434.

31. Kirkels JH, van Echteld CJA, Ruigrok TJC: Intracellular magnesium during myocardial ischemia and reperfusion: Consequences for postischemic recovery. *J Mol Cell Cardiol* 1989;21:1209–1218.

32. Gao WD, Backx PH, Azan-Backx M, Marban E: Myofilament Ca^{2+} sensitivity in intact versus skinned rat ventricular muscle. *Circ Res* 1994;74: 408–415.

33. Reimer KA, Jennings RB, Hill ML: Total ischemia in dog hearts, in vitro. 2. High energy phosphate depletion and associated defects in energy metabolism, cell volume regulation, and sarcolemmal integrity. *Circ Res* 1981;49:901–911.

34. Schaper W, Binz K, Sass S, Winkler B: Influence of collateral blood flow and of variations in MVO_2 on tissue ATP content in ischemic and infarcted myocardium. *J Mol Cell Cardiol* 1987;19:19–37.

35. Schaper W: Experimental infarcts and the microcirculation, in Hearse DJ, Yellon DM (eds): *Therapeutic Approaches to Myocardial Infarct Size Limitation.* New York, Raven Press, 1984, pp 79–90.

36. Maroko PR, Kjekshus JK, Sobel BE, et al: Factors influencing infarct size following experimental coronary artery occlusions. *Circulation* 1971;43: 67–82.

37. Schaper J, Schaper W: Time course of myocardial necrosis. *Cardiovasc Drugs Ther* 1988;2:17–25.

38. Jennings RB, Reimer KA, Steenbergen C: Myocardial ischemia revisited. The osmolar load, membrane damage, and reperfusion. *J Mol Cell Cardiol* 1986;18:769–780.

39. Rose A, Opie LH, Bricknell O: Evaluation of histologic criteria of early experimental myocardial infarction. Comparison with biochemical and electrocardiographic parameters. *Arch Pathol* 1976;100: 516–571.

40. Lochner A, de Villiers M: Phosphatidylcholine biosynthesis in myocardial ischemia. *J Mol Cell Cardiol* 1989;21:151–163.

41. Heathers GP, Yamada KA, Kanter EM, Corr PB: Long-chain acylcarnitines mediate the hypoxia-induced increase in α_1-adrenergic receptors on adult canine myocytes. *Circ Res* 1987;61:735–746.

42. Van der Vusse GJ, Roemen ThHM, Prinzen FW, et al: Uptake and tissue content of fatty acids in dog myocardium under normoxic and ischemic conditions. *Circ Res* 1982;50:538–546.

43. Maupoil V, Rochette L, Tabard A, et al: Evolution of free radical formation during low-flow ischemia and reperfusion in isolated rat heart. *Cardiovasc Drugs Ther* 1990;4:791–796.

44. Opie LH. Hypothesis: Glycolytic rates control cell viability in ischemia. *J Appl Cardiol* 1988;3: 407–414.

45. Opie LH, Bricknell OL: Role of glycolytic flux in effect of glucose in decreasing fatty acid–induced release of lactate dehydrogenase from isolated coronary ligated rat heart. *Cardiovasc Res* 1979;13: 693–702.

46. Weiss J, Hiltbrand B: Functional compartmentation of glycolytic versus oxidative metabolism in isolated rabbit heart. *J Clin Invest* 1985;75:436–447.

47. Lopaschuk GD, Wall SR, Olley PM, Davies NJ: Etomoxir, a carnitine palmitoyltransferase I inhibitor, protects hearts from fatty acid–induced ischemic injury independent of changes in long-chain acylcarnitine. *Circ Res* 1988;63:1036–1043.

47A. Clarke B, Wyatt KM, May GR, McCormack JG: On the roles of long-chain acyl carnitine accumulation and impaired glucose utilization in ischaemic contracture development and tissue damage in the guinea-pig heart. *J Moll Cell Cardiol* 1996;28: 171–181.

48. Randle PJ, Garland PB, Hales CN, Newsholme EA: The glucose fatty acid cycle: Its role in insulin sensitivity and the metabolic disturbances of diabetes mellitus. *Lancet* 1963;1:785–789.

49. Bricknell OL, Opie LH: Effects of substrates on tissue metabolic changes in the isolated rat heart during underperfusion and on release of lactate dehydrogenase and arrhythmias during reperfusion. *Circ Res* 1978;43:102–115.

50. Braunwald E, Kloner RA: The stunned myocardium: Prolonged, postischemic ventricular dysfunction. *Circulation* 1982;66:1146–1149.

51. Nayler WG, Elz JS: Reperfusion injury: Laboratory artifact or clinical dilemma. *Circulation* 1986;74: 215–221.

52. Jolly SR, Kane WJ, Bailie MB, et al: Canine myocardial reperfusion injury: Its reduction by the combined administration of superoxide dismutase and catalase. *Circ Res* 1984;54:277–285.

53. Opie LH: Reperfusion injury and its pharmacological modification. *Circulation* 1989;80:1049–1062.

54. Allshire A, Piper M, Cuthbertson KSR, Cobbold PH: Cytosolic free Ca^{2+} in single rat heart cells

during anoxia and reoxygenation. *Biochem J* 1987; 244:381–385.

55. Berlin JR, Cannell MB, Lederer WJ: Cellular origins of the transient inward current in cardiac myocytes. Role of fluctuations and waves of elevated intracellular calcium. *Circ Res* 1989;65:115–126.

56. Opie LH, Coetzee WA: Role of calcium ions in reperfusion arrhythmias. Relevance to pharmacological intervention. *Cardiovasc Drugs Ther* 1988;2: 623 636.

57. Coetzee WA, Opie LH: Effects of components of ischemia and metabolic inhibition on delayed afterdepolarizations in guinea-pig papillary muscle. *Circ Res* 1987;61:157–165.

58. Thandroyen FT, McCarthy J, Burton K, Opie LH: Ryanodine and caffeine prevent ventricular arrhythmias during acute myocardial ischemia and reperfusion in rat heart. *Circ Res* 1988;62:306–314.

59. du Toit EF, Opie LH: Antiarrhythmic properties of specific inhibitors of sarcoplasmic reticulum calcium ATPase in the isolated perfused rat heart after coronary artery ligation. *J Am Coll Cardiol* 1994;23: 1505–1510.

60. Yamada M, Hearse DJ, Curtis MJ: Reperfusion and readmission of oxygen. Pathophysiological relevance of oxygen-derived free radicals to arrhythmogenesis. *Circ Res* 1990;67:1211–1224.

61. Hearse DJ. Stunning: A radical re-view. *Cardiovasc Drugs Ther* 1991;5:853–876.

62. Ambrosio G, Jacobus WE, Bergman CA: Preserved high-energy phosphate metabolic reserve in globally "stunned" hearts despite reduction of basal ATP content and contractility. *J Mol Cell Cardiol* 1987;19: 953–964.

63. Kusuoka H, Porterfield JK, Weisman HF, et al: Pathophysiology and pathogenesis of stunned myocardium: Depressed Ca^{2+}-activation of contraction as a consequence of reperfusion-induced cellular calcium overload in ferret hearts. *J Clin Invest* 1987;79:950–961.

64. Becker LC, Levine JH, DiPaula AF, et al: Reversal of dysfunction in postischemic stunned myocardium by epinephrine and postextrasystolic potentiation. *J Am Coll Cardiol* 1986;7:580–589.

65. du Toit EF, Opie LH: Inhibitors of Ca^{2+}-ATPase pump of sarcoplasmic reticulum attenuate reperfusion stunning in isolated rat heart. *J Cardiovasc Pharmacol* 1994;24:678–684.

66. Bolli J, Jeroudi MO, Patel BS, et al: Marked reduction of free radical generation and contractile dysfunction by anti-oxidant therapy begun at the time of reperfusion: Evidence that myocardial "stunning" is a manifestation of reperfusion injury. *Circ Res* 1989;65:607–622.

67. Zweier JL, Flaherty JT, Weisfeldt ML: Direct measurement of free radical generation following reperfusion of ischaemic myocardium. *Proc Natl Acad Sci USA* 1987;84:1404–1407.

68. Kloner RA: Do neutrophils mediate the phenomenon of stunned myocardium? *J Am Coll Cardiol* 1989;13:1164–1166.

69. Schaper W: Molecular mechanisms in "stunned" myocardium. *Cardiovasc Drugs Ther* 1991;5: 925–932.

70. Dennis SC, Coetzee WA, Cragoe EJ Jr, Opie LH: Evidence for a role for Na^+/H^+ exchange in the genesis of reperfusion arrhythmias in isolated rat hearts. *Circ Res* 1990;66:1156–1159.

71. Tani M, Neely JR: Role of intracellular Na^+ in Ca^{2+} overload and depressed recovery of ventricular function of reperfused ischemic rat hearts. Possible involvement of H^+–Na^+ and Na^+–Ca^{2+} exchange. *Circ Res* 1989;65:1045–1056.

72. Chin TK, Spitzer KW, Philipson KD, Bridge JHB: The effect of exchanger inhibitory peptide (XIP) on sodium–calcium exchange current in guinea-pig ventricular cells. *Circ Res* 1993;72:497–503.

73. Bajaj AK, Cobb MA, Virmani R, et al: Limitation of myocardial reperfusion injury by intravenous perfluorochemicals. Role of neutrophil activation. *Circulation* 1989;79:645–656.

74. Tubau JF, Rahimtoola SH: Hibernating myocardium: A historical perspective. *Cardiovasc Drugs Ther* 1992;6:267–271.

74A. Conversano A, Walsh JF, Geltman EM, Perez JE, Bergmann SR, Gropler RJ: Delineation of myocardial stunning and hibernation by positron emission tomography in advanced coronary artery disease. *Am Heart J* 1996;131:440–450.

75. Thornton JD, Liu GS, Olsson RA, Downey JM: Intravenous pretreatment with α_1-selective adenosine analogues protects the heart against infarction. *Circulation* 1992;85:659–665.

76. Baxter GF, Marber MS, Patel VC, Yellon DM: Adenosine receptor involvement in a delayed phase of myocardial protection 24 hours after ischemic preconditioning. *Circulation* 1994;90:2993–3000.

77. Opie LH: The ever expanding spectrum of ischemic left ventricular dysfunction. *Cardiovasc Drugs Ther* 1994;8:297–304.

4

Acute Ischemic Syndromes: Coronary Pathophysiology and Angiographic Correlations

John A. Ambrose, MD, and Craig Hjemdahl-Monsen, MD

The acute ischemic syndromes include the following clinical conditions: acute myocardial infarction (both Q wave and non-Q wave), unstable angina, and sudden ischemic death. Each syndrome can be specifically defined, although their presentations often overlap. The clinical distinction between non-Q wave and Q wave infarction may in some cases be only the absence of Q waves on the electrocardiogram. In other cases, non-Q wave infarction may be difficult to distinguish clinically from unstable angina except for the absence of an elevated creatine phosphokinase and the presence of reversible electrocardiographic changes in patients with unstable angina. Acute sudden ischemic death is often preceded by angina-like chest pain and acute myocardial infarction.

Not only is there an overlap in their clinical presentations, but data from a number of different disciplines suggest a common pathophysiologic mechanism in these syndromes (1). The results of pathologic, angiographic, angioscopic, biochemical, and therapeutic trials indicate the importance of thrombus formation secondary to disruption of an atherosclerotic plaque as the main mechanism underlying these syndromes. The occurrence of minor or major plaque fissuring and the formation of intraintimal and/or intraluminal thrombosis result in a spectrum of clinical presentations that depend on such factors as the severity and acuteness of luminal obstruction, the duration of total coronary occlusion, the presence or absence of collaterals, and the metabolic demands of the heart (1–3) (Fig. 4–1). In this chapter we consider the pathophysiology of these acute ischemic syndromes with special emphasis on their angiographic findings. As any discussion of pathophysiology of these acute syndromes must begin with the pathologic substrate, we must first consider the growth and development of the atherosclerotic plaque and the mechanisms involved in plaque disruption.

DEVELOPMENT OF ATHEROSCLEROTIC PLAQUE

Development of the atherosclerotic plaque can be divided into two distinct phases. The first phase is slow and insidious. During this period there is accretion of plaque material over a period of many years, during which there may be no symptoms (4); however, slow progression of coronary artery disease can result in symptoms when significant narrowing occurs within the coronary artery. Initial manifestations usually occur with exertion when there is an increase in myocardial oxygen demand

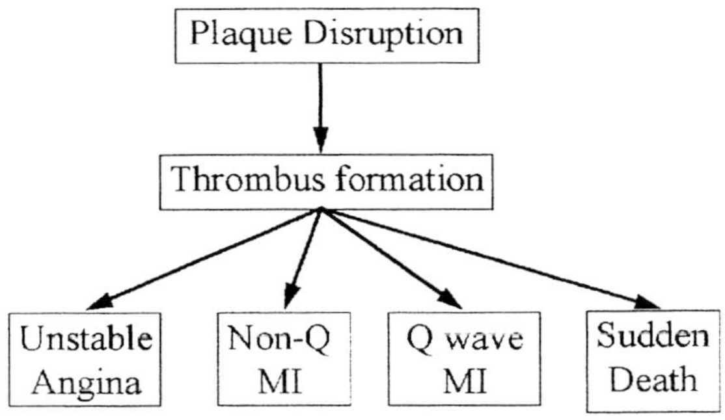

Outcome dependent on:

- amount of obstruction before and after plaque disruption
- the suddenness of the onset of obstruction
- duration of total occlusion
- ability to acutely recruit collaterals
- myocardial O_2 demands

Figure 4–1.

and an imbalance in the supply/demand ratio. The second phase of atherosclerosis involves more rapid and dramatic changes in the progression of the underlying coronary plaque. This rapid progression, which results from platelet and thrombus formation following plaque fissuring, is responsible for the development of an acute coronary syndrome or over time may be incorporated into the plaque as a fibroatheroma (5). The process of plaque disruption and thrombus formation results in a "complex plaque"—the common pathologic substrate for these syndromes.

Phase I

As our objective in this chapter is not to discuss the factors leading to the very early development of atherosclerosis, we begin this part with only a brief discussion of the early lesions of atherosclerosis. The earliest lesion of atherosclerosis is referred to as the fatty streak. Grossly, the fatty streak appears as an area of yellowish discoloration. This yellow discoloration is due to the presence of lipid, usually in the form of cholesterol and cholesterol ether. The lipid is located within foam cells, which are derived from monocytes/macrophages or smooth muscle cells. Fatty streaks are commonly found in children and young adults in both the aorta and the coronary arteries. They generally are found at points of turbulence in the coronary arteries (especially at bifurcations). The predilection for formation of fatty streaks on the wall opposite a flow divider has been observed in the coronary tree as well as in the carotid and brachiocephic bifurcations (6–8). It is at these locations that the coronary arteries are subjected to various hydrodynamic stresses because of the flow of blood. Collectively, the hydrodynamic forces constitute the rheology of the blood, which is determined by various factors including wall shear stress and pulsatile blood flow. Wall shear stress is a frictional force acting on the surface of the vessel and depends on blood flow velocity, viscosity, and vessel lumen size (9). Some fatty streaks progress into the more advanced lesions of atherosclerosis called fibroatheromas (10). In patients with risk factors for coronary artery disease, that is, smoking, increased cholesterol, positive family history, and hypertension, progression to the more advanced lesions of atherosclerosis may be accelerated (11). Microscopically, the fibroatheroma contains the characteristic lesion of atherosclerosis, which is intimal smooth muscle cell proliferation (12). Activated smooth muscle cells within the plaque are capable of ingesting cholesterol and also assuming the histologic characteristics of foam cells. Various amounts of intracellular and extracellular cholesterol, mostly in the form of cholesterol and cholesterol ester, are found within these lesions. These activated smooth muscle cells are surrounded by collagen, elastic fibers, and proteoglycan. Fibroatheromas are characteristically covered by a fibrous cap composed of smooth muscle cells and connective tissue.

Phase II

The rapid progression of an atherosclerotic plaque represents the second phase of atherosclerosis (see also Ch. 20). Formerly, rapid progression of an atherosclerotic lesion was felt to be related to the process of plaque hemorrhage (13). Vasa vasorum are more developed in advanced atherosclerotic plaques (14). Damage to the vasa vasorum with intraplaque hemorrhage was felt to be the primary pathogenic mechanism leading to thrombus formation. More recent data indicate that hemorrhage into a plaque is an uncommon cause of intraluminal thrombus formation. In at least 75% of cases of intracoronary thrombus, careful pathologic analyses reveal the presence of a disruption of the fibrous cap to the atherosclerotic plaque (15) (vida infra). After disruption, the atheromatous gruel beneath the fibrous cap is exposed to the flow of blood. Exposed collagen fibers formerly within the plaque serve as a strong stimulus for the attachment and aggregation of platelets, especially when deep portions of the vessel wall are exposed (16). There may be an acute increase in shear forces, which can also magnify the extent of platelet accumulation (17). As platelets adhere to the undersurface of the exposed plaque and become activated, three pathways for platelet aggregation can be stimulated: adenosine diphosphate, thromboxane, and thrombin/collagen (18). Activation of the coagulation pathway generates the formation of thrombin. With activation of the coagulation system, red cells and fibrin attach to the mass of platelets. Characteristically, in arterial thrombi the head of the thrombus is rich in platelets, while the tail of the thrombus contains red cells and fibrin (19). Tissue factor may be exposed with plaque disruption and lead to thrombus formation by directly activating the intrinsic and extrinsic coagulation pathways.

Although the formation of a thrombus after plaque disruption may acutely occlude the lumen, initially there may be a change in plaque geometry related to disruption itself or to the presence of intraluminal thrombus. The net effect is an increase in the bulk of the plaque. Humoral factors released during platelet activation may also potentiate thrombus formation. Vasospasm occurring at the site of a ruptured plaque can reduce or even halt the flow of blood to the coronary artery (20). Stasis of blood promotes further thrombus formation. The process of plaque disruption and thrombus formation does not necessarily lead to the development of an acute coronary syndrome but may be a mechanism for subclinical plaque progression. In a recent study 26% of plaques in a group of stable patients without previous evidence of acute coronary syndromes were found to have complex plaque characteristics (21).

MECHANISMS OF PLAQUE DISRUPTION

It has been suggested that plaque disruption represents a random event in the coronary arteries (22). All plaques, however, do not have the same propensity for disruption. Pathologic analyses indicate that lipid content contributes to the propensity of a plaque to undergo disruption (23) (Fig. 4–2). Typically, there is a lipid core underlying a fibrous cap. Disruption with thrombus formation usually occurs at a point where the cap has been thinned. Plaques with a lipid volume of greater than 40% may have the greatest likelihood of undergoing disruption (24). In a study examining atherectomy specimens, lipid-rich plaques were also more commonly associated with rest angina and post–myocardial infarction culprit lesions than in stable lesions that were usually fibrous (25). As lipid volume contributes to instability, removal of lipid may promote plaque stability (26). This has been suggested by the results of several lipid lowering trials that showed a discrepancy between the small amount of angiographic plaque regression and the larger reduction in clinical events with therapy (27, 28). Loree et al suggest a possible mechanism. The form in which

Mechanism of Plaque Disruption

I. "Vulnerable" Plaque
- lipid-rich
- thinned fibrous cap
- inflammation
- mild to moderate stenosis

II. Plaque "Triggers"
- External
  - circumferential wall stress
  - abnormal rheology
- Internal
  - localization of stress related to structural configuration
  - Inflammation

Figure 4–2. Mechanism of Plaque Disruption

the lipid exists within the lipid pool may play a role in its propensity to disrupt (29). The ratio of liquid cholesterol to cholesterol crystals within the plaque contributes to the stiffness of the lipid pool. Increasing stiffness by decreasing this ratio theoretically decreases plaque rupture, while increasing this ratio increases the chances of plaque rupture. Efforts to lower serum cholesterol may act to decrease this ratio by selective removal of the cholesterol in the liquid form, thus stiffening the lipid pool and decreasing clinical events.

The site of plaque disruption appears, by computer analysis, to be found at the point of maximal wall shear stress in the majority of cases (30). Stress on the plaque is related to several factors. The reduction in the vessel lumen by the plaque results in increased flow velocity, which is associated with high wall shear stress. Other hydrodynamic factors such as pulsatile blood flow and the bending and twisting motions of the coronary arteries may also contribute to the likelihood of a plaque to disrupt. Wide inflow and outflow angles promoting flow separation may also contribute to disruption. In mild to moderate lesions, circumferential tension or wall stress is greater than in more severe lesions where the radius is smaller [wall stress = (pressure × radius) / cap thickness]. In the presence of a sudden increase in intracavitary pressure, particularly when the cap is thin, a "vulnerable" plaque may disrupt (31). The structural configuration of the plaque also localizes the stress. As the lipid pool has little tensile strength, stress is displaced to the fibrous cap and particularly to the lateral edge, where there is less cap support (23, 32).

Although increased lipid pools under a thinned out fibrous cap at sites of increased wall stress are prone to plaque disruption, pathologic studies in patients dying following acute myocardial infarction also indicate the importance of an inflammatory process underlying the plaque's propensity to disrupt (33, 34). Disrupted plaques contain localized accumulations of macrophages and activated T-lymphocytes at the site of disruption. Recent information has shown that the activated T-cells may trigger the macrophages to produce metalloproteinases, which may degrade the fibrous cap. T-cells also produce gamma interferon, which interferes with collagen synthesis and may further weaken the cap (34). The presence of an inflammatory reaction in patients with unstable angina has been noted by the presence of increased levels of cell surface glycoproteins (CD11/CD18 receptors) on granulocytes and monocytes obtained from the coronary sinuses of these patients (35). These receptors become up-regulated in response to chemotactic factors associated with inflammatory reactions, and thus suggesting an associated inflammatory state perhaps within the coronary tree or in the microcirculation in patients with unstable angina (36). In another study, monocyte and neutrophil activation in unstable angina was found to be due to interactions between platelets and leukocytes (37).

Once a plaque has become disrupted, the amount of thrombus material that forms is due to a complex interaction related to the extent of vessel wall injury, tissue factor and other thrombogenic substances within the plaque, the hypercoagulability of blood, and hemodynamic factors such as vasospasm (38,32). Deep injury to a plaque with exposure of the media (myocardial infarction) results in more extensive thrombus formation than superficial plaque injury (unstable angina). Lipid-rich plaque is more thrombogenic than other plaque components when evaluated experimentally (39).

Before considering further the evidence for plaque disruption with thrombus formation as the underlying anatomic–pathophysiologic link among the acute coronary syndromes, it must be understood that particularly in the case of unstable angina, this pathophysiology probably explains a majority but not all patients presenting with this clinical diagnosis. It is clear from the multiple definitions of unstable angina that it represents a heterogeneous clinical syndrome with the potential for several different pathogenic substrates. The classification of Braunwald is helpful in understanding the heterogeneity in definition and probably pathogenesis (40). Not all patients classified as unstable angina have an underlying plaque disruption and thrombus. In a study of patients with unstable angina involving analysis of atherectomy specimens from patients without angiographic evidence of intraluminal thrombus, Flugelman et al found that an abundance of smooth muscle cells was associated with plaque material obtained from culprit lesions in unstable angina patients (41). Thrombus and plaque rupture occurred in only one-third of these patients. They proposed that smooth muscle cell proliferation may be an alternative mechanism for development of unstable angina in some patients. In other patients with a clinical diagnosis of unstable angina, increased oxygen demands or secondary causes such as congestive heart failure or anemia are occasionally responsible. Other clinical studies of unstable angina indicate normal or nonobstructive coronary artery disease in 10% to 15% of cases.

ANATOMIC–PATHOPHYSIOLOGIC LINKS BETWEEN THE ACUTE CORONARY SYNDROMES

The particular clinical syndrome developing after plaque disruption depends on a number of interacting factors, including the amount of obstruction before and after plaque disruption; the suddenness of the onset of the obstruction; the duration of total coronary occlusion; and the ability to acutely recruit collaterals quickly (2). In discussing the different syndromes it is also important to distinguish, when possible, the pathogenesis of the particular syndrome from the mechanisms responsible for ischemia, infarction, and sudden death. One way to simplify some of these mechanisms is to consider ischemia in terms of the supply/demand ratio. Additionally, it cannot be overemphasized that these syndromes should be considered as a continuous spectrum of disease differing quantitatively in the amount of ischemia/necrosis resulting from plaque disruption. In sudden ischemic death these same pathologic changes may result in a fatal arrhythmia. In the next section we present a working hypothesis to explain the pathophysiology of these different syndromes.

Q WAVE MYOCARDIAL INFARCTION

Clinically, myocardial infarction can be divided into Q wave and non-Q wave infarction. Although this distinction is not the same as that between transmural and nontransmural myocardial infarction, it is nevertheless useful. Clinically, patients with non-Q wave infarction usually have less myocardial necrosis that patients with Q wave infarction, and their in-hospital prognosis is significantly better (42). Q wave infarction usually results from a sudden total occlusion of a coronary artery that cannot immediately recruit sufficient collaterals to the distal coronary bed to limit the extent of necrosis. There is a sudden and profound cessation of myocardial blood flow without a measurable increase in myocardial oxygen demand. In approximately 15% to 30% of cases, coronary arteriography within 6 hours of infarction shows not total occlusion but a severe obstruction, often with diminished distal coronary flow (43). In these cases intermittent total occlusion is the most likely explanation for the development of infarction.

In patients with acute transmural infarction, intracoronary thrombus can be found in nearly all cases on careful pathologic examination (5,19,44, 45). Earlier studies indicating that thrombus was the effect rather than the cause of infarction have been refuted (46,47). Serial histologic analysis usually indicated rupture or fissuring of atherosclerotic plaques at the site of thrombus formation (48).

Patients with Q wave myocardial infarction lie on one end of the spectrum of acute coronary syndromes, with unstable angina at the other end. The substrate of a disrupted atherosclerotic plaque is seen in 75% of cases, and superficial intimal injury in the remaining 25% (49). The extent of lysable thrombus in Q wave myocardial infarction is greater than in unstable angina (50). This is apparent from the results of clinical trials of thrombolytic therapy, which show clinical benefit with therapy only in acute myocardial infarction (51,52). Despite the proposed similarity of pathologic substrate in acute myocardial infarction and in unstable angina, the clinical presentations are obviously different, which may in part be due to differences in the amount and type of thrombus present at the site of the disrupted plaque, leading to total occlusion in acute myocardial infarction and a severe but non-occlusive lesion in unstable angina (38). Thrombus at sites of arterial vessel injury is platelet rich, whereas thrombus found extending distal to the site of plaque disruption is red cell and fibrin rich. This results in a different appearance to the thrombus, which has been noted angioscopically by Mizuno et al (53). Thrombus seen in the coronary arteries in patients with unstable angina was pale, whitish-gray in 71%, whereas thrombus seen in the coronary arteries of patients with myocardial infarction was red or mixed white and red. This gross descriptive difference is similar to pathologic descriptions of platelet thrombus (grayish-white) and fibrin thrombus (red or mixed white and red) (54,55).

In addition to vessel wall injury, alterations in coagulation and blood flow contribute to the high incidence of total obstruction of coronary flow secondary to thrombus in acute myocardial infarction. Certain risk factors such as elevated fibrinogen and Factor VII levels (56,57) correlate with the risk of acute myocardial infarction. Cigarette smoking, which can increase fibrinogen levels and increase platelet aggregation, is also known to be a risk factor for myocardial infarction (58). The demonstration that aspirin can reduce the incidence of myocardial infarction further suggests the importance of platelet aggregation as a risk factor for myocardial infarction (59). The diurnal variation in the onset of myocardial infarction, which is increased in the morning hours and may be associated with an increase in platelet aggregability after assuming the upright position, is also consistent with this hypothesis (60). Transient decreases in blood flow provoked by vasoconstrictor substances or even distal embolization of thrombotic material may result in further thrombus formation. Increased vasomotion at the site of plaque disruption may contribute to the formation of a stasis (i.e., fibrin-rich) thrombus; thus only a small amount thrombus may be initially necessary for an acute myocardial infarction to occur in the presence of a dynamic stenosis (61).

Another interesting pathologic feature of acute myocardial infarction is the frequent finding of a plaque of only mild to moderate severity existing prior to the clinical event. This has been repeatedly demonstrated by angiographic studies in acute myocardial infarction (see below). In patients with sudden disruption of such a mild or moderate plaque and the formation of an occlusive thrombus, the distal coronary bed may be unable to recruit collaterals immediately. The result will be complete infarction of the territory subtended by the coronary artery or possibly even sudden ischemic death.

UNSTABLE ANGINA

As usually defined, unstable angina refers to either the new onset of low-workload or rest angina (class III or IV or angina unrelated to exertion according to the Canadian Heart Classification) or an increase in the frequency and severity of previously stable angina. When plaque disruption with thrombus formation results in unstable angina, in most cases a severe stenosis, more than 70% but less than 100% occlusive, will be found in the ischemia-related artery (62). Data from thrombolytic trials in unstable angina suggest that in the majority of patients with less than total coronary occlusion (approximately 90% of patients with unstable angina have a patent ischemia-related artery at angiography) there is little angiographic benefit with thrombolytics, probably because of the absence or paucity of lysable, fibrin thrombus (63–65). We have suggested that the amount of intraluminal fibrin-rich thrombus formation in unstable angina is an important distinction from myocardial infarction (50). There are at least four possible mechanisms for the lack of lysable thrombus in unstable angina:

1. The thrombus formation in unstable angina develops slowly after plaque disruption. Pathologic data from a selected number of patients dying after a bout of unstable angina and in whom intracoronary thrombus was present show layering of thrombotic material at the site of plaque disruption (66). Therefore, chronic, subacute, and acute thrombus formation may be present before clinical symptoms begin. Furthermore, there may be a hiatus between the clinical presentation of unstable angina and the administration of thrombolytic therapy. By the time a thrombolytic agent is administered, much of the thrombus could already be organized.

2. After plaque disruption the initial thrombus formation may be located underneath the fibrous cap. The initial event may therefore be a change in geometry of a plaque with little intracoronary thrombus actually exposed and therefore amenable to thrombolysis.
3. As demonstrated experimentally, a superficial plaque fissure or ulcer rather than a disruption into the media may be responsible for transient thrombus formation (67). This could be the pathogenic mechanism in some patients with unstable angina. As the thrombus is only transient, at any given moment there is little acute thrombus.
4. As already discussed, the composition of the thrombus in unstable angina is predominately platelet rich or a white thrombus, in contrast to the predominantly fibrin-rich or red thrombus found in acute Q wave myocardial infarction. Therefore, the thrombus tail is missing. As mentioned earlier, the amount of thrombus forming is related to an interaction of several variables. In unstable angina, the stimulus for thrombus formation is less intense than in acute myocardial infarction, and thrombolytic therapy is not beneficial for these platelet-rich thrombi.

The mechanisms of ischemia in unstable angina are undoubtedly related to the presence of the pathogenic substrate–plaque disruption with thrombus. These ischemic mechanisms are related to either decreased supply, increased demand, or a combination of the two. Transient decreases in supply may be related to several factors. Transient episodes of platelet aggregation and/or thrombus formation may be followed by endogenous lysis and/or embolization (3). An imbalance between vasoconstrictor substances released from activated platelets and vasodilator substances from the endothelium (68) can also lead to ischemia. An inflammatory reaction that has been identified in unstable angina (35, 69) could also play a role in causing ischemia either through elaboration of a tissue factor like procoagulant, through other inflammatory mediators that can lead to neutrophil–platelet interactions (70,71) or directly. Elevations of C-reactive protein have been shown to predict a poor outcome in patients with unstable angina (72). Patients with elevated levels were found to have more recurrent ischemic episodes than those patients with low levels of this acute-phase reactant. Thus inflammation could have pathogenic, ischemic, and prognostic importance in unstable angina. Finally, the myocardial oxygen demands can also play a role in ischemia in unstable angina. Once a new lesion develops in the coronary arteries, even small changes in myocardial demand may precipitate ischemia as a result of the change in the supply/demand ratio (73).

NON-Q WAVE MYOCARDIAL INFARCTION

Non-Q wave infarction is defined as the presence of myocardial necrosis without the presence of Q waves on a 12-lead electrocardiogram. Pathologically, this does not necessarily imply that the infarction was nontransmural (see Ch. 18). When compared with Q wave infarction, however, the amount of myocardial necrosis is usually less with non-Q wave infarction (42). Pathogenetically, this syndrome falls between unstable angina and Q wave infarction. The ischemic episode is more prolonged than that in Q wave infarction. In subendocardial necrosis (not to be confused with non-Q wave myocardial infarction—a clinical diagnosis) the incidence of occlusive thrombi at autopsy is infrequent, occurring in as few as 13% of cases (44). In these hearts extensive coronary atherosclerosis usually is present, suggesting decreased perfusion as the pathogenic mechanism in some cases; however, small thrombi or fissures could be missed if pathologic analysis were performed late after infarction. Although there have been no large pathologic analyses in patients with non-Q wave myocardial infarction, angiographic studies suggest an incidence of plaque disruption and thrombus formation similar to that found in unstable angina. Non-Q wave infarction probably develops under one of three conditions: (i) There may be a new and persistent total occlusion of an infarct-related artery with some recruitable collaterals. (ii) There may be a transient total occlusion with spontaneous reopening of the infarct-related artery so that necrosis is limited. (iii) In some patients with diffuse disease with or without collaterals, an episode of transient hypotension or relative hypoperfusion in relation to myocardial oxygen demands could result in subendocardial necrosis, regionally or globally. As most infarct-related arteries are patent after non-Q wave infarction (60–80% patency rate), spontaneous reperfusion with a shorter duration of total coronary occlusion differentiates this syndrome from that of Q wave myocardial infarction in the majority of patients.

SUDDEN ISCHEMIC DEATH

Sudden death related to ischemic heart disease occurs in at least two subgroups of patients. In the first group there is resting left ventricular dysfunction with scarring and an arrhythmic substrate. This arrhythmic substrate provides the proper conditions for the development of malignant ventricular arrhythmias. In the second group, there is an acute coronary lesion with intracoronary thrombus formation. In pathologic studies, undoubtedly there is overlap between this latter group of patients and patients dying after acute myocardial infarction. Furthermore, at least one-third of patients who survive an episode of sudden death are found to have had acute myocardial infarction (74). In sudden ischemic death, the incidence of intracoronary thrombi is variable. Some studies found it infrequently (75,76). Davies and Thomas found an acute evolving arterial lesion in 95% of cases and a recent intraluminal thrombus in 74% (15). As many patients with sudden death have a scarred left ventricle with an arrhythmic substrate, acute coronary lesions are not a necessary prerequisite. In a subsequent publication, Davies et al studied an additional 168 cases of ischemic sudden death (77). Patients with single-vessel disease, acute myocardial infarction, or a recent history suggestive of clinical ischemia were more likely to have coronary thrombosis than patients with a scarred left ventricle, old myocardial infarction and three-vessel disease.

How acute thrombus formation leads to a terminal arrhythmia is unclear, but it may be related to a sudden and total cessation in blood flow and/or embolization of platelet and/or thrombotic material to the distal coronary bed (66).

ANGIOGRAPHIC CORRELATIONS AND PATHOGENESIS OF THE ACUTE CORONARY SYNDROMES

There are abundant angiographic data correlating pathoanatomy of the coronary arteries with the hypothesis described above. Angiographic analysis of a number of variables on coronary arteriography, including the morphology of plaques, the presence of intracoronary filling defects indicating thrombus, and the angiographic as well as the clinical response to thrombolytic agents, has added significantly to our knowledge and understanding of these syndromes.

Angiographic Correlations in Q Wave Myocardial Infarction

DeWood et al demonstrated the presence of intracoronary thrombus in the early hours after acute myocardial infarction (78). Eighty-four percent of patients had total coronary occlusion of the infarct-related artery within 6 hours of the onset of infarction. This percentage decreased to 63% when angiography was performed 12 to 24 hours after therapy. Thrombus formation in acute myocardial infarction has also been amply demonstrated by the uniform success in lysing occlusive thrombi in patients presenting within hours of infarction (79–83). A variety of thrombolytic agents have been employed including streptokinase, recombinant tissue plasminogen activator (t-PA), urokinase, and anisoylated plasminogen streptokinase activator complex (APSAC). Reperfusion or patency rates of about 60% to 80% have been reported in studies in which these agents were either given intravenously or directly into the coronary artery (see Chs. 19, 20, and 22). Lower recanalization rates have been demonstrated for some of these agents, especially those with fibrin nonselectivity. Recanalization rates also diminish as time increases from the onset of symptoms (84). Older thrombi may be more resistant to the usual doses of thrombolytic therapy.

Although total occlusion of the infarct-related artery is usually found when angiography is performed within hours of infarction, 15% to 30% of patients will have less than total occlusion, often with diminished antegrade flow.

Coronary Morphology

In patients in whom successful thrombolysis has been carried out and in patients with acute or recent myocardial infarction and a patent infarct-related artery, the morphology of coronary stenoses reveals eccentric and irregular plaques in the majority of cases (85). Sixty-six percent of patients with patent infarct-related arteries after Q wave myocardial infarction were found to have these lesions, which are similar to those found in unstable angina (type II eccentric or complex lesions). Wilson et al studied patent arteries after recent myocardial infarction and noted an irregularity in the lesion that suggested an ulceration or plaque rupture had played a role (86). An "ulceration index" was defined that incorporated this irregularity. Lesions responsible for myocardial infarction were found to have a significantly different ulceration index compared with those for patients with stable angina. Utilizing videodensitometric techniques, Brown et al found a distinct translucency superimposed on a less translucent plaque in patient infarct-related arteries after successful thrombolysis (87). The authors felt that this translucency on angiography represented nonlysed thrombus superimposed on an atherosclerotic plaque (Fig. 4–3).

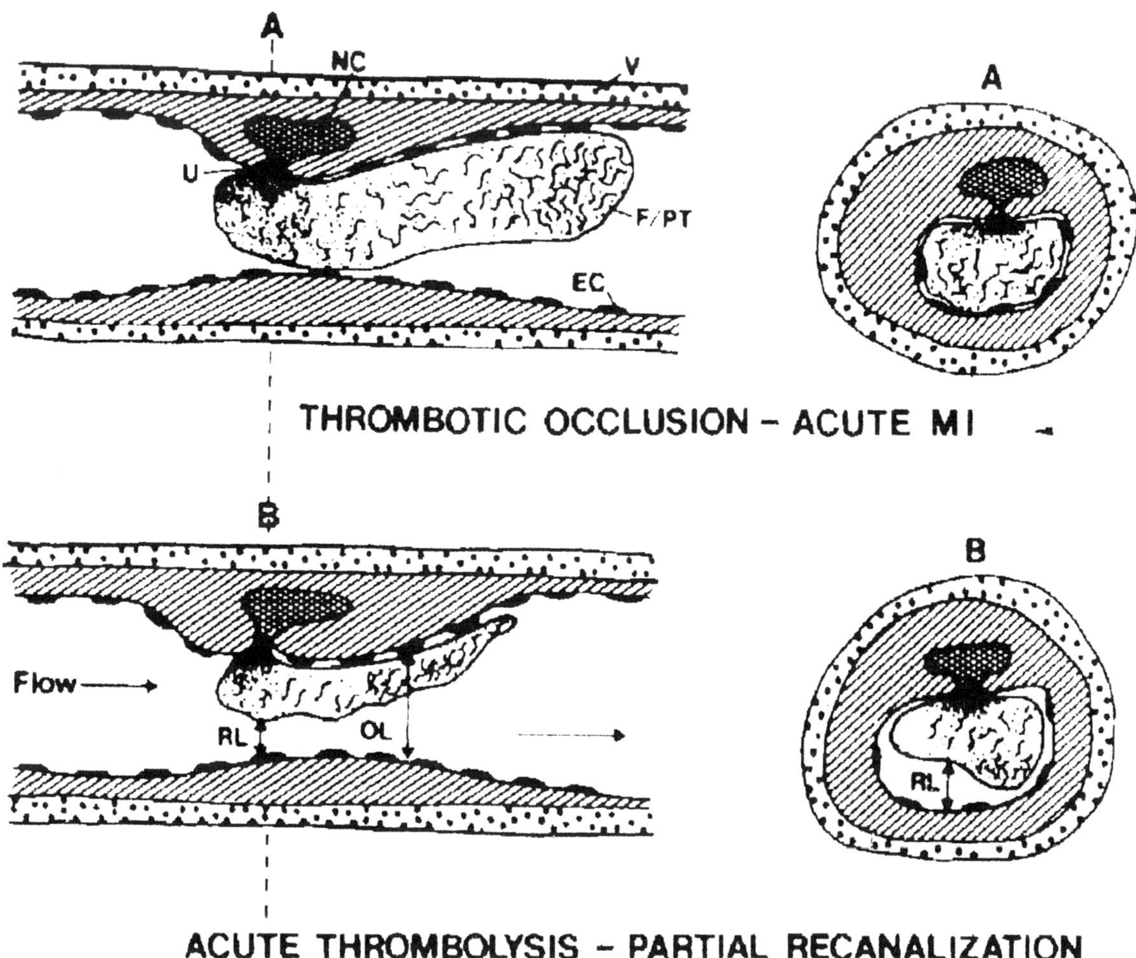

Figure 4–3.

The irregular morphology seen following lytic therapy is also subject to remodeling over a short period of time. In a study comparing coronary lesion morphology in 72 patients with acute myocardial infarction on day 1 to day 8 following intravenous streptokinase, Davies et al found irregular and eccentric lesions as well as globular and linear filling defects on day 1 (88). Using Wilson's ulceration index, patients restudied on day 8 had a reduction in the ulceration index and had fewer number of globular filling defects if maintained on heparin. In the APRICOT (Antithrombotics in the Prevention of Reocclusion in Coronary Thrombolysis) study, the infarct-related stenoses were noted to show dynamic changes in the 3 months following infarction, with nearly half of the complex lesions becoming smooth, and also an increase in the minimal lumen diameter (89). Wilson's ulceration index has also been found to be a critical determinant of clinical instability (90). Those patients with a higher ulceration index required urgent medical intervention including angioplasty or bypass surgery in the days following thrombolysis, whereas those patients with a low index stabilized on medical therapy. Thrombus and complex lesions seen angiographically have also been corroborated by angioscopic data (53,91).

Angiographic Progression of Coronary Disease and Myocardial Infarction

There have been a number of interesting observations concerning the severity of the atherosclerotic plaque responsible for myocardial infarction. Of the 32 patients studied by Brown et al, after successful thrombolysis, in 32% the underlying stenosis was felt to be less than 50% and in 66% the underlying stenosis was less than 60% (87). Selected patients in whom angiography was performed before and after infarction as well as studies analyzing the size of the atherosclerotic lesion after successful thrombolysis indicate that mild or moderate lesions are often the site of subsequent myocardial infarction. Ambrose et al found that 48% of myocardial infarctions evolve from lesions less than 50% on initial angiography (92); Little et al found less than 50% lesions in 66% of patients prior to infarction (93). In another study, Giroud et al found that the most severe stenosis was a poor predictor of intervening acute myocardial infarction. Although 50% of patients had stenoses >50% severity on initial angiography (excluding total occlusion), the lesion responsible for the intervening myocardial infarction was <50% in 78% of cases (94). In a similar study evaluating disease progression with or without infarction, Nobuyoshi et al found new myocardial infarction in 23 of 39 patients with coronary segments <50% narrowed on initial angiography (95). (Table 4–1).

These results differ from patients who were restudied and found to have a new total coronary occlusion but without an intervening infarction. In this latter group of patients a severe lesion (>70%) is usually present at the site of subsequent new total occlusion (92) (Fig. 4–4). A prospective 5-year angiographic study at the Mayo Clinic yielded similar conclusions. The majority of subsequent infarct-related lesions were not hemodynamically significant at the time of the initial study. In contrast, total occlusions tended to involve more severely narrowed vessels but often did *not* result in clinical infarctions (96).

Angiographic studies after successful thrombolysis often show moderate coronary stenoses in the infarct-related artery. In both the Thrombolysis In Myocardial Infarction (TIMI) and the Thrombolysis After Myocardial Infarction (TAMI) trials, approximately 10% to 15% of patients were found to have less than 50% narrowing within 48 hours of successful thrombolysis (97,98) (see Ch. 22). Hackett et al, utilizing quantitative techniques immediately after thrombolysis, found that nearly 60% of patients had lesions between 50% and 75% occlusive (99). As pathologically it may be difficult to quantify the degree of underlying stenosis after

Table 4–1. Angiographic Evolution to Myocardial Infarction

Study	n	Initial angiographic stenosis ≤50%	51–70%	>70%
Ambrose et al (92)	23	48	30	22
Little et al (93)	29	66	31	3
Nobuyoshi et al (95)	39	58	15	26
Giroud et al (94)	92	78	9	13
Hackett et al (99)	10	90	10	0

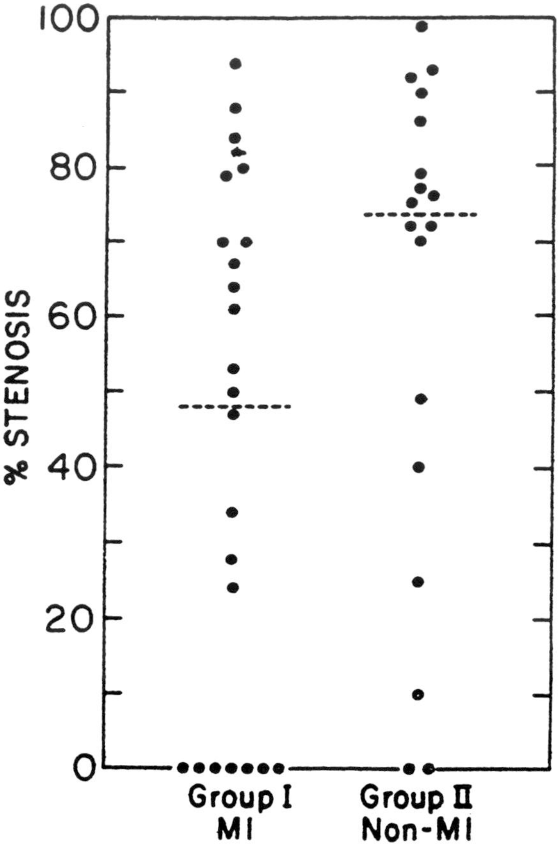

Figure 4–4.

plaque disruption, this latter angiographic analysis may overestimate the severity of the underlying plaque before infarction (48). Furthermore, in some cases residual thrombus may be present, which may also overestimate the size of the underlying plaque (67). This is suggested by the results of the APRICOT study, which would suggest that ongoing dissolution of thrombus may occur in the months following initial thrombolysis, in the presence of antithrombotic therapy (89).

From analysis of these angiographic data, it is impossible to know how frequently mild to moderate lesions are the site of subsequent infarction because of patient selection. Furthermore, not all the angiographic data support the notion that myocardial infarction develops from less than severe lesions. Moise et al found new coronary occlusions in 31% of 313 patients restudied after medical therapy for coronary artery disease (100). In their analysis a new occlusion was strongly associated with an interim infarction. The best predictor of infarction was the presence, on initial study, of at least an 80% narrowing of an artery supplying a nonakinetic left ventricular segment. In 54% of arteries, however, the site of occlusion was either distal to or in a different segment of the same artery remote from the 80% narrowing. Analysis of patients in the CASS Registry with left anterior descending coronary artery lesions found that the quantitative severity of coronary lesions was the most important factor directly related to subsequent anterior infarction (101). Unfortunately, repeat angiography was not performed, and the culprit lesion responsible for infarction could not be accurately determined. Additionally, in nearly half of the patients the myocardial infarction was non-Q wave. Finally, in patients with coronary artery disease and coronary insufficiency, Neill et al found new total occlusion in 9 of 30 severely stenotic lesions (80% to 95% narrowing) on follow-up angiography 4 months after the acute event (102). Five of thirty-four patients had an interim infarction in the distribution of the new occlusion; however, six additional patients with progression of coronary disease from a severe narrowing to total occlusion did not develop Q wave infarction after occlusion. In these patients it is likely that collaterals prevented or limited the size of the infarction. While we cannot be sure how frequently mild lesions precede an acute infarction, it is likely that a majority of cases of large infarcts are preceded by lesions that cannot acutely recruit collaterals after sudden and total coronary occlusion. Thus angiographic studies suggest these have less than 70% diameter reduction prior to infarction.

Angiographic Correlations in Unstable Angina

Early studies on the extent of coronary artery disease in patients with either unstable or stable angina found no significant differences in both the number of diseased vessels and in percentage stenosis (103,104). Other investigators have noted some interesting angiographic findings, however. In one study of unstable angina with crescendo angina and both rest and exertional pain, the incidence of left main narrowing was quite high (25%) (105).

Studies in unstable angina have indicated a variable number of patients with single-, double-, and triple-vessel disease. Single-vessel disease can be found in 12% to 52% of patients (106,107). These differences likely reflect patient selection. For example, younger patients with unstable angina are likely to have single- or double-vessel disease; three-vessel disease is more common in elderly patients.

Coronary Morphology

Because quantitative variables could not differentiate unstable angina from stable angina, the first systematic evaluation of coronary morphology on angiography was done in unstable angina (108). With respect to angiographic variables, morphology refers specifically to the symmetry and irregularity of a coronary stenosis seen in orthogonal views. With careful attention to these morphologic features, Ambrose et al evaluated the coronary morphology of obstructive coronary stenoses in 110 patients with either stable or unstable angina (Fig. 4–5). In patients with unstable angina, an asymmetric or eccentric narrowing with a narrow neck and/or irregular borders was observed in 54% of lesions compared with only 7% of lesions in patients with stable angina. When the stenosis responsible for the acute syndrome could be identified on the basis of clinical or ventriculographic criteria, this specific morphology was observed in 71% of ischemia-producing lesions. This lesion was called a type II eccentric lesion (complex lesion) to distinguish it from the smooth eccentric (type I) or concentric lesion commonly seen

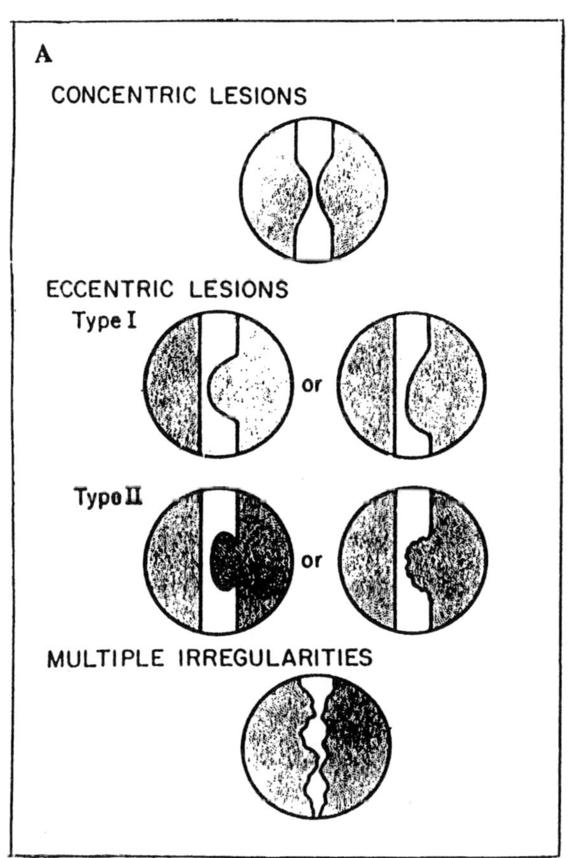

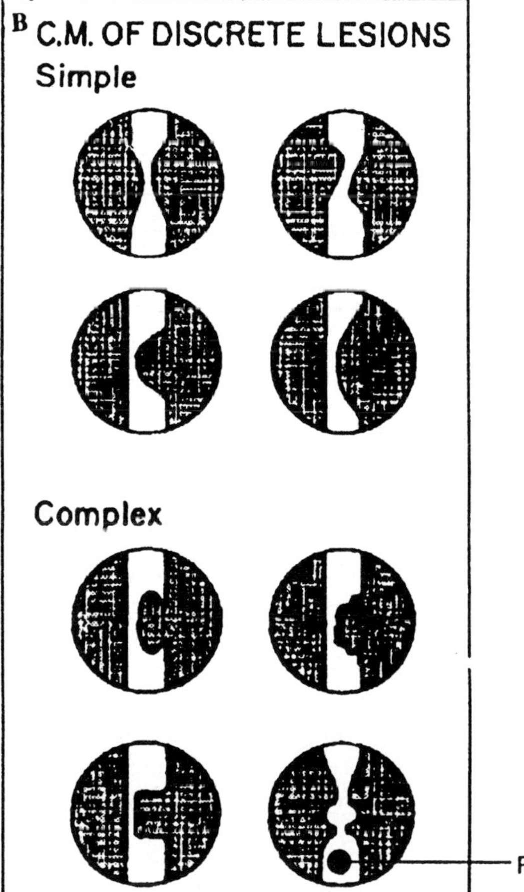

Figure 4–5.

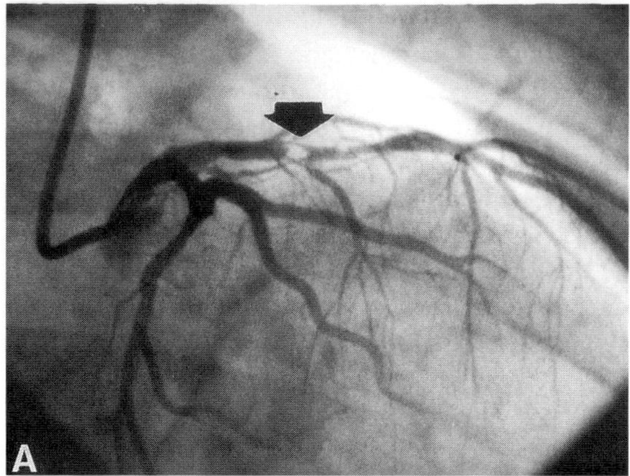

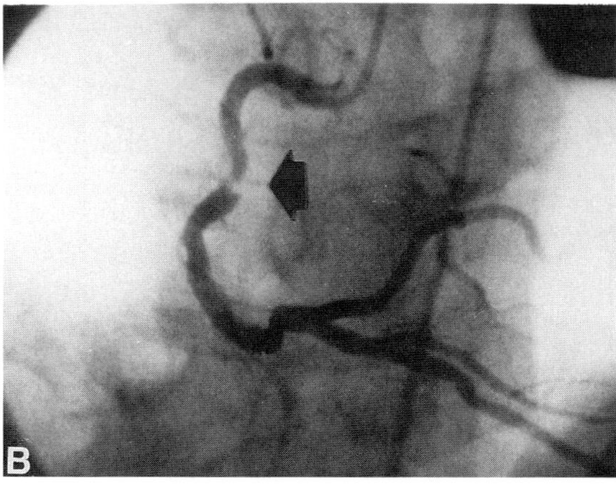

Figure 4–6.

in patients with stable angina (Fig. 4–6). These findings have been corroborated by other investigators, although these lesions were called "T" lesions, complex plaques, or intracoronary thrombi (109,110). The irregular borders and overhanging edges noted on angiography may be the angiographic equivalent of intracoronary thrombus or a disrupted plaque by pathologic examination. Results of postmortem angiography in patients dying after myocardial infarction or after bypass surgery were reported by Levin and Fallon (111). Complex lesions that were eccentric and had irregular borders demonstrated plaque disruption with occlusive or mural thrombi on pathologic examination in approximately 80% of cases.

At about the same time that the angiographic observations of coronary morphology in unstable angina were being made, a number of other studies reported the incidence of intraluminal thrombus at angiography in unstable angina (112–115). Angiographically, thrombus was defined as a radiolucent area of filling defect at or distal to a coronary stenosis. The reported prevalence of this angiographic finding varied between 1% and 52%. The variation and occurrence of intracoronary thrombi may be the result of several clinical features, including the duration of unstable angina and the timing of angiography after the last episode of rest pain. The more acute the clinical syndrome, the more likely thrombus will be found on angiography. Patients with a long history of severe disabling angina who are admitted to the hospital with a slight increase in symptoms and a diagnosis of unstable angina would be less likely to have an intracoronary thrombus than a patient with the new onset of angina occurring at rest.

Probably the most important factor relating to the incidence of intracoronary thrombus in unstable angina has been the angiographic definition of thrombus. There has been no standardized definition for the presence of intracoronary thrombus, especially when the ischemia-related artery was less than 100% occluded. Patent ischemia-related arteries are found in approximately 90% of patients at angiography after an episode of rest pain (116,117). As a consequence, there is marked overlap between the definition of a complex lesion and the definition of an intracoronary thrombus. The thrombus present in unstable angina may consist of a mural, laminar component at the site of disruption of the plaque and may or may not have a fibrin-rich tail that appears as a filling defect proximal or distal to the lesion. A useful definition of intracoronary thrombus that we have used in our studies has been the presence of a radiolucent filling defect visualized in multiple projections and located either proximal or distal to a significant stenosis. The filling defect should be surrounded by contrast on at least three sides (Fig. 4–7). Although the distinction between a complex lesion and an intracoronary thrombus may be semantic, as both contain thrombus, it has been our experience that proximal or dis-

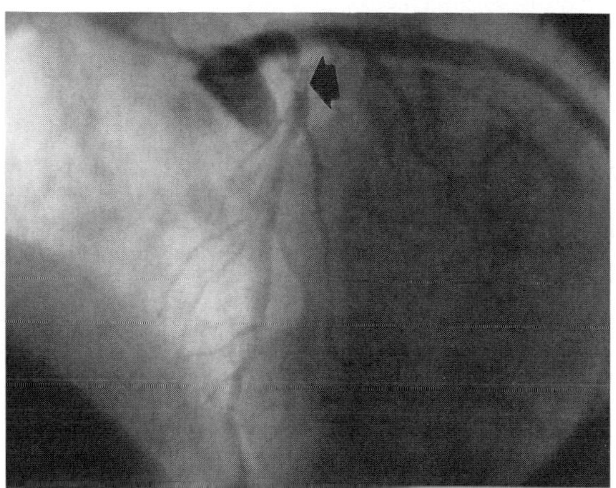

Figure 4–7.

tal filling defects increase the incidence of sudden closure at the time of angioplasty. The presence of a complex lesion is also associated with a somewhat higher sudden closure rate than noncomplex lesions (118). Finally, these proximal or distal filling defects are seen more commonly after myocardial infarction than with unstable angina (2,119).

Angiographic Response to Thrombolytic Therapy in Unstable Angina

Thrombolytic therapy has been proven to be effective in acute myocardial infarction; however, there does not appear to be a role for thrombolytic therapy in unstable angina. Several small studies have been published with variable angiographic as well as clinical results (63 65, 115, 120–122). In some patients clinical improvement occurred after thrombolysis (120); however, this often was unrelated to the angiographic change in percentage stenosis (121). Studies such as the UNASEM trial, which randomized to intravenous anistreplase (APSAC) or placebo, reported a significant angiographic improvement with thrombolysis only if initially totally occluded arteries were included in the analysis (123). Similar angiographic improvement has been seen in other studies as well, when the pretreatment angiogram showed totally or subtotally occluded arteries (65,122). Other studies utilizing quantitative techniques before and after thrombolysis showed no angiographic improvement. Ambrose et al (63) and Topol et al (64) found no significant differences in percentage stenosis after thrombolysis.

The Thrombolysis in Myocardial Infarction (TIMI-III) trial has perhaps settled the controversy on the use of thrombolytic therapy for most patients with unstable angina or non-Q wave myocardial infarction. In the TIMI-IIIA study, 306 patients were randomized to receive intravenous t-PA or placebo and were studied angiographically before and after therapy (124). A substantial improvement in the culprit stenosis was seen in 15% of t-PA treated patients and in 5% of the patients receiving placebo. However, the clinical relevance of this observation was not observed in the larger TIMI-IIIB study, which assessed the potential benefit of t-PA compared with placebo as well as an early invasive versus conservative treatment strategy in 1,473 patients (125). In this study there was no difference between t-PA and placebo for the combined endpoint of death, myocardial infarction, or failure of initial therapy at 6 weeks. In fact, fatal and nonfatal myocardial infarction after randomization occurred more frequently in the t-PA treated patients, as well as several intracranial hemorrhages. Therefore, the investigators concluded that the addition of t-PA to the treatment regimen in unstable angina and non-Q wave myocardial infarction was of no benefit and may be harmful. Thus, although thrombolysis is accepted therapy in patients with acute myocardial infarction, the prognosis may be worse with its use in unstable angina. Waters and Lam reviewed the results of randomized, placebo-controlled trials where heparin was given in the placebo arm (126). The combination of a thrombolytic and heparin resulted in a higher rate of acute myocardial infarction than placebo and heparin.

Response to Other Modalities in Unstable Angina

Although thrombolytics have been found to be of little benefit and possibly harmful as therapy in unstable angina, the use of antithrombins and antiplatelet therapy has recently gained interest. There are presently little data that has systematically evaluated the angiographic effects of these therapies. However, Topol et al studied the use of hirudin in patients with angiographic thrombus comparing heparin alone versus four different regimens of intravenous hirudin. Angiographic follow-up showed there was more angiographic resolution of thrombus in the patients randomized to receive hirudin (127).

The clinical benefits of antithrombotic therapy and antiplatelet therapy in unstable angina are well known (128–131). There is a growing interest in other agents that affect thrombin generation because of the association of increased thrombin levels and cardiac events, the limitations of current antithrombotic medications, and the involvement of thrombin in both platelet aggregation and the clotting cascade (132). Recent experience with a new antithrombin (Hirulog) showed a reproducible prolongation of the activated partial thromboplastin time (aPTT), and a fall in fibrinopeptide A levels in patients with unstable angina (133). Similar studies with the thrombin inhibitor argatroban showed a prolongation of aPTT, and a fall in fibrinopeptide A levels while on therapy (134). However, following a 4-hour infusion of argatroban in a group of patients with unstable angina, there was a rebound of the thrombin–antithrombin III complex levels that was associated with recurrent angina.

The effects of antiplatelet therapy in unstable angina pectoris may in part be due to inhibition of thrombin generation that has been reported to be increased in patients with unstable angina (135,136). Aspirin DL-lysine was found to decrease thrombin generation as measured by a fall in thrombin–antithrombin III complex levels (137). The responsiveness of platelets to thrombin-induced platelet aggregation may be an important factor in coronary disease progression. Lam et al (138) found increased disease progression over a two year period in patients found to have platelet hyperaggregability.

Inhibition of platelet aggregation by the glycoprotein (GP) IIb/IIIa receptor antagonist (c7E3 Fab), a monoclonal antibody fragment, was found to reduce episodes of ischemia in patients with unstable angina, compared with a placebo treated group. Angiographic improvements seen with the monoclonal antibody, however, were not significant, possibly due to the small size of the patient group treated (139). Other studies with this group of agents in the acute management on unstable angina are ongoing, and the results should be available within the next year. For coronary intervention, the c7E3 Fab monoclonal antibody fragment was evaluated in the EPIC (Evaluation Prevention of Ischemic Complications) trial. There was a 35% reduction in composite endpoints (death, myocardial infarction, or urgent revascularization) with bolus and 12-hour infusions. In the subgroup of patients with unstable angina, the reduction in composite endpoints was 71% (140).

Angiographic Progression of Coronary Disease in Unstable Angina

A major angiographic feature of patients with unstable angina is the occurrence of angiographic progression of coronary disease. Moise et al demonstrated significant progression of coronary artery disease by assessing the coronary angiograms of patients with unstable angina who had previously undergone angiography and compared them with those of a group of control patients with stable angina (141). Seventy-six percent of patients with a diagnosis of new unstable angina had progression of coronary artery disease on their second angiogram, compared with 33% of control patients. In 38% of unstable patients the progression to obstructive coronary lesions occurred from previously "healthy" segments. Ambrose et al also noted angiographic progression of stenosis severity in a group of patients with unstable angina who had undergone prior angiography (142). Again, progression was found in about 75% of patients, and in 72% of these patients the "culprit" lesion was less than 50% obstructed on the initial angiogram. These data are quite similar to the findings of progression of coronary disease in myocardial infarction. In both syndromes mild to moderate plaques are frequently the site of subsequent acute syndromes. In "stabilized" patients with recent unstable angina awaiting angioplasty, Chen et al noted significant disease progression, particularly of complex plaques, over an 8-month period. Progression was frequently clinically associated with a coronary event and angiographically with development of a new total occlusion (143).

Angiographic Correlations in Non-Q Wave Myocardial Infarction

The angiographic features of patients with non-Q wave infarction fall somewhere between those of patients with unstable angina and those of patients with Q wave myocardial infarction (see Ch. 18). The number of vessels involved in patients with non-Q wave infarction is similar to that in patients with unstable angina and Q wave infarction (144). Total occlusion is seen more frequently than in unstable angina but less often than in acute Q wave myocardial infarction (116,144,145). Angiography performed within days of non-Q wave infarction indicates total coronary occlusion in 20% to 40% of patients. In patients with patent infarct-related arteries, angiographic morphology is also similar to that seen in unstable angina (116). In approximately two thirds of infarct-related arteries, a complex lesion (type II eccentric plaque) is seen. This further supports the similar mechanism underlying the pathophysiology of the acute coronary syndromes. What appears different from unstable angina is the presence of more intracoronary thrombus (filling defects) in non-Q wave myocardial infarction (119).

Serial studies in patients with non-Q wave infarction indicate a significant progression in lesion severity in the majority of patients in whom a prior angiogram was available for review. Although Little et al found that progression occurred from lesions that were often less than 50% occlusive (93), our findings in a small group of patients indicate that a severe stenosis can sometimes be present (92). Klein and colleagues compared the preinfarct angiogram to a postinfarct angiogram for a group of patients with Q wave and non-Q wave infarctions (146). Patients with non-Q wave infarction had either a severe preexisting stenosis prior to infarction, a minimal luminal narrowing (<20% stenosis), or no stenosis prior to infarction. As discussed in the preceding section, there may be two populations of patients with non-Q wave infarction. Patients who present initially with total coronary occlusion have an underlying severe stenosis. When occlusion occurs, collaterals are present to limit infarction. In the second group of patients with patent infarct-related arteries at angiography (60% to 80% of patients with non-Q wave infarction), intermittent total occlusion of a lesion that has progressed from a less than significant stenosis is found.

Angiographic Correlations in Sudden Cardiac Death

Because of the small number of survivors, there are few angiographic data to demonstrate the link to patients with sudden death. Furthermore, pathologic and clinical studies in patients with sudden death obviously deal with different subgroups. Clinical studies analyze patients who survive! In 64 out-of-hospital survivors of ischemic death, Weaver et al found at least one-vessel disease at angiography in 94% of patients and a 61% incidence of multivessel disease (147). Sixty-seven percent of patients had at least one total occlusion. More than two-thirds had some degree of left ventricular dysfunction.

The incidence of complex or acute lesions on angiography in survivors of sudden death has been reported in two small studies. Stevenson et al, using angiographic criteria similar to those of Ambrose et al, found complex lesions in 64% of survivors without inducible ventricular tachycardia compared with only 25% of patients with inducible ventricular tachycardia (148). Additionally, Lo et al found eccentric irregular or irregular lesions in 50% of survivors of sudden death without ventricular tachycardia compared with only 19% of patients with inducible ventricular tachycardia (149). Those without inducible tachycardia would be less likely to have a long-term substrate for the induction of ventricular arrhythmias. In these patients it is likely that a sudden ischemic event led to the malignant ventricular arrhythmias. Although these studies indicate a higher incidence of complex lesions in ischemic death, both studies excluded patients with acute myocardial infarction. This latter group obviously would have a high incidence of complex lesions on angiography and also on pathologic examination. The exclusion of patients with myocardial infarction is in part responsible for the low incidence of complex lesions on angiography after sudden death in comparison with more recent autopsy studies.

CONCLUSIONS

Coronary pathophysiology in the acute coronary syndromes reveals a spectrum of ischemia starting with unstable angina and continuing through non-Q wave infarction, Q wave infarction, and sudden cardiac death. All syndromes in the majority of cases share the same pathogenetic substrate of plaque disruption and thrombus formation. Differences among the syndromes are related to the suddenness and degree of the onset of the obstruction, the duration of total coronary occlusion, and the ability to acutely recruit collaterals. Angiographic analyses reveal a preponderance of complex lesions and/or intracoronary thrombi.

The clinical manifestations of ischemia and/or infarction in these syndromes are directly or indirectly related to this pathogenetic substrate. In unstable angina, ischemia is related to transient decreases in blood flow and/or transient increases in myocardial oxygen demand. These transient decreases in supply may be related to intermittent thrombus formation with spontaneous lysis or embolization and/or changes in vasomotor tone. Once a new coronary lesion has developed, small increases in myocardial oxygen demand can potentially precipitate episodes of ischemia. In new total obstructions of a coronary artery resulting from acute thrombus formation, Q wave myocardial infarction usually develops unless collaterals can be recruited immediately to limit infarct size or the vessel is opened medically or spontaneously. In a significant proportion of patients with Q wave infarction, the underlying atherosclerotic plaque is only mild to moderate prior to the clinical event. In non-Q wave infarction, the degree of ischemia/necrosis falls between that of unstable angina and that of Q wave infarction. Finally, sudden ischemic death is often precipitated by plaque disruption with thrombus formation, but there is overlap between this group and patients dying after myocardial infarction. The terminal event in sudden ischemic death is often a malignant ventricular arrhythmia. It has been postulated that a sudden cessation in blood flow and/or embolization of thrombotic material may set up the conditions that lead to the terminal arrhythmia.

REFERENCES

1. Gorlin R, Fuster V, Ambrosse JA: Anatomic–physiologic links between acute coronary syndromes. *Circulation* 1986;74:6–9.
2. Ambrose JA: Coronary angiographic findings in the acute coronary syndromes in unstable angina, in Bleifeld W, Braunwald WE, Hamm C (eds): *Unstable Angina.* Berlin/Heidelberg, Springer-Verlag, pp
3. Ambrose JA, Hjemdahl-Monsen CE: Arteriographic anatomy and mechanisms of myocardial ischemia in unstable angina. *J Am Coll Cardiol* 1987;9:1397–1402.
4. Fuster V: Pathogenesis of atherosclerosis, in Spittell JA Jr (ed): *Clinical Medicine.* Philadelphia, Harper & Row, 1981, pp 1–22.
5. Chandler AB, Chapman I, Erhardt LR, et al: Coronary thrombosis in myocardial infarction: Report of a workshop on the role of coronary thrombosis in the pathogenesis of acute myocardial infarction. *Am J Cardiol* 1974;34:823–832.
6. Fox B, James K, Morgan B, Seed A: Distribution of fatty and fibrous plaques in young human coronary arteries. *Arteriosclerosis* 1983;48:139–145.
7. Kjaernes M, Svindland A, Walloe L, Wille SO: Location of early atherosclerotic lesions in an arterial bifurcation in humans. *Acta Pathol Microbiol Immunol Second Sect A* 1981;89:35–40.
8. Zairns CK, Giddens DP, Bharadvaj BK, Sottiurai VS, Mabon RF, Glagov S: Carotid bifurcation atherosclerosis. Quantitative correlation of plaque location with flow velocity profiles and wall shear stress. *Circ Res* 1983;53:502–514.
9. Bird RB, Steward WE, Lighfoot EN: *Transport Phomena.* New York. John Wiley & Sons, 1960, p 780.
10. Stary HC: Evolution and progression of atherosclerotic lesions in coronary arteries of children and young adults. *Arteriosclerosis* 1989;9(Suppl I):119–132.
11. Fuster V, Kottke BA: Atherosclerosis. A. Pathogenesis, pathology, and presentation of atherosclerosis, in Brandenburg RO (ed): *Cardiology: Fundamentals and Practice.* Chicago, Year Book Medical Publishers 1987, pp 951–971.
12. Ross R: The pathogenesis of atherosclerosis—an update. *N Engl J Med* 1986;314:488–500.
13. Chapman I: Morphogenesis of occluding coronary artery thrombosis. *Arch Pathol* 1965;80:256–261.

14. Barger CA, Beeuwkes R III, Lainey LL, Silverman KJ: Hypothesis: Vasa vasorum and neovascularization of human coronary arteries—a possible role in the pathophysiology of atherosclerosis. *N Engl J Med* 1984;310:1137–1140.

15. Davies MJ, Thomas A: Thrombosis and acute coronary lesions in sudden cardiac ischemic death. *N Engl J Med* 1984;310:1137–1140.

16. Crowley JG, Pierce RA: The affinity of platelets for subendothelium. *Am J Surg* 1981;47:529 532.

17. Badimon L, Badimon JJ, Ballvez A, et al: Incidence of arterial damage and wall shear rate on platelet deposition: Ex vivo study in a swine model. *Arteriosclerosis* 1986;6:312–320.

18. Colman RW, Walsh PN: Mechanisms of platelet aggregation, in Colman RW, Hirsh J, Marder VJ, Salzman EW (eds): *Hemostasis and Thrombosis.* Philadelphia, JB Lippincott, 1987, pp 594–605.

19. Constantinides P: Plaque fissures in human coronary thrombosis. *J Atheroscler Res* 1966;6:1–17.

20. Hackett D, Davies G, Chierchia S, Maseri A: Intermittent occlusion in acute myocardial infarction. Value of combined thrombolytic and vasodilator therapy. *N Engl J Med* 1987;317:1055–1059.

21. Chester MR, Chen L, Kaski JC: Angiographic evidence for frequent "silent" plaque disruption in patients with stable angina. *J Am Coll Cardiol* 1995;2:428A.

22. Falk E: Plaque rupture with severe pre-existing stenosis precipitating coronary thrombosis. Characteristics of coronary atherosclerotic plaques underlying fatal occlusive thrombi. *Br Heart J* 1983;50:127–134.

23. Richardson PD, Davies MJ, Born GVR: Influence of plaque configuration and stress distribution on fissuring of coronary atherosclerotic plaques. *Lancet* 1989;2:941–944.

24. Davies MJ, Richardson PD, Woolk N, et al: Risk of thrombosis in human atherosclerotic plaque. Role of extracellular lipid, macrophage and smooth muscle content. *Br Heart J* 1993;69:377–381.

25. Sharma SK, Fyle B, Bongu R, et al: Lipid rich plaques with thrombus are common in unstable rest angina: Observations from atherectomy tissue analysis. *J Am Coll Cardiol* 1995;25:281A.

26. Brown BG, Zhao XQ, Sacco DE, Albers JJ: Lipid lowering and plaque regression: New insights into prevention of plaque disruption and clinical events in coronary disease. *Circulation* 1993;87:1781–1791.

27. Brown G, Albers JJ, Fisher LD, et al: Regression of coronary artery disease as a result of intensive lipid lowering therapy in men with high levels of apolipo-protein B. *N Engl J Med* 1990;323:1289–1298.

28. Watts GF, Lewis B, Brunt JNH, et al: Effects on coronary artery disease of lipid lowering diet, or diet plus cholestyraminie, in the St. Thomas Atherosclerosis Regression Study (STARS). *Lancet* 1992;339:563–569.

29. Loree HM, Tobias BJ, Gebson LJ, et al: Mechanical properties of model atherosclerotic lesion lipid pools. *Athero and Thromb* 1994;14:230–234.

30. Cheng GC, Loree HM, Kamm RD, Fishbein MC, Lee RT. Distribution of circumferential stress in ruptured and stable atherosclerotic lesions. *Circulation* 1993;87:1179–1187.

31. MacIsaac AI, Thomas JD, Topol EJ: Toward the quiescent coronary plaque. *J Am Coll Cardiol* 1993;22:1228–1241.

32. Fuster V: Lewis A. Conner Memorial Lecture. Mechanisms leading to myocardial infarction: Insights from studies of vascular biology. *Circulation* 1994;90:2126–2126.

33. Van der Wal AC, Becker AE, Van der Loos CM, Das PK: Site of intimal rupture or erosion of thrombosed coronary atherosclerotic plaques is characterized by an inflammatory process irrespective of the dominant plaque morphology. *Circulation* 1994;89:36–44.

34. Libby P: Molecular bases of the acute coronary syndromes. *Circulation* 1995;91:2844–2850.

35. Mazzone A, DeServi S, Ricevuti G, et al: Increased expression of neutrophil and monocyte adhesion molecules in unstable coronary artery disease. *Circulation* 1993;88:358–363.

36. de Servi S, Mazzone A, Ricevuti G, Specchia G: Site of leukocyte activation in unstable angina. *J Am Coll Cardiol* 1995;25:312A.

37. Ott I, Neumann FJ, Gawaz M, Schomig A: Platelet–leukocyte interaction in patients with unstable angina. *J Am Coll Cardiol* 1995;25:312A.

38. Ambrose JA: Plaque disruption and the acute coronary syndromes of unstable angina and myocardial infarction: If the substrate is similar, why is the clinical presentation different? *J Am Coll Cardiol* 1992;19:1653–1658.

39. Fernandez-Ortiz A, Badimon JJ, Falk E, et al: Characterization of the relative thrombogenicity of therosclerotic plaque components: Implications for consequences of plaque rupture. *J Am Coll Cardiol* 1994;23:1562–1569.
40. Braunwald E: Unstable angina; a classification. *Circulation* 1989;80:410–414.
41. Flugelman MY, Virmani R, Correa R, et al: Smooth muscle cell abundance and fibroblast growth factors in coronary lesions of patients with nonfatal unstable angina. A clue to the mechanism of transformation from the stable to the unstable clinical state. *Circulation* 1993;88:2493–2500.
42. Gibson RS: Clinical, functional and angiographic distinctions between Q wave and non-Q wave myocardial infarction: Evidence of spontaneous reperfusion and implications for intervention trials. *Circulation* 1987;75(Suppl V): V-128–V-138.
43. Rentrop KP, Feit F, Sherman W, Thorton JC: Serial angiographic assessment of coronary artery obstruction and collateral flow in acute myocardial infarction; report from the second Mount Sinai–New York University Reperfusion Trial. *Circulation* 1989;80:1166–1175.
44. Davies MH, Woolf N, Robertson WB: Pathology of acute myocardial infarction with particular reference to occlusive coronary thrombi. *Br Heart J* 1976;38:659–664.
45. Freifeld AG, Schuster EH, Bulkley BH: Nontransmural versus transmural myocardial infarction. *Am J Cardiol* 1983;75:423–432.
46. Roberts WC, Buja LM: The frequency and significance of coronary arterial thrombi and other observations in fatal acute myocardial infarction. *Am J Med* 1972;52:425–443.
47. Erhardt LR, Lundman T, Mellstedt H: Incorporation of 125I-labelled fibrinogen into coronary arterial thrombi in acute myocardial infarction in man. *Lancet* 1973;387–390.
48. Davies MH, Thomas AC: Plaque fissuring: The cause of acute myocardial infarction, sudden ischaemic death, and crescendo angina. *Br Heart J* 1985;53:363–373.
49. Davies MJ: Thrombosis and coronary atherosclerosis, in Julian D, Kubler W, Norris RM, Swan HJC, Collen D, Verstraete M, (eds): *Thrombolysis in Cardiovascular Disease.* New York, Marcel Dekker, 1989, pp 25–43.
50. Ambrose JA, Alexopoulos D: Thrombolysis in unstable angina: Will the beneficial effects of thrombolytic therapy in myocardial infarction apply to patients with unstable angina? *J Am Coll Cardiol* 1989;13:1666–1671.
51. GISSI (Gruppo Italiano per lo Studio della Strptochinasi nell' Infarccto Miocardico): Effectiveness of intravenous thrombolytic treatment in acute myocardial infarction. *Lancet* 1986;1:397–401.
52. ISIS-2 (Second International Study of Infarct Survival) Collaborative Group: Randomised trial on intravenous streptokinase, oral aspirin, both, or neither among 17,187 cases of suspected acute myocardial infarction: ISIS-2. *Lancet* 1988;2: 349–360.
53. Mizuno K, Satomura K, Miyamoto A, et al: Angioscopic evaluation of the character of coronary thrombus in acute coronary syndromes. *N Engl J Med* 1992;326:287–291.
54. Pasternack RC, Braunwald E, Sobel BE: Acute myocardial infarction, in Anderson JR (ed): *Heart Diseases,* 3rd ed. Philadelphia, WB Saunders, 1988, pp 1222–1313.
55. Anderson JR: Pathological thrombosis, in Anderson JR (ed): *Muer's Textbook of Pathology,* 12th ed. New York, Edward Arnold, 1985, pp 1012–1013.
56. Wilhelmsen L, Svardsudd K, Korsan-Bengtsen K, Larsson B, Welin L, Tibblin G: Fibrinogen as a risk factor for stroke and myocardial infarction. *N Engl J Med* 1984;311:501–505.
57. Meade TW, Mellows S, Brozovic M, et al: Haemostatic function and ischemic heart disease: Principal results of the Northwick Park Heart Study. *Lancet* 1986;2:533–537.
58. Hawkins R: Smoking, platelets and thrombosis. *Nature* 1972;236:450–452.
59. Ridker PM, Manson JE, Buring JE, Muller JE, Hennekens CH: Circadian variation of acute myocardial infarction and the effect of low-dose aspirin in a randomized trial of physicians. *Circulation* 1990;82:897–902.
60. Brexinski DA, Tofler GH, Muller JE, et al: Morning increase in platelet aggregability: Association with assumption of the upright posture. *Circulation* 1988;78:35–40.
61. Santamore WP, Yelton BW, Ogilby JD: Dynamics of coronary occlusion in the pathogenesis of myocardial infarction. *J Am Coll Cardiol* 1991;18: 1397–1405.
62. Ambrose JA: Coronary arteriographic analysis and angiographic morphology. *J Am Coll Cardiol* 1989;13:1492–1494.

63. Ambrose JA, Hjemdahl-Monsen C, Borrico S, et al: Quantitative and qualitative effects of intracoronary streptokinase in unstable angina and non-Q wave infarction. *J Am Coll Cardiol* 1987;9: 1156–1165.

64. Topol EJ, Nicklas JM, Kander NH, et al: Coronary revascularization after intravenous tissue plasminogen activator for unstable angina pectoris: Results of a randomized, double-blind, placebo-controlled trial. *Am J Cardiol* 1988;62: 368–371.

65. De Zwaan C, Bar FW, Janssen JHA, et al: Effects of thrombolytic therapy in unstable angina: Clinical and angiographic results. *J Am Coll Cardiol* 1988;12:301–309.

66. Falk E: Unstable angina with fatal outcome: Dynamic coronary thrombosis leading to infarction and/or sudden death. *Circulation* 1985;71:699–708.

67. Fuster V, Badimon L, Cohen M, et al: Insights into the pathogenesis of acute ischemic syndromes. *Circulation* 1988;77:1213–1220.

68. Conti CR: Coronary-artery vasoconstriction. *Curr Opinion Cardiol* 1988;3:468–479.

69. Neri Serneri GG, Albate R, Gori AM, et al: Transient intermittent lymphocyte activation is responsible for the instability of angina. *Circulation* 1992;86:790–797.

70. Entman ML, Ballantyne DM: Inflammation in acute coronary syndromes. *Circulation* 1993;88: 800–803.

71. Bazzoni G, Dejana E, Del Maschio A: Platelet–neutrophil interactions; possible relevance in the pathogenesis of thrombosis and inflammation. *Haematologica* 1991;76:491–499.

72. Liuzzo G, Biasucci LM, Gallimore JR, et al: The prognostic value of C-reactive protein and serum amyloid a protein in severe unstable angina. *N Engl J Med* 1994;331:417–424.

73. Langer A, Freeman MR, Armstrong PW: ST segment shift in unstable angina: Pathophysiology and association with coronary anatomy and hospital outcome. *J Am Coll Cardiol* 1989;13: 1495–1502.

74. Cobb LA, Werner JA, Trobaugh GB: Sudden cardiac death. I. A decade's experience with out-of-hospital resuscitation. II. Outcome of resuscitation, management, and future direction. *Mod Conc Cardiolvasc Dis* 1980;49:31–42.

75. Warnes CA, Roberts WC: Sudden coronary death: Relation of amount and distribution of coronary narrowing at necropsy to previous symptoms of myocardial ischemia, left ventricular scarring and heart weight. *Am J Cardiol* 1984;54: 65–73.

76. Baroldi G, Falzi G, Mariani F: Sudden coronary death: A postmortem study in 208 selected cases compared to 97 "control" subjects. *Am Heart J* 1979;98:20–31.

77. Davies MH, Bland JM, Hangartner JRW, et al: Factors influencing the presence or absence of acute coronary artery thrombi in sudden ischaemic death. *Eur Heart J* 1989;10:203–208.

78. DeWood MA, Spores J, Notske RN, et al: Prevalence of total coronary occlusion during the early hours of transmural myocardial infarction. *N Engl J Med* 1980;303:897–902.

79. Verstraete M, Bory M, Collen D, et al. Randomized trial of intravenous recombinant tissue-type plasminogen activator versus intravenous streptokinase in acute myocardial infarction. *Lancet* 1985;1:842–847.

80. The TIMI Study Group: The thrombolysis in myocardial infarction (TIMI) trial. *N Engl J Med* 1985;312:932–936.

81. Neuhaus KL, for the GAUS Study Group: Intravenous recombinant tissue plasminogen activator (rt-PA) and urokinase in acute myocardial infarction: Results of the German Activator Urokinase Study (GAUS). *J Am Coll Cardiol* 1988;12: 581–587.

82. Bonnier HJRM, Visser RF, Klomps HC, Hoffmann HJML, and the Dutch Invasive Reperfusion Study Group: Comparison of intravenous anisoylated plasminogen streptokinase activator complex and intracoronary streptokinase activator complex and intracoronary streptokinase in acute myocardial infarction. *Am J Cardiol* 1988;62: 25–30.

83. Rentrop P, Blanke H, Karsch KR, et al: Selective intracoronary thrombolysis in acute myocardial infarction and unstable angina pectoris. *Circulation* 1981;63:307–317.

84. Topol EJ: Thrombolysis, in Topol EJ (ed): *Textbook of Interventional Cardiology.* Philadelphia, WB Saunders, 1990, p 77.

85. Ambrose JA, Winters SL, Arora RR, et al: Coronary angiographic morphology in myocardial infarction: A link between the pathogenesis of unstable angina and myocardial infarction. *J Am Coll Cardiol* 1985;6:1233–1238.

86. Wilson RF, Holida MD, White CW: Quantitative angiographic morphology of coronary stenosis leading to myocardial infarction or unstable angina. *Circulation* 1986;73:286–293.

87. Brown BG, Gallery CA, Badger RS, et al: Incomplete lysis of thrombus in the moderate underlying atheroscleroslerotic lesion during intracoronary infusion of streptokinase for acute myocardial infarction: Quantitative angiographic observations. *Circulation* 1986;73:653–661.

88. Davies SW, Marchant B, Lyons JP, et al: Coronary lesion morphology in acute myocardial infarction: Demonstration of early remodeling after streptokinase treatment. *J Am Coll Cardiol* 1990;16: 1079–1086.

89. Veen G, Meijer A, Werter CJPJ, et al: Dynamic changes of culprit lesion morphology and severity after successful thrombolysis for acute myocardial infarction: An angiographic follow up study. *J Am Coll Cardiol* 1994;23:147A.

90. Davies SW, Marchant B, Lyons JP, et al: Irregular coronary lesion morphology after thrombolysis predicts early clinical instability. *J Am Coll Cardiol* 1991;18:669–674.

91. Forrester JS, Litvack F, Grundfest W, Hickey A: A perspective of coronary disease seen through the arteries of living man. *Circulation* 1987;75:505–513.

92. Ambrose JA, Tannenbaum MA, Alexopoulos D, et al: Angiographic progression of coronary artery disease and the development of myocardial infarction. *J Am Coll Cardiol* 1988;12:56–62.

93. Little WC, Constantinescu M, Applegate RJ, et al: Can coronary angiography predict the site of a subsequent myocardial infarction in patients with mild to moderate coronary artery disease? *Circulation* 1988;78:1157–1166.

94. Giroud D, Li JM, Urban P, Meier B, Rutishauser W: Relation of the site of acute myocardial infarction to the most severe coronary arterial stenosis at prior angiography. *Am J Cardiol* 1992; 69:729–732.

95. Nobuyoshi M, Tanaka M, Nosaka H, et al: Progression of coronary atherosclerosis: Is coronary spasm related to progression? *J Am Coll Cardiol* 1991;18:914–910.

96. Webster MWI, Chesebro JH, Smith HC, et al: Myocardial infarction and coronary artery occlusion: A prospective 5-year angiographic study. *J Am Coll Cardiol* 1990;15:218A.

97. The TIMI Study Group: Comparison of invasive and conservative strategies following intravenous tissue plasminogen activator in acute myocardial infarction: Results of the thrombolysis in myocardial infarction (TIMI) II trial. *N Engl J Med* 1989; 320:618–628.

98. Topol EJ, Califf RM, George BS, et al: A randomized trial of immediate versus delayed elective angioplasty after intravenous tissue plasminogen activator in acute myocardial infarction. *N Engl J Med* 1987;317:581–583.

99. Hackett D, Davies G, Maseri A: Pre-existing coronary stenoses in patients with first myocardial infarction are not necessarily severe. *Br Heart J* 1988;9:1317–1323.

100. Moise A, Lesperance J, Theroux P, et al: Clinical and angiographic predictors of a new total coronary occlusion in coronary artery disease: Analysis of 313 non-operated patients. *Am J Cardiol* 1984;54:1176–1181.

101. Ellis S, Alderman E, Cain K, et al: Prediction of risk of anterior myocardial infarction by lesion severity and measurement method of stenoses in the left anterior descending coronary distribution: A CASS Registry study. *J Am Coll Cardiol* 1988;11: 908–916.

102. Neill WA, Wharton TP, Fluri-Lundeen J, Cohen IS: Acute coronary insufficiency—coronary occlusion after intermittent ischemic attacks. *N Engl J Med* 1980;302:1157–1162.

103. Fuster V, Frye RL, Connolly DC, et al: Arteriographic patterns early in the onset of the coronary syndromes. *Br Heart J* 1975;37:1250–1255.

104. Alison HW, Russell RO Jr, Mantle JA, et al: Coronary anatomy and arteriography in patients with unstable angina pectoris. *Am J Cardiol* 1978;41: 204–209.

105. Plotnick GD, Greene HI, Carliner NH, et al: Clinical indicators of left main coronary artery disease in unstable angina. *Ann Int Med* 1979;91: 149–153.

106. Victor MF, Likoff MJ, Mintz GS, Likoff W: Unstable angina pectoris of new onset; a prospective clinical and arteriographic study of 75 patients. *Am J Cardiol* 1981;47:228–232.

107. Conti CR, Brawley RK, Griffith LSC, et al: Unstable angina pectoris: Morbidity and mortality in 57 consecutive patients evaluated angiographically. *Am J Cardiol* 1973;32:745–750.

108. Ambrose JA, Winters SL, Stern A, et al: Angiographic morphology and the pathogenesis of unstable angina pectoris. *J Am Coll Cardiol* 1985;5:609–616.

109. Haft JI, Goldstein JE, Niemiera ML: Coronary arteriographic lesion of unstable angina. *Chest* 1987;92:609–612.

110. Williams AE, Freeman MR, Chisholm RJ, et al: Angiographic morphology in unstable angina pectoris. *Am J Cardiol* 1988;62:1024–1027.

111. Levin DC, Fallon JT: Significance of the angiographic morphology of localized coronary stenoses. Histopathologic correlation. *Circulation* 1982; 66:316–320.

112. Bresnahan DR, Davis DR, Holmes DR Jr, Smith HC: Angiographic occurrence and clinical correlates of intraluminal coronary artery thrombus: Role of unstable angina. *J Am Coll Cardiol* 1985;6:285–289.

113. Vetrovec GW, Cowley MJ, Overton H, Richardson DW: Intracoronary thrombus in syndromes of unstable myocardial ischemia. *Am Heart J* 1981; 102:1202–1208.

114. Capone G, Wolf NM, Meyer B, Meister SG: Frequency of intracoronary filling defects by angiography in angina pectoris at rest. *Am J Cardiol* 1985;56:403–406.

115. Mandlekorn JB, Wolf NM, Singh S, et al: Intracoronary thrombus in nontransmural myocardial infarction in unstable angina pectoris. *Am J Cardiol* 1983;52:1–6.

116. Ambrose JA, Hjemdahl-Monsen CE, Borrico S, et al: Angiographic demonstration of a common link between unstable angina pectoris and non-Q wave acute myocardial infarction. *Am J Cardiol* 1988;61:244–247.

117. Cowley MJ, DiSciascio G, Rehr RB, Vetrovec GW: Angiographic observations and clinical relevance of coronary thrombus in unstable angina pectoris. *Am J Cardiol* 1989;63:108E–113E.

118. Mehran R, Ambrose JA, Bongu RM, et al: Angioplasty of complex lesions in ischemic rest angina. Results of the TAUSA trial. *J Am Coll Cardiol,* in press.

119. Rivera W, Sharaf BL, Miele NJ, et al: Coronary anatomy in patients who present with non-Q wave myocardial infarction differs from unstable angina pectoris: A report from TIMI 3B. *Circulation* 1994;90:I-438.

120. Gold HK, Johns JA, Leinbach RC, et al: A randomized, blinded, placebo-controlled trial of recombinant human tissue-type plasminogen activator in patients with unstable angina pectoris. *Circulation* 1987;75:1192–1199.

121. Vetrovec GW, Leinbach RC, Gold HK, Cowley MJ: Intracoronary thrombolysis in syndromes of unstable ischemia: Angiographic and clinical results. *Am Heart J* 1982;104:946–952.

122. Gotoh K, Minamino R, Katoh O, et al: The role of intracoronary thrombus in unstable angina: Angiographic assessment and thrombolytic therapy during ongoing angina attacks. *Circulation* 1988;77:526–534.

123. Bar FW, Verheugt FW, Col J, et al: Thrombolysis in patients with unstable angina improves the angiographic but not the clinical outcome. Results of UNASEM, a multicenter, randomized, placebo-controlled, clinical trial with anistreplase. *Circulation* 1992;86:131–137.

124. The TIMI III Investigators: Early effects of tissue-type plasminogen activator added to conventional therapy on the culprit coronary lesion in patients presenting with ischemic cardiac pain at rest. Results of the Thrombolysis in Myocardial Ischemia (TIMI IIIA) Trial. *Circulation* 1993;87:38–52.

125. The TIMI III Investigators: Effects of tissue plasminogen activator and a comparison of early invasive and conservative strategies in unstable angina and non-Q wave myocardial infarction. Results of the TIMI IIIB Trial. Thrombolysis in Myocardial Ischemia. *Circulation* 1994;89:1545–1556.

126. Waters D, Lam JY: Is thrombolytic therapy striking out in unstable angina? *Circulation* 1992;86:1642–1644.

127. Topol EJ, Fuster V, Harrington RA, et al: Recombinant hirudin for unstable angina pectoris. A multicenter, randomized angiographic trial. *Circulation* 1994;89:1557–1566.

128. Ouimet TP, McCans J: Aspirin, heparin, or both to treat acute unstable angina. *N Engl J Med* 1988;319:1105–1115.

129. Lewis HD, Davis JW, Archibald DG: Protective effects of aspirin against acute myocardial infarction and death in men with unstable angina: Results of a Veterans Administration cooperative study. *N Engl J Med* 1983;309:396–403.

130. Cairns JA, Gent M, Senger J: Aspirin, sulfinpyrazone, or both in unstable angina: Results of a Canadian multicenter trial. *N Engl J Med* 1985; 313:1369–1375.

131. Telford AM, Wilson C: Trial of heparin versus atenolol in prevention of myocardial infarction in intermediate coronary syndrome. *Lancet* 1981;1: 1225–1228.

132. Willerson JT, Casscells W: Thrombin inhibitors in unstable angina: Rebound or continuation of angina after argatroban withdrawal? *J Am Coll Cardiol* 1993;21:1048–1051.

133. Lidon RM, Theroux P, Juneau M, Adelman B, Maraganore J: Initial experience with a direct antithrombin, Hirulog, in unstable angina. *Circulation* 1993;88:1495–1501.

134. Gold HK, Torres FW, Garabedian HD, et al: Evidence for a rebound coagulation phenomenon after cessation of a 4-hour infusion of a specific thrombin inhibitor in patients with unstable angina pectoris. *J Am Coll Cardiol* 1993;21: 1039–1047.

135. Serneri GGN, Gensini GF, Crnobali M, et al: Association between time of increased fibrinopeptide A levels in plasma and episodes of spontaneous angina: A controlled prospective study. *Am Heart J* 1987;113:672–678.

136. Theroux P, Latour JG, Leger-Gauthier C, Lara JD: Fibrinopeptide A and platelet factor levels in unstable angina pectoris. *Circulation* 1987;75:156–162.

137. Yasu T, Oshima S, Imanishi M, et al: Effects of aspirin DL-lysine on thrombin generation in unstable angina pectoris. *Am J Cardiol* 1993;71:1164–1168.

138. Lam JYT, Latour JG, Lesperance J, Waters D: Platelet aggregation, coronary artery disease progression and future coronary events. *Am J Cardiol* 1994;73:333–338.

139. Simoons ML, Jan de Boer M, van den Brand MJBM: Randomized trial of a GPIIb/IIIa platelet receptor blocker in refractory unstable angina. *Circulation* 1994;89:596–603.

140. Lincoff MA, Califf RM, Anderson K, Weisman HF, Topol EJ, for the EPIC Investigators: Striking clinical benefit with platelet GP IIb/IIIa inhibition by c7E3 among patients with unstable angina: Outcome in the EPIC trial. *Circulation* 1994;4(2):I21.

141. Moise A, Theroux P, Taigmans Y, et al: Unstable angina and progression of coronary atherosclerosis. *N Engl J Med* 1983;309:685–689.

142. Ambrose JA, Winters SL, Arora RR, et al: Angiographic evolution of coronary artery morphology in unstable angina. *J Am Coll Cardiol* 1986;7: 472–478.

143. Chen L, Chester MR, Redwood S, Huang J, Leatham E, Kaski JC: Angiographic stenosis progression and coronary events in patients with "stabilized" unstable angina. *Circulation* 1995;91: 2319–2324.

144. Huey BL, Gheorghiade M, Crampton RS, et al: Acute non-Q wave myocardial infarction associated with early ST segment elevation: Evidence for spontaneous coronary reperfusion and implications for thrombolytic trials. *J Am Coll Cardiol* 1987;9:18–25.

145. DeWood MA, Stifter WF, Simpson CS, et al: Coronary arteriographic findings soon after non-Q wave myocardial infarction. *N Engl J Med* 1986;315:417–423.

146. Decanay S, Kennedy HJ, Uretz E, Parrillo JE, Klein LW: Morphological and quantitative angiographic analyses of progression of coronary stenoses. A comparison of Q-wave and non-Q wave myocardial infarction. *Circulation* 1994;90: 1739–1746.

147. Weaver WD, Lorch GS, Alvarez HA, Cobb LA: Angiographic findings and prognostic indicators in patients resuscitated from sudden cardiac death. *Circulation* 1976;54:895–900.

148. Stevenson WG, Wiener I, Yeatman L, et al: Complicated atherosclerotic lesions: A potential cause of ischemic ventricular arrhythmias in cardiac arrest survivors who do not have inducible ventricular tachycardia? *Am Heart J* 1988;116:1–6.

149. Lo Y-SA, Cutler JE, Balke K, et al: Angiographic coronary morphology in survivors of cardiac arrest. *Am Heart J* 1988;115:781–785.

5

Triggers of Onset of Acute Myocardial Infarction

Mylan C. Cohen, MD, MPH, and James E. Muller, MD

INTRODUCTION

Advances made in the interpretation of the pathologic and angiographic findings accompanying myocardial infarction described in Chapters 2 to 4, and documentation of a prominent circadian variation of infarction onset, suggest that the onset of myocardial infarction is, in most cases, triggered by activities of the patient. If triggering occurs with such frequency, improved understanding of its mechanism could lead to improved treatment of coronary artery disease and generation of insights that may contribute to prevention of both initial and recurrent myocardial infarction. Although triggering appears to be a new topic of interest, the concept has strong historical roots.

HISTORY OF THE TRIGGERING CONCEPT

In their original clinical description of acute myocardial infarction in 1910, Obraztsov and Strazhesko noted, "Direct events often precipitated the disease; the infarct began in one case on climbing a high staircase, in another during an unpleasant conversation, and in a third during emotional distress associated with a heated card game" (1). Their view, that infarction was triggered, was challenged in the 1930s as larger studies revealed that myocardial infarction often occurred without an obvious precipitating event. Authors argued for (2,3) and against (4,5) the belief that triggers were frequent. The controversy was eventually suspended for many years as Master's conclusion, based on retrospective questionnaires, that "Coronary occlusion takes place irrespective of the physical activity being performed or the type of rest taken," gained widespread acceptance (6). However, studies conducted with modern epidemiologic methods and the insight provided by new understanding of the pathogenesis of myocardial infarction indicate that the original concept of Obraztsov and Strazhesko may be correct. The recent documentation of increased infarction onset in the morning hours (7) has revitalized investigation of triggering.

MORNING INCREASE OF MYOCARDIAL INFARCTION

That myocardial infarction does not occur randomly throughout the day, but shows prominent circadian variation with increased morning frequency,

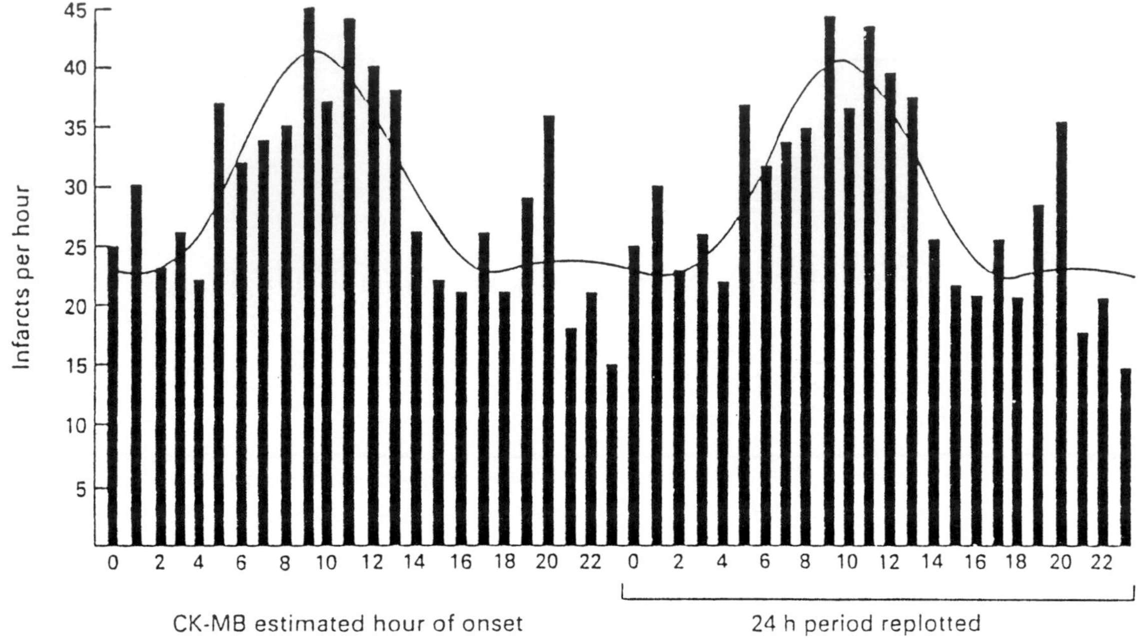

Figure 5–1. The number of infarctions beginning during each of the 24 hours of the day is plotted on the left side of the figure. On the right, the identical data are plotted again to permit appreciation of the relation between the end and the beginning of the day. A two-harmonic regression equation for the frequency of onset of myocardial infarction has been fitted to the data (curved line). A prominent circadian rhythm is present, with a primary peak incidence of infarction at 9 AM and a secondary peak at 8 PM. *Reprinted with permission* (7).

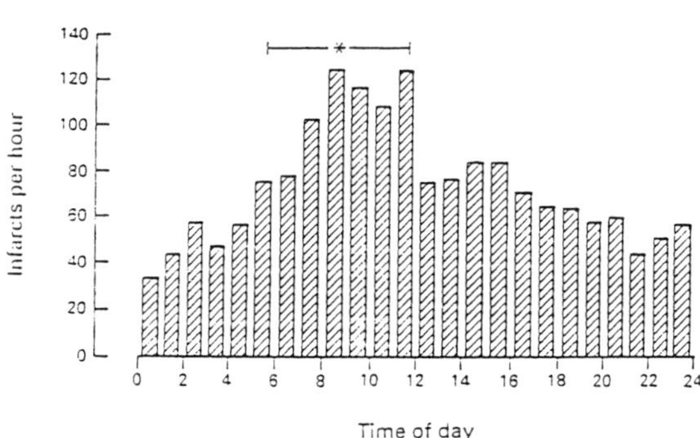

Figure 5–2. Bar graph of incidence of myocardial infarction of 1,741 patients of the ISAM (Intravenous Streptokinase in Acute Myocardial Infarction) Study. There is a marked circadian variation ($p < 0.001$) with a peak during the morning hours. Myocardial infarction occurred 1.8 times more frequently between 6 AM and 12 noon compared with the average of other quarters of the day. The risk of myocardial infarction in the afternoon and evening was approximately equally distributed, whereas during the night a trough period occurred in the incidence of myocardial infarction. *Reprinted with permission* (8).

supports the concept that daily activities are important triggers. Evidence obtained from the Multicenter Investigation of the Limitation of Infarct Size (MILIS) (7) (Fig. 5–1) and from the Intravenous Streptokinase in Acute Myocardial Infarction (ISAM) study (8) (Fig. 5–2) clearly demonstrates that myocardial infarction is at least three times more likely to begin in the morning than in the late evening. Both studies determined the onset of myocardial infarction objectively, based on the time of first appearance of creatine kinase in the plasma. Their finding is supported by a larger number of studies (9) that used onset of pain as the marker for time of myocardial infarction onset. These earlier studies received limited attention, however, because delayed reporting of myocardial infarction onset, which might have started while the patient was sleeping, was thought to explain the increased morning incidence. More detailed analysis has indicated that the morning increase in myocardial infarction is attenuated in subgroups receiving beta-adrenergic blockade and may be altered in the elderly, diabetics, smokers, and those with prior infarction (7,10).

In a refinement of the original reports on circadian variation, Goldberg et al reported that the increased incidence of myocardial infarction in the morning occurs in the first few hours after awakening (11).

Additionally, sudden cardiac death, a condition often caused by coronary thrombosis, has a similar circadian pattern (12–15), a finding that reinforces the finding that nonfatal myocardial infarction has a prominent morning increase in onset. Furthermore, stroke, a third condition often caused by occlusive arterial thrombosis, has a similar morning increase (16,17).

EPIDEMIOLOGIC EVIDENCE THAT ACTIVITIES TRIGGER ONSET

Sumiyoshi et al reported on activities prior to onset in 416 patients with infarction admitted to the National Heart Center of Japan from 1977 to 1985 (18). Fifty-three percent of patients without prior angina reported their infarct began during moderate to heavy exercise, emotional stress, or excitement. In an effort to obtain control data, information was collected on the frequency of emotional and physical stress during the same month 1 year prior to infarction and compared with the frequency of stress in the month immediately prior to infarction. Although the frequency of stress in the month prior to infarction was significantly higher than that reported during the control period (58% versus 34%, $p < 0.01$), recall bias complicates interpretation of the finding. Additionally, our group has reviewed reporting of possible triggers of infarction by 849 patients enrolled in the MILIS. This study revealed that 48.5% reported a possible trigger and 13.6% reported two or more triggers (19). The possible triggers included emotional upset (18.8%), moderate physical activity (14.4%), heavy physical activity (8.7%), lack of sleep (8.0%), overeating (6.9%), sexual activity (1.2%), surgery (0.4%), and miscellaneous (6.6%). These data are comparable with the findings of Sumiyoshi et al (18).

However, it is not the report of the activities themselves, but the collection of appropriate control data that poses the greatest obstacle to clarifying the role of potential trigger activities in the onset of infarction. To overcome the methodologic problems involved in collection of such data, Maclure has developed a case-crossover design; in this design, each patient serves as his or her own control for relatively recent activities (20). A study entitled "Determinants of the Onset of Myocardial Infarction," funded by the National Heart, Lung and Blood Institute, currently utilizes this method. More than 1,800 patients with infarction have been interviewed to determine their activities in the hours immediately before infarction onset and in a control period 24 hours earlier. The relative risk for an MI is calculated as the observed frequency of the activity during a designated hazard period (the hour prior to the MI) compared with its expected frequency based on the individual's usual frequency of exertion. With the use of this method, it has now been demonstrated that heavy exertion (exertion estimated to be ≥6 METs) produced a 5.9-fold increase in risk (95% confidence interval: 4.6–7.7) of MI in the subsequent hour (21) (Fig. 5–3). The risk of MI onset during heavy exertion was significantly higher in those who were sedentary (107-fold) compared with those who regularly exercised (2-fold) (Fig. 5–4). Willich et al found similar results in a German population (22).

Although there is abundant anecdotal evidence that psychological stress may trigger onset of MI, there have been no controlled studies of this acute phenomenon. Prior studies of anger, hostility, and type A personality as risk factors for MI have focused on chronic risk and have yielded controversial and sometimes contradictory results (23). In the ONSET study, data on outbursts of anger were collected in 1,623 patients. Anger corresponding to levels greater than 4 in a 7-level self-report anger scale was reported by 14% of patients within 26 hours prior to MI onset. Using the same study design described above for the study of physical exertion, we found that the risk of MI onset was significantly elevated in the 2 hours following an outburst of anger, with a relative risk of 2.0 (95% confidence interval: 1.7–3.2) (24).

Sexual activity has also been documented to trigger myocardial infarction (25). The relative risk of an MI occurring in the hour after sexual activity

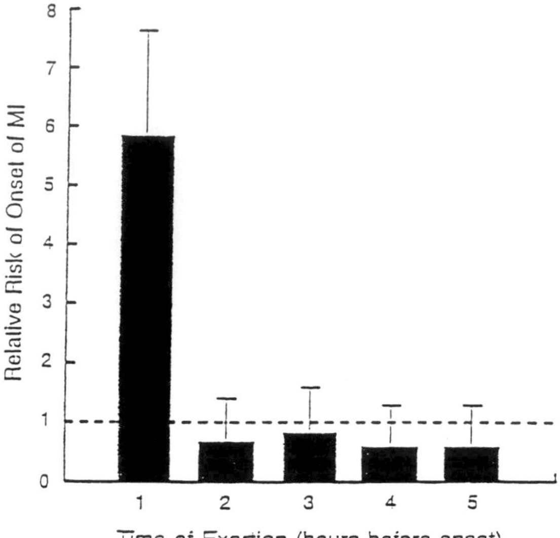

Figure 5–3. Time of onset of myocardial infarction after an episode of heavy physical exertion (induction time). Each of the five hours before the onset of myocardial infarction was assessed as an independent hazard period, and exertion during each hour was compared with that during the control period. Only exertion during the hour immediately before the onset of myocardial infarction was associated with an increase in the relative risk, suggesting that the induction time for myocardial infarction is less than one hour. The T bars indicate the 95% confidence limits. The dotted line indicates the baseline risk. *Reprinted with permission* (21).

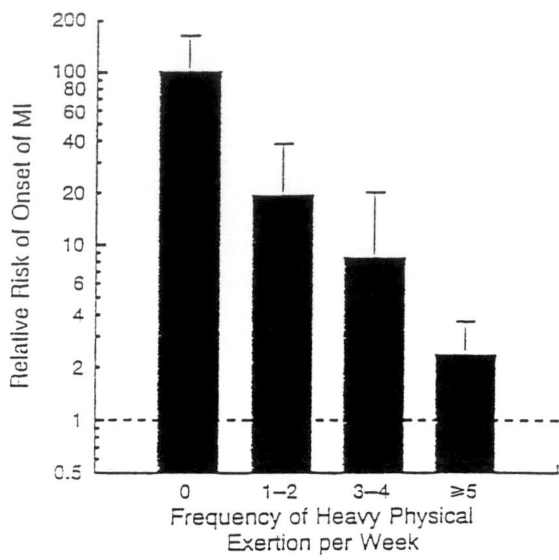

Figure 5–4. Modification of the relative risk of myocardial infarction by usual frequency of heavy exertion (defined as ≥6 METs). The relative risks for heavy physical exertion are shown for subgroups of patients whose habitual frequency of heavy physical exertion is less than 1, 1 to 2, 3 to 4, and 5 or more episodes per week. Note that the relative risk is presented on a logarithmic scale. Sedentary individuals experienced an extreme relative risk (107), while those who exerted themselves 5 or more times per week had an increase in risk only 2.4 times over baseline ($p < 0.001$). Error bars indicate 95% confidence intervals. *Reprinted with permission* (21).

is 2.1 compared with baseline risk. While this documentation of an elevated relative risk might lead to concern over sexual activity in patients in rehabilitation programs, the data actually provide grounds for reassurance of such patients. The relative risk was not elevated in those with a history of cardiac disease compared with those without. In addition, since the baseline absolute risk of an MI in any given hour is extremely low (approximately 10 chances in 1 million per hour for a patient with a prior MI), doubling of baseline risk would produce only a small increase in absolute risk and should not be a factor in the decision of an asymptomatic patient to engage in sexual activity.

Finally, the progress made in identifying triggers of MI in controlled studies makes it possible to estimate the percentage of all infarctions that are triggered. As shown in Fig. 5–5, the recognized triggers

Percent of MI's that are Triggered

(1,700 patient interviews in the NHLBI MI Onset Study)

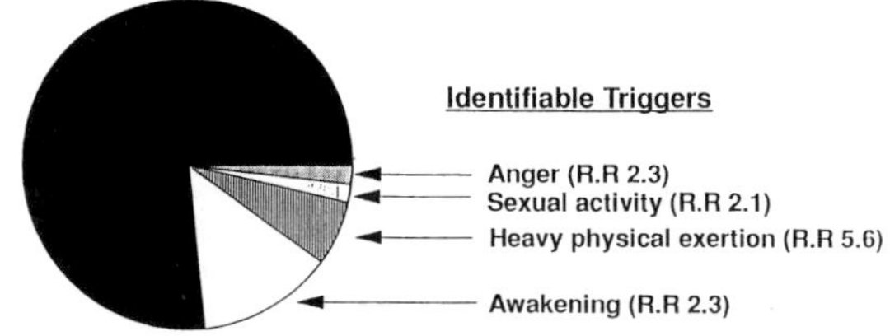

At least 245,000 MI's per year are triggered.

Figure 5–5. Percent of MIs that are triggered.

of awakening, physical exertion, anger, and sexual activity account for 15% to 20% of MIs, or almost 250,000 MIs annually in the United States. This undoubtedly represents an underestimate of triggering, and it indicates the importance of understanding triggering mechanisms.

AUTOPSY AND ANGIOGRAPHIC DATA PERTINENT TO TRIGGERING MECHANISMS

In 1980, DeWood et al convincingly showed that occlusive coronary artery thrombosis is the cause of most Q wave myocardial infarctions (26). Furthermore, coronary angiographic and angioscopic studies have demonstrated a high frequency of nonocclusive coronary thrombosis in patients with unstable angina (27,28). The underlying cause of thrombus formation links these observations to the concept of triggering. While examining serial histologic sections of occluded coronary arteries, Constantinides discovered that thrombus had formed over a ruptured atherosclerotic plaque in all cases he examined (29). A recent angiographic study supports this pathologic finding; contrast media out pouching, indicative of plaque rupture, was observed in patients who had undergone successful thrombolysis (30).

Two mechanisms of plaque rupture have been proposed (see Ch. 4): Constantinides has advanced the concept that the rupture occurs from the lumen *into the plaque* (29), while Barger et al have proposed that rupture may occur from the plaque *into the lumen* (31). The latter theory is based on the presence of extensive vasa vasorum in atherosclerotic plaques. Since these vessels may originate proximal to a coronary stenosis, under certain conditions their pressure could exceed that in the coronary lumen distal to the stenosis, leading to explosive rupture of the plaque into the lumen. Richardson et al (32) have recently reported that in 63% of cases, rupture of the plaque occurred at the junction of a lipid pool with normal tissue. Presence of a lipid core, a thin fibrous cap, and macrophage activity seem to be important factors that predispose an atherosclerotic plaque to disrupt (33). The recent finding that there is a spectrum of lesions from fibrous plaques composed predominantly of smooth muscle cells to lipid-rich lesions with numerous macrophages leads to the concept that inflammatory mechanisms modulate plaque morphology (34–36). Intrinsic plaque characteristics and extrinsic factors that predispose and initiate plaque rupture remain areas of intense investigation (37).

Although autopsy studies generally reveal severe atherosclerotic stenosis at the base of a fatal coronary thrombus (38), there is angiographic evidence that in many patients surviving a myocardial infarction, the degree of stenosis is relatively mild and obstructive thrombus accounts for the majority of the obstruction to blood flow. Brown et al reported that the degree of "original" stenosis in patients with myocardial infarction observed following treatment with streptokinase was <60% in two-thirds of the cases (39). Little et al recently studied the extent of prior stenosis at sites in the coronary arteries that subsequently became totally occluded. In two-thirds of the patients with mild to moderate coronary disease, the site of occlusion had less than a 50% stenosis on the preinfarction angiogram (40). Haft et al have also described "catastrophic" progression of coronary lesions (41), which presumably results from episodes of thrombosis. Rapold et al have reported signs of increased activity of the clotting system and platelets in patients with infarction later found to have no angiographically visible coronary atherosclerosis (42). These findings may explain the absence of prior symptoms in many patients presenting with acute myocardial infarction, and they indicate that attempts to identify and modify triggers of thrombus formation may have great clinical benefit (43).

MORNING INCREASE OF PHYSIOLOGICAL PROCESSES THAT MIGHT TRIGGER MYOCARDIAL INFARCTION

Morning accentuation of physiologic processes to which vulnerable atherosclerotic plaques are exposed, alone or in combination, could account for the morning increase in myocardial infarction onset (Figs. 5–1 and 5–2) through a variety of mechanisms.

The morning arterial pressure surge (44) could initiate plaque rupture. The coronary arterial tone increase (45) could worsen the flow reduction produced by a fixed stenosis. The arterial pressure increase and the coronary tone increase could result in increased shear stress (force directed against the endothelium resulting from increased coronary blood flow velocity) (46) predisposing to plaque rupture and increased platelet deposition (47). The increase in blood viscosity (48), increased platelet aggregability (49) (resulting from assumption of the upright posture) (50), and an insufficient countervailing increase in circulating t-PA activity (51–53) could produce a state of relative hypercoagulability. Such a thrombotic tendency could increase the likelihood that an otherwise harmless mural thrombus overlying a small plaque fissure would propagate and occlude the coronary lumen. Although serum cortisol levels are falling during the period of increased disease onset, they are increased above basal levels (54). This increase could enhance the sensitivity of the coronary arteries to the vasoconstrictor effects of catecholamines (55), which have a prominent surge after assumption of the upright posture (50).

Although a 24-hour periodicity of disease onset (Figs. 5–1 and 5–2) and physiologic processes is well established, the degree to which this periodicity results from a true, endogenous circadian rhythm versus the daily rest–activity cycle is only partially characterized. Cortisol secretion, for example, is well known to be an endogenous circadian process not dependent on daily activity (54), while the morning platelet aggregability increase is abolished if the subjects remain at bedrest (49,56). The rest–activity cycle appears to be a major determinant of disease onset, since adjustment for time of awakening shows that infarction onset (11) and increased transient ischemia (57) follow awakening, but such adjustment could also align the population for their endogenous circadian rhythms.

Although the peak incidence of disease onset occurs in the morning, it is likely that similar physiologic processes trigger disease onset at other times of the day. The peak morning incidence of infarct onset probably results from the synchronization of the population for triggers in the morning, while a secondary evening peak in infarct onset observed in the MILIS data may result from synchronization of the population for an additional trigger, such as the evening meal. For other periods of the day, exposure of the population to potential triggers is random, and no other prominent peaks of incidence are observed.

OTHER POTENTIAL TRIGGERING CYCLES

The circadian (24-hour) cycle is not the only cycle that may provide clues to triggering of disease onset; weekly (58,58a) and yearly (59–61) variation in the frequency of myocardial infarction have been reported. Thompson et al reported an excess frequency of myocardial infarction in men on Monday and a relatively high frequency on Saturday (58). In industrialized societies, work is organized on a weekly schedule with Mondays and Saturdays as transitions from leisure to work or work to leisure. The stress of adjustment to a change in activity may induce myocardial infarction.

Mortality from ischemic heart disease increases in the winter (59–61). Interestingly, the seasonal variation in heart disease mortality has been confirmed in the Southern Hemisphere with peak mortality occurring during June, July, and August (61–64). The reversal of seasonality between the hemispheres makes it likely that environmental factors underlie the observations (64).

"The heart does not like the cold," observed Vuori in his review of the effects of cold on the heart (65). Anderson and Rochard (66) observed that in men over 65 years, a 4.4°C decline in temperature within 24 hours was associated with a 16% increase in the number of sudden coronary deaths; an 8.3°C decline in temperature was associated with a 25% increase in sudden coronary death (Fig. 5–6). Their report also adds control data and quantitation to the well-accepted belief, based on anecdotes (67), that snow shoveling causes infarction. They found that on days when there was snowfall of

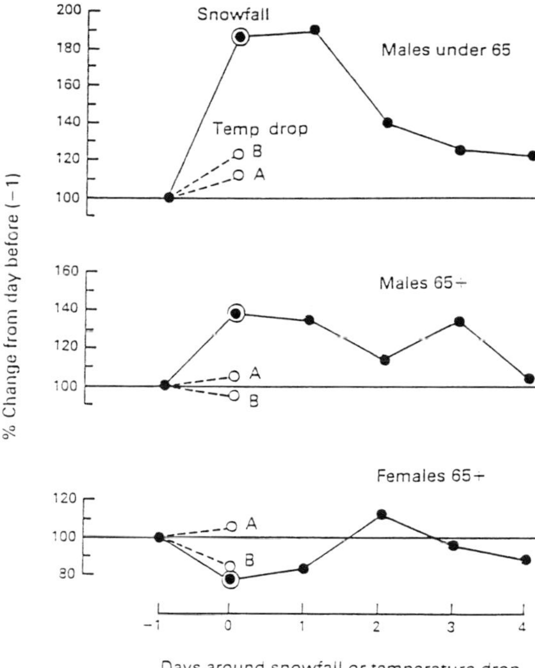

Figure 5–6. Daily rates of sudden death from ischemic heart disease (coroner's cases) in metropolitan Toronto expressed as percentages of rates on day preceding cold snap (temperature drop of 4.4°C to 8.3°C [A] or 8.8°C to 18.3°C [B]) or snowfall of 10.2 cm or more. *Reprinted with permission (66).*

10.2 cm or more, the mean daily rate of sudden death from ischemic heart disease in men under the age of 65 years was 2.67, or 88% higher than the base rate of 1.42 reported the day before the snowfall. The increase persisted for 1 day after the snowfall and decreased over the following 3 days, until by the fourth day, the incidence was only 25% higher than baseline (66). Giaconi et al have reported an annual increase in systemic arterial pressure during the winter months (68). Thus the winter increase in arterial pressure and ischemic heart disease onset appears to have a parallel relationship to the morning increase in arterial pressure and disease onset. Other parallel relationships are likely to be identified as this line of research is pursued.

There may also be unusual mechanisms of disease onset occurring in only a minority of the population, such as postural hypotension, which has been suggested as a trigger of stroke onset, causing decreased perfusion (69). Other possible triggering changes are those associated with acute infectious diseases (70,71).

TIMING AND TRIGGERS OF TRANSIENT MYOCARDIAL ISCHEMIA

Transient myocardial ischemia is more frequent and more easily studied than the cardiovascular catastrophes of myocardial infarction, sudden cardiac death, and stroke. Continuous Holter monitoring eliminates bias resulting from unobserved periods, allowing precise determination of the timing of transient myocardial ischemia. Such studies have consistently demonstrated a peak incidence of ischemic episodes between 6 AM and 12 noon (57,72,73). Furthermore, Rocco et al adjusted the time of ischemia for wake time; he demonstrated the increase in frequency occurs in the first 4 hours after awakening and initiating the day's activities (73), a finding similar to that reported for myocardial infarction onset (11).

Investigations of the possible triggers of transient ischemia have attempted to identify activities or pathophysiologic processes that occur immediately prior to ischemic episodes. When potential mental, as well as physical, causes of ischemia are considered, over half of transient ischemic episodes are preceded by possible triggering activities (74). Gottdiener et al recently demonstrated that patients with ischemia during mental stress testing also have increased ischemia during sedentary activities in daily life (75). In another recent study, Parker et al showed that delay of morning activity delays the onset of the transient ischemia peak (76).

ABILITY OF AGENTS THAT BLOCK POTENTIAL TRIGGERING PROCESSES TO PREVENT MYOCARDIAL INFARCTION

The theories advanced above are indirectly supported by the demonstrated efficacy of aspirin therapy and beta-adrenergic blockade in preventing myocardial infarction (77,78). Aspirin, presumably acting primarily as an antiplatelet agent, is thought to reduce the occurrence of sudden death and myocardial infarction by preventing coronary thrombosis. In the Physicians Health Study aspirin reduced the overall incidence of myocardial infarction by 44% (77). In a detailed analysis of this beneficial effect, Ridker et al found that aspirin exerted a selective effect—a 59% reduction—during the morning interval when platelet activity is increased (79). This prevention of infarction by elimination of a potential triggering mechanism—a platelet activity surge—supports the assertion that platelet activity surges are harmful, suggests that increased basal platelet activity in individuals is an unrecognized risk factor for infarction, and demonstrates the potential value of identifying triggering processes.

Beta-adrenergic blocking agents have been shown to prevent myocardial infarction and sudden cardiac death even though these agents do not have potent antithrombotic or antiarrhythmic properties. A clue to the mechanism is provided by the observations in the MILIS and the ISAM databases that beta-blockade eliminated the morning peak in incidence of myocardial infarction (7,8) (Fig. 5–7). Additionally, in the Beta Blocker Heart Attack Trial there was a morning increase in sudden cardiac death in the placebo group but not in the group randomly assigned to beta-blockade therapy, suggesting that the beneficial effect was achieved by blockade of the morning surge in sympathetic activity (80). A recent study has demonstrated that nadolol modifies hemodynamic responses to potential mental and physical triggers (81). Beta-blockade, but not a short-acting calcium blocker, has been shown to attenuate the morning increase in silent myocardial ischemia (82), and a recent review has summarized the inability of previously available calcium blocker preparations to provide a cardioprotective effect (83). It has been suggested that the beta blockers may prevent rupture of atherosclerotic plaques, just as they are considered to exert a beneficial effect in dissecting aneurysm by prevention of rupture of the aortic wall. With increased knowledge of triggering mechanisms, it is likely that the impressive gains already achieved by aspirin and beta-blockade therapy can be increased.

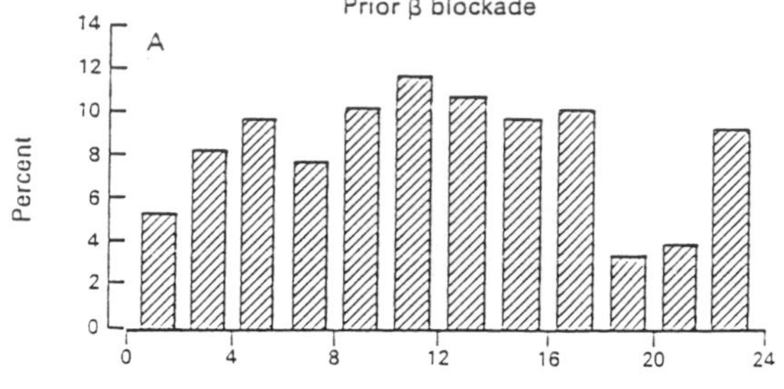

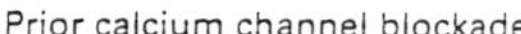

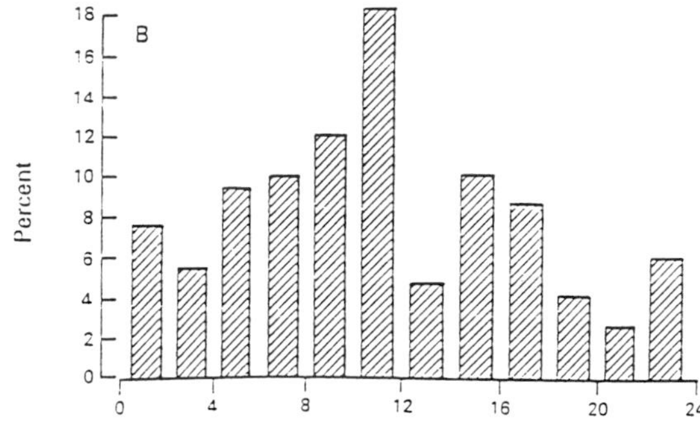

Figure 5–7. **A:** Bar graph of the incidence of myocardial infarction in the group of 206 patients in the ISAM Study receiving beta-adrenergic blocker therapy before their myocardial infarction. Morning incidence of myocardial infarction did not increase. Percentage of myocardial infarctions per 2-hour interval is indicated on the y axis, and the time of day is indicated on the x axis (military time). **B:** Bar graph of the incidence of myocardial infarction in the group of 147 patients receiving calcium antagonists before their myocardial infarction. Morning incidence of myocardial infarction increased ($p < 0.01$) similar to that observed in the total study population. *Reprinted with permission* (8).

GENERAL THEORY OF TRIGGERING OF CORONARY THROMBOSIS

The new information on triggering has provided the basis for a general theory of onset of coronary thrombosis (84). The hypothesis presented in Fig. 5–8 adds the concept of triggering activities to the general scheme of the role of thrombosis in the acute coronary syndromes advanced by Falk, Davies and Thomas, Fuster, Willerson, and others (37,38,85–88). It involves three important new concepts: *triggers, acute risk factors,* and *vulnerable plaques.*

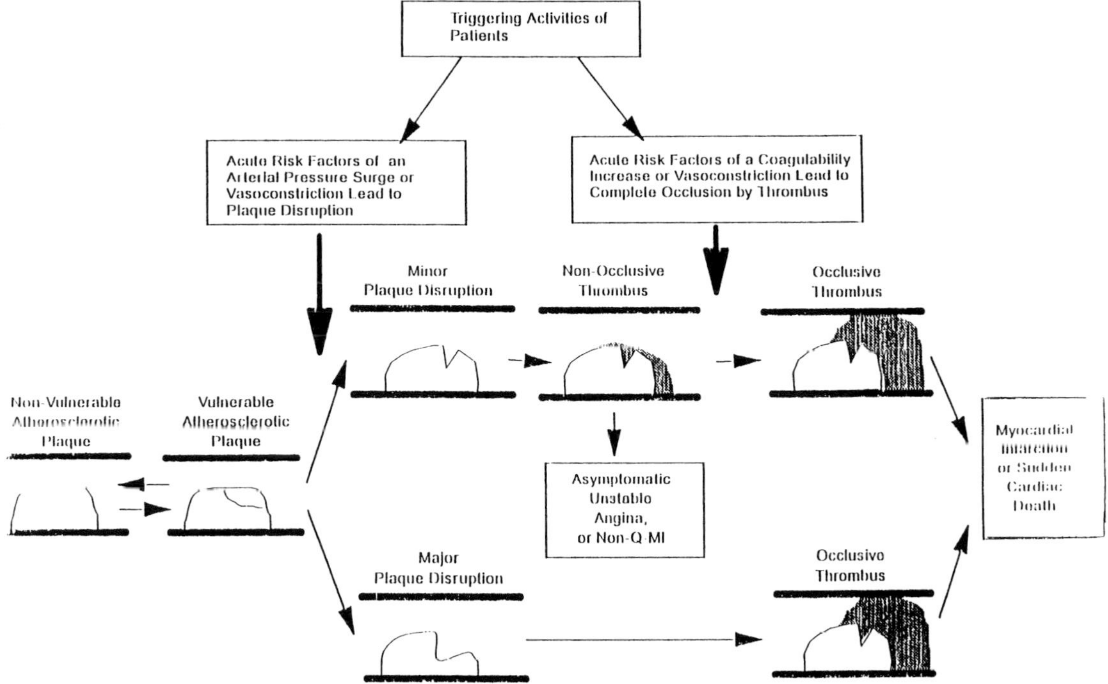

Figure 5–8. Illustration of a hypothetical method by which daily activities may trigger coronary thrombosis. Three triggering mechanisms are presented: (1) physical or mental stress producing hemodynamic changes leading to plaque rupture, (2) activities causing a coagulability increase, and (3) stimuli leading to vasoconstriction. The scheme depicting the role of coronary thrombosis in unstable angina, myocardial infarction, and sudden cardiac death has been well described by numerous authors. The novel portion of this figure is the addition of triggers. See text for detailed discussion. *Reprinted with permission* (84).

It is postulated that onset occurs when a "vulnerable" atherosclerotic plaque disrupts and occlusive thrombus formation occurs. Hemodynamic stresses may cause the disruption of the plaque; hemostatic and vasoconstrictive forces may then determine if the resultant thrombus is occlusive.

It is proposed that the initial step in the process is the development, with advancing age, of a vulnerable atherosclerotic plaque. Plaque vulnerability is defined functionally as the susceptibility of a plaque to disruption. Development of such vulnerability is a poorly understood process, but presumably it is a dynamic, potentially reversible disorder caused by several factors including changes in plaque constituents or its blood supply via vasa vasorum, and/or changes in the functional integrity of the overlying endothelium due in part to increased macrophage activity and thinning of the plaque collagen cap. The new catheterization laboratory techniques of intracoronary angioscopy and ultrasound may, in the future, permit detection of vulnerable plaques prior to their disruption.

Onset of MI might begin when a physical or mental stress produces a hemodynamic change that is sufficient to disrupt a vulnerable plaque. Vasoconstrictive and thrombogenic forces might then lead to coronary occlusion. Shear forces may also play an important role in thrombus formation, as suggested by Folts (88) and others.

The finding that disrupted plaques without thrombi are sometimes observed at autopsy in patients dying of noncardiac disease suggests that, in some cases, acute plaque disruption may not be the initial step in disease onset (89). In such patients the trigger may lead to occlusive thrombosis by causing an increase in thrombotic tendency, or vasoconstriction, in the presence of a previously nonthrombogenic plaque. It is also possible that the plaques became disrupted at the time of death, an occurrence perhaps more likely during a violent death. These possibilities underscore the need for studies of the lesions causing disease onset in living patients.

A synergistic combination of triggering activities may account for thrombosis in a setting in which each activity alone may not exceed the threshold for causation of infarction. For example, the combination of physical exertion (producing a minor plaque disruption) followed by cigarette smoking (producing an increase in coronary artery vasoconstriction and a relatively hypercoagulable state) (90) may be needed to cause occlusive thrombosis and disease onset. Also, the response to a potential trigger of a healthy individual may differ from that observed in an individual with a condition predisposing to MI. Exaggerated or paradoxical responses may be observed. For example, hypertensives demonstrate a greater increase in forearm vascular resistance after infusion of norepinephrine than normals (91). Patients with atherosclerosis may demonstrate a paradoxical vasoconstrictor response in response to acetylcholine infusion (92), and an impaired increase in fibrinolytic potential with exercise (93).

The findings of circadian variation and triggering have also led to the concept of an acute risk factor that supplements the traditional concept of a chronic risk factor. The acute risk factor is defined as the pathophysiologic change (vasoconstrictive, hemodynamic, or hemostatic) potentially leading to occlusive coronary thrombosis. The acute risk factor results from a combination of an external stress (physical or mental) and the individual's reactivity to that stress. While the extent of atherosclerosis changes slowly with time (chronic risk factor), hemodynamic, vasoconstrictive, and prothrombotic forces (acute risk factors) may be rapidly generated by external stresses.

SIGNIFICANCE

The primary immediate value of recognition of the circadian variation of acute onset of myocardial infarction is the emphasis that can be placed on pharmacologic protection during the morning hours for patients already receiving anti-ischemic therapy. Although no scientific studies have been performed to test the hypothesis, it seems reasonable that long-acting anti-ischemic agents would have an advantage over short-acting agents in providing protection against myocardial infarction in the morning when the effects of short-acting agents taken the night before may begin to wear off.

Even complete elimination of the morning increase in onset of myocardial infarction by effective therapy would prevent only a small fraction of the total morbidity and mortality caused by this disease. Although the incidence of disease onset is greatest in the 6 AM to noon period, the majority of infarcts occur at other times of the day, and their prevention requires a broader approach. For this reason, it is likely that the primary significance of the recognition of circadian variation of disease onset is the support it provides for the broader concept that the onset of infarction *at any time of the day* is frequently triggered by activities of the patient. This concept provides a number of clues to the mechanisms of disease onset—clues that suggest a value of studies ranging from the epidemiologic to the molecular level.

On the epidemiologic level, studies must be conducted in which patients who experience a nonfatal myocardial infarction are interviewed to determine if the event had an identifiable trigger. Since potentially triggering activities occur frequently without producing an event, the studies must be controlled for the frequency of potential triggers at times when an event did not occur.

The certainty with which an activity can be identified as a trigger will also vary in individual cases. In a patient whose plaque is only slightly vulnerable, the activity required to produce disease onset may be extreme, and the activity can be recognized as a trigger by its intensity. Other features that may aid in the recognition of an activity as a trigger are its occurrence immediately before the event, its ability to produce physiologic changes likely to trigger thrombosis, and its absence as part of the patient's routine activity. However, in a patient with an extremely vulnerable plaque, even nonstrenuous, routine, daily activities such as eating a heavy meal may be sufficient to trigger the cascade leading to infarction (94). In such instances, it may be impossible to identify the triggering activity even though it was present. Thus, the group of patients with *identifiable* triggers will be a subset of those in whom external triggering actually occurred.

On the clinical level, increased study of the relationship between daily activities and potentially triggering physiologic responses could clarify the manner in which these processes cause disease onset.

On the basic science level, there is a need for complete characterization of the control mechanisms of potentially adverse and beneficial physiologic processes. With improved understanding of these mechanisms, clinicians may eventually be able to eliminate unnecessary and potentially detrimental surges in arterial pressure, vasoconstriction, and coagulability that contribute to disease onset, and to increase the activity of potentially beneficial processes such as the fibrinolytic system. The factors determining plaque vulnerability require further characterization. The reduction in clinical events recently achieved by marked lowering of plasma cholesterol (94) might result not only from a reduced tendency to coronary artery stenosis, but also from a reduction in the formation of lipid pools within plaques that might increase the susceptibility of a plaque to rupture (32).

Greater understanding of triggering mechanisms should facilitate progress in the prevention of myocardial infarction. The means of prevention would not be to eliminate potential triggering activities—an undesirable and unattainable goal—but to design regimens that can be evaluated in randomized studies for their ability to sever the linkage between a potential triggering activity and development of myocardial infarction.

REFERENCES

1. Obraztsov VP, Strazhesko ND: The symptomatology and diagnosis of coronary thrombosis, Vorobeva VA, Konchalovski MP (eds): *Works of the First Congress of Russian Therapists.* Comradeship Typography of A. E. Mamontov, 1910, pp 26–43.
2. Fitzhugh G, Hamilton BE: Coronary occlusion and fatal angina pectoris. Study of the immediate causes and their prevention. *JAMA* 1993;100:475–480.
3. Sproul J: A general practitioner's views on the treatment of angina pectoris. *N Engl J Med* 1936;215: 443–452.
4. Parkinson J, Bedford DE: Cardiac infarction and coronary thrombosis. *Lancet* 1928;1:4–11.
5. Phipps C: Contributory causes of coronary thrombosis. *JAMA* 1936;106:761–762.
6. Master AM: The role of effort and occupation (including physicians) in coronary occlusion. *JAMA* 1960;174:942–948.
7. Muller JE, Stone PH, Turi ZG, et al, and the MILIS Study Group: Circadian variation in the frequency of onset of acute myocardial infarction. *N Engl J Med* 1985;313:1315–1322.
8. Willich SN, Linderer T, Wegscheider K, et al, and the ISAM Study Group: Increased morning incidence of myocardial infarction in the ISAM Study: Absence with prior beta-adrenergic blockade. *Circulation* 1989;80:853–858.
9. Thompson DR, Blandford RL, Sutton TW, Marchant PR: Time of onset of chest pain in acute myocardial infarction. *Int J Cardiol* 1985;7:139–146.
10. Hjalmarson A, Gilpin E, Nicod P, et al: Differing circadian patterns of symptom onset in subgroups of patients with acute myocardial infarction. *Circulation* 1989;80:267–275.
11. Goldberg R, Brady P, Muller JE, et al: Time of onset of symptoms of acute myocardial infarction. *Am J Cardiol* 1990;66:140–144.
12. Muller JE, Ludmer PL, Willich SN, et al: Circadian variation in the frequency of sudden cardiac death. *Circulation* 1987;75:131–138.
13. Willich SN, Levy D, Rocco MB, Tofler GH, Stone PH, Muller JE: Circadian variation in the incidence of sudden cardiac death in the Framingham Heart Study Population. *Am J Cardiol* 1987;60: 801–806.
14. French AJ, Dock W: Fatal coronary arteriosclerosis in young soldiers. *JAMA* 1944;124:1233–1237.
15. Moritz AR, Zamcheck N: Sudden and unexpected deaths of young soldiers. Diseases responsible for such deaths during World War II. *Arch Pathol* 1946; 42:459–494.
16. Tsementzis SA, Gill JS, Hitchcock ER, Gill SK, Beevers DG: Diurnal variation of and activity during the onset of stroke. *Neurosurgery* 1985;17:901–904.
17. Marler JR, Price TR, Clark GL, et al: Morning increase in onset of ischemic stroke. *Stroke* 1989;20: 473–476.

18. Sumiyoshi T, Haze K, Saito M, Fukami K, Goto Y, Hiramori K: Evaluation of clinical factors involved in onset of myocardial infarction. *Jpn Circ J* 1986;50: 164–173.
19. Tofler GH, Stone PH, Maclure M, et al, and the MILIS Study Group: Analysis of possible triggers of acute myocardial infarction (MILIS Study). *Am J Cardiol* 1990;66:22–27.
20. Maclure M: The case-crossover design: A method for studying transient effects on the risk of acute events. *Am J Epidemiol* 1991;133:144–153.
21. Mittleman MA, Maclure M, Tofler GH, et al, for the Determinants of Myocardial Infarction Onset Study Investigators: Triggering of acute myocardial infarction by heavy physical exertion: Protection against triggering by regular exertion. *N Engl J Med* 1993; 329:1677–1683.
22. Willich SN, Lewis SM, Lowel H, Arntz HR, Schubert F, Schroder R: Physical exertion as a trigger of acute myocardial infarction. Triggers and mechanisms of Myocardial Infarction Study Group. *N Engl J Med* 1993;329:1684–1690.
23. Eaker ED: Use of questionnaires, interviews and psychological tests in epidemiologic studies of coronary heart disease. *Eur Heart J* 1988;9:698–704.
24. Mittleman MA, Maclure M, Sherwood JB, et al: Triggering of acute myocardial infarction onset by episodes of anger. *Circulation* 1995;92:1720–1725.
25. Muller JE, Maclure M, Mittleman M, Sherwood J, Tofler GH, for the ONSET Study Investigators: Risk of myocardial infarction doubles in the two hours after sexual activity but absolute risk remains low. *Circulation* 1993;88(Suppl I):I-509.
26. DeWood MA, Spores J, Notske R, et al: Prevalence of total coronary occlusion during the early hours of transmural myocardial infarction. *N Engl J Med* 1980;303:897–902.
27. Ambrose JA, Winters SL, Stern A, et al: Angiographic morphology and the pathogenesis of unstable angina pectoris. *J Am Coll Cardiol* 1985;5: 609–616.
28. Sherman CT, Litvack F, Grundfest W, et al: Coronary angioscopy in patients with unstable angina pectoris. *N Engl J Med* 1986;315:913–919.
29. Constantinides P: Plaque fissure in human coronary thrombosis. *J Atheroscler Res* 1966;6:1–17.
30. Nakagawa S, Hanada Y, Koiwaya Y, Tanaka K: Angiographic features in the infarct-related artery after intracoronary urokinase followed by prolonged anticoagulation: Role of ruptured atheromatous plaque and adherent thrombus in acute myocardial infarction in vivo. *Circulation* 1988;78: 1335–1344.
31. Barger AC, Beeuwkes R, Lainey LL, Silverman KJ: Hypothesis: Vasa vasorum and neovascularization of human coronary arteries. *N Engl J Med* 1984; 310: 175–177.
32. Richardson PD, Davies MJ, Born GVR: Influence of plaque configuration and stress distribution on fissuring of coronary atherosclerotic plaques. *Lancet* 1989;2:941–944.
33. Falk E: Why do plaques rupture? *Circulation* 1992;86 (Suppl III):III-30–III-42.
34. van der Wal AC, Becker AE, van der Loos CM, Das PK: Site of intimal rupture or erosion of thrombosed coronary atherosclerotic plaques is characterized by an inflammatory process irrespective of the dominant plaque morphology. *Circulation* 1994;89: 36–44.
35. Fernandez-Ortiz A, Badimon JJ, Falk E, et al: Characterization of the relative thrombogenecity of atherosclerotic plaque components: Implications for consequences of plaque rupture. *J Am Coll Cardiol* 1994;23:1562–1569.
36. Alexander RW: Inflammation and coronary artery disease. *N Engl J Med* 1994;331:468–469.
37. Fuster V, Badimon L, Badimon JJ, Chesebro JH: The pathogenesis of coronary artery disease and the acute coronary syndromes. *N Engl J Med* 1992;326: 242–250.
38. Falk E: Plaque rupture with severe pre-existing stenosis precipitating coronary thrombosis. *Br Heart J* 1983;50:127–134.
39. Brown BG, Gallery CA, Badger RS, et al: Incomplete lysis of thrombus in the moderate underlying atherosclerotic lesion during intracoronary infusion of streptokinase for acute myocardial infarction: Quantitative angiographic observations. *Circulation* 1986;73:653 661.
40. Little WL, Constantinescu M, Applegate RJ, et al: Can coronary angiography predict the site of a subsequent myocardial infarction in patients with mild-to-moderate coronary artery disease? *Circulation* 1988;78:1157–1166.
41. Haft JI, Haik BJ, Goldstein JE: Catastrophic progression of coronary artery lesions, the common

mechanism for coronary disease progression (abstract). *Circulation* 1987;76(Suppl IV):IV–168.

42. Rapold HJ, Haeberli A, Kuemmerli H, Weiss M, Baur HR, Straub WP: Fibrin formation and platelet activation in patients with myocardial infarction and normal coronary arteries. *Eur Heart J* 1989;10: 323–333.
43. Oliver MF: Prevention of coronary heart disease—propaganda, promises, problems, and prospects. *Circulation* 1986;73:1–9.
44. Millar-Craig MW, Bishop CN, Raferty EB: Circadian variation in blood pressure. *Lancet* 1978;1: 795–797.
45. Fujita M, Franklin D: Diurnal changes in coronary blood flow in conscious dogs. *Circulation* 1987;76: 488–491.
46. Vita JA, Treasure CB, Ganz P, Cox DA, Fish RD, Selwyn AP: Control of shear stress in the epicardial coronary arteries of humans: Impairment by atherosclerosis. *J Am Coll Cardiol* 1989;14:1193–1199.
47. Badimon L, Badimon JJ: Mechanisms of arterial thrombosis in nonparallel streamlines: Platelet thrombi grow on the apex of stenotic severely injured vessel wall: Experimental study in pig model. *J Clin Invest* 1989;4:1134–1144.
48. Ehrly AM, Jung G: Circadian rhythm of human blood viscosity. *Biorheology* 1973;10:577–583.
49. Tofler GH, Brezinski DA, Schafer AI, et al: Concurrent morning increase in platelet aggregability and the risk of myocardial infarction and sudden cardiac death. *N Engl J Med* 1987;316:1514–1518.
50. Brezinski DA, Tofler GH, Muller JE, et al: Morning increase in platelet aggregability: Association with assumption of the upright posture. *Circulation* 1988; 78:35–40.
51. Rosing DR, Brakman P, Redwood DR, et al: Blood fibrinolytic activity in man: Diurnal variation and the response to varying intensities of exercise. *Circ Res* 1970;27:171–184.
52. Andreotti F, Davies GJ, Hackett DR, et al: Major circadian fluctuations in fibrinolytic factors and possible relevance to time of onset of myocardial infarction, sudden cardiac death, and stroke. *Am J Cardiol* 1988;62:635–637.
53. Speiser W, Langer W, Pschaick A, et al: Increased blood fibrinolytic activity after physical exercise: Comparative study in individuals with different sporting activities and in patients after myocardial infarction taking part in a rehabilitation sports program. *Thromb Res* 1988;51:543–555.
54. Weitzman ED, Fukushima D, Nogeire C, Roffwarg H, Gallagher TF, Hellman L: Twenty-four hour pattern of the episodic secretion of cortisol in normal subjects. *J Clin Endocrinol* 1971;33:14–22.
55. Sudhir K, Jennings GL, Esler MD, et al: Hydrocortisone-induced hypertension in humans: Pressor responsiveness and sympathetic function. *Hypertension* 1989;13:416–421.
56. Winther K, Hillegass W, Tofler GH, et al: Effects of platelet aggregation and fibrinolytic activity during upright posture and exercise in healthy men. *Am J Cardiol* 1992;70:1051–1055.
57. Nademanee K, Intarachot V, Josephson MA, Singh BN: Circadian variation in occurrence of transient overt and silent myocardial ischemia in chronic stable angina and comparison with Prinzmetal's angina in men. *Am J Cardiol* 1987;60:494–498.
58. Thompson DR, Pohl JEE, Sutton TW: Acute myocardial infarction and day of the week. *Am J Cardiol* 1992;69:266–267.
58a. Willich SN, Lowel H, Lewis M, Hormann A, Arntz HR, Keil U. Weekly variation of acute myocardial infarction. Increased Monday risk in the working population. *Circulation* 1994;90:87–93.
59. Bull GM: Meteorological correlates with myocardial and cerebral infarction and respiratory disease. *Br J Prev Soc Med* 1973;27:108–113.
60. Rose G: Cold weather and ischaemic heart disease. *Br J Prev Soc Med* 1966;20:97–100.
61. Ornato JP, Siegel L, Craren EJ, Nelson N: The seasonal incidence of death due to acute myocardial infarction. *Cor Art Dis* 1990;1:199–203.
62. Scragg R: Seasonal variation of mortality in Queensland. *Community Health Stud* 1982;6: 120–129.
63. Marshall RJ, Scragg R, Bourke P: An analysis of the seasonal variation of coronary heart disease and respiratory disease mortality in New Zealand. *Int J Epidemiol* 1988;17:325–331.
64. Douglas AS, Russell D, Allan TM: Seasonal, regional and secular variations of cardiovascular and cerebrovascular mortality in New Zealand. *Aust NZ J Med* 1990;20:669–676.
65. Vuori I: The heart and the cold. *Ann Clin Res* 1987;19:156–162.

66. Anderson TW, Rochard C: Cold snaps, snowfall and sudden death from ischemic heart disease. *Can Med Assoc J* 1979;121:1580–1583.
67. Muller JE, Tofler GH, Edelman E: Probable triggers of onset of acute myocardial infarction. *Clin Cardiol* 1989;12:473–475.
68. Giaconi S, Ghione S, Palombo C, et al: Seasonal influences on blood pressure in high normal to mild hypertensive range. *Hypertension* 1989;14:22–27.
69. Dobkin BH: Orthostatic hypotension as a risk factor for symptomatic occlusive cerebrovascular disease. *Neurology* 1989;39:30–34.
70. Spodick DH, Flessas AP, Johnson MM: Association of acute respiratory symptoms with onset of acute myocardial infarction: Prospective investigation of 150 consecutive patients and matched control patients. *Am J Cardiol* 1984;53:481–482.
71. Saikku P, Leinonen M, Tenkanen L, et al: Chronic *Chlamydia pneumoniae* infection as a risk factor for coronary heart disease in the Helsinki Heart Study. *Ann Intern Med* 1992;116:273–278.
72. Selwyn AP, Shea M, Deanfield JE, Wilson R, Horlock P: Character of transient ischemia in angina pectoris. *Am J Cardiol* 1986;58:21B–25B.
73. Rocco MB, Barry J, Campbell S, et al: Circadian variation of transient myocardial ischemia in patients with coronary artery disease. *Circulation* 1987;75:395–400.
74. Barry J, Selwyn AP, Nabel EG, et al: Frequency of ST-segment depression produced by mental stress in stable angina pectoris from coronary artery disease. *Am J Cardiol* 1988;61:989–993.
75. Gottdiener JS, Krantz DS, Howell RH, et al: Induction of silent myocardial ischemia with mental stress testing: Relation to the triggers of ischemia during daily life activities and to ischemic functional severity. *J Am Coll Cardiol* 1994;24: 1645–1651.
76. Parker JD, Testa MA, Jimenez AH, et al: Morning increase in ambulatory ischemia in patients with stable coronary artery disease. Importance of physical activity and increased cardiac demand. *Circulation* 1994;89:604–614.
77. The Steering Committee of the Physicians' Health Study Research Group: Final report on the aspirin component of the ongoing Physicians' Health Study. *N Engl J Med* 1989;321:129–135.
78. Beta-Blocker Heart Attack Trial Research Group: A randomized trial of propranolol in patients with acute myocardial infarction. Mortality results. *JAMA* 1982;247:1707–14.
79. Ridker PM, Manson JE, Buring JE, Muller JE, Hennekens CH: Circadian variation of acute myocardial infarction and the effect of low-dose aspirin in a randomized trial of physicians. *Circulation* 1990;82: 897–902.
80. Peters RW, Muller JE, Goldstein S, Byington R, Friedman LM: Propranolol and the morning increase in the frequency of sudden cardiac death (the BHAT Study) *Am J Cardiol* 1989;63: 1518–1521.
81. Jimenez AH, Tofler GH, Chen X, Stubbs ME, Solomon HS, Muller JE: Effects of nadolol on hemodynamic and hemostatic responses to potential mental and physical triggers of myocardial infarction in subjects with mild systemic hypertension. *Am J Cardiol* 1993;72:47–52.
82. Mulcahy D, Keegan J, Cunningham D, et al: Circadian variation of total ischemic burden and its alteration with anti-anginal agents. *Lancet* 1988;2: 755–759.
83. Held Ph, Yusuf S, Furberg CD: Calcium channel blockers in acute myocardial infarction and unstable angina: An overview. *Br Med J* 1989;299: 1187–1192.
84. Muller JE, Abela GS, Nesto RW, Tofler GH: Triggers, acute risk factors, and vulnerable plaques: The lexicon of a new frontier. *J Am Coll Cardiol* 1994;23: 809–813.
85. Davies MJ, Thomas AC: Thrombosis and acute coronary artery lesions in sudden cardiac ischemic death. *N Engl J Med* 1984;310:1137–1140.
86. Ip JH, Fuster V, Badimon L, Badimon J, Taubman MB, Chesebro JH: Syndromes of accelerated atherosclerosis: Role of vascular injury and smooth muscle cell proliferation. *J Am Coll Cardiol* 1990;15: 1667–1687.
87. Willerson JT, Campbell WB, Winniford MD, et al: Conversion from chronic to acute coronary artery disease: Speculation regarding mechanisms (editorial). *Am J Cardiol* 1984;54:1349–1354.
88. Coller BS, Folts JD, Smith SR, Scudder LE, Jordan R: Abolition of in vivo platelet thrombus formation in primates with monoclonal antibodies to the platelet GPIIb/IIIA receptor. Correlation with bleeding time, platelet aggregation, and blockade of GPIIb/IIIa receptors. *Circulation* 1989;80: 1766–1774.

89. Arbustini E, Grass M, Diegoli M, et al: Coronary thrombosis in non-cardiac death. *Cor Art Dis* 1993;4: 751–759.
90. Belch JJF, McArdle BM, Burns P, Lowe GDO, Forbes CD: The effects of acute smoking on platelet behaviour, fibrinolysis, and haemorheology in habitual smokers. *Thromb Haemost* 1984; 51:6–8.
91. Egan B, Schork N, Panis R, Hinderliter A: Vascular structure enhances regional resistance responses in mild essential hypertension. *J Hypertens* 1988;6: 41–48.
92. Ludmer PL, Selwyn AP, Shook TL, et al: Paradoxical vasoconstriction induced by acetylcholine in atherosclerotic coronary arteries. *N Engl J Med* 1986; 315:1046–1051.
93. Khann PK, Seth HN, Balasubramanian V, Hoon RS: Effect of submaximal exercise on fibrinolytic activity in ischemic heart disease. *Br Med J* 1975;2: 910–912.
94. Brown G, Albers JJ, Fisher LD, et al: Regression of coronary artery disease as a result of intensive lipid-lowering therapy in men with high levels of apolipoprotein B. *N Engl J Med* 1990;323:1289–1298.

6

The Changing Natural History and Prognosis of Acute Myocardial Infarction

Robin M. Norris, MD, FRCP, FRACP

Mortality from coronary heart disease continues to fall. Figures 6–1a and b show that age-adjusted death rates from ischemic heart disease have declined in the United States in both sexes by approximately 65% from the peak levels of 25 years ago (2, 80, 81). The decline has been steady at about 4% per year from 1968 to 1992, and there is no evidence that the rate has slowed.

Data from most but not all other countries show a similar but smaller decline. Thus mortality has fallen by approximately 30% in the United Kingdom, and the decline started nearly 10 years later than in the U.S.A. However in some countries in Eastern Europe, mortality rates from coronary heart disease are increasing (Figures 6–2a and 6–2b).

How much of the decline in mortality rate in Western countries can be explained by improvement in prognosis after acute myocardial infarction? Between 1985 and 1990 mortality from coronary heart disease fell by 25% for both men and women in the Minneapolis and St. Paul metropolitan area. This was explained by both a declining incidence of myocardial infarction in the population and the improved survival of patients with myocardial infarction (103). The decline in incidence is consistent with continuing improvements in the risk-factor profile in regard to cardiovascular disease. It is likely that the marked improvement in both short-term and long-term survival among patients hospitalized for myocardial infarction results from the greater use of newer forms of therapy which have been shown to be of benefit e.g. acute reperfusion, aspirin, anticoagulants, beta-blockers etc.

In discussing changes in the natural history and prognosis of acute myocardial infarction it is appropriate to take as a starting point the decade of the 1960s. At that time mortality from ischemic heart disease was at its peak, and attitudes toward treatment of acute myocardial infarction tended to be nihilistic. The earlier wave of enthusiasm for anticoagulants (3) was being replaced by skepticism (4), cardiopulmonary resuscitation was a novelty, coronary care units were still in the experimental phase and established in only a few hospitals (5), and little attention was paid to risk factors, particularly for patients with established ischemic heart disease.

SHORT-TERM AND HOSPITAL COURSE OF ACUTE MYOCARDIAL INFARCTION

During a one-year period, 1966–67, we described the mortality of all 757 patients with acute myo-

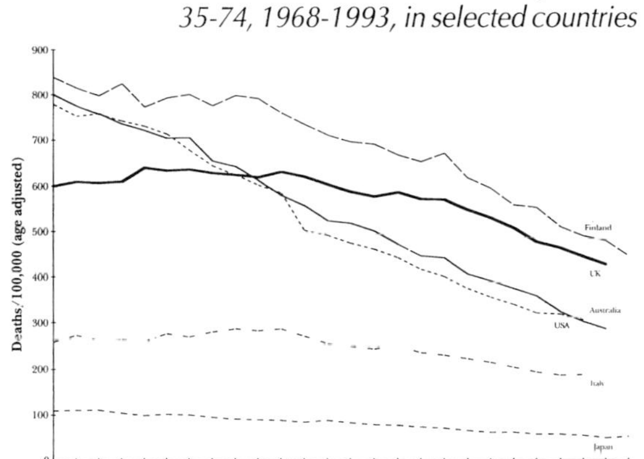

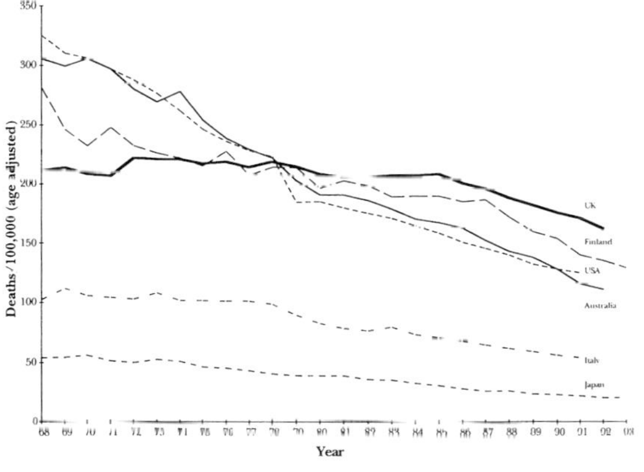

Figure 6–1. Death rates from coronary heart disease (A) in men and (B) in women aged 35–74 years in selected countries. Reproduced with permission from British Heart Foundation, Coronary Heart Disease Statistics 1996.

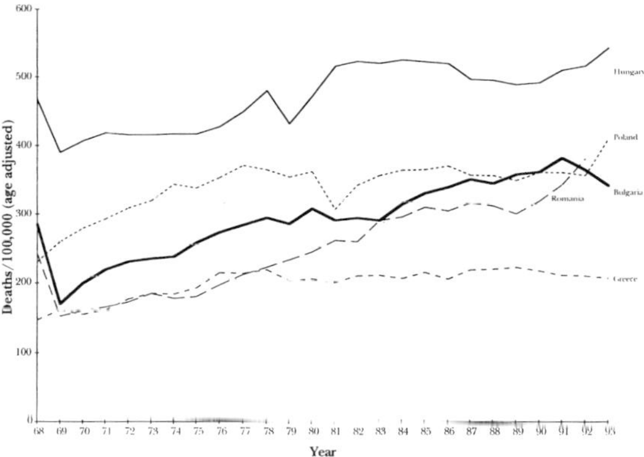

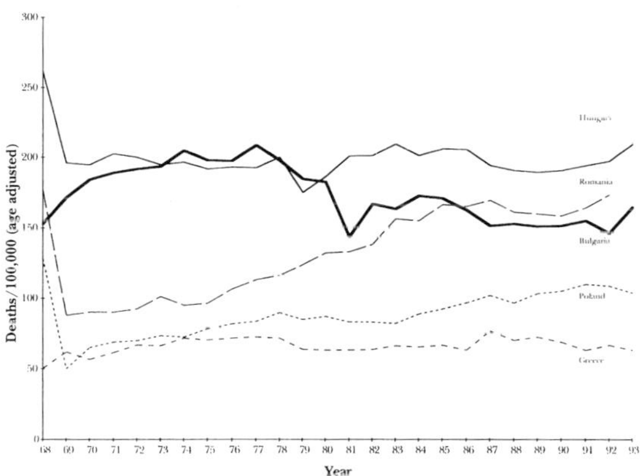

Figure 6–2. Death rates from coronary heart disease (A) in men and (B) in women aged 35–74 years in selected East European countries in which rates are rising. Reproduced with permission from British Heart Foundation, Coronary Heart Disease Statistics, 1996.

cardial infarction who were admitted to hospitals in Auckland, New Zealand (6–8), and we followed their progress at 3 years (9), 6 years (10), and 15 years (11) after the index infarction. During that year there was no coronary care unit in Auckland, and although 6 patients were resuscitated from ventricular fibrillation at one of the participating hospitals, they were considered as having died for the purposes of the mortality analysis. Twenty-six percent of these patients died in hospital (6); hospital mortality for patients under 70 years of age was 22% (7). Fifty-two percent of these deaths were due to arrhythmias or presumed arrhythmias, and of these, two-thirds occurred from the fourth day of hospital admission onward (6). This pattern of mortality was similar to that which had been described from other centers during the pre–coronary care era (12,13).

Although introduction of coronary care units during the 1960s and early 1970s was a revolution in treatment that was enthusiastically adopted by most cardiologists (5,14), the value of hospital-based coronary care was contested by some studies of the patients who were randomized to home or hospital care (15,16). The weaknesses of these studies were that only a proportion of patients who were originally seen could be treated at random, and that randomization was carried out on patients who had already survived several hours after the onset on infarction. In 1996 no one would doubt the efficacy of early hospital-based coronary care, together with prehospital coronary care carried out by trained paramedics (17). By comparing patients treated in a coronary care unit with a group treated in our hospital wards during the year before the coronary care unit opened, we were able to show that hospital mortality was reduced significantly (from 31% to 12%) by coronary care for that group of patients (about one-third of the total) who had infarction of moderate severity as judged by a coronary prognostic index (8).

Total hospital mortality for patients under 70 years of age was reduced from 22% to 17% in our coronary care unit during 1967–1968 (8), and mortality declined further to 13% by 1977–1979 (18). The major reason for this decline was the reduction in "arrhythmic" deaths resulting from ventricular fibrillation from 52% to 12% of all deaths (Fig. 6–3) (19). In the early years of coronary care, mortality from cardiac failure and cardiogenic shock was not considered to have been reduced, and this was our own experience, as shown in Fig. 6–3. Moreover the early wave of enthusiasm for prophylactic antiarrhythmic treatment for prevention of ventricular fibrillation (5) waned when it was shown, through tape recordings of arrhythmias, that the relationship between so-called "warning arrhythmias" and ventricular fibrillation was frequently absent (20); of 13 randomized clinical trials of intravenous lidocaine for prevention of ventricular fibrillation, only 2 showed a positive result (21). A later meta-analysis of the results of 11 randomized controlled trials showed a small reduction in the incidence of ventricular fibrillation as a result of the use of lidocaine; however, this was offset by an increase in the incidence of asystole (22,23) (see Chs. 3 and 14). Thus, during the early 1970s, it appeared that the coronary care unit reduced mortality predominantly through electrocardiographic monitoring, close observation by nurses, and effective use of the defibrillator.

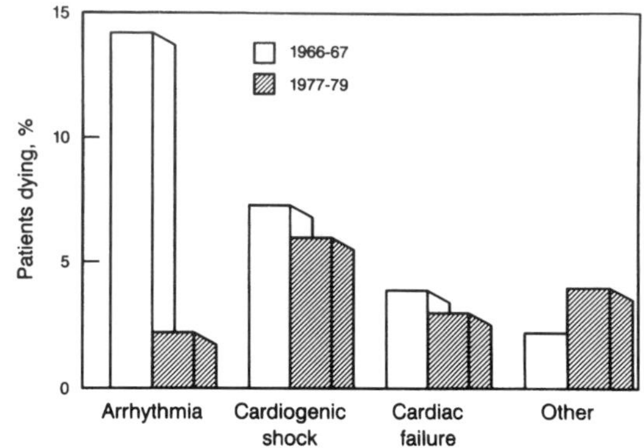

Figure 6–3. Comparison of mortality from arrhythmia, cardiogenic shock, cardiac failure, and other causes (principally cardiac rupture) in 767 patients admitted to hospitals in Auckland during 1966–1967, before the opening of coronary care units (6), with mortality of 574 patients treated in the coronary care unit at Green Lane Hospital during 1977–1979 (18). *Reproduced from Myocardial Infarction: Its Presentation, Pathogenesis, and Treatment. Edinburgh, Churchill Livingstone, 1982, with permission.*

During the 1970s, however, two major developments set the stage for further reductions in hospital mortality from acute myocardial infarction. First, use of the Swan–Ganz catheter allowed classification of acute myocardial infarction into hemodynamic subsets (24) and allowed prognosis to be predicted accurately by the patient's hemodynamic status (25). It was shown that the heart undergoing infarction functions best at a moderately high filling pressure (26), and that when the filling pressure is low (as with right ventricular infarction) the patient should be treated with transfusion, not diuretics (27). Although relatively few lives have probably been saved by the use of the Swan–Ganz catheter, and mortality may even have been increased by its indiscriminate use (28), the concepts introduced have been invaluable.

The second major development during the 1970s comprised the initial attempts to treat the process of myocardial infarction itself, not just its complications. The idea that myocardial infarct size could be limited by reduction of myocardial oxygen demand (29) or by restoration of oxygen supply by reperfusion (30) originated in the experimental animal laboratory, and it was not until some years later that evidence for limitation of infarct size by use of intravenous beta blockers was reported in randomized clinical trials in patients (31,32) (see Ch. 12). Later, a very large clinical trial of intravenous beta-blockade, the First International Study of Infarct Survival (ISIS-I) (33), showed that hospital mortality was modestly reduced by intravenous administration of atenolol (from about 5% to 4%) in that subset of patients who did not have contraindications to beta-blockade on admission to the coronary care unit. Retrospective analysis of the ISIS I data showed that the reduction in mortality obtained by use of atenolol may have been achieved by prevention of cardiac rupture on the first day after infarction (34); however, intravenous beta-blockade, rather surprisingly, never became popular, and the results reported in a large trial of intravenous metoprolol given in conjunction with thrombolysis were equivocal and difficult to interpret (35,36). Thus reduction of myocardial oxygen demand by intravenous beta-blockade has not been a factor in the decline in early mortality from acute myocardial infarction that has occurred since the 1960s. By contrast, reduction of mortality by administration of oral beta blockers for 1 to 3 years after completion of the index infarct (37–39) has almost certainly been a factor in the improvement in late mortality that has occurred over the same period (see Ch. 12).

Notwithstanding the preceding points, we (18,40) and others (41,42) reported a continued decline in hospital mortality for patients treated in coronary care units during the 1970s and early 1980s. The reason for this decline is uncertain. It may have resulted from the increasing experience gained in the treatment of arrhythmias in the coronary care unit and the better understanding and more prompt treatment of the hemodynamic complications (43). It is also possible that the decline was illusory and due to case selection.

The next breakthrough in the treatment of myocardial infarction was the use of thrombolytic therapy (see Ch. 19). The success of intracoronary streptokinase (44) was followed by reports of equivalent benefit from intravenous streptokinase, both in reduction of mortality rate (45,46) and in limitation of myocardial damage in survivors (47). Later, similar benefits were shown for tissue plasminogen activator, the naturally occurring activator of the fibrinolytic system, made by recombinant DNA technology (48,49).

Controversy followed about the relative advantages of streptokinase (SK) and recombinant tissue-type plasminogen activator (r-tPA). Although the initial study showed a clear advantage for r-tPA with respect to patency of the infarct-related coronary artery at 90 minutes after administration (50), two subsequent large international multicenter trials (51,52) failed to show a corresponding advantage for t-PA over SK in mortality reduction. Because of continued uncertainty, a third large international trial (GUSTO) was mounted; this included a subset of patients studied by angiography, and r-tPA was given in an accelerated dosage regimen with intravenous heparin. This study, which included 41,021 patients, showed a clear advantage for accelerated t-PA with heparin in preventing 1 further death for every 100 patients treated (53). The angiographic substudy, which recruited 2,431 patients (54), confirmed what had long been suspected but never formally proved; both reduction in mortality from acute myocardial infarction and preservation of left ventricular function depend on early restoration of flow through the infarct-related artery. Even though accelerated r-tPA restored flow more rapidly than SK, its efficacy was not ideal; only 54% of patients had complete reperfusion at 90 minutes after starting infusion of the drug.

If the best currently available thrombolytic drug is still imperfect, would mechanical revascularization by balloon angioplasty be even better? Two reports have claimed that it is (55,56), but the treatment is available in so few centers that it is unlikely to have a global impact on survival. Although accelerated t-PA with aspirin is now the treatment of choice in most U.S. centers, streptokinase is still favored in most other countries worldwide because of its lesser cost and slightly better safety profile (53). The aim now is to improve thrombolytic therapy further with a continued search for better thrombolytic and adjuvant agents and, even more important, to improve triage and reduce delay from the time that symptoms start to the time of administration of treatment.

What has been the effect of thrombolytic therapy on early survival from hospitalized myocardial infarction? A meta-analysis of the results of all comparative trials of thrombolytic drugs versus placebo that involved more than 1,000 patients (58,600 in all) has been published recently (57). Results showed that although patients of all age groups received benefit, age rather than thrombolytic therapy was still the most important prognostic factor. Thirty-five-day mortality for the under 65 year age group who received thrombolytic therapy ($n = 17{,}993$) was 5.5%; for those in the under 75 year age group ($n = 26{,}480$) it was 8.0%, and for patients of all ages ($n = 29{,}315$) it was 9.6%. Most of the large trials of course included many patients who were shown not to benefit from thrombolytic therapy. Those trials with entry restricted to patients who benefit the most (those with prolonged chest pain and ST segment elevation treated within 6 hours of onset) tended to show an even lower mortality rate within the range 3–5% for patients under 70 years of age (35,58,59).

Not only is mortality reduced by thrombolytic therapy, but morbidity has also been decreased. The incidence of cardiac failure, ventricular fibrillation, and severe conduction disturbances requiring transvenous pacing have all been reduced, with consequent reduction in the length of hospital stay in many cases. Figure 6–4 shows that the proportion of patients with left ventricular ejection fraction ≤40% at 3 to 4 weeks after infarction [a group with a known high late mortality rate (60)] was reduced from about 20% to under 10% as a result of thrombolysis.

Assuming a 5% 30-day mortality rate for patients under 70 years of age who present within 6 hours of onset of infarction with ST segment elevation and are appropriately treated with thrombolytic therapy, the dotted line in Fig. 6–5 shows the remarkable decline in mortality that is now, in theory, achievable. In many parts of the world, unfortunately, mortality is nowhere near as low as this. This is shown by the continuous line in Fig. 6–5, and reasons for the disparity are discussed in the next section.

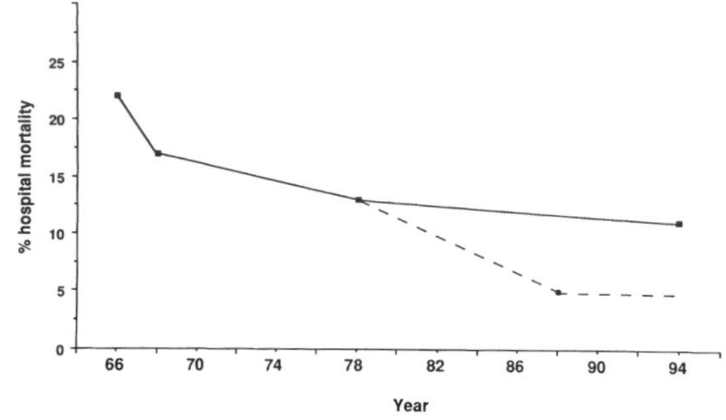

Figure 6–4. Introduction of thrombolysis reduced the proportion of patients with ejection fraction ≤40% measured at 3 to 4 weeks after the first transmural myocardial infarction from approximately 20% to less than 10%. Patients studied between 1977 and 1982 were consecutive male patients under 60 years of age who were enrolled in a study of prognosis and coronary surgery (60); those studied between 1984 and 1986 and from 1986 to 1988 took part in trials of thrombolysis (47, 47a). All patients had an ejection fraction ≤40% after a first transmural myocardial infarction. SK = streptokinase, t-PA = tissue plasminogen activator.

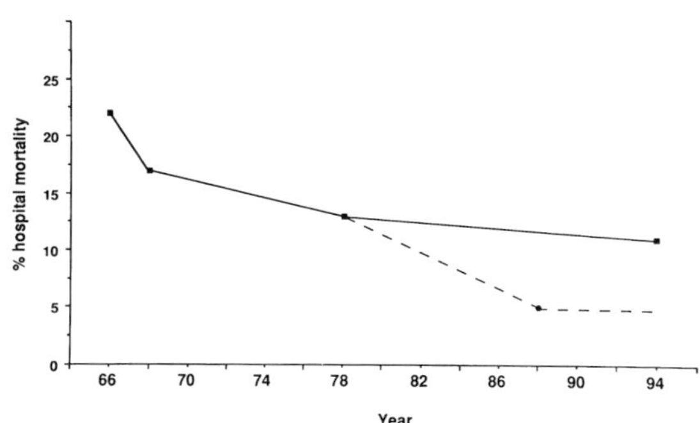

Figure 6–5. Decline in hospital mortality from acute myocardial infarction from 1966 to the present. Mortality percentages refer to patients under 70 years of age and are based on experience with (from left to right) 545 patients treated outside a coronary care unit during 1966–1967 (6), 300 patients treated after opening of a coronary care unit during 1967–1968 (8), and 574 patients treated in a coronary care unit during 1977–1979 (18). The dotted line to the right shows the expected mortality rate of patients treated appropriately with early thrombolytic therapy, while the continuous line shows an estimate of hospital mortality, based on data from UK hospitals during 1994–95, for unselected patients with acute myocardial infarction (see text for details).

HOSPITAL MORTALITY FROM ACUTE MYOCARDIAL INFARCTION IN THE "REAL WORLD"; POSSIBLE DIFFERENCES BETWEEN EUROPE AND NORTH AMERICA

It has been suggested that patients admitted to trials with unrestrictive entry conditions such as ISIS are representative of the generality of hospital patients with myocardial infarction. Unfortunately, however, this is not the case. Patients entered into clinical trials are younger and are less likely to have co-morbidity than the generality of patients, while critically ill patients, including these who die in the emergency room, tend not to be entered (61,62). However, the suggestion (63) that patients not entered into clinical trials have a mortality rate five times as high as those who are entered is almost certainly an overestimate because of the incorrect assumption that elderly patients are ineligible for thrombolytic therapy (57).

Truer estimates of mortality are provided by community epidemiological surveys such as the ongoing Monitoring Trends in Cardiovascular Disease (MONICA) study (64,65) and our own United Kingdom Heart Attack Study (UKHAS) (62,66), and by hospital-based registries such as those which have been set up to monitor the use of thrombolytic therapy (67–69) or of management strategies in general (70–73). Comparisons of the results of these studies suggest important and interesting geographical differences in the treatment and outcome of acute myocardial infarction.

With respect to treatment, it appears that thrombolytic therapy is used in only 30–35% of patients in the United States (67,68) and Denmark (69), and the proportion in the United States and Canada is no higher in early survivors of infarction severe enough to have caused left ventricular dysfunction (73). In the United Kingdom, on the other hand, about 50% of patients receive thrombolytic therapy (74), although the proportion may be lower in hospitals that do not participate in clinical trials (75). However, invasive investigation leading to revascularization is undertaken more frequently in the United States than in Canada (73), and much more frequently than in the United Kingdom, (75a, 75b and unpublished data from the UK Heart Attack Study).

Early mortality rates reported from large consecutive unselected groups of hospitalized patients treated during the thrombolytic era are shown in Table 6–1. This shows the marked effect of increasing age to worsen prognosis and emphasizes the unreliability of comparisons between different groups of patients with differing cutoff points for age. Even so, a remarkable disparity between mortality rates reported from different countries is suggested, with rates at or below 5% for patients under 65 years in the United States and Canada (similar to those reported from the thrombolytic trials), but much higher rates in the United Kingdom, Germany, and

Table 6–1. Hospital Mortality from Acute Myocardial Infarction in the Thrombolytic Era

			Mortality rate by age							
			All ages		<75		<70		<65	
Reference	Country	Year	No of cases	%M*	No of cases	%M	No of cases	%M	No of cases	%M
68	USA	1990–93	240,989	11	174,373	6.8	140,791	5.4		4.2
67	USA	1988–91	6,270	10	4357	6.6			2,620	3.6
71a	Canada	1992		8	547	5.5			318	2.5
71	Canada	1991	19,748	17.1			10,913	8.9		
70	Canada	1990–92	3,178	9.9	2,917	8.4	2,435	6.9		
66	UK	1994–95			2,428	19.0	1,735	14.2	1,177	10.7
72	Germany	1988–89	338	28.7			193	19.2		
69	Denmark		1,881	23	1,258	18.1	943	15.2	652	13.3

*M = mortality

Denmark. Some of these differences can be explained by differing definitions and conditions. Thus the Seattle group (67) excluded patients who had been resuscitated from cardiac arrest outside hospital and those developing infarction while they were in hospital for another condition. Again, it is possible that the high hospital mortality rates found by the MONICA investigators (64) were due in some cases to inclusion of patients who had experienced out of hospital arrest and were pronounced dead in hospital. Removal of those cases from our UK series that would have been excluded from the Seattle series reduced our in hospital mortality rates from 19.0% to 12.3% for patients under 75 years of age and from 10.7% to 5.8% for those aged under 65 years. For both age groups mortality was significantly greater in the United Kingdom than in Seattle.

It seems highly likely that geographical differences in hospital mortality rates exist, at least between Europe and North America. The possibility merits urgent investigation with international comparisons using standardized diagnostic criteria. If such differences are confirmed, reasons should be sought. As stated earlier, differing use of thrombolytic therapy seems an unlikely reason. Possibly the much more aggressive use of angiography and invasive revascularization in the United States than in many European centers may be part of the explanation.

DECLINING MORTALITY FROM ACUTE MYOCARDIAL INFARCTION

Has mortality from myocardial infarction been reduced? Advances in therapeutics, like those in other branches of science, tend to come not gradually but stepwise. The greatest step forward in the treatment of acute myocardial infarction occurred during the 1960s with the introduction of closed chest cardiopulmonary resuscitation, defibrillators, and coronary care units. Another occurred during the 1980s with thrombolytic therapy and direct angioplasty. These advances take a long time (up to 10 years) to be promulgated and implemented to the stage that mortality rates are reduced globally. Thus it is probably unrealistic to expect any change from comparisons made within a time span of less than 10 years unless some radical improvement in management has been adopted and fully implemented over the intervening period.

Studies taking the long-term view do indeed show a decline in mortality, at least in North America. A meta-analysis published in 1991 (76) showed that average in-hospital mortality decreased from 29% during the 1960s to 21% during the 1970s and to 16% during the 1980s. Allowing for the lack of an age cutoff in most of the studies, these figures are comparable with those which we found and which are shown in Fig. 6–4. Similarly, administrative data from all general hospitals in Ontario, Canada (71), showed a 22.3% hospital mortality in 1981, which had declined to 16.3% in 1991. Figures from the Minnesota Heart Study (77,103) showed a significant decline (from 18% to 12% in men) from 1970 to 1980, no significant decline (from 12% to 13%) between 1980 and 1985, but a marked decline (from 13% to 10%) between 1985 and 1990. In one coronary care unit in Gothenburg, Sweden, hospital mortality declined from 18.5% in 1979 to 11.8% in 1990 (78). However, no clear trends for in-hospital case fatality rates could be seen in Worcester, Massachusetts, between 1975 and 1988 (79). Official figures for fatality rates from acute myocardial infarction in the United States confirm the downward trend (80,81). For men aged under 65 years, case fatality was 7.7% in 1984, 5.9% in 1987, and 5.0% in 1990.

LATE SURVIVAL AFTER MYOCARDIAL INFARCTION

Useful data for comparison with later studies are provided by the group of patients treated initially during the pre-coronary care era in Auckland, New Zealand. When followed at a median of 3 years after infarction and discharge from hospital during 1966, the mortality rate of 545 patients was 33% at 3 years and 16% at 1 year; for 413 patients under 70 years of age, mortality was 28% at 3 years and 14% at 1 year (9). By 6 years after infarction, mortality had risen to 48% for all patients and to 42% for those under 70 years of age (10), and after 15 years of follow-up, mortality was 75% and 68%, respectively (11). Survival could be predicted at each of these follow-up surveys by use of a coronary prognostic index (9), which was based on, in addition to age, indirect measurements of the amount of left ventricular myocardial damage sustained (heart size and lung field congestion at the time of the index infarct, and whether the index infarct had been first or recurrent).

To determine whether prognosis had changed as a result of the general use of coronary care units and the development of secondary prevention by coronary surgery and beta blockers—which had not been available or widely prescribed during the 1960s—we followed a group of 203 patients under 70 years of age who had been discharged from Green Lane Hospital during 1981–1982 and compared them with 191 patients who had been discharged during 1966–1967 (82) (Fig. 6–6). Three-year mortality was 14% for the 1981–1982 patients compared with 25% for 1966–1967 patients (p = 0.02). One-year mortality for the 1981–1982 patients was 6.5%. Moreover, it could be shown from calculation of the coronary prognostic indices that the prognosis should have been worse in 1981–1982 than it had been in 1966–1967. Late survival had been improved to a similar extent for all categories of coronary prognostic index. We hypothesized (83) that the improvement could be explained in terms of the known effects of the four major improvements in secondary prevention of ischemic heart disease that had occurred between 1966 and 1981: (i) routine treatment in coronary care units for patients with a reinfarction, (ii) development of coronary surgery, (iii) use of beta blockers for routine therapy after infarction, and (iv) recognition of cigarette smoking as a reversible risk factor. If this hypothesis was correct, there would be no need to postulate any change in the natural history of ischemic heart disease between 1966 and 1981.

Since 1985, the development of thrombolytic therapy, in addition to reducing early mortality rates, has resulted in a significant improvement in left ventricular function for surviving patients (47,49) (see Fig. 6–4). As left ventricular function, apart from age, is the most important prognostic factor for long-term survival, it would be expected

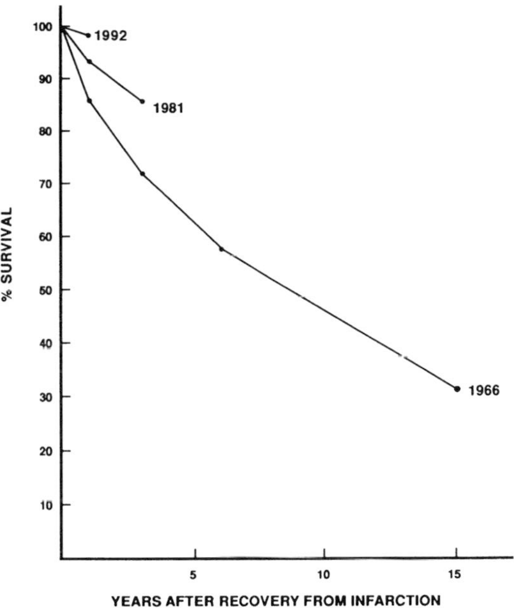

Figure 6–6. Decline in mortality after recovery from myocardial infarction between 1966 and 1981. Both survival curves refer to patients under 70 years of age. The lower curve describes the fate of all 545 patients admitted to Auckland during 1966 and followed at 3 years (9), 6 years (10), and 15 years (11) after the index infarction. The middle curve refers to 203 patients admitted during 1981 (82). The only contemporary study of unselected patients, including those unsuitable for thrombolytic therapy (upperline) is a one-year follow-up of 2266 Canadian patients (70). This shows a late mortality of 5.1% which represents a probable further improvement in the 1990's.

that long-term survival, in addition to early survival, should be improved as a result of thrombolysis. Here again, however, evidence is conflicting, with the suggestion that reported figures may be biased by case selection. Follow-up of from 1 to 6 years from patients treated in trials with r-tPA or streptokinase in which recruitment was limited by age, and selection criteria were carefully defined, show an annual mortality rate for hospital survivors of between 2% and 4% (84–88). On the other hand, a meta-analysis of results from nine trials conducted mainly in Europe, most of which had liberal entry criteria and no age restriction, and all of which enrolled more than 1,000 patients, showed a mortality rate at a mean follow-up of 1.9 years of 11.3% (89). Moreover, no additional benefit of fibrinolytic therapy over placebo could be shown in ISIS-II survivors between 35 days and 4 years of follow-up (90). No recent series appears to have been reported of long-term follow-up of consecutive patients treated both inside and outside clinical trials with and without thrombolytic therapy. Until this is done, no firm conclusions on the impact of thrombolytic therapy or indeed any other form of therapy on long-term survival after myocardial infarction can be made. Nonetheless the Canadian myocardial infarction study (CAMI) in which 43% patients received thrombolytic therapy does demonstrate a substantial improvement in one-year post-discharge mortality of 5.3% for patients under 75 years of age recruited into the study between 1990 and 1992 (70). Moreover during 1 year after hospital discharge, only 1.7% of patients aged ≤75 yrs and 1.9% of patients of all ages died of a presumed arrhythmic death.

RELATIONSHIP BETWEEN DECLINE IN MORTALITY FROM ACUTE MYOCARDIAL INFARCTION AND DECLINE IN COMMUNITY MORTALITY FROM ISCHEMIC HEART DISEASE

In projecting the reduction in mortality from acute infarction obtained by use of thrombolytic therapy or indeed from other more recently discovered therapies (91,92) to their likely community impact, it is clear that the benefits describe what is achievable rather than what has actually been achieved. The major factor acting against thrombolytic therapy is delay in its institution; when delay can be minimized to 1–2 hours, mortality reduction is greater and cardiac damage in surviving patients is less than that which has been reported from the large-scale trials (93,94). Factors contributing to delay need to be carefully analyzed and fully understood if therapeutic advances are to be turned to community benefit. Patients can delay in reporting symptoms because of lack of knowledge of their significance, or more frequently because of the psychological mechanism of denial. Community campaigns have aimed to reduce patient delay by public education (95–98); some success has been claimed in reducing delay times and, consequently, in reducing the severity of completed infarcts (95–97), although it appears that campaigns conducted intensively over a short period of time may not be effective (98). The problem of hospital delay in starting thrombolytic therapy, which was on average more than 1 hour in the GUSTO trial (53), can be addressed by the institution of "fast track" regimens in which "door to needle times" can be reduced to as little as 31 minutes by administration in the accident and emergency department rather than the coronary care unit (99).

Again, as has been stated previously, thrombolytic therapy is applicable to, at most, 50% of hospitalized patients. Patients who are ineligible because of co-morbidity, bleeding risk, or atypical ECG appearances have a much higher mortality rate than those who are eligible (62,100). Further initiatives are necessary for improving the hospital treatment of patients who are unsuitable for thrombolytic therapy.

Mortality rates for patients treated in hospital can never, however, be related to decline in community mortality so long as community and hospital mortality rates are not compared simultaneously in defined populations. In the United Kingdom, the decline in community mortality has been considerably less over the last 30 years than has been the case in the United States (1,2). We have been comparing community with hospital mortality in Brighton, England, since 1993, and in Brighton, South Glamorgan, and York during 1994–95. Early results from the Brighton and United Kingdom Heart Attack Studies (66) showed a distressingly high out-of-hospital mortality rate from acute heart attack (myocardial infarction plus sudden cardiac death). In Brighton during 1993, total case fatality for persons under 75 years of age was 48%. Of all cardiac deaths, 75% occurred outside hospital, and this proportion was higher (86%) for people under 65 years of age than for those aged 65–74 years (71%). These out-of-hospital to in-hospital ratios were, if anything, higher than those which were reported 20–25 years ago (101,102). Mortality figures from Brighton, York, and South Glamorgan in 1994–95 were similar to those which we had found in Brighton during 1993, and there were no important differences among the three centers.

Data such as these show the impossibility of using hospital data to assess community mortality and morbidity. Moreover, they show what may easily be forgotten, that in terms of saving lives, resuscitation from ventricular fibrillation, particularly when this is extended to the out-of-hospital scene, is more important than thrombolytic therapy. Resuscitation of more patients from ventricular fibrillation rather than salvage of myocardium by early reperfusion must be the major aim of community programs to reduce delay. From the figures it would appear that improvements in hospital therapy have had at best a limited impact on community mortality rates in the United Kingdom. No similar studies in the United States could be identified at the time of writing of this chapter, but such studies are urgently needed. Apart from improvements in primary prevention, improvements in identification and triage of patients at risk could have contributed to the greater decline in mortality from ischemic heart disease in the United States than has occurred in most other countries. This possibility awaits investigation.

CONCLUSION

The last 25 years have shown enormous advances in the treatment of acute myocardial infarction. Given early access to treatment, hospital mortality rates can be reduced to 25% or less of those which pertained during the 1960s. Given state of the art therapy, careful follow-up, and an aggressive strategy toward invasive investigations and revascularization in selected cases, long-term mortality can probably be reduced to a near-similar degree.

The problem in 1996, however, is not a lack of therapeutic options, but a failure, in many parts of the world, to implement the advances that have been made. The problem of medically unattended sudden cardiac death is seemingly the most intractable, and it is the area in which the least progress has been made. Public education to reduce delay in hospital admission times and stronger efforts toward secondary prevention for patients with known coronary heart disease are two areas in which improvements are possible. However, the continuing decline in community mortality in the United States and elsewhere suggests that therapeutic advances are indeed being gradually implemented.

REFERENCES

1. American heart Association: *Heart and Stroke facts: 1995 Statistical Supplement.*
2. British Heart Foundation/Coronary Prevention Group Statistics Database. *British Heart Foundation, London,* 1996;23–24.
3. Wright IS, Marple CD, Beck DF: Report of the committee for the evaluation of anticoagulants in the treatment of coronary thrombosis with myocardial infarction (a progress report on the statistical analysis of the first 800 cases studied by this committee). *Am Heart J* 1948;36:801–815.
4. Medical Research Council: Assessment of short-term anticoagulant administration after cardiac infarction: Report of the working party on anticoagulant therapy in coronary thrombosis. *Br Med J* 1969;1:335–342.
5. Lown B, Fakhro AM, Hood WB, Thorn SW: The coronary care unit. *JAMA* 1967;199:188–198.
6. Norris RM, Bensley KE, Caughey DE, Scott PJ: Hospital mortality in acute myocardial infarction. *Br Med J* 1968;3:143–146.
7. Norris RM, Brandt PWT, Caughey DE, et al: A new coronary prognostic index. *Lancet* 1969;1:274–278.
8. Norris RM, Brandt PWT, Lee AJ: Mortality in a coronary-care unit analysed by a new coronary prognostic index. *Lancet* 1969;1:278–281.
9. Norris RM, Caughey DE, Deeming LW, et al: Coronary prognostic index for predicting survival after recovery from acute myocardial infarction. *Lancet* 1970;1:485–488.
10. Norris RM, Caughey DE, Mercer CJ, Scott PJ: Prognosis after myocardial infarction. Six year follow-up. *Br Heart J* 1974;36:786–790.
11. Merrilees MA, Scott PJ, Norris RM: Prognosis after myocardial infarction: Results of 15 year follow-up. *Br Med J* 1984;288:355–359.
12. Honey GE, Truelove SC: Prognostic factors in myocardial infarction. *Lancet* 1957;1:1155–1161.
13. Killip T: In Meltzer LE, Kitchell JR (eds): *The Current Status of Intensive Coronary Care.* New York, American College of Cardiology, 1966.

14. Goble AJ, Sloman G, Robinson JS: Mortality reduction in a coronary care unit. *Br Med J* 1966; 1:1005–1009.
15. Mather HG, Morgan DC, Pearson NG, et al: Myocardial infarction: A comparison between home and hospital care for patients. *Br Med J* 1976; 1:925–929.
16. Hill JD, Hampton JR, Mitchell JR: A randomized trial of home-versus-hospital management for patients with suspected myocardial infarction. *Lancet* 1978;1:837–841.
17. Baum RS, Alvarez H, Cobb LA: Survival after resuscitation from out-of-hospital ventricular fibrillation. *Circulation* 1974;50:1231–1235.
18. Norris RM, Sammel NL: Predictors of late hospital death in acute myocardial infarction. *Progr Cardiovasc Dis* 1980;23:129–140.
19. Norris RM: *Myocardial Infarction: Its Presentation, Pathogenesis and Treatment.* Edinburgh, Churchill Livingstone, 1982, p 41.
20. Lie KI, Wellens HJ, Downar E, Durrer D: Observations on patients with primary ventricular fibrillation complicating acute myocardial infarction. *Circulation* 1975;52:755–759.
21. Noneman JW, Rogers JF: Lidocaine prophylaxis in acute myocardial infarction. *Medicine* 1978;57: 501–515.
22. MacMahon S, Collins R, Yusuf S: The effects of lidocaine on ventricular fibrillation and asystole following suspected acute myocardial infarction. *Circulation* 1986(Suppl II):II–43.
23. Yusuf S, Wittes J, Friedman L: Overview of results of randomized clinical trials in heart disease. 1. Treatment following myocardial infarction. *JAMA* 1988;260:2088–2093.
24. Forrester JS, Diamond G, Chatterjee K, Swan HJ: Medical therapy of acute myocardial infarction by application of hemodynamic subsets. *N Eng J Med* 1976;295:1404–1413.
25. Weber KT, Janicki JS, Russell RO, Rackley CE: Identification of high risk subsets of acute myocardial infarction. Derived from the myocardial infarction research unit cooperative study data bank. *Am J Cardiol* 1978;41:197–203.
26. Crexells C, Chatterjee K, Forrester JS, et al: Optimal level of filling pressure of the left side of the heart in acute myocardial infarction. *N Engl J Med* 1973;289: 1263–1266.
27. Cohn JN, Guika NH, Broder MI, Limas CJ: Right ventricular infarction. Clinical and hemodynamic features. *Am J Cardiol* 1974;33:209–214.
28. Gore JM, Goldberg RJ, Spodick DH, et al: A community-wide assessment of the use of pulmonary artery catheters in patients with acute myocardial infarction. *Chest* 1987;92:721–727.
29. Maroko PR, Kjekshus JK, Sobel BE, et al: Factors affecting infarct size following experimental coronary artery occlusions. *Circulation* 1971;43:67–82.
30. Ginks WR, Sybers HD, Maroko PR, et al: Coronary artery reperfusion. II. Reduction of myocardial infarct size at 1 week after the coronary occlusion. *J Clin Invest* 1972;51:2717–2723.
31. Peter T, Norris RM, Clarke ED, et al: Reduction of enzyme levels by propranolol after acute myocardial infarction. *Circulation* 1978;57:1091–1095.
32. Norris RM, Clarke ED, Sammel NL, et al: Protective effects of propranolol in threatened myocardial infarction. *Lancet* 1978;2:907–909.
33. ISIS-I (First International Study of Infarct Survival) Collaborative Group: A randomised trial of intravenous atenolol among 16027 cases of suspected acute myocardial infarction: ISIS I. *Lancet* 1986; 2:57–66.
34. ISIS-I (First International Study of Infarct Survival) Collaborative Group: Mechanisms for the early mortality reduction provided by beta-blockade started early in acute myocardial infarction. *Lancet* 1988;1: 921–923.
35. The TIMI Study Group: Comparison of invasive and conservative strategies after treatment with intravenous tissue plasminogen activator in acute myocardial infarction. *N Engl J Med* 1989;320: 618–627.
36. Norris RM: Letter to the editor. *New Engl J Med* 1989;321:612.
37. The Norwegian Multicenter Study Group: Timolol-induced reduction in mortality and reinfarction in patients surviving acute myocardial infarction. *N Engl J Med* 1981;304:801–807.
38. Beta-Blocker Heart Attack Research Group: A randomized trial of propranolol in patients with acute myocardial infarction. *JAMA* 1982;247: 1717–1724.
39. The Beta-Blocker Pooling Project Research Group: Subgroup findings from randomized trials in post infarction patients. *Eur Heart J* 1988;9:8–16.
40. Norris RM, Barnaby PF, Brown MA, et al: Prevention of ventricular fibrillation during acute myocardial infarction by intravenous propranolol. *Lancet* 1984;2:883–886.
41. O'Rourke MF, Walsh B, Fletcher M, Crowley A: Impact of the new generation coronary care unit. *Br Med J* 1976;2:837–839.

42. Hunt D, Sloman G, Christie D, Penington C: Changing patterns and mortality of acute myocardial infarction in a coronary care unit. *Br Med J* 1977;1:795–798.
43. Geddes JS, Adgey AAJ, Pantridge JF: Prevention of cardiogenic shock. *Am Heart J* 1980;99:243–254.
44. Kennedy JW, Ritchie JL, Davis KB, et al: Western Washington randomized trial of intracoronary streptokinase in acute myocardial infarction. *N Engl J Med* 1983;309:1477–1482.
45. GISSI Trial Group: Effectiveness of intravenous thrombolytic treatment in acute myocardial infarction. *Lancet* 1986;1:397–401.
46. ISIS-II (Second international study of infarct survival) Collaborative Group: Randomised trial of intravenous streptokinase, oral aspirin, both or neither among 17187 cases of suspected acute myocardial infarction. ISIS II. *Lancet* 1988;2: 349–359.
47. White HD, Norris RM, Brown MA, et al: Effect of intravenous streptokinase on left ventricular function and early survival after acute myocardial infarction. *N Engl J Med* 1987;317:850–855.
47a. White HD, Rivers JT, Maslowski AH et al: Effect of intravenous streptokinase as compared with that of tissue plasminogen activator on left ventricular junction after tissue myocardial infarction. *N Engl J Med* 1989;320:817–821.
48. Wilcox RG, Olsson CG, Skene AM, et al: Trial of tissue plasminogen activator for mortality reduction in acute myocardial infarction. *Lancet* 1988;2: 525–533.
49. O'Rourke M, Baron D, Keogh A, et al: Limitation of myocardial infarction by early infusion of recombinant tissue-type plasminogen activator. *Circulation* 1988;77:1311–1315.
50. Chesebro JH, Knatterud G, Roberts R, et al: Thrombolysis in myocardial infarction (TIMI) trial, Phase I: A comparison between intravenous tissue plasminogen activator and intravenous streptokinase. *Circulation* 1987;76:142–154.
51. The International Study Group: In-hospital mortality and clinical course of 20,891 patients with suspected acute myocardial infarction randomised between alteplase and streptokinase with or without heparin. *Lancet* 1990;336:71–75.
52. ISIS-III (Third International Study of Infarct Survival) Collaborative Group. ISIS III: A randomised comparison of streptokinase vs tissue plasminogen activator vs anistreplase and of aspirin plus heparin vs aspirin alone among 41,299 cases of suspected acute myocardial infarction. *Lancet* 1992;339: 753–770.
53. The GUSTO Investigators: An international randomized trial comparing four thrombolytic strategies for acute myocardial infarction. *N Engl J Med* 1993;329:673–682.
54. The GUSTO Angiographic Investigators: The effects of tissue plasminogen activator, streptokinase, or both, on coronary artery patency, ventricular function, and survival after acute myocardial infarction. *N Engl J Med* 1993;329:1615–1622.
55. Grines CL, Browne KF, Marco J, et al: A comparison of immediate angioplasty with thrombolytic therapy for acute myocardial infarction. *N Engl J Med* 1993;328:673–679.
56. Zyjlstra F, Jan de Boer M, Hoemtje JCA, et al: A comparison of immediate coronary angioplasty with intravenous streptokinase in acute myocardial infarction. *N Engl J Med* 1993;328:680–684.
57. Fibrinolytic Therapy Trialists' Collaborative Group: Indications for fibrinolytic therapy in suspected acute myocardial infarction: Collaborative overview of early mortality and major morbidity results from all randomised trials of more than 1,000 patients. *Lancet* 1994;343:311–322.
58. Van de Werf F, Arnold ER: Intravenous tissue plasminogen activator and size of infarct, left ventricular function and survival in acute myocardial infarction. *Br Med J* 1988;297:1374–1379.
59. Rivers JT, White HD, Cross DB, et al: Reinfarction after thrombolytic therapy followed by conservative management: Incidence and effect of smoking. *J Am Coll Cardiol* 1990;16:340–348.
60. White HD, Norris RM, Brown MA, et al: Left ventricular end-systolic volume as the major determinant of survival after recovery from myocardial infarction. *Circulation* 1987;76:44–51.
61. Col NF, Gurwitz JH, Alpert JS, Goldberg RJ: Frequency of inclusion of patients with cardiogenic shock in trials of thrombolytic therapy. *Am J Cardiol* 1994;73:149–157.
62. Dixon G, on behalf of the UK Heart Attack Study Group: Mortality inside and outside clinical trials. *Br Heart J* 1995;73:P48.
63. Cragg DR, Freidman HZ, Bonema JD et al: Outcome of patients with acute myocardial infarction who are ineligible for thrombolytic therapy. *Ann Intern Med* 1991;115:173–177.
64. Löwel H, Dobson A, Keil V, et al: Coronary heart disease fatality in four countries: A community study. *Circulation* 1993;88:2524–2531.

65. Tunstall-Pedoe H, Kuulasmaa K, Amoytel P, et al: Myocardial infarction and coronary deaths in the World Health Organization MONICA project. Registration procedures, event rates and case-fatality rates in 38 populations from 21 countries in four continents. *Circulation* 1994;90:583–612.

66. Norris RM, on behalf of the UKHAS Group: Mortality from ischaemic heart disease outside hospital: More bad news from the UK Heart Attack Study. *Br Heart J* 1995;73:P50.

67. Maynard C, Weaver WD, Litwin PE, et al: Hospital mortality in acute myocardial infarction in the era of reperfusion therapy (the Myocardial Infarction Triage and Intervention Project). *Am J Cardiol* 1993; 72:877–882.

68. Rogers WJ, Bowlby LJ, Chandra NC, et al: Treatment of myocardial infarction in the United States (1990–93). Observations from the National Registry of Myocardial Infarction. *Circulation* 1994;90: 2103–2114. Also personal communication from Dr. Rogers.

69. Steffensen, Grande P, Clemmensen P, Sandoe E: Long-term prognosis in patients with acute myocardial infarction in relation to eligibility for intravenous thrombolytic therapy. *Circulation* 1994;90: I–500. Also personal communication from Dr Steffensen.

70. Rouleau JL, Talajic M, Sussex B, et al. Myocardial infarction patients in the 1990's—their risk factors, stratification and survival in Canada; the Canadian assessment of myocardial infarction (CAMI) study. *JACC* 1996;27:1119–1127.

71. Naylor CD, Chen E: Population-wide mortality trends among patients hospitalized for acute myocardial infarction: The Ontario experience 1981–1991. *J Am Coll Cardiol* 1994;24:1431–1438.

71a. Le Feurre CA, Connally SJ, Cairns JA, et al: Comparison of mortality from acute myocardial infarction between 1980, 1987 and 1992 in a geographically-defined state population. *Circulation* 1993; 88(Suppl I);I:508.

72. Klein HH, Hengstenberg C, Peuckert M, Jurgensen R: Comparisons of death rates from acute myocardial infarction in two different periods (1977–78 versus 1988–89). *Am J Cardiol* 1993;71: 518–523.

73. Rouleau JL, Moyé LA, Pfeffer MA, et al: A comparison of management patterns after acute myocardial infarction in Canada and the United States. *N Engl J Med* 1993;328:779–784.

74. Norris RM, Dixon GF, Roy S: What proportion of patients with myocardial infarction should receive thrombolytic therapy? *Br Heart J* 1994;71:P40.

75. Ketley D, Woods KL: Impact of clinical trials on clinical practice: example of thrombolysis for acute myocardial infarction. *Lancet* 1993;342:891–894.

75a. El Gaylani NK on behalf of the UK Heart Attack Study investigators: Coronary angloplasty is underused in the management of acute myocardial infarction *Heart* 1996;75:28.

75b. Beatt KJ, Huehns TY, Amency R et al: Is the "Wait and see" strategy for invasive investigation post-myocardial infarction flawed? *Heart* 1996;75:P51.

76. de Vreede JJM, Gorgells APM, Verstraaten MP, et al: Did prognosis after acute myocardial infarction change during the past 30 years? A meta-analysis. *J Am Coll Cardiol* 1991;18:698–706.

77. McGovern PG, Folsom AR, Sprajka M, et al: Trends in survival of hospitalized myocardial infarction patients between 1970 and 1985. The Minnesota Heart Survey. *Circulation* 1992;85: 172–179.

78. Dellborg M, Eriksson P, Riha M, Swedberg K: Declining hospital mortality in acute myocardial infarction. *Eur Heart J* 1994;15:5–9.

79. Goldberg RJ, Gorak EJ, Yarzebski J, et al: A community wide perspective of sex differences and temporal trends in the incidence and survival rates after acute myocardial infarction and out of hospital deaths caused by coronary heart disease. *Circulation* 1993;87: 1947–1953.

80. Gillum RF: Acute myocardial infarction in the United States 1970–83. *Am Heart J* 1987;113: 804–811.

81. Gillum RF: Trends in acute myocardial infarction and coronary heart disease death in the United States. *J Am Coll Cardiol* 1994;23:1273–1277.

82. Stewart AW, Fraser J, Norris RM, Beaglehole R: Changes in severity of myocardial infarction and 3 year survival rates after myocardial infarction in Auckland 1966–67 and 1981–82. *Br Med J* 1988; 297:517–519.

83. Norris RM, Stewart AW, Fraser JR, Beaglehole R: Improved prognosis after myocardial infarction 1981 versus 1966. *Circulation* 1988;78(Suppl II): 468.

84. Simoons ML, Vos J, Tijssenn JGP, et al: Long-term benefit of early thrombolytic therapy in patients with acute myocardial infarction: A 5 year follow-up of a trial conducted in the Interuniversity Car-

diology Institute of the Netherlands. *J Am Coll Cardiol* 1989;14: 1609–1615.

85. Califf RM, Topol EJ, George BS, et al: One-year outcome after therapy with tissue plasminogen activator: Report from the Thrombolysis and Angioplasty in Myocardial Infarction trial. *Am Heart J* 1990;119:777–785.

86. Taylor GJ, Moses H, Katholi RE, et al: Six-year survival after coronary thrombolysis and early revascularization after acute myocardial infarction. *Am J Cardiol* 1992;70:26–30.

87. Arnold AER, Simoons ML, Van de Werf F: Recombinant tissue-type plasminogen activator and immediate angioplasty in acute myocardial infarction. One year follow-up. *Circulation* 1992;86: 111–120.

88. Williams DO, Braunwald E, Knatterud G, et al: One-year results of the Thrombolysis in Myocardial Infarction (TIMI) Phase II trial. *Circulation* 1992; 85:533–542.

89. Fibrinolytic Therapy Trialists Collaborative Group: R Collins Personal Communication, 1995.

90. Baigent C, Collins R: ISIS-2: 4 year mortality follow-up of 17,187 patients after fibrinolytic and anti-platelet therapy in suspected acute myocardial infarction. *Circulation* 1993;88:1–291.

91. Pfeffer MA, Braunwald E, Moyé LA, et al: Effect of captopril on mortality and morbidity in patients with left ventricular dysfunction after myocardial infarction. *N Engl J Med* 1992;327:669–677.

92. The SOLVD Investigators: Effects of enalapril on mortality and the development of heart failure in asymptomatic patients with reduced left ventricular ejection fractions. *N Engl J Med* 1992; 327:685–691.

93. Weaver WD, Cerqueira M, Hallstrom AP, et al: Prehospital-initiated vs hospital-initiated thrombolytic therapy. The Myocardial Infarction Triage and Intervention trial. *JAMA* 1993;270:1211–1216.

94. Rawles J: Halving of mortality at 1 year by domiciliary thrombolysis in the Grampian region early anistreplase trial (GREAT). *J Am Coll Cardiol* 1994;23:1–5.

95. Rowley JM, Hill JD, Hampton JR, Mitchell JRA: Early reporting of myocardial infarction: Impact of an experiment in patient education. *Br Med J* 1982;284:1741–1746.

96. Eppler E, Eisenberg MS, Schaeffer S, et al: 911 and emergency department use for chest pain: Results of a media campaign. *Ann Emerg Med* 1994;24: 202–208.

97. Blohm M, Herlitz J, Hartford M, et al: Consequence of a media campaign focusing on delay in acute myocardial infarction. *Am J Cardiol* 1992;69: 411–413.

98. Bett N, Aroney G, Thompson P: Impact of a natioanl educational campaign to reduce patient delay in possible heart attack. *Aust NZ J Med* 1993;23: 157–161.

99. Birkhead JS: Time delay in provision of thrombolytic treatment in six district hospitals. *Br Med J* 1992;305:445–448.

100. Lee HS, Cross SJ, Rawles JM, Jennings KP: Patients with suspected myocardial infarction who present with ST depression. *Lancet* 1993;342: 1204–1207.

101. Armstrong A, Duncan B, Oliver MF, et al: Natural history of acute coronary attacks: A community study. *Br Heart J* 1972;34:67–80.

102. Kinlen LJ: Incidence and presentation of myocardial infarction in an English community. *Br Heart J* 1973; 35:616–622.

103. McGovern PG, Pankow JS, Shahar E, et al. Recent trends in acute coronary heart disease. Mortality, morbidity, medical care and risk factors. *NEJM* 1996;334:884–890.

PART II

Clinical Presentations and Diagnostic Techniques

7

Acute Myocardial Infarction: Clinical Presentations and Diagnosis

Harlan M. Krumholz, MD, and Jeanne Y. Wei, MD, PhD

Acute myocardial infarction is a major cause of mortality and morbidity in atherosclerosis-prone societies (1–3). Each year approximately 1.5 million Americans suffer a myocardial infarction, and more than 400,000 individuals will likely die from it this year (1–3). Few life-threatening diseases are encountered by physicians as commonly as acute myocardial infarction.

Myocardial infarction, as seen by the pathologist, is the morphologic manifestation of irreversible cell death in an area of the heart that is caused by a prolonged, and often abrupt, mismatch between the supply of oxygen and nutrients in the blood and the metabolic needs of the myocardial cells (4–7) (see Ch. 3 for further details). The most common cause of this condition is the sudden interruption of blood flow in an epicardial coronary artery by a thrombus formed in an area with atherosclerotic disease (4–12).

Acute myocardial infarction, from the clinician's perspective, may include a broad range of clinical manifestations (13–36). The various electrocardiographic patterns, laboratory findings, and imaging studies that suggest the presence of myocardial necrosis are discussed in depth in Chapters 8 through 11. The clinical presentation of acute myocardial infarction, which may be subtle or obvious, results from the interplay of many factors including the location of the infarct, the extent of the damage, and the onset of the infarct in relation to the time of presentation.

The spectrum of clinical presentations of acute myocardial infarction can present a challenge for the most astute physician. Even the lay public is familiar with the significance of unrelenting, crushing substernal chest pain. Nevertheless, clinical presentations of acute myocardial infarction vary widely and the correct diagnosis may at times be elusive. A familiarity with the various guises of myocardial infarction is among the most fundamental knowledge that is required by the clinician.

Many acute infarcts are not diagnosed at the time they occur. The diagnosis may be missed because these infarctions occur silently or because the symptoms may be overlooked or misinterpreted (37,38). A report from the Framingham Study revealed that among their greater than 5,000 participants, more than 25% of the myocardial infarctions were discovered through the appearance of new diagnostic evidence during routine biennial examinations. Although half of these infarcts were truly silent, the others were associated with symptoms (37). Among 7,331 Japanese-American men in Hawaii, 33% of transmural infarctions and 22% of all nonfatal infarctions were clinically unrecognized (38). The diagnosis of acute myocardial infarction is also missed in many hospitalized patients. A study of autopsies performed at a large community hospital revealed that the correct antemortem diagnosis of acute myocardial infarction was made in only 53% of the cases (39). Of note, cardiologists failed to make the diagnosis in 38% of the cases.

The clinical diagnosis of acute myocardial infarction may be difficult to make initially because some very helpful information—including serial electrocardiograms, cardiac enzymes, and imaging studies—are not available during the first few hours of a patient's presentation. In the era of acute reperfusion, time is of the essence and the decision to introduce or withhold such therapy must usually be made on the basis of history, examination, and a single electrocardiogram. Although the definitive diagnosis might not be established for a number of hours, a presumptive diagnosis may be entertained on the basis of history and physical examination. In practice, the patient interview and the physical examination, despite their limitations, often determine whether the patient is sent home with reassurance or is admitted to the cardiac care unit (40–42).

This chapter considers the varied presentations of acute myocardial infarction and focuses on the ability of the physician's keen senses and general acumen to make the presumptive diagnosis of acute myocardial infarction.

THE CLINICAL HISTORY

The clinical history plays two important roles in the presumptive diagnosis of myocardial infarction. First, the history reveals the patient's own "story," the cornerstone to the early presumptive diagnosis of myocardial infarction. Second, the history establishes the presence of risk factors for coronary artery disease (the most common antecedent condition of acute myocardial infarction) or for other conditions that place the patient at risk for acute myocardial infarction. The persuasiveness of the patient's story and the likelihood that the patient has an underlying condition predisposing him or her to an acute myocardial infarction combine to produce a probability that the patient has sustained an infarct.

The patient's story includes the timing and character of the symptoms. In a series of 777 elderly hospitalized patients, aged 65 to 100 years, the presentation of acute myocardial infarction changed substantially with increasing age. Chest pain or discomfort became less common with increasing age; syncope, stroke, and acute confusion became more common. Shortness of breath, the most frequently reported symptom in the absence of chest pain, was equally common at all ages. The authors conclude that "atypical" presentations are common in the very old (43–45).

In addition, the predictive value of classic features of acute myocardial infarction (including a pressure-like quality of pain, of substernal location, or typical pattern of pain radiation) is much lower among older patients than younger patients (57–59). As a consequence, elderly patients who present to the emergency room with chest discomfort are more likely to be admitted to the hospital, and a larger percentage of them, compared with younger patients, subsequently "rule out" for acute myocardial infarction (60).

TIMING

Prodromal symptoms, that is, those symptoms that precede the onset of acute myocardial infarction, occur commonly but are not a reliable finding (46). The most predictive prodrome is an unstable pattern of angina. Stowers and Short interviewed 180 patients in the hospital with acute myocardial infarction and questioned them about prodromal symptoms in the 2 months preceding the current hospital admission. Two-thirds of the patients remembered having prodromal symptoms, and most of these patients described either the onset or an intensification of attacks of pain in the chest (47). Fewer patients, 13% of the total, noted other symptoms, particularly tiredness or shortness of breath. Other prodromal symptoms occurred rarely.

Patients with preinfarction angina may sometimes have smaller, less severe infarcts (48). Kloner and his colleagues reported that, in the TIMI 4 trials, patients who presented with a history of angina at any time prior to their acute myocardial infarction had a significantly lower likelihood of in-hospital death, severe congestive heart failure, or shock, had smaller creatine kinase–determined infarct size, and were less likely to have Q waves on their electrocardiogram (49). In a recent study, Hofgren and colleagues prospectively evaluated the presence of prodromal symptoms in 914 patients admitted to the coronary care unit with suspected myocardial infarction, of which half ruled in for an infarction. Prodromal chest pain was reported by 57%, and other symptoms were reported by 61%. Tiredness was the most common symptom other than chest pain. Women reported prodromal symptoms other than chest pain significantly more commonly than men. The presence of prodromal symptoms did not differentiate patients who were subsequently diagnosed with an acute myocardial infarction. Moreover, the prodromal symptoms were not correlated with the size or location of the infarction (50). The time of day may also be associated with the risk of acute myocardial infarction, with a peak incidence between 6 AM and 12 noon (51,52) (see Ch. 5). Myocardial infarction commonly occurs after a period of heavy exertion, particularly among individuals who do not exercise very frequently (53,54). The time of day when the symptoms begin may not always help with the diagnosis. Although occurrence in the morning is the most common, acute myocardial infarction can occur at any time (see Ch. 5).

SYMPTOMS

Symptoms are insensitive and nonspecific indicators of acute myocardial infarction. Perhaps a quarter of all acute infarcts occur without symptoms (18,37–39). Even when symptoms are present, they often cannot be reliably differentiated from ischemia without infarction or even nonischemic pain. Nevertheless, the timing and character of symptoms play an important role in the presumptive diagnosis of acute myocardial infarction.

Typical Versus Atypical Symptoms

The symptoms of acute myocardial infarction can be considered as either typical, that is, frequently associated with myocardial infarction, or atypical, that is, less commonly associated with myocardial infarction. The classic hallmark symptom of acute myocardial infarction is chest pressure or pain. Patients may, however, present with symptoms that appear primarily pulmonary, neurologic, gastrointestinal, or even renal. Such symptoms as nausea, vomiting, syncope, focal neurologic deficits, abdominal pain, and dyspnea can sometimes lead the clinician away from the timely diagnosis of acute myocardial infarction, especially if they occur in the absence of chest pain (15–17, 55–57).

Chest Pain

Chest pain or pressure is the most common presenting symptom of an acute myocardial infarction. The chest discomfort is similar to classic angina except that the pain is usually unrelenting and severe (1,14,15). It often cannot be relieved with rest or sublingual nitroglycerin and lasts 30 minutes or longer. Like angina, the discomfort is characteristically substernal in location, radiating to the arms or lower jaw, presurelike in character, and not pleuritic (15).

The nature of the chest pain in relation to previous symptoms is important. Chest pain which is the same as that during a prior myocardial infarction or worse than prior angina is an important predictor of complication within 24 hours of presentation among patients who come to the emergency department with acute chest pain (90). Nevertheless, the absence of these symptoms do not preclude the diagnosis of acute myocardial infarction.

Patients with an acute myocardial infarction who do not present with chest pain are at risk of not being treated appropriately. In a study of more than 16,000 Medicare beneficiaries hospitalized with acute myocardial infarction in Alabama, Connecticut, Iowa and Wisconsin, the absence of chest pain was associated with patients eligible for aspirin who were not treated (91).

Atypical symptoms are also associated with inappropriate triage decisions. In a prospective study of emergency room patients who presented with acute chest pain, 4% of the patients with a subsequent diagnosis of acute myocardial infarction were sent home. These patients were much more likely to have less typical symptoms, and not to have a previous history of myocardial infarction or angina than a comparable group of patients who were admitted to the hospital (42).

The severity of chest discomfort is not correlated with the amount of myocardium at risk (61). The site of the myocardial infarction does not always correspond to the location of the chest discomfort. In addressing this issue, Pasceri and colleagues (48) reported that pain location, severity, and duration were similar in patients with anterior and inferior Q wave infarctions. The location of the chest pain or pressure may give some information about the location among patients who have had a previous infarction. Patients who had an infarction in the same area as the previous infarct had discomfort in the same location, whereas two-thirds of the patients with an infarct in another region had the symptom in a different location (48). The resolution of chest pain or pressure with medical therapy does not always predict a patent infarct artery (62). In fact, even patients with chest discomfort that is relieved by conventional medical therapy tend to benefit from thrombolytic therapy if they meet electrocardiographic criteria for the therapy (61–63).

Other Symptoms

A variety of other symptoms may be associated with acute myocardial infarction. Dyspnea, or worsening heart failure, is the most common other symptom. This may occur alone or in conjunction with chest pain or pressure. The presentation of a patient with pulmonary edema should initiate a search for a precipitant. Myocardial infarction is a common cause of pulmonary edema (1,64).

Nausea and vomiting are commonly associated with acute myocardial infarction, although these symptoms are insensitive and nonspecific. Herlihy and colleagues (65), found that nausea or vomiting in association with chest pain in patients admitted to the cardiac care unit increased the probability of a subsequent diagnosis of myocardial infarction. Similar conclusions were drawn from a study by Logan and associates of 227 patients admitted to the cardiac care unit in which the presence of nausea, vomiting, belching, and sweating increased the likelihood of an infarction (66). Nausea has been associated with inferior infarctions and the subsequent development of Q waves on the electrocardiogram (48,65,66). Thus these gastrointestinal symptoms, although generally nonspecific, are helpful in patients in whom the diagnosis of myocardial infarction is suspected.

The ability of gastrointestinal symptoms to predict the location of an infarct is less clear. In the study by Herlihy and colleagues, nausea was not a good predictor of an inferior wall infarction but it was associated with larger peak creatine kinase activity levels (65). Another study reported that the incidence of gastrointestinal symptoms was higher in patients with inferior infarctions compared with anterior infarctions (70% versus 48%) (48). Whether nausea implies a larger infarct size is not clearly established. As nausea and vomiting may also be signals of coronary reperfusion, the higher peak creatine kinase activity associated with nausea and vomiting may actually be the result of creatine kinase washout associated with coronary reperfusion and not the consequence of larger infarcts (33,63–69).

Confusion, agitation, stroke, sudden death, syncope, psychosis, weakness, peripheral embolism, and palpitations are other occasional presentations of myocardial infarction (39–56). Physicians should consider the possibility of acute myocardial infarction in patients who present with these conditions in the absence of an obvious etiology, and these atypical presentations should not lure physicians away from the diagnosis of myocardial infarction.

The importance of these atypical features (Table 7–1) in elderly patients should be emphasized (43,57–59). Acute myocardial infarction associated with syncope, acute confusion, and stroke occur commonly in octogenarians, in whom "atypical" symptoms are the rule. Dyspnea is a prominent symptom in elderly patients, and chest pain and diaphoresis decline substantially in frequency with advancing age (see Table 7–1).

Silent or nonclinically detected myocardial infarctions tend to occur more commonly in patients without prior angina pectoris, in those with diabetes or hypertension, and in the elderly (1, 37–39,

Table 7–1. Atypical Symptoms of Myocardial Infarction in the Elderly

	Percentage of Patients With Symptom		
Symptom	Aged 65–74 Years	Aged 75–84 Years	Aged ≥85 Years
Chest pain	78	60	38
Dyspnea	41	44	43
Sweating	34	23	14
Syncope	3	18	18
Confusion	3	8	19
Stroke	2	7	7

Modified from Bayer et al (43), with permission.

42–45). This may reflect differences in pain threshold, perhaps resulting from neuropathy, receptor resetting, and/or decreased sensory innervation.

RISK FACTORS

The interpretation of the history in the diagnosis of acute infarction will be tempered by the presence or absence of cardiac risk factors, which in themselves reflect the prevalence of coronary artery disease and infarction. In a patient population with a high prevalence of coronary artery disease, typical symptoms are powerful predictors. In a population with a very low prevalence of disease, however, even typical symptoms may not strongly suggest the diagnosis of myocardial infarction.

Atherosclerotic coronary artery disease is by far the most common precursor of an acute infarct (1–7). Patients with traits, or risk factors, associated with an increased risk of developing coronary artery disease are more likely to suffer an acute myocardial infarction compared with individuals without these traits. In addition, a patient who has had clinical manifestations of coronary artery disease is at even greater risk of myocardial infarction.

It should be noted, however, that patient do not always accurately report a history of prior myocardial infarction and independent verification is important (92). In a study of 3,703 patients admitted to a coronary care unit, a history of a prior myocardial infarction could only be substantiated in 60%. Most of the false positive reports were related to previous hospitalizations, including unstable angina.

While knowledge about other risk factors, such as elevated homocysteine levels, is growing, the major risk factors remain, at least for the moment, hypertension, cigarette smoking, family history, diabetes mellitus, hypercholesterolemia, and male sex (70–72). The presence of these traits in a patient presenting for evaluation must be determined. In addition, a history of any previous manifestations of coronary artery disease should be sought.

The Multiple-Risk Factor Intervention Trial (MRFIT) confirmed the strong association between serum cholesterol and coronary artery disease (71). Men in the highest decile of cholesterol (greater than 263 mg/dl) had a fourfold higher risk than those in the lowest decile (less than 168 mg/dl). With increasing age, however, the importance of total serum cholesterol may decrease (73). The relationship between elevated blood pressure and coronary artery disease is strong at all ages (70–74). There is a continuous increase in the risk of coronary artery disease with increasing systolic blood pressure and diastolic blood pressure. In the MRFIT, subjects with a diastolic blood pressure in the range 90 to 104 mm Hg had about twice the risk of death from coronary artery disease than normotensive subjects. The risk of death from coronary artery disease also increased with increasing systolic blood pressure. Subjects with systolic blood pressure greater than 175 mm Hg had about eight times the risk of death from coronary artery disease than did subjects with a systolic blood pressure under 125 mm Hg (71).

In the MRFIT, smokers died twice as often of coronary artery disease than nonsmokers (71). Patients with diabetes also are at increased risk of suffering from coronary artery disease (71). The rate of death from coronary artery disease for diabetics may be more than three times higher than that for nondiabetics (71). Family history makes an independent contribution to an individual's risk of developing coronary heart disease before the age of 60 years. Family history is also a strong risk factor for death from coronary heart disease. This risk factor is strongest in younger individuals. A recent study of the Swedish Twin Registry demonstrated that the importance of family history becomes less pronounced in older age (75). Another issue with regard to family history is the reliability of the information. Investigators from Belfast reported patients commonly do not accurately report their family history of coronary disease. The sensitivity, specificity, and positive predictive value for reports of myocardial infarction in first degree relatives were 67%, 97%, and 71% (76). Nonsmoking, nondiabetic subjects without hypercholesterolemia (<220 mg/dl) and hypertension (diastolic blood pressure <90 mm Hg) had an 18-fold lower risk of death from coronary artery disease than smoking, diabetic, hypertensive, hypercholesterolemic individuals (71).

Male sex is another important trait associated with coronary artery disease as coronary artery disease rates in women tend to lag behind those for men by about 10 to 15 years (57,71,77). Age in itself is a major risk factor for coronary artery disease (70–72). The preponderance of all deaths from heart disease occur in individuals 65 years old or older (57–59,70,71).

UNUSUAL CAUSES OF ACUTE MYOCARDIAL INFARCTION

The recreational use of cocaine and other cardiostimulants has been associated with an increased incidence of myocardial ischemia and infarction, even in patients without significant coronary artery disease (78). Patients with endocarditis or left-sided thrombi are at risk of embolization into a coronary artery. Patients with coronary spasm can occasionally have a myocardial infarction (79). Pregnancy confers a small risk of coronary artery dissection and subsequent myocardial infarction (77). Other unusual causes include ergot therapy, serum sickness, wasp stings, cardiac trauma, blast injury, and "allergic" coronary vasospasm (80). Invasive cardiac procedures, for example, coronary angiography, have become important precipitants of acute infarction.

PHYSICAL EXAMINATION

A careful physical examination provides valuable clues to the presence and severity of an evolving myocardial infarction. The evaluation begins with an assessment of the hemodynamic status of the patient. Myocardial ischemia and necrosis are important causes of hemodynamic decompensation. In addition, the pattern and extent of the hemodynamic abnormality may provide a clue to the infarct location and, possibly, the patient's prognosis (19–21). Clinicians should interpret the findings of physical examination with care. Gadsboll and colleagues examined 102 patients with acute myocardial infarction and correlated symptoms and signs to findings of vascular congestion on chest x-ray, reduced left or right radionuclide ventricular ejection fractions, enlarged ventricular volumes, or hemodynamic evidence of ventricular dysfunction. The three physicians who independently examined the patients frequently disagreed on the presence of the physical signs of heart failure. In addition, these signs did not reliably predict the radiographic, radionuclide, or hemodynamic measures of ventricular performance (64).

Vital Signs

In the first hours after an acute infarct, the temperature is usually normal. The heart rate may be fast, slow, or normal, and the rhythm may be regular or irregular. Blood pressure may be high, low, or normal. The respiratory rate may be normal; in the presence of pulmonary edema, however, it is markedly abnormal. Abnormal vital signs may be the result of the myocardial infarction (bradycardia in an inferior infarction) or may be related to the cause of myocardial infarction (hypertensive crisis or atrial fibrillation with a rapid ventricular response). During the first moments of a patient's presentation, the physical examination should focus less on the diagnosis of acute myocardial infarction and more on the assessment and treatment of the patient's hemodynamic status. Once it is established that the patient has a normal blood pressure and pulse and is hemodynamically stable, the evaluation can proceed with all deliberate speed. If, however, the patient is hypotensive, prompt treatment should be initiated to support the blood pressure.

Hemodynamic compromise does not necessarily imply the presence of myocardial dysfunction. The physician should determine the etiology of the hypotension from among the various types of shock, including obstructive, oligemic, distributive, and cardiogenic shock. Obstructive shock occurs when factors extrinsic to the myocardium and valves prevent adequate filling of the chambers to allow sufficient forward output, for example, pulmonary embolus. Oligemic shock, also termed hypovolemic shock, is the consequence of massive blood loss. Hypovolemic shock or hypotension complicating acute myocardial infarction is particularly common in the elderly, who may be extremely sensitive to preload reduction (80). The latter may be the consequence of vomiting, diaphoresis, deficient intake as a result of nausea, administration of narcotics, diuretics, or antianginal drugs, among others (55–59,81–83). Distributive shock is the result of abnormal volume of distribution from an inappropriately low systemic vascular resistance. This can occur from sepsis, toxins, endocrine disorders, neurologic disorders, and anaphylaxis. Cardiogenic shock usually results from pump failure or acute regurgitation or rupture.

Perhaps 10% of patients presenting with acute myocardial infarction will have cardiogenic shock (1,84–87). Shock may also be associated with cardiac arrhythmias, myocarditis, cardiomyopathies, acute mitral regurgitation, acute myocardial rupture, and aortic stenosis. It may also be a cause of acute myocardial infarction in that hypotension and poor perfusion may lead to a mismatch in myocardial supply and demand. A diagnosis of shock other than cardiogenic does not therefore exclude the presence of an acute infarct.

Vital signs provide strong prognostic information. The mean arterial pressure was the most important prognostic variable in a recent multivariable analysis of predictors of 30-day outcomes in a large sample of Medicare beneficiaries (93). Tachypnea and the presence of shock also had independent prognostic value. Low systolic blood pressure (<110 mm Hg) is associated with a higher risk of complications within 24 hours of admission (90).

General Appearance

Patients evolving a myocardial infarction may appear gravely ill or fairly robust. Pale skin and diaphoresis in a patient clenching a fist over the chest (Levine's sign) while describing her or his chest discomfort is helpful in suggesting the presence of myocardial necrosis.

Jugular Venous Pulse

Patients with acute myocardial infarction may present with normal or elevated neck veins. The height of the jugular venous pulse is a valuable parameter in that it provides information on the patient's central venous pressure and assists in the location of the site of the presumptive myocardial infarction. Moreover, the character of the venous waveform may provide a clue to other unsuspected pathology (19).

The neck veins may provide information about the location of the acute infarct. Identification of right ventricular infarction is important because it has consequences for treatment, especially in the hypotensive patient (see Ch. 17). Right ventricular infarction causes characteristic hemodynamic changes, including an elevation in right-sided filling pressure relative to that of the left side. The physical examination may also have value in excluding hemodynamically significant right ventricular infarction. In a prospective study of patients with inferior myocardial infarction who were evaluated by physical examination and right heart catheterization, an elevated jugular venous pressure was observed in 7 of 8 patients with right ventricular infarction and 14 of 45 patients without right ventricular infarction ($p < 0.01$). In addition, Kussmaul's sign was seen in all patients with right ventricular infarction (88). Therefore, the absence of both an elevated jugular venous pulse and

Kussmaul's sign in patients with an inferior myocardial infarction would make the presence of a hemodynamically significant right ventricular infarction less likely (88).

Lungs

A normal pulmonary examination is not unusual at the presentation of an acute myocardial infarction (19). An examination of the lungs, however, is important in determining the presence of pulmonary edema (see Ch. 24). Diffuse crackles, wheezes, or coarse breath sounds are a clue to interstitial edema. The presence of rales above the bases bilaterally is associated with a significantly higher risk of adverse events within 24 hours of admission (90). The absence of pulmonary finding with markedly elevated neck veins may suggest a right ventricular infarction.

Heart

Findings on the cardiac examination may reveal evidence of underlying cardiac pathology and even suggest whether the etiology is ischemic. Evanescent findings that wax and wane with episodes of pain suggest that a component of reversible ischemia is responsible. Abnormal findings that suggest chronic disease are clues to the patient's antecedent chronic cardiac condition. In addition, the cardiac examination may provide evidence of complications of the acute infarct. Careful documentation of the cardiac examination at presentation helps with the patient's initial assessment and allows for later comparison with findings that may evolve over subsequent days.

Palpation, an often overlooked component of the physical examination, may provide information about the size of the heart and its movement. Right ventricular enlargement is characterized by a prominent parasternal heave. Left ventricular enlargement is often associated with a laterally displaced apical impulse. A ventricular aneurysm is suggested by a systolic bulging of the apex and may occur in an anterior myocardial infarction. Gallops may also be felt as a presystolic impulse or an early diastolic impulse.

Auscultation can provide an abundance of information, even in this technologic age. The clinician needs to focus on the presence of a rub, gallop, or murmur. The presence of a rub is a helpful finding in a patient with atypical symptoms. A loud three-component rub in a young person with chest pain would tend to steer the clinician away from concerns about ischemic heart disease and toward the pericardium. Nonetheless, one should caution against a false sense of security, as friction rubs may be the consequence of an acute myocardial infarction, especially transmural infarcts. Some investigators feel that an atrial gallop, the S_4, is invariably found in myocardial infarction. Transient gallops suggest the presence of reversible ischemia. The presence of an S_3 may herald the onset of hemodynamic decompensation. The presence of an S3 gallop on admission is associated with a significantly worse 30-day mortality (93).

The presence of murmurs should be sought and documented. It is also helpful to know if the murmur had been heard previously. New murmurs must be characterized as they may suggest the presence of one of the dreaded complications of acute myocardial infarction, including papillary muscle rupture, ventricular septal defect, or free wall perforation.

Abdomen

The abdomen should be assessed for evidence of pathology as well as possible signs of right-sided heart failure. In particular, the size and character of the liver should be examined. A large, tender liver may suggest the presence of hepatic congestion and elevated right-sided heart pressures. A pulsatile liver suggests the presence of severe tricuspid regurgitation. Acute tricuspid regurgitation in the context of a right ventricular infarction may require surgical repair (89). As most any upper abdominal pathology can masquerade as acute myocardial infarction, a thorough examination is necessary. An equally important aspect of the examination is the identification of concomitant diseases that could affect prognosis and therapy (for example, abdominal aortic aneurysm and vascular bruits).

Extremities

Edema in the extremities may suggest the presence of right-sided heart failure. Unilateral swelling or tenderness raises the possibility of a thrombus. Cyanosis in the extremities suggests either sluggish blood flow or generalized arterial desaturation. Clubbing may suggest that the condition is chronic. Cool extremities in a hypotensive patient suggest shock with an elevated systemic vascular resistance.

Central Nervous System

The patient's mental status and the presence of any focal neurologic deficits should be determined. Confusion is a common atypical symptom of myocardial infarction, especially in the elderly (43–45, 57–59). One investigator has suggested that baseline altered mental status accounts for the large number of atypical presentations in the elderly, as confused patients are unlikely to communicate their symptoms well. Ischemic heart disease deserves to be in the differential diagnosis of patients presenting with confusion. Moreover, an inability to obtain a clear history is a probable contraindication to thrombolytic therapy, particularly because it is essential to exclude recent trauma such as falls. Focal neurologic deficits must also be sought in these patients. Stroke is commonly associated with acute myocardial infarction and is often part of the presentation. A previous stroke often signals the presence of vascular disease and may increase the clinician's suspicion of coronary artery disease. The presence of a focal neurologic deficit may deter the physician from using a thrombolytic agent. Documentation of the patient's status on presentation provides for possible comparison later.

SIGNS OF RISK FACTORS FOR MYOCARDIAL INFARCTION

Skin examination may reveal the presence of xanthomas in patients with severe hyperlipidemia. The tendons of the fingers, toes, wrists, ankles, as well as the skin of the elbows and knees, are common sites for xanthomas. Xanthelasma may be found in the skin of the upper and lower eyelids. In addition the skin may hold clues to the diagnosis of endocarditis, and evidence of embolic phenomena should be sought. Examination of the head may reveal exophthalmos and suggest the diagnosis of thyrotoxicosis. Fundoscopic examination can demonstrate the presence of chronic hypertension, diabetes mellitus, hypercholesterolemia, and atherosclerosis. The fundus can also reveal evidence of endocarditis (Roth spots).

The neck examination should focus on the thyroid and on the arterial and venous pulses. Examination of the carotid pulse may provide an assessment of the presence of aortic valve pathology. The quality of the pulses and the presence of bruits can also provide some indication of the presence of atherosclerotic disease. A thorough examination of the other arterial pulses may reveal evidence of diffuse atherosclerotic disease.

ATYPICAL CARDIAC ENZYME PATTERNS

In addition to differences in the presentation of acute myocardial infarction in the elderly, the cardiac enzyme profile may also be altered with advanced age (see Ch. 8). In the acute infarct setting, the finding of a transiently elevated myocardial fraction of creatine kinase (CK MB isoenzyme) in the presence of normal total creatine kinase level (with a typical infarct creatine kinase curve) tends to occur twice as often in patients aged 70 years and older than in younger patients (32,36,55–57). These events of CK MB elevation usually occur in concert with several other clinical findings typically associated with acute infarction and likely represent definite myocardial injury, which should be considered part of the spectrum of nontransmural, non–Q wave myocardial infarction (32,36). It is possible that a lower total creatine kinase level may represent smaller amounts of necrosis, decreased numbers of myocytes or myofibers in the myocardium, an altered isoenzyme distribution (increased CK MB fraction), or other changes in the older heart. There may be an increased incidence of smaller, non–Q wave infarcts in the elderly.

SUMMARY

There is a broad spectrum of clinical presentations of acute myocardial infarction. Although history and physical examination may not be the most sensitive or specific indicators of an acute infarct, they provide the basis for important triage and treatment decisions early in the course of a patient's evaluation. The goals of the history and the physical examination are to make a diagnosis, assess immediate therapy, determine the presence and severity of risk factors for coronary artery disease, and identify concomitant medical disease that could affect prognosis and therapy.

REFERENCES

1. Pasternak RC, Braunwald E, Sobel BE: Acute myocardial infarction, in Braunwald E (ed): *Acute Myocardial Infarction,* 4th ed. Philadelphia, WB Saunders, 1992, pp 1200–1292.
2. American Heart Association: *1995 Heart and Stroke Facts,* Statistical Supplement. Dallas, American Heart Association Center, 1995, pp 1–2.
3. Peli S, Fayerweather E: Trends in the incidence of myocardial infarction and in associated mortality and morbidity in a large employed population, 1957–1983. *N Engl J Med* 1985;312:1005.
4. Fuster V, Badimon L, Badimon JJ, et al: The pathogenesis of coronary artery disease and the acute coronary syndromes. *N Engl J Med* 1992;326: 242–250, 310–318.
5. Bloor CM: *Cardiac Pathology.* Philadelphia, JB Lippincott, 1978, p 176–221.
6. Buja LM, Willerson JT: Clinicopathologic correlates of acute ischemic heart disease syndromes. *Am J Cardiol* 1981;47:343–56.
7. Andersen HR, Falk E, Nielsen D: Clinical first myocardial infarction: Coronary artery disease and old infarcts in 53 consecutive fatal cases from a coronary care unit. *Am J Cardiovasc Pathol* 1989;2:315–319.
8. Blumgart HL, Schlesinger MJ, Davis D: Studies on the relation of the clinical manifestations of angina pectoris, coronary thrombosis, and myocardial infarction to the pathologic findings with particular reference to the significance of the collateral circulation. *Am Heart J* 1940;19:1–91.
9. Warnes CA, Roberts WC: Morphologic findings in sudden coronary death: A comparison of those with and those without previous symptoms of myocardial ischemia. *Cardiol Clin* 1986;4:607–615.
10. Friedberg CK, Horn H: Acute myocardial infarction not due to coronary artery occlusion. *JAMA* 1939;112:1675–1679.
11. Silver MD, Baroldi G, Mariani F: The relationship between acute occlusive coronary thrombi and myocardial infarction studied in 100 consecutive patients. *Circulation* 1980;61:219–27.
12. DeWood MA, Spores J, Notske R, et al: Prevalence of total coronary occlusion during the early hours of transmural myocardial infarction. *N Engl J Med* 1980;303:897–902.
13. Feldman RL: Coronary thrombosis, coronary spasm and coronary atherosclerosis and speculation on the link between unstable angina and acute myocardial infarction, editorial. *Am J Cardiol* 1987;59:1187–90.
14. Harper RW, Kennedy G, DeSanctis RW, Hutter AM Jr: The incidence and pattern of angina prior to acute myocardial infarction: A study of 577 cases. *Am Heart J* 1979;97:178–83.
15. Baker P: Suspected myocardial infarction: Early diagnostic value of analgesic requirements. *Br Med J* 1985;290:27.
16. Ingram DA, Fulton RA, Portal RW, Aber CP: Vomiting as a diagnostic aid in acute ischemic cardiac pain. *Br Med J* 1980;281:636–7.
17. Uretsky BF, Farquhar DS, Borezin A, Hood WB: Symptomatic myocardial infarction without chest pain: Prevalence and clinical course. *Am J Cardiol* 1977;40:498–503.
18. Sullivan W, Vlodaver Z, Tuna N, et al: Correlation of electrocardiographic and pathologic findings in healed myocardial infarction. *Am J Cardiol* 1978;42: 724–32.
19. Chizner MA: Bedside diagnosis of the acute myocardial infarction and its complications. *Curr Probl Cardiol* 1982;7:1–86.
20. Stein PD, Sabbah HN, Barr I: Intensity of heart sounds in the evaluation of patients following myocardial infarction. *Chest* 1979;75:679–84.
21. Riley CP, Russell RO Jr, Rackley CE: Left ventricular gallop sound and acute myocardial infarction. *Am Heart J* 1973;86:598–602.
22. Galve E, Garcia-Del-Castillo H, Evangelista A, et al: Pericardial effusion in the course of myocardial infarction: Incidence, natural history, and clinical relevance. *Circulation* 1986;73:294–9.

23. Sobel BE, Shell WE: Serum enzyme determinations in the diagnosis and assessment of acute myocardial infarction. *Circulation* 1972;45:471–82.
24. Lott JA: Serum enzyme determinations in the diagnosis of acute myocardial infarction: An update. *Hum Pathol* 1984;15:706–16.
25. Klarlund K, Pedersen BK, Theander TG, Andersen V: Depressed natural killer cell activity in acute myocardial infarction. *Clin Exp Immunol* 1987;70: 209–216.
26. Weidner N: Laboratory diagnosis of acute myocardial infarct. Usefulness of determination of lactate dehydrogenase (LDH)-1 level and the ratio of LDH-1 to total LDH. *Arch Pathol Lab Med* 1982;106: 375–77.
27. Fuchs J, Weinberger I, Teboul A, et al: Plasma viscosity and hematocrit in the course of acute myocardial infarction. *Eur Heart J* 1987;8:1195–1200.
28. Ong L, Reiser P, Coromilas J, et al: Left ventricular function and rapid release of creatine kinase MB in acute myocardial infarction: Evidence for spontaneous reperfusion. *N Engl J Med* 1983;309:1–6.
29. Bain RJ, Poeppinghaus VJ, Jones GM, Peaston MJ: Cortisol level predicts myocardial infarction in patients with ischemic chest pain. *Int J Cardiol* 1989; 25:69–72.
30. Blanke H, von Hardenberg D, Cohen M, et al: Patterns of creatine kinase release during acute myocardial infarction after nonsurgical reperfusion: Comparison with conventional treatment and correlation with infarct size. *J Am Coll Cardiol* 1984;3:675–80.
31. Roberts R, Gowda KS, Ludbrook PA, Sobel BE: Specificity of elevated serum MB creatine phosphokinase activity in the diagnosis of acute myocardial infarction. *Am J Cardiol* 1975;36:433–7.
32. Heller GV, Blaustein AS, Wei JY. Implications of elevated myocardial isoenzymes in the presence of normal serum creatinine kinase activity. *Am J Cardiol* 1983;51:24–27.
33. Wei JY, Markis JE, Malagold M, Grossman W: Time course of serum cardiac enzymes after intracoronary thrombolytic therapy. *Arch Intern Med* 1985;145: 1596–1600.
34. Turi ZG and cooperating investigators from the MILIS Study Group: Electrocardiographic, enzymatic and scintigraphic criteria of acute myocardial infarction as determined from study of 726 patients. *Am J Cardiol* 1985;55:1463–1465.
35. Flaherty JT, Becker LC, Bulkley BH, et al: A randomized prospective trial of intravenous nitroglycerin in patients with acute myocardial infarction: Benefits of early treatment. *Circulation* 1983;68: 576–588.
36. Hong RA, Licht JD, Wei JY, et al: Elevated CK-MB with normal total creatine kinase in suspected myocardial infarction: Associated clinical findings and early prognosis. *Am Heart J* 1986;111:1041–7.
37. Kannel WB, Abbott RD: Incidence and prognosis of unrecognized myocardial infarction. An update on the Framingham Study. *N Engl J Med* 1984;311: 1144–1147.
38. Yano K, MacLean CJ: The incidence and prognosis of unrecognized myocardial infarction in the Honolulu, Hawaii, heart program. *Arch Intern Med* 1989; 149:1528–1532.
39. Zarling EJ, Sexton H, Milnor PJ: Failure to diagnose acute myocardial infarction. The clinicopathologic experience at a large community hospital. *JAMA* 1983;250:2835–2837.
40. Hoffman JR, Igarashi E: Influence of electrocardiographic findings on admission decisions in patients with acute chest pain. *Am J Med* 1986;80: 1184–1186.
41. Risoe C, Kirkeby OJ: Initial presentation of acute myocardial infarction and the relation to short-term clinical course. *Scand J Prim Health Care* 1986;4: 29–31.
42. Lee TH, Rouan GW, Weisberg MC, et al: Clinical characteristics and natural history of patients with acute myocardial infarction sent home from the emergency room. *Am J Cardiol* 1987;60:456–459.
43. Bayer AJ, Chadha JS, Farag RR, Pathy MS: Changing presentation of myocardial infarction with increasing old age. *J Am Geriatr Soc* 1986;34: 263–266.
44. Goldberg RJ, Gore JM, Gurwitz JH, et al: The impact of age on the incidence and prognosis of initial acute myocardial infarction. The Worcester Heart Attack Study. *Am Heart J* 1989;117:543–9.
45. Day JJ, Bayer AJ, Pathy MS, Chadha JS: Acute myocardial infarction: Diagnostic difficulties and outcome in advanced old age. *Age Ageing* 1987;16: 239–243.
46. Klaeboe G, Otterstad J, Winsnes T, Espeland N: Predictive value of prodromal symptoms in myocardial infarction. *Acta Med Scand* 1987;222: 27–30.
47. Stowers M, Short D: Warning symptoms before major myocardial infarction. *Br Heart J* 1970;32: 833–838.

48. Pasceri V, Cianflone D, Finochiarrio ML, et al: Relation between myocardial infarction site and pain location in Q-wave acute myocardial infarction. *Am J Cardiol* 1995;75:224–227.
49. Kloner RA, Shook T, Przyklenk K, et al: Previous angina alters in-hospital outcome in TIMI 4. A clinical correlate to preconditioning. *Circulation* 1995;91:37–45.
50. Hofgren C, Karlson BW, Herlitz J: Prodromal symptoms in subsets of patients hospitalized for suspected acute myocardial infarction. *Heart Lung* 1995;24:3–10.
51. Muller JE, Stone PH, Turi ZG, et al: Circadian variation in the frequency of onset of acute myocardial infarction. *N Engl J Med* 1985;313:1315–1322.
52. Tofler GH, Muller JE, Stone PH, et al: Modifiers of possible timing and possible triggers of acute myocardial infarction in the Thrombolysis in Myocardial Infarction Phase II (TIMI II) Study Group. *J Am Coll Cardiol* 1992;20:1049–1055.
53. Mittleman MA, Maclure M, Tofler GH, et al: Triggering of acute myocardial infarction by heavy physical exertion: Protection against triggering by regular exertion. *N Engl J Med* 1993;329:1677–1683.
54. Willich SN, Lewis M, Lowel H, et al: Physical exertion as a trigger of acute myocardial infarction. *N Engl J Med* 1993;329:1684–1690.
55. Black DA: Mental state and presentation of myocardial infarction in the elderly. *Age Ageing* 1987;16:125–127.
56. Lipsitz LA, Pluchino FC, Wei JY: The prevalence and prognosis of minimally elevated creatine kinase—MB activity in elderly patients with syncope. *Arch Intern Med* 1987;147:1321–1323.
57. Wei JY, Gersh BJ: Heart disease in the elderly. *Curr Probl Cardiol* 1987;12:1–65.
58. O'Rourke RA, Chatterjee K, Wei JY: Atherosclerotic coronary heart disease in the elderly. *J Am Coll Cardiol* 1987;10:52A–56A.
59. Krumholz HM: The clinical challenges of myocardial infarction in the elderly. *West J Med* 1989;151:304–310.
60. Solomon CG, Lee TH, Cook EF, et al: Comparison of clinical presentation of acute myocardial infarction in patients older than 65 years of age to younger patients: The Multicenter Chest Pain Study experience. *Am J Cardiol* 1989;63:772–776.
61. Christian TF, Gibbons RJ, Hopfenspirger MR, et al: Severity and response of chest pain during thrombolytic therapy for acute myocardial infarction: An indicator of myocardial salvage and infarct size. *J Am Coll Cardiol* 1993;22:1311–1316.
62. Califf RM, O'Neill W, Stack RS, et al: Failure of simple clinical measurements to predict perfusion status after intravenous thrombolysis. *Ann Intern Med* 1988;108:658–662.
63. Cox DA, Rogers WJ, Aguirre FV, et al: Effect on outcome of the presence or absence of chest pain at initiation of recombinant tissue plasminogen activator therapy in acute myocardial infarction. *Am J Cardiol* 1994;73:729–736.
64. Gadsboll N, Hoilund-Carlsen P, Nielsen G, et al: Symptoms and signs of heart failure in patients with myocardial infarction: Reproducibility and relationship to chest x-ray, radionuclide ventriculography and right heart catheterization. *Eur Heart J* 1989;10: 1017–1028.
65. Herlihy T, McIvor ME, Cummings CC, et al: Nausea and vomiting during acute myocardial infarction and its relation to infarct size and location. *Am J Cardiol* 1987;60:20–22.
66. Logan R, Wong F, Barclay J: Symptoms associated with myocardial infarction: Are they of diagnostic value? *NZ Med J* 1986;99:276–278.
67. Wei JY: Nausea and vomiting during acute myocardial infarction. *Am J Cardiol* 1988;62:178–179.
68. Wei JY, Markis JE, Malagold M, Braunwald E: Cardiovascular reflexes stimulated by reperfusion of ischemic myocardium in acute myocardial infarction. *Circulation* 1983;67:796–801.
69. Wei JY, Markis JE, Braunwald E: Coronary reperfusion stimulates cardiac reflexes. *Int J Cardiol* 1984;5:537–540.
70. Yano K, Reed SM, McGee DL: Ten-year incidence of coronary heart disease in the Honolulu heart program. Relationship to biologic and lifestyle characteristics. *Am J Epidemiol* 1984;119:653.
71. Multiple-Risk Factor Intervention Trial Research Group: Multiple-risk factor intervention trial: Risk factor changes in mortality results. *JAMA* 1982;248:1465.
72. Selhub J, Jacques PF, Bostom AG, et al: Association between plasma homocysteine concentrations and extracranial carotid-artery stenosis. *N Engl J Med* 1995;332:286–291.
73. Krumholz HM, Seeman TE, Merrill SS, et al: Lack of association between cholesterol and coronary heart disease mortality and morbidity and all-cause mortality in persons older than 70 years. *JAMA* 1994;272:1335–1340.

74. SHEP Cooperative Research Group: Prevention of stroke in antihypertensive drug treatment in older persons with isolated systolic hypertension. *JAMA* 1991;265:3255–3264.
75. Mahrenberg ME, Risch N, Berkman LF, et al: Genetic susceptibility to death from coronary heart disease in a study of twins. *N Engl J Med* 1994;330:1041–1046.
76. Kee F, Robo JY, Nicaud V, et al: Reliability of reported family history of myocardial infarction. *Br Med J* 1993;307:1528–1530.
77. Wei JY, Bulkley BH: Myocardial infarction before age 36 years in women: Predominance of apparent nonatherosclerotic events. *Am Heart J* 1982; 104:561.
78. Smith H, Liberman HA, Brody SL, et al: Acute myocardial infarction temporally related to cocaine use. Clinical, angiographic, and pathophysiologic observations. *Ann Intern Med* 1988;108:131 134.
79. Wei JY, Genecin A, Greene HL, Achuff SC: Coronary artery spasm with ventricular fibrillation during thyrotoxicosis: Response to attaining euthyroid state. *Am J Cardiol* 1979;43:335–339.
80. Gersh BJ, Clements IP, Chesebo JH: Acute myocardial infarction: Diagnosis and prognosis, in Brandenburg RO, Fuster V, Giuliani ER, et al (eds): *Cardiology: Fundamentals and Practice.* Chicago, Year Book Medical Publishers, 1987, pp 1116–1152.
81. Shannon RP, Wei JY, Rosa RM, et al: The effect of age and sodium depletion on cardiovascular response to orthostasis. *Hypertension* 1986;8:438–442.
82. Wei JY: Cardiovascular drugs in the elderly: Antianginal agents. *Drug Ther* 1987;17:31–43.
83. Wei JY: Aging and cardiovascular drugs. *Primary Cardiol* 1987;13:64–68.
84. Wei JY, Hutchins GM, Bulkley BH: Papillary muscle rupture in fatal acute myocardial infarction: A potentially treatable form of cardiogenic shock. *Ann Intern Med* 1979;59:588–592.
85. Weintraub RM, Wei JY, Thurer RL: Surgical repair of remediable post-infarction cardiogenic shock in the elderly: Early and long-term results. *J Am Geriatr Soc* 1986;34:389–392.
86. Weiss JL, Wei JY, Kappleman NB: Ventricular septal defect complicating myocardial infarction. *J Hopkins Med J* 1977;141:95–100.
87. Weintraub RM, Thurer RL, Wei JY, Aroesty JM: Repair of post-infarction VSD in the elderly: Early and long-term results. *J Thorac Cardiovasc Surg* 1983;85:191–196.
88. Dell'Italia LJ, Starling MR, O'Rourke RA: Physical examination for exclusion of hemodynamically important right ventricular infarction. *Ann Intern Med* 1984;101:797–798.
89. Silverman BD, Carabajal NR, Chorches MA, Taranto AI: Tricuspid regurgitation and acute myocardial infarction. *Arch Intern Med* 1983;143: 434–436.
90. Goldman L, Cook EF, Johnson PA, Brand DA, Rouan G, Lee TH: Prediction of the need for intensive care in patients who come to emergency departments with acute chest pain. *N Engl J Med* 1996;334:1498–504.
91. Krumholz HM, Radford MJ, Ellerbeck EF, Hennen J, Meehan TP, Petrillo M, Wang Y, Kresowik TF, Jencks SF: Aspirin in the treatment of acute myocardial infarction in elderly Medicare beneficiaries: patterns of use and outcomes. *Circulation* 1995;92: 2841–7.
92. Rosamond WD, Sprafka JM, McGovern PG, Nelson M, Luepker RV: Validation of self-reported history of acute myocardial infarction: experience of the Minnesota Heart Survey Registry. *Epidemiology* 1995;67–9.
93. Normand ST, Glickman ME, Sharma VRK, McNeil BJ. Using admission characteristics to predict short-term mortality from myocardial infarction in elderly patients. *JAMA* 1996;275:1322–8.

8

Biochemical Detection of Acute Myocardial Infarction

Allan S. Jaffe, MD

Since the 1950s, when aspartate amino transferase (AST, previously known as SGOT) was first used diagnostically for the detection of acute myocardial injury (1), the use of changes in biochemical markers in plasma for the diagnosis of acute myocardial infarction has increased substantially. At present, the diagnosis of acute myocardial infarction will, in general, not be made even in the classic clinical setting in the absence of biochemical confirmation. In some instances the electrocardiogram (ECG) may not reflect myocardial injury, and because the clinical presentations of patients with ischemic heart disease are extremely variable, at times elevations in the molecular markers of myocardial injury are the only evidence of infarction. This has led some to suggest that the presence of increases in plasma markers alone may be sufficient for the diagnosis of infarction (2). This advocacy presumes an in-depth understanding on the part of the diagnostician of the issues related to the measurement and the sensitivity and specificity of each molecular marker used for diagnostic purposes.

In addition to their diagnostic importance, these markers can be used to estimate size of infarction if their release and clearance from plasma, their concentration in myocardium, their volume of distribution, and the extent to which they are depleted from myocardium after myocardial injury can be determined. Such estimates have been shown to correlate closely with those derived morphologically, especially in the absence of thrombolysis (3–5).

In the context of thrombolysis, both the kinetics of release of macromolecules from the heart and their diagnostic uses change. Early definitive confirmation of infarction by plasma markers in candidates for thrombolysis would be most helpful, and substantial investigative attempts are proceeding in that direction (6–9). In addition, since recanalization alters the rate of release of these molecular markers, it appears that their rate of change in plasma can be used to determine whether or not coronary recanalization has been induced (10–12). Finally, if the kinetics of release of these markers after thrombolysis can be defined, the ability to use release over time as an indicator of the size of myocardial infarction in patients treated with thrombolytic agents may be possible. Since the kinetics of release and perhaps the percentage of any given marker that appears in blood compared with that depleted from heart may be altered by thrombolysis (13), definition and correction for this factor will be essential to definition of the relationship between the extent of infarction documented biochemically and treatment with and without thrombolytic agents.

CHARACTERISTICS OF MOLECULAR MARKERS USED FOR THE DETECTION OF MYOCARDIAL INJURY (14)

The characteristics of the macromolecule measured will determine its optimal use diagnostically. Markers that are relatively small, such as myoglobin (molecular weight 17,800 daltons), are released more rapidly from myocardium and cleared more rapidly from plasma than are larger macromolecules (15,16). The advantage of these markers is that because they are cleared rapidly, they normally are present only in low levels in plasma; and thus their rapid release is more easily detectable, permitting earlier diagnosis. On the other hand, because of the rapid clearance, the diagnostic window for detection of myocardial injury with small molecules such as myoglobin is narrow. Furthermore, because myoglobin is present in skeletal muscle as well, elevations in plasma are not specific for cardiac injury (17). High molecular weight markers such as lactate dehydrogenase (LD; previously known as LDH, with a molecular weight of 135,000 daltons) are released more slowly and disappear from plasma more slowly (18). Accordingly, the diagnosis of myocardial injury is made later, but the time window during which diagnostic changes can be detected is much broader, permitting the application of diagnostic criteria over many days. The measurement of relatively tissue-specific LD isoenzymes has in recent years improved the specificity of diagnosis based on LD, but newer markers such as the troponins are likely to be still more specific (19). Myosin light chain fragments and the troponins have intermediate molecular weights (20,000 to 27,000 daltons) and are released rapidly from myocardium due to an immediately releasable "cytosolic pool" (20–22). Continuing release of structurally bound protein is slow, and thus this marker remains elevated for many days (21–24). These markers (especially cardiac troponin I and T) have improved specificity for myocardium and thus will become important diagnostic markers.

At present, the MB isoenzyme of creatine kinase (CK) still is the diagnostic marker of choice. Its molecular weight, which has been reported to be from 78,500 to 85,100 daltons (25), is associated with relatively early release from myocardium and an intermediate clearance time relative to myoglobin and LD, which permits a diagnostic window of roughly 6 to 36 hours depending on the extent of myocardial damage (26,27). The specificity of MBCK (also written CK MB) for myocardium is high, although not as high as the troponins (19). The specificity of all of these markers for myocardial tissue and thus for defining specific tissue injury will be discussed subsequently for each marker.

Whether these molecule markers are released in response to irreversible myocardial injury only or in response to reversible injury as well is controversial. Because these macromolecules are components of myocytes, it has been presumed that in the absence of disruption of the cell membrane, they will not be released. It is further presumed that the release of myocardial cellular constituents should be a marker of cell death. This has been substantiated in part by experimental studies where the release of CK parallels histologic evidence of myocardial injury (28–30). It is also consistent with the inability to provoke CK release despite overt ischemia in most patients with unstable angina (31) or ischemia induced with exercise stress testing (32). However, in experimental studies small amounts of CK released into lymph, coronary sinus effluent, or plasma have been detected in the absence of characteristic histologic evidence of myocardial injury (33,34). Whether detection of minute quantities of CK is indicative of release from reversibly damaged tissue or results from difficulties in detecting small amounts of myocardial necrosis is unclear. Small amounts of enzyme released from irreversibly injured cells in different locations could lead to detectable quantities in body fluid, despite an insufficient contiguous mass of injured tissue to permit detection by morphometric analysis. Clinical studies to resolve this issue are difficult in humans, but there is a corollary in skeletal muscle. Elevations in skeletal muscle enzymes are common in response to exercise. Although the concept that release of enzymes during exercise is indicative of muscle necrosis is distressing, with extremely strenuous exercise, marked enzyme release and muscle necrosis does occur (35,36). By analogy, this finding supports the concept that the release of macromolecules from myoctyes within the heart is indicative of myocardial injury. It may well be that the use of markers that require degradation from structural proteins prior to release will lead to an answer to this controversy in the future (21,22). At present, although scientific disagreement continues to exist, the finding of increases in levels of macromolecules that are tissue-specific for myocardial injury, in the absence of laboratory and clinical circumstances known to induce false or real elevations not due to infarction (e.g., myocarditis), should be considered indicative of myocardial injury.

CREATINE KINASE

At present, the marker of diagnostic choice is the MB isoenzyme of CK. Creatine kinase catalyzes the transfer of a high-energy phosphate group from ATP to creatine to produce creatine phosphate (CP) (37). Creatine phosphate is thought to be the substrate most readily available when there is a sudden increase in energy utilization. ATP in mitochondria donate high-energy phosphate molecules in response to the action of the mitochondrial CK isoenzyme on creatine, resulting in the production of CP (38). The CP then diffuses into the cytosol, where cytosolic CK catalyzes the removal of the high-energy phosphate to produce ATP (39).

The relative efficiency of various forms of CK in high-energy phosphate transport is unclear, but three distinct isoenzymes (40) and a mitochondrial form (41) are known to exist. The three isoenzyme forms are all dimers consisting of 39,000 to 42,500 dalton subunits that are synthesized in the cytosol of the cell (42). Single chains are inactive. These isoenzymes are composed of either two M units (MMCK), two B subunits (BBCK), or one M and one B unit (MBCK). In general, BBCK is found in high abundance in brain, MM is abundant in skeletal muscle, and MB is most prevalent in the heart (43). Mitochondrial CK has a separate structure and is not formed from M and B chains. In addition, multiple isoforms representing minor post-translational modifications of the amino terminus of the M and B chains have been described (44–46).

Creatine kinase is inactivated and proteolysed in lymph (47). Thus varying proportions of CK will reach the plasma depending on the tissue that has been injured, blood flow, and local lymphatic perfusion. CK clearance is not affected by heart rate, blood pressure, or cardiac output (48). CK is not excreted with the urine and is not influenced by changes in renal or hepatic blood flow (49). Hypothyroidism reduces CK clearance and exogenously administered thyroid accelerates clearance (50). Nonspecific reticuloendothelial blockade also retards CK clearance (51).

Isoforms of both MMCK and MBCK have been described. Three isoforms of MMCK are known to exist, with the tissue isoform designated as MM_3 (52–54). MM_3 has lysines at the amino terminus of both M chains and is virtually the only isoform detected in tissue. After release into plasma, carboxypeptidase N cleaves first one, and subsequently both terminal lysines (54,55). This generates an intermediate form, designated MM_2, in which a lysine is present at the aminoterminus of only one M chain, and an ultimate conversion product, MM_1, which is devoid of lysines on the M chains. These structural changes are associated with a change in charge, permitting the isoforms to be separated by methods that separate proteins by charge, such as electrophoresis (44–46,52–54). MM_3 migrates more slowly toward the anode, MM_2 with intermediate speed, and MM_1 the most quickly and the furthest. Isoforms of MBCK also have been described. In theory, four such isoforms exist, since it is known that the tissue isoform has lysines present on both M and B chains (56). Thus, in addition to the tissue form, there should be a form in which the M lysine is removed and the B lysine remains, a form in which the B chain lysine has been removed but the M chain lysine remains, and an ultimate conversion product with both lysines absent. Controversy exists as to whether or not all four forms that can be produced in hybridization experiments (56) occur in vivo. Most investigators have only reported two forms (57,58); however, it is now clear that at least three forms circulate in vivo: the tissue form; a lysine negative B, lysine positive M chain variant that co-migrates with the tissue form; and a form without lysines on either carboxyl terminal, which migrates with the lysine negative M, lysine positive B chain form. It is unclear if significant amounts of the lysine negative M, lysine positive B chain form exist in plasma. It is also now clear that, in contrast to MMCK, cleavage of the B chain terminal lysine is favored (59,60).

Distribution of Creatine Kinase Isoenzymes in Tissue

Creatine kinase is a ubiquitous protein, found in most tissues (43). MMCK is the predominant isoenzyme found in muscle. Skeletal muscle has been reported to contain as much as 12,000 IU/gm and as little as 225 IU/gm of CK activity. Although some studies (61–63), predominantly those based on the assay of CK activity, failed to detect MBCK in skeletal muscle (Fig. 8–1), it has become clear with the use of more sensitive techniques to measure the mass of CK protein that a substantial proportion of skeletal muscles contain trace amounts (1% to 3%) of MBCK (64,65) and, in rare instances, even more. Because of the large quantity of CK in skeletal muscle, this amount, which is small in percentage terms, is substantial in absolute terms compared with the amount in myocardium (roughly 15% of total CK, or approximately 240 IU/g) (66). However, in general, modest degrees of skeletal muscle damage in the absence of a chronic myopathic process do not result in detectable increases in MBCK in plasma. For example, intramuscular injections and instrumentation during cardiac catheterization or during uncomplicated angioplasty results in elevations of total but not MBCK (67,68).

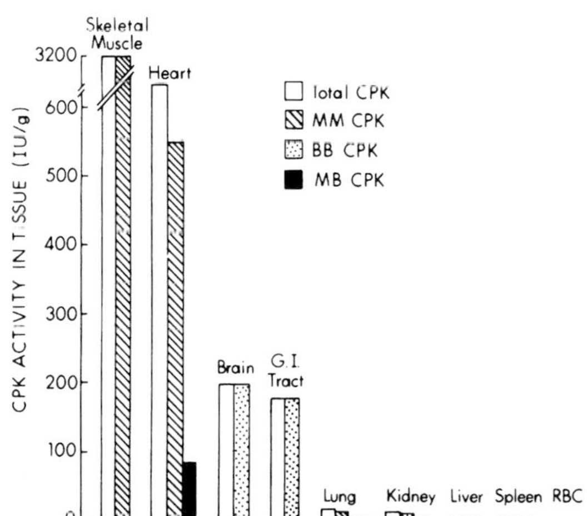

Figure 8–1. Total and MBCK activity from extracts of human tissue obtained at operation. With activity assays, very little if any MBCK is detected in tissue other than the heart. Minor amounts have been found with more sensitive techniques based on detection of CK protein. *Reproduced from Roberts et al (61), with permission.*

When skeletal muscle is damaged, it regenerates B chains in response to injury (69). This is thought to represent a return to "ontogeny," since during early fetal development BBCK is the predominant CK isoenzyme in skeletal muscle (70,71). By birth, MM predominates. When injury occurs, an increased number of B chains are in proximity to a high concentration of M chains, which results in high levels of MBCK in the regenerating muscle. This phenomenon has been described in response to chronic and acute muscle injury (72–78) and extremely strenuous exercise (35,36,79,80), and it is likely the partial explanation for elevations in MBCK plasma in patients with hypothyroidism (81) and renal disease (82) as well. Thus, when severe and especially continuing muscle injury is present, substantial quantities of MBCK can be released into plasma, confounding the diagnosis of acute infarction. Recently, it has been shown that even the small amounts of MBCK in skeletal muscle can confound diagnosis in patients with acute and chronic muscle disease, patients with renal failure, individuals after extreme exercise (19), perioperative patients (83), and those with possible blunt thoracic trauma (84).

Human myocardium contains approximately 1,600 IU/gm of CK activity (49). It is thought to contain 15% to 30% MBCK (66). Controversy exists as to whether or not the MBCK found in heart occurs as a consequence of chronic or acute muscle injury or is a normal constituent (85). At present, judging from autopsy data (86), data from other primates (87), and the ability to make the diagnosis of acute infarction based on a rising and falling pattern of MBCK even in the patient whose myocardium was thought to be totally normal before injury (88), it appears that MBCK usually resides in myocardium. However, it may be that the amount of MBCK in the heart increases in response to myocardial injury (89). We have observed percentages of MBCK as high as 50% of CK protein in some hearts (unpublished data), suggesting that a reparative process similar to the one documented in skeletal muscle may occur in myocardium. Although this response to injury would improve the sensitivity of detection of acute infarction in some patients, it could confound comparative measurements of infarct size in many others.

Tissues such as brain, gastrointestinal tract, prostate, and uterus are known to contain substantial quantities of BBCK (43). With older assays that measured the B subunit, there was ambiguity in ascribing increases in assay values to increases in MBCK because of the possibility that BBCK had been released from other tissues.

On occasion, tumors have been reported to contain high concentrations of B chains; such reports are unusual (90–93).

Techniques of Measurement

Samples for assay of CK activity and/or mass can be collected as either serum or plasma. In plasma, EDTA has been shown to preserve CK activity and particularly isoform proportions optimally (94,95). All samples for measurement of activity should be maximally reduced with β mecaptoethanol to protect against oxidation of sulfhydryl groups in the active center of the compound and loss of activity. The thiol groups donated by mecaptoethanol protect in part against this loss of activity (96).

Assays for CK activity are based on the coupled enzyme system developed by Oliver (97) and improved by Rosalki and others (98–100). It uses one of two reactions, the so-called "reverse reaction":

$$\text{Phosphocreatine} + \text{ADP} \xrightarrow{\text{CK}} \text{Creatine} + \text{ATP}$$

$$\text{ATP} + \text{Glucose} \xrightarrow{\text{HK}} \text{Glucose-6-phosphate} + \text{ADP}$$

$$\text{Glucose-6-phosphate} + \text{NADP} \xrightarrow{\text{G-6-PDH}}$$

$$\text{6-Phosphogluconate} + \text{NADPH}$$

or a variant of this procedure, the so-called "forward reaction":

$$\text{Creatine} + \text{ATP} \xrightarrow{\text{CK}} \text{Phosphocreatine} + \text{ADP}$$

$$\text{ADP} + \text{Phosphoenolpyruvate} \xrightarrow{\text{PK}} \text{ATP} + \text{Pyruvate}$$

$$\text{Pyruvate} + \text{NADH} \xrightarrow{\text{LDH}} \text{Lactate} + \text{NAD}$$

The rate of change in the absorbance from either NADH to NAD (101) or from NADP to NADPH is proportional to CK activity (97–100). Fluorescence is detected by absorption of ultraviolet light absorption at 340 nm. Both the forward and reverse reactions will proceed if ATP is added to the reaction mixture at the critical time, even in the absence of CK. Commercially available assay kits employ inhibitors of adenylate kinase, which is in high concentration in erythrocytes and is the most common extraneous source of ATP (102). Nonetheless, gross hemolysis, if present, can produce sufficient ATP, so that inhibition is not total and spurious elevations can occur (102). Since the activity of CK is temperature dependent, the temperature at which the assay has been accomplished must be reported.

Correction factors for temperature are as follows (98).:

37 to 30°C,	0.58
30 to 25°C,	0.68
37 to 25°C,	0.39

Nonimmunoassay Isoenzyme Procedures

Most isoenzyme assays relied on the separation of CK isoenzymes by charge. Of late, sensitive monoclonal antibodies to MBCK have become available, which have reduced substantially our reliance on these methods (103,104). Nonetheless, electrophoretic methods remain essential to the quality control of all assay methods. Although multiple modifications exist, in general the sample is diluted to a CK activity of roughly 300 IU/L, applied to a gel, and electrophoresed (105). BBCK moves closest to the anode, MMCK stays close to the origin, and MBCK migrates to an intermediate position (106). Mitochondrial CK, if present, migrates in the opposite direction (107). The gel is then overlayed with reagents for either the forward or backward reaction, and fluorescence is determined by ultraviolet light at a fixed reaction time presumed to be at equilibrium. The gel can then be read qualitatively by comparison with standards electrophoresed concomitantly, or it can be read semiquantitatively using scanning at that cytometry. Electrophoresis with cellulose acetate has a sensitivity of 10 to 12 IU/L, or roughly the upper limit of the normal range (63,108). Electrophoresis on agarose permits detection of isoenzymes at levels of approximately 5 IU/L, well within the normal range (109).

Although the electrophoretic method has provided reliable data for many years, it is far from perfect. Macrokinases, including IgG bound to CK (macro CK 1) or aggregates of mitochondrial CK (macro CK 2), are also detected (110,111). The migration of macro CK 1 is similar to that of MBCK and in the absence of appropriately placed controls can be confused with this isoenzyme. Macro CK 2 tends to migrate near MMCK and can cause confusion with respect to the semiquantitation of activity. In addition, naturally fluorescing compounds such as bilirubin, pyridoxine, benzodiazepines, antidepressants, aspirin in high doses, and antibiotics can cause artifactual bands (112). This is particularly a problem in samples from patients with renal failure in which artifactual bands (those that are still present after electrophoresis with the absence of CP) that migrate in the region of MBCK and BBCK are common (Fig. 8–2).

The method also is cumbersome, and its use requires skilled personnel, making it less popular than

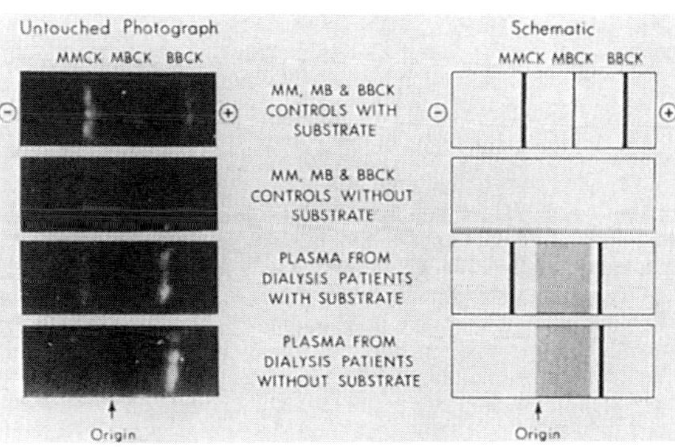

Figure 8–2. Normal migration of creatine kinase isoenzymes (**top**), and their lack of presence in the absence of specific substrate (creatine phosphate) (**second panel from top**). Plasma from a patient supported with chronic renal dialysis has a band that migrates close to that shown for MBCK, but it is still present even in the absence of creatine phosphate. Thus it is artifactual. Such bands are common in patients with renal failure. *Reproduced from Jaffe et al (82), with permission.*

automated methods. However, the availability of assays based on the use of MBCK monoclonal antibodies have made other automated assays obsolete (103,104).

Macrokinases also are collected in the fractions extracted by many of these assays as MBCK or B subunit activity (110,111). Their presence, although rare, can confound results.

Immunoassay Procedures

Techniques based on monoclonal antibodies that recognize unique epitopes mostly on the M chain and that do not cross-react with the MM or BB isoenzyme are now in use with most assays. These techniques provide for very rapid determination of MBCK mass (5 to 7 minutes) and avoid some of the interferences from other substances encountered with activity assays. However, as with any assay, interferences can occur (113).

The ability to provide quality for these new techniques based on CK mass, with activity assays and electrophoresis, is essential at this time. With mass assays there is generally a close correlation between CK activity and protein concentration, except when levels of MBCK are very high (i.e., in patients with thrombolysis), where modest discordances have been observed (114). One might speculate that the inactivation of CK can occur in myocardium when oxygen free radical scavengers are present (115) or inactivation in the circulation might reduce the specific activity of MBCK, but an increase in specific activity is instead observed. The reason for this increase is unclear, but it could be due to the interaction of plasmin with the epitope on MBCK for monoclonal antibody binding or the format of the assays. Rarely, if ever, do these differences cause diagnostic confusion (114). Thus radioimmunoassays based on monoclonal antibodies have replaced most other assays. However, comparison of results with those of electrophoretic methods and activity assays, to provide quality control, is still prudent.

Separation of Isoforms

Creatine kinase isoforms originally were recognized after separation by electrophoresis (44,45). More recently, more rapid methods such as high-voltage electrophoresis (116), immunoblotting (117), and chromatofocusing (118) have been developed. Techniques based on extraction of either the lysine-rich tissue isoform or of the ultimate lysine negative conversion product (MM_1) with monoclonal antibodies would be extremely attractive. Although strategies employing isoforms are biologically attractive, the presently available techniques for measurement are not yet sufficiently facile to permit widespread clinical application.

Creatine kinase MB also has isoforms (44,45). At present, a rapid electrophoretic method is used to obtain semiquantitative results with adequate sensitivity and specificity, but only two of the four isoforms can be resolved (57,58). Thus it may be some time before a facile technique that results in the separation of all of the MBCK isoforms can be routinely applied in the clinical environment (59,60). Furthermore, at the levels recommended for diagnosis, which require only tiny amounts of activity (only 1 IU/L), some groups have questioned the analytic reliability of the separations (119).

Diagnosis of Acute Myocardial Infarction with Creatine Kinase

Soon after the onset of acute myocardial infarction, levels of CK begin to increase. Levels of the tissue isoforms rise to a perceptibly elevated degree very early because conversion and clearance is rapid, which results in very low physiologic levels of these isoforms in plasma, and because all the new enzyme released is in this form. Accordingly, patients should manifest increased levels of tissue isoforms (6–9,120) very early after the onset of acute infarction (Fig. 8–3). Data from studies of MMCK suggest that a strategy in which both MM isoforms and MBCK are measured can detect acute infarction by analysis of the initial plasma sample in most patients. Forty-seven of fifty consecutive patients (94%) admitted to the hospital who ultimately were documented to have acute infarction were detected by analysis of MM isoforms and MBCK (7). This included the diagnosis of 3 of 4 patients admitted within 2 hours and 12 of 13 admitted within 4 hours who had normal levels of MBCK (mean = 4.6 ± 0.6 IU/L). Levels of MBCK were helpful in diagnosing patients who presented more than 16 hours after the onset of infarct, at a time when isoform proportions had returned to normal in 33%. Thus, in the long view, once more convenient techniques for measurement are developed, the measurement of MMCK isoforms should allow the early rapid diagnosis of acute infarction (7). Recently, data obtained by analysis of levels of MB isoforms and what is presumed to be the tissue isoform have indicated that earlier detection of acute infarction than that with MBCK is also achievable with MBCK isoforms. MBCK isoform levels begin to rise at 2 to 4 hours after infarction and are diagnostic in nearly 90% by 4 to 6 hours, a time when MBCK activity is elevated in only approximately 50% of patients. MBCK activity does not achieve a sensitivity of 90% until 10 to 12 hours (121,122). The difference between MBCK activity and MB isoforms may have been accentuated by the use of MBCK activity measurements rather than mass measurements, which rise earlier (123–125). Thus isoforms may permit the earlier diagnosis of acute infarction. Recently, MBCK isoforms were used to evaluate 1,110 consecutive patients who presented with possible acute myocardial infarction (122). With 6 hours of serial sampling, 95.7% of the 121

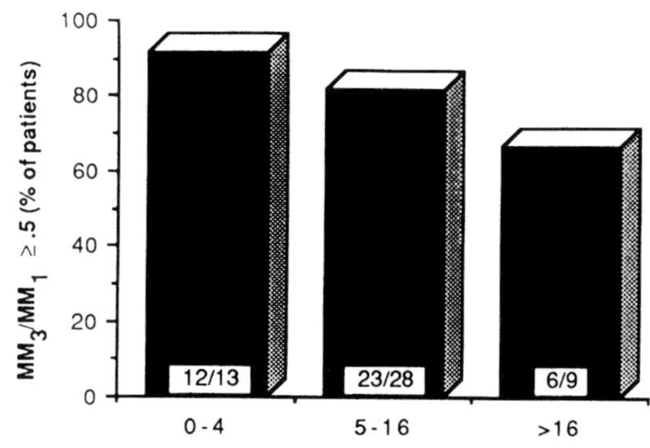

Figure 8–3. Sensitivity of criteria based on isoform proportions with respect to the interval of time from the onset of acute infarction to the time of acquisition of initial plasma sample. MM isoform sensitivity is highest very early after the onset of infarction. Six of the eight patients in whom isoform proportions were not abnormal presented between 5 and 16 hours and had elevated levels of MBCK. Thus total sensitivity for detection of infarction was 47 of 50 (94%). *Reproduced from Abendschein et al (7), with permission.*

patients with acute infarction were detected (Fig. 8–4). The average time to an increased isoform measurement was 1.22 ± 1.17 hours, and nearly half (41%) of these patients had elevations in the first sample, a mean of 3.25 ± 1.7 hours after the onset of symptoms. These data were in contrast to the results of MBCK activity measurements, which were only elevated in 48% of patients after 6 hours of measurements. Importantly, the specificity of this analysis for exclusion of infarction after 6 hours was 93.9% for hospitalized patients and 96.2% for those sent home. The mean time for this analysis was 1.22 ± 1.17 hours. The false-positive incidence was 3.8%. This study clearly documents that the diagnosis of acute infarction can be made earlier with MBCK isoforms. What remains to be determined is the extent to which false positive diagnoses were minimized by astute patient selection, given that false positive elevations of MB isoforms are observed in patients with skeletal muscle injury and head trauma (126). Such a report should not be surprising since one might suspect that the very sensitive criteria used, which relies on as little as 1 IU of MBCK and a ratio of MB2 to MB1 >1.5, would easily be met by even the small amounts of MBCK present in skeletal muscle. This is despite the fact that MBCK isoforms are more specific for infarction than are MM isoforms. In the study in which initial samples were analyzed for MM isoforms, there was a 23% false-positive rate (7).

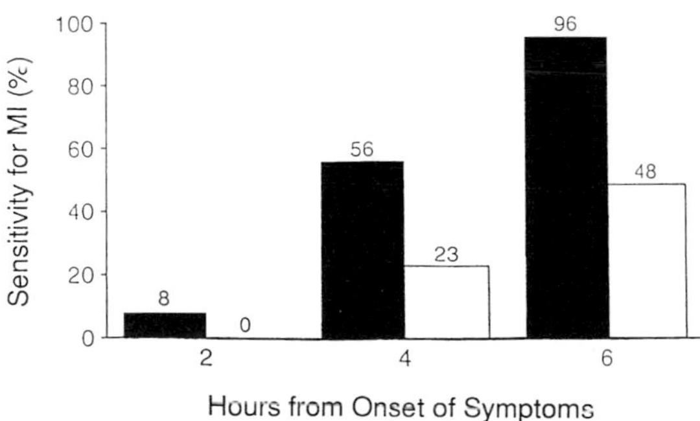

Figure 8–4. Comparison of the sensitivity of MBCK (light bars) and MBCK isoforms (dark bars) for the early detection of acute myocardial infarction. Infarction was subsequently confirmed by evaluation of serial measurements of MBCK. *Reproduced from Puleo et al (122), with permission.*

Total CK and MBCK rise in plasma in the bulk of patients between 6 and 10 hours after the onset of infarction and, in the absence of thrombolysis, usually peak at 24 hours (26,27,127). In general, peak MBCK level occurs slightly earlier than the peak with total CK. MBCK also appears to be cleared from blood slightly more rapidly than total CK (127) (Fig. 8–5). The time to peak for smaller infarctions is shorter (27). Since many of these smaller infarctions are non-Q wave infarctions, some have interpreted this finding as suggesting that myocardial injury with non-Q wave infarction is caused by transient thrombotic occlusion and subsequent spontaneous thrombolysis and reperfusion causing more rapid washout of CK. This is only one possibility. The more prompt egress of total CK and MBCK into plasma in patients with recanalization is reflected by accelerated washout of these enzymes, so that, in general, levels have risen into the abnormal range by 2 hours after successful treatment (128).

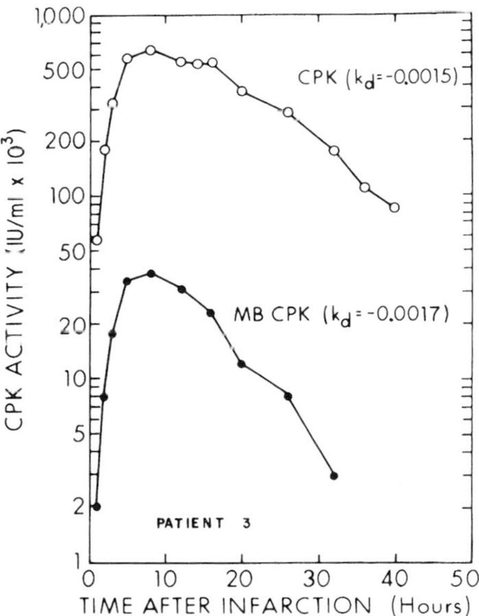

Figure 8–5. Total plasma and MB time–activity curves from a patient with acute myocardial infarction. The curves and the relative percentage of MB with respect to total CK are reasonably constant. MBCK disappears slightly more rapidly. *Reproduced from Roberts et al (106), with permission.*

The relationship between the amounts of total CK and MBCK in plasma reflects their distribution in tissue, since it appears that MBCK and MMCK are released equally from myocardium during infarction. MBCK in plasma should then be approximately 15% of total CK in the absence of coronary recanalization. However, in patients with large infarctions there is noncardiac release of MMCK, which diminishes the relative percentage of MBCK with respect to total CK in plasma (127). Accordingly, percentages of MB range from 1% to 21% of total CK, suggesting that the use of percentage criteria for the diagnosis of infarction are not well advised (129). In the appropriate clinical setting, any elevation of MBCK above baseline, associated with a rising and falling pattern compatible with infarction, in the absence of other conditions known to be associated with elevations with MBCK, should be considered indicative of infarction.

Conditions that may be associated with elevated MBCK in the absence of acute infarction include the following:

1. *Laboratory artifacts.* Artifacts can occur with electrophoresis due to hemolysis, hyperbilirubinemia, or drugs (102,112). They also occur when macrokinases are present and in patients with renal failure (82,110,111). These artifacts are rare, with modern assays based on monoclonal antibodies. The possibility that such increases are artifactual should be suspected by the clinician who understands the methods of measurement of CK and the clinical circumstances under which elevations occur. Patients in whom macro CK 1 is detected most often manifest very marked increases in the percentage of MBCK with respect to total CK. These individuals are usually older, are more frequently women, and are often chronically ill. The estimated incidence in hospitalized patients is said to be 1.6%, but this is likely an overestimate. Macro kinase CK 2 is also associated with chronic disease and the severely ill patient (110,111). The concomitant use of drugs, laboratory artifacts, and the state of the sample when it is sent to the laboratory (with or without hemolysis) must be noted to permit accurate interpretation (112). Other considerations necessary to avoid artifacts with the electrophoretic method include a high level of laboratory quality control and experienced technicians.
2. Immunoassays can cross-react with circulating immunoglobulins and some may detect macrokinases as well. Recently, false-positive elevations due to the presence in vivo of atypical forms of alkaline phosphatase have been reported when reagents that contain alkaline phosphatase have been used to stabilize the assay reagents (114). In general, such results are easy to identify and yield MB determinations in excess of those for total CK. These findings can be definitively unmasked by electrophoresis.
3. Myocyte necrosis, even in the absence of infarction, will lead to increases in MBCK. Thus myocarditis, severe pericarditis with myocardial involvement (129,130), electrical injury (whether induced by accident or with recurrent countershocks of 400 joules or more) (131,132), and myocardial contusion will result in increases in MBCK (74,75,133). Since in many cases concomitant muscle injury may be present, as stated above the use of the relative percentage of MBCK with respect to total CK may be misleading (19)—the small amount of MBCK released with cardiac injury may be quite modest compared with the massive amount of CK released when there is extensive muscle damage, as with thoracic trauma. Thus, when concomitant massive skeletal muscle injury is present and there is a suspicion of concomitant myocardial injury, acceptance of relatively lower MBCK/total CK ratios or the use of alternative methods may be necessary. In a large study of trauma victims, the percentage of MBCK with respect to total CK did not distinguish between those patients with and without myocardial contusion (133). This is likely because patients with myocardial contusion had a greater mass of skeletal muscle damaged as well. Thus, when myocardial injury not related to infarction may be present, methods of evaluation over and above enzymatic measures may be necessary.
4. As indicated above, small amounts of MBCK can be released in response to skeletal muscle

injury. Because the amount, if any, of MBCK released is small, this rarely causes diagnostic confusion. There are, however, conditions in which this can occur. Patients with myopathies of a variety of sorts can have quite marked elevations in MBCK in their muscles and therefore, with muscle injury, increased MBCK in plasma as well (19,73–75,77,78,129,134). Very high percentages of MBCK with respect to total CK have been described in patients with polydermatomyositis, even in the absence of any evidence of cardiac involvement (19,134). In patients who have suffered massive rhabdomyolysis due to trauma or a crush injury; in those who have chronic myopathy including polydermatomyositis, myotonias, ALS, or Duchenne's muscular dystrophy; or in highly trained athletes' participation in major physical exertion, substantial amounts of MBCK can be released into plasma (73–78). In general, such elevations are detected in plasma for longer periods than are increases due to acute myocardial infarction, likely because of the continuing release that generally characterizes skeletal muscle injury. Thus persistent elevations in MBCK and the lack of a rising and falling characteristic of the enzyme changes of acute infarction should alert the clinician to the possibility that elevations are related to underlying skeletal muscle disease.

Detection of this type of false-positive elevation was in the past thought to be simple because overt skeletal muscle damage was thought to be invariably present. It is now clear that many patients with perioperative infarction can also be difficult to diagnose until markers that are virtually totally specific for myocardium, such as cardiac troponin I, become available (83). It also is possible that more modest degrees of exercise in less well-trained athletes or subtle chronic myopathies such as those associated with intermittent alcohol use could lead to elevations. Although in theory this is a possibility, at present there is little information to support this concept. Accordingly, these patients should be considered to have acute infarction unless there is substantial clinical evidence to the contrary.

5. In addition to artifactual bands detected on electrophoresis, a small percentage of patients with renal failure are known to have modest elevations of MBCK in plasma that are chronic and persistent (82). This is likely due to some degree of chronic skeletal muscle myopathy associated with abnormalities in parathyroid hormone and calcium and a nonspecific abnormality in CK clearance related to reticuloendothelial dysfunction.
6. Patients with hypothyroidism also are known to have increased levels of MBCK in plasma that probably result from skeletal muscle myopathy, alterations in the clearance of CK, and perhaps cardiac infiltration by mucopolysaccharide as well. Exogenously administered thyroid hormone increases the disappearance rate of CK through the reticuloendothelial system in laboratory animals, and hypothyroidism reduces clearance (50,51,81).
7. On rare occasions tumors that contain MBCK or BBCK can lead to increases in MBCK. In general, in this situation levels are persistently elevated and do not manifest a rising and falling pattern (90–93).

Enzymatic documentation has become the essential component for the diagnosis of acute infarction. When properly timed (every 6 hours) samples are obtained, the absence of absolute increases in MBCK excludes the diagnosis. However, since at times the onset of acute infarction can be difficult to ascertain and therefore the appropriateness of the timing of sample acquisition problematic, confirmation with additional biochemical tests (see below) may be necessary to exclude infarction. Conversely, a typical rise and fall in MBCK should be considered highly indicative of acute infarction, even in the presence of an atypical presentation. Other causes, including artifactual technical increases and the presence of other disease states known to cause elevations of MBCK, must be considered.

The diagnosis of acute infarction should not be made unless MBCK increases to above the absolute range of normal. The upper limit of normal will vary from institution to institution depending on the assay employed, biologic variability, the fact that values for MBCK have a logarithmic distribution, and the less precise technical accuracy of these assays at the lower end of the reference range (26). The American Association of Clinical Chemistry is moving to standardize the normal range of all MBCK assays in the hope of simplifying comparisons of assay results (135).

Some patients, especially the elderly, may have increases in plasma MBCK despite total CK activity within the normal range. These patients frequently have concomitant increases in other molecular markers of myocardial injury. Often ECG changes are present (136–138). Although the prognosis for such patients is quite good, it is not as good as that of individuals in whom MBCK elevations are not documented, suggesting that some component of infarction has occurred (138).

MBCK is consistently elevated after cardiac surgery because even small amounts of surgical manipulation of the heart are sufficient to induce release (139). Accordingly, despite a variety of algorithms devised to detect perioperative infarction in cardiothoracic surgery patients, plasma MBCK values do not provide for reliable diagnosis.

Detection of reinfarction (i.e., extension of infarction) is more problematic. During the period in which MBCK is rising, detection of reinfarction by analysis for this isoenzyme is impossible. Once MBCK has returned to normal, reelevation of its plasma level and similar criteria to that used initially can be employed. However, while MBCK is declining, the diagnosis of reinfarction is again difficult because the small amounts of enzyme released may simply blunt the downslope of the CK time or mass–activity curve rather than inducing a new discrete increase. Accordingly, it has been suggested that when MBCK is elevated but values are declining, a 25% increase from previous values in two samples should be the criteria for recurrent injury (140).

Detection of Coronary Recanalization

Coronary recanalization and myocardial reperfusion induce characteristic changes in the amount and pattern of enzyme release from injured myocardium. Although definitive studies are lacking, it appears that the release ratio (the amount of enzyme that appears in plasma compared with that depleted from myocardium) doubles in response to early recanalization (after 2 hours of occlusion in the dog) (13). It is likely that the release ratio is a continuum that depends on the time from the onset of symptoms to that of coronary recanalization. Although this poses a problem for the calculation of infarct size, the augmented amount of enzyme and its very rapid release in response to the return of nutritive perfusion permit strategies to be developed based on changes in enzyme kinetics that might allow for the detection of recanalization.

Studies based on changes in total CK thus far have not yielded reliable results for the vast majority of patients (12,141). If the time to peak CK is 4 hours or less, it is highly predictive of the presence of recanalization. Unfortunately, the time to peak CK in most patients falls between 4 and 16 hours, a period during which accuracy of the time to peak CK is between 40% and 60%. Although ways of deconvoluting the total CK may be developed, more interest has been focused on the very early detection of recanalization than on waiting for peak levels. Very early detection does not appear possible with total CK (12).

Results with MBCK have been somewhat more promising (128,142), and even criteria for very early application have been proposed. Criteria based on a 2.2-fold increase in MBCK over the first 90 minutes for patients with inferior infarction and a 2.5-fold increase during the initial 90 minutes for patients with anterior infarction were reported to be highly accurate predictors of the presence of coronary recanalization. With the use of rapid radioimmunoassays, such determinations can now easily be made in a timely fashion and can be used to determine which patients might be considered for rescue angioplasty (128). However, comparison of criteria based on MBCK with those based on isoforms (see below) suggests that earlier determinations (i.e., at 1 hour) are not nearly as precise with MBCK (12).

Changes in isoforms of MMCK and in values of myoglobin have been used to detect coronary recanalization (10–12,116, 143–145). In experimental animals with coronary stenosis, the rate of rise in enzyme release retains its accuracy as a marker of recanalization far better than the time to peak values or the slope of the disappearance rate (10). Although the detection of recanalization based on the clearance of activity during the downslope has been proposed and has reasonable diagnostic accuracy in patients (116), the rate of rise in enzyme release provides for earlier detection. The rate of rise in the MMCK tissue isoform (MM_3) between treatment and 60 minutes permits the classification of patients into those with and without coronary recanalization by 60 minutes after treatment. Seventeen of eighteen patients with recanalization and 11 of 12 without were properly identified with this technique, even though the mean time to coronary recanalization in most studies is 40 ± 20 minutes. Thus, some patients were likely to have experienced recanalization after the 60-minute sample had been obtained (11). Recent data from a large national cooperative trial suggest that 92% of patients with coronary recanalization can be identified using a rate of rise of the tissue isoform of MMCK of >0.18%/min and an absolute value >54% (146). In that study, an additional 30% of patients (false negatives) also would have been identified by those criteria. Unfortunately, these optimistic results were not confirmed in the recent report from the TAMI group (147).

Data for the rate of rise in MMCK isoforms provide comparable accuracy with those based on the rate of rise in myoglobin (12). Preliminary results in small numbers of patients with MBCK isoforms suggests that comparable sensitivity may be achievable with MB isoforms (116). However, concomitant measurement of the rates of change of both MM and MBCK isoforms may permit identification of individuals who recanalize and reocclude (Fig. 8–6). Using a criteria of a rate of rise >0.18%/min, a subset of patients who met this criteria with MBCK isoforms but not MMCK isoforms were identified. In half of these patients, the rate of rise of MMCK isoforms was >0.18%/min during the next hour (those shown to recanalized at catheterization) and in half it remained below this level (the group found to be occluded at catheterization and thought to have reoccluded). Patients who were persistently occluded did not manifest a substantial rise in either of the isoforms (148).

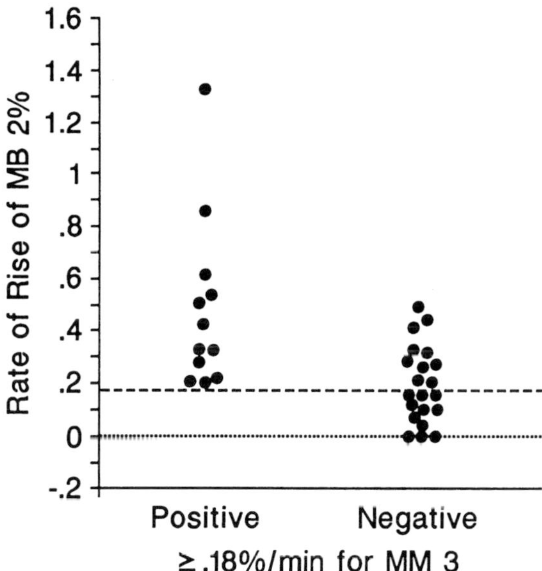

Figure 8–6. Values for the rate of rise of MMCK (abscissa) and MBCK (ordinate) isoforms 1 hour after treatment. Using a criteria for recanalization of >0.18%/minute, there were 10 patients in whom there was discordance between criteria based on MMCK and those based on MBCK. In 5 who recanalized, MBCK criteria were more sensitive, and criteria were met with MMCK during the next hour. In 5 who had occluded infarct-related arteries, MMCK criteria were not met after 1 hour, suggesting that this combination of criteria can be used to identify patients who reocclude. *Reproduced from Jaffe et al (148), with permission.*

Measurement of Infarct Size

Determinations of the extent of infarction based on levels of MBCK in experimental studies have documented that approximately 85% of the CK found in myocardium is depleted in response to myocardial injury (149). Of this percentage, roughly 15% reaches the circulation unless coronary recanalization is induced, in which circumstance the percentage appears to at least double (13). The remainder of the CK is hydrolyzed either locally or in lymph (47). Since the amount of enzyme depleted from the heart is directly proportional to the size of the myocardial infarction as long as a predictable relationship exists between the amount of CK depleted and the amount that reaches the plasma, serial values allow for summation of enzyme values and extrapolation mathematically to the amount depleted and, therefore, to infarct size. Extensive modeling of the volume of distribution and multiple determinations of the disappearance of CK have facilitated calculations (49). An excellent correlation has been found in experimental animals and in three clinical studies between enzymatic infarct size and morphometric infarct size at autopsy (Fig. 8–7). Enzymatic estimates also are closely correlated with ejection fraction (150), hemodynamics (7), the incidence of ventricular arrhythmias (151), and prognosis (152,153).

In the setting of coronary recanalization, enzyme kinetics are altered. Specifically, the amount of enzyme released into plasma (15%) relative to that depleted from myocardium (still 85%) (154) doubles in animals in which recanalization is achieved 2 hours after coronary occlusion (13). Thus comparisons between patients undergoing recanalization and those who do not receive such treatment can be problematic. It is reasonable to assume that higher peak total enzyme level should occur with recanalization than in its absence. Thus data suggesting that lesser peak levels are present can be considered evidence of a reduction in myocardial injury. However, caution is necessary because late recanalization may not affect the release ratio, but only accelerate the rate of rise in enzyme release. Therefore, comparisons of peak enzyme levels in more homogeneous groups of patients (i.e., those only with early recanalization or those only without recanalization) may be more relevant.

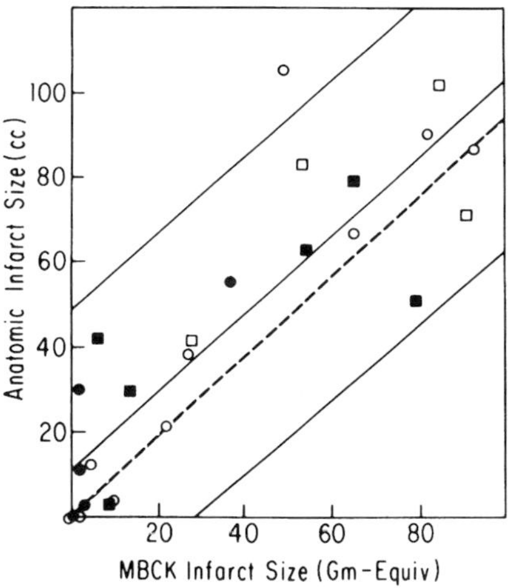

Figure 8–7. Relationship between anatomic and MBCK estimates of infarct size. Open symbols represent recent infarcts (≤16 days), and enclosed symbols, older infarcts. Solid lines represent the regression line and the 95% confidence limits for prediction of anatomic infarct size from the enzymatic estimates. Spearman correlation coefficient = 0.871, n = 25. *Reproduced from Hackel et al (3), with permission.*

MYOGLOBIN

Myoglobin, a heme protein with a molecular weight of 17,800 daltons, is believed to function as a reservoir for oxygen because of its ability to bind oxygen. Initially it was even confused with hemoglobin. It is found in both skeletal and cardiac muscle but not in smooth muscle (155). Isoenzymes have not been described, and it is presumed that cardiac and skeletal muscle myoglobin are identical, but this has not been proven definitively. Because of its small molecular weight, myoglobin is rapidly released from myocardium, reaching peak plasma levels by approximately 10 hours, and is cleared rapidly, returning to the normal range within 24 hours (16,156–161). Myoglobin clearance is biexponential and in experimental models is approximately 10 minutes after a bolus injection and 38 ± 3 minutes after the onset of coronary recanalization when renal function is normal (16). Because of its early release, myoglobin is a very early marker of myocardial injury, and its use to facilitate the early diagnosis of acute infarction has been advocated by some (156–163). In these studies, up to 65% of patients with subsequently documented acute infarction have elevated levels of myoglobin in their initial plasma samples (159,162). An intermittent pattern of myoglobin release, the so-called staccato pattern, has been described in substantial numbers of patients in whom abrupt rises and falls in plasma levels occur during the upslope portion of the myoglobin time–mass curve (164,165). This phenomenon is probably related to transient occlusion and reperfusion with intermittent release of enzymes rather than alterations in renal clearance, and it is ablated by treatment with thrombolytic agents (166). However, since myoglobin is cleared by the kidney, even minor perturbations in glomerular filtration rate may lead to false or augmented increases in plasma levels (17,167). The fact that myoglobin also is abundant in skeletal muscle reduces further its specificity for myocardial injury (168,169). In some studies as many as 50% of patients who subsequently fail to meet criteria for acute infarction have elevated levels of myoglobin at the time of admission (163). Whether this is because myoglobin is more sensitive to small amounts of necrosis or exceedingly prone to false-positive increases due to concomitant skeletal muscle release or abnormal renal clearance is unclear. Recently, attempts have been made to improve the specificity of myoglobin measurements by the concomitant measurement of carbonic anhydrase 3. Carbonic anhydrase 3 is another small molecule that is released rapidly when skeletal muscle injury occurs. However, only tiny amounts exist in heart. Thus a strategy where increases of myoglobin associated with increases in carbonic anhydrase 3 are attributed to skeletal muscle injury and those without elevations of carbonic anhydrase 3 to cardiac release has been proposed (170). How well such criteria perform and whether the consistency of the relationships will allow for diagnosis in patients with both skeletal muscle injury and cardiac involvement is unclear.

This lack of specificity is less critical for the determination of coronary recanalization. Because of its small size and rapid clearance from the circulation, myoglobin is ideally suited for this task. In experimental studies, myoglobin appears comparable with MMCK isoforms in its ability to detect coronary recanalization, with a change from 25% to 100% of peak levels in 48 ± 27 minutes (171). In patients, the suggested increase in myoglobin over 2 hours of 4.6 times (145) appears to lack sensitivity, especially in patients in whom myoglobin is already elevated (12). However, when a >3 ng/ml/min rate of change in myoglobin in samples obtained between pretreatment and 60 minutes is used as a criterion, myoglobin and isoform data are comparable for predicting recanalization, both with high sensitivity and specificity (12).

Recently, a novel approach to detecting coronary patency prior to treatment has been reported. In 72 patients with acute infarction, a ratio of the initial myoglobin value to the initial CK value of >5.0 was found to be indicative of a patent infarct-related vessel. The sensitivity, specificity, and predictive accuracy for this criteria were 75%, 96%, and 92% respectively for the 56 patients with occluded vessels and the 16 with patent infarct-related arteries (172).

At present, rapid assays are commercially available in radioimmunoassay format for the determination of serum myoglobin (173,174).

LACTATE DEHYDROGENASE ENZYMES

Lactate dehydrogenase (now known as LD) is a tetramer with a molecular weight of 135,000 daltons. It exists ubiquitously in many tissues and catalyzes the reversible reduction of pyruvate to lactate as the last step of glycolysis. There are both "M" (muscle) and "H" (heart) subunits that give rise to five isoenzymes. Most tissues contain all five isoenzymes. The heart contains predominantly LD1 and to a lesser extent LD2. Red cells, kidney, brain, stomach, and pancreas are other important sources of LD1, and LD5 predominates in skeletal muscle and liver (17,26). Previously, HBDH, a marker of the action of LD1 on α-ketobutyrate, was measured as a surrogate for LD1 (175). At present, most laboratories simply measure LD isoenzymes independently. The ratio of LD1 to LD2 also appears to reduce the biologic variability between individuals (176). Because the proportion of LD1 to LD2 in heart is greater than 1, ratios of LD1 and LD2 in normal individuals have been placed at <0.76. Ratios >0.76 have been considered by some as suggestive of acute infarction. Unfortunately, there is substantial variability even among normal individuals, who on occasion may have LD1/LD2 ratios >0.76. Thus the exact cutoff at which normal may be distinguished from abnormal is unclear. Use of a ratio of >0.76 has better sensitivity but lacks specificity, whereas use of a ratio of 1 has less sensitivity but better specificity (18). Fortunately, LD testing is rarely necessary and is only used when the time course of infarction is such that CK enzyme values likely have returned to normal. Under these circumstances the LD1 to LD2 ratio may be helpful since LD activity rises to an abnormal level at about 10 hours after the onset of infarction, reaches a peak 24 to 48 hours thereafter, and remains elevated for 10 to 14 days (18). Since both troponin T and I are elevated in plasma for many days after acute cardiac insults, it is likely that eventually the assay of these proteins will replace the need to measure LD (21,22).

False-positive increases in LD1 and LD2 suggestive of infarction can occur in response to skeletal muscle injury in a manner analogous to that described for MBCK (177). In the absence of chronic or acute skeletal muscle injury, LD4 and LD5 are found in these muscles. Hemolysis, renal disease, and gastrointestinal abnormalities can also cause the release of substantial amounts of LD1 (177). LD is cleared by the reticuloendothelial system (18).

It has been presumed that the release ratio (the percentage of LD depleted from the heart that is released into plasma) remains constant with or without thrombolysis. Thus comparisons of peak LD levels as surrogates for infarct size have been made (178). The validity of this approach awaits further experimental and clinical validation.

TROPONINS

There are three distinct troponin polypeptides designated as T, I, and C, which regulate the calcium-mediated interaction of actin and myosin (179,180). Each has tissue specific isoforms (181–185). From the diagnostic prospective, the importance of the troponins is that there are tissue-specific forms, especially of I and T, which are the products of separate genes. Different isoforms of troponin I and T are present in slow twitch, fast twitch, and cardiac muscle (182,183,185). Troponin C has only fast and slow twitch forms. The slow twitch form is expressed in heart, which means that elevations of troponin C are unlikely to have high specificity for cardiac release (184).

Most of the troponin that exists in heart is tightly bound to the contractile apparatus, but there is a small percentage (2–6%) that is available in a more rapidly releasable pool, perhaps in the cytosol (22,186,187). This early releasable "cytosolic pool" permits early rapid release of the marker. The structural pool takes many days to be degraded and is responsible for the pronged release observed after myocardial damage.

Specificity

Cardiac troponin I (cTnI) is not expressed in skeletal muscle during embryogenesis, although the skeletal muscle form is expressed in the heart during the developmental stages of life (188). However, after birth, only the cardiac form is expressed in myocardium (188,189). Even in models of skeletal muscle injury, cTnI is not reexpressed (189–191). Thus, from first principles, elevations in cardiac troponin I should be highly specific for myocardial injury. Elevations are not observed in marathon runners (19,192), individuals involved in ultra exercise (193), patients with acute or chronic skeletal muscle disease, or patients with renal failure unless cardiac damage is present as well (19,194).

The specificity of cardiac troponin T is less well established. Both cardiac and skeletal muscle TnT are expressed during embryogenesis in both heart and skeletal muscle. Thus, in models of experimental muscle injury in the rat, the cardiac form is reexpressed in skeletal muscle and the skeletal muscle form in heart (185,195,196). Whether this occurs in humans is unknown, although given the troponins are highly conserved across species lines, the likelihood of similar behavior in human skeletal muscle is greater for the troponins than for some other proteins. Some of the difficulty in defining the specificity of cTnT has been related to the changing assays that have been utilized. The original polyclonal assay clearly had substantial cross-reactivity with the skeletal muscle form (197,198). A more recent assay predicated on monoclonal antibodies has less cross-reactivity, but the antibody used in the tag position is still not totally specific (199). Thus it is possible that material that is captured in association with cTnT by the specific capture antibody could be labeled by the less than perfectly specific second antibody. Recently, an assay that utilized two separate monoclonal antibody with separate epitopes for cTnT has been devised (200). Once an analytically specific assay is available, it should be possible to determine with more precision the real specificity of cardiac troponin T and whether or not elevations observed are related to subtle degrees of myocardial injury or are false-positive elevations and a lack of cardiac specificity. The issue of the specificity of troponin T is a critical issue since despite several studies in patients with skeletal muscle injury (201) and/or after extreme exercise that have failed to show elevations (202), elevations but have been reported in patients with polydermatomyositis (203), renal failure (194), and in boxers (204). In the latter two situations, elevations of cTnI were not observed.

Preliminary studies suggest that both of the troponins are cleared rapidly, supporting the concept that it is degradation and release from the structural pool that leads to the persistent elevations. Initial studies with cTnT suggest that if one samples long enough, almost all the troponin that is released from the heart can be accounted for by serum values. This suggests that the release ratio for the "structural pool" may be near unity (22). Since the release ratio is altered by thrombolysis with most other markers (13), if confirmed, this fact would allow for direct measurements of infarct size in both thrombolysed and nonthrombolysed patients by serial measurements of cTnT. Despite the suggestion that the release ratio is near unity, the time course of release of cTnT and cTnI is altered in response to thrombolysis. This is thought due to more rapid washout of the early releasable pool (22). With both markers, an increased rate of rise in protein concentration is observed, indicative of more rapid washout (22,205,206).

Detection of Acute Myocardial Infarction

There are substantial problems in evaluating any new approach to the diagnosis of acute myocardial infarction. New markers often are developed to overcome difficulties in the present diagnostic methods. However, often the present methods are at least in part, still the "gold standard." Thus it is very difficult for a marker of myocardial injury to claim to be more sensitive than the traditional gold standard, MBCK. In addition, although we know from developmental biology and from studies of specificity that elevations of cTnT and cTnI are more specific than MBCK for cardiac damage, because MBCK is still relied on for the diagnosis of acute infarction, it is difficult to ask clinicians to ignore elevations. This reality should be kept in mind as one begins to evaluate the results of studies that often rely on the "clinicians" diagnosis or the WHO standards of meeting at least two of three criteria including chest pain, ECG changes, and elevations of MBCK.

In a series of 188 patients admitted with suspicion of acute myocardial infarction, cTnT was elevated in 86 of the 89 diagnosed with infarction by the staff of the coronary care unit (187). The three patients in whom cTnI was not elevated included one who went to surgery after an initial sample with a marginally elevated MBCK, and two others with minor elevations in MBCK, which declined slowly; this is often a marker of release of MBCK from skeletal muscle. Thus the sensitivity of cTnI compared with MBCK as in other studies (207) was high (86 of 89, or 97%). In the 99 patients in whom infarction was excluded clinically, elevations of cTnI were found in 5. All of these patients had suffered multiple episodes of chest discomfort prior to admission, and cTnI may have been elevated due to infarction that occurred prior to admission because elevations of cTnI persist for many days. Thus, in this study a high degree of comparability was observed. Judging from peak values and the kinetics of release, it appeared that there was more cTnI than MBCK released early in patients with infarction, suggesting that cTnI may have the potential to be more sensitive than MBCK, but this issue was not studied definitively. However, such a finding would be consistent with the fact that there is 13 times more cTnI per gram of myocardium than MBCK (187,207). A biphasic pattern of cTnI release, which is thought to be due to release first of the early releasable pool and then release of the structural pool, is observed in some patients (207).

Early detection of acute infarction is not markedly facilitated by cTnI since it rises with about the same time course as MBCK (21,207). However, in patients in whom there is suspicion of myocardial injury and concomitant skeletal muscle damage, there is a clear advantage to the use of cTnI. cTnI facilitates the diagnosis of myocardial contusion by avoiding difficulties with spurious elevations due to chest wall trauma in patients in whom there is suspicion of contusion (84). In addition, in perioperative patients cTnI is more accurately detected (83). In a study of 96 patients undergoing vascular surgery and 12 undergoing spinal surgery, samples for MBCK and cTnI were obtained serially. An echocardiogram taken preoperatively and an echocardiogram taken prior to discharge were used to define the presence or absence of myocardial damage, which was considered to be present if new regional dysfunction was present. Eight patients had perioperative infarction diagnosed by serial echocardiography. All eight had elevations of cTnI (Fig. 8–8). Six of these patients had elevations in MBCK as well. However, an additional 19 patients without infarction also had elevations in MBCK compared with only 1 for cTnI. The use of MBCK as a percentage of total CK improved specificity from 19 to 1 but further reduced sensitivity so that only 5 of the 8 patients with perioperative infarction were detected. Thus overall accuracy was far better with cTnI, which suggests that in situations where there was the possibility of concomitant skeletal muscle damage that the use of cTnI will be preferable to the use of MBCK. However, if measurement of cardiac troponin I is substituted for MBCK, it must be recognized that because cTnI persists in plasma, elevations can not be used to estimate the time of onset of infarction (187). This may be important in the Emergency Department in relation to decisions about where to admit patients or how long to keep them in the hospital. Thus it is likely that some conjoint role for both MBCK and cTnI will develop.

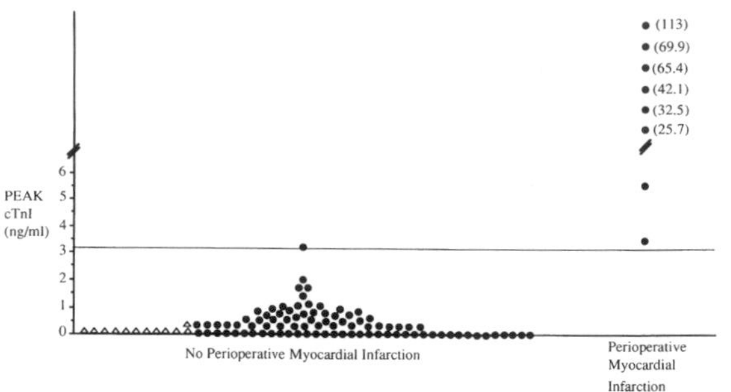

Figure 8–8. Values of cardiac troponin I in patients with (on the right) and without (on the left) myocardial infarction. In contrast to values of MBCK, which were commonly elevated in the absence of infarction, cTnI manifested very high specificity. *Reproduced from Adams et al (83), with permission.*

Comparative studies also have been done with cTnT and suggest that it, too, has at least comparable and perhaps even superior sensitivity to MBCK for the diagnosis of acute infarction. There has been substantial variability in the criteria utilized for the diagnosis of infarction, which has ranged from the limit of detectability (0.1 ng/ml) (22) to, in some of the original studies, values of 0.5 ng/ml (197). The higher values were suggested for use with the initial assay, which used polyclonal sera; subsequent assays utilizing more specific antibodies have defined a level of 0.1 or 0.2 ng/ml as indicative of acute infarction (208,209). Obviously, as indicated above, the use of "conventional criteria" for the diagnosis of acute infarction may have put cTnT at a disadvantage. Regardless, the sensitivity of cTnT has always been found to be very high, in some studies 100% from 10 hours to roughly 5 days (197,198). Elevations of cTnT in plasma occur at approximately the same time or perhaps slightly earlier after the onset of acute infarction than those of MBCK (197). In some studies, cTnT was increased in 50% of patients in the initial sample (210). These early elevations likely represent infarction prior to admission, which led to the detection of persistent elevations or the insensitivity of MBCK activity measurements. It is unlikely that cTnT often rises substantially more rapidly than MBCK given what is known of its kinetics of release (197,198). cTnT remains elevated for up to 10 days and thus is clearly better than measurement of MBCK for the retrospective diagnosis of acute infarction (197,198). It also commonly manifests a biphasic pattern of release (198) that reflects the early releasable and structural pools respectively (Fig. 8–9). In at least some patients, new increases in cTnT were observed in the absence of increases in MBCK, leading to suggestions that cTnT may be more sensitive than MBCK (209). Thus a very high percentage of patients with acute myocardial infarction are sensitively detected by measurements of cTnT. Issues of specificity remain to be totally adjudicated, since in some studies substantial numbers of patients who are critically ill in the absence of acute cardiovascular illness have been observed

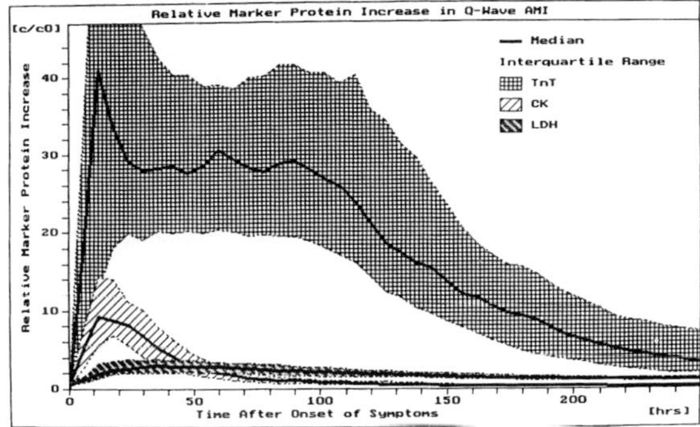

Figure 8–9. Biphasic release of cardiac troponin T after acute myocardial infarction. Initial release is predominantly from the "cytosolic pool." Subsequent release is indicative of degradation of structurally bound protein. A similar pattern has been described with cardiac troponin I as well. *Reproduced from Katus et al (198), with permission.*

to have increases in cTnT as well (211). Whether such increases represent undetected and unsuspected infarction or a lack of biologic and/or analytic specificity is unclear. This is a particularly important issue in patients undergoing noncardiac surgery, where frequent minor increases in cTnT have been reported and presumed to be due to acute cardiac injury (201).

Patients who are critically ill can be more easily evaluated by measurement of troponins given their high cardiac specificity. In a study of critically ill medical patients, 32 of 209 patients had elevations of cTnI suggestive of myocardial injury. In only one-third was the diagnosis made by the physicians caring for the patients. Patients with elevated cTnI had a 40% mortality rate compared to 14% for those with normal values (201a).

An interesting subset of patients are those with unstable angina. It has recently been reported that a substantial percentage of these patients have elevated levels of cTnT on admission (209). Patients with elevated levels of cTnT and unstable angina have a substantially worse prognosis with more deaths, more myocardial infarctions, and a greater need for mechanical revascularization than do those without such elevations. It may be that elevations represent small amounts of necrosis below the level of detection observed with MBCK and therefore subtle degrees of "microinfarction." On the other hand, they may simply represent infarction that has occurred in the days prior to admission at a time when elevations of cTnT may persist. It is not surprising that patients with a component of infarction and unstable angina would have a worse prognosis than those with unstable angina alone. Nonetheless, there appears to be substantial data that looking at high-risk patients for the presence of cTnT may be worthwhile since elevations, regardless of whether they represent increased sensitivity for infarction or cardiac injury occurring in the days prior to presentation, seem to be markers of increased risk. It has been reported that when one utilizes electrocardiographic triage, and specifically the presence of ST segment changes, that the independent prognostic significance of elevations in cTnT disappears (212). However, recent data confirmed that the increased risk conferred by elevations of cTnT is independent of electrocardiographic changes in patients with unstable angina (212a). Furthermore, preliminary data with cTnI in patients with unstable angina suggests that elevations in cTnI confer similar prognostic implications (212b).

Recently, the prognostic significance of an elevated troponin at the time of presentation was reported in patients with both Q wave and non-Q wave myocardial infarction (212c).

The Detection of Coronary Recanalization

Preliminary data with cTnI have documented changes in kinetics similar to that seen with other markers, namely, a rapid increase in the appearance of the marker in plasma that suggests it may be useful for the detection of coronary recanalization (206).

cTnI has also been studied and has been reported to have diagnostic sensitivity similar to other markers utilized for this purpose (22,207).

Calculation of Infarct Size

Preliminary data in experimental animals suggest a release ratio of near unity, which would allow cTnT to be utilized as a marker of infarct size (22). Preliminary clinical studies have supported this concept, and cTnT has been correlated to ejection fraction and scintigraphic measurement of infarct size (213–215).

REFERENCES

1. Karmen A, Wroblewski F, Ladue JS: Transaminase activity in human blood. *J Clin Invest* 1954;34: 126–133.
2. Roberts R: The two out of three criteria for the diagnosis of infarction: Is it passe? *Chest* 1984;86: 511–513.
3. Hackel DB, Reimer KA, Ideker RE, et al: Comparison of enzymatic and anatomic estimates of myocardial infarct size in man. *Circulation* 1984;70: 824–835.
4. Bleifeld W, Mathey D, Hanrath P, Buss H, Effert S: Infarct size estimated from serial serum creatine phosphokinase in relation to left ventricular hemodynamics. *Circulation* 1977;55:303–311.
5. Grande P, Hansen BF, Christiansen C, Naestoft J: Estimation of acute myocardial infarct size in man by serum CK-MB measurements. *Circulation* 1982; 65:756–764.
6. Jaffe AS, Serota H, Grace A, Sobel BE: Diagnostic changes in plasma creatine kinase isoforms early after the onset of acute myocardial infarction. *Circulation* 1986;74:105–109.
7. Abendschein D, Seacord LM, Nohara R, Sobel BS, Jaffe AS: Prompt detection of myocardial injury by assay of creatine kinase isoforms in initial plasma samples. *Clin Cardiol* 1988;11:661–664.
8. Morelli RL, Carlson CJ, Emilson B, et al: Serum creatine kinase MM isoenzyme sub-bands after acute myocardial infarction in man. *Circulation* 1983;67:1283–1289.
9. Wu AHB, Gornet TG, Wu VH, et al: Early diagnosis of acute myocardial infarction by rapid analysis of creatine kinase iso-enzyme-3 (CK-MM) subtypes. *Clin Chem* 1987;33:358–362.
10. Nohara R, Myears DW, Sobel BE, et al: Optimal criteria for rapid detection of myocardial reperfusion by creatine kinase MM Isoforms in the presence of residual high grade coronary stenosis. *J Am Coll Cardiol* 1989;14:1067–1073.
11. Seacord LM, Abendschein DR, Nohara R, Hartzler G, Sobel BE, Jaffe AS: Detection of reperfusion within one hour after coronary recanalization by analysis of isoforms of the MM creatine kinase isoenzyme in plasma. *Fibrinolysis* 1988;2:151–156.
12. Abendschein DA, Ellis AK, Eisenberg PR, Klocke FJ, Sobel BE, Jaffe AS: Prompt detection of coronary recanalization by analysis of rates of change of concentrations of macromolecular markers in plasma. *Cor Art Dis* 1991;2:201–212.
13. Vatner SF, Baig H, Manders WT, et al: TI Effects of coronary artery reperfusion on myocardial infarct size calculated from creatine kinase. *J Clin Invest* 1978;61:1048–1056.
14. Adams JE, Abendschein DR, Jaffe AS: Biochemical markers of myocardial injury: Is MB creatine kinase the choice for the 1990s? *Circulation* 1993;88: 750–763.
15. Granadier E, Keidar S, Kahana L, et al: The roles of serum myoglobin, total CPK, and CK-MB isoenzyme in the acute phase of myocardial infarction. *Am Heart J* 1983;105:408–416.
16. Klocke FJ, Copley DP, Krawszyk JA, Reichlin M: Rapid renal clearance of immunoreactive canine plasma myoglobin. *Circulation* 1982;65:1522–1528.
17. Roberts R: Myoglobinemia as an index to myocardial infarction. *Ann Intern Med* 1977;87:788–789.
18. Vasudevan G, Mercer DW, Varat MA: Lactic dehydrogenase isoenzyme determination in the diagnosis of acute myocardial infarction. *Circulation* 1978; 57:1055–1057.
19. Adams JE III, Bodor GS, Davila-Roman VG, et al: Cardiac troponin I: A marker with high specificity for cardiac injury. *Circulation* 1993;88:101–106.
20. Zak R, Martin AF, Reddy K, Rabinowitz M: Control of protein balance in hypertrophied cardiac muscle. *Circ Res* 1976;38:145–150.
21. Bodor GS, Porter S, Landt Y, Ladenson JH: The development of monoclonal antibodies and an assay for cardiac troponin-I with preliminary results in suspected myocardial infarction. *Clin Chem* 1992;11: 2203–2214.
22. Katus HA, Remppis A, Scheffold T, Diederich KW, Kuebler W: Intracellular compartmentation of cardiac troponin T and its release kinetics in patients with reperfused and nonreperfused myocardial infarction. *Am J Cardiol* 1991;67:1360–1367.
23. Larue C, Calzolari C, Bertinchant J, Leclerq F, Grolleau R, Pau B: Cardiac-specific immunoenzymometric assay of troponin I in the early phase of acute myocardial infarction. *Clin Chem* 1993;39: 972–979.
24. Samarel AM, Ferguson AG, Vanderheid RS, Daveson R, Ganote CE: Release of unassembled rat cardiac myosin light chain following calcium paradox. *Circ Res* 1986;58:166–171.
25. Bais R, Edward JB: Creatine kinase. *CRC Crit Rev Clin Lab Sci* 1982;16:291–335.
26. Sobel BE, Shell WE: Serum enzyme determinations in the diagnosis and assessment of myocardial infarction. *Circulation* 1972;45:471–482.

27. Cox DA, Stone PH, Muller JE, et al: Prognostic implications of an early peak in plasma MB creatine kinase patients with acute myocardial infarction. *J Am Coll Cardiol* 1987;10:979–990.

28. Hirzel HO, Sonnenblick EH, Kirk ES: Absence of a lateral border zone of intermediate creatine phosphokinase depletion surrounding a central infarct 24 hours after acute coronary occlusion in the dog. *Circulation* 1977;41:673–683.

29. Siegel RJ, Said JW, Shell WE, et al: Identification and localization of creatine kinase B and M in normal, ischemic and necrotic myocardium: An immunohistochemical study. *J Mol Cell Cardiol* 1984;16: 95–103.

30. Ahmed SA, Williamson JR, Roberts R, et al: The association of increased plasma MBCPK activity and irreversible ischemic myocardial injury in the dog. *Circulation* 1976;54:187–193.

31. Klein MS, Ludbrook PA, Mimbs JW, et al: Perioperative mortability rate in patients with unstable angina selected by exclusion of myocardial infarction. *J Thorac Cardiac Surg* 1977;73:253–257.

32. Klein MS, Weiss AN, Roberts R, Coleman RE: Technetium-99 stannous pyrophosphate scintigrams in normal subjects, patients with exercise-induced ischemia and patients with a calcified valve. *J Am Coll Cardiol* 1977;39:360–363.

33. Michael LH, Hunt JR, Weilbaecher D, et al: Creatine kinase and phosphorylase in cardiac lymph: Coronary occlusion and reperfusion. *Am J Physiol* 1985;248(3 Pt 2):350–359.

34. Heyndrickx GR, Amano J, Kenna T, et al: Creatine kinase release not associated with myocardial necrosis after short periods of coronary artery occlusion in conscious baboons. *J Am Coll Cardiol* 1985;6: 1299–1303.

35. Apple FS, Rogers MA, Sherman WM, et al: Profile of creatine kinase isoenzymes in skeletal muscles of marathon runners. *Clin Chem* 1984;30:413–416.

36. Siegel AJ, Silverman LM, Evans WJ: Elevated skeletal muscle creatine kinase MAB isoenzyme levels in marathon runners. *JAMA* 1983;250: 2835–2837.

37. Lehmann H: Uber die Enzymatische Synthese der Kreatinphosphoraure durch Umesterung der Phosphobrenztraubensaure. *Biochem Z* 1935;281: 271–291.

38. Jacobus WE, Lehninger A: Creatine kinase of rat heart: Mitochondrial coupling of creatine phosphorylation to electron transport. *J Biol Chem* 1973;248: 4803–4810.

39. Bessman S, Carpenter C: The creatine–creatine phosphate energy shuttle. *Annu Rev Biochem* 1985; 54:831–862.

40. Burger A, Richterich R, Aebi H: Die Heterogenital der kreatin-kinase. *Biochem Z* 1964;339:305.

41. Jacobs H, Heldt HW, Klingenberg M: High activity of creatine kinase in mitochondria from muscle and brain and evidence for a separate mitochondrial isoenzyme of creatine kinase. *Biochem Biophys Res Commun* 1964;16:516–521.

42. Dawson DM, Eppenberger HM, Kaplan NO: Creatine kinase: Evidence for a dimeric structure. *Biochem Biophys Res Commun* 1965;21:346–353.

43. Neumeier D: Tissue specific and subcellular distribution of creatine kinase isoenzymes, in H. Lang (ed): *Creatine Kinase Isoenzymes.* Berlin, Heidelberg, Springer-Verlag, 1981, pp 85–131.

44. Wevers RA, Delsing M, Klein A, et al: Post-synthetic changes in creatine kinase isoenzymes. *Clin Chim Acta* 1978;86:323–327.

45. Wevers RA, Olthuis HP, Van Niel JC, et al: A study on the dimeric structure of creatine kinase. *Clin Chim Acta* 1977;75:377–385.

46. Hashimoto H, Grace AM, Billadello JJ, et al: Non denaturing quantification of subforms of canine MM creatine kinase isoenzymes (isoforms) and their interconversion. *J Lab Clin Med* 1985;103:470–484.

47. Clark GL, Robinson AK, Gucap DR, et al: Effects of lymphatic transport of enzymes on plasma creatine kinase time activity curves after myocardial infarction in dogs. *Circ Res* 1978;43:162–169.

48. Mimbs JW, Yolas DE, Miller JG, et al: Detection of myocardial infarction in vitro based on altered elevation of ultrasound. *Circ Res* 1977;41:192–198.

49. Roberts, R: Enzymatic estimation: Creatine kinase, in Wagner GS (ed): *Myocardial Infarction Measurement and Intervention.* The Hague, Boston, London, Martinus Nijhoff, 1982, 107–142.

50. Karlsberg RP, Roberts R: Effect of altered thyroid function on plasma creatine kinase clearance in the dog. *Am J Physiol* 1978;235(6):E614–618.

51. Sobel BE, Markham J, Karlsberg RP, et al: The nature of disappearance of creatine kinase from the circulation and its influence on enzymatic estimation of infarct size. *Circ Res* 1977;41(6):836–844.

52. Billadello JJ, Roman DG, Grace AM, et al: The nature of post-translational formation of MM creatine kinase isoforms. *J Biol Chem* 1985;260: 14988–14992.

53. Leon CA, Young JB, Puleo PR, et al: Quantification of myocardial creatine kinase subforms in

biopsies from patients undergoing cardiac transplantation. *J Am Coll Cardiol* 1986;7:80A.

54. Abendschein DR, Serota H, Plummer TH Jr, et al: Conversion of MM creatine kinase isoforms in human plasma by carboxypeptidase. *NJ Lab Clin Med* 1987;110:798–806.
55. Perryman MB, Knell JD, Roberts R: Carboxypeptidase-catalyzed hydrolysis of C-terminal lysine: Mechanism for in vivo production of multiple forms of creatine kinase in plasma. *Clin Chem* 1984;30:662–664.
56. Billadello JJ, Fontanet HL, Strauss AW, et al: Characterization of MB creatine kinase isoform conversion in vitro and in vivo in dogs. *J Clin Invest* 1989; 83(5):1637–1643.
57. Puleo PR, Guadagno PA, Roberts R, et al: Sensitive rapid assay of subforms of creatine kinase MB in plasma. *Clin Chem* 1989;35:1452–1455.
58. Christenson RH, Ohran EM, Clemmense P, et al: Characteristics of creatine kinase-MB and MB isoforms in serum after reperfusion in acute myocardial infarction. *Clin Chem* 1989;3511: 2179–2185.
59. Prager NA, Suzuki T, Jaffe AS, Sobel BE, Abendschein DR: The nature and time course of generation of isoforms of MB creatine kinase in vivo. *J Am Coll Cardiol* 1992;20:414–419.
60. Kanemitsu F, Okigaki T: Creatine kinase MB isoforms for early diagnosis and monitoring of acute myocardial infarction. *Clinica Chemica Acta* 1992; 206:191–199.
61. Roberts R, Gowda KS, Ludbrook PA, et al: Specificity of elevated serum MB creatine phosphokinase activity in the diagnosis of acute myocardial infarction. *Am J Cardiol* 1975;36:433–437.
62. Yasmineh WG, Ibrahim GA, Abbasnezhad MA, et al: Isoenzyme distribution of creatine kinase and lactate dehydrogenase in serum and skeletal muscle in Duchenne muscular dystrophy, collagen disease, and other muscular disorders. *Clin Chem* 1978;24: 1985–1989.
63. Roberts R, Henry PD, Witteveen SAGT, et al: Quantification of serum creatine phosphokinase isoenzyme activity. *Am J Cardiol* 1974;33:650–654.
64. Tsung JS, Tsung SS: Creatine kinase isoenzymes in extracts of various human skeletal muscles. *Clin Chem* 1986;32:1568–1510.
65. Wilhelm AH, Albers KM, Todd JK: Creatine phosphokinase isoenzyme distribution in human skeletal and heart muscles. *IRCS Med Sci* 1976;4: 418–420.
66. Sobel BE, Markham J, Roberts R: Factors influencing enzymatic estimates of infarct size. *J Am Coll Cardiol* 1977;39:130–132.
67. Rosenblum AM, Ludbrook PA, Jaffe AS: Significance of elevated MB creatine kinase in patients after cardiac catheterization. *Cardiac Catheter Diagn* 1984;10:547–552.
68. Spadaro JJ, Ludbrook PA, Tiefenbrunn AJ, Kurnik PB, Jaffe AS: Paucity of subtle myocardial injury after angioplasty delineated with MB CK. *Cathet and Cardiovasc Diagn* 1986;12:230–234.
69. Sadeh M, Stern LZ, Czyzewski K, et al: Alterations of creatine kinase, ornithine decarboxylase, and transglutaminase during muscle regeneration. *Life Sci* 1984;34:483–488.
70. Tzvetanova E: Creatine kinase isoenzymes in muscle tissue of patients with neuromuscular diseases and human fetuses. *Enzyme* 1971;12:279–288.
71. Foxall CD, Ermery AE: Changes in creatine kinase and its isoenzymes in human fetal muscle during development. *J Neurol Sci* 1975;24:483–492.
72. Jaffe AS, Garfinkel BT, Ritter CS, Sobel BE: Plasma MB creatine kinase after vigorous exercise in professional athletes. *Am J Cardiol* 1984;53: 856–858.
73. Keshgegian AA, Feinberg NV: Serum creatine kinase MB isoenzyme in chronic muscle disease. *Clin Chem* 1984;30:575–578.
74. Shahanglan S, Ash OW, Wahlstrom NO, et al: Creatine kinase and lactate dehydrogenase isoenzymes in serum of patients suffering burns, blunt trauma, or myocardial infarction. *Clin Chem* 1984;30: 1332–1338.
75. Goto I, Nagamine M, Katsuki S: Creatine phosphokinase isoenzymes in muscles. *Arch Neurol* 1969;20: 422–429.
76. McBride JW, Labrosse KR, McCoy HG, et al: Is serum creatine kinase-MB in electrically injured patients predictive of myocardial injury? *JAMA* 1986;255:764–776.
77. Jockers-Wretou E, Grabert K, Muller E, et al: Serum creatine kinase isoenzyme pattern in nervous system atrophies and neuromuscular disorders. *Clin Chim Acta* 1976;73:183–186.
78. Silverman LM, Mendell JR, Sahenk Z, et al: Significance of creatine phosphokinase isoenzymes in Duchenne dystrophy. *Neurology* 1976;26:561–564.
79. Staubli M, Roessler B, Hochi HP, et al: Creatine kinase and creatine kinase MB in endurance runners and in patients with myocardial infarction. *Eur J Appl Physiol* 1985;54:40–45.

80. Siegel AJ, Silverman LM, Holman BL: Normal results of post-race thallium-201 myocardial perfusion imaging in marathon runners with elevated serum MB creatine kinase levels. *Am J Med* 1985;79: 431–434.

81. Chemnitz G, Schmidt E, Schmidt FW: Creatine kinase and isoenzymes in hypothyroidism, in Lang H (ed): *Creatine Kinase Isoenzymes.* Berlin, Heidelberg, Springer-Verlag, 1981, pp 183–185.

82. Jaffe AS, Ritter C, Meltzer V, Harter H, Roberts R: Unmasking artifactual increases in creatine kinase isoenzymes in patients with renal failure. *J Lab Clin Med* 1984;104:193–202.

83. Adams JE, Sicard G, Allan BT, et al: More accurate diagnosis of perioperative myocardial infarction with measurement of cardiac troponin I. *N Engl J Med* 1994;330:670–674.

84. Adams JE, Davila-Roman VG, Bessey PQ, Blake DP, Ladenson, JH, Jaffe AS: Improved detection of cardiac contusion with cardiac troponin I. *Am Heart J*, in press. 1996;131:308–312.

85. Ingwall JS, Kramer MF, Fifer MA, et al: The creatine kinase system in normal and diseased human myocardium. *N Engl J Med* 1985;313.1050–1054.

86. Marmor A, Margolis T, Alpan G, et al: Regional distribution of the MB isoenzyme of creatine kinase in the human heart. *Arch Pathol Lab Med* 1980;104: 425–427.

87. Yasmineh WG, Pyle RB, Nicolott DM: Rate of decay and distribution volume of MB isoenzyme of creatine kinase, intravenously injected into the baboon. *Clin Chem* 1976;22:1095–1097.

88. Baraka M, Deveaux N, Frank R, et al: Creatine kinase MB isoenzyme activity after endocardial catheter fulguration (abstract). *Circulation* 1987; 76(Suppl IV):IV-174.

89. Ingwall JS: The hypertrophied myocardium accumulates the MB-creatine kinase isozyme. *Eur Heart J* 1984;5(Suppl F):129–139.

90. Hoag GN, Franks CR, DeCoteau WE: Creatine kinase isoenzymes in serum of patients with cancer of various organs (letter). *Clin Chem* 1978;24(9):1654.

91. Lamar W, Woodard L, Statland BE: Clinical implications of creatine kinase-BB isoenzyme (letter). *N Engl J Med* 1978;299(15):834–835.

92. Zweig MH, Silverman LM, Dermer GB, Van-Steirteghan AC: Serum creatine kinase isoenzyme BB as an indicator of active metastatic disease (letter). *Clin Chem* 1979;25(6):1190–1191.

93. Silverman LM, Dermer GB, Zweig MH, Van-Steirteghem AC, Tokes ZA: Creatine kinase BB: A new tumor-associated marker. *Clin Chem* 1979;25: 1432–1435.

94. George S, Ishikawa Y, Perryman MB, et al: Purification and characterization of naturally occurring and in vitro induced multiple forms of MM creatine kinase. *J Biol Chem* 1984;259:2667–2674.

95. Abendschein DR, Fontanet HL, Nohara R: Optimized preservation of isoforms of creatine kinase MM isoenzyme in plasma specimens and their rapid quantification by semi-automated chromatofocusing. *Clin Chem,* 1990;36:723–727.

96. Morin LG: Creatine kinase: Stability, inactivation, reactivation. *Clin Chem* 1977;23(4):646–652.

97. Oliver IT: A spectrophotometric method for the determination of creatine phosphokinase and myokinase. *Biochem J* 1955;61:116–122.

98. Rosalki SB: An improved procedure for serum creatine phosphokinase determination. *J Lab Clin Med* 1967;69(4):696–705.

99. Nielsen L, Ludwiggen B: Improved method for determination of creatine kinase. *J Lab Clin Med* 1963;62:159–168.

100. Swanson JR, Wilkinson JH: Measurement of creatine kinase activity in serum, in Cooper GR, King JS Jr (eds): *Standard Methods of Clinical Chemistry,* vol 7. New York Academic Press, 1972, pp 33–42.

101. Tanzer ML, Gilvarg C: Creatine and creatine kinase measurement. *J Biol Chem* 1959;234: 3201 3204.

102. Greenson JK, Farber SJ, Dubin SB: The effect of hemolysis on creatine kinase determination. *Arch Pathol Lab Med* 1989;113:184–185.

103. Vaidya HC, Maynard Y, Dietzler DN, et al: Direct measurement of creatine kinase MB activity in serum after extraction with a monoclonal anti body specific to the MB isoenzyme. *Clin Chem* 1986;32:657–663.

104. Landt Y, Vaidya HC, Porter SE, et al: Semi-automated direct colorimetric measurement of creatine kinase isoenzyme MB activity after extraction from serum by use of a CK-MB specific monoclonal antibody. *Clin Chem* 1988;34:575–581.

105. Morin LG: Evaluation of current methods for creatine kinase isoenzyme fractionation. *Clin Chem* 1977; 23:205–210.

106. Rosalki SB: Creatine phosphokinase isoenzymes. *Nature* 1965;207:414.

107. Roberts R, Grace AM: Purification of mitochondrial creatine kinase. *J Biol Chem* 1980;255: 2870–2877.

108. Allard D, Cabrol D: Electrophoretic study of creatine phosphokinase isoenzymes in human and rabbit tissues. *Pathol Biol* 1970;18(19):847–850.
109. Hennrich N: Differentiation of creatine kinase isoenzymes by non immunological methods, in Lang H (ed): *Creatine Kinase Isoenzymes.* Berlin, Heidelberg, Springer-Verlag, 1981, pp 41–48.
110. Urdal P, Landaas S: Macro creatine kinase BB in serum, and some data on its prevalence. *Clin Chem* 1979;25:461–465.
111. Lang H, Wurzburg U: Creatine kinase, an enzyme of many forms. *Clin Chem* 1982;28: 1439–1447.
112. Aleyassine H, Tonks DB: Albumin-bound fluorescence: A potential source of error in fluorometric assay of creatine kinase BB isoenzyme (letter). *Clin Chem* 1978;24:1849–1850.
113. Butch AW, Goodnow TT, Brown WS, et al: Stratus automated creatine kinase-MB assay evaluated; identification and elimination of falsely increased results associated with a high molecular-mass form of alkaline phosphatase. *Clin Chem* 1989;35:2048–2053.
114. Eisenberg PR, Shaw D, Schaab C, Jaffe AS: Concordance of creatine kinase-MB activity and mass. *Clin Chem* 1989;35:440–443.
115. Cerutti PA, Fridovich I, McCord JM: Oxy-radicals in molecular biology and pathology. Proceedings of an Upjohn–UCLA Symposium, 1988, pp 27–35.
116. Puleo PR, Perryman MB, Bresser MA, et al: Creatine kinase isoform analysis in the detection and assessment of thrombolysis in man. *Circulation* 1987;75:1162–1169.
117. Grace AM, Gualdoni J, Strauss AW, et al: Quantification of isoforms of plasma MM creatine kinase (CK) with an immunoblot procedure. *Cathet Cardiovasc Diagn* 1987;13:26–32.
118. Nohara R, Sobel BE, Jaffe AS, Abendschein DR: Quantitative analysis of isoforms of creatine kinase MM in plasma by chromatofocusing with on-line monitoring of enzyme activity. *Clin Chem* 1988;34(2):235–239.
119. Bhayana V, Cohoe S, Leung FY, Jabolonsky G, Henderson AR: Diagnostic evaluation of creatine kinase-2 mass and creatine kinase-3 and -2 isoform ratios in early diagnosis of acute myocardial infarction. *Clin Chem* 1993;39:488–495.
120. Hashimoto H, Abendschein DR, Strauss AW, et al: Early detection of myocardial infarction in conscious dogs by analysis of plasma MM creatine kinase isoforms. *Circulation* 1985;71:363–369.
121. Puleo PR, Guadagno A, Roberts R, et al: Early diagnosis of acute myocardial infarction based on assay for subforms of creatine kinase-MB. *Circulation* 1990;82:759–764.
122. Puleo PR, Meyer D, Wathen C, et al: Use of a rapid assay of subforms of creatine kinase MB to diagnose or rule out acute myocardial infarction. *N Engl J Med* 1994;331:561–566.
123. Mair J, Artner-Dworzak E, Dienstl A, et al: Early detection of acute myocardial infarction by measurement of mass concentration of creatine kinase-MB. *Am J Cardiol* 1991;68:1545–1550.
124. Collinson PO, Rosalki SB, Kuwana T, et al: Early diagnosis of acute myocardial infarction by CK-MB mass measurements. *Ann Clin Biochem* 1992;29: 43–47.
125. Marin MM, Teichman SL: Use of rapid serial sampling of creatine kinase MB for the very early detection of myocardial infarction in patients with acute chest pain. *Am Heart J* 1992;123:354–361.
126. Wu AH, Wang XM, Gornet TG, Ordonez Llanos J: Creatine kinase MB isoforms in patients with skeletal muscle injury: Ramifications for early detection of acute myocardial infarction. *Clin Chem* 1992;38(12): 2396–2400.
127. Roberts R, Ambos HD, Sobel BE: Estimation of infarct size with MB rather than total CK. *Int J Cardiol* 1983;2(5–6):479–492.
128. Garabedian BD, Gold HK, Yasuda T, et al: Detection of coronary artery reperfusion with creatine kinase-MB determinations during thrombolytic therapy: Correlation with acute angiography. *J Am Coll Cardiol* 1988;11:729–734.
129. Jaffe AS, Pierce GF, Ladenson JH: Elevations in MB creatine kinase which are not indicative of acute myocardial infarction. *Primary Cardiol* 1985;11:61–70.
130. Lott JA, Stang JM: Serum enzymes and isoenzymes in the diagnosis and different diagnosis of myocardial ischemia and necrosis (review). *Clin Chem* 1980;26:1241–1250.
131. Ehsani A, Ewy GA, Sobel BE: Effects of electrical countershock on serum creatine phosphokinase (CPK) isoenzyme activity. *Am J Cardiol* 1976;37: 12–18.
132. Reiffel JA, Gambino SR, McCarthy DM, et al: Direct current cardioversion. Effect on creatine kinase, lactic dehydrogenase and myocardial isoenzymes. *JAMA* 1978;239:122–124.
133. Potkin RT, Werner JA, Trobaugh GB, et al: Evaluation of noninvasive rests of cardiac damage in

suspected cardiac contusions. *Circulation* 1982;66: 627–631.

134. Larca LJ, Coppola JT, Honig S: Creatine kinase MB isoenzyme in dermatomyositis: A noncardiac source. *Ann Int Med* 1981;94:341–343.

135. Vaidya H, Apple F, Boches F, et al: Standardization of creatine kinase-MB (CKMB) mass immunoassay. *Clin Biochem Revs* 1993;14:337.

136. Dillon MC, Calbreath DF, Dixon AM, et al: Diagnostic problem in acute myocardial infarction: CK-MB in the absence of abnormally elevated total creatine kinase levels. *Arch Intern Med* 1982; 142:33–38.

137. Heller GV, Blaustein AS, Wei JY: Implications of increased myocardial isoenzyme level in the presence of normal serum creatine kinase activity. *Am J Cardiol* 1983;51:24–27.

138. Salim Y, Collins R, Lin L, et al: Significance of elevated MB isoenzyme with normal creatine kinase in acute myocardial infarction. *Am J Cardiol* 1987;59: 245–250.

139. Klein MS, Coleman RE, Weldon CS, et al: Concordance of electrocardiographic and scintigraphic criteria of myocardial injury after cardiac surgery. *J Thorac Carciovasc Surg* 1976;71:934–937.

140. Muller JE, Rude RE, Baunwald E, et al: Myocardial infarct extension: Incidence, outcome, and risk factors in the MILIS study. *Ann Intern Med* 1988;108:1–6.

141. Gore JM, Roberts R, Ball SP, et al: Peak creatine kinase as a measure of effectiveness of thrombolytic therapy in acute myocardial infarction. *Am J Cardiol* 1987;59:1234–1238.

142. Lawrence O, Coromilas J, Zimmerman JM, et al: A physiologically based model of creatine kinase-MB release in reperfusion of acute myocardial infarction. *Am J Cardiol* 1989;64:11–15.

143. Apple FS, Sharkey SW, Werdick M, et al: Analyses of creatine kinase isoenzymes and isoforms in serum to detect reperfusion after acute myocardial infarction. *Clin Chem* 1987;33:507–511.

144. Morelli RL, Emilson B, Rapaport E: MM-CK subtypes diagnose reperfusion early after myocardial infarction. *Am J Med Sci* 1987;293:139–149.

145. Ellis AK, Little T, Masud ARZ, et al: Early noninvasive detection of successful reperfusion in patient with acute myocardial infarction. *Circulation* 1988;78: 1352–1357.

146. Abendschein DR, Puleo PR, Cannon CP, and the TIMI IV and V investigators: Noninvasive detection of early coronary artery patency based on plasma MM and MB creatine kinase isoforms. *Circulation* 1992;86:1–267.

147. Christenson RH, Ohman EM, Topol EJ, et al: Creatine kinase MM and MB isoforms in patients receiving thrombolytic therapy and acute angiography. *Clin Chem* 1995;41:844–852.

148. Jaffe AS, Eisenberg PR, Abendschein DR: Conjoint use of MM and MB creatine kinase isoforms for detection of coronary recanalization. *Am Heart J* 1994;127:1461–1466.

149. Roberts R, Henry PD, Sobel BE: An improved basis for enzymatic estimation of infarct size. *Circulation* 1975;52:743–754.

150. Rogers WJ, McDaniel HG, Smith LR, et al: Correlation of CPK-MB and angiographic estimates of infarct size in man. *Circulation* 1977;56: 199–205.

151. Roberts R, Husain R: Relation between infarct size and ventricular arrhythmia. *Br Heart J* 1975; 37:1169–1175.

152. Sobel BE, Bresnahan GF, Shell WE, et al: Estimation of infarct size in man and its relation to prognosis. *Circulation* 1972;46:640–648.

153. Geltman EM, Ehsani AA, Campbell MK, et al: The influence of location and extent of myocardial infarction on long-term ventricular dysrhythmia and mortality. *Circulation* 1979;60:1805–1814.

154. Roberts R, Ishikawa Y: Enzymatic estimation of infarct size during reperfusion. *Circulation* 1983; 68(Suppl I):I-83–I-89.

155. Kagen LJ. *Myoglobin: Biochemical, Physiological and Clinical Aspects.* New York, Columbia University Press, 1973.

156. Keller P, Munscher P, Pheiffer G: Immunologischer Myoglobinnachweis beim Herzinfarkt. *Therapiewoche* 1976;26:1–8.

157. Miyoski K, Saito S, Kawai H, et al: Radioimmunoassay for human myoglobin: Methods and results in patients with skeletal muscle or myocardial disorders. *J Lab Clin Med* 1978;93:341–352.

158. Sonnemaker RE, Daniels DL, Craig WE, et al: Serum myoglobin determination: Laboratory and clinical evaluation. *J Nucl Med* 1979;20:120–124.

159. Kagan L, Scheidt S, Roberts L, et al: Myoglobinemia following acute myocardial infarction. *Am J Med* 1975;58:177–182.

160. Tommaso CL, Salzeider K, Arif M, et al: Serial myoglobin vs CPK analysis as an indicator of uncomplicated myocardial infarction size and its use in assessing early infarct extension. *Am Heart J* 1970;99:149–154.

161. Norregaard-Hansen K, Lind KE, Vind Ludvigsen C, et al: Serum myoglobin compared with creatine kinase in patients with acute myocardial infarction. *Acta Med Scand* 1980;207:265–270.
162. Cairns JA, Missirlis E, Walker WH: Usefulness of serial determinations of myoglobin and creatine kinase in serum compared for assessment of acute myocardial infarction. *Clin Chem* 1983;29(3): 469–473.
163. Almog C, Isakov A, Ayalon D, Burke M, Shapira I: Serum myoglobin in detection of myocardial necrosis in patients with "coronary insufficiency." *Clin Cardiol* 1987;10:347–349.
164. Kagen L, Scheidt S, Butt A: Serum myoglobin in myocardial infarction: The "staccato phenomenon." *Am J Med* 1977;62.
165. Loogna E, Sylvent C, Groth T, Mogensen L: Complexity of enzyme release during acute myocardial infarction in a controlled study with early nifedipine treatment. *Eur Heart J* 1985;6:114–119.
166. Gasser RNA, Hauptlorenz S, Dworzak E, et al: The typical staccato phenomenon of myoglobin in acute myocardial infarction disappears under thrombolytic treatment. *Fibrinolysis* 1987;1: 177–182.
167. Groth T, Hakman M, Sylven C. Prediction of myocardial infarct size from early serum myoglobin observations. *Scand J Clin Lab Invest* 1987;47: 599–603.
168. Norregaard-Hansen R, Petersen R, Hangaard J, et al: Early observations of S-myoglobin in the diagnosis of acute myocardial infarction: The influence of discrimination limit, analytical quality, patient's sex and prevalence of disease. *Scand J Clin Lab Invest* 1986;46:561–569.
169. Roxin LE, Cullhed J, Groth T, et al: The value of serum myoglobin determinations in the early diagnosis of acute myocardial infarction. *Acta Med Scand* 1984;215:417–425.
170. Vaananen HK, Syrjala H, Ragkila P, et al: Serum carbonic anhydrase III and myoglobin concentration in acute myocardial infarction. *Clin Chem* 1990;36:635–638.
171. Ellis AK, Little T, Zaki Masud AR, Klocke FJ: Patterns of myoglobin release after reperfusion of injured myocardium. *Circulation* 1985;72:639–647.
172. Abe J, Yamaguchi T, Isshiki T, et al: Myocardial reperfusion can be predicted by myoglobin/ creatine kinase ratio of a single blood sample obtained at the time of admission. *Am Heart J* 1993; 126:279–285.
173. Stone MJ, Willerson JT, Gomez-Sanchez CE, Waterman MR: Radioimmunoassay of myoglobin in human serum. Results in patients with myocardial infarction. *J Clin Invest* 1975;56: 1334–1339.
174. Rosano TG, Kenny MA: A radioimmunoassay for human serum myoglobin: Method development and normal values. *Clin Chem* 1977;23:69–95.
175. Van Der Laarse A, Hermens WT, Hollaar L: Assessment of myocardial damage in patients with acute myocardial infarction by serial measurement of serum a-hydroxybutyrate dehydrogenase levels. *Am Heart J* 1984;107:248–260.
176. Moses GC, Henderson AR: Biological variation of lactate dehydrogenase isoenzyme-1/isoenzyme-2 ratio. *Clin Chem* 1985;31:1072–1073.
177. Lott JA: Serum enzyme determinations in the diagnosis of acute myocardial infarction. *Human Pathol* 1984;15:706–716.
178. Simoons ML, Serruys PW, Van Den Brand M, et al: Early thrombolysis in acute myocardial infarction: Limitation of infarct size and improved survival. *J Am Coll Cardiol* 1986;7:717–728.
179. Eisenberg E, Kielley WW: Troponin–tropomyosin complex. *J Biol Chem* 1974;249:4742–4748.
180. Potter JD, Gergely J: Troponin, tropomyosin, actin interaction in the calcium regulation of muscle contraction. *Biochemistry* 1974;13:2697–2703.
181. MacGeoch C, Barton PJ, Vallins WJ, Bhavsar P, Spurr NK: The human cardiac troponin I locus: Assignment to chromosome 19p13.2-19q13.2. *Hum Genet* 1991;88:101–104.
182. Wilkinson JM, Grand RJA: Comparison of amino acid sequence of troponin I from different striated muscles. *Nature* 1978;271:31–35.
183. Wade R, Eddy R, Shows TB, Kedes L: cDNA sequence, tissue specific expression and chromosomal mapping of the human slow-twitch skeletal muscle isoform of troponin I. *Genomics* 1990;7: 346–357.
184. Schreier T, Kedes L, Gahlmann R: Cloning, structural analysis, and expression of the human slow twitch skeletal muscle/cardiac troponin C gene. *J Biol Chem* 1990;265:21247–21253.
185. Anderson PAW, Malouf NN, Oakeley AE, Pagani ED, Allen PD: Troponin T isoform expression in humans: A comparison among normal and failing adult heart, fetal heart and adult and fetal skeletal muscle. *Circulation* 1991;69:1226–1233.
186. Martin AF: Turnover of cardiac troponin subunits. *J Biol Chem* 1981;256:964–968.

187. Adams JE III, Schechtman KB, Landt Y, Ladenson JH, Jaffe AS: Comparable detection of acute myocardial infarction by creatine kinase MB isoenzyme and cardiac troponin I. *Clin Chem* 1994;40: 1291–1295.

188. Toyota N, Shimada Y: Differentiation of troponin in cardiac and skeletal muscles in chicken embryos as studied by immunofluorescence microscopy. *J Cell Biol* 1981;91:497–504.

189. Saggin L, Gorza L, Ausoni S, Schiaffino S: Troponin I switching in the developing heart. *J Biol Chem* 1989;264:16299–16302.

190. Wilkinson JM, Grand RJA: Comparison of amino acid sequence of troponin I from different striated muscles. *Nature* 1978;271:31–35.

191. Bhavsar P, Dhoot GK, Cumming DVE, Butler-Brown GS, Yacoub MH, Barton OJR: Development expression of troponin I isoforms in fetal human heart. *FEBS Lett* 1991;292:5–8.

192. Cummins P, Young A, Auckland ML, Michie CA, Stone PCW, Shepstone BJ: Comparison of serum cardiac specific troponin I with creatine kinase, creatine kinase-MB isoenzyme, tropomyosin, myoglobin and C-reactive protein release in marathon runners: Cardiac or skeletal muscle trauma? *Eur J Clin Invest* 1987;17:317–324.

193. Dávila-Román V, Guest TM, Rowe WJ, Tuteur PG, Ladenson JH, Jaffe AS: Ultra exercise induces right ventricular dysfunction. *J Am Coll Cardiol* 1995;260A.

194. Bhayana V, Gougoulias T, Cohoe S, Henderson AR: Discordance between results for serum troponin T and I in renal disease. *Clin Chem* 1995;41:312–317.

195. Schwartz K, de la Bastie D, Bouveret P, Oliviero P, Alonso S, Buckingham M: Alpha skeletal muscle actin mRNA accumulate in hypertrophied adult rat hearts. *Circ Res* 1986;59:551–555.

196. Saggin L, Gorza L, Ausoni S, Schiaffino S: Cardiac troponin T in developing, regenerating and denervated rat skeletal muscle. *Development* 1990;110: 547–554.

197. Mair J, Artner-Dworzak E, Lechleitner P, et al: Cardiac troponin T in diagnosis of acute myocardial infarction. *Clin Chem* 1991;37:845–852.

198. Katus HA, Remppis A, Neumann FJ, et al: Diagnostic efficiency of troponin T measurements in acute myocardial infarction. *Circulation* 1991;83: 902–912.

199. Katus HA, Looser S, Hallermayer K, et al: Development and in vitro characterization of a new immunoassay of cardiac troponin T. *Clin Chem* 1992;38: 386–393.

200. Katus HA, Muller-Bardorf M, Hallermayr K, et al: Development and characterization of an improved rapid enzyme immunoassay specific for cardiac troponin T. *J Am Coll Cardiol* 1994;abst:77A.

201. Katus HA, Schoeppenthau M, Tanzeem A, et al: Non-invasive assessment of perioperative myocardial cell damage by circulating cardiac troponin T. *Br Heart J* 1991;65:259–264.

201a. Guest TM, Ramanathan AV, Schechtman KB, Ladenson JH, Jaffe AS. Myocardial injury in critically ill medical patients: A surprisingly frequent complication. *JAMA* 1995;273:1945–1949.

202. Collinson PO, Stubbs PJ: The prognostic value of serum troponin T in unstable angina. *N Engl J Med* 1992;327:1760–1761.

203. Kobayashi S, Tanaka M, Tamura N, Hashimoto H, Hirose S: Serum cardiac troponin T in polymyositis/dermatomyosistis (letter). *Lancet* 1992;340:726.

204. Mair J, Wohlfarter T, Koller A, Mayr M, Artner-Dworzak E, Puschendorf B: Serum cardiac troponin T after extraordinary endurance exercise (letter). *Lancet* 1992;340:1048.

205. Mair J, Puschendorf B, Michel G: Clinical significance of cardiac contractile proteins for the diagnosis of myocardial injury. *Adv Clin Chemistry;* 31:63–98.

206. Mair J, Artner-Dworzak E, Lechleitner P, et al: Cardiac troponin T in diagnosis of acute myocardial infarction. *Clin Chem* 1991;37:845–852.

207. Cummins B, Auckland M, Cummins P: Cardiac-specific troponin I radioimmunoassay in the diagnosis of acute myocardial infarction. *Am Heart J* 1987;113:1333–1344.

208. Gerhardt W, Katus HA, Ravkilde J, et al: S-troponin T and mass concentration of S-CKMB as markers of ischemic myocardial injury. *Clin Chem* 1991;37: 1405–1411.

209. Hamm CW, Ravkilde J, Gerhardt W, et al: The prognostic value of serum troponin T in unstable angina. *N Engl J Med* 1992;327:146–150.

210. Bakker AJ, Koelemay MJW, Gorgels JPMC, et al: Troponin T and myoglobin at admission: Value of early diagnosis of acute myocardial infarction. *Eur Heart J* 1994;15:45–53.

211. Wu AHB, Valdes R, Apple F, et al: Cardiac troponin T immunoassay for diagnosis of acute myocardial infarction. *Clin Chem* 1994;40:900–907.

212. Ravkilde J, Nissen H, Horder M, Thygesen K: Independent prognostic value of serum creatine kinase isoenzyme MB mass, cardiac troponin T and myosin light chain levels in suspected acute myocardial infarction. *J Am Coll Cardiol* 1995;25:574.

212a. Lindahl B, Venge P, Wallentin L, for the FRISC Study Group: Relation between troponin T and the risk of subsequent cardiac event in unstable coronary artery disease. *Circulation* 1996;93: 1651–1656.

212b. Galvani M, Ottani F, Ladenson JH, et al: Adverse influence of elevated cardiac troponin I in unstable angina. *Circulation* 1995;92:I–598 (abstract).

212c. Ohman EM, Armstrong P, Califf RM, et al. Risk stratification in acute ischaemic syndromes using serum troponin T. *Eur Heart J* 1995;16:179 (abstract).

213. Katus HA: Troponin T analysis in ischemic heart disease. *Clin Chem* 1992;38:919.

214. Wagner I, Mair J, Fridrich L, et al: Cardiac troponin T release in acute myocardial infarction is associated with scintigraphic estimates of myocardial scar. *Cor Art Dis* 1993;4:537–544.

215. Omura T, Teragaki M, Tani T, et al: Estimation of infarct size using serum troponin T concentration in patients with acute myocardial infarction. *Jpn Circ J* 1993;57:1062–1070.

APPENDIX: RECOMMENDATIONS FOR THE USE OF SERUM ENZYME ASSAYS IN THE DIAGNOSIS OF ACUTE MYOCARDIAL INFARCTION*

1. A single set of cardiac enzyme values in the emergency room is not sufficiently sensitive to exclude myocardial infarction. Although a single, markedly positive MBCK value will greatly increase the probability of acute infarction, data are insufficient to support or reject a policy whereby low-risk patients, who otherwise would be sent home, would be observed until one or more MBCK values are obtained.

2. If myocardial infarction is suspected, then samples of total CK and MBCK levels should be measured on admission and about 12 and 24 hours later, although condensed versions of this strategy may ultimately prove to be equally efficacious and more cost effective. If myocardial infarction may have occurred more than 24 hours before admission, and if CK and MBCK levels are not diagnostic, a total LD level should be ordered. If the total LD level is elevated, an assay of LD isoenzymes should be obtained. If the first LD1/LD2 ratio is only slightly less than 1.0, a second assay is probably indicated.

3. If chest pain recurs after admission, CK and MBCK assays should be done at 0, 12, and 24 hours. "Surveillance" enzyme assays are not recommended in asymptomatic patients without electrocardiographic changes.

4. Routine use of enzyme assays other than those for CK, MBCK, and LD isoenzymes is not recommended.

5. If more than 2 hours may pass before CK isoenzymes will be assayed, the serum sample should be preserved on ice.

6. Strategies including MBCK assays can be used to diagnose myocardial infarction in the setting of noncardiac surgery and cardiac catheterization and after electrical countershock.

7. In the setting of cardiac surgery, myocardial infarction cannot be diagnosed by elevations in MBCK unless extremely persistent (more than 12 hours); new Q waves appear on the electrocardiogram; or regional defects on technetium pyrophosphate scintigraphy are detected.

8. False-positive elevation of MBCK can be minimized by diluting samples with marked elevations of total CK; detecting isoenzyme variants that masquerade as MBCK on column chromatography assays by retesting the sample on an electrophoretic assay if the clinical presentation is atypical for myocardial infarction; or considering other sources of MBCK (for example, myocarditis, renal failure, neuromuscular diseases, trauma) if a true elevation of MBCK levels is found in the absence of a typical rise and fall of CK and MBCK levels and other evidence for myocardial infarction.

---

*Adapted from Lee TH, Goldman L: Serum enzyme assay in the diagnosis of acute myocardial infarction. Ann Intern Med 1986;105:221–233, with permission.

9

New Insights into the Electrocardiogram of Acute Myocardial Infarction

Ashish Parikh, MD, and Prediman K. Shah, MD

Recent interventional approaches in the management of acute myocardial infarction have not only reduced postinfarct morbidity and mortality but have also provided important and new insights into the electrocardiographic (ECG) changes following acute myocardial infarction (MI). The evolution and application of thrombolytic therapy and coronary angioplasty, now widely used in the management of acute MI, made it possible to correlate ECG changes in acute MI to coronary anatomy, myocardial function, and perfusion. In this chapter, some of the newer and important insights that have been gained during this period are briefly discussed.

ACUTE INFERIOR MYOCARDIAL INFARCTION: "UPS AND DOWNS" OF PRECORDIAL ST SEGMENTS

Precordial ST Depression

Precordial ST segment depression occurs in nearly 50% to 70% of patients with acute inferior MI and generally resolves over the subsequent 48 to 72 hours in the majority, with persistent ST depression remaining in about 16% of cases (1–18). ST segment depression is most commonly noted in leads V_1, V_2, and V_3 and in some patients it is associated with ST depression in leads 1 and aVL as well (9,19) (Fig. 9–1).

Most, but not all, studies have shown that as a group, patients with precordial ST depression have larger infarcts than their counterparts without ST depression, as evidenced by higher peak CK release; more extensive wall motion abnormalities; larger defect size by thallium-201, technetium-99*m*, and positron emission tomography (PET); and higher QRS scores of infarct size (2,4–6,8–10,14,18–24) (Fig. 9–2). Similarly, global left ventricular function as reflected by the ejection fraction and hemodynamic state is depressed to a greater extent in patients with ST depression than in those without (2,4,7,8,9,14, 18–20), although some have failed to confirm these findings (5,10,23,25–27). Consistent with these findings, most studies have shown that patients with precordial ST depression have a worse prognosis than their counterparts without ST depression. Thus patients with ST depression, in comparison with those without, develop postinfarction complications such as congestive heart failure, recurrent or persistent ischemia, arrhythmias and conduction abnormalities, and death more frequently, especially if ST depression is marked or persistent (2–4,6–8,28–30). The presence of maximal ST segment depression in precordial leads V_4–V_6 compared with leads V_1–V_3 has

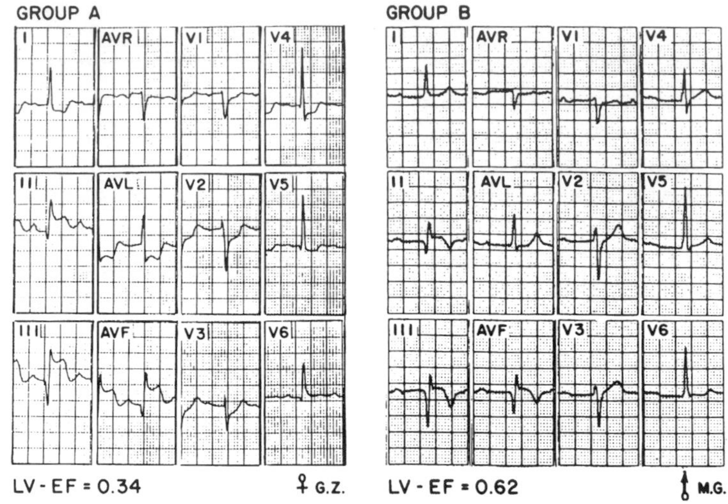

Figure 9–1. Twelve-lead ECG from two patients with acute inferior MI: **A.** With precordial ST depression. **B.** Without precordial ST depression. Note the depressed left ventricular ejection fraction (LVEF) in the patient with precordial ST segment depression. *Adapted from Shah et al (2), with permission.*

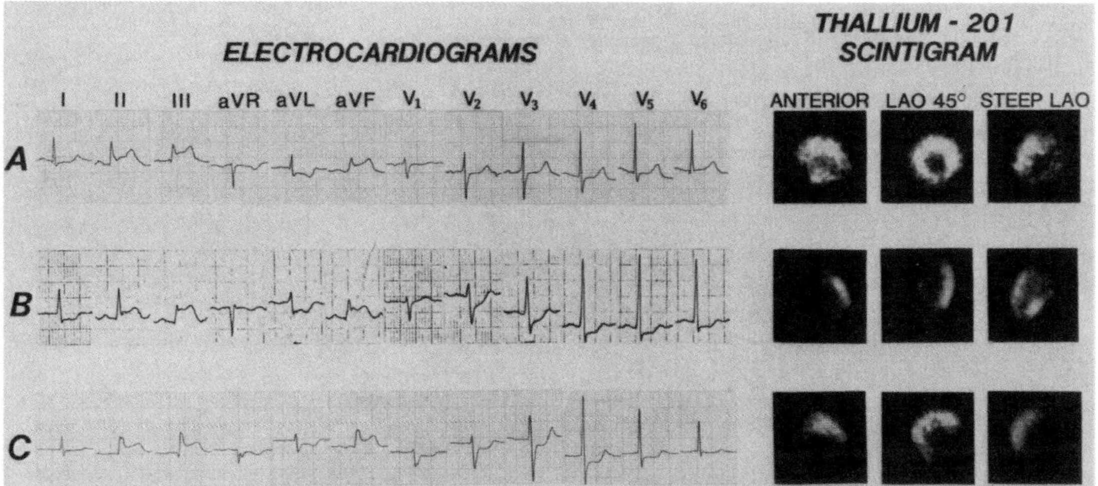

Figure 9–2. Twelve-lead ECG and corresponding thallium-201 scintigrams from three representative patients with acute inferior MI: **A.** No precordial ST segment depression and normal posterolateral and septal thallium-201 uptake. **B.** Precordial ST segment depression leads V_1 to V_6 and a large thallium-201 perfusion defect of the ventricular septum. **C.** Precordial ST segment depression in leads V_2 to V_6 and a thallium-201 perfusion defect of the posterolateral wall. Note the reduced thallium-201 uptake of the inferior wall in all three scintigrams. LAO = left anterior oblique. *Adapted from Lew et al (13), with permission.*

been shown to be particularly associated with high mortality (31,31a). A particularly large data bank study from the Duke University Group and the Gusto-1 trial demonstrated a significantly higher short-term as well as long-term (1 to 5 years) mortality rate in patients with, compared with those without, precordial ST segment depression (22,22a). Some investigators, however, have failed to confirm adverse prognostic implications of precordial ST segment depression (5,16,19,27,32).

Mechanism(s) of Precordial ST Depression

There is no firm agreement about the factor(s) that determines the presence and magnitude or absence of precordial ST depression in acute inferior MI. Two factors to which such ST depression has been attributed are discussed here.

Multivessel Disease and Specifically Left Anterior Descending Coronary Artery Disease

The presence of precordial ST depression has been attributed by some to concomitant anterior or anteroseptal ischemia presumably related to multivessel disease and to left anterior descending coronary artery (LAD) disease in particular. In support of this explanation, the greater prevalence of multivessel disease with ST depression has been emphasized by some (1,7,9) but not confirmed by others (4,10,13,22). The prevalence of left anterior descending coronary artery disease has been reported to be 12% to 93% in the group with ST depression and 10% to 68% in those without ST depression (1,3–5,7–15). The prevalence of left anterior descending coronary artery disease appears to be higher in patients with severe ST depression (>3 mm) and in those in whom ST depression occurs after or persists beyond the first 6 hours or so (7,11). The bulk of data does not support a role for multivessel disease or left anterior descending coronary artery disease as a frequent cause of precordial ST segment depression in acute inferior MI. Some reports, however, do suggest that at least in some patients, left anterior descending coronary artery disease and ischemia at a distance (in the left anterior descending coronary artery disease distribution) may be contributing to the precordial ST segment depression. Using positron emission tomography (PET), Billadello and his colleagues detected anterior ischemia in three of nine patients with precordial ST depression, and all three of these patients had left anterior descending coronary artery disease; however, three of five patients with ST depression and left anterior descending artery disease did not have ischemia in the anterior wall on PET (21).

Posterolateral and Inferoseptal Involvement with a Larger Inferior Infarct

Several lines of evidence support the thesis that in most patients with acute inferior MI, precordial ST depression is related to a larger inferior infarct, with contiguous involvement of the posterolateral wall and/or the inferoseptal wall. The findings of a greater extent and severity of regional wall motion abnormality of the inferior wall, a higher frequency of wall motion and perfusion abnormalities of the inferoseptal as well as the posterolateral wall, and a greater frequency of evolution of an acute posterior MI pattern on a 12-lead ECG in patients with precordial ST depression, compared with those without, support this explanation (4,7,9,13,17–20,23,26,27,29,32,33–36).

Precordial ST Segment Elevation

A small number of patients with an acute inferior MI show concomitant ST segment elevation in precordial leads, most frequently affecting leads V_1 and V_2, but at times involving additional left-sided precordial leads as well (37,38). In a consecutive series, this pattern was noted in less than 10% of patients with an acute inferior MI (38). These precordial ST segment elevations have been shown to result from concomitant right ventricular infarction as documented by scintigraphic evidence of right ventricular necrosis and right ventricular systolic dysfunction (38) (see Ch. 17). Precordial ST elevation resulting from right ventricular infarction can be distinguished from ST elevation resulting from acute anterior MI when the magnitude of ST elevation declines progressively from lead V_1 and V_2, but at times involving additional left-sided precordial leads as well (37,38). In some patients predominant right ventricular infarction may occur as a result of occlusion of a right ventricular marginal branch, in which case precordial ST elevation may be the only ECG abnormality (Fig. 9–3). Similarly, in a patient with a prior acute inferior MI, reocclusion of a right coronary artery may produce a similar pattern.

Composite Explanation for the "Ups and Downs" of Precordial ST Deviations

On the basis of our clinical observations in 1985 we postulated that precordial ST depression in acute inferior MI was largely a reciprocal phenomenon caused by inferior infarction. Its magnitude was influenced by two opposing influences: posterolateral or inferoseptal extension of the left ventricular infarct tended to exaggerate the reciprocal ST depression, whereas infarction of the right ventricle, an anteriorly located cardiac chamber, tended to attenuate the precordial ST depression by producing a rightward and anteriorly directed ST vector (13,39). Within this conceptual framework, the magnitude and direction of the precordial ST shift would depend on the size of inferior and posterolateral infarction and the presence and extent of concomitant right ventricular involvement. Evidence to support this concept was derived from an experimental study as well as a more detailed analysis of ECG data from patients with acute inferior MI (38,39). In the canine model, where the circumflex coronary artery supplies the inferior wall of the left ventricle and the right coronary artery exclusively supplies the right ventricle, occlusion of the circumflex artery was associated with inferior ST elevation and anterior lead ST depression, whereas right coronary artery occlusion was associated with anterior ST elevation. Combined occlusion of both vessels was associated with inferior ST elevation and attenuation or elimination of anterior ST depression (38). Similarly, in patients, when the magnitude of the precordial ST shift was related to the magnitude of the inferior ST elevation, the correlation was poor ($r = -0.46$); however, on elimination of data for patients with right ventricular infarction and those with posterolateral infarction, the correlation improved substantially to $r = -0.89$ ($p < 0.001$) (39). The slope relating inferior ST elevation to precordial ST shift was significantly influenced by the presence of posterolateral infarction and right ventricular infarction. Thus the magnitude of precordial ST depression for any given magnitude of inferior ST elevation was greater in the presence of posterolateral infarction than in its absence, and conversely, the magnitude of precordial ST depression for any magnitude of inferior ST elevation was less in the presence of right ventricular infarction than in its absence (39) (Figs. 9–4 and 9–5).

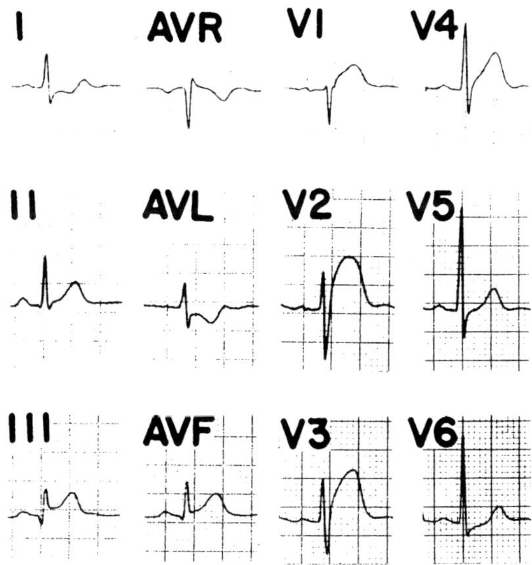

Figure 9–3. Twelve-lead ECG of a patient with acute inferior MI. Note, in addition to the inferior ST elevation, the concomitant ST elevations in precordial leads V_1 to V_3, indicative of right ventricular infarction.

In conclusion, data strongly support the thesis that the "ups" and "downs" of the precordial ST segments in acute inferior MI are determined by reciprocal factors related to the size of the inferior infarction as well as the involvement of the adjacent posterolateral wall and/or the inferoseptal wall. This reciprocal influence may be attenuated or reversed by concomitant infarction of the right ventricle, which tends to produce a rightward and anteriorly directed ST vector. Furthermore, as a group, patients with precordial ST depression have worse clinical outcome related to a larger extent of ischemia/infarction. Concomitant ischemia of the anterior wall ap-

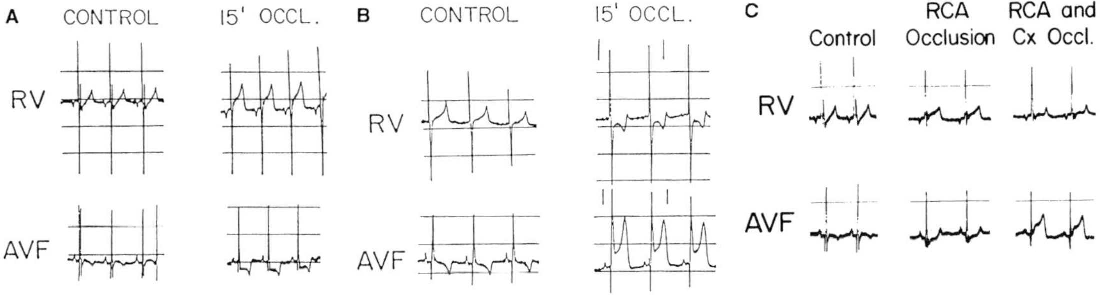

Figure 9–4. Effect of 15-minute occlusion of the right coronary artery, circumflex artery, or both on the ECG of a dog recorded anteriorly over the right ventricle and in an inferior lead. Note that the reciprocal ST depression over the anterior (right ventricular) lead produced by circumflex occlusion is abolished by simultaneous occlusion of the right coronary artery. *Adapted from Lew et al (39), with permission.*

pears to play a role in only a minority proportion of patients with precordial ST depression (see Ch. 17).

ACUTE ANTERIOR MYOCARDIAL INFARCTION: "UPS AND DOWNS" OF INFERIOR ST SEGMENTS

Analogous to the patients with acute inferior MI, 37% to 62% of patients with an acute anterior MI have concomitant ST segment depression in one or more inferior leads (5,16,22,25,28,30,32,40,41) (Fig. 9–6). Few studies, however, have addressed the clinical significance of inferior ST segment changes in acute anterior MI. In 1984, Jugdutt and his colleagues studied left ventricular function and clinical course of patients who had survived 3 months after an acute anterior MI (42). Those patients with concomitant inferior ST segment depression had worse left ventricular function and a more complicated clinical course than patients without inferior ST segment depression (34). This was attributed to the higher prevalence of multivessel coronary artery disease in patients with inferior ST segment depression. Stimulated by our analysis of patients with acute inferior MI, we postulated that the direction and magnitude of inferior ST segments in acute anterior MI may be determined by the net result of two opposing forces: (i) reciprocal effects of anterior ST elevation, tending to produce inferior ST depression, and (ii) concomitant ischemia of the inferior wall, tending to attenuate or even reverse the direction of inferior ST segments. Using our thrombolysis database, we investigated this hypothesis in a cohort of consecutive patients with acute anterior MI undergoing thrombolysis in whom coronary anatomy was defined by angiography, myocardial perfusion was determined by thallium scintigraphy, and left ventricular function was determined by radionuclide or contrast ventriculography. Two groups of patients were identified: (i) patients with scintigraphic evidence of concomitant inferior wall ischemia/infarction in whom coronary angiography revealed either a relatively long left anterior descending artery that wrapped around the left ventricular apex to supply a portion of the inferior wall, or an old inferior infarction with the previously occluded posterior descending artery supplied by collaterals from the LAD; (ii) patients without evidence of concomitant inferior wall ischemia/infarction in whom the left anterior descending artery tended to be relatively short, failing to continue beyond the left ventricular apex. All patients without inferior wall ischemia/infarction had inferior lead ST segment depression that was greater in magnitude (in absolute terms as well as relative to the magnitude of precordial ST segment elevation) compared with the patients with evidence of inferior ischemia/infarction. Furthermore, 30% of patients with concomitant inferior ischemia had either isoelectric or elevated inferior ST segments. These observations are consistent with the clinicopathologic studies of Meyers et al, who found inferior ST depression in patients with infarction limited to the

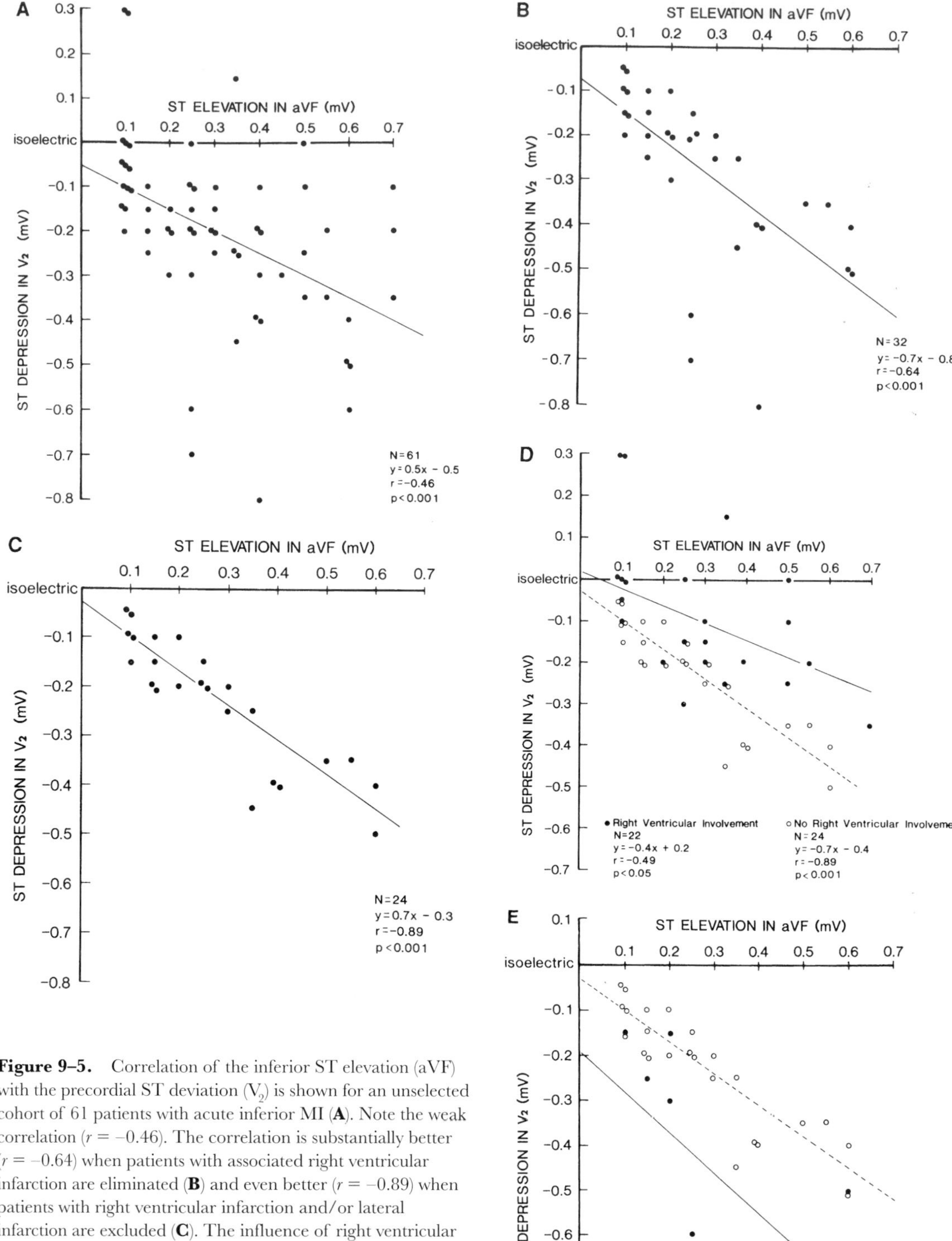

Figure 9–5. Correlation of the inferior ST elevation (aVF) with the precordial ST deviation (V_2) is shown for an unselected cohort of 61 patients with acute inferior MI (**A**). Note the weak correlation ($r = -0.46$). The correlation is substantially better ($r = -0.64$) when patients with associated right ventricular infarction are eliminated (**B**) and even better ($r = -0.89$) when patients with right ventricular infarction and/or lateral infarction are excluded (**C**). The influence of right ventricular infarction (**D**) and lateral infarction (**E**) on the slope and regression of this relationship is also shown. Note that for any given level of inferior ST elevation, the magnitude of precordial ST depression is less when there is right ventricular infarction; conversely, presence of lateral infarction exaggerates the degree of precordial ST depression for any given level of inferior ST elevation. *Adapted from Lew et al (39), with permission.*

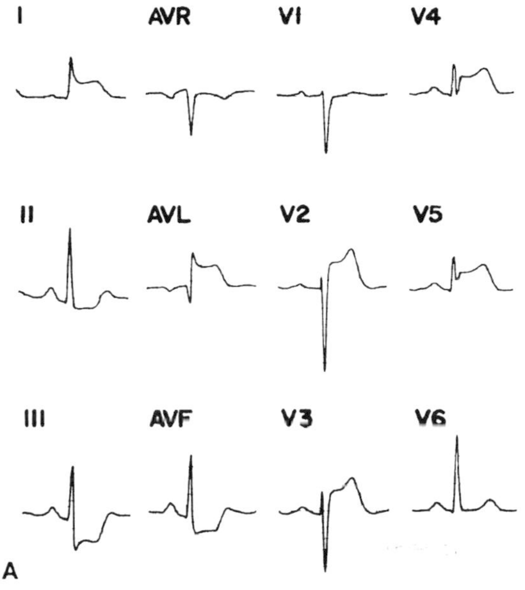

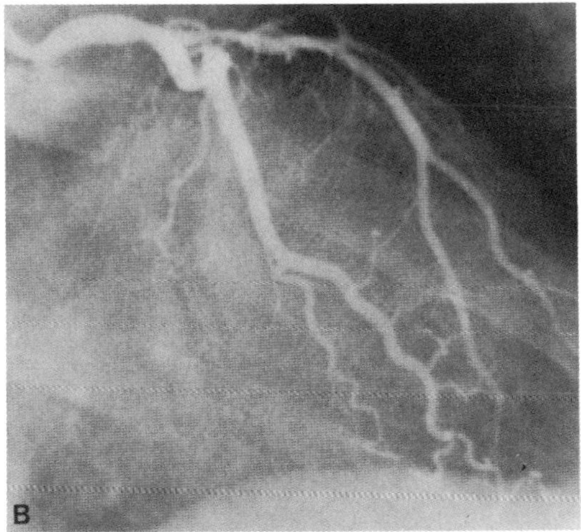

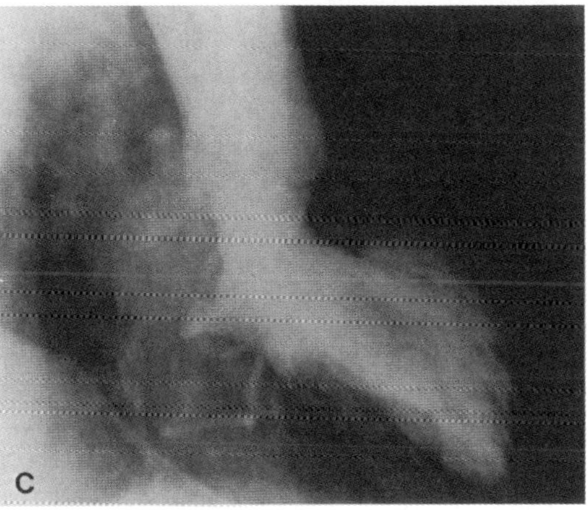

Figure 9–6 **A.** Twelve-lead ECG of a patient with acute anterior MI with inferior ST depression. **B.** The left coronary angiogram (after thrombolytic therapy) of the same patient shows that the left anterior descending artery is relatively short and does not extend beyond the apex of the left ventricle to supply the inferior wall. **C.** End-systolic frame of the left ventriculogram of the same patient demonstrating anterior wall asynergy without inferior wall involvement. *Adapted from Lew et al (41), with permission.*

anterior wall and noted the absence of such depression when the anterior infarct continued around the apex to involve other inferior wall or when there was an associated old posterior infarction (43). In addition, the magnitude of inferior ST depression correlated poorly with the precordial ST elevation ($r = -0.18$) until patients with inferior ischemia/infarction were eliminated ($r = -0.5, p < 0.01$). Patients with a proximal left anterior descending artery occlusion tended to have greater precordial ST elevation and correspondingly a greater inferior ST depression (Figs. 9–7 and 9–8).

It thus appears that the inferior lead ST segment depression during an acute anterior MI is primarily a reciprocal manifestation of precordial ST segment elevation, a conclusion supported by experimental observations and clinical and clinicopathologic correlations (41–44). Inferior ST depression is exaggerated by a more proximal site of left anterior descending artery occlusion, indicating a more severe and a larger anterior infarct associated with a greater degree of precordial ST segment elevation and subject to attenuation (or even replacement by elevation) by concomitant inferior wall ischemia/infarction, analogous to the way precordial ST depression in acute inferior MI is attenuated or reversed by concomitant ischemia/infarction of the right ventricle. The observations of Pichler et al, who noted poorer left ventricular function, and of Jugdutt and colleagues, who noted worse left ventricular function and prognosis in patients with anterior MI and inferior ST depression, can thus be explained on the basis of a larger anterior infarction in patients with inferior ST segment depression rather than concomitant inferior ischemia/infarction (28,42,45) (Figs. 9–9 and 9–10).

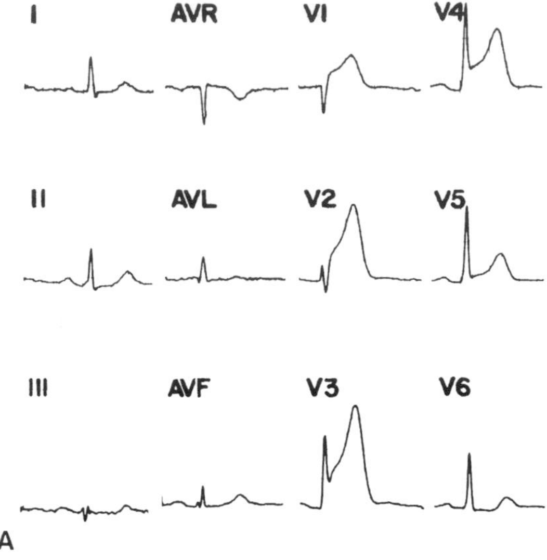

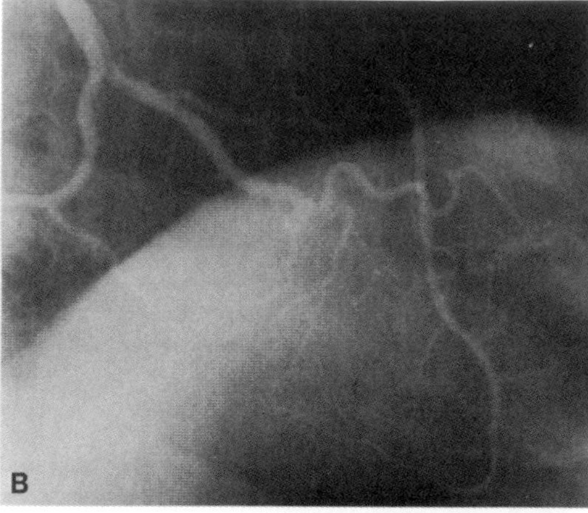

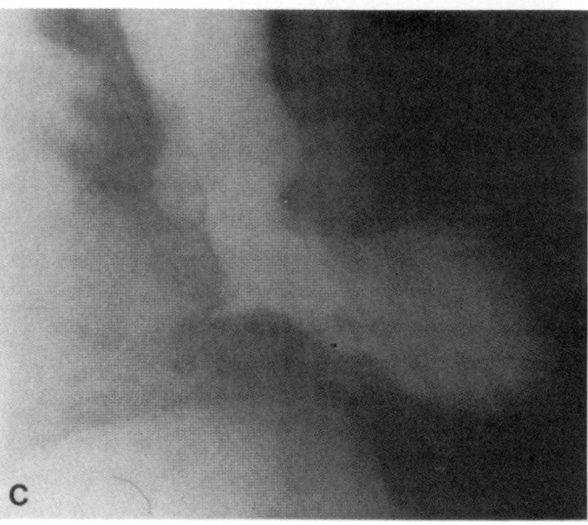

Figure 9–7 **A.** Twelve-lead ECG of a patient with acute MI without inferior ST abnormalities. **B.** Left coronary angiogram (after thrombolytic therapy) of the same patient demonstrating a long left anterior descending artery that wraps around the apex of the left ventricle to supply part of the inferior wall. **C.** End-systolic frame of the left ventriculogram of the same patient showing asynergy of anterior as well as inferior walls. *Adapted from Lew et al (41), with permission.*

RECIPROCAL ELECTROCARDIOGRAPHIC CHANGES IN ISCHEMIA AND INFARCTION

The electrical activity of a single myocardial region may be approximated by a single current dipole, and the validity of this model for representing ST segment responses to acute MI has been established in experiments (46,47). The electrical field generated by a single-dipole source is characterized by direct as well as reciprocal potentials corresponding to the head and tail end of the dipole, respectively. In this single-dipole model, the maximum potential is analogous to the primary ST elevation recorded in leads directly overlying the injured myocardium, whereas the minimum potential corresponds to the reciprocal ST depression observed over remote leads overlying opposite sites on the torso (46,47). These theoretic principles derived from the electrical dipole models have been further validated in experimental models of myocardial injury as well as in humans with the use of body surface isopotential maps (48–50). These observations indicate that reciprocal ST segment depression in response to primary ST segment elevation is to be expected as a biophysical phenomenon with a sound theoretic basis. In the clinical situation, expression and magnitude of such reciprocal changes depend on a number of factors, such as lead placement relative to location of primary site of injury, magnitude and size of the primary site of injury, and the modifying influence of additional and contiguous areas of myocardial injury.

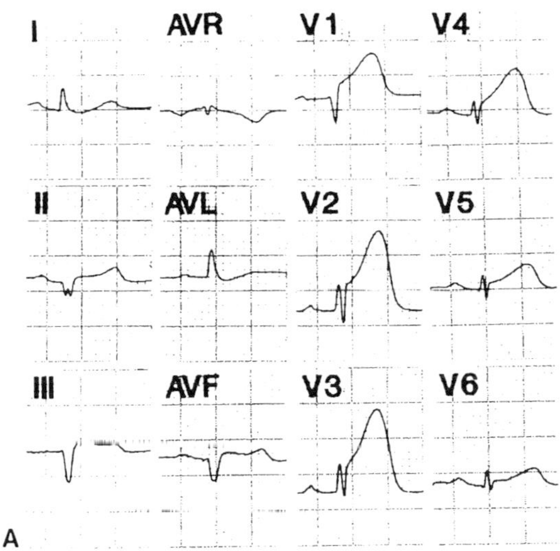

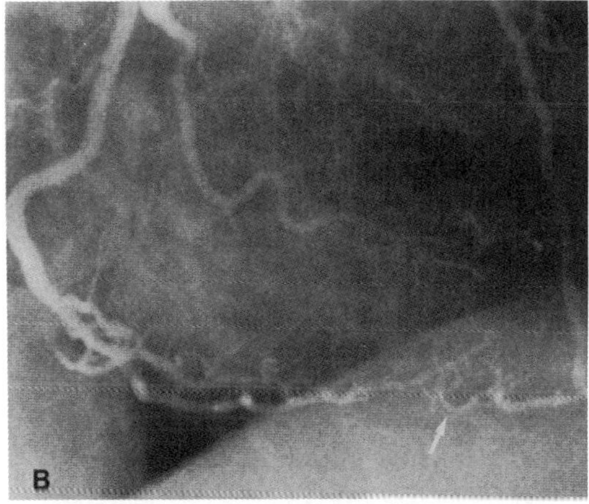

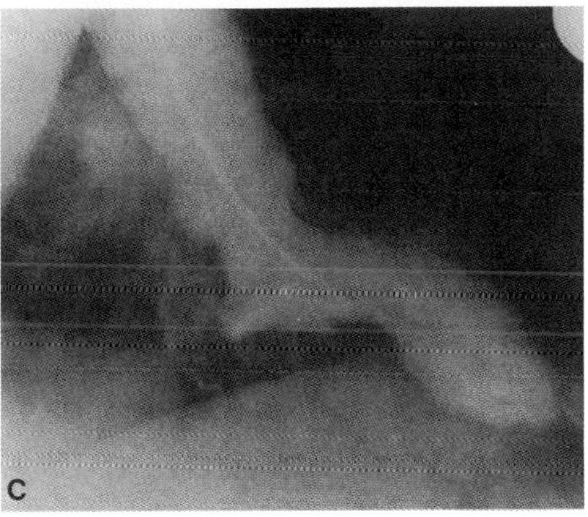

Figure 9–8. Twelve-lead ECG of a patient with acute anterior MI demonstrating ST segment elevation in precordial leads. Note Q waves in inferior leads from a prior inferior infarction. In addition to precordial ST elevation, there is ST segment elevation in inferior leads as well. **B.** Left coronary angiogram (performed after thrombolytic therapy) of the same patient demonstrating a previously occluded right coronary artery filled by collaterals from the left anterior descending artery. **C.** End-systolic frame of the left ventriculogram of the same patient demonstrating anterior as well as inferior asynergy. *Adapted from Lew et al (41), with permission.*

ELECTROCARDIOGRAM IN RIGHT VENTRICULAR INFARCTION

Right ventricular infarction occurs in 40% to 50% of patients with an acute inferior MI, and its presence can have important clinical, hemodynamic, and prognostic implications (51–53) (see Ch. 17). It is almost always due to occlusion of the right coronary artery at or proximal to its right ventricular marginal branch.

The first ECG diagnosis of right ventricular MI was reported by Erhardt et al, who showed that ST segment elevation in right-sided precordial leads V_{3R} and V_{4R} was a reliable sign of right ventricular infarction as verified at autopsy (54) (Fig. 9–11). Since then, these findings have been confirmed by several other investigators (55–60). The sensitivity and specificity of ST elevation in right-sided precordial leads, especially lead V_{4R}, for the diagnosis of right ventricular MI is well over 90% (54–60). These ST changes tend to be most prominent in the early hours of acute MI, and then to dissipate over the subsequent 24 hours or so. A rightward and anterior displacement of the ST segment vector by ischemic injury to the anteriorly located right ventricular free wall is considered the basis for these ECG findings in right ventricular infarction. In 1985 our group reported ST segment elevation in V_1 and left precordial leads in patients with acute inferior MI and associated right ventricular infarction (38). These precordial ST changes could easily be mistaken for signs of acute anterior MI, especially when the ST elevation extends as far as lead

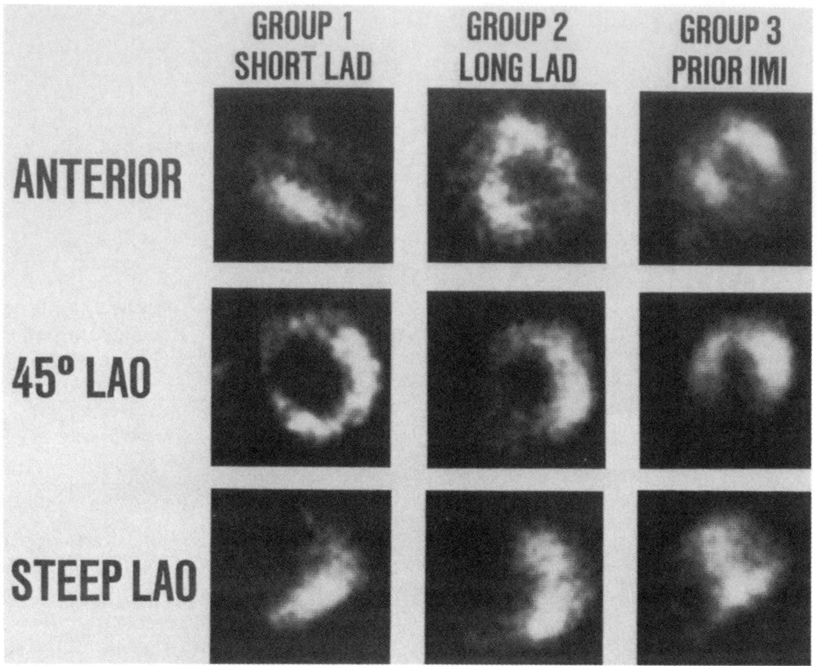

Figure 9–9. Thallium-201 scintigrams of three representative patients: (1) with an acute anterior MI and a short left anterior descending artery, (2) with a long left anterior descending artery, and (3) with a prior acute inferior MI and a new acute anterior MI with left > right collaterals. Note that in the patient with a short left anterior descending artery, there is decreased thallium uptake into the anterolateral and septal walls and normal uptake into the inferior and posterolateral walls, whereas in the other two patients, in addition to decreased uptake of thallium into the anterolateral and septal walls, there is decreased thallium uptake into the inferior and/or posterolateral wall, indicating concomitant inferior or posterior ischemia. *Adapted from Lew et al (41), with permission.*

V_5 or V_6. These findings were, however, noted in only a minority of patients (<10%) despite the 40% to 50% prevalence of right ventricular infarction in patients with an acute inferior MI. The reasons for this discrepancy can be understood when the unifying concept discussed earlier is applied. On the basis of these principles, the direction of precordial ST segments in acute inferior MI is subject to two opposing influences: right ventricular infarction tends to elevate the ST segments, and inferior and posterolateral infarction tends to produce reciprocal ST depression. Thus, in patients with acute inferior MI with concomitant right ventricular infarction, the tendency for right ventricular current of injury to elevate the precordial ST segments would be opposed by the reciprocal effects of inferoposterior current of injury and vice versa, such that left-sided precordial ST segment elevation would occur only when right ventricular involvement predominated and the inferoposterior injury was small. More frequently, however, concomitant right ventricular injury would simply attenuate the magnitude of precordial ST depression. Review of our clinical data showed that occlusion of the proximal right coronary artery is frequently associated with right ventricular infarction and less precordial ST depression, both in absolute terms as well as relative to the degree of inferior ST elevation, than occlusion of the distal right coronary artery or circumflex coronary artery, where right ventricular infarction does not generally occur (56). Thus a ratio of precordial to inferior ST change was found to be an additional useful sign of proximal right coronary artery occlusion and concomitant right ventricular infarction. Specifically, an ST depression in V_2 of 50% or less of the magnitude of ST elevation in aVF was 80% sensitive and 90% specific for the diagnosis of right ventricular infarction resulting from proximal right coronary artery occlusion (56) (Fig. 9–12).

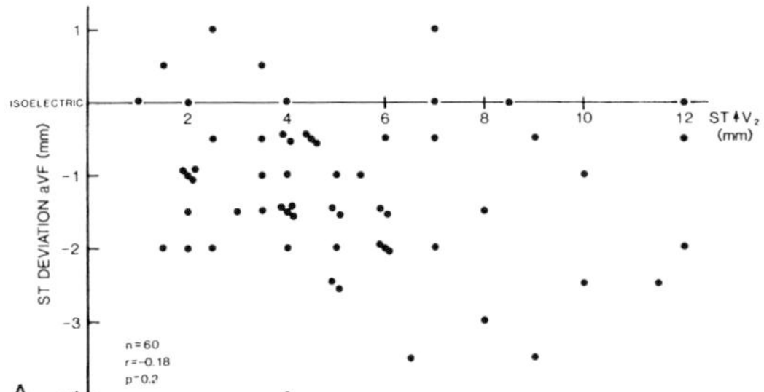

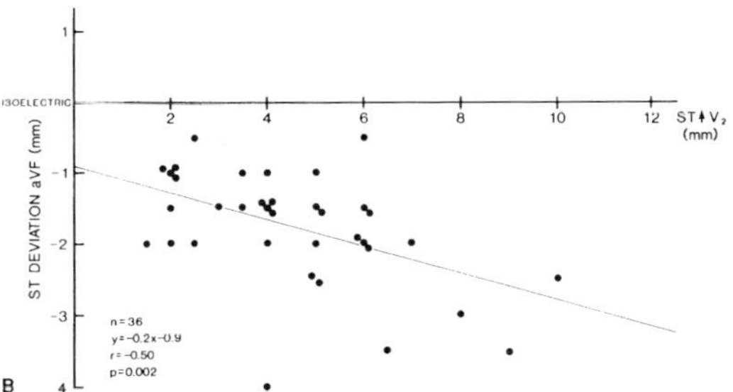

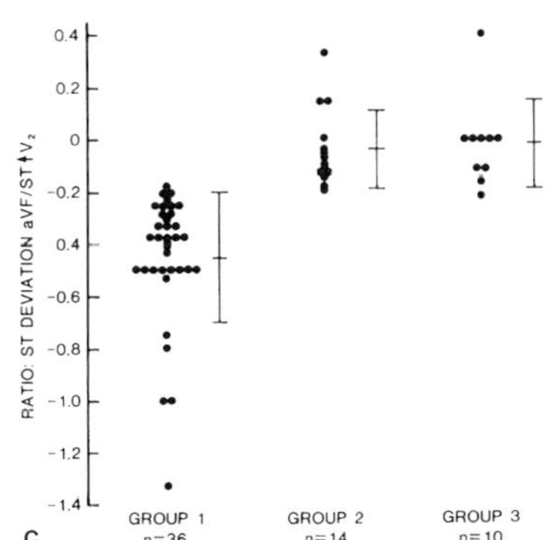

Figure 9–10 **A.** Poor correlation between inferior (aVF) ST deviation and precordial (V_2) ST elevation in patients with acute anterior MI with $r = -0.18$ (not significant). **B.** After exclusion of patients with scintigraphic and ventriculographic signs of concomitant inferior ischemia, the correlation of inferior ST change with precordial ST elevation improves to $r = -0.50$ ($p < 0.01$). **C.** Ratio of inferior ST depression to precordial ST elevation for patients with an acute anterior MI with a short left anterior descending artery and no signs of inferior ischemia (group 1), with a long "wraparound" left anterior descending artery and signs of inferior ischemia (group 2), and with an additional old inferior infarction and left anterior descending artery to posterior descending collaterals (group 3). Note that group 1 patients have a significantly lower ratio compared with the patients in the other two groups. *Adapted from Lew et al (41), with permission.*

INFERIOR MYOCARDIAL INFARCTION: CIRCUMFLEX CORONARY ARTERY OCCLUSION VERSUS RIGHT CORONARY ARTERY OCCLUSION

Acute inferior MI results from right coronary artery occlusion in 50% to 70% of cases, with most of the remaining cases resulting from circumflex occlusion and, rarely, from occlusion of a left anterior descending artery that wraps around the apex to supply a portion of the inferior wall. The ECG diagnosis of circumflex coronary occlusion as a cause of acute MI can be particularly difficult, as about 38% of cases have minimal to no acute ST segment shifts (61). In addition, when circumflex occlusion produces inferior ST elevation, differentiation from right coronary artery occlusion can be difficult. A retrospective and prospective analysis of our thrombolysis database has shown that when inferior ST segment elevation is present during an acute inferior MI, the presence of circumflex occlusion is suggested by the concomitant presence of ST segment elevation in one or more lateral leads (V_5, V_6, aVL) in association with an isoelectric or elevated ST in lead 1. The sensitivity and specificity of these ECG findings are 80% and 90%, respectively (62). These observations have been confirmed by Huey et al (61) in a prospectively studied group of patients with acute MI in the same study; evolution of a posterior infarct pattern in V_1 was highly specific for circumflex occlusion (96%), although the sensitivity was only 21% (61) (Fig. 9–13). Although the possible existence of reciprocal ST segment elevation as a mirror image of the ST segment depression on the opposite side of the heart has been hypothetically considered to be possible, in fact only one documented case of ST segment elevation in leads V_1–V_3 along with marked ST segment depression in lateral leads (I, aVL, V_5, and V_6) resulting from posterior infarction (angiographically confirmed circumflex coronary occlusion) has been described in which the precordial ST segment elevation was attributed to reciprocal effect of posterior ST segment depression (63).

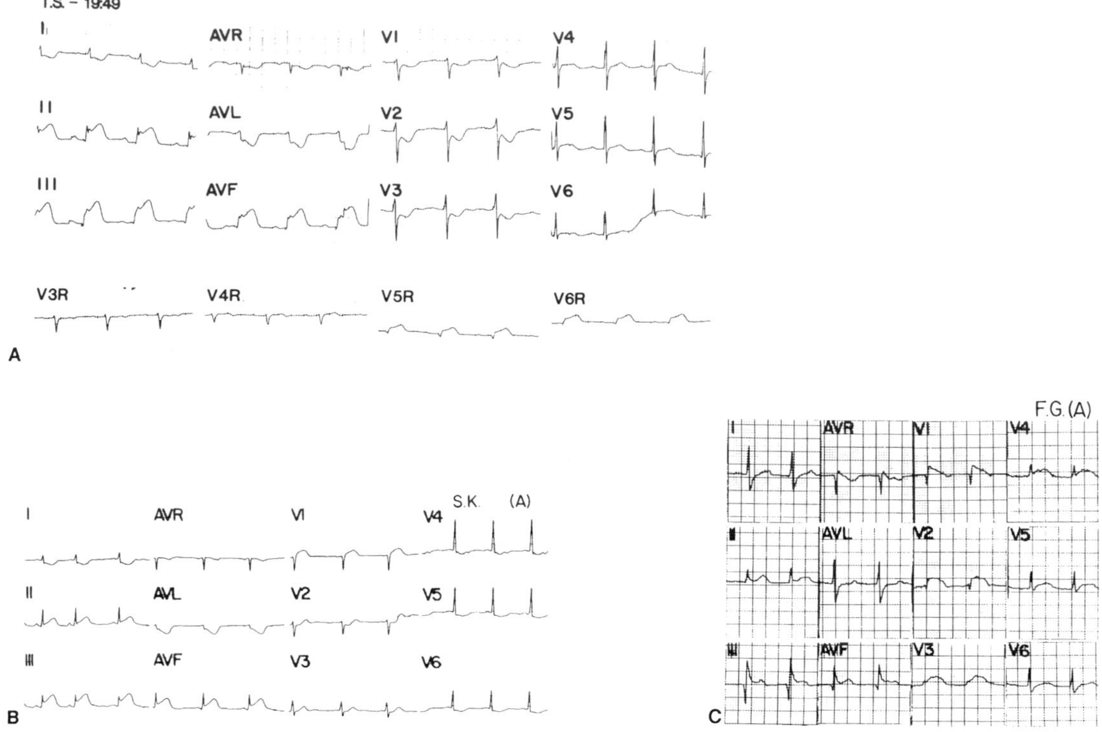

Figure 9–11. Examples of ECG findings in three different patients with acute inferior MI and associated right ventricular infarction. The signs of right ventricular infarction are ST segment elevation in right-sided precordial leads V_{5R} and V_{6R} (**A**), ST segment elevation in lead V_1 (**B**), and ST segment elevation in V_1, V_2, V_3, V_4, and V_5 (**C**). The patient represented in **C** had extensive right ventricular infarction with very little involvement of the left ventricle.

DIAGNOSIS OF MYOCARDIAL INFARCTION IN THE PRESENCE OF LEFT BUNDLE BRANCH BLOCK

An accurate diagnosis of myocardial infarction in the presence of complete left bundle branch block continues to pose difficulties. In left bundle branch block, the initial forces are directed from right to left and either superiorly or inferiorly. When the inferiorly directed forces predominate, a QS complex may be recorded in the precordial leads, simulating the appearance of an anterior infarction, whereas if the initial vector is oriented to the left and superiorly, a QS complex may be produced in the inferior leads, simulating a pattern of inferior infarction. A number of criteria have been suggested as being useful in the ECG diagnosis of acute myocardial infarction in the presence of left bundle branch block, but the results have been inconsistent and conflicting (64–75). The discrepant results are due in part to the different criteria used for confirmation of the underlying myocardial infarction, which have included historical data, autopsy findings, perfusion defects on thallium-201 scintigraphy, abnormalities of regional wall motion, abnormal serum creatine kinase levels, and review of prior ECGs during normal conduction (64–75). In a 1988 report from the MILIS study group, the validity of many of the previously reported criteria were tested in a relatively small cohort of 35 patients who presented with a left bundle branch block and symptoms suggestive of acute MI (76). Of these 35 patients, 24 had an acute MI and or a previously documented myocardial infarction. The diagnosis of acute MI was based on serial enzyme

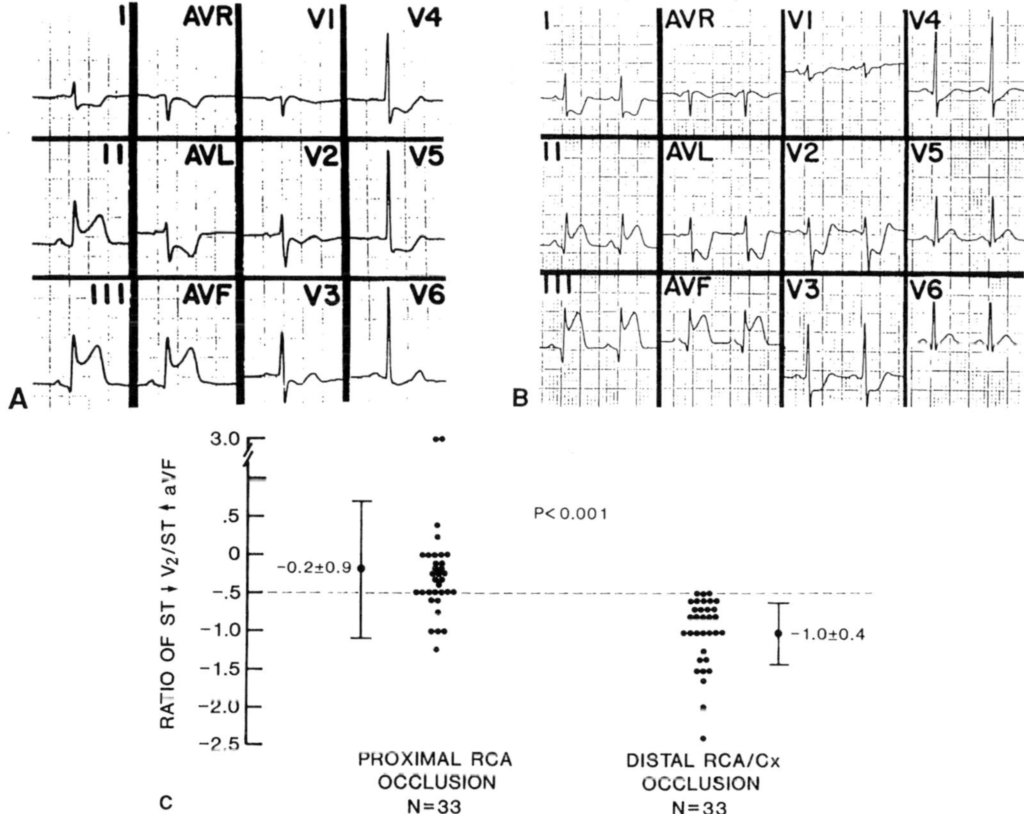

Figure 9–12 **A.** Twelve-lead ECG of a patient with proximal right coronary artery occlusion. Note that the magnitude of precordial ST depression in lead V_2 is less than 50% of the ST elevation in lead aVF, reflecting attenuation of reciprocal precordial ST depression by simultaneous right ventricular ischemia. **B.** Twelve-lead ECG of a patient with distal right coronary artery occlusion demonstrating inferior ST elevation and precordial ST depression; the magnitude of ST depression in lead V_2 is almost equal to the magnitude of ST elevation in lead aVF, reflecting unattenuated reciprocal precordial ST depression in the absence of right ventricular ischemia. **C.** Comparison of the distributions of the ratio of ST depression in lead V_2 to ST elevation in lead aVF in 33 patients with proximal right coronary artery occlusion (with right ventricular involvement) and 33 patients with distal right coronary artery occlusion or circumflex coronary artery occlusion (without right ventricular involvement). Note that a ratio of <0.5 separates the patients without right ventricular involvement from those with right ventricular involvement. *Adapted from Lew et al (56), with permission.*

elevations, whereas a prior MI was documented by prior ECG changes and cardiac enzyme elevations. The remaining 11 patients had neither an acute nor a prior MI. The sensitivity, specificity, and predictive value of these criteria are summarized in Table 9–1. As can be seen, the most useful criteria were Q waves in at least two leads (I, aVL, V_5, V_6); R wave regression from V_1 to V_4; notching of the upstroke of the S wave in at least two of leads V_3, V_4, and V_5 (Cabrera's sign); and primary ST–T wave changes in two or more adjacent leads. These criteria were highly specific (90% to 100%) but relatively insensitive (<40%) for the diagnosis of myocardial infarction. ST segment elevation of 2 mm or more concordant to the main QRS deflection or more than 7 mm discordant to the main QRS deflection has also been suggested as a useful sign of acute MI in the presence of left bundle branch block. In a report by Wackers this sign, compared with all other ECG findings, was the most sensitive (54%) and most specific (97%) sign of acute MI in the presence of left bundle branch block (77). In

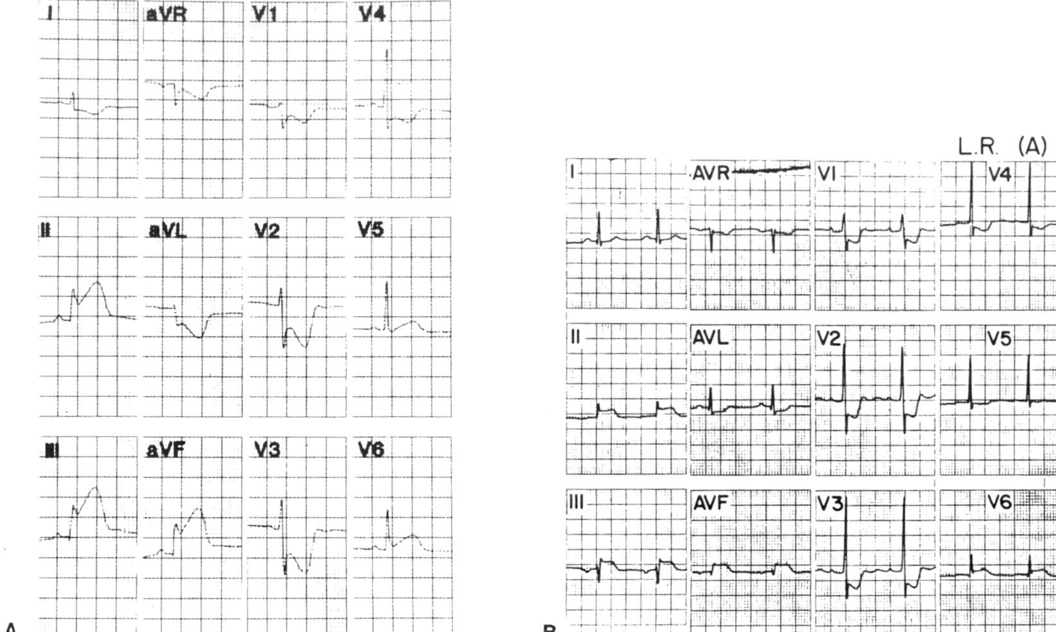

Figure 9–13 **A.** Twelve-lead ECG of a patient with acute inferior MI resulting from a right coronary artery occlusion. Note that in addition to inferior lead ST elevation, there is a slightly elevated ST in V_6 with ST depression in leads 1 and aVL. **B.** Twelve-lead ECG of a patient with acute inferior MI resulting from circumflex coronary artery occlusion. Note that the ST elevation in inferior leads and in lead V_6 is similar to that observed in the patient with right coronary artery occlusion. In contrast, however, the patient with the circumflex coronary artery occlusion has an isoelectric ST segment in lead 1. Also of note is the relatively tall R wave compared with the S wave in lead V_1 in the patient with circumflex coronary artery occlusion. *Adapted from Lew et al (41), with permission.*

the same report Wackers also noted that serial ECG changes that involved the QRS and/or the ST segments during the first 48 hours, often disappearing by 4 to 5 days, were even more reliable signs (sensitivity 67%) of acute MI in patients with left bundle branch block than any individual or combination of other specific ECG criteria examined (77). Recent data from the Gusto-I trial have provided additional information regarding the diagnosis of acute myocardial infarction in presence of left bundle branch block (Ref 72a). Of the 26,033 North American patients, 131 (0.5%) had left bundle branch block with their acute myocardial infarction. The three EKG findings with independent value in the diagnosis of acute myocardial infarction in these patients were: ≥1 mm ST segment elevation that was concordant in direction to the QRS complex, ≥1 mm ST segment depression in leads V_1, V_2, V_3, ≥5 mm ST segment elevation that was discordant in direction with QRS complex. These simple criteria may be valuable in identifying acute myocardial infarction in the setting of left bundle branch block; however, limited sensitivity of these criteria continue to warrant the policy that patients with signs and symptoms highly suggestive of acute myocardial infarction but presenting with a left bundle branch block should be considered candidates for reperfusion therapy unless specific contraindication exist.

In conclusion, the diagnosis of acute of previous MI in the presence of left bundle branch block is at best difficult if not impossible because of the poor sensitivity of the ECG criteria. The high specificity of some of the criteria suggests that at least in some

Table 9–1. Sensitivity, Specificity, and Predictive Value of ECG Criteria in Identifying Myocardial Infarction in the Presence of Left Bundle Branch Block

ECG Criteria	Sensitivity (%)	Specificity (%)	Positive Predictive Value (%)	Negative Predictive Value (%)
Q wave (≥30 ms): I, aVL, V_5, V_6[a]	20.8	100	100	36.7
Q wave (any size): I, aVL, V_5, V_6[a]	29.2	90.9	87.5	37
R wave regression: V_1–V_4	20.8	100	100	36.7
R wave regression: V_1–V_4[b]	19	100	100	37
Late-notching S wave: V_3, V_5	29.2	90.9	87.5	37
Early-notching S wave: V_3–V_5[a]	8.3	100	100	33.3
ST and T wave changes[a]	25	90.9	85.7	37.5
ST changes only[a]	16.7	90.9	80	33.3
T wave changes only[a]	29.2	72.7	70	32
ST or T wave changes[a]	33.3	72.7	72.2	33.3
Chapman's sign: I, aVL, V_5, V_6[a]	20.8	72.7	62.5	29.6
S wave: V_5, V_6 (≥40 ms)[a]	29.2	81.8	77.8	34.6
QS pattern: V_1–V_4	12.5	81.8	60	30
QS pattern: V_1–V_4	9.5	80	66.7	32.1
Q wave inferior leads (≥30 ms)[a]	8.3	100	100	33.3
Q wave inferior leads (≥30 ms)[b]	4.8	100	100	33.3
Q wave inferior leads (any size)[a]	12.5	100	100	34.4
Q wave: lead III (>30 ms)	16.7	54.6	44.4	23.1
Notching R wave inferior leads[a]	16.7	90.9	80	33.3
Notching S wave: aVF	33.3	72.7	72.7	33.3

[a] Present in two or more leads.

[b] Excluding patients with left-axis deviation.

Adapted from Hands et al (76), with permission.

patients, such a diagnosis can be made with confidence when certain ECG findings are present.

ROLE OF THE ELECTROCARDIOGRAM IN THE DIAGNOSIS OF REPERFUSION DURING THROMBOLYTIC THERAPY

Reperfusion therapy with intravenous thrombolytic agents has reemerged in the past decade as an effective means of reducing infarct size, preserving ventricular function and topography, reducing electrical instability, and reducing morbidity and mortality in patients with an acute evolving myocardial infarction (78–80). Conversely, failure of reperfusion has been shown to portend a substantial increase in morbidity and mortality (81). Since the outcome of patients who fail to reperfuse with thrombolytic therapy may be improved with additional interventions such as rescue PTCA (see Ch. 22), it becomes clinically important to recognize reperfusion or its failure at the bedside so that acute angiography and additional intervention can be applied to those who fail thrombolysis, sparing patients who have reperfused unnecessary acute invasive intervention. While urgent coronary angiography can effectively distinguish an open from a closed culprit artery, its routine application for this purpose is seriously limited because of logistic reasons, costs, invasive nature with attendant risk of periaccess complications, the snapshot nature of angiographic evaluation, and the fact that epicardial vessel patency may exist despite lack of nutritive flow at the level of downstream microcirculation (no reflow phenomenon). Therefore, several investigators have evaluated a number of noninvasive, nonangiographic markers to determine the success or failure of reperfusion, and among these techniques, electrocardiographic monitoring is most suitable for routine bedside application.

ELECTROCARDIOGRAPHIC MARKERS OF REPERFUSION

Rapid and Progressive Decrease in ST Segment Elevation

Several investigators have assessed the value of a decrease in ST segment elevation following thrombolytic therapy as a potential marker of reperfusion at the bedside (82–89) (Table 9–2). The results have been somewhat contradictory. Careful analysis has, however, shown that when ST segment trend is monitored continuously or at 5–15 minute intervals during the first 2–3 hours after initiation of thrombolytic therapy, successful reperfusion is indicated by a progressive and rapid decrease in the magnitude of ST segment elevation (by ≥50% of maximum elevated value achieved within 45–60 minutes from the onset of first noticeable decrease in ST elevation) (89). Decrease in ST segment elevation also occurs with natural evolution of acute myocardial infarction, even with a persistently occluded culprit artery; however, the decrease in ST segment elevation after reperfusion is about 5 times faster than the rate of decline associated with natural evolution of myocardial infarction (85). It is important to note that despite reperfusion, the ST segment does not fully return to isoelectric state in about 70% of patients (89). Furthermore, in about 50% of cases of successful reperfusion, the final resolution of ST segment elevation is preceded by marked transient fluctuations of ST segment elevation; these dynamic changes are not evident when ST segments are sampled at only two points in time, namely, one before and another at a fixed time after initiation of treatment (89). In addition to rapid and progressive ST segment resolution, reperfusion is also associated with rapid early inversion of T waves in the leads showing ST segment elevation (90). Failure of progressive and rapid ST segment resolution or resolution followed by reelevation is associated with a totally or nearly totally occluded culprit artery (TIMI flow grades 0 and 1). Patients with an open culprit artery but with sluggish flow (TIMI flow grade 2) frequently show no ST segment or only partial ST segment resolution, often with ongoing symptoms of ischemia.

Some investigators have reported results suggesting a limited usefulness of ST segment resolution as a marker of reperfusion (83,84). However, these apparent discrepancies can be attributed to differences in methodology and criteria used: (i) Inclusion of patients with TIMI flow grade 2 in the reperfused category. Several studies have documented that the clinical outcome of patients with TIMI grade 2 flow is virtually identical to that of patients with TIMI grade 0 flow or failed reperfusion, and therefore they should not be lumped with patients with TIMI flow grade 3 (81). (ii) Imprecise definition of ST segment resolution as improved, resolved, or unchanged without quantitative assessment. (iii) "No reflow phenomenon," wherein angiography reveals a patent vessel but physiologically there is no nutrient flow to the ischemic myocardium due to compromise of the microcirculation. Here the culprit vessel may be angiographically patent, yet signs and symptoms of ischemia (i.e., ST segment elevation) may not have improved. (iv) Inadequate frequency of ST segment sampling (comparison of one pretreatment EKG with one posttreatment EKG done at a fixed time after initiation of thrombolytic therapy), thereby missing transient pre and post therapy fluctuations in ST segments that frequently precede final ST segment resolution.

Importance of Frequent/Continuous Monitoring of ST Segments

Over the past 14 years of bedside observations conducted in several hundred patients with acute evolving myocardial infarction receiving thrombolytic therapy, we have observed several dynamic phenomena affecting the ST segment before and during the first 2–3 hours after initiation of lytic therapy:

1. Decrease in ST elevation before initiation of lytic therapy, suggesting spontaneous reperfusion (Fig. 9–14).
2. Marked worsening of ST segment elevation, and often of ischemic symptoms as well, minutes before initiation of therapy, suggesting progression of a subtotal occlusion to total occlusion (Fig. 9–15).

Table 9–2. Summary of Studies of ST Segment Analysis for the Diagnosis of Reperfusion

Study	No. of patients	Chest pain,[a] h	Catheterization time[b]	Quantitative ST segment?	No. of leads[c]	ST segment elevation[d]	ST segment criteria	Sensitivity, %	Specificity, %	Frequent ECG/Holter monitoring?	Differentiation of TIMI 2 and 3 flow?
Clemmensen et al (82)	53	6	90 min	Yes	12	J	>20% improved	88	80	NS	No
Califf et al (83)	386	6	90 min	No	2	NA	Improved/ resolved	53	76	No	No
Kircher et al (84)	56	6	90 min	No	2/12	NA	Improved	52	88	No	No
Krucoff et al (85)	46	24	Acute IC	Yes	2–3	J + 60 ms	Steady state	89	82	Yes	Yes
Richardson et al (86)	188	6	6 d	Yes	1/12	J + 20 ms	−2 mm	67	80	Yes	No
Saran et al (87)	45	4	90 min	Yes	1/12	J	>25% improved	97	43	No	No
Hogg et al (88)	45	6	90 min	Yes	1	J	> 50% improved	93	100	Yes	NS
Shah et al (89)	82	6	4–24	Yes	3–4	J	> 50% improved	100	69 (100)*	Yes	Yes

Modified from Ohman M et al: Myocardial salvage after reperfusion. J Electrocardiography 25 (suppl):23, 1992.

[a]Maximum duration of chest pain prior to treatment

[b]Time to perform cardiac catheterization after thrombolysis

[c]Quantitative ST segment measurement during thrombolysis?

[d]The point from which the ST segment elevation is measured

*If patients with reocclusion prior to coronary angiography but after initial reperfusion are excluded

NA = not applicable, NS = not specified.

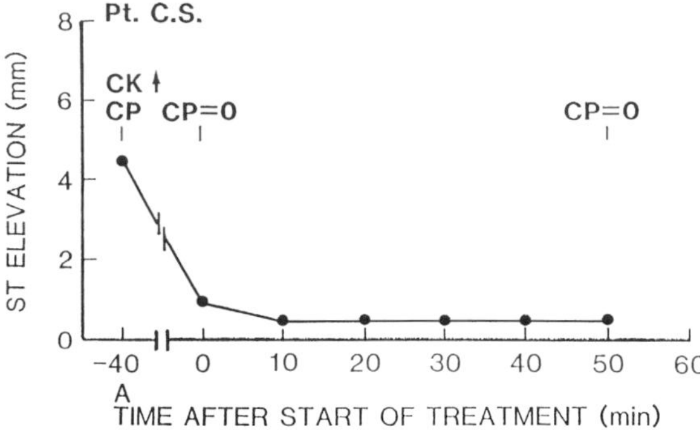

Figure 9–14. Time course of ST segment elevation in a selected patient with manifestations of spontaneous reperfusion. Between the time of admission (A) and the time at which thrombolytic therapy was initiated (time 0), both the chest pain (CP) and ST elevation improved markedly. Plasma creatine kinase (CK) and MBCK activities increased before therapy was begun. *Adapted from Shah et al (89), with permission.*

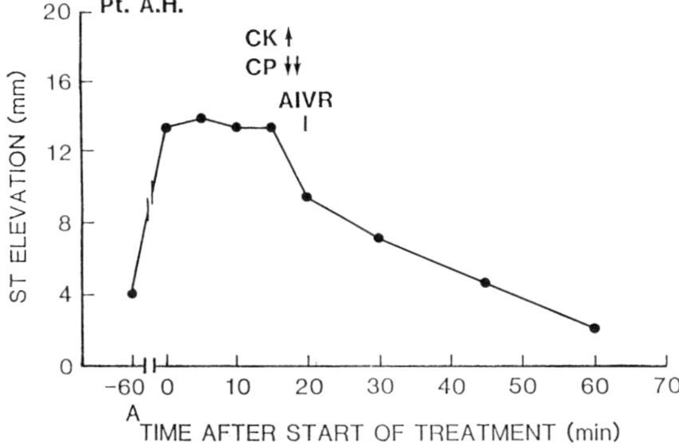

Figure 9–15. Time course of ST elevation in a selected lead of a patient who had a marked increase in ST segment elevation between the time of admission (A) and the time at which thrombolytic therapy was begun (time 0). During thrombolysis ST elevation was relatively stable for 15 minutes and then decreased rapidly and progressively along with a decrease in chest pain (CP). The marked increase in ST elevation observed between admission and before initiation of lytic therapy shows the potential for serious error when the diagnosis of reperfusion is made from only 2 EKGs (one on admission and one at a fixed time, e.g., 90 minutes, after the start of lytic therapy). AIVR = accelerated idioventricular rhythm. *Adapted from Shah et al (89), with permission.*

3. Episodes of transient decrease and then reelevation of ST segments following lytic therapy, suggesting intermittent opening and closing of culprit artery (Fig. 9–16).
4. Marked, transient, and paradoxic increase in ST elevation and chest pain followed, in minutes, by a rapid resolution of both, indicating reperfusion (ST segment paradox) (91–96) (Fig. 9–17). This paradox has been attributed to (a) progression from subtotal to total coronary occlusion, (b) transient occlusion of the microcirculation from vasospasm and/or fragmented thrombi embolizing downstream, or (c) reperfusion injury. Some studies have suggested that such an ST paradox is a marker of extensive damage and imparts an unfavorable prognosis (95,96), while others have indicated it to be a marker of favorable outcome (93).

These dynamic changes in ST segments would not be apparent with limited sampling and only become apparent with frequent or continuous monitoring of ST segments. In general, studies that have utilized continuous or frequent ST segment monitoring have demonstrated a high level of accuracy of ST segment resolution as a marker of reperfusion. If ST segments are assessed only at two fixed time points, as has been done in some studies (83,84), the maximum ST segment elevation and, therefore, a decline of 50% or more in ST segment elevation may be missed. This is well illustrated in Fig. 9–16, where despite successful reperfusion confirmed at coronary angiography, the ST segment at 90 minutes posttreatment would have been considered unchanged from the pretreatment value, leading to an erroneous conclusion that reperfusion had not occurred.

Many of the nonangiographic markers of reperfusion are based on the principle of restoration of flow with accelerated washout and termination of ischemia regardless of whether flow is antegrade or retrograde, and therefore total coronary occlusion with adequate collateral flow could produce clinical and electrocardiographic signs of reperfusion in the face of a total occluded culprit artery, thus contributing to the apparent discrepancy.

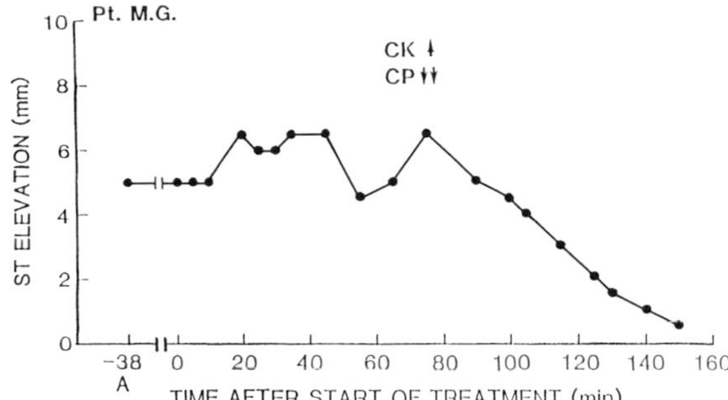

Figure 9–16. A selected lead from a patient receiving thrombolytic therapy, showing the typical fluctuations in magnitude of ST elevation that occur during therapy. Changes in chest pain (CP) paralleled changes in ST segment elevation. A = admission, CK = creatine kinase. *Adapted from Shah et al (89), with permission.*

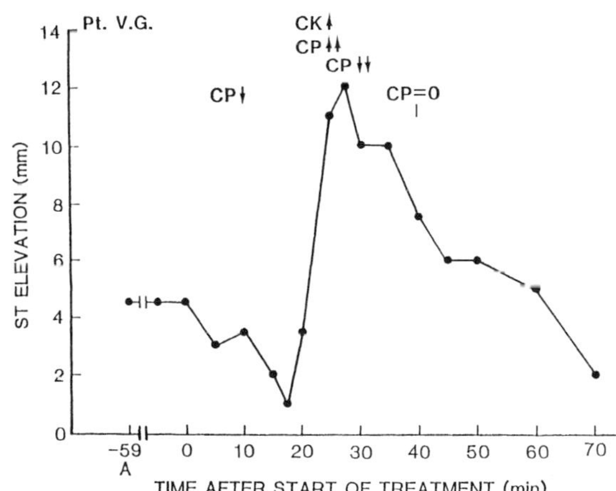

Figure 9–17. A selected lead from a patient receiving thrombolytic therapy, showing the dramatic worsening of ST segment elevation just before the onset of final rapid and progressive resolution of ST elevation (ST segment paradox). A = admission, CK = creatine kinase, CP = chest pain. *Adapted from Shah et al (89), with permission.*

Prognostic Importance of Early Resolution of ST Segment Elevation Following Thrombolytic Therapy in Acute Myocardial Infarction

Data from two large randomized trials of thrombolytic therapy have shown that early resolution of ST segment elevation is associated with a significantly lower early and long-term mortality compared with only partial or no ST segment resolution (97,98) (Tables 9–3 and 9–4). In the ISAM study, failure of resolution of ST segment was the most powerful (p = 0.0001) independent predictor of early mortality (97). These findings further underscore the additional value of ST segment monitoring in patients undergoing thrombolytic therapy.

Table 9–3. Effect of Early ST Segment Resolution Within 3 Hours of Treatment with Streptokinase on Mortality in Patients with Acute Myocardial Infarction Included in the ISAM Trial

	Magnitude of early ST segment resolution		
	>70%	<70%–>30%	<30%–0%
	(*N* = 679)	(*N* = 475)	(*N* = 362)
3-week mortality	2.2%	3.4%	8.6%

Data adapted from (97).

Table 9–4. The Effect of Early ST Segment Resolution at 4 Hours Following Treatment with Streptokinase or t-PA on Clinical Outcome in Patients with Acute Myocardial Infarction Included in the GISSI Trial

	Magnitude of ST segment resolution	
	>50%	<50%
	N = 4,951	*N* = 2,475
Composite endpoint*	16.2%	22.9%
30-day mortality	3.5%	7.4%
6-month mortality	5.7%	9.9%

(* = death, clinical heart failure, ejection fraction < 35%, injured myocardial segment > 45%, QRS score > 10).

Data adapted from (98).

REPERFUSION ARRHYTHMIAS

Accelerated Idioventricular Rhythm (AIVR)

Nonsustained or sustained ventricular tachycardia at rates of less than or equal to 120 beats per minute, also called *accelerated idioventricular rhythm (AIVR),* is a common arrhythmia in patients with acute myocardial infarction. Several studies have shown that reperfusion is accompanied by AIVR in up to 50% of patients, especially detected when continuous or frequent EKG monitoring is used (89,99). Classic AIVR has been defined as a ventricular rhythm occurring at 50 to 120 beats per minute starting after a long pause, resulting in a long coupling interval. This rhythm is usually regular and is terminated by the capture of ventricle by the sinus node. In a prospective study of 87 patients receiving intravenous or intracoronary thrombolysis for acute myocardial infarction, Gorgels et al showed that classic AIVR occurred in 50% of patients with reperfusion and in only 7% of patients without reperfusion (100). In contrast, another form of ventricular arrhythmia, *slow ventricular tachycardia,* also occurring at irregular rates of 50 to 120 beats per minute but starting with a premature ventricular beat and a short coupling interval, was not associated with reperfusion. Some of the reported discrepancy about value of AIVR as a marker of reperfusion may have resulted from lumping together of classic AIVR with slow ventricular tachycardia. In our experience, AIVR is a specific but relatively insensitive indicator of reperfusion, occurring in only in 50% of reperfused patients.

Cardioinhibitory (Bezold–Jarisch) Reflex

Several investigators have shown that sudden appearance of sinus bradycardia accompanied by hypotension can signal reperfusion of the artery supplying inferior wall of the myocardium, i.e., in most instances, the right coronary artery. This phenomenon is believed to be a type of Bezold–Jarisch reflex provoked by stimulation of cardiac baroreceptors with increased vagal input and withdrawal of sympathetic tone (101). This phenomenon is observed in 23–65% of cases of right coronary artery reperfusion, thus providing corroborative evidence of reperfusion (89,102). The transient bradycardia and hypotension can lead to sudden and precipitous clinical and hemodynamic deterioration, but the changes tend to be transient and respond to trendenlenberg position and atropine. In rare instances, a malignant form of this syndrome may be resistant to therapy, leading to a fatal outcome.

Signal-Averaged Electrocardiography (SAECG) for Detection of Late Potential

Signal-averaged EKG has been used to detect late potentials as markers of increased vulnerability for inducible and spontaneous ventricular arrhythmias following acute myocardial infarction. Several studies have demonstrated that in patients with acute myocardial infarction a patent infarct-related artery is associated with a reduced frequency of positive late potentials compared with patients with persistent occlusion (103,104). Tranchesi et al (105) have recently examined the significance of late potentials in a SAECG as a marker of reperfusion. In 54 patients with acute myocardial infarction and an angiographically documented occlusion, a baseline SAECG was recorded before initiation of thrombolysis. A coronary angiogram and SAECG were recorded again 90 minutes after r-tPA infusion. In 50% of the patients with successful reperfusion the late potentials disappeared after reperfusion (from 16/35 to 8/35; $p = 0.03$), whereas in patients with a closed artery there was no change in the prevalence of positive late potentials (8/19 before to 7/19 after attempted but failed thrombolysis). These preliminary findings, while interesting, demonstrate the limited accuracy of late potentials and their changes following lytic therapy for the bedside diagnosis of reperfusion.

Online Vectorcardiography

Recently, continuous vectorcardiography has been used to assess changes in the QRS and ST segment vector as a marker of reperfusion (106). The QRS vector difference can be described as the total change within the QRS complex, and the ST vector magnitude is the deviation of ST segment 20 msec after the termination of QRS complex, measured and added in X,Y,Z vectorcardiographic leads (X,Y,Z). Dellborg et al (106) used a computerized system for online dynamic analysis of QRS complex and ST segment changes in 21 patients presenting with acute myocardial infarction. All of these patients had interventions attempting reperfusion either by thrombolysis or angioplasty. Based on a previous study, prospectively defined criteria were used to predict reperfusion. Reperfusion defined by TIMI grade 2 or 3 flow was tentatively identified by an increase of the QRS vector difference by ≥0.1 uV/min from start of vectorcardiographic monitoring or a decrease in ST vector magnitude >0.83 uV/min. Subjective blinded evaluation of the QRS vector trend curve was also done in addition to the prospectively determined parameters, the rapid pattern being suggestive of reperfusion. Prospectively determined criteria for QRS vector difference correctly classified 15 of 16 patients with a patent vessel and 2 of the 5 patients with a persistently occluded vessel at coronary angiography. On the other hand, the ST vector magnitude change was not very sensitive and missed the diagnosis of reperfusion in 30% of patients. While this technique appears promising based on preliminary results, the full potential of this approach needs to be defined in larger series of patients.

In conclusion, bedside recognition of reperfusion in patients presenting with acute myocardial infarction associated with ST segment elevation can be best accomplished at the present time by assessment of objective signs of termination of ischemia (i.e., rapid decrease in ST segment elevation). Since ST segments may dramatically fluctuate before and during thrombolytic therapy, an accurate determination of progressive decrease (by 50%) relative to the highest ST segment elevation requires frequent (every 5–15 minutes) or continuous monitoring of ST segments (either a selected lead or all 12 leads). Although other bedside signs such as AIVR and Bezold–Jarisch reflex also indicate reperfusion, their limited sensitivity restricts their usefulness. Biochemical markers, related to accelerated washout associated with reperfusion, while promising, are still limited in their usefulness because the results are difficult to obtain in a timely fashion. Acute coronary angiography, while useful, is neither practical nor may it turn out to be the gold standard for reperfusion. Since the goal of reperfusion is to achieve termination of ongoing ischemia, noninvasive markers of ischemia termination may be a better standard than the anatomic evidence obtained on coronary angiography. The favorable prognostic impact of early ST segment resolution in the ISAM and GISSI-2 trials supports the clinical relevance and importance of signs of ischemia termination.

REFERENCES

1. Chaitman BR, Waters DD, Corbara F, Bourassa MG: Prediction of multivessel disease after inferior myocardial infarction. *Circulation* 1978;57:1085–1090.
2. Shah PK, Pichler M, Berman DS, et al: Noninvasive identification of a high risk subset of patients with acute inferior myocardial infarction. *Am J Cardiol* 1980;46:915–921.
3. Salcedo JR, Baird MG, Chambers R, Beanlands DS: Significance of reciprocal ST segment depression in anterior precordial leads in acute inferior myocardial infarction: Concomitant left anterior descending coronary artery disease? *Am J Cardiol* 1981;48: 1003–1008.
4. Gibson RS, Crampton RS, Watson DD, et al: Precordial ST-segment depression during acute inferior myocardial infarction: Clinical, scintigraphic and angiographic correlations. *Circulation* 1982;66: 732–741.
5. Croft CH, Woodward W, Nicod P, et al: Clinical implications of anterior ST segment depression in patients with acute inferior myocardial infarction. *Am J Cardiol* 1982;50:428–436.
6. Gelman JS, Saltups A: Precordial ST segment depression in patients with inferior myocardial infarction: Clinical implications. *Br Heart J* 1982;48: 560–565.
7. Haraphongse M, Jugdutt BL, Rossall RE: Significance of precordial ST-segment depression in acute transmural inferior infarction: Coronary angiographic findings. *Cathet Cardiovasc Diagn* 1983;9: 143–151.

8. Jenning SK, Reid DS, Julian DG: "Reciprocal" depression of the ST segment in acute myocardial infarction. *Br Med J* 1983;287:634–637.
9. Roubin GS, Shen WF, Nicholson M, et al: Anterolateral ST segment depression in acute inferior myocardial infarction: Angiographic and clinical implications. *Am Heart J* 1984;107: 1177–1182.
10. Cohen M, Blanke H, Karsh KR, et al: Implications of precordial ST segment depression during acute inferior myocardial infarction. Arteriographic and ventriculographic correlations during the acute phase. *Br Heart J* 1984;52:497–501.
11. Tendera M, Campbell WB: Significance of early and later anterior precordial ST segment depression in inferior myocardial infarction. *Am J Cardiol* 1984;54:994–996.
12. Little WC, Rogers EW, Sodums MT: Mechanism of anterior ST segment depression during acute inferior myocardial infarction. *Ann Intern Med* 1984;100:226–229.
13. Lew AS, Weiss AT, Shah PK, et al: Precordial ST segment depression during acute inferior myocardial infarction: Early thallium-201 scintigraphic evidence of adjacent posterolateral or inferoseptal involvement. *J Am Coll Cardiol* 1985;5: 203–209.
14. Berland J, Cribier A, Behar P, Letac B: Anterior ST depression in inferior myocardial infarction: Correlation with results of intracoronary thrombolysis. *Am Heart J* 1986;111:481–488.
15. Kouvras G, Spyropoulou M, Bacoulas G: The significance of persistent precordial ST segment >0.1 mV depression in acute inferior myocardial infarction. *Angiology* 1986;37:57–62.
16. Wasserman AG, Ross AM, Bogaty D, et al: Anterior ST segment depression during acute inferior myocardial infarction: Evidence for the reciprocal change theory. *Am Heart J* 1983;106:516–520.
17. Brymer JF, Khaja F, Marzilli M, Goldstein S: "Ischemia at a distance" during intermittent coronary artery occlusion: A coronary anatomic explanation. *J Am Coll Cardiol* 1985;6:41–45.
18. Ruddy TD, Yasuda T, Gold HK, et al: Anterior ST segment depression in acute inferior myocardial infarction as a marker of greater inferior, apical, and posterolateral damage. *Am Heart J* 1986;112: 1210–1216.
19. Ong L, Valdellon B, Coromilas J, et al: Precordial ST segment depression in inferior myocardial infarction. Evaluation by quantitative thallium-201 scintigraphy and technetium-99m ventriculography. *Am J Cardiol* 1983;51:734–739.
20. Goldberg HL, Borer JS, Jacobstein JG, et al: Anterior ST segment depression in acute inferior myocardial infarction: Indicator of posterolateral infarction. *Am J Cardiol* 1981;48:1009–1015.
21. Billadello JJ, Smith JL, Ludbrook PA, et al: Implications of "reciprocal" ST segment depression associated with acute myocardial infarction identified by positron tomography. *J Am Coll Cardiol* 1983;2: 616–624.
22. Ferguson DW, Pandian N, Kroschos M, et al: Angiographic evidence that reciprocal ST-segment depression during acute myocardial infarction does not indicate remote ischemia: Analysis of 23 patients. *Am J Cardiol* 1984;53:55–62.
22a. Peterson ED, Hathaway WR, Zabel KM, Pieper KS et al: Prognostic significance of precordial ST segment depression during inferior myocardial infarction in the thrombolytic era: results in 16,521 patients. *J of Am Coll Cardiol* 1996;28:305–312.
23. Ruddy TD, Yasuda T, Gold HK, et al: Correlations of regional wall motion and myocardial perfusion in patients with and without anterior precordial ST segment depression during acute inferior myocardial infarction. *Am J Noninv Cardiol* 1987;1:81–87.
24. Rutledge JC, Amsterdam EA, Bogren H, Arons D: Anterior ST segment depression associated with acute inferior myocardial infarction: Clinical, hemodynamic and angiographic correlates. *Am J Noninv Cardiol* 1987;1:290–295.
25. Camara EJN, Chandra N, Ouyang P, et al: Reciprocal ST change in acute myocardial infarction: Assessment by electrocardiography and echocardiography. *J Am Coll Cardiol* 1983;2: 251–257.
26. Boden WE, Bough EW, Korr KS, et al: Inferoseptal myocardial infarction: Another cause of precordial ST-segment depression in transmural inferior wall myocardial infarction? *Am J Cardiol* 1984;54: 1216–1223.
27. Mukharji J, Murray S, Lewis SE, et al: Is anterior ST depression with acute transmural inferior infarction due to posterior infarction? *J Am Coll Cardiol* 1984;4:28–34.
28. Pichler M, Shah PK, Peter T, et al: Wall motion abnormalities and electrocardiographic changes in acute transmural myocardial infarction: Implica-

tions of reciprocal ST segment depression. *Am Heart J* 1983;106:1003–1009.

29. Hlatky MA, Califf RM, Lee KL, et al: Prognostic significance of precordial ST segment depression during inferior acute myocardial infarction. *Am J Cardiol* 1985;55:325–329.

30. Akhras F, Upward J, Jackson G: Reciprocal change in ST segment in acute myocardial infarction: Correlation with findings on exercise electrocardiography and coronary angiography. *Br Med J* 1985;290: 1931–1934.

31. Hasdai D, Sclarovsky S, Solodky A, Sulkes J, Strasberg B, Birnbaum Y: Prognostic significance of maximal precordial ST-segment depression in right (V_1 to V_3) versus left (V_4 to V_6) leads in patients with inferior wall acute myocardial infarction. *Am J Cardiol* 1994;74:1081–1084.

31a. Birnbaum Y, Herz I, Selarovsky S et al: Prognostic significance of precordial ST segment depression on admission electrocardiogram in patients with inferior myocardial infarction. *J of Am Coll Cardiol* 1996;28:313–318.

32. Katz R, Conroy RM, Robinson K, Mulcahy R: The etiology and prognostic implications of reciprocal electrocardiographic changes in acute myocardial infarction. *Br Heart J* 1986;55:423–427.

33. Gibson RS, Taylor GJ, Watson DD, et al: Prognostic significance of resting anterior thallium-201 defects in patients with inferior myocardial infarction. *J Nucl Med* 1980;231:1015–1021.

34. Boden WE, Kleiger RE, Gibson RS, et al: Electrocardiographic evolution of posterior acute myocardial infarction: Importance of early precordial ST segment depression. *Am J Cardiol* 1987;59: 782–787.

35. Putini RL, Natale E, Ricci R, et al: Dipyridamole echocardiography evaluation of acute inferior myocardial infarction with concomitant anterior ST segment depression. *Eur Heart J* 1993;14: 1328–1333.

36. Wong CK, Freedman SB, Gautovich G, Bailey BP, Bernstein L, Kelly DT: Mechanism and significance of precordial ST-segment depression during inferior wall acute myocardial infarction associated with severe narrowing of the dominant right coronary artery. *Am J Cardiol* 1993;71: 1025–1030.

37. Chou T, Van der Bel-Kahn J, Allen J, et al: Electrocardiographic diagnosis of right ventricular infarction. *Am J Med* 1981;70:1175–1180.

38. Geft IL, Shah PK, Rodriguez L, et al: ST elevations in leads V_1 to V_5 may be caused by right coronary artery occlusion and acute right ventricular infarction. *Am J Cardiol* 1984;53:991–996.

39. Lew AS, Maddahi J, Shah PK, et al: Factors that determine the direction and magnitude of precordial ST segment deviations during inferior wall acute myocardial infarction. *Am J Cardiol* 1985;55: 893–898.

40. Quyyumi AA, Rubens MB, Richards AF, et al: Importance of "reciprocal" electrocardiographic changes during occlusion of left anterior descending coronary artery. *Lancet* 1986;1:347–350.

41. Lew AS, Hod H, Cercek B, et al: Inferior lead ST segment changes during acute anterior myocardial infarction: A marker of the presence or absence of concomitant inferior wall ischemia. *J Am Coll Cardiol* 1987;10:519–526.

42. Haraphongse M, Tanornsup S, Jugdutt BI: Inferior ST segment depression during acute anterior myocardial infarction: Clinical and angiographic correlations. *J Am Coll Cardiol* 1984;4:467.

43. Meyers GB, Klein HA, Hiratzka T: Correlation of electrocardiographic and pathologic findings in an anteroposterior infarction. *Am Heart J* 1949;37: 205–236.

44. Crawford MH, O'Rourke RA, Grover GL: Mechanism of inferior electrocardiographic ST segment depression during acute anterior myocardial infarction in a baboon model. *Am J Cardiol* 1984;54: 1114–1117.

45. Fletcher WO, Gibbons RJ, Clements IP: The relationship of inferior ST depression, lateral ST elevation, and left precordial ST elevation to myocardium at risk in acute anterior myocardial infarction. *Am Heart J* 1993;126:526–535.

46. Mirvis DM: Physiologic bases for anterior ST segment depression in patients with acute inferior wall myocardial infarction. *Am Heart J* 1988;116: 1308.

47. Mirvis DM, Keller FW, Ideker RE, et al: Equivalent generator properties of acute ischemic lesions in the isolated rabbit heart. *Circ Res* 1978;42: 676–685.

48. Mirvis DM: Body surface distributions of repolarization potentials after acute myocardial infarction: I. Isopotential and isoarea mapping. *Circulation* 1980;62:878–887.

49. Mirvis DM: Body surface distributions of repolarization potentials after acute myocardial infarction:

II. Relationship between isopotential mapping and ST segment potential summation methods. *Circulation* 1981;63:623–631.

50. Longhead MG, Walker SJ, Lavercombe PS, et al: Prognosis of anterior ST depression in inferior infarction determined by body surface mapping. *Circulation* 1986;74(Suppl II):II–273.
51. Cohn JN, Guiha NH, Broder MI, et al: Right ventricular infarction: Clinical and hemodynamic features. *Am J Cardiol* 1974;33:209–214.
52. Shah PK, Maddahi J, Berman DS, et al: Scintigraphically detected predominant right ventricular dysfunction in acute myocardial infarction: Clinical and hemodynamic correlates and implications for therapy and prognosis. *J Am Coll Cardiol* 1986;6: 1264–1272.
53. Shah PK, Maddahi J, Staniloff H, et al: Variable spectrum and prognostic implications of left and right ventricular ejection fractions in patients with and without clinical heart failure after acute myocardial infarction. *Am J Cardiol* 1986;58:387–393.
54. Erhardt LR, Sjogren A, Wahlberg I: Single right sided precordial lead in the diagnosis of right ventricular involvement in inferior myocardial infarction. *Am Heart J* 1976;91:571–576.
55. Croft CH, Nicod P, Corbett JR, et al: Detection of acute right ventricular infarction by right precordial electrocardiography. *Am J Cardiol* 1982;50: 421–427.
56. Lew AS, Laramee P, Shah PK, et al: Ratio of ST segment depression in V_2 to ST segment elevation in a V_F: An aid to early diagnosis of concomitant right ventricular involvement during inferior myocardial infarction. *Am J Cardiol* 1986;57:1047–1051.
57. Klein HO, Tordijman T, Ninio R, et al: The early recognition of right ventricular infarction: Diagnostic accuracy of the electrocardiographic V_{4R} lead. *Circulation* 1983;67:558–565.
58. Braat SH, Brugada P, DeZwann C, et al: Value of electrocardiogram in diagnosing right ventricular involvement in patients with acute inferior wall myocardial infarction. *Br Heart J* 1983;49: 368–371.
59. Lopez-Sendon J, Coma-Canella I, Alcasena S, et al: Electrocardiographic findings in acute right ventricular infarction: Sensitivity and specificity of electrocardiographic alterations in right precordial leads V_{4R}, V_{3R}, V_1 and V_3. *J Am Coll Cardiol* 1985;6: 1273–1279.
60. Braat SH, Brugada P, den Dulk K, et al: Value of lead V_{4R} for recognition of the infarct coronary artery in acute inferior myocardial infarction. *Am J Cardiol* 1985;53:1538–1541.
61. Huey BL, Beller GA, Kaiser DL, Gibson RS: A comprehensive analysis of myocardial infarction due to left circumflex artery occlusion: Comparison with infarction due to right coronary artery and left anterior descending artery occlusion. *J Am Coll Cardiol* 1988;12:1156.
62. Bairey CN, Shah PK, Lew AS, et al: Electrocardiographic differentiation of occlusion of the left circumflex vs. right coronary arteries as a cause of inferior acute myocardial infarction. *Am J Cardiol* 1987;60:456–459.
63. Kataoka H, Tamura A, Mikuriya Y: Central precordial reciprocal ST-segment elevation in posterolateral myocardial infarction. *Am Heart J* 1993; 125:1202–1204.
64. Dressler W, Roesler H, Schwager A: The electrocardiographic signs of myocardial infarction in the presence of bundle branch block. *Am Heart J* 1950;39:217–242.
65. Bersoain-Santander M, Gomez-Ebensperguer G: Electrocardiographic diagnosis of myocardial infarction in cases of complete left bundle branch block. *Am Heart J* 1960;60:886–897.
66. Wackers FJ: Complete left bundle branch block: Is the diagnosis of myocardial infarction possible? *Int J Cardiol* 1983;2:521–529.
67. Doucet P, Walsh TJ, Massie E: A vectorcardiographic and electrocardiographic study of left bundle branch block. *Am J Cardiol* 1966;17: 171–179.
68. Rhoads DV, Edwards JE, Pruitt RD: The electrocardiogram in the presence of myocardial infarction and intraventricular block of the left bundle-branch type. *Am Heart J* 1961;62:735–745.
69. Haveldo C, Sohi GS, Flowers NC, Horan LG: The pathological correlates of the electrocardiogram: Complete left bundle branch block. *Circulation* 1982;65:445–451.
70. Chapman MG, Pearce ML: Electrocardiographic diagnosis of myocardial infarction in the presence of left bundle branch block. *Circulation* 1957;16: 558–571.
71. Horan LG, Flowers NC, Tollesson WJ, Thomas JR: The significance of diagnostic Q waves in the presence of bundle branch block. *Chest* 1970;58: 214–220.
72. Luy G, Bahl OP, Massie E: Intermittent left bundle branch block. A study of the effects of left bundle

branch block on the electrocardiographic patterns of myocardial infarction and ischemia. *Am Heart J* 1973;85:332–340.

72a. Sgarbossa EB, Pinski SL, Barbegelata A, Underwood DA, Gates KB, Topol EJ, Califf RM, Wagner GS: Electrocardiographic diagnosis of evolving acute myocardial infarction in the presence of left bundle branch block: GUSTO-1 Investigators. New England J of Med: 1996; 334(*): 381–487.

73. Rodriguez MI, Anselmi A, Sodi-Pallares D: The electrocardiographic diagnosis of septal infarctions. *Am Heart J* 1953;43:525–544.

74. Pantridge JF: Observations on the electrocardiogram and ventricular gradient in complete left bundle branch block. *Circulation* 1951;3: 589–599.

75. Wasserburger RH, White DH, Lindsay ER: Noninfraction QS complexes in leads 2, 3, and aVF as seen in the WPW syndrome and LBBB. *Am Heart J* 1962;64:617–624.

76. Hands ME, Cook F, Stone PH, et al: Electrocardiographic diagnosis of myocardial infarction in the presence of complete left bundle branch block. *Am Heart J* 1988;116:23–31.

77. Wackers FJT: The diagnosis of myocardial infarction in the presence of left bundle branch block. *Cardiol Clin* 1987;5:393 401.

78. Gruppo Italiano per lo Studio della Sopravvivenza nell'Infarto Miocardico: GISSI-2: A factorial randomised trial of alteplase versus streptokinase and heparin versus no heparin among 12 490 patients with acute myocardial infarction. *Lancet* 1990;336: 65–71.

79. ISIS-3 (Third International Study of Infarct Survival) Collaborative Group: ISIS-3: A randomised comparison of streptokinase vs antistreplase and of aspirin plus heparin vs aspirin alone among 41 299 cases of suspected acute myocardial infarction. *Lancet* 1993;339:753–770.

80. The GUSTO Investigators: An international randomized trial comparing four thrombolytic strategies for acute myocardial infarction. *N Engl J Med* 1993;329:673–682.

81. The GUSTO Investigators: The effects of tissue plasminogen activator, streptokinase, or both on coronary-artery patency, ventricular function and survival after acute myocardial infarction. *N Engl J Med* 1993;329(22):1615–1622.

82. Clemmensen P, Ohman EM, Sevilla DC, et al: Changes in standard electrocardiographic ST segment elevation predictive of successful reperfusion in acute myocardial infarction. *Am J Cardiol* 1990; 66:1407.

83. Califf RM, O'Neil, Stack RS, et al: Failure of simple clinical measurements to predict perfusion status after intravenous thrombolysis. *Ann Intern Med* 1988;108:658.

84. Kircher BJ, Topol EJ, O'Neil WW, et al: Prediction of infarct coronary artery recanalization after intravenous thrombolytic therapy. *Am J Cardiol* 1987;59:513.

85. Krucoff MW, Green CE, Satler LF, et al: Non invasive detection of coronary artery patency using continuous ST segment monitoring. *Am J Cardiol* 1986;57:916.

86. Richardson SG, Morton P, Murtagh JG, et al: Relation of coronary arterial patency and left ventricular function to electrocardiographic changes after streptokinase treatment during acute myocardial infarction. 1988;61:961.

87. Saran RK, Been M, Furniss SS, et al: Reduction in ST segment elevation after thrombolysis predicts either coronary reperfusion or preservation of left ventricular function. *Br Heart J* 1990; 64:113.

88. Hogg KJ, Hornung RS, Howie CA, et al: Electrocardiographic prediction of coronary artery patency after thrombolytic treatment in acute myocardial infarction: Use of ST segment as a noninvasive marker. *Br Heart J* 1988;60:275.

89. Shah PK, Cercek B, Lew A, et al: Angiographic validation of bedside markers of reperfusion. *J Am Coll Cardiol* 1993;21:55–61.

90. Matezky S, Barabash GI, Shahar A, et al: Early T wave inversion after thrombolytic therapy predicts better coronary perfusion: Clinical and angiographic study. *J Am Coll Cardiol* 1994;24: 378–383.

91. Sato H, Kodama K, Masuyama T, Nanto S, Komamura K, Inoue M: Acute electrocardiographic changes associated with successful coronary thrombolysis in acute myocardial infarction. *Jpn Circ J* 1987;51:265–274.

92. Shah PK, Cercek B, Ganz W: Marked transient ST segment elevation during thrombolytic therapy: A marker of impending reperfusion. *Circulation* 1992; 86(Suppl 1):I-268.

93. Shechter M, Rabinowitz B, Beker B, et al: Additional ST segment elevation during the first hour of thrombolytic therapy: An electrocardiographic sign

predicting favorable clinical outcome. *J Am Coll Cardiol* 1992;20:1460–1464.

94. Kondo M, Tamura K, Tanio H, Shimono Y: Is ST-segment re-elevation associated with reperfusion an indicator of marked myocardial damage after thrombolysis? *J Am Coll Cardiol* 1993;21: 62–67.

95. Dissmann R, Linderer T, Goerke M, von Ameln H, Rennhak U, Schroder R: Sudden increase of the ST segment elevation at time of reperfusion predicts extensive infarcts in patients with intravenous thrombolysis. *Am Heart J* 1993;126: 832–839.

96. Milida T, Oda H, Toeda T, Higuma N: Additional ST-segment elevation immediately after reperfusion and its effect on myocardial salvage in anterior wall acute myocardial infarction. *Am J Cardiol* 1994;73:851–855.

97. Shroder R, Dissmann R, Bruggemann T, et al: Extent of early ST segment elevation resolution: A simple but strong predictor of outcome in patients with acute myocardial infarction. *J Am Coll Cardiol* 1994;24:384–391.

98. Mauri F, Maggioni AP, Franzosi MG, et al: A simple electrocardiographic predictor of the outcome of patients with acute myocardial infarction treated with a thrombolytic agent. *J Am Coll Cardiol* 1994;24:600–607.

99. Cercek B, Lew A, Laramee P, et al: Time course and characteristics of ventricular arrhythmias after reperfusion in acute myocardial infarction. *Am J Cardiol* 1987;60:214–218.

100. Gorgels APM, Vos MA, Letsch IS, et al: Usefulness of accelerated idioventricular rhythm as a marker for myocardial necrosis and reperfusion during thrombolytic therapy in acute myocardial infarction. *Am J Cardiol* 1988;61:231–235.

101. Wei JY, Markis JE, Malagold M, et al: Cardiovascular reflexes stimulated by reperfusion of ischemic myocardium in acute myocardial infarction. *Circulation* 1983;67:796–801.

102. Esente P, Giambartolomei A, Gensini G, et al: Coronary reperfusion and Bezold–Jarisch reflex (bradycardia and hypotension). *Am J Cardiol* 1983; 52:221–224.

103. Hong M, Peter T, Peters W, et al: Relation between acute ventricular arrhythmias, ventricular late potentials and mortality in acute myocardial infarction. *Am J Cardiol* 68:1403–1409.

104. Vatterot PJ, Hammill SC, Bailey KR, et al: Late potentials on signal averaged electrocardiograms and patency of infarct related artery in survivors of acute myocardial infarction. *J Am Coll Cardiol* 1991;17:330–337.

105. Trachesi B, Verstrate M, Van de Werf F, et al: The assessment of coronary reperfusion through the analysis of signal averaged surface electrocardiograms before and after coronary thrombolysis. *Circulation* 1990;82(4, Suppl III):III–254.

106. Delborg M, Topol E, Swedberg K: Dynamic QRS complex and ST segment vectorcardiographic monitoring can identify vessel patency in patients with acute myocardial infarction treated with reperfusion therapy. *Am Heart J* 122:943–948.

10

Echocardiography in Acute Myocardial Infarction

Jae K. Oh, MD, and Rick A. Nishimura, MD

The role of echocardiography in acute myocardial infarction has evolved as the management strategy of acute myocardial infarction has changed (1–6). Two-dimensional echocardiography visualizes the entire left and right ventricular myocardium in multiple tomographic planes, allowing assessment of global and regional myocardial function (7). This provides information about diagnosis and prognosis and may aid in the decision about acute intervention (2,4). In the critically ill patient, two-dimensional echocardiography has proven invaluable in determining the cause of hemodynamic compromise, be it left ventricular dysfunction or the mechanical complications of myocardial infarction. Doppler echocardiography with color flow imaging heightens the sensitivity of detecting these mechanical complications, especially if used in conjunction with transesophageal echocardiography (6,8,9). In addition, the ability of Doppler echocardiography for noninvasive assessment of blood flow velocities within cardiac chambers, across valves, and in great vessels allows the determination of hemodynamic variables, such as cardiac output, diastolic filling pattern, left ventricular filling pressure, and pulmonary artery pressures. (10,11)

Its current clinical role can be classified into the following areas: (i) diagnosis and exclusion of acute myocardial infarction in patients with prolonged chest pain and nondiagnostic electrocardiogram, (ii) estimation of the myocardium at risk and final infarct size, (iii) monitoring of acute reperfusion therapy (thrombolysis and/or angioplasty), (iv) detection of infarct complications, (v) evaluation of myocardial viability, and (vi) determination of prognosis. Therefore, at the various clinical stages of acute myocardial infarction, echocardiography plays an important role by providing anatomical, functional, and hemodynamic information.

The technological advances in echocardiographic equipment over the past decade have resulted in high-resolution images and smaller portable machines, which can easily be moved to a patient's bedside. Information necessary for clinical decision making is immediately available, and the noninvasive nature of the examination allows repeated examinations. Echocardiography is widely available throughout all centers that practice acute care medicine, and there is little overhead once the equipment has been purchased.

There is information contained in echocardiographic images that has not yet been fully explored and may provide valuable data in the future. Areas of investigation include computerized analysis of wall motion, myocardial perfusion imaging using contrast echocardiography, tissue characterization, and intra-arterial visualization of plaque severity and structure.

WALL MOTION ANALYSIS

The diagnosis of myocardial ischemia and/or infarction by echocardiography is based on the detection of decreased or absent myocardial wall thickening. In 1935 Tennant and Wiggers (12) first described an immediate cessation of myocardial thickening after the ligation of a coronary artery in a canine model. Analysis of LV wall thickening has subsequently been shown to be an early sensitive marker of myocardial ischemia (13). This was initially described by M-mode echocardiography, which could detect thickening of the myocardium directly (14–16), but provided only a one-dimensional "ice pick" view of the myocardium. Two-dimensional echocardiography overcame this limitation by providing the ability to examine the entire myocardium utilizing multiple tomographic planes (7). In the canine model, significant changes occur on two-dimensional echocardiographic imaging within minutes of acute occlusion of coronary arteries (17–20). These consist of a decrease in wall thickening or the affected area of myocardium that soon evolves to dyskinesis. Hypokinesis is present in the adjacent segments (21). These changes begin 15 to 20 seconds after the occlusion and are maximal 10 to 20 minutes after the onset of occlusion. Similar results have been found in humans for the affected region of myocardium during the transient ischemia of balloon inflation with percutaneous transluminal coronary angiography (22).

It should be, however, emphasized that the left ventricular myocardium becomes akinetic when 20% to 25% of the transmural wall thickness is involved with myocardial ischemia or infarction. This was termed as a "threshold phenomenon" by Lieberman et al. (19), indicating that transmural myocardial infarction cannot be differentiated readily from nontransmural myocardial infarction involving more than the threshold of 20% to 25% of the LV wall thickness. This concept becomes important in the understanding of myocardial viability, infarct expansion, and LV volume measurement as the most important prognostic indicators after myocardial infarction.

Multiple studies have been done in the presence of myocardial infarction in humans, correlating the site of wall motion abnormality on two-dimensional echocardiography with electrocardiograms and pathologic specimens (23–26). The extent of the wall motion abnormality seen on two-dimensional echocardiography, however, frequently overestimates the true extent of the area of infarction, both in the experimental mode (20,21) and in humans (27). This discrepancy may be the result of several factors. A hypothesis by Wyatt et al. (28) suggested that infarcted muscle fibers may act as a parallel mechanical resistor and impede contraction in adjacent, normally perfused segments (the "parallel fiber hypothesis"). Ischemia of the border zone may cause a wall motion abnormality in the absence of true infarction (21). The recently proposed concept of "stunned myocardium" may also contribute to the overestimation of infarct size by two-dimensional echocardiography (29,30) because recovery of wall motion abnormalities may take days to months after successful reperfusion. "Ischemia at a distance" may also lead to overestimation of the extent of infarction in that areas of myocardium remote from the infarct develop wall motion abnormalities as a result of (i) interruption of collateral channels by occlusion of the feeding vessels or (ii) increase in oxygen demand in noninfarcted myocardium perfused by a second critically narrowed vessel (31). Despite these caveats, two-dimensional echocardiography has emerged as a standard noninvasive method for the detection and determination of the extent of wall motion abnormalities in patients with acute coronary syndromes.

The most commonly used method of wall motion analysis by two-dimensional echocardiography is a qualitative one that uses a subjective visual interpretation of wall motion. The presence of a wall motion abnormality, as well as its extent and severity, is readily detected by an experienced echocardiographer. Many factors are involved in this interpretation. As with other imaging modalities used to assess regional wall motion, such as radionuclide angiography and cineangiography, endocardial motion is an important factor in determining the presence or absence of wall motion abnormalities.

Two-dimensional echocardiography provides the additional information of true wall thickening in addition to endocardial motion. The visual assessment also incorporates the effect of translation and rotation of the heart, as the heart will move its center of mass during a systolic contraction as well as rotate around its long axis, so that spatial displacement of the entire heart is present throughout the cardiac cycle. In addition, there is both spatial and temporal heterogeneity of contraction. Even in normal hearts, all parts of the myocardium do not demonstrate equal contraction (32). There is less vigorous contraction at the base compared with the apex, and the posterior wall contracts more vigorously than the other walls. Temporal heterogeneity refers to the concept that there is variability in the temporal sequence of myocardial contraction so that different areas of the myocardium will contract and relax at different times (33,34). All of these concepts are taken into consideration when analyzing the myocardium for wall motion abnormalities. Despite the complexity of factors contributing to interpretation of wall motion abnormalities, the visual assessment by two-dimensional echocardiography has become a well-established technique for wall motion analysis. It compares favorably with other modalities, such as cineangiography (35–37) and radionuclide angiography (38,39) for assessing regional wall motion. The limitation of two-dimensional echocardiography is in the ability to visualize all segments of the myocardium because of poor ultrasound penetration in certain patients, for example, those with chronic obstructive pulmonary disease, obesity, or chest deformities. Prospective studies have, however, shown that more than 90% of all segments of the myocardium are adequately seen in patients with coronary artery disease (40,41).

The visual assessment of wall motion is qualitative, describing the presence or absence of wall motion and its location. To provide a semiquantitative measure of the extent of myocardium involved by abnormally contracting myocardium, a wall motion score index has evolved (37,38,42–44). The entire left ventricular myocardium is divided into several segments. The exact number and location of the segments vary with each laboratory. Figure 10–1 demonstrates one of these models, in which a

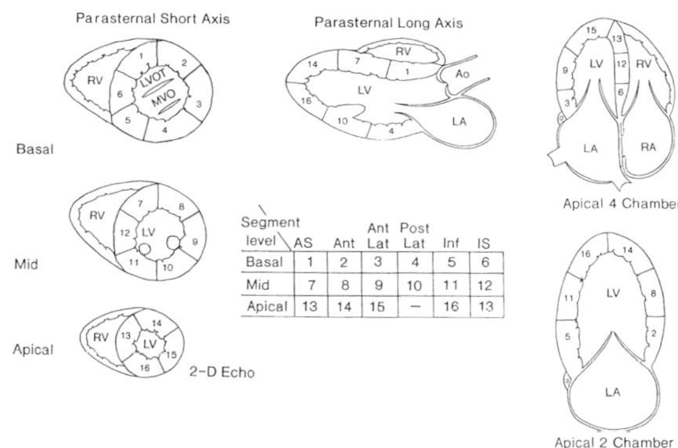

Figure 10–1. Sixteen-segment model for regional wall motion analysis recommended by the American Society of Echocardiography. The LV is divided into 16 segments: six segments from basal level, six segments from mid-papillary muscle level, and four segments from the apical level. All 16 segments are visualized from tomographic planes of two-dimensional echocardiography. According to contractility, each segment is given a wall motion score. Segment 13 (apical septum) should be used only once, depending on the coronary anatomy. *From OhJK, et al: The Echo Manual, Boston: Little, Brown, 1994.*

16-segment division of the left ventricle is obtained, which the American Society of Echocardiography (ASE) has recommended (45). The echocardiographer examines each individual segment and assigns the segment a score that indicates the contractility of that particular segment. The absolute number of the score varies with the laboratory, but ASE recommendations are as follows: 1 = normal, 2 = hypokinetic, 3 = akinetic, 4 = dyskinetic, and 5 = aneurysm. The numbers assigned to each segment are then added together and divided by the number of segments to obtain a wall motion score index. In this particular model, a wall motion score index of 1 indicates a normally contracting myocardium, and a wall motion score becomes larger as more myocardium is involved with infarction.

The wall motion score index is an excellent indicator of overall regional function. Because coronary artery disease involves the ventricle in a segmental manner, the wall motion score index provides more information than the ejection fraction in terms of overall left ventricular function. As discussed later, the wall motion score index has been shown to be a prognostic indicator in the acute myocardial infarction (40–42,44), postmyocardial infarction (43,44), and chronic coronary artery disease (37). Because it also indicates the proportion of myocardium involved during myocardial infarction, it may have important implications in the immediate decision for acute intervention (2,4).

The wall motion score index can be utilized to estimate the amount of myocardium at risk in patients with acute myocardial infarction and the extent of final infarct size after treatment with thrombolysis or angioplasty. Currently, perfusion defect determined by technetium sestamibi radionuclide imaging is a standard reference for these measurements. To correlate the wall motion score index with the perfusion defect, two-dimensional echocardiography was performed at the same time of technetium sestamibi injection before and several days after acute reperfusion therapy (either thrombolysis or PTCA) in patients with acute transmural myocardial infarction (46). The overall correlation was satisfactory both at the initial examination prior to reperfusion therapy (hence, myocardium at risk) and at predismissal study (myocardial infarct size). However, the correlation was poor in patients with inferior wall myocardial infarction.

The advent of digital analysis has greatly enhanced the usefulness of two-dimensional echocardiography in coronary artery disease (47). By transferring the video images of a two-dimensional echocardiogram through an analog-to-digital converter, a complete cardiac cycle in real time is stored in digital format. This information can be stored on either a floppy or hard disk for prompt image retrieval. Various display formats allow comparison of images in a side-by-side format, so that the same tomographic image of the myocardium at two different times can be seen simultaneously (Fig. 10–2). This has markedly enhanced the ability of a visual analysis of wall motion to detect subtle changes over time. This type of system is useful for following the natural history of wall motion in acute myocardial infarction, assessing changes of myocardial function in response to acute intervention, and providing the ability to detect new wall motion changes in diagnostic tests, such as stress echocardiography.

Digital technology will contribute to the application of quantitative echocardiography. The "continuous loop" playback capabilities enhance the detection of endocardial borders, which is not possible because of ultrasound "dropout" in still frame images. Quantitative analysis of left ventricular volume mass and ejection fraction (45,48–51) is made much easier by digital imaging and may provide valuable information on a patient with acute myocardial infarction (52).

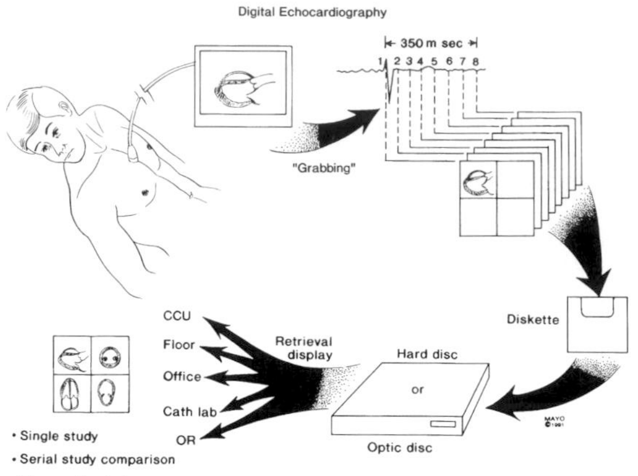

Figure 10–2. Digital echocardiography. Echocardiographic images are digitized, and desired segments of representative cardiac cycles are captured. Eight (in this diagram) separate sequential images (50 msec between two images, 7 intervals, giving a total of 350 msec of the cardiac cycle) are grabbed onto eight separate cells. Each cell can also be split into two or four compartments to contain multiple images. The onset and duration of image capture can be manipulated. Once the capturing is completed, the digitized image can be stored on a diskette or in the central hard disk (or optic disk), which can store multiple studies depending on its capacity. The central station is connected to multiple terminals, where the digitized study can be retrieved to review or to compare with previous studies. CCU = coronary care unit; OR = operating room. *From OhJK, et al: The Echo Manual, Boston: Little, Brown, 1994.*

Quantitative analysis of wall motion has been limited to the investigative laboratory in the past (17,18,53,54). Multiple problems emerge in attempts to quantitate regional wall motion because of the complexity of regional wall motion (that is, translation, rotation, temporal heterogeneity, and spatial heterogeneity), as discussed previously. Use, however, of a floating epicardial center of mass (55) and the center line method (56) show promise and may provide a means by which quantitation of regional wall motion will become possible in the future. Other methods for quantitation of wall motion, such as endocardial surface mapping (57–60) and end-systolic radius-to-thickness ratio (52), also show promise. Quantitation of wall motion will be especially useful in providing assessment of changes in regional ventricular function and response to acute intervention, because two-dimensional echocardiography is a method that lends itself to repeated measurements.

USE OF WALL MOTION ANALYSIS IN THE DIAGNOSIS AND EXCLUSION OF ACUTE MYOCARDIAL INFARCTION

Not all patients with prolonged chest pain due to myocardial ischemia or infarction present with a typical electrocardiogram or enzymatic findings. More than 50 percent of patients with myocardial infarction show nonspecific findings on the initial electrocardiogram obtained (61,62). The patient's description and intensity of chest pain cannot be correlated with the presence or extent of myocardial ischemia or infarction. Since we do not yet have a more sensitive diagnostic test that can be performed promptly in the emergency room, most of these patients with chest pain syndrome (with nondiagnostic electrocardiogram and prolonged chest pain) are admitted to the hospital with less than 30 percent chance of detecting myocardial infarction in them (63). Use of a rapid assay of subforms of creatine kinase (CK), MB has been found to be reliable in detecting myocardial infarction within the first 6 hours after the onset of chest pain syndromes (64). However, the sensitivity of CK-MB subform assays may not be satisfactory if the assays are obtained within 4 hours from the onset of chest pain. Perfusion imaging technique has been also utilized in the emergency room to detect perfusion defect in patients with chest pain syndrome with good sensitivity on the specificity (65). However, this technique requires a 2- to 3-hour delay in detecting perfusion defect. The main advantage of echocardiography is the ability to perform echocardiographic examination in the emergency room and the immediate availability of the echocardiographic findings (66,67). As discussed earlier, myocardial contractility diminishes or ceases immediately with ischemia or infarction, manifested as regional wall motion abnormalities that are readily identified in most of the patients by two-dimensional echocardiography. Therefore, it is an attractive concept to utilize the presence of regional wall motion abnormalities as a marker of myocardial infarction in patients with prolonged chest pain and nondiagnostic electrocardiogram, and patient triage can be based on the echocardiographic information. Several studies confirmed the utility of echocardiography in this setting. Studies from the University of Virginia (67) and the University of Cincinnati (68) showed that the absence of left ventricular wall motion abnormalities practically excludes subsequent detection of myocardial infarction and the presence of regional wall motion abnormalities has a high sensitivity for detecting myocardial infarction, although positive predictive value was only 31 percent since the regional wall motion abnormalities are not specific for acute myocardial infarction. Therefore, if the patient triage is based on the presence and absence of regional wall motion abnormalities on echocardiographic examination, this may result in more than 30 percent reduction in hospital admission without increasing the number of patients with acute myocardial infarction dismissed from the emergency room. This triage scheme incorporating the use of two-dimensional echocardiography in the emergency room will reduce estimated total cost by 24 percent (67). Once regional wall motion abnormalities are detected in patients with prolonged chest pain but nondiagnostic electrocardiogram, the patients are admitted to the hospital for further observation and evaluation. Whether these patients with regional wall motion abnormalities and no diagnostic electrocardiogram can benefit from urgent coronary angiography and possibly reperfusion therapy has not been adequately evaluated in large trials. Occasionally, echocardiography may be useful in detecting nonischemic underlying etiology for chest pain syndromes such as pulmonary embolism, valvular heart disease, cardiomyopathies, pericardial disease, or aortic dissection. The incidence of these findings is probably small, but the treatment with an anticoagulation or thrombolytic therapy in a subset of these patients (aortic dissection or cardiac tamponade) may result in a disastrous clinical outcome. However, the above approach requires availability of prompt echocardiographic examination and interpretation in the emergency room, which is the main limitation to utilizing echocardiography in this clinical setting. Recently, transmission of digitized real-time echocardiographic images has been accomplished via existing telephone line to a laptop computer, and this approach will improve the utilization of echocardiography (69).

MONITORING OF ACUTE REPERFUSION THERAPY BY ECHOCARDIOGRAPHY

Two-dimensional echocardiographic analysis of regional wall motion abnormalities has a limited diagnostic utility in the presence of a classic history and ST elevation in ECG; however, the amount of myocardium at risk can be reasonably estimated by calculating wall motion score index. Using the 16-segment model, wall motion score index greater than 1.8 usually suggests more than 20% perfusion defect (46) and increased complication unless wall motion abnormalities reverse with reperfusion therapy. The initial two-dimensional echocardiographic assessment can be used to compare subsequent regional wall motion abnormalities and wall motion score index after reperfusion therapy to monitor its effects on myocardial contractility (30,70,71). Several factors determine whether or not a patient will benefit from acute reperfusion therapy with thrombolysis or PTCA. The time from the onset of pain to the intervention is important. The amount of myocardium at risk from the affected artery may also determine who will have the greatest benefit from acute interventional therapy. Patients with a large proportion of myocardium at risk will probably derive more benefit from reperfusion therapy than those patients with a small proportion of myocardium at risk. Because aggressive interventional therapy poses a small but finite risk, the decision of whether or not to intervene must be made on the basis of the risk-to-benefit ratio. Two-dimensional echocardiographic determination of the area of myocardium at risk, as estimated by the percentage of abnormally contracting myocardium, may aid in this decision-making process (2–4). If there is a question of another cause of chest pain, especially in those in whom thrombolytic therapy may be detrimental (that is, aortic dissection, pericarditis), two-dimensional echocardiography will be of benefit. Current investigative work on tissue characterization by analysis of ultrasonic back scatter may aid in the decision for thrombolytic therapy in the future by distinguishing between infarcted and viable myocardium (72,73). The noninvasive nature of echocardiography makes it a useful modality for assessing changes in wall motion after reperfusion therapy. Echocardiographic studies performed before thrombolysis was introduced showed a variable change in wall motion after myocardial infarction. Such factors will have to be taken into consideration when future studies are performed.

When a patient presents with transmural acute myocardial infarction (ST elevation in the ECG), underlying LV myocardium is akinetic or dyskinetic. Once the myocardium is successfully reperfused within an appropriate time frame (usually within 4 hours), it may become more contractile on subsequent two-dimensional echocardiographic studies (70,71). Serial echocardiographic studies demonstrated that the improvement in regional myocardial contractility is evident within 24 to 48 hours, and improvement continues until several days to months (30,70,71). Therefore, serial two-dimensional echocardiographic imaging is useful in detecting reperfused myocardial segment, especially using digital echocardiography by which serial images of the same tomographic planes can be compared side by side. This apparent value of serial echocardiographic imaging after reperfusion therapy has not been well appreciated due to the cost of repeated examinations and lack of physician's hands-on skills in obtaining echocardiographic images in these patients. Persistent akinesis does not always indicate failed reperfusion. Unless reperfusion therapy achieves recovery of more than 75% of transmural thickness involved with infarction, the myocardium may remain akinetic, although the more myocardium is reperfused, the less tendency exists to develop infarct expansion. When the myocardium remains akinetic while being viable, low-dose dobutamine may be helpful to unravel its viability; this is discussed later in this chapter (77).

EVALUATION OF COMPLICATIONS OF ACUTE MYOCARDIAL INFARCTION

The incidence and mortality of cardiogenic shock after acute myocardial infarction have remained similar at 7.5% and 80%, respectively from 1975 to 1988 in a community-based study (78). The incidence of shock in patients treated with thrombolysis was 5.7% (79). Since the patients who have cardiogenic shock after myocardial infarction have a poor prognosis unless there is a reversible cause, it is of paramount clinical importance to identify the underlying etiology promptly, based on which proper treatments can be given. It is essential that a fast and accurate diagnosis be made in the critically ill patient so that proper treatment is instituted. Two-dimensional and Doppler echocardiography with color flow imaging have been shown to be useful in prompt identification of the cause of hemodynamic compromise in these patients, specifically in looking for mechanical complications (1,6). In addition, transesophageal echocardiography has provided a new window to the heart by which the heart can be easily visualized, especially in the critically ill patient in whom a precordial echocardiogram may not be possible (9,80–85a). The presence of normal systolic function in a critically ill patient should immediately lead one to suspect a mechanical complication. An international registry from 19 centers of the 251 patients with cardiogenic shock after myocardial infarction showed that severe left ventricular failure was the cause of shock in 85%, RV infarct in 2%, and mechanical complication in 8%. When cardiogenic shock is caused by ventricular failure, revascularization of the culprit coronary artery as well as other medical treatments including intravenous inotropic agents and afterload reducer increase the chance of the patient's survival.

Right ventricular infarct and failure may result in significant hypotension and low output, which requires judicious management of fluid therapy, inotropic support, maintenance of atrioventricular synchrony, and cautious reduction of pulmonary vascular resistance (86,87). Although right ventricular infarct may be diagnosed by clinical examination, ST elevation in the right precordial ECG leads, and characteristic hemodynamic pressure tracing, two-dimensional echocardiography can reliably diagnose this entity by the presence of enlarged right ventricle with hypokinesis or akinesis of the underlying myocardium (88,89). The diagnosis of right ventricular infarction by two-dimensional echocardiography has been made in 40% to 65% of all patients with inferior myocardial infarction (90,91). The area of involvement of the right ventricle is most commonly the free lateral wall (84%), followed by the diaphragmatic (66%), apical (40%), and septal (10%) walls (92). The findings on two-dimensional echocardiography compare favorably with those from radionuclide angiography in right ventricular infarction (89–91), with a higher sensitivity and specificity than physical examination or electrocardiography (91). In some patients, the predominant abnormality may be severe tricuspid regurgitation resulting from coexistent right tricuspid papillary muscle involvement and annulus dilation from the right ventricular infarction, which can be readily identified by two-dimensional echocardiography and Doppler echocardiography (93). Diastolic filling of the right ventricle is abnormal in patients with right ventricular infarction (94,95). The tricuspid valve velocity curve in patients with right ventricular infarction demonstrates a lower initial filling velocity and a higher velocity with atrial contraction, which has been attributed to impaired relaxation (94). Occasionally, hypoxemia may be a predominant manifestation of RV infarct due to right to left shunt via the patent foramen ovale as right atrial pressure increases. This complication can be easily diagnosed by contrast echocardiography (96) or color flow imaging, especially in conjunction with transesophageal echocardiography (Fig. 10–3).

Other causes of cardiogenic shock may be reversible if there is early recognition and intervention is undertaken. Rupture of the papillary muscle, ventricular septum, or free wall may cause the acute onset of cardiogenic shock (97). In these situations, it is usually associated with preserved left ventricular function and a limited extent of coronary artery disease (98,99). The prognosis for these patients is therefore excellent if the underlying mechanical problem can be promptly treated (100–104).

Rupture of the papillary muscle can be diagnosed by two-dimensional echocardiography by

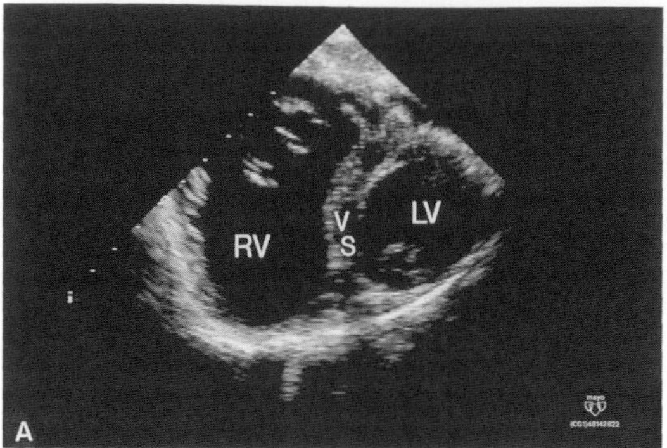

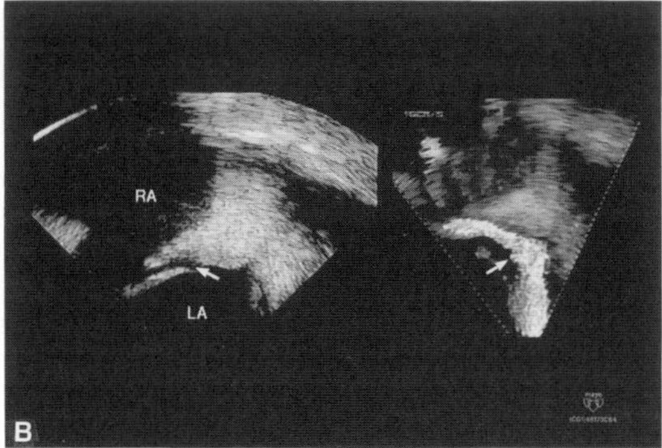

Figure 10–3. **A.** Transgastric transesophageal echocardiographic view of right ventricle (RV) and left ventricle (LV). The RV is markedly dilated due to right ventricular infarct. In real time, severe hypokinesis or akinesis of the right ventricular free wall is easily seen. VS = ventricular septum. **B.** Longitudinal view of the patent foramen ovale (indicated by an arrow in left) in a patient with right ventricular infarct. Right atrium (RA) is dilated due to right ventricular infarct and right atrial pressure elevation, and there is a gap (arrow) between the fossa ovalis and the superior fatty limbus. Color flow imaging (right) indicates continuous flow from the RA to left atrium (LA) resulting in significant hypoxemia in this patient with right ventricular infarct.

direct visualization of the affected papillary muscle (6,97). Partial papillary muscle rupture can be identified by a tear in the papillary muscle with the remaining part of the muscle still intact (105) (Fig. 10–4). This results in significant mitral regurgitation as a result of the instability of the attachment of the mitral valve chordal apparatus and portends the possibility of further hemodynamic deterioration if the papillary muscle ruptures completely. A complete papillary muscle rupture can be identified by visualizing the entire head of the papillary muscle as swinging free from the myocardium (98,106). (Figs. 10–5, 10–6, Color Plate 5). This results in a flail mitral valve leaflet and severe mitral regurgitation. Even if direct visualization of the papillary muscle is not possible, a large spatial extent of a mitral regurgitation jet into the left atrium on Doppler echocardiography with color flow imaging provides evidence for papillary muscle rupture or dysfunction. Continuous-wave Doppler echocardiography

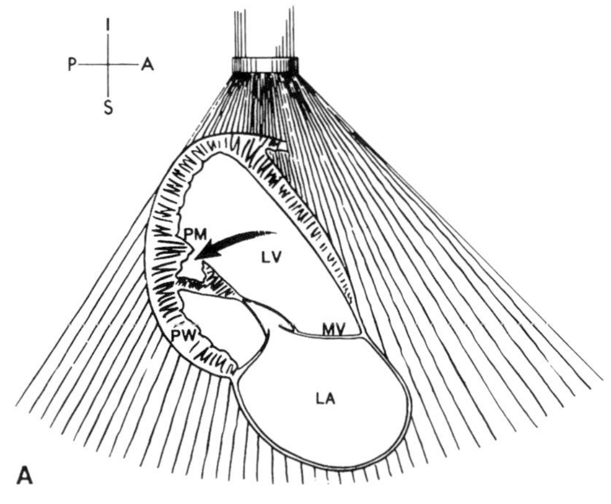

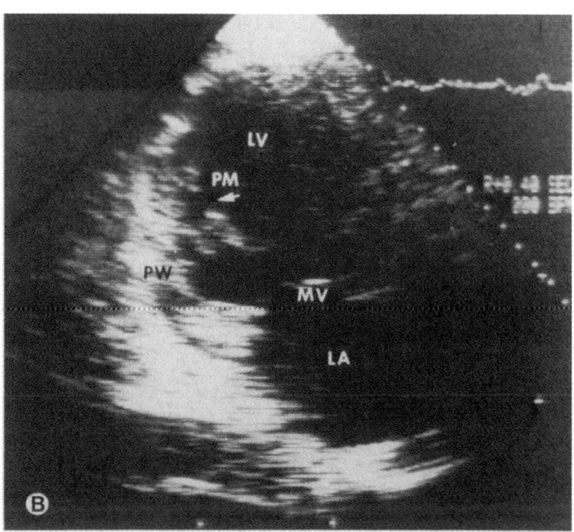

Figure 10–4. Two-dimensional echocardiographic diagnosis of a partial posteromedial papillary muscle rupture. **A,** Schematic diagram. **B,** Apical long-axis view demonstrating the site of the partial papillary muscle rupture (arrow). LA = left atrium, LV = left ventricle, MV = mitral valve, PM = papillary muscle, PW = posterior wall.

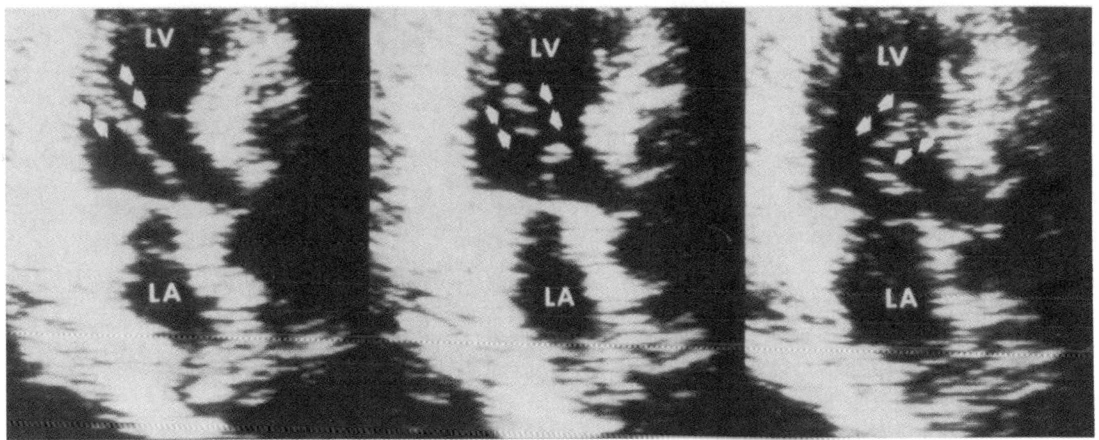

Figure 10–5. Two-dimensional echocardiographic still frames of complete papillary muscle rupture. Posteromedial papillary muscle can be seen freely mobile within left ventricular cavity (arrows). Severe mitral regurgitation was present. LA = left atrium, LV = left ventricle.

of the mitral regurgitation jet may aid indirectly because it reflects the instantaneous gradient between the left ventricle and left atrium during systole (107). Because papillary muscle rupture results in acute, severe mitral regurgitation in a noncompliant, high-pressure left atrium, there is rapid equilibration of left ventricular and left atrial pressure through systole. This results in a mitral velocity curve by continuous-wave Doppler echocardiography of a lower velocity than would be expected in chronic mitral regurgitation (<4 m/s) with a rapidly tapering decelerating of velocity. The patients with acute severe mitral regurgitation due to papillary muscle rupture develop significant respiratory distress, and transthoracic echocardiography may not be satisfactory. Transesophageal echocardiography in this clinical situation should be able to detect mitral valve abnormalities and severe mitral regurgitation in all patients (8,9). Pulmonary vein is always accessible to transesophageal echocardiography, and systolic flow reversible in pulmonary vein complements the diagnosis of severe mitral

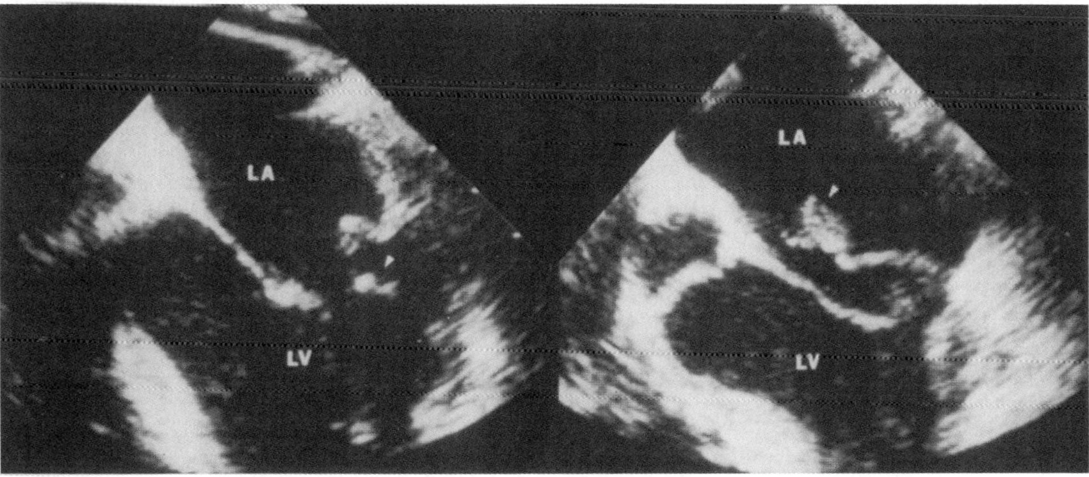

Figure 10–6. Transesophageal echocardiogram demonstrating complete papillary muscle rupture. Entire head of papillary muscle (arrowheads) is shown during diastole (left) and systole (right). There is a complete lack of coaptation of the mitral valve. LA = left atrium, LV = left ventricle.

regurgitation. In this urgent clinical setting, the mitral value is usually replaced, but in selected cases, the ruptured papillary muscle may be repaired with the help of intraoperative transesophageal echocardiography.

Ventricular septal defect (VSD) occurs in 1% to 3% of all patients with acute myocardial infarction and results in progressive hemodynamic deterioration unless surgically corrected. Infarct VSD is diagnosed by demonstration of a disrupted ventricular septum with left-to-right shunt (108–117). The defect is always located in the region of the thinned myocardium with akinesis to dyskinesis. The diagnosis can be established 90% of the cases by transthoracic 2D-Doppler-color flow imaging (Fig. 10–7, Color Plate 6). Transesophageal echocardiogram may be necessary in a small subgroup of patients with a suboptimal transthoracic study (6,9,118) (Figs. 10–8, 10–9). Prognosis of infarct VSD is poorer when the location is in the inferior septum and it is associated with RV infarct. The location and characteristics of VSD, and RV involvement, are clearly determined by echocardiography. Peak flow velocity across the VSD measured by continuous wave Doppler may be used to estimate right ventricular systolic pressure. Coexistent septal aneurysms and severe mitral regurgitation can be identified, which is important information for surgical management of these patients (110).

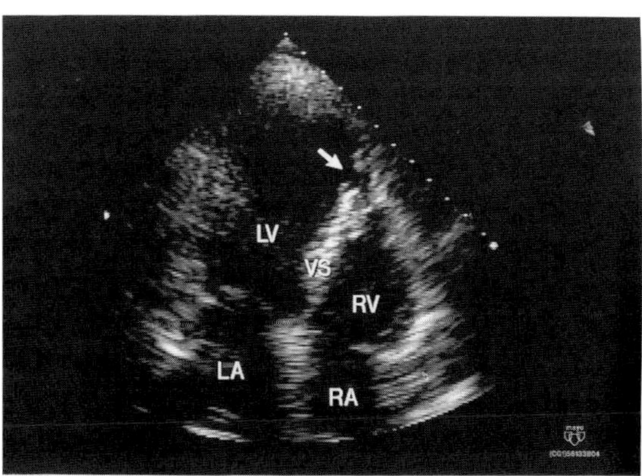

Figure 10–7. Apical four-chamber view of a patient with anterior apical myocardial infarction. Entire apex was thinned with akinesis to dyskinesis with a tear (arrow). This is a typical example of ventricular septal defect in patients with transmural anterior apical myocardial infarction.

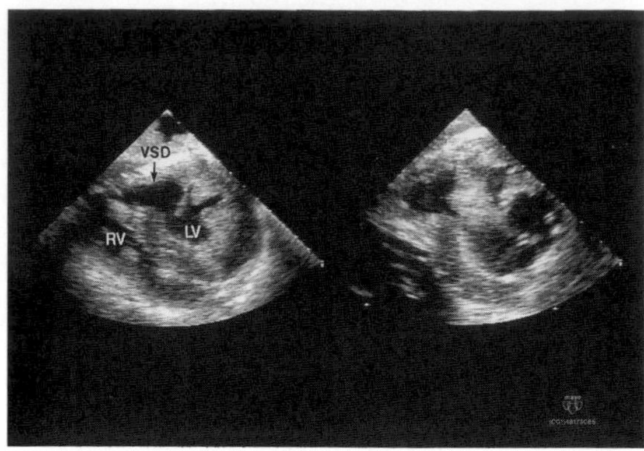

Figure 10–8. Transverse four-chamber view of transesophageal echocardiography. In this patient, basal septum had a defect not well seen by transthoracic echocardiogram, but transesophageal echocardiography shows clear ventricular septal defect, indicated by an arrow.

The most typical clinical presentation of papillary muscle rupture and VSD after acute myocardial infarction is a new systolic murmur with progressive, sometimes abrupt, hemodynamic deterioration. Another important, but not well appreciated, clinical entity that also presents with new systolic murmur and hypotension is dynamic LVOT obstruction in previously hypertensive patients with apical infarct and hyperdynamic basal

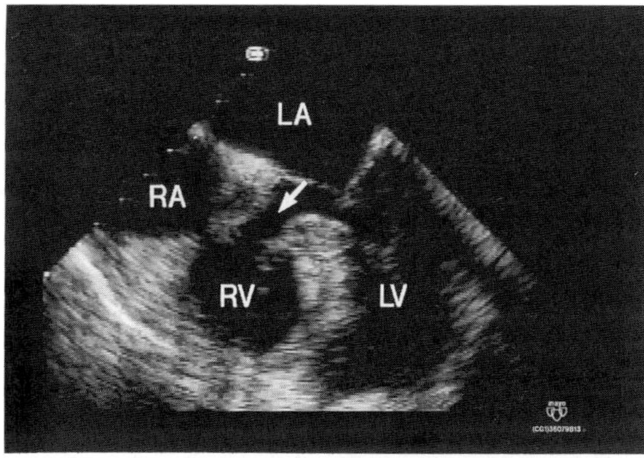

Figure 10–9. Transesophageal echocardiography shows short-axis view of the left ventricle demonstrating a large defect in the inferior septum typical of postinfarct ventricle septal defect (VSD). A muscle flap is also seen in the left ventricular side as a remnant of septal tear. Color flow imaging clearly shows a large shunt from the left ventricle (LV) to right ventricle (RV). This patient sustained a small inferior wall transmural myocardial infarction.

function. This can be reliably diagnosed by 2D/Doppler echocardiography.

Most patients with free wall rupture usually present as the acute onset of electrical–mechanical dissociation. A subset of patients, however, present subacutely with hypotension, recurrent chest pain, and/or emesis (119). Detection of free wall rupture in these patients enables surgical repair with survival rate of more than 50% (120). The transthoracic two-dimensional echocardiogram may not be able to show the site of the rupture but will demonstrate a pericardial effusion with 2D and Doppler echocardiographic characteristics of pericardial tamponade. Presence of pericardial effusion alone is not sufficient to diagnose subacute free wall rupture, since it is relatively common after acute myocardial infarction. Blood clot in the pericardial cavity increases echodensity, which is more suggestive of free wall rupture (120). Because an acute rupture may result in a loculated effusion, it is safest to utilize an echo-directed pericardiocentesis for emergency treatment (121). In rare instances, a pseudoaneurysm will form after a free wall rupture contained within a limited portion of the pericardial space (most frequently in the lateral wall). It may be difficult to identify a pseudoaneurysm on two-dimensional echocardiography if the defect is small and contained. With pulsed-wave Doppler and color flow imaging, however, the velocity of moving red blood cells can be identified in an extracardiac space, which itself communicates with the left ventricle, indicating the presence of a pseudoaneurysm (Fig. 10–10, Color Plate 4).

Pericardial effusion on two-dimensional echocardiography is seen in up to 26% of patients with myocardial infarction. It is more common in patients with larger regions of myocardium involved by the infarction (122). The short-term prognosis is poorer in patients in whom pericardial effusion has developed than in those who did not have pericardial effusion, and this is related to the extent of infarction. Hemodynamically significant cases of pericardial effusion are less frequent, usually seen in less than 4% of all patients with myocardial infarction. Recently, Doppler echocardiography has provided insight into the pathophysiologic process that occurs in pericardial tamponade (123,124). It is thought that the primary pathophysiology involves a dissociation between intrathoracic and intracardiac pressures and an enhanced ventricular interaction between the left and right ventricles. There are discrete Doppler echocardiographic parameters reflected in these events, including a decrease in the initial mitral velocity with inspiration, a prolongation of the isovolumic relaxation period with inspiration, a decrease in the tricuspid valve initial velocity with expiration, and a loss of diastolic forward flow and reversal flow in the hepatic vein during expiration. Serial Doppler studies provide a noninvasive modality for follow-up of patients with pericardial effusion to determine when early hemodynamic indices of pericardial tamponade appear. When early tamponade is present, a two-dimensional-directed pericardiocentesis can be used to remove the pericardial fluid safely.

Two-dimensional echocardiography has become a most practical and reliable imaging modality for detection of left ventricular thrombus (125–127) (Fig. 10–12). It is important to differentiate thrombus from aberrant chordae or artifacts that are frequently seen. The appearance of thrombus is that of a nonhomogeneous echodensity with a margin distinct from the underlying wall, which itself is dyskinetic (125,128). With these criteria, two-dimensional Doppler echocardiography has a sensitivity of 95% and a specificity of 86% in detecting rhombus compared with pathologic study (129). In prospective studies of patients with myocardial infarction, it has been shown

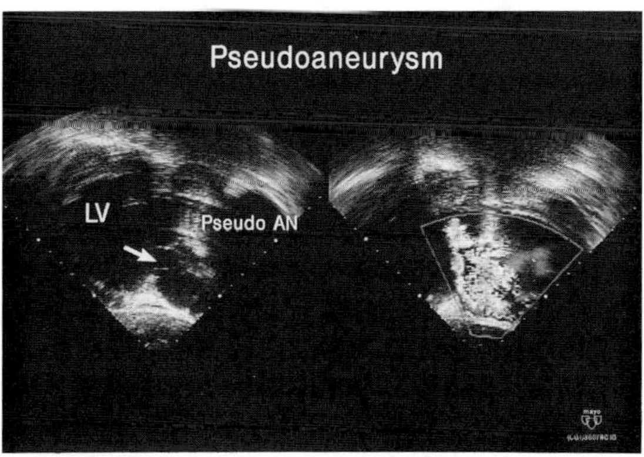

Figure 10–10. Transesophageal echocardiographic example of pseudoaneurysm due to the rupture of the left ventricular free wall at the inferolateral wall (arrow). Color flow imaging showed significant flow from the left ventricle to the pseudoaneurysm (AN).

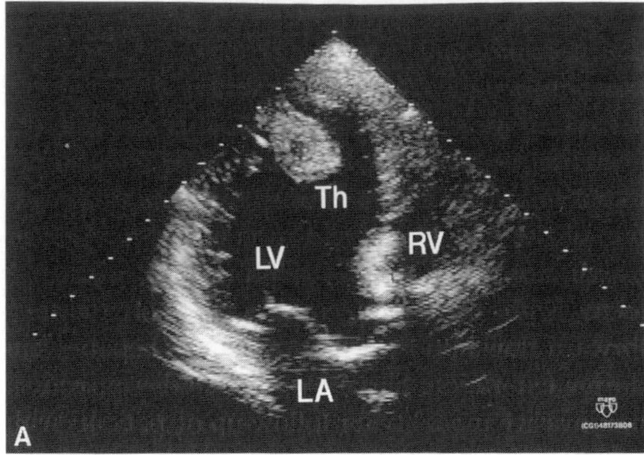

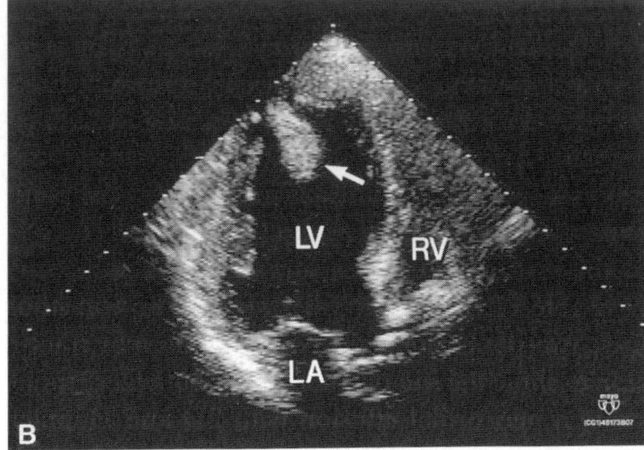

Figure 10–12. A. Example of a pedunculated mobile apical thrombus (TA) in a patient with an anteroapical infarct. **B.** The mobile nature of the thrombus can be appreciated by varying shapes of the thrombus into separate frames. This appearance suggests a high probability of embolization. *Boston: From OhJK, et al: The Echo Manual, Little, Brown, 1994, p 80.*

that left ventricular thrombi will be present in up to 30% to 40% of patients with anterior apical myocardial infarctions, although infrequently in patients with inferior myocardial infarctions (127,130,131). If apical dyskinesis is present, thrombus will be present in almost 50% of patients (127). Although left ventricular thrombus is commonly seen on two-dimensional echocardiography, there is only a 3% to 5% overall incidence of systemic emboli after myocardial infarction (132–134). Attempts have therefore been made to identify patients with detected thrombus at risk for systemic embolic events based on the ultrasonic characteristics of the thrombus (135–137). Protrusion of the thrombus into the left ventricular cavity is a sensitive predictor of thromboembolic events with an 88% sensitivity and an 82% specificity. The presence of a mobile thrombus is not as sensitive but is highly specific in predicting thromboemboli. The risk of developing a thromboembolic event with laminated thrombus with a smooth convex surface is low. Serial follow-up echocardiograms have shown that most left ventricular thrombi decrease in size or spontaneously resolve within 1 to 3 months (130,131,137). Up to 25% of patients continue to have thrombi at 2 years (131). Earlier reports had demonstrated a high mortality when thrombus developed, especially in the early hospital stay (130), however, emerging data suggest that left ventricular thrombus may protect against myocardial rupture (135). This becomes important because thrombolytic therapy may affect the incidence and outcome of patients with thrombus (138,139).

ECHOCARDIOGRAPHIC ASSESSMENT OF HEMODYNAMICS IN ACUTE MYOCARDIAL INFARCTION

Management of the critically ill patient rests on accurate determination of the hemodynamic status. Physical examination alone may be inaccurate in determining the filling pressures and cardiac output of a critically ill patient. Right-sided heart catheterization with a balloon-tipped catheter and thermodilution cardiac output has been able to provide information for management and determination of prognosis in the critically ill patient. Hemodynamic subsets have been used to direct treatment as well as determine prognosis (140). Right-side heart catheterization is, however, an invasive procedure with known complications (141).

Doppler echocardiography has enabled the noninvasive measurement of blood flow velocities within the cardiac chambers, across valves, and in great vessels (10,142). By the application of hydrodynamic principles, blood flow velocities can accurately measure volumetric flow (143). The application of a modification of the Bernoulli equation has allowed derivation of intracardiac pressures (144). Finally, recent insight into diastolic filling of the left and right ventricles obtained by Doppler echocardiography may provide valuable information regarding the filling pressures of the heart (11).

Volumetric flow, or cardiac output, can be accurately measured by Doppler echocardiography (143,145–147). The concept of deriving volumetric flow uses the hydrodynamic principle of laminar flow through a rigid tube. With knowledge of the area of the tube and the velocity at which flow proceeds through the tube, the volumetric flow rate can be determined from the product of these two parameters. Two-dimensional echocardiography can measure a valve orifice or diameter of great-vessel, thus providing the cross-sectional area of the region. Pulsed-wave or continuous-wave Doppler echocardiography can measure the velocity of blood flow over time. The time–velocity integral, which is the area underneath the time–velocity curve, can be multiplied by the area through which the blood flows, providing a measurement of stroke volume. Multiplication of the stroke volume by the heart rate provides an estimate of cardiac output.

Many sites have been used to determine volumetric flow rate by Doppler echocardiography (143). These include the tricuspid valve, the mitral valve, the mitral annulus, the pulmonary outflow tract, the left ventricular outflow tract, the aortic valve, and the ascending aorta. There are multiple assumptions that go into deriving volumetric flow from Doppler echocardiography: assumption of laminar flow; assumption of a fixed cross-sectional area; and assumption of a zero angle of incidence between the Doppler beam and the blood flow velocity. Despite these assumptions, there have been excellent correlations between Doppler-derived cardiac output and other conventional measures of cardiac output.

The most accurate location for determination of cardiac output by Doppler echocardiography is the left ventricular outflow tract (142,143). In this region, the blood flow velocity attains a more laminary profile compared with other regions, and the cross-sectional area changes little with time. This location may be difficult to examine in the critically ill patient. It is the continuous-wave Doppler echocardiogram of the ascending aorta that provides useful information in the patients who are technically difficult to image (145,146). This method requires measurement of the ascending aorta at the sinotubular junction. A continuous-wave Doppler beam is directed from the suprasternal notch down inferiorly and to the right to obtain the maximal blood velocity in the ascending aorta. Although absolute cardiac output measurement is not as accurate as when measured in the left ventricular outflow tract, this method provides a semiquantitative estimate of whether or not the cardiac output is high or low. In addition, changes in stroke volume can be accurately measured because the changes in the time–velocity integral correlate well with changes in true cardiac output.

Intracardiac pressures can be measured by continuous-wave Doppler echocardiography (142,144). The modified Bernoulli equation is utilized for this; the pressure gradient between two cardiac chambers is determined by squaring the velocity and multiplying by a constant of 4 (pressure gradient = $4 \times \text{velocity}^2$). If the pressure in one chamber is assume or measured, the pressure in the other chamber can then be calculated. Tricuspid regurgitation is present in 80% to 90% of patients studied by Doppler echocardiography. The peak systolic velocity of the tricuspid regurgitation jet can be used to calculate the instantaneous gradient between the right ventricle and right atrium (148). By assuming the right atrial pressure, judged by clinical examination of the jugular venous pressure, one can determine the right systolic pressure. If there is no right ventricular outflow obstruction, this will approximate the pulmonary artery systolic pressure, giving a measure of the degree of pulmonary hypertension. Mitral regurgitation is frequently present in patients with myocardial infarction (149–152), and the peak systolic velocity of the mitral regurgitation jet will indicate the pressure gradient between the left atrium and left ventricle during systole (103). If there is no left ventricular outflow obstruction, the cuff blood pressure can be used to estimate the left ventricular systolic pressure, and a noninvasive assessment of left atrial pressure can thus be made.

There has been great interest in using Doppler echocardiography to determine diastolic filing of both the left and right ventricles (11,153,154). This can be evaluated by studying the flow velocities obtained by pulsed-wave Doppler echocardiography of mitral inflow, pulmonary veins, tricuspid inflow, and the hepatic and superior vena cava (11). Diastolic function is a complex sequence of interrelated events that has been difficult to study in the past (155,156). When the Doppler flow velocities are viewed as a reflection of the relative changes in left atrial and left ventricular pressure relationships, however, information can be obtained about the diastolic filling properties of the ventricle (11,157). This is demonstrated in Fig. 10–13, in which the normal mitral flow velocity and the corresponding left atrial and left ventricular pressure contours are shown. The initial early diastolic velocity begins at a point of pressure crossover, as the left ventricular pressure decreases below the left atrial pressure owing to continued myocardial relaxation and diastolic suction of the left ventricle. This pressure gradient between the left atrium and left ventricle generates a "driving pressure" across the mitral valve that results in acceleration of the mitral flow velocity. After this decrease in left ventricular pressure, the left ventricular pressure increases because of the viscoelastic forces of the myocardium, pericardial restraint, and ventricular interaction. The left ventricular pressure will approximate or even exceed left atrial pressure, resulting in deceleration of flow velocity. During mid-diastole, there is continued forward flow because of inertial forces, despite the absence of a measurable pressure gradient. At atrial contraction, the left atrial pressure increases relative to the left ventricular pressure and results in a late acceleration of mitral flow velocity (11,155).

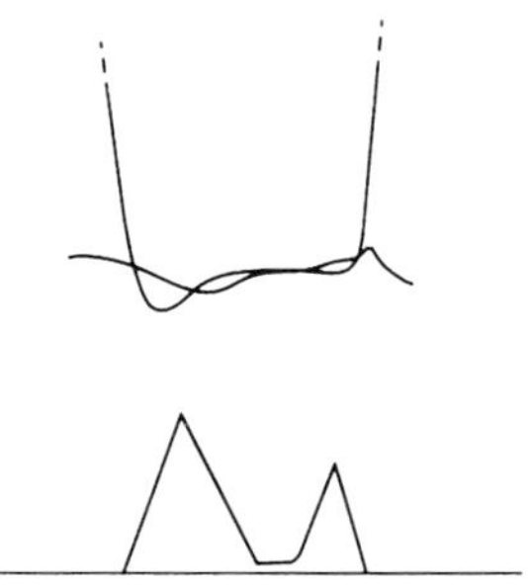

Figure 10–13. The schematic diagram of left atrial and left ventricle pressures (top) and simultaneous mitral flow velocity curve (bottom); see text for details. *Reproduced from Nishimura et al. (10) with permission of the Mayo Foundation.*

In the presence of impaired relaxation, there will be a lower peak early gradient between the left atrium and left ventricle and a decrease in the left atrial–left ventricular gradient in mid-diastole. Because less filling is present in early diastole, there will be a larger amount of filling with atrial contraction. Relaxation will be prolonged in the presence of myocardial ischemia, and if filling pressures do not increase, the mitral flow velocity will consist of a low E, prolonged deceleration time, and low E/A ratio.

In patients who have a decrease in compliance, there is a rapid increase in left ventricular pressure early in diastole because of a large rapid filling wave in the left ventricular pressure trace. This rapid increase in left ventricular pressure results in shortening of the deceleration time because the left atrial–left ventricular pressure gradient is decreasing more rapidly. The E velocity will be high because of the high driving pressure across the mitral valve resulting from a high initial left atrial pressure. With these conceptual relationships in mind between the pressure contours and the mitral flow velocities, it is then possible to determine the type of left ventricular filling based on the mitral flow velocities.(Figs. 10–14, 10–15).

In the presence of a high preload of the left ventricle, there will be an increase in left atrial pressure, relative to the left ventricular pressure, in early diastole. This results in a higher initial driving pressure across the mitral valve and a more rapid decline in pressure gradient between the left atrium and left ventricle. Subsequently, the E velocity will be high and the deceleration time will shorten. Conversely, a lower preload results in a lower driving pressure across the mitral valve and a slower decline in pressure gradient between the left atrium and left ventricle. This results in a low initial E velocity and prolongation of the deceleration time. These concepts can be used in the management of the critically ill patient (157a). If a patient has a high E velocity and

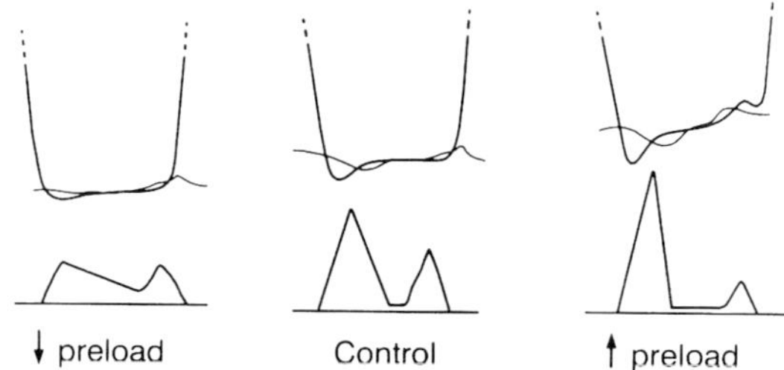

Figure 10–14. Schematic diagram of left ventricular and left atrial pressure traces (top) and simultaneous mitral inflow velocities (bottom) in low preloading condition, control state, and high preload condition. For an explanation, see text. *Reproduced from Nishimura et al. (10), with permission of the Mayo Foundation.*

short deceleration time (<150 ms), the preload of the heart is most likely increased and the wedge pressure is high (157b). Conversely, if the initial E velocity is low and the deceleration time is prolonged (>300 ms), the preload is low (157c). The velocity pattern in the pulmonary vein can provide further information regarding LV filling and LA pressure (158,158a). As the LV filling pressure increases, the systolic component of pulmonary vein forward flow decreases. Flow duration of mitral A velocity and pulmonary vein (PV) atrial flow reversal also provides an insight into the status of LV diastolic pressure and LA pressure. When those pressures are normal, the duration of mitral A velocity is at least equal or usually longer than that of pulmonary vein atrial flow reversal. With elevation of pressures, mitral A velocity duration becomes shorter and pulmonary vein atrial flow reversal lasts longer. When the difference is greater than 50 msec (PV flow reversal − MV A flow duration), LV end-diastolic pressure is elevated with a high sensitivity (159,160).

It has been well appreciated that high filling pressure or S_3 after myocardial infarction portends a poor prognosis. Hence, it is expected that restrictive diastolic filling pattern on Doppler echocardiography indicates a similarly poor prognosis. When diastolic filling was determined within 24 hours of admission to the coronary care unit with acute myocardial infarction, shortened deceleration time (<160 msec) indicative of restrictive filling and high filling pressure could predict the presence or development of congestive heart failure and death due to low cardiac output (Table 10–1) (161). As heart failure is treated, diastolic filling pattern becomes less restrictive by Doppler echocardiography.

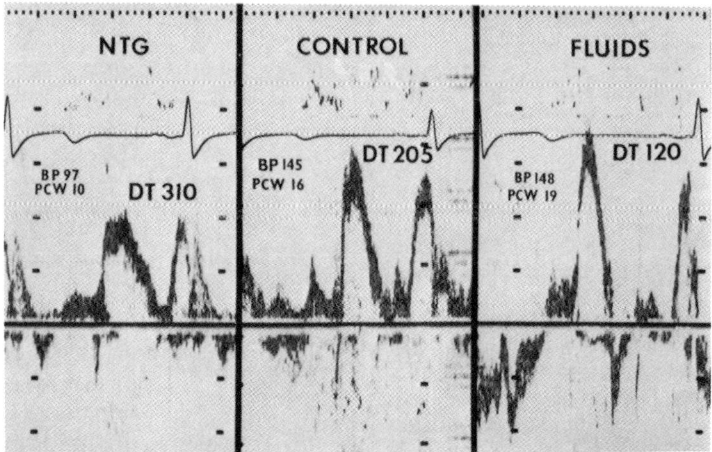

Figure 10–15. Actual mitral inflow velocities from a patient who underwent a decrease in preload with nitroglycerin (NT) and an increase in preload with 500 cc of normal saline. BP = blood pressure. DT = deceleration time. PCWP = pulmonary capillary wedge pressure. As there is a progressive increase in pulmonary capillary wedge pressure, there is an increase in E velocity and decrease in deceleration time.

Table 10–1. Patient Characteristics as a Function of Deceleration Time.

	DT > 160 msec (n = 35)	DT ≤ 160 msec (n = 27)	P
Men (no.)	28	21	—
Age (yr)	63 ± 12	63±8	—
HR (beats/min)	72±13	80±14	0.03
SBP (mm Hg)	118±26	107±16	0.04
DBP (mm Hg)	68±10	62±10	0.03
Clinical heart failure [no. (%)]			
At admission	2 (6)	13 (48)	0.0001
During hospitalization	4 (11)	19 (70)	<0.0001
Death	1 (3)	4 (15)	0.086
LVEF (%)	58±14	41±16	0.0003
WMSI	1.63±0.41	2.05±0.47	<0.001
LVEDP (mm Hg)*	21±8	29±8	0.006
E 0.54±0.15	0.69±0.21	0.002	
A 0.62±0.18	0.48±0.16	0.003	
E/A	0.95±0.35	1.52±0.49	<0.0001

A, Peak velocity of late filling wave caused by atria contraction; E, peak velocity of early rapid filling wave; E/A, E to A ratio; DBP, diastolic blood pressure; DT, deceleration time of E velocity; HR, heart rate; LVEDP, left ventricular end-diastolic pressure; LVEF, left ventricular ejection fraction; SBP, systolic blood pressure; WMSI, wall motion score.

**From OhJK, et al: J Am Soc Echocardiogr 1992;5:497–503.*

PROGNOSTIC EVALUATION: STRESS ECHOCARDIOGRAPHY AND EVALUATION OF MYOCARDIAL VIABILITY

Echocardiography is an excellent technique for prediction of prognosis in the setting of acute myocardial infarction by assessing global and regional left ventricular function. In the early M-mode era, it was shown that an enlarged left ventricular dimension and a delayed mitral valve closure predicted subsequent in-hospital mortality. Many studies of two-dimensional echocardiography have shown that the wall motion score index, as a measure of the degree of abnormally functioning myocardium, is a predictor of subsequent complications, such as congestive heart failure, ventricular arrhythmias, and mortality (39–43).

Patients who present in congestive heart failure have worse wall motion score indices than those who appear clinically stable at admission. As expected, these patients have a much poorer prognosis during the remainder of their hospital stay. The advantage of the wall motion score index is that it can predict the onset of complications in patients who appear clinically stable at presentation (40,41). In one study, a complication developed in 79% of patients who were in Killip class I at dismissal but had a wall motion score index ≥2, as opposed to less than 18% of patients who had a wall motion index <2 (41). These findings are important in this era of cost containment and its influence on length of hospital stay. There is a tendency to decrease the number of hospital days in which a patient is being monitored if he or she appears clinically stable at presentation to the hospital. If, however, a high incidence of complications will eventually develop in a subset of these patients, and they can be identified by a worse wall motion score index, then the hospital stay of these patients should not be shortened. Acute recanalization during myocardial infarction has altered the incidence of in-hospital complications and mortality. The previous studies assessing the value of wall motion in predicting prognosis may therefore not necessarily be applicable when thrombolytic therapy is available, since wall motion score index improves significantly with successful reperfusion (30,70,71). Further studies need to be performed in this area.

Three pathophysiologic processes may occur while the patient is in the hospital, and they predict an increased incidence of complications: (i) infarct extension, (ii) ischemia at a distance, and (iii) infarct expansion. All three may be identified by two-dimensional echocardiography (162–164). Infarct extension refers to infarction of an area of myocardium adjacent to the initial infarcted segment; it is associated with a 2.5 times increase in hospital mortality and a 30% decrease in 1-year survival (163). On two-dimensional echocardiography, there is a larger area of wall motion abnormality at the site of the initial infarction. The sensitivity and specificity for identification of an infarct extension in one study were 77% and 100%, respectively. Ischemia at a distance indicates the occurrence of ischemia, infarction, or both at site remote from the initial infarction. Remote area from the initial infarct location is usually hyperdynamic during early period of acute myocardial infarction unless there is a significant stenosis of the coronary artery supplying the remote myocardial segment. This may be visualized as areas of regional wall motion abnormalities that are not involved with the initial infarct on two-dimensional echocardiography and is indicative of a critical stenosis in a noninfarcted vessel (40). When this is seen on two-dimensional echocardiography, there is a higher incidence of recurrent angina, reinfarction, shock, and death. Infarct expansion or ventricular remodeling occurs in more than 70% of patients who die from myocardial infarction (164). Progressive thinning and dilation of the infarcted segment are present as a result of the disruption of cells within the region of infarct (164). Two-dimensional echocardiography can visualize this dilation as well as assess myocardial thickness. These findings of infarct expansion have been shown to occur in 29% of patients presenting with myocardial infarction within 3 to 14 days and are associated with a high in-hospital mortality (162) as well as an increased incidence of cardiac rupture (165,166).

The prognosis of a patient after dismissal from the hospital after myocardial infarction depends on several variables: presence or absence of ventricular arrhythmias, left ventricular function, progressive ventricular dilation, and residual ischemia. As in the acute myocardial infarction setting, the wall motion score index has been shown by numerous investigators to predict complications in the 1- to 2-year period after dismissal from the hospital (38,43,44,167). The worse the wall motion score index, the greater the amount of myocardial dysfunction, and the poorer the prognosis. Therefore, a predismissal two-dimensional echocardiogram may be used to stratify high-risk patients after myocardial infarction. Although more difficult and time consuming, determination of left ventricular size and volume is more prognostic than wall motion score index alone. We expect variable degree of ventricular expansion for a given wall motion score index depending on the extent of transmural wall thickness involvement with myocardial infarction. Myocardial segments with nontransmural involvement tend to dilate much less than the transmurally infarcted segments, although their wall motions are similarly akinetic. Serial echocardiographic measurements after acute myocardial infarction in the SAVE trial demonstrated that LV dilatation was significantly greater in patients who developed cardiac events compared with that of the patients with no event (168). A major limitation of echocardiographic determination of LV size and volume is that it is not feasible in all patients. Better delineation of the endocardium with the help of contrast or high resolution echocardiography, and automatic border detection may facilitate this important clinical application in future (Figs. 10–16, 10–17).

Of the patients who have remained clinically stable throughout the hospitalization after myocardial infarction, it is important to identify those who may have latent residual ischemia. Low-level exercise testing has been used to identify such patients who have not manifested clinical signs of ischemia during the hospitalization (169,170). The predictive accuracy of exercise testing has been increased by the simultaneous use of imaging modalities that examine wall motion or perfusion before and during exercise. Although there is a growing wealth of information concerning the prognostic value of radionuclide exercise studies (both tomographic thallium and sestamibi imaging), these modalities are not available in all centers treating patients with myocardial infarction.

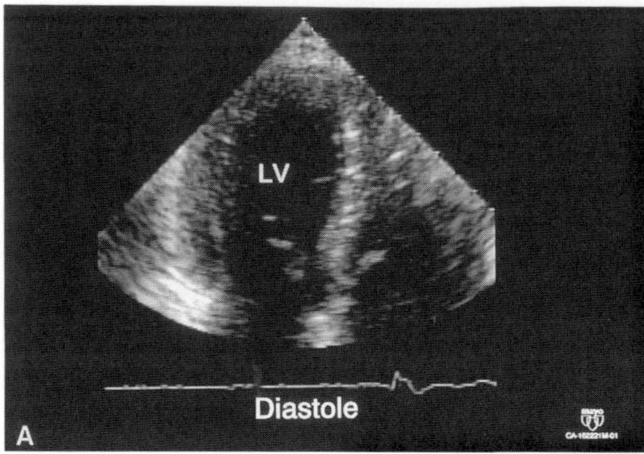

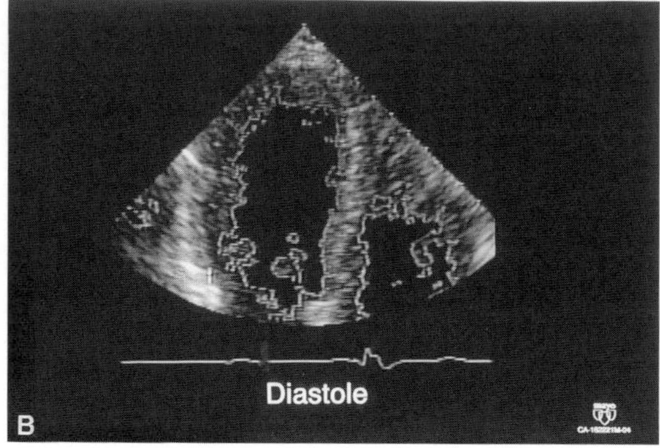

Figure 10–16. **A.** Transthoracic apical four-chamber view showing left ventricular cavity during diastole. **B.** Acoustic quantification (AQ) is applied to the same image as in **A.** Due to the difference in back scatter from the endocardium and from the left ventricular cavity with blood, where significant difference in the back scatter takes place endocardial boundary is defined and connected throughout the region of interest, and it can be used for estimating change in the left ventricular cavity size and volume.

In chronic coronary heart disease, two-dimensional echocardiography has been used in conjunction with treadmill or bicycle stress testing, allowing visualization of global systolic performance and regional wall motion before, during, and immediately after exercise (170–176). The ability of exercise echocardiography to identify exercise-induced ischemia has compared well with that of thallium scanning and radionuclide angiography (177–180). The advent of digitized imaging, allowing side-by-side viewing of preexercise and postexercise images, has made exercise echocardiography into an accurate, reproducible, and easily applicable modality. As opposed to earlier studies, with the newer high-resolution ultrasound equipment, adequate images for analysis can be obtained in more than 90% of patients.

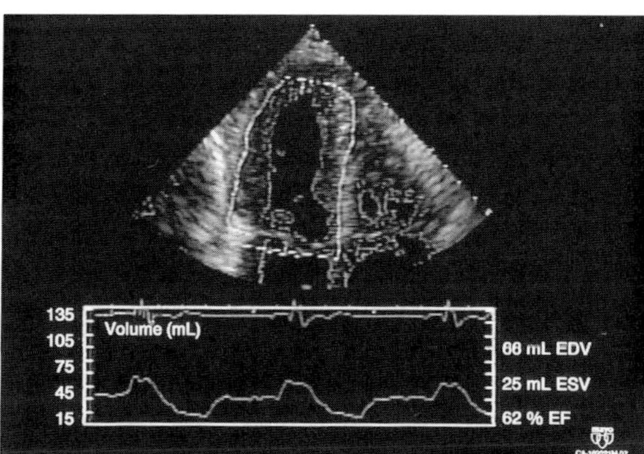

Figure 10–17. From the real-time, automatic border detection of the left ventricular endocardium, end-diastolic and end-systolic volumes are instantaneously determined, so that the ejection fraction can be calculated. In this example, end-diastolic volume of 66 ml and end-systolic volume of 25 ml were calculated, providing an ejection fraction of 62 percent.

In the patient who has had a myocardial infarction and who has resting regional wall abnormalities, there are certain criteria for a positive exercise echocardiographic test: new regional wall abnormalities in a previously normal segment, or marked worsening of wall motion in an area separate from a stable wall motion abnormality. Worsening of a single abnormal segment does not constitute a positive result. With these criteria, the addition of two-dimensional echocardiographic imaging in one study has increased the sensitivity compared with routine electrocardiography from 65% to 95% and specificity from 55% to 80% in predicting ischemic events after myocardial infarction (181). Similarly, the sensitivity and specificity in another study were increased from 55% to 70% and from 67% to 95% in predicting multivessel disease in survivors of myocardial infarction disease (182). Data on exercise echocardiography after myocardial infarction have been limited (181–183a); however, the wide availability of echocardiography will lead to wider utilization of exercise echocardiography in the future.

There are patients who are not able to exercise properly after myocardial infarction because of either orthopedic limitation or generalized disability. Transvenous atrial pacing (184,185) with echocardiographic monitoring has been proposed as a method for evaluating these patients after myocardial infarction (186,187). Transesophageal pacing has been used as a noninvasive modality for increasing heart rate, and the combination of transesophageal pacing and echocardiographic imaging has been useful in these nonambulatory patients after myocardial infarction. However, these modalities are rarely used in clinical practice. Instead, pharmacological stress echocardiography is increasingly utilized as an alternative stress agent. Among several available pharmacological agents, dobutamine is the most reliable and commonly used agent in conjunction with echocardiographic detection of regional wall motion abnormalities (188–190).

Dobutamine stress echocardiography is most helpful soon after myocardial infarction to detect viable myocardium. As discussed earlier in the chapter, the reperfused myocardium soon after acute transmural myocardial infarct may remain akinetic for a period of time (stunned myocardium). Dobutamine at a low dose (10 to 20 mic/kg/min) brings out the contractility of myocardium, and the augmentation of myocardial contractility with infusion of low-dose dobutamine has a reasonable correlation with viability detected by PET and predicts recovery of myocardial contractility, especially after revascularization (74–77, 191–194).

Dobutamine stress echocardiography was performed in the CCU as early as 3 days after infarction in patients with reperfusion therapy, and it was shown to have high sensitivity and specificity for detecting reversible myocardial dysfunction. The most recent study (77) showed that at least in hibernating myocardium, biphasic response predicted recovery of myocardial function after revascularization. During low-dose dobutamine, recruitment of contractile reserve improves wall motion of the dysfunctional myocardium. However, as the dobutamine dose is increased, myocardial ischemia occurs, resulting in worsening of wall motion. Dipyridamole infusion has been used as a pharmacological stress agent in conjunction with echocardiography, mostly in Italy. A large-scale multicenter EPIC (Echo Persantine Italian Cooperative) study (195) showed that dipyridamole stress echocardiography is safe early after uncomplicated myocardial infarction and allows effective risk stratification. However, it does not appear to show any advantage, over dobutamine stress echocardiography. Viable myocardium can be also identified by contrast echocardiography in patients with poor LV function after myocardial infarct (196). However, clinical utility of identifying viable myocardium by low-dose dobutamine or contrast echocardiography requires further clinical investigation (196a,196b).

FUTURE DIRECTIONS

Several areas of investigation in ultrasonography may prove beneficial in the management of a patient with myocardial infarction. There are three areas of special interest in this era of interventional cardiology: contrast echocardiography, tissue characterization, and intravascular ultrasonography.

Contrast echocardiography is an attempt to evaluate perfusion of the myocardium by imaging the heart before and after injection of a contrast solution (196). It has been shown that injection of contrast medium into a coronary artery produces a change in the ultrasonographic appearance of the myocardium, that is, more intensive echoreflectance resulting in a brighter white myocardial image. The area of ultrasonographic change in the myocardium with a selective coronary injection has been shown to be proportional to the area perfused by the coronary artery injected (197–199). By using digitized subtraction images before and after injection of contrast medium, time–intensity curves can be constructed for a region of interest of the myocardium. Analysis of these time–intensity curves has produced parameters that predict coronary flow and myocardial perfusion in animals (200–202). Use of sonicated Renografin results in uniform small microbubbles that cross capillary networks (203,204), and it has been shown to be safe in humans (205,206). Current work is being done with selective coronary injections of sonicated contrast medium, examining time–intensity curves under different flow reserve conditions in humans. The ideal contrast agent would be one that could be injected intravenously, could cross the pulmonary capillary bed, and could be imaged as it enters the coronary circulation. This would provide a noninvasive measure of the amount of myocardium perfused and the degree of perfusion in viable myocardium. A most recent study showed that myocardial contrast echocardiography during cardiac catheterization could define viable myocardial segments in patients with poor LV systolic function caused by myocardial infarction (200). However, not all segments with contrast pattern achieve functional recovery after revascularization. Further studies are needed to determine whether myocardial contrast echocardiography can be used to define management strategies that can favorably alter the outcome in such patients (200). There are numerous new contrast agents being tested, but no one particular agent has been identified as the most useful clinically. A new innovative means to image myocardial contrast agent is "second harmonic" imaging. A preliminary study demonstrated that coronary flow reserve could be determined noninvasively using this contrast imaging (207).

Tissue characterization examines the ultrasonographic characteristics of the myocardium to provide information about myocardial function and viability. Before the advent of two-dimensional echocardiography, it was empirically noted that an increase in echodensity occurred in areas of old myocardial infarction on M-mode echocardiography (208). The increase in acoustic reflections was thought to result from an increase in hydroxyproline synthesis and an increase in collagen content (209). The concept of differing echodensities then evolved into a color-encoded two-dimensional system, and this was found to be useful in detecting old myocardial infarction in animals and humans (209–211). To detect the more rapid changes that occur during ischemia and reperfusion, much of the current work in tissue characterization has focused on ultrasonographic attenuation and back scatter (212–215). It is thought that changes in both myocardial structure and function cause alterations in the physical properties of the tissue that can be quantitated with changes in frequency-dependent ultrasonographic attenuation and back scatter. This is based on the changes in integrated back scatter that occur during the cardiac cycle (213,214). In the presence of ischemia and reperfusion, this cyclic variation of integrated back scatter becomes abnormal but recovers faster than wall thickening in reversible injured myocardium (215). This could have important implications for assessing the effect of acute reperfusion in myocardial infarction in terms of tissue viability.

Intravascular ultrasonography utilizes high-frequency ultrasound transducers mounted on the tip of a catheter inserted directly into an artery (216–218). It carries a minimal risk, and coronary spasm is the most frequent event from a multicenter survey (219). This produces high-resolution images of arterial structure and can quantitate absolute lumen area and determine the type of atherosclerosis plaque present (220–223). Intracoronary thrombus, medial hemorrhage, and plaque dissection that are associated with acute coronary syndrome may be visualized by intravascular ultrasonography (224). This modality, therefore, has the potential for determining severity of a stenosis, guiding interventional catheter-based therapy (225,226), assessing the results of catheter-based therapy, and possibly predicting the response to the different types of catheter-based therapies. Clinical utility of intracoronary imaging has not been, however, established in the setting of acute myocardial infarction.

SUMMARY

Two-dimensional echocardiography and Doppler echocardiography are able to provide valuable information in the patient with myocardial infarction from diagnosis to prognosis. Imaging of wall motion abnormalities is useful in diagnosis and prognosis of a patient, as well as in assessing the need for acute intervention. In the critically ill patient, the cause of the hemodynamic compromise as well as hemodynamic variables can be assessed by the combination of two-dimensional and Doppler echocardiography, especially using a transesophageal window.

Reperfusion attempt by thrombolysis or angioplasty has become a routine practice in patients with acute myocardial infarction. Echocardiography is useful in estimating the amount of myocardium at risk and final infarct size. Furthermore, viability of dysfunctional myocardium can be assessed by dobutamine echocardiography, contrast echocardiography, or a combination of both. Finally, patients' prognosis can be determined by combination of systolic and diastolic function evaluation by 2D/Doppler echocardiography. Echocardiography is, therefore, an essential diagnostic adjunct in patients with acute myocardial infarction to optimize myocardial salvage and to improve patients' long-term survival.

REFERENCES

1. Reeder GS, Seward JB, Tajik AJ: The role of two-dimensional echocardiography in coronary artery disease: A critical appraisal. *Mayo Clin Proc* 1982;57: 247–258.
2. Kloner RA, Parisi AF: Acute myocardial infarction: Diagnostic and prognostic applications of two-dimensional echocardiography (editorial). *Circulation* 1987;75:521–524.
3. Quinones MA: Echocardiography in acute myocardial infarction. *Cardiol Clin* 1984;2:123–134.
4. Oh JK, Miller FA, Shub C, et al: Evaluation of acute chest pain syndromes by two-dimensional echocardiography: Its potential application in the selection of patients for acute reperfusion therapy. *Mayo Clin Proc* 1987;62:59–66.
5. Broderick TM, et al: Comparison of regional and global left ventricular function by serial echocardiograms after reperfusion in acute myocardial infarction. *J Am Soc Echocardiogr* 1989;2:315–323.
6. Kishon Y, et al: Evolution of echocardiographic modalities in detection of postmyocardial infarction ventricular septal defect and papillary muscle rupture: Study of 62 patients. *Am Heart J* 1993;126: 667–675.
7. Tajik AJ, Seward JB, Hagler DJ, et al: Two-dimensional real-time ultrasonic imaging of the heart and great vessels: Technique, image orientation, structure identification, and validation. *Mayo Clin Proc* 1978;53:271–303.
8. Seward JB, Khandheria BK, Oh JK, et al: Transesophageal echocardiography: Technique, anatomic correlations, implementation, and clinical applications. *Mayo Clin Proc* 1988;63:649–680.
9. Oh JK, et al: Transesophageal echocardiography in critically ill patients. *Am J Cardiol* 1990;66: 1492–1495.
10. Nishimura RA, Miller FA Jr, Callahan MJ, et al: Doppler echocardiography: Theory, instrumentation, technique, and application. *Mayo Clin Proc* 1985; 60:321–343.
11. Nishimura RA, Abel MD, Hatle LK, Tajik AJ: Assessment of diastolic function of the heart: Background and current applications of Doppler echocardiography: II. Clinical Studies. *Mayo Clin Proc* 1989;64:181–204.
12. Tennant R, Wiggers CJ: The effect of coronary occlusion on myocardial contraction. *Am J Physiol* 1935;112:351–361.
13. Wyatt HL, Forrester JS, Tyberg JV, et al: Effect of graded reduction in regional coronary perfusion on regional and total cardiac function. *Am J Cardiol* 1975;36:185–192.
14. Kerber RE, Abboud FM: Echocardiographic detection of regional myocardial infarction: An experimental study. *Circulation* 1973;47:997–1005.
15. Corya BC, Rasmussen S, Knoebel SB, et al: Echocardiography in acute myocardial infarction. *Am J Cardiol* 1975;36:1–10.
16. Kerber RE, Marcus ML, Abboud FM: Echocardiography in experimentally-induced myocardial ischemia. *Am J Med* 1977;63:21–28.
17. Pandian NG, Kerber RE: Two-dimensional echocardiography in experimental coronary stenosis: I. Sensitivity and specificity in detecting transient myocardial dyskinesis: Comparison with sonomicrometers. *Circulation* 1982;66:597–602.
18. Pandian NG, Kieso RA, Kerber RE: Two-dimensional echocardiography in experimental coronary stenosis: II. Relationship between systolic wall thinning and regional myocardial perfusion in severe coronary stenosis. *Circulation* 1982;66: 603–611.
19. Lieberman AN, Weiss JL, Jugdutt BI, et al: Two-dimensional echocardiography and infarct size: Relationship of regional wall motion and thickening to the extent of myocardial infarction in the dog. *Circulation* 1981;63:739–746.
20. Wyatt HL, Meerbaum S, Heng MK, et al: Experimental evaluation of the extent of myocardial dysynergy and infarct size by two-dimensional echocardiography. *Circulation* 1981;63:607–614.
21. Homans DC, Asinger R, Elsperger KJ, et al: Regional function and perfusion at the lateral border of ischemic myocardium. *Circulation* 1985;71:1038–1047.
22. Alam M, Khaja F, Bryumer J, et al: Echocardiographic evaluation of left ventricular function during coronary artery angioplasty. *Am J Cardiol* 1986;57: 20–25.

23. Teichholz LE, Cohen MV, Sonnenblick EH, Gorlin R: Study of left ventricular geometry and function by B-scan ultrasonography in patients with and without asynergy. *N Engl J Med* 1974;291:1220–1226.
24. Heger JJ, Weyman AE, Wann LS, et al: Cross-sectional echocardiography in acute myocardial infarction: Detection and localization of regional left ventricular asynergy. *Circulation* 1979;60: 531–538.
25. Heger J, Weyman AE, Noble R, et al: An analysis of the site, extent, and hemodynamic consequences of acute myocardial infarction by cross-sectional echocardiography (abstract). *Circulation* 1977;56 (Suppl III): III–152.
26. Heger JJ, Weyman AE, Wann LS, et al: Cross-sectional echocardiographic analysis of the extent of left ventricular asynergy in acute myocardial infarction. *Circulation* 1980;61:1113–1118.
27. Weiss JL, Bulkley BH, Hutchins GM, Mason SJ: Two-dimensional echocardiographic recognition of myocardial injury in man: Comparison with postmortem studies. *Circulation* 1981;63:401–408.
28. Wyatt HL, Forrester JS, da Luz PL, et al: Functional abnormalities in nonoccluded regions of myocardium after experimental coronary occlusion. *Am J Cardiol* 1976;37:366–372.
29. Braunwald E, Kloner RA: The stunned myocardium prolonged, post-ischemic ventricular dysfunction. *Circulation* 1982;66:1146–1149.
30. Oh JK, Gersh BJ, Nassef LA Jr, et al: Effects of acute reperfusion on regional myocardial function: Serial two-dimensional echocardiography assessment. *Int J Cardiol* 1989;22:161–168.
31. Schuster EH, Bulkley BH: Ischemia at a distance after acute myocardial infarction: A cause of early postinfarction angina. *Circulation* 1980;62:509–515.
32. Haendchen RV, Wyatt HL, Maurer G, et al: Quantitation of regional cardiac function by two-dimensional echocardiography: I. Patterns of contraction in the normal left ventricle. *Circulation* 1983;67: 1234–1245.
33. Gibson DG, Doran JH, Traill TA, Brown DJ: Regional abnormalities of left ventricular wall movement during isovolumic relaxation in patients with ischemic heart disease. *Eur J Cardiol* 1978;7(Suppl): 251–264.
34. Weyman AE, Franklin TD Jr, Hogan RD, et al: Importance of temporal heterogeneity in assessing the contraction abnormalities associated with acute myocardial ischemia. *Circulation* 1984;70:102–112.
35. Kisslo JA, Robertson D, Gilbert BW, et al: A comparison of real-time, two-dimensional echocardiography, and cineangiography in detecting left ventricular asynergy. *Circulation* 1977;55:134–141.
36. Ohuchi Y, Kuwako K, Umeda T, Machii K: Real-time, phased-array, cross-sectional echocardiographic evaluation of left ventricular asynergy and quantitation of left ventricular function: A comparison with left ventricular cineangiography. *Jpn Heart J* 1980;21:1–15.
37. Shiina A, Tajik AJ, Smith HC, et al: Prognostic significance of regional wall motion abnormality in patients with prior myocardial infarction: A prospective correlative study of two-dimensional echocardiography and angiography. *Mayo Clin Proc* 1986;61: 254–262.
38. Van Reet RE, Quinones MA, Poliner LR, et al: Comparison of two-dimensional echocardiography with gated radionuclide ventriculography in the evaluation of global and regional left ventricular function in acute myocardial infarction. *J Am Coll Cardiol* 1984;3:243–252.
39. Bhatnagar SK, Al-Yusuf AR, Nawaz MK, et al: Left ventricular function of survivors of a first complicated acute myocardial infarction. A prehospital discharge cross-sectional echocardiographic study. *Int J Cardiol* 1988;19:67–80.
40. Gibson RS, Bishop HL, Stamm RB, et al: Value of early two-dimensional echocardiography in patients with acute myocardial infarction. *Am J Cardiol* 1982;49:1110–1119.
41. Nishimura RA, Tajik AJ, Shub C, et al: Role of two-dimensional echocardiography in the prediction of in-hospital complications after acute myocardial infarction. *J Am Coll Cardiol* 1984;4:1080–1087.
42. Horowitz RS, Morganroth J: Immediate detection of early high-risk patients with acute myocardial infarction using two-dimensional echocardiographic evaluation of left ventricular regional wall motion abnormalities. *Am Heart J* 1982;103:814–822.
43. Bhatnagar SK, Moussa MAA, Al-Yusuf AR: The role of prehospital discharge two-dimensional echocardiography in determining the prognosis of survivors of first myocardial infarction. *Am Heart J* 1985;109:472–477.
44. Kan G, Visser CA, Koolen JJ, Dunning AJ: Short and long term predictive value of admission wall motion score in acute myocardial infarction: A cross sectional echocardiographic study of 345 patients. *Br Heart J* 1986;56:422–427.

45. Schiller NB, Shah PM, Crawford M, et al: Recommendations for quantitation of the left ventricle by two-dimensional echocardiography. *J Am Soc Echocardiogr* 1989;2:358–367.

46. Oh JK, Gibbons RJ, Christian TF, et al: Correlation of regional wall motion abnormalities detected by two-dimensional echocardiography with perfusion defect determined by technetium-99m sestamibi imaging in patients treated with reperfusion therapy during acute myocardial infarction. *Am Heart J* 1996; 131(1):32–7.

47. Feigenbaum H: Digital recording, display, and storage of echocardiograms. *J Am Soc Echocardiogr* 1988; 5:378–383.

48. Tortoledo FA, Quinones MA, Fernandez CG, et al: Quantification of left ventricular volumes by two-dimensional echocardiography: A simplified and accurate approach. *Circulation* 1983;67:579–584.

49. Quinones MA, Waggoner AD, Reduto LA, et al: A new, simplified, and accurate method for determining ejection fraction with two-dimensional echocardiography. *Circulation* 1981;64:744–753.

50. Starling MR, Crawford MH, Sorensen SG, et al: Comparative accuracy of apical biplane cross-sectional echocardiography and gated equilibrium radionuclide angiography for estimating left ventricular size and performance. *Circulation* 1981;63: 1075–1084.

51. Baran AO, Rogal GJ, Nanda NC: Ejection fraction determination without planimetry by two-dimensional echocardiography: A new method. *J Am Coll Cardiol* 1983;1:1471–1478.

52. Zoghbi WA, Charlat ML, Bolli R, et al: End-systolic radius to thickness ratio: An echocardiographic index of regional performance during reversible myocardial ischemia in the conscious dog. *J Am Coll Cardiol* 1987;10:1113–1121.

53. Parisi AF, Moynihan PF, Folland ED, Feidman CL: Quantitative detection of regional left ventricular contraction abnormalities by two-dimensional echocardiography: II. Accuracy in coronary artery disease. *Circulation* 1981;63:761–767.

54. Force T, Kemper AJ, Bloomfield P, et al: Non–Q wave perioperative myocardial infarction: Assessment of the incidence and severity of regional dysfunction with quantitative two-dimensional echocardiography. *Circulation* 1985;72:781–789.

55. Zoghbi WA, Charlat ML, Bolli R, et al: Quantitative assessment of left ventricular wall motion by two-dimensional echocardiography: Validation during reversible ischemia in the conscious dog. *J Am Coll Cardiol* 1988;11:851–860.

56. Zoghbi WA, Haichin RN, Cheirif J, et al: Echocardiographic quantitation of regional wall motion in the thrombolysis in acute myocardial infarction (TIMI) trial-phase II: Preliminary observations (abstract). *J Am Coll Cardiol* 1988;11:195A.

57. Wilkins GT, Southern JF, Choong CY, et al: Correlation between echocardiographic endocardial surface mapping of abnormal wall motion and pathologic infarct size in autopsied hearts. *Circulation* 1988;77: 978–987.

58. Guyer DE, Gibson TC, Gillam LD, et al: A new echocardiographic model for quantifying three-dimensional endocardial surface area. *J Am Coll Cardiol* 1986;8:819–829.

59. Guyer DE, Foale RA, Gillam LD, et al: An echocardiographic technique for quantifying and displaying the extent of regional left ventricular dyssynergy. *J Am Coll Cardiol* 1986;8:830–835.

60. Visser CA, Lie KI, Kan G, et al: Detection and quantification of acute, isolated myocardial infarction by two-dimensional echocardiography. *Am J Cardiol* 1981;47:1020–1025.

61. Short D: The earliest electrocardiographic evidence of myocardial infarction. *Br Heart J* 1970;32: 6–15.

62. Blanke H, Cohen M, Schlueter GU, Karsch KR, Rentrop KP: Electrocardiographic and coronary arteriographic correlations during acute myocardial infarction. *Am J Cardiol* 1984;54:249–255.

63. Weigarten SR, Ermann B, Riedinger MS, et al: Selecting the best triage rule for patients hospitalized with chest pain. *Am J Med* 1989;87:494–500.

64. Puleo PR, Meyer D, Wathen C, et al: Use of a rapid assay of subforms of creatine kinase MB to diagnose or rule out acute myocardial infarction. *N Engl J Med* 1994;331:561–566.

65. Hilton TC, Thompson RC, Williams HJ, et al: Technetium-99m sestamibi myocardial perfusion imaging in the emergency room evaluation of chest pain. *J Am Coll Cardiol* 1994;23:1016–1022.

66. Oh JK, et al: Role of two-dimensional echocardiography in the emergency room. *Echocardiography* 1985;3:217–226.

67. Sabia P, et al: Value of regional wall motion abnormality in the emergency room diagnosis of acute myocardial infarction: A prospective study using two-dimensional echocardiography. *Circulation* 1991;84(Suppl I):85–92.

68. Gibler WB, Runyon JP, Levy RC, et al: A rapid diagnostic and treatment center for patients with chest pain in the emergency department. *Ann Emerg Med* 1995;25:1–8.
69. Trippi JA, Lee KS, Kopp G, et al: Emergency echocardiography telemedicine: an efficient method to provide 24-hour consultative echocardiography. *J Am Coll Cardiol* 1996;27:1748–52.
70. Asinger RW, Mikell FL, Elsperger KJ, et al: Serial changes in left ventricular wall motion by two-dimensional echocardiography following anterior myocardial infarction. *Am Heart J* 1988;116: 50–58.
71. Bourdillon PDV, Broderick TM, Williams ES, et al: Early recovery of regional left ventricular function after reperfusion in acute myocardial infarction assessed by serial two-dimensional echocardiography. *Am J Cardiol* 1989;63:641–646.
72. Miller JG, Perez JE, Sobel BE: Ultrasonic characterization of myocardium. *Prog Cardiovasc Dis* 1985;28: 85–110.
73. Molunski MR, Mohr GA, Perez JE, et al: Ultrasonic tissue characterization with integrated backscatter: Acute myocardial ischemia, reperfusion, and stunned myocardium in patients. *Circulation* 1989;80: 491–503.
74. Pierard LA, et al: Identification of viable myocardium by echocardiography during dobutamine infusion in patients with myocardial infarction after thrombolytic therapy: Comparison with positron emission tomography. *J Am Coll Cardiol* 1990;15: 1021–1031.
75. Cigarroa CG, et al: Dobutamine stress echocardiography identifies hibernating myocardium and predicts recovery of left ventricular function after coronary revascularization. *Circulation* 1993;88: 430–436.
76. Watada H, Ito H, Oh H, et al: Dobutamine stress echo predicts reversible dysfunction and quantitates the extent of irreversibly damaged myocardium after reperfusion of anterior myocardial infarction. *J Am Coll Cardiol* 1994;24:624–630.
77. Afridi I, Kleiman NS, Raizner AE, et al: Dobutamine echocardiography in myocardial hibernation. Optimal dose and accuracy in predicting recovery of ventricular function after coronary angioplasty. *Circulation* 1995;91:663–670.
78. Goldberg RJ, Gore JM, Alpert JS, et al: Cardiogenic shock after acute myocardial infarction. *N Engl J Med* 1991;325:1117–1122.
79. Hochman JS, Boland J, Sleeper LA, et al: Current spectrum of cardiogenic shock and effect of early revascularization on mortality. Results of an international registry. *Circulation* 1995;91:873–881.
80. Foster E, Schiller NB: The role of transesophageal echocardiography in critical care: UCSF experience. *J Am Soc Echocardiogr* 1992;5:368–374.
81. Hwang JJ, Shyu KG, Chen JJ, et al: Usefulness of transesophageal echocardiography in the treatment of critically ill patients. *Chest* 1993;104: 861–866.
82. Chenzbraun A, Pinto FJ, Schnittiger I, et al: Transesophageal echocardiography in the intensive care unit: Impact on diagnosis and decision-making. *Clin Cardiol* 1994;17:438–444.
83. Pearson AC, Castello R, Labovitz AJ: Safety and utility of transesophageal echocardiography in the critically ill patient. *Am Heart J* 1990;119:1083.
84. Font VE, Obarski TP, Klein AL, et al: Transesophageal echocardiography in the critical care unit. *Cleve Clin J Med* 1991;58:315–322.
85. Khoury AF, Afridi I, Quinones MA, Zoghbi WA: Transesophageal echocardiography in critically ill patients: Feasibility, safety, and impact on management. *Am Heart J* 1994;127:1363–1371.
86. Zehender M, Kasper W, Kauder E, et al: Right ventricular infarction as an independent predictor of prognosis after acute inferior myocardial infarction. *N Engl J Med* 1993;328:981–988.
87. Kinch JW, Ryan TJ: Right ventricular infarction. *N Engl J Med* 1994;330:1211–1217.
88. D'Arcy B, Nanda NC: Two-dimensional echocardiographic features of right ventricular infarction. *Circulation* 1982;65:167–173.
89. Panidis IP, Ren J-F, Kotler MN, et al: Two-dimensional echocardiographic estimation of right ventricular ejection fraction in patients with coronary artery disease. *J Am Coll Cardiol* 1983;2:911–918.
90. Arditti A, Lewin RF, Hellman C, et al: Right ventricular dysfunction in acute inferoposterior myocardial infarction: An echocardiographic and isopic study. *Chest* 1985;87:307–314.
91. Bellamy GR, Rasmussen HH, Nasser FN, et al: Value of two-dimensional echocardiography, electrocardiography, and clinical signs in detecting right ventricular infarction. *Am Heart J* 1986;112: 304–309.
92. Lopez-Sendon J, Garcia-Fernandez MA, Coma-Canella I, et al: Segmental right ventricular function after acute myocardial infarction: Two-dimen-

sional echocardiographic study in 63 patients. *Am J Cardiol* 1983;51:390–396.

93. Vatterott PJ, Nishimura RA, Gersh BJ, Smith HC: Severe isolated tricuspid insufficiency in coronary artery disease. *Int J Cardiol* 1987;14:295–301.

94. Fujii J, Yazaki Y, Sawada H, et al: Noninvasive assessment of left and right ventricular filling in myocardial infarction with a two-dimensional Doppler echocardiographic method. *J Am Coll Cardiol* 1985;5: 1155–1160.

95. Isobe M, Yazaki Y, Takaku F, et al: Right ventricular filling detected by pulsed Doppler echocardiography during the convalescent stage of inferior wall acute myocardial infarction. *Am J Cardiol* 1987;59: 1245–1250.

96. Lin SS, Oh JK, Tajik AJ, et al: Right-to-left shunts in patients with severe hypoxemia; transesophageal contrast echocardiography study. *J Am Coll Cardiol* 1995;17A(901–53).

97. Vlodaver Z, Edwards JE: Rupture of ventricular septum or papillary muscle complicating myocardial infarction. *Circulation* 1977;55:815–822.

98. Nishimura RA, Schaff HV, Shub C, et al: Papillary muscle rupture complicating acute myocardial infarction: Analysis of 17 patients. *Am J Cardiol* 1983;51:373–377.

99. Radford MJ, Johnson RA, Daggett WM Jr, et al: Ventricular septal rupture: A review of clinical and physiological features and an analysis of survival. *Circulation* 1981;64:545–553.

100. Nishimura RA, Schaff HV, Gersh BJ, et al: Early repair of mechanical complications after acute myocardial infarction. *JAMA* 1986;256:47–50.

101. Montoya A, McKeever L, Scanlon P, et al: Early repair of ventricular septal rupture after infarction. *Am J Cardiol* 1980;45:345–348.

102. Lemery R, Smith HC, Giuliani ER, Gersh BJ: Prognosis in rupture of the ventricular septum after acute myocardial infarction and role of early surgical intervention. *Am J Cardiol* 1992;70: 147–151.

103. Califf RB, Bengston JR: Cardiogenic shock. *N Engl J Med* 1994;330:1724–1730.

104. Kishon Y, Oh JK, Schaff HV, et al: Mitral valve operation in post-infarction papillary muscle rupture: Immediate results and long-term follow-up of 22 patients. *Mayo Clin Proc* 1992;67: 1023–1030.

105. Nishimura RA, Shub C, Tajik AJ: Two-dimensional echocardiographic diagnosis of partial papillary muscle rupture. *Br Heart J* 1982;48: 598–600.

106. Patel AM, Miller FA, Khandheria BK, et al: Role of transesophageal echocardiography in the diagnoses of papillary muscle rupture secondary to myocardial infarction. *Am Heart J* 1989;6: 1330–1333.

107. Nishimura RA, Tajik AJ: Determination of left-sided pressure gradients by utilizing Doppler aortic and mitral regurgitation signals: Validation by simultaneous dual catheter and Doppler studies. *J Am Coll Cardiol* 1988;11:317–321.

108. Scanlan JG, Seward JB, Tajik AJ: Visualization of ventricular septal rupture utilizing wide-angle two-dimensional echocardiography. *Mayo Clin Proc* 1979;54:381–384.

109. Farcot JC, Boisante L, Rigaud M, et al: Two dimensional echocardiographic visualization of ventricular septal rupture after acute anterior myocardial infarction. *Am J Cardiol* 1980;45:370–377.

110. Rogers EW, Glassman RD, Feigenbaum H, et al: Aneurysms of the posterior intraventricular septum with ventricular septal defect. *Chest* 1980;78: 741–746.

111. Bishop HL, Gibson RS, Stamm RB, et al: Role of two-dimensional echocardiography in the evaluation of patients with ventricular septal rupture postmyocardial infarction. *Am Heart J* 1981;102: 965–971.

112. Drobac M, Gilbert B, Howard R, et al: Ventricular septal defect after myocardial infarction: Diagnosis by two-dimensional contrast echocardiography. *Circulation* 1983;67:335–341.

113. Richards KL, Hoekenga DE, Leach JK, Blaustein JC: Doppler cardiographic diagnosis of interventricular septal rupture. *Chest* 1979;76:101–103.

114. Eisenberg PR, Barzilai B, Perez JE: Noninvasive detection by Doppler echocardiography of combined ventricular septal rupture and mitral regurgitation in acute myocardial infarction. *J Am Coll Cardiol* 1984;4: 617–620.

115. Recusani F, Raisaro A, Sgalambro A, et al: Ventricular septal rupture after myocardial infarction: Diagnosis by two-dimensional and pulsed Doppler echocardiography. *Am J Cardiol* 1984;54: 277–281.

116. Miyaake K, Okamota M, Kinoshita N, et al: Doppler echocardiographic features of ventricular septal rupture in myocardial infarction. *J Am Coll Cardiol* 1985;5:182–187.

117. Smith G, Endresen K, Sivertssen E, Semb G: Ventricular septal rupture diagnosed by simultaneous cross-sectional echocardiography and Doppler ultrasound. *Eur Heart J* 1985;6:631–636.

118. Sohn DW, Shin GJ, Oh JK, et al: Role of transesophageal echocardiography in hemodynamically unstable patients. *Mayo Clin Proc* 1995;70: 925–931.

119. Oliva PB, Hammill SC, Edwards WD: Cardiac rupture, a clinically predictable complication of acute myocardial infarction: Report of 70 cases with clinicopathologic correlations. *J Am Coll Cardiol* 1993;22:720–726.

120. Lopez-Sendon J, Gonzalez A, de sa Lopez E, et al: Diagnosis of subacute ventricular wall rupture after acute myocardial infarction: Sensitivity and specificity of clinical, hemodynamic and echocardiographic criteria. *J Am Coll Cardiol* 1992;19: 1145–1153.

121. Callahan JA, Seward JB, Tajik AJ, et al: Pericardiocentesis assisted by two-dimensional echocardiography. *J Thorac Cardiovasc Surg* 1983;85: 877–879.

122. Pierard LA, Albert A, Henrard L, et al: Incidence and significance of pericardial effusion in acute myocardial infarction as determined by two-dimensional echocardiography. *J Am Coll Cardiol* 1986;8:517–520.

123. Appleton CP, Hatle LK, Popp RL: Cardiac tamponade and pericardial effusion: Respiratory variation in transvalvular flow velocities studied by Doppler echocardiography. *J Am Coll Cardiol* 1988;11:1020–1030.

124. Burstow DJ, Oh JK, et al: Cardiac tamponade: Characteristic pulsed-wave Doppler observations. *Mayo Clin Proc* 1989;64:312–324.

125. Reeder GS, Tajik AJ, Seward JB: Left ventricular mural thrombus: Two-dimensional echocardiographic diagnosis. *Mayo Clin Proc* 1981;56:82–86.

126. DeMaria AN, Bommer W, Neumann A, et al: Left ventricular thrombi identified by cross-sectional echocardiography. *Ann Intern Med* 1979;90:14–18.

127. Asinger RW, Mikell FL, Elspeger J, Hodges M: Incidence of left ventricular thrombosis after acute transmural myocardial infarction: Serial evaluation by two-dimensional echocardiography. *N Engl J Med* 1981;305:297–302.

128. Asinger RW, Mikell FL, Sharma B, et al: Observations on detecting left ventricular thrombus with two dimensional echocardiography: Emphasis on avoidance of false positive diagnoses. *Am J Cardiol* 1981; 47:145–156.

129. Stratton JR, Lighty GW Jr, Pearlman AS, Ritchie JL: Detection of left ventricular thrombus by two dimensional echocardiography: Sensitivity, specificity, and causes of uncertainty. *Circulation* 1982; 66: 156–166.

130. Spirito P, Bellotti P, Chiarella F, et al: Prognostic significance and natural history of left ventricular thrombi in patients with acute anterior myocardial infarction: A two-dimensional echocardiographic study. *Circulation* 1985;72:774–780.

131. Nihoyannopoulos P, Smith GC, Maseri A, Foale RA: The natural history of left ventricular thrombus in myocardial infarction: A rationale in support of masterly inactivity. *J Am Coll Cardiol* 1989;14:903–911.

132. Hilden T, Iversen K, Raaschou F, Schwartz M: Anticoagulants in acute myocardial infarction. *Lancet* 1961;2:327–331.

133. Veterans Administration Hospital Investigators: Anticoagulants in acute myocardial infarction: Results of a cooperative clinical trial. *JAMA* 1973; 225:724–729.

134. Haugland JM, Asinger RW, Mikell FL, et al: Embolic potential of left ventricular thrombi detected by two-dimensional echocardiography. *Circulation* 1984;70:588–598.

135. Stratton JR, Resnick AD: Increased embolic risk in patients with left ventricular thrombi. *Circulation* 1987;75:1004–1011.

136. Visser CA, Kan G, Meltzer RS, et al: Embolic potential of left ventricular thrombus after myocardial infarction: A two dimensional echocardiographic study of 119 patients. *J Am Coll Cardiol* 1985;5:1276–1280.

137. Jugdutt BI, Sivaram CA, Wortman C, et al: Prospective two dimensional echocardiographic evaluation of left ventricular thrombus after embolism after acute myocardial infarction. *J Am Coll Cardiol* 1989;13:554–564.

138. Held AC, Gore JM, Paraskos J, et al: Impact of thrombolytic therapy on left ventricular mural thrombi in acute myocardial infarction. *Am J Cardiol* 1988;62:310–311.

139. Eigler N, Mauer G, Shah PK: Effect of early systemic thrombolytic therapy on left ventricular mural thrombus formation in acute anterior myocardial infarction. *Am J Cardiol* 1984;54: 261–263.

140. Forrester JS, Diamond G, Chatterjee K, Swan HJC: Medical therapy of acute myocardial infarction by application of hemodynamic subsets. *N Engl J Med* 1976;295:1356–1362, 1404–1413.

141. Foote GA, Schabel SI, Hodges M: Pulmonary complications of flow-directed balloon-tipped catheter. *N Engl J Med* 1974;290:927–931.

142. Hatle L, Angelsen B: *Doppler Ultrasound in Cardiology: Physical Principles and Clinical Applications.* Philadelphia, Lea & Febiger, 1982.

143. Zoghbi WA, Quinones MA: Determination of cardiac output by Doppler echocardiography: A critical appraisal. *Herz* 1986;11:258–268.

144. Nishimura RA, Tajik A: Measurement of intracardiac pressures. State of the art—1986. *Herz* 1986;11:283–290.

145. Nishimura RA, Callahan MJ, Schaff HV, et al. Noninvasive measurement of cardiac output by continuous-wave Doppler echocardiography: Initial experience and review of the literature. *Mayo Clin Proc* 1984;59:484–489.

146. Chandraratna PA, Nanna M, McKay C, et al: Determination of cardiac output by transcutaneous continuous-wave ultrasonic Doppler computer. *Am J Cardiol* 1984;53:234–237.

147. Nishimura RA: Another measurement of cardiac output: Is it truly needed? *J Am Coll Cardiol* 1989;13:1393–1394.

148. Currie PJ, Seward JB, Chan KL, et al: Continuous wave Doppler determination of right ventricular pressure: A simultaneous Doppler catheterization study in 127 patients. *J Am Coll Cardiol* 1985;6:750–756.

149. Izumi S, Miyatake K, Beppu S, et al: Mechanism of mitral regurgitation in patients with myocardial infarction: A study using real-time two dimensional Doppler flow imaging and echocardiography. *Circulation* 1987;76:777–785.

150. Barzilai B, Gessler C Jr, Perez JE, et al: Significance of Doppler-detected mitral regurgitation in acute myocardial infarction. *Am J Cardiol* 1988;61: 220–223.

151. Lehmann, KG, et al: Mitral regurgitation in early myocardial infarction: Incidence, clinical detection, and prognostic implications. *Ann Intern Med* 1992;117.10–17.

152. Tcheng JE, et al: Outcome of patients sustaining acute ischemic mitral regurgitation during myocardial infarction. *Ann Intern Med* 1992;117: 18–24.

153. Labovitz AJ, Pearson AC: Evaluation of left ventricular diastolic function: Clinical relevance and recent Doppler echocardiographic insights. *Am Heart J* 1987;114:836–851.

154. DeMaria AN, Wisenbaugh T: Identification and treatment of diastolic dysfunction: Role of transmitral Doppler recordings. *J Am Coll Cardiol* 1987; 9:1106–1107.

155. Gaasch WH, Cole JS, Quinones MA, Alexander JK: Dynamic determinants of left ventricular diastolic pressure volume relations in man. *Circulation* 1975;51:317–323.

156. Brutsaert DL, Rademakers FE, Sys SU: Triple control of relaxation: Implications in cardiac disease. *Circulation* 1984;69:190–196.

157. Nishimura RA, Abel MD, Housmans PR, et al: Mitral flow velocity curves as a function of different loading conditions: Evaluation by intraoperative transesophageal echocardiography. *J Am Soc Echocardiogr* 1989;2:79–87.

157a. Heidenreich PA, Stainback RF, Redberg RF, et al: Transesophageal echocardiography predicts mortality in critically ill patients with unexplained hypotension. *J Am Coll Cardiol* 1995;26:152–8.

157b. Giannuzzi P, Imparato A, Temporelli PL, et al: Doppler-derived mitral deceleration time of early filling as a strong predictor of pulmonary capillary wedge pressure in postinfarction patients with left ventricular systolic dysfunction. *J Am Coll Cardiol* 1994;23:1630–7.

157c. Cecconi M, Manfrin M, Zanoli R, et al: Doppler echocardiographic evaluation of left ventricular end-diastolic pressure in patients with coronary artery disease. *J Am Soc Echocardiogr* 1996;9: 241–50.

158. Nishimura RA, Abel MD, Hatle LK, Tajik AJ: Relationship of pulmonary vein to mitral flow velocities by transesophageal Doppler echocardiography: Effect of different loading conditions. *Circulation* 1990;981:1488–1497.

158a. Kuecherer HF, Kusumoto F, Muhuideen IA, et al. Pulmonary venous flow patterns by transesophageal pulsed Doppler echocardiography: relation to parameters of left ventricular systolic and diastolic function. *Am Heart J* 1991;122: 1683–93.

159. Rossvoll O, Hatle LK: Pulmonary venous flow velocities recorded by transthoracic Doppler, relations to LV diastolic pressures. *J Am Coll Cardiol* 1993;21:1687–1696.

160. Appleton CP, Galloway JM, Gonzalez MS, Gaballa M, Basnight MA: Estimation of left ventricular filling pressures using two-dimensional and Doppler echocardiography in adult cardiac patients: Additional value of analyzing left atrial size, left atrial ejection fraction and the difference in the duration of pulmonary venous and mitral flow velocities at atrial contraction. *J Am Coll Cardiol* 1993;22:1972–1982.

161. Oh JK, Ding ZP, Gersh BJ, et al: Restrictive left ventricular diastolic filling identifies the patients with heart failure after acute myocardial infarction. *J Am Soc Echocardiogr* 1992;5:497–503.

162. Eaton LW, Weiss JL, Bulkley BH, et al: Regional cardiac dilatation after acute myocardial infarction: Recognition by two-dimensional echocardiography. *N Engl J Med* 1979;300:57–62.

163. Maisel AS, Ahnve S, Gilpin E, et al: Prognosis after extension of myocardial infarct: The role of Q wave or non Q wave infarction. *Circulation* 1985;71:211–217.

164. Hutchins GM, Bulkley BH: Infarct expansion versus extension: Two different complications of acute myocardial infarction. *Am J Cardiol* 1978; 41:1127–1132.

165. Schuster EH, Bulkley BH: Expansion of transmural myocardial infarction: A pathophysiologic factor in cardiac rupture. *Circulation* 1979;60: 1532–1538.

166. Jugdutt BI, Michorowski BL: Role of infarct expansion in rupture of the ventricular septum after acute myocardial infarction: A two-dimensional echocardiographic study. *Clin Cardiol* 1987;10: 641–652.

167. Nishimura RA, Reeder GS, Miller FA Jr, et al: Prognostic value of predischarge 2-dimensional echocardiogram after acute myocardial infarction. *Am J Cardiol* 1984;53:429–432.

168. St. John Sutton M, Pfeffer MA, Plappert T, et al: Quantitative two dimensional echocardiographic measurements are major predictors of adverse cardiovascular events after acute myocardial infarction. The protective effects of captopril. *Circulation* 1994;89:68–75.

169. Theroux P, Waters DD, Halphen C, et al: Prognostic value of exercise testing soon after myocardial infarction. *N Engl J Med* 1979;301: 341–345.

170. Koppes GM, Kruyer W, Beckmann CH, Jones FG: Response to exercise early after uncomplicated acute myocardial infarction in patients receiving no medication: Long-term follow-up. *Am J Cardiol* 1980;46:764–769.

171. Wann LS, Faris JV, Childress RH, et al: Exercise cross-sectional echocardiographic in ischemic heart disease. *Circulation* 1979;60:1300–1308.

172. Morganroth J, Chen CC, David D, et al: Exercise cross-sectional echocardiographic diagnosis of coronary artery disease. *Am J Cardiol* 1981;47: 20–26.

173. Maurer G, Nanda NC. Two-dimensional echocardiographic evaluation of exercise-induced left and right ventricular asynergy. Correlation with thallium scanning. *Am J Cardiol* 1981;48: 720–727.

174. Crawford MH, Amon KW, Vance WS. Exercise 2-dimensional echocardiography: Quantitation of left ventricular performance in patients with severe angina pectoris. *Am J Cardiol* 1983;51:1–6.

175. Limacher MC, Quinones MA, Poliner LR, et al: Detection of coronary artery disease with exercise two-dimensional echocardiography. Descriptionof a clinically applicable method and comparison with radionuclide ventriculography. *Circulation* 1983;67:1211–1218.

176. Heng MK, Simard M, Lake R, et al: Exercise two-dimensional echocardiography for diagnosis of coronary artery disease. *Am J Cardiol* 1984;54:502–507.

177. Robertson WS, Feigenbaum H, Armstrong WF, et al: Exercise echocardiography: A clinically practical addition in the evaluation of coronary artery disease. *J Am Coll Cardiol* 1983;2: 1085–1091.

178. Quinones MA, Verani MS, Haichin RM et al: Exercise echocardiography versus^{201} T1 single photon emission computed tomography in evaluation of coronary artery disease: analysis of 292 patients. *Circulation* 1992;85:1026–1031.

179. Pozzoli MM, Fioretti PM, Salustri A, et al: Exercise echocardiography and technetium-99m MIBI single-photon emission computed tomography in the detection of coronary artery disease. *Am J Cardiol* 1991;67:350–355.

180. Roger VL, Pellikka PA, Oh JK, et al: Stress echocardiography. Part I. Exercise echocardiography: tech-

niques, implementation, clinical applications and correlations. *Mayo Clin Proc* 1995;70:5–15.

181. Ryan T, Armstrong WF, O'Donnell JA, Feigenbaum H: Risk stratification after acute myocardial infarction by means of exercise two-dimensional echocardiography. *Am Heart J* 1987;114: 1305–1316.

182. Jaarsma W, Visser CA, Kupper AJF, et al: Usefulness of two-dimensional exercise echocardiography shortly after myocardial infarction. *Am J Cardiol* 1986;57:86–90.

183. Applegate RJ, Dellitalia LJ, Crawford MH: Usefulness of two-dimensional echocardiography during low-level exercise testing early after uncomplicated acute myocardial infarction. *Am J Cardiol* 1987;60:10–14.

183a. Quintana M, Lindvall K, Ryden L, et al: Prognostic value of predischarge exercise stress echocardiography after acute myocardial infarction. *Am J Cardiol* 1995;76:1115–1121.

184. McKay RG, Aroesty JM, Heller GV, et al: The pacing stress test reexamined: Correlation of pacing induced hemodynamic changes with the amount of myocardium at risk. *J Am Coll Cardiol* 1984;3:1469–1481.

185. Heller GV, Aroesty JM, McKay RG, et al: The pacing stress test: A reexamination of the relation between coronary artery disease and pacing induced electrocardiographic changes. *Am J Cardiol* 1984;54:50–55.

186. Tzivoni D, Gottlieb S, Keren A, et al: Early right atrial pacing after myocardial infarction: I. Comparison with early treadmill testing. *Am J Cardiol* 1984;53:414–417.

187. Tzivoni D, Gottlieb S, Keren A, et al: Early right atrial pacing after myocardial infarction: II. Results in 77 patients with predischarge angina pectoris, congestive heart failure, or age older than 70 years. *Am J Cardiol* 1984;53:418–420.

188. Sawada SG, Segar DS, Ryan T, et al: Echocardiographic detection of coronary artery disease during dobutamine infusion. *Circulation* 1991;83: 1605–1614.

189. Marwick T, Willemart B, D'Hondt AM, et al: Selection of the optimal nonexercise stress for the evaluation of ischemic regional myocardial dysfunction and malperfusion: Comparison of dobutamine and adenosine using echocardiography and 99mTc-MIBI single photon emission computed tomography. *Circulation* 1993;87: 345–354.

190. Pellikka PA, Roger VL, Oh JK, Miller FA, Seward JB, Tajik AJ: Stress echocardiography. Part II. Dobutamine stress echocardiography: Techniques, implementation, clinical applications, and correlations. *Mayo Clin Proc* 1995;70:16–27.

191. Smart SC, Sawada S, Ryan T, et al: Low-dose dobutamine echocardiography detects reversible dysfunction after thrombolytic therapy of acute myocardial infarction. *Circulation* 1993;88: 405–415.

192. Sklenar J, Ismail S, Villanueva FS, et al: Dobutamine echocardiography for determining the extent of myocardial salvage after reperfusion. An experimental evaluation. *Circulation* 1994;90: 1502–1512.

193. Barilla F, Gheorghiade M, Alam M, Khaja F, Goldstein S: Low-dose dobutamine in patients with acute myocardial infarction identifies viable but not contractile myocardium and predicts the magnitude of improvement in wall motion abnormalities in response to coronary revascularization. *Am Heart J* 1991;122:1522–1531.

194. Previtali M, Poli A, Lanzarini L, et al: Dobutamine stress echocardiography for assessment of myocardial viability and ischemia in acute myocardial infarction treated with thrombolysis. *Am J Cardiol* 1993;72:124G–130G.

195. Picano E, Pingitore A, Sicari R, et al: Stress echocardiographic results predict risk of reinfarction early after uncomplicated acute myocardial infarction: large-scale multicenter study. Echo Persantine International Cooperative (EPIC) Study Group. *J Am Coll Cardiol* 1995;26(4): 908–13.

196. Feinstein SB: Myocardial perfusion imaging: Contrast echocardiography today and tomorrow. *J Am Coll Cardiol* 1986;8:251–253.

196a. Chan RKM, Lee KJ, Calafiore P, et al: Comparison of dobutamine echocardiography and positron emission tomography in patients with chronic ischemic left ventricular dysfunction. *J Am Coll Cardiol* 1996;27:1601 7.

196b. Arnese M, Cornel JH, Salustri A, et al: Prediction of improvement of regional left ventricular function after surgical revascularization: a comparison of low-dose dobutamine echocardiography with T1-201 single-photon emission computed tomography. *Circulation* 1995;91:2748–52.

197. Kaul S, Pandian NG, Okada RD, et al: Contrast echocardiography in acute myocardial ischemia: I. In vivo determination of total left ventricular "area of risk." *J Am Coll Cardiol* 1984;4:1272–1282.

198. Kaul S, Glasheen WP, Oliner JD, Kelly P, Gascho JA: Relation between anterograde blood flow through a coronary artery and the size of the perfusion bed it supplies: Experimental and clinical implications. *J Am Coll Cardiol* 1991;17: 1403–1413.

199. Sabia PJ, Powers ER, Jayaweera AR, Ragosta M, Kaul S: Functional significance of collateral blood flow in patients with recent acute myocardial infarction: A study using myocardial contrast echocardiography. *Circulation* 1992;85:2080–2089.

200. Camarano G, Ragosta M, Gimple LW, Powers ER, Kaul S: Identification of viable myocardium with contrast echocardiography in patients with poor left ventricular systolic function caused by recent or remote myocardial infarction. *Am J Cardiol* 1995;75:215–219.

201. Kemper AJ, Force T, Kloner R, et al: Contrast echocardiographic estimation of regional myocardial blood flow after acute coronary occlusion. *Circulation* 1985;72:1115–1124.

202. Cheirif J, Zoghbi WA, Bolli R, et al: Assessment of regional myocardial perfusion by contrast echocardiography: II. Detection of changes in transmural and subendocardial perfusion during dipyridamole-induced hyperemia in a model of critical coronary stenosis. *J Am Coll Cardiol* 1989;14:1555–1565.

203. Feinstein SB, Shah PM, Bing RJ, et al: Microbubble dynamics visualized in the intact capillary circulation. *J Am Coll Cardiol* 1984;4:595–600.

204. Cheirif J, Yamamoto H, Zoghbi WA, et al: Demonstration of physiological transit time of sonicated meglumine diatrizoate in a microvascular preparation. *J Cardiovasc Ultrasonogr* 1987;6: 245–247.

205. Moore CA, Smucker ML, Kaul S: Myocardial contrast echocardiography in humans: I. Safety—a comparison with routine coronary arteriography. *J Am Coll Cardiol* 1986;8:1066–1072.

206. Cheirif J, Zoghbi WA, Raizner AE, et al: Assessment of myocardial perfusion in humans by contrast echocardiography: I. Evaluation of regional coronary reserve by peak contrast intensity. *J Am Coll Cardiol* 1988;11:735–743.

207. Mulvagh SL, Foley DA, Klarich KK, Aeschbacher BC, Tei C, Seward JB: Visualization of coronary arteries and measurement of coronary blood flow with transthoracic echocardiography after intravenous administration of a new echocardiographic contrast agent. *J Am Coll Cardiol* 1995;special issue:228A (752–6).

208. Rasmussen S, Corya BC, Feigenbaum H, Knoebel SB: Detection of myocardial scar tissue by M-mode echocardiography. *Circulation* 1978; 57:230–237.

209. Parisi AF, Nieminen M, O'Boyle JE, et al: Enhanced detection of the evolution of tissue changes after acute myocardial infarction using color-encoded two-dimensional echocardiography. *Circulation* 1982;66:764–770.

210. Skorton DJ, Melton HE, Jr, Pandian NG, et al: Detection of acute myocardial infarction in closed chest dogs by analysis of regional two-dimensional echocardiographic gray-level distributions. *Circ Res* 1983;52:36–44.

211. Chandraratna PAN, Ulene R, Nimalasuriya A, et al: Differentiation between acute and healed myocardial infarction by signal averaging and color encoding two-dimensional echocardiography. *Am J Cardiol* 1985;56:381–384.

212. Mimbs JW, Yuhas DE, Miller JG, et al: Detection of myocardial infarction in vitro based on altered attenuation of ultrasound. *Circ Res* 1977;41: 192–198.

213. Sagar KB, Rhyne TL, Warltier DC, et al: Intramyocardial variability in integrated backscatter: Effects of coronary occlusion and reperfusion. *Circulation* 1987;75:436–442.

214. Fitzgerald PJ, McDaniel MD, Rolett EL, et al: Two-dimensional ultrasonic tissue characterization: Backscatter power, endocardial wall motion, and their phase relationship for normal, ischemic, and infarcted myocardium. *Circulation* 1987;76: 850–859.

215. Wickline SA, Thomas LJ III, Miller JG, et al: Sensitive detection of the effects of reperfusion on myocardium by ultrasonic tissue characterization with integrated backscatter. *Circulation* 1986;74: 389–400.

216. Yock PG, Johnson EL, Linker DT: Intravascular ultrasound: Development and clinical potential. *Am J Cardiac Imaging* 1988;2:185–193.

217. Pandian NG: Intravascular and intracardiac ultrasound imaging: An old concept, now on the road to reality. *Circulation* 1989;80:1091–1094.

218. Pandian NG, Kreis A, Brockway B, et al: Ultrasound angioscopy: Real-time, two-dimensional, intraluminal ultrasound imaging of blood vessels. *Am J Cardiol* 1988;62:493–494.

219. Nishimura RA, Edwards WD, Warnes CA, et al: Intravascular ultrasound. Pathologic correlation: Lessons for the future (abstract). *Circulation* 1989;80(Suppl II):II-580.

220. Hodgson JM, Reddy KG, Suneja R, Nair RN, Lesnefsky EJ, Sheehan HM: Intracoronary ultrasound imaging: Correlation of plaque morphology with angiography, clinical syndrome and procedural results in patients undergoing coronary angioplasty. *J Am Coll Cardiol* 1993;21:35–44.

221. Tobis JM, Mallery J, Mahon D, et al: Intravascular ultrasound imaging of human coronary arteries in vivo: Analysis of tissue characterization with comparison to in vitro histological specimens. *Circulation* 1991;83:913–926.

222. Nissen SE, Gurley JC, Grines CL, et al: Intravascular ultrasound assessment of lumen size and wall morphology in normal subjects and patients with coronary artery disease. *Circulation* 1991;84:1087–1099.

223. Fitzgerald PJ, Ports TA, Yock PG: Contribution of localized calcium deposits to dissection after angioplasty: An observational study using intravascular ultrasound. *Circulation* 1992;86:64–70.

224. Mizuno K, Satomura K, Miyamoto A, et al: Angioscopic evaluation of coronary-artery thrombi in acute coronary syndromes. *N Engl J Med* 1992;326:287–291.

225. Ellis SG, DeCesare NB, Pinkerton CA, et al: Relation of stenosis morphology and clinical presentation to the procedural results of directional coronary atherectomy. *Circulation* 1991;84:644–653.

226. Safian RD, Gelbfish JS, Eray RE, Schnitt SJ, Schmidt DA, Baim DS: Coronary atherectomy: Clinical, angiographic, and histologic findings and observations regarding potential mechanisms. *Circulation* 1990;82:69–79.

11

Radionuclide Imaging in Acute Myocardial Infarction

George A. Beller, MD, FACC

Radionuclide imaging techniques performed at rest or with exercise or pharmacologic stress have proven clinically useful in the evaluation of patients with suspected or proven acute myocardial infarction (1–4). These noninvasive modalities can assist in the diagnosis of acute infarction, determination of myocardial "area at risk" distal to an occluded coronary artery, assessment of the efficacy of coronary reperfusion strategies, in distinguishing irreversible from reversible regional left ventricular asynergy in the infarct zone, determination of infarct size, and identification of inducible ischemia within or remote from the infarct zone. The emergence of quantitative single-photon emission computed tomographic (SPECT) imaging and the introduction of new technetium-99*m* (^{99m}Tc)-labeled perfusion imaging agents have enhanced accuracy of infarct size determination and improved the process of risk stratification. Both rest and redistribution thallium-201 (^{201}Tl) imaging and positron emission tomography (PET) imaging of flow and myocardial metabolism have permitted a more accurate assessment of myocardial viability in postinfarction patients, leading to better selection of patients who would benefit most from revascularization. Both conventional SPECT imaging techniques and PET can identify stunned and hibernating myocardium in patients with acute infarction.

Equilibrium or first-pass radionuclide angiography provides the capability to serially evaluate global and regional left ventricular function noninvasively after acute infarction. This permits identification of patients with significant left ventricular dysfunction after infarction who may be at high risk for an adverse outcome after hospital discharge, particularly if extensive regional asynergy reflects irreversible myocardial injury. Echocardiography is, perhaps, better suited for the comprehensive assessment of global and regional left ventricular function after infarction, and dobutamine stress echocardiography has yielded useful clinical information relative to preserved viability in the region of infarction. Table 11–1 lists the various nuclear cardiology techniques presently available or under investigation that have clinical applicability in patients with acute myocardial infarction.

PRINCIPLES AND TECHNIQUES OF MYOCARDIAL PERFUSION IMAGING

Introduction

There are presently two major approaches to imaging of regional myocardial blood flow with ra-

Table 11–1. Radionuclide Imaging Techniques in Patients With Acute Myocardial Infarction

1. Detection, localization and sizing of acute infarction
   a. SPECT thallium-201 or technetium-99*m* sestamibi imaging at rest
   b. Indium-111 antimyosin antibody imaging
   c. Technetium-99*m* pyrophosphate imaging
2. Assessment of myocardial viability
   a. Rest and delayed SPECT thallium-201 imaging
   b. Rest SPECT technetium-99*m* sestamibi imaging
   c. Iodine-123 phenylpentadecanoic acid (IPPA) imaging
   d. Positron emission tomography of perfusion and metabolism
3. Evaluation of left ventricular function
   a. First-pass radionuclide angiography
   b. Equilibrium gated radionuclide angiography
4. Detection of residual ischemia and multivessel coronary artery disease
   a. Exercise SPECT thallium-201 or technetium-99*m* sestamibi imaging
   b. Dipyridamole, adenosine or dobutamine thallium-201 or technetium-99*m* sestamibi imaging

SPECT = single-photon emission computed tomography.

dionuclides. These are ^{201}Tl or ^{99m}Tc sestamibi imaging using planar or SPECT techniques and PET with either rubidium-82 (^{82}Rb), nitrogen-13 ammonia ($^{13}NH_3$), or oxygen-15 water. These radionuclides concentrate in myocardium in proportion to blood flow and the myocardial extraction fraction for each tracer (5–12). When these agents are administered intravenously, their uptake by heart muscle approximates the fraction of the cardiac output perfusing the total myocardial mass. These perfusion tracers must first traverse the capillary wall, interstitial space, and muscle cell membrane before entering the cell, where they either equilibrate with a monovalent cation pool (for example, ^{201}Tl, ^{82}Rb) or bind to mitochondrial membranes (^{99m}Tc sestamibi). Both passive and active transport processes are operative.

For the radionuclide monovalent cations, the active transport system involves adenosine triphosphate (ATP)-dependent sodium–potassium exchange mechanisms. A diminution in regional blood flow, a functional or structural alteration in cell membrane transport activity, or a lack of ATP production would result in abnormally reduced uptake of ^{201}Tl, ^{82}Rb, or $^{13}NH_3$. Sarcolemmal membrane injury or irreversible alterations in intracellular metabolism would affect the myocardial uptake of ^{99m}Tc-labeled agents such as sestamibi and tetrofosmin, which do not require Na^+, K^+, -ATPase activity for myocardial sequestration. When the radionuclide monovalent cations and ^{99m}Tc-labeled perfusion agents are administered under conditions of myocardial ischemia or infarction, those regions that are either underperfused, irreversibly injured, or scarred appear as initial "defects" in tracer uptake on both planar or tomographic images.

Instrumentation

The majority of nuclear cardiology laboratories currently employ SPECT imaging, rather than planar imaging, for myocardial perfusion scintigraphy. Single-photon emission computed tomographic imaging yields images of tomograms of the heart without significant interference of activity from noncardiac or overlapping myocardial regions (13–15). The tomographic approach is an improvement over the planar approach in contrast resolution and assists in the enhanced detection of small regions of hypoperfusion (for example, subendocardial infarction). Because SPECT images are free of background, defect contrast is higher, and the size of defects is made greater by tomographic reconstructed views. With this improvement in contrast resolution is some loss in spatial resolution.

Tomographic SPECT imaging is best accomplished with a large field-of-view gamma camera equipped with a low-energy, general-purpose collimator. Detector orbits can be elliptical or circular and can either be 180° or 360° arcs. The 180° orbit is characterized by high spatial and contrast resolution, whereas the 360° orbit is associated with enhanced field uniformity. Typically, in a 180° orbit, the camera makes 32 or 64 stops for 40 seconds, acquiring each image. Each of the projections is corrected for field nonuniformity and for misalignment of the mechanical center of rotation with respect to the reconstruction matrix.

After the orbit is complete, the series of images taken at different angles around the patient are "back projected" into the transverse axial images, which are slices that are oriented perpendicular to the axis of rotation. Transverse tomograms are reconstructed from the apex of the heart to the base.

Typically, short-axis, horizontal long-axis, and vertical long-axis tomograms are reconstructed. Figure 11–1 is an example of normal SPECT ^{99m}Tc sestamibi tomograms in a patient with chest pain. This study was acquired utilizing a three-headed SPECT camera. This three-headed system has certain advantages, including extremely high resolution, and by using fan-beam or cone-beam collimators, both spatial resolution and sensitivity are enhanced (16). In the future, attenuation correction will be possible employing the SPECT technique (17).

Sensitivity and specificity of SPECT perfusion imaging are enhanced by employing quantitative computer-assisted analyses (18). One of the most common approaches for quantitating myocardial perfusion on SPECT imaging is two-dimensional polar maps (19). These polar maps are constructed by mapping sequential maximal-count circumferential profiles, ranging from apex to base of the heart, into successive rings on the polar map. The apex is placed in the center of the map, and the base is displayed at the periphery. This polar map is also referred to as a bull's-eye plot, which consists of

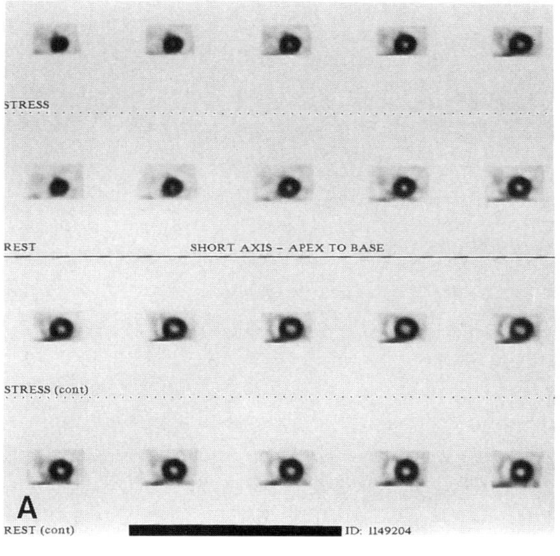

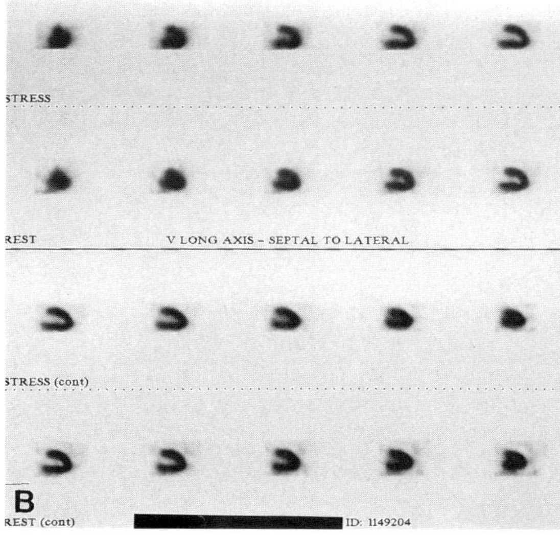

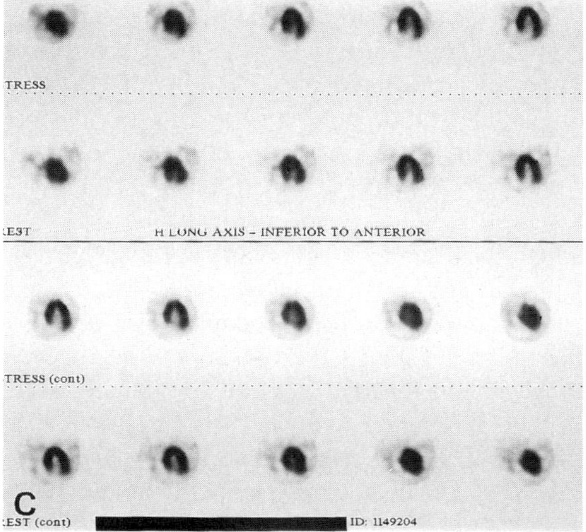

Figure 11–1. **A.** Stress and rest short-axis ^{99m}Tc sestamibi tomograms from apex (upper left images) to base (lower right images) in a normal patient. **B.** Stress and rest vertical long-axis tomograms from the septum (upper left images) to the lateral wall (lower right images) in the same normal patient. **C.** Stress and rest horizontal long-axis tomograms from inferior (upper left images) to superior (lower right images) projections in the same normal patient.

a series of 15 concentric circles made up from the 15 profiles interpreted from the 12 slices from apex to base. Bull's-eyes are constructed for stress and delayed images and can be normalized using normal patient databases, or regional activity can be expressed as a percent of maximal activity in the bull's-eye plot. Mean values and standard deviations are derived from the normal population for each of the angular locations in each of the 15 profiles. Comparing each patient's bull's-eye with a gender-matched normal file results in the conversion of the bull's-eye into a standard deviation map displaying pixels color-coded to the number of standard deviations away from normal. Color Plate 7 shows a bull's-eye polar map display of a patient with a significant left anterior descending coronary artery obstruction. The resting bull's-eye plot shows partial reversibility of this defect.

Technetium-99*m*-labeled perfusion agents can be utilized in conjunction with the SPECT technique to obtain gated tomograms where end-systolic and end-diastolic images can be viewed for assessment of systolic thickening (20,20a). Areas of hypoperfusion that show preserved systolic thickening on gated tomograms indicate presence of resting viability. Color Plate 8 shows a normal gated ^{99m}Tc sestamibi SPECT study where end-diastolic images are shown on the left columns and end-systolic images are shown in the right columns. Note the uniform systolic thickening in all myocardial regions. Normal thickening is indicated by enhanced brightness of the myocardial walls as well as by diminution in the left ventricular cavity size at end-systole.

Gated tomography is also valuable in differentiating artifact from scar, particularly in women who display some persistent hypoperfusion in the anterior wall on stress and rest images. Such diminution of activity could represent artifact from breast attenuation or a prior myocardial scar. Demonstration of normal systolic thickening of the anterior wall on gated tomograms would provide evidence that the defect is artifactual and due to breast attenuation. Similarly, there is often evidence for a reduction in tracer activity in the high posterobasal segment that is secondary to attenuation of activity. Demonstration of normal systolic thickening of the posterior wall, in a patient demonstrating persistent diminution in activity in this region on both stress and rest images, would lend support to the determination of artifact rather than posterior wall scar.

Radionuclide Imaging Agents

Thallium-201

Thallium-201 is still the most commonly utilized agent for myocardial perfusion imaging, both in patients with chest pain and in patients with a recent myocardial infarction. Thallium-201 is a metallic element in group IIIA of the periodic table. It decays by electron capture with a 73-hour half-life. Its principal photo peaks are at 135 and 167 keV, and it emits mercury x-rays of 69 to 83 keV. The 80-keV x-ray is at the low end of the energy spectrum for resolution with a gamma scintillation camera. Thus scintigraphy is most often undertaken with a high-resolution, low-energy collimator and a gamma scintillation camera.

After intravenous injection, the early myocardial uptake of ^{201}Tl is directly proportional to regional blood flow and the extraction of ^{201}Tl by the myocardium (5,6,21,22). The extraction fraction, defined as the percentage of the dose of ^{201}Tl extracted by the myocardium in the first pass through the heart after intracoronary injection, is in the range of 85%. As with all other diffusible radionuclides, at high myocardial blood flow, the extraction of ^{201}Tl diminishes (23,24). There is a slight diminution in extraction of ^{201}Tl with acidosis and hypoxemia (6). Drugs such as propranolol and digitalis have little effect on myocardial extraction.

Extraction of ^{201}Tl (as well as ^{99m}Tc sestamibi) is unaltered in stunned myocardium characterized by postischemic dysfunction after reperfusion or by a chronic low-flow state resulting in ischemic alterations in systolic function (Fig. 11–2) (25–29). Similarly, extraction of ^{201}Tl is not altered by transient decreases in coronary perfusion pressure as long as sarcolemmal membrane integrity remains intact (29). All data available to date suggest that extraction of ^{201}Tl by the myocardial cell is not appreciably diminished until irreversible membrane injury occurs (30). Thus, in the absence of necrosis or severe ischemia, defects observed on myocardial scintigrams reflect alterations in blood flow rather

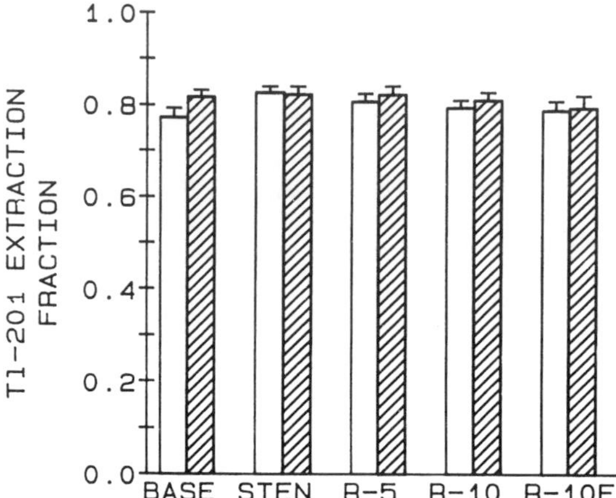

Figure 11–2. First-pass ^{201}Tl extraction fraction in control (open bars) and stunned (cross-hatched bars) dogs. The stunned group underwent ten, 5-minute transient left anterior descending coronary artery (LAD) occlusions interspersed by 10 minutes of reflow. (BASE = baseline; STEN = critical stenosis; R-5 = after the fifth transient occlusion and reflow; R-10 = after the tenth transient occlusion and reflow; R-10E = 40 minutes after the tenth reperfusion.) At R-10 in the stunned dogs, complete absence of thickening in the LAD perfusion zone was evident. Note that no alteration of ^{201}Tl extraction fraction is observed compared with the sham-operated control animals (open bars). *Reprinted from Moore et al (26), with permission.*

than metabolic dysfunction of the membrane transport system in the presence of intact perfusion. When defects are observed with resumption of normal blood flow (for example, after reperfusion), one can deduce that irreversible cellular injury has occurred or that there is a persistent abnormality in microcirculatory nutrient flow or abnormal flow reserve because of endothelial dysfunction. For example, persistence of abnormal myocardial uptake of ^{201}Tl can be seen soon after successful coronary angioplasty and has been attributed to reversible alterations in endothelial function (abnormal flow reserve) or alterations in flow at the microcirculatory level (31–33).

Following the initial myocardial uptake phase after intravenous injection, there is a continuous exchange of myocardial ^{201}Tl and ^{201}Tl in the blood pool that recirculates from the systemic compartment (21,29,34–38). Thallium-201 is continually washing out of normally perfused myocardium and replaced by recirculating ^{201}Tl from residual activity in the blood pool (24). This process of continuous exchange forms the basis of the phenomenon designated as ^{201}Tl "redistribution." Redistribution or delayed defect resolution is observed when the radionuclide is administered during transient underperfusion of the myocardium or with a chronic reduction in myocardial blood flow (rest redistribution) (28,39).

With respect to myocardial imaging in patients, redistribution is designated as either "total" or "partial" resolution of early defects as assessed by repeat imaging at 2½ to 4 hours after ^{201}Tl administration. For example, when ^{201}Tl is injected during peak exercise or after dipyridamole-induced vasodilation, a heterogeneity of ^{201}Tl uptake will be observed if one vessel is perfused by a significantly stenotic artery and the other major coronary arteries have no significant narrowings. When the resting state is achieved soon after exercise, there is a restoration of relatively homogeneous flow to normal myocardium and to myocardium perfused by the stenotic artery. This delayed redistribution occurs because ^{201}Tl is washed out of the normal myocardium and accumulates or exhibits slow washout from the previously underperfused or ischemic segment.

In the instance of dipyridamole or adenosine infusion, there may be a transmural coronary steal in the stenotic region, where flow absolutely decreases in subendocardial layers with a minimal increase in the subepicardial zones (40–42). Total transmural flow may be unchanged; however, flow in the distribution of normally perfused myocardium will increase three- to fivefold. When ^{201}Tl or any other radionuclide is injected under these conditions of flow heterogeneity, a defect in the stenotic region will be noted (40). Delayed redistribution of ^{201}Tl occurs after dipyridamole-induced ischemia, comparable with what is observed with exercise stress.

Some patients may not demonstrate substantial evidence for delayed redistribution until 12 to 24 hours after ^{201}Tl administration (43,44). This observation is of clinical importance, as some defects that appear to be persistent at 2 to 4 hours actually represent viable myocardium and not scar or recent necrosis. Recently, the ability to distinguish between reversible ischemia and scar by ^{201}Tl scintigraphy has been enhanced by the administration of a second resting dose of ^{201}Tl after the 4-hour redistribution image has been obtained (45–49). The reinjection of this second dose in the resting state has yielded results that are comparable with or superior to those achieved with 24-hour redistribution imaging (50). Some persistent defects on 4-hour redistribution images that have some residual viability will show total or partial defect resolution after the repeat resting injection.

Thallium-201 redistribution over time, when the tracer is injected in the resting state, can be observed under conditions of a chronic reduction in regional blood flow as with a severe coronary stenosis (39,51–56). The mechanism for "rest redistribution" with chronic underperfusion is both a diminution in the initial uptake of ^{201}Tl after intravenous injection and a decrease in the intrinsic ^{201}Tl washout rate. There is a significantly slower washout of ^{201}Tl over time from myocardial zones perfused by the high-grade stenosis compared with the washout from the nonischemic region. These disparate washout rates from hypoperfused and normal myocardium result in near normalization of ^{201}Tl activity at approximately 3 to 4 hours. Figure 11–3 depicts an example of rest ^{201}Tl redistribution on serial myocardial images.

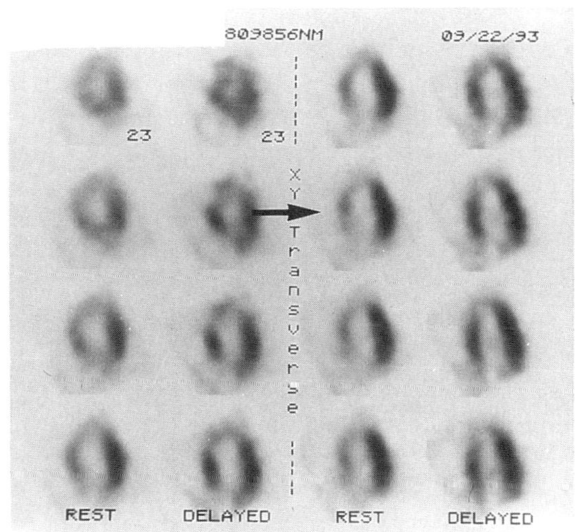

Figure 11–3. Rest and delayed rest ^{201}Tl horizontal long-axis tomograms in a patient with a severe left anterior descending coronary artery stenosis and asynergy of the anterior wall, apex, and septum. Note the initial reduction in ^{201}Tl activity in the anteroseptal region on the resting image (arrow), which shows substantial rest ^{201}Tl redistribution on the delayed image.

As previously mentioned, when ^{201}Tl is administered intravenously under conditions of a myocardial scar or acute necrosis, a persistent defect, defined as no change in defect magnitude or size on serial imaging, can be observed. Partial redistribution can be seen when there is a mixture of necrosis and ischemic myocardium in the presence of some preserved antegrade flow or physiologically relevant collateral flow. It should again be emphasized that some mild persistent defects, where ^{201}Tl activity is reduced by no more than 50% compared with nonischemic activity, may represent hypoperfused but viable areas of myocardium (53,57). If such mild persistent defects are observed in the presence of intact regional systolic function and lack of Q waves on the electrocardiogram, the presence of viable myocardium should be suspected.

Reverse ^{201}Tl redistribution is defined as the appearance of a defect for the first time on delayed images, when the initial uptake appeared relatively homogeneous. This type of defect pattern is being observed more frequently with the advent of thrombolytic therapy (58). When ^{201}Tl is injected during exercise testing in a patient who previously underwent successful reperfusion with a thrombolytic agent or after angioplasty, there may be significant exercise-induced enhancement of blood flow in the subepicardial regions of the infarct zone that remain viable. This increased uptake in the hyperemic epicardial region prevents the identification of the zone of subendocardial necrosis. There is subsequently more rapid ^{201}Tl clearance from this epicardial zone compared with normal zone washout, which then yields a significant defect for the first time in the infarct region on the delayed scintigrams. Reverse redistribution may also represent an artifact secondary to normal ^{201}Tl washout from an area of apical thinning, which would yield the "false" appearance of a defect in this region on the delayed image.

Technetium-99m Sestamibi

Technetium-99*m* sestamibi (^{99m}Tc hexakis 2-methoxyisobutyl isonitrile) is a ^{99m}Tc-labeled isonitrile. It is a lipophilic cationic ^{99m}Tc complex that, like ^{201}Tl, is taken up by the myocardium in proportion to regional blood flow (7–9,27,28,59,–61).

Technetium-99*m* sestamibi demonstrates negligible redistribution after transient myocardial ischemia, and separate injections of the radionuclide are required during stress and rest to distinguish between ischemia and irreversible myocardial injury (17,60). Figure 11–4 depicts exercise and rest ^{99m}Tc sestamibi SPECT images in a patient with a severe proximal stenosis of the left anterior descending coronary artery.

Although the first-pass myocardial extraction of ^{99m}Tc sestamibi is less efficient than that of ^{201}Tl, the relative myocardial uptakes of both tracers are similar under physiologic flow conditions (62).

The absence of significant redistribution and the relatively slow myocardial clearance of ^{99m}Tc sestamibi are favorable characteristics for SPECT studies, in which data acquisition requires 30 minutes (63–65). Postexercise imaging is performed 30 minutes and resting imaging is performed 60 minutes after injection of ^{99m}Tc sestamibi, to permit liver and pulmonary activity to clear sufficiently for optimum visualization of the myocardium. Intracellular transport of ^{99m}Tc sestamibi involves passive distribution across plasma and mitochondrial membranes. After an equilibrium state is reached, ^{99m}Tc sestamibi is sequestered largely within mitochondria by the large negative transmembrane potentials (66,67). When plasma or mitochondrial membrane potentials are depolarized, net uptake of ^{99m}Tc sestamibi is inhibited and the radionuclide cannot be retained. Mitochondrial membrane depolarization is the feature of irreversible myocyte injury. Metabolic derangements simulating ischemia or hypoxia result in diminished ^{99m}Tc sestamibi uptake. Technetium-99*m* sestamibi retention in myocardial cells depends on viability of both mitochondrial and plasma membranes (66,67,68). Under constant flow conditions, sodium cyanide, a cytochrome C oxidase inhibitor, and Triton X-100, a sarcolemmal membrane detergent, reduces peak

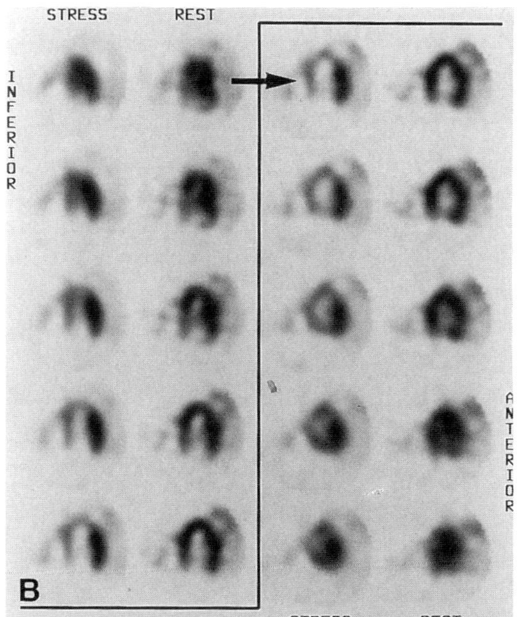

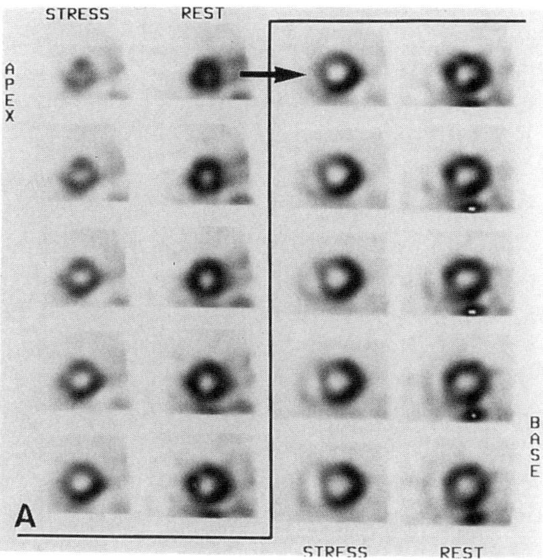

Figure 11–4. A. Stress and rest short-axis tomograms depicting a reversible anteroseptal defect (arrow). The defect extends from the apical slices (upper left) to the basilar slices (lower right). This patient had a significant stenosis of the left anterior descending coronary artery. **B.** Horizontal long-axis ^{99m}Tc sestamibi tomograms in the same patient whose short-axis tomograms are shown in **A.** Note the severe defect in the septum (arrow), which demonstrates complete reversibility on the resting study. The tomograms are displayed from the inferior region (upper left) to the anterior region (lower right).

accumulation of 99^{m}Tc sestamibi and results in loss of cellular retention of the agent.

Beller et al (69) showed that, in intact dogs, 99^{m}Tc sestamibi cellular retention depends on myocardial viability. Technetium-99*m* sestamibi was administered intravenously to dogs at baseline under normal conditions, after which the left anterior descending coronary artery was occluded for 3 hours and then reperfused for another 3 hours. In animals occluded for 3 hours, a subsequent 3-hour period of reflow resulted in loss of 99^{m}Tc sestamibi in the endocardial zone of the ischemic region to 40% of the nonischemic level (Fig. 11–5). This loss corresponded to sustained elevation of coronary sinus 99^{m}Tc sestamibi activity during the reflow period. Thus an ischemic insult causing myocardial membrane injury causes myocytes to "dump" 99^{m}Tc sestamibi into the coronary sinus venous effluent.

Further evidence that myocardial 99^{m}Tc sestamibi uptake depends on cellular viability is that

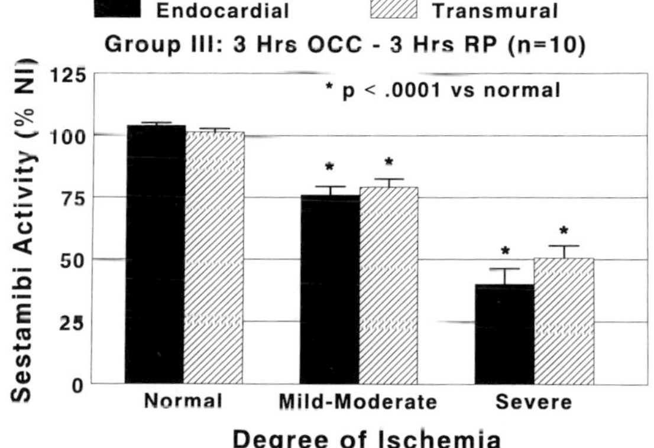

Figure 11–5. Endocardial and transmural ^{99m}Tc sestamibi activity (percent nonischemic [NI]) in 10 dogs that underwent total occlusion of the left anterior descending coronary artery for 3 hours (Hrs) followed by 3 hours of reperfusion (RP). Myocardial samples were grouped with respect to the degree of hypoperfusion during the phase of total occlusion. In these experiments, ^{99m}Tc sestamibi was administered intravenously prior to coronary occlusion. Note the significant loss of ^{99m}Tc sestamibi activity after occlusion and reperfusion in zones subjected to severe ischemia. This loss in myocardial activity corresponded to a significant efflux of ^{99m}Tc sestamibi in the coronary sinus. These experiments suggest loss of intracellular retention of ^{99m}Tc sestamibi following a severe ischemic insult. *Reprinted from Beller et al (69), with permission.*

such uptake is not significantly affected either by myocardial stunning or by sustained low-flow ischemia ("short-term hibernation"). Experiments performed in dogs with a 50% reduction in left anterior descending coronary artery flow demonstrate almost comparable 99^{m}Tc sestamibi and ^{201}Tl uptake in the asynergic zone perfused by the severely stenotic vessel (61). Despite severe systolic dysfunction, 99^{m}Tc sestamibi uptake was greater than 50% of normal uptake in the perfusion zone of the left anterior descending artery. Thus postischemic dysfunction attributed to stunning or sustained low-flow ischemia does not appear to substantially affect 99^{m}Tc sestamibi uptake as long as myocardial cells remain viable.

Technetium-99m Teboroxime

Technetium-99*m* teboroxime is a neutral lipophilic agent that is in the class of compounds designated as boronic acid adducts of technetium oximes (BATO compounds) (70–74). Technetium-99*m* teboroxime uptake is not dependent upon active sarcolemmal membrane transport, and images predominantly reflect regional blood blow. It has an extremely short myocardial half-life, approximately 12 minutes. This mandates a rapid SPECT acquisition protocol (75). Serial 99^{m}Tc teboroxime imaging may be useful for determining if reflow was accomplished following reperfusion therapy (76). This agent cannot be employed for assessment of myocardial viability and should be considered solely for the noninvasive assessment of regional myocardial blood flow.

Technetium-99m Tetrofosmin

Technetium-99*m* tetrofosmin is a cationic complex that has been synthesized and proven useful as a myocardial perfusion agent (77–79). This complex shows good myocardial uptake with rapid clearance from blood and liver and little uptake in the lungs. Uptake of 99^{m}Tc tetrofosmin in the myocardium is proportional to regional myocardial blood flow (78). Preliminary experimental data have shown that 99^{m}Tc tetrofosmin imaging at rest can distinguish irreversible myocardial injury from viable myocardium during sustained low-flow ischemia (80). In this experimental model of short-term hibernation, 99^{m}Tc tetrofosmin uptake was significantly lower than ^{201}Tl uptake and comparable with 99^{m}Tc sestamibi uptake as assessed in previous experiments.

Technetium-99m NOET

Technetium 99*m*-NOET is a new neutral cardiac imaging agent that is taken up in the myocardium in proportion to blood flow and, like ^{201}Tl, shows delayed redistribution after intravenous injection (80a,80b). SPECT imaging has yielded comparable diagnostic information to ^{201}Tl when both agents have been studied with exercise stress in the same patients (80b).

Perfusion Imaging Agents for Positron Emission Tomography

Positron emission tomography performed in conjunction with administration of ^{82}Rb or $^{13}NH_3$ has been used for detecting coronary artery disease with much success (81,82). Rubidium-82 is obtained directly from a generator; a cyclotron is not required. Because of its short half-life (75 seconds), it is well-suited for repeated serial myocardial imaging. Studies have demonstrated that the sensitivity for detecting significant coronary artery disease by PET with ^{82}Rb or $^{13}NH_3$ is greater than 90%. Monitoring ^{82}Rb kinetics after intravenous injection may also permit detection of myocardial viability (83). This perfusion imaging technique is still limited to a few regional centers with available technology and is still undergoing clinical investigation.

Oxygen-15-labeled water can also be used with PET for assessment of myocardial blood flow (84). Oxygen-15 water is a positron-emitting flow tracer that is independent of metabolism with respect to myocardial uptake. It has an ultrashort half-life of 2 minutes, requiring large doses of activity to be administered. Oxygen-15 water is not only concentrated in the myocardium but also distributed into the blood pool; therefore, blood pool activity must be accurately subtracted to assess myocardial oxygen-15 water uptake. The blood pool subtraction utilizing oxygen-15 carbon monoxide blood pool imaging is required. The subject inhales 40 to 50 mCi of oxygen-15-labeled carbon monoxide to label the blood pool. The blood pool activity is subtracted from myocardial oxygen-15 activity, yielding an image outlining oxygen-15 activity in the left ventricular myocardium.

PRINCIPLES AND TECHNIQUES OF IMAGING OF VENTRICULAR FUNCTION

The advent of nuclear cardiology techniques has allowed the evaluation of global and segmental ventricular function through gated cardiac blood pool imaging using either the *first-pass* or the *equilibrium* method (13,85). With radionuclide angiography, the cause of heart failure can usually be determined. A diffuse uniform diminution in left ventricular wall motion suggests primary dilated cardiomyopathy, whereas depressed global left ventricular function with segmental wall motion abnormalities suggests ischemic heart disease. Measurement of ventricular volumes both at rest and during exercise, as well as the determination of right and left ventricular ejection fractions, can be undertaken using this imaging approach.

"First-Pass" Radionuclide Angiography

"First-pass" radionuclide angiography employs rapidly acquired image frames to observe the fate of a bolus of ^{99m}Tc as it traverses the venous system to the right side of the heart, pulmonary artery, lungs, left atrium, and left ventricle (86). Several cardiac cycles can be sampled continuously as the bolus of ^{99m}Tc passes through the right and then the left ventricle. Time–activity curves are generated by measuring radioactive counts in the blood pools over time. Ejection fraction values are obtained by dividing the stroke counts (end-diastolic counts minus end-systolic counts) by the end-diastolic counts. It is also possible to approximate end-systolic and end-diastolic ventricular volumes, pulmonary blood volume, and segmental wall motion using this first-pass technique. The radionuclide angiography approach is well suited for detection of left-to-right intracardiac shunts employing a computer program called "gamma variate analysis" (87). Finally, "first-pass" radionuclide angiography can be performed both at rest and during exercise stress.

Equilibrium Radionuclide Angiography

Unlike first-pass studies, gated equilibrium radionuclide angiography is performed after thorough mixing of ^{99m}Tc-labeled red blood cells within the intravascular compartment. As the ^{99m}Tc remains within the blood pool, serial imaging studies can be acquired over several hours. Acquisition of the images is synchronized with the QRS complex on the electrocardiogram. By employment of this multigated acquisition approach, each cardiac cycle is divided into multiple frames. Usually, acquisition is gated to the R wave on the electrocardiogram. All the cycles within a given RR interval range are added together for an imaging interval ranging from 3 to 10 minutes. The images derived depict the average cardiac cycle during this period of data collection. From these "resultant" images, both regional wall motion and global ventricular function can be evaluated. A relative volume curve is derived from the series of images by assessing changes in radioactivity that occur within the cardiac chambers during the cardiac cycle. As with the first-pass study, the gated equilibrium study can be displayed as an endless-loop cine format in which frames are displayed in a movie mode. This average cardiac cycle is displayed over and over again and simulates the beating heart, comparable to what is observed with a contrast ventriculogram. The ejection fraction of the left ventricle is calculated in a manner similar to that described for the first-pass technique. Regional systolic function can be visually evaluated, or a "regional" ejection fraction derived by computer processing.

A nonimaging nuclear probe or "nuclear stethoscope" can also be applied in patients for assessing left ventricular function (88). This device is placed over the region of the left ventricle and yields time–activity curves but generates no images. It requires optimum positioning on the chest wall for reliable left ventricular functional measurements. Recently, an ambulatory variant of this nuclear probe (VEST) has been introduced that permits monitoring of left ventricular function during normal activity (89,90).

PRINCIPLES AND TECHNIQUES OF MYOCARDIAL INFARCT-AVID IMAGING

Another nuclear cardiology technique that has been utilized in patients with acute myocardial infarction is infarct avid scintigraphy. The principle behind this approach is that the radiopharmaceutical administered is sequestered in zones of recently infarcted myocardium and can be localized on gamma camera images as "hot spots." Formerly, the most commonly used infarct-avid imaging agent was ^{99m}Tc stannous pyrophosphate, which reached maximal intensity in the necrotic region 48 to 72 hours after onset of infarction (91). This technique was shown to be most clinically useful when patients presented later than 24 hours after the onset of chest pain, when enzymes and the electrocardiogram may be nondiagnostic.

A new infarct-avid imaging technique involves the scintigraphic detection and quantification of myocardial necrosis after intravenous injection of radiolabeled myosin-specific antibody (92–95). It is based on the principle that myosin-specific antibodies will bind to intracellular myosin when plasma membrane integrity has been altered by ischemic damage. Studies have shown that the location of radiolabeled antimyosin antibody corresponds precisely to histochemically delineated zones of myocardial infarction. As with ^{99m}Tc pyrophosphate, one has to wait at least 24 hours after administration of the radiopharmaceutical to allow blood pool clearance of the agent before discrete uptake can be accurately imaged. Indium-111 (^{111}In) antimyosin and ^{201}Tl imaging can be undertaken simultaneously to separate regions of necrosis from peri-infarction ischemia. It has been proposed that this dual imaging approach may be useful for identifying patients with acute myocardial infarction who have additional regions of myocardium at risk, particularly in the distribution of vessels reperfused by thrombolytic agents but where there is a residual high-grade stenosis (96).

IMAGING OF MYOCARDIAL METABOLISM

Regional myocardial metabolism can be noninvasively assessed utilizing either PET tracers such as fluorine-18, 2-deoxyglucose (FDG) or carbon-11 acetate (97). Fluorine-18, 2-deoxyglucose is a glucose analog that is initially taken up in myocardial cells and is trapped by conversion to FDG 6-phosphate. Fluorine-18, 2-deoxyglucose 6-phosphate is impermeable to the cell membrane and remains within the cells at high concentrations for more than 40 to 60 minutes. The magnitude of FDG activity on PET images is indicative of the rate of myocardial glucose consumption. Under conditions of ischemia, there is increased FDG uptake, presumably reflecting the substrate utilization in the glycolytic pathway. Carbon-11 acetate and dynamic PET imaging have been utilized for the evaluation of regional myocardial oxidative metabolism (98). After being extracted intracellularly, carbon-11 acetate is converted to acetyl-CoA, enters the tricarboxylic acid cycle, and is then oxidized to carbon dioxide and water. The slope of the rapid-clearance curve component of carbon-11-labeled carbon dioxide from the heart correlates well with myocardial oxygen consumption. This rapid-clearance component is referred to as K_1.

Iodine-123 phenylpentadecanoic acid (IPPA) is the most clinically applicable agent to evaluate regional myocardial fatty acid utilization using SPECT methodology (99,99a). The metabolism of IPPA follows a biexponential clearance curve. The clearance of the tracer is reduced in zones of low-flow ischemia, reflecting reduced beta oxidation and more incorporation into intracellular triglycerides (Fig. 11–6). Zones of necrosis show reduced IPPA uptake, and washout is rapid.

In the sections to follow, clinical applications of these nuclear cardiology techniques are reviewed. Although all have provided substantial information in research studies, not all have proven clinically useful or cost-effective in evaluation of patients with acute infarction.

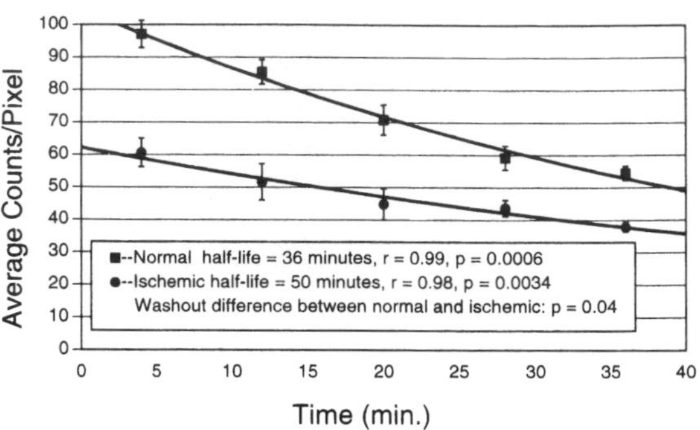

Figure 11–6. Myocardial clearance from normal (top curve) and ischemic zones (lower curve) in a representative patient receiving iodine-123 phenylpentadecanoic acid (IPPA) for the assessment of myocardial viability. Note that the clearance of the tracer is reduced in the zone of low-flow ischemia, which may reflect reduced beta oxidation. *Reprinted from Hansen (99), with permission.*

DETECTION, LOCALIZATION, AND SIZING OF ACUTE MYOCARDIAL INFARCTION

Resting Thallium-201 Scintigraphy

Resting ^{201}Tl scintigraphy can be undertaken in the acute phase of a suspected or even clinically evident myocardial infarction; however, whether an apparent ^{201}Tl defect is new and due to acute myocardial necrosis or old and due to prior infarction with subsequent scarring cannot be determined. An exception might be when a prior imaging study is available for comparison. van der Wieken et al (100) have suggested that resting myocardial ^{201}Tl scintigraphy could be performed in the emergency room, in patients presenting with chest pain and nondiagnostic electrocardiograms, to diagnose acute infarction. These investigators found that if the acute-phase scintigram was unequivocally normal, the chance of a subsequent infarction being confirmed by other variables was in the range of 1%. Overall, acute ^{201}Tl scans showing a defect had a 99% sensitivity and an 80% specificity for detecting acute infarction within 24 hours if "equivocal" scan readings were considered to be within normal limits. Not all patients presenting with chest pain with an abnormal resting scintigram demonstrate subsequent evidence of acute myocardial infarction. Certain patients with unstable angina (51,52,101) or those receiving ^{201}Tl in the midst of an episode of coronary vasospasm may also exhibit abnormal resting perfusion (102). Nevertheless, it is probably important that these patients also be admitted into an acute care unit for further observation and management.

Wackers et al (103) showed that the frequency of positive scans in patients presenting with suspected acute infarction was significantly higher in patients (90 of 96) studied within 24 hours after onset of symptoms than in those (75 of 104) studied later. Patients studied serially showed a diminution in the size of the ^{201}Tl defect, perhaps related to resolution of peri-infarction resting ischemia with enhanced antegrade perfusion or development of coronary collaterals. Thus the sensitivity of ^{201}Tl scintigraphy for detection of infarction is greater the earlier the images are obtained after onset of symptoms. Right ventricular infarction can be identified on exercise ^{201}Tl scintigraphy by demonstration of absent or diminished ventricular ^{201}Tl uptake on initial scintigraphy.

Myocardial ^{201}Tl scintigraphy can be employed for localization of infarction to the vascular region supplied by the three major coronary arteries. A defect in the middle and upper anteroseptal regions is nearly 100% specific for an obstruction in the left anterior descending coronary artery. Similarly, defects noted in the upper posterolateral wall on the 45° left anterior oblique projection are highly specific for left circumflex coronary artery occlusion. Defects localized to the apex may be in the vascular-risk region of any of the three major arteries. Approximately 90% of inferior wall defects demonstrated on the anterior projection image will be associated with right coronary narrowing.

Single-photon emission computed tomographic ^{201}Tl imaging is superior to planar ^{201}Tl imaging for detection and sizing of acute myocardial infarction. One study showed that planar imaging was less sensitive than SPECT imaging in detecting anterior (87% versus 96%), inferior (73% versus 97%), and nontransmural (47% versus 87%) infarctions (104). Enhanced sensitivity was restricted to detecting smaller infarcts when the peak creatine kinase (CK) activity was ≤1,000 IU/L. For such infarcts, planar imaging yielded positive scans in 44% of patients compared with an 89% detection rate with SPECT. Specificity was 92% for the two techniques. Similar findings were reported by Ritchie and coworkers (105), who reported an 87% sensitivity for SPECT ^{201}Tl imaging compared with 63% for planar imaging for detection of infarction. As expected, peak CK levels were lower in patients who had infarctions detected only by the SPECT technique.

Myocardial infarctions caused by acute occlusion of the left circumflex coronary artery are better detected by resting myocardial perfusion imaging than by conventional 12-lead electrocardiography. Huey et al (106) found that only 48% of patients with a circumflex-related infarction had evidence for significant ST segment elevation in any of the conventional electrocardiographic (ECG) leads, when presenting on hospital admission. The size of the perfusion abnormality in the posterolateral wall in these patients was substantially larger than predicted from the magnitude of abnormal changes on the electrocardiogram. In that study, ^{201}Tl defect size in the distribution of an occluded circumflex vessel was comparable with the defect size seen with patients having left anterior descending coronary artery occlusion (Fig. 11–7A). Interestingly, the probability of a future cardiac event after hospital discharge was comparable in patients with a left anterior descending, left circumflex, or right coronary infarct-related vessel (Fig. 11–7B).

The presence of coronary collaterals to an occluded infarct-related vessel may limit the perfusion defect size on resting scintigraphy compared with patients without collaterals. Imamura et al (107) found that ^{201}Tl defect size was smaller in patients with angiographic coronary collaterals, compared with patients without collaterals, seen on angiography.

In the patient with an acute inferior myocardial infarction by ECG criteria, an associated initial anterior wall defect at rest with subsequent "rest redistribution" suggests the presence of multivessel

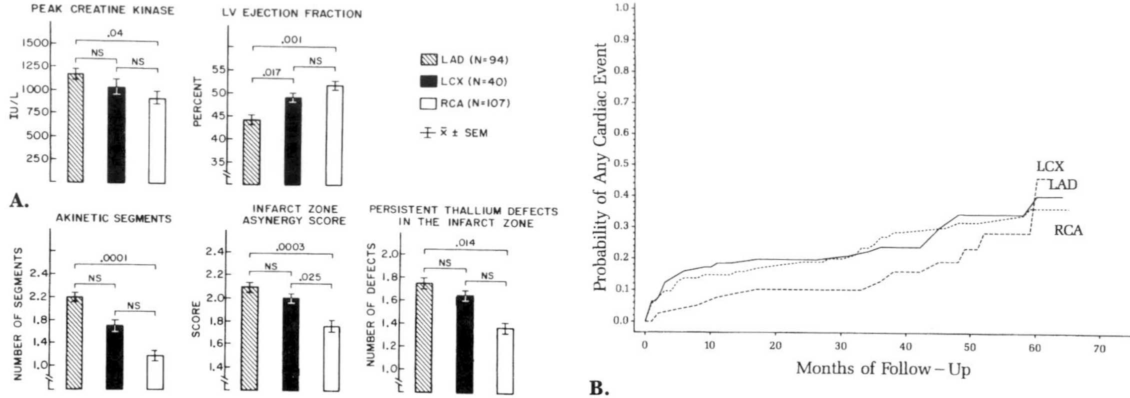

Figure 11–7. **A.** Measures of infarct size based on identity of the infarct-related coronary artery in 241 patients <65 years of age who underwent resting radionuclide angiography and submaximal exercise planar ^{201}Tl scintigraphy prior to discharge. LAD = left anterior descending coronary artery; LCX = left circumflex coronary artery; LV = left ventricular; RCA = right coronary artery. **B.** Probability of a cardiac event (death, reinfarction, or unstable angina requiring bypass surgery or angioplasty) in the 241 patients stratified by the infarct-related vessel as depicted in **A.** *Reprinted from Huey et al (106), with permission.*

coronary artery disease (108). These scan findings also suggest that the left anterior descending lesion is high grade because of abnormal resting blood flow. It has been reported by our group (108) that patients with an inferior infarction who demonstrate resting anterior wall redistribution defects have a higher prevalence of future cardiac events than patients with inferior myocardial infarction who have only persistent defects in the inferior wall and inferoapical region (see Ch. 17). Hakki et al (109) studied the relative value of rest ^{201}Tl scintigraphy, radionuclide ventriculography, and 24-hour Holter monitoring for evaluating prognosis after acute myocardial infarction. All three tests proved to be important predictors of survival by univariate Cox survival analysis; the ^{201}Tl score, however, was the only important predictor by multivariate analysis. The predictive power of the ^{201}Tl score was comparable to that of combined ejection fraction and Holter monitoring. As expected, patients with the largest perfusion defects were at the highest risk of cardiac death during the first year after infarction. These findings are not surprising, as previous experimental and clinical data (110) indicated that the extent of myocardial hypoperfusion on ^{201}Tl scintigrams accurately reflected myocardial infarct size.

It has been known for some time that infarct size is an important prognostic variable in survivors of acute infarction. In the study by Prigent et al (110), SPECT ^{201}Tl and histologic infarct size were highly correlated ($r = 0.93$). Another study showed that a perfusion abnormality of 33% or more of the left ventricular circumference separates high-risk and low-risk patients (111). In a study of myocardial infarction survivors without heart failure, those patients who subsequently died had larger absolute ^{201}Tl defects in terms of percentage area of the left ventricle and more severe defects than patients who remained asymptomatic during the follow-up period (Fig. 11–8) (112) (see Chs. 30–31). The resting ejection fraction did not differentiate between event and nonevent groups. Increased right ventricular ^{201}Tl uptake at rest is a marker of significant left ventricular dysfunction and identifies a subset of patients with a worse prognosis (113).

Clinicopathologic studies have been performed in patients who died from an acute myocardial infarction and who had previously undergone resting ^{201}Tl imaging during the acute phase. Wackers et al (114) correlated the scintigraphic location and estimated size of infarction in vivo with postmortem findings. There was good agreement (91%) between scintigraphic and postmortem location of in-

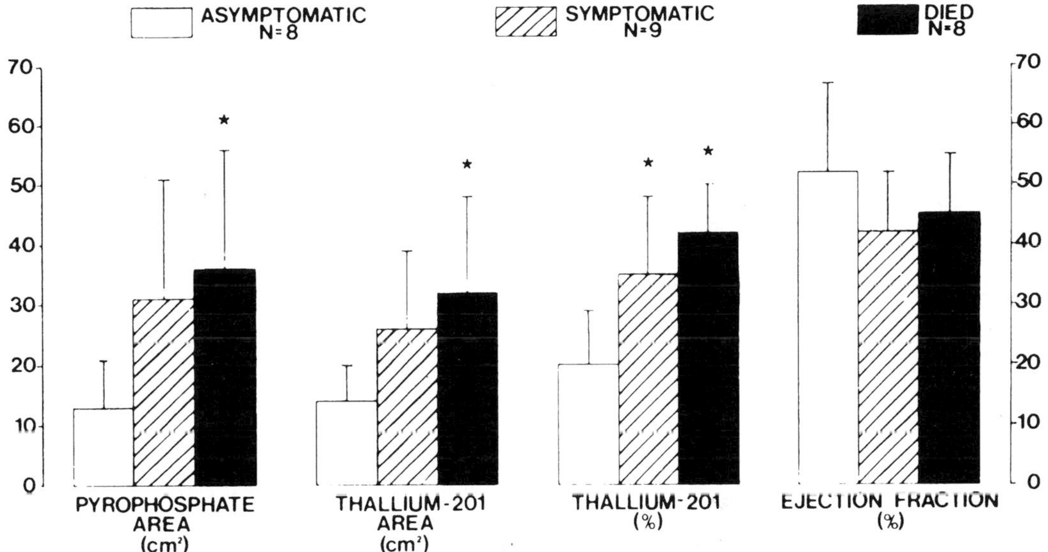

Figure 11–8. Scintigraphic parameters of acute infarction related to late prognosis. The percent perfusion abnormality on ^{201}Tl scintigraphy appeared to best separate asymptomatic survivors from symptomatic survivors and those who died. *Reprinted from Botvinick et al (112), with permission.*

farction. The size of infarction determined from computer-processed drawings of postmortem slices of the heart correlated well with size determined from the scintiscans. In this study, the ^{201}Tl scan provided more precise location of infarction than the electrocardiogram, and the size of the scintigraphically abnormal area reflected the extent of necrosis. Tamaki and coworkers (115) showed that when ^{201}Tl scintigraphic infarct size was compared with the accumulated MBCK isoenzyme release, infarct volume determined from SPECT images correlated closely with MBCK release ($r = 0.89$). Mahmarian et al (116) found a better correlation between anterior compared with inferior infarction defect size on ^{201}Tl scintigrams with CK release into the serum. This finding may be attributed to the release of CK from the infarcted right ventricle in patients with acute occlusion of the right coronary artery.

Thus these data clearly indicate that the extent of myocardial ^{201}Tl perfusion abnormalities represents an accurate reflection of the degree of ischemic damage, particularly when SPECT images are quantitated. Those patients with the largest defects have the most unfavorable prognosis.

Resting Radionuclide Angiography

Regional wall motion abnormalities detected by radionuclide angiography (or echocardiography) are not specific for acute myocardial necrosis in patients presenting with chest pain. Patients with acute infarction, old infarction, or acute regional ischemia without necrosis exhibit regional systolic wall motion abnormalities. Radionuclide angiography often demonstrates a reduced right ventricular ejection fraction and right ventricular asynergy in patients with acute inferior infarction (117) (see Ch. 17). Right ventricular systolic function usually recovers in the subacute and chronic phase of infarction (see Ch. 17).

Localization of acute myocardial infarction can be accomplished by resting radionuclide angiography in patients without a prior history of myocardial damage. One of the best prognostic measurements that can be derived by radionuclide angiography in acute infarction patients is the left ventricular ejection fraction (118). In the Multicenter Postinfarction Research Group study comprising 799 patients with acute infarction who underwent predischarge radionuclide angiography, the 1-year cardiac mortality rate increased exponentially as the resting left ventricular ejection fraction fell below 40% (Fig. 11–9A) (118). The importance of the left ventricular ejection fraction as a prognostic variable in postinfarction patients has been sustained in patients receiving thrombolytic therapy (119,120). Postinfarction patients treated with a thrombolytic agent, however, may have an improved survival rate at any level of left ventricular ejection fraction, compared with infarction patients treated in the prethrombolytic era (Fig. 11–9B). Simoons et al (121) showed that mortality exceeded 50% at 5 years in patients who received thrombolytic therapy but were discharged with an ejection fraction of less than 30% (Fig. 11–10). In contrast, patients with an ejection fraction of greater than 40% experienced an annual mortality of approximately 2%. The resting left ventricular ejection fraction at discharge and at 6 weeks was comparable in postinfarction patients receiving thrombolytic therapy on admission who were randomized to a "conservative" strategy and those randomized to a "invasive" strategy in the Thrombolysis in Myocardial Infarction (TIMI)-IIB study (122). At 6 weeks, baseline left ventricular ejection fraction was 51% in the 796 patients randomized to the invasive strategy and 50% in patients randomized to the "conservative" strategy.

Rogers et al (123) investigated the variables predictive of a good functional outcome following thrombolytic therapy in the TIMI-II pilot study. In patients assigned to the 18- to 48-hour angioplasty group, variables independently predicting survival were a resting left ventricular ejection fraction of greater than 50%, fewer leads with ST segment elevation on admission, younger age, rapid normalization of ST segments with dramatic relief of chest pain during tissue plasminogen activator (t-PA) infusion, absence of arrhythmias within the first 24 hours of treatment initiation, no prior infarction, and being a nonsmoker at entry.

Infarct artery patency has been consistently reported to be associated with better regional ventricular function after thrombolytic therapy. White et al (124) found that when the left ventricular ejection fraction was ≥50% after thrombolytic therapy, only occluded infarct-related arteries with TIMI grade 0, 1, or 2 flow supplying greater than 25% of the left ventricle affected prognosis in an adverse manner. If the left ventricular ejection fraction were less than 50%, an occluded infarct-related artery was an adverse prognostic variable whatever its myocardial distribution. Data from the GUSTO trial (125) indicate that TIMI grade 3 flow in the infarct vessel after front-loaded t-PA infusion results in a higher left ventricular ejection fraction (61 ± 14%) compared with TIMI grades 0 and 1 flow (56 ± 14% and 54 ± 12%, respectively). Mortality in 30 days was 4% among patients with a 90-minute left ventricular ejection fraction value greater than 45%,

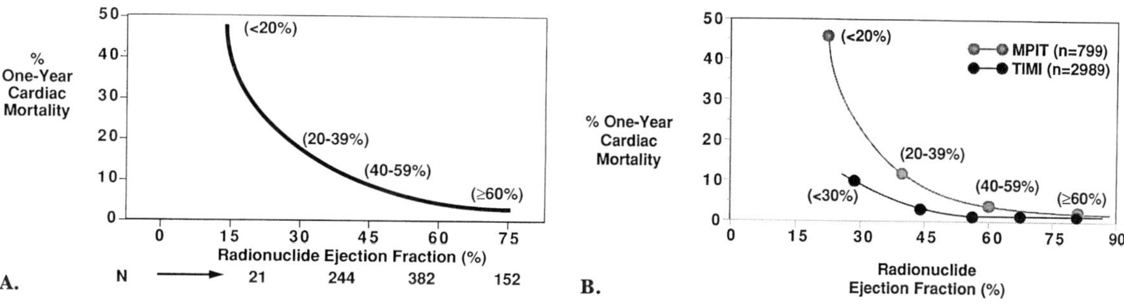

Figure 11–9. The resting radionuclide ejection fraction versus one-year cardiac mortality in patients in the Multicenter Postinfarction Research Group study comprising 799 patients with acute infarction who underwent predischarge radionuclide angiography. *Adapted from the Multicenter Postinfarction Research Group (118), with permission.* **B.** Radionuclide ejection fraction for the 2,989 patients enrolled in the TIMI-II trial in which all patients received thrombolytic therapy versus one-year cardiac mortality rate shown with the curve of the radionuclide ejection fraction versus one-year mortality rate for the Multicenter Postinfarction Research Trial (MPIT) depicted in **A.** Mortality rate is lower at any given value of ejection fraction in the TIMI-II patients. *Reprinted from Bonow (119), with permission.*

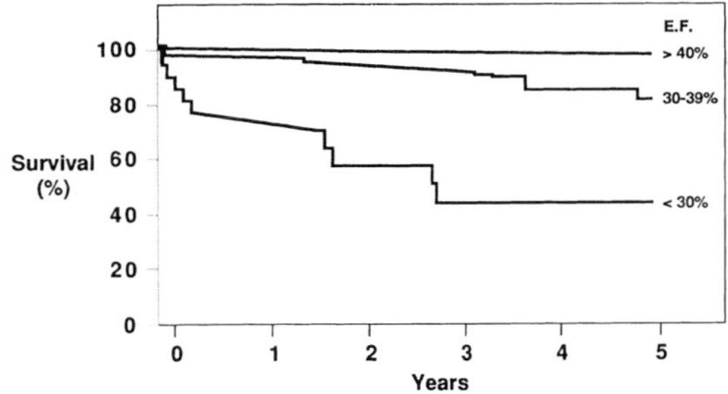

Figure 11–10. Survival rate during follow-up versus the predischarge left ventricular ejection fraction (E.F.) in patients who received thrombolytic therapy on admission. Note that patients who had a predischarge ejection fraction of <30% had nearly a 50% mortality during five years of follow up. *Reprinted from Simoons et al (121), with permission.*

but 15% among those with a left ventricular ejection fraction greater than 15%. In 542 patients reported by Harrison et al (126), patients with TIMI grade 0 flow were less likely to improve function than were patients with patent infarct-related arteries. Interestingly, the correlation between time to reperfusion and improvement in function was not strong.

An open artery after coronary angioplasty performed for postinfarction ischemia is associated with a significantly lower mortality over the next 5 years compared to patients whose infarct-related arteries were closed at the end of angioplasty (4.9% versus 19.4%) (126a). This survival benefit was most apparent in patients with a left ventricular ejection fraction of <50%.

More recently, direct angioplasty has been advocated as an alternative to thrombolytic therapy for rapidly accomplishing infarct artery patency in patients with acute infarction (see Ch. 22). However, Grines et al (127) found that left ventricular ejection fraction was comparable in patients randomized to direct angioplasty and randomized to t-PA (53% for both).

Extensive asynergy may be the result of new damage and prior scar rather than secondary to acute necrosis alone. Such patients show a depressed ejection fraction. Many may not manifest significant symptomatic heart failure. An infarct patient presenting in Killip class I or II who has a left ventricular ejection fraction below 40% has a high likelihood of subsequently developing heart failure or cardiogenic shock in the coronary care unit (128). Patients with a non–Q wave myocardial infarction tend to have more hypokinesis in the infarct zone than akinesis or dyskinesis and have a higher resting ejection fraction (129). This is expected, as postmortem studies in these patients demonstrate a lesser degree of necrosis (see Ch. 18). Patients with anterior infarction have a greater depression of left ventricular ejection fraction than inferior infarction patients (130). Patients with an initially low or decreasing ejection fraction have a significantly greater incidence of early mortality and left ventricular dysfunction than those patients whose ejection fraction is normal or improves to normal after admission.

Resting radionuclide angiography can aid in determining the presence or absence of certain complications associated with acute myocardial infarction, such as left ventricular aneurysm, pseudoaneurysm, mitral regurgitation, ventricular septal rupture, and ischemia remote from the infarct (see Ch. 16) (131–133). The resting gated blood pool scan is particularly well suited for recognition of aneurysmal left ventricular dilation, which most often can be distinguished from pseudoaneurysms or akinetic myocardial segments that may not be suitable for surgery.

For overall assessment of regional myocardial dysfunction in acute infarction, two-dimensional echocardiography permits more complete evaluation of a larger number of segments than radionuclide angiography (see Ch. 10). Radionuclide angiography has an advantage in that more accurate global measurements of left ventricular function can be made because the ejection fraction calculation is based on changes in relative counts in the left ventricular blood pool, and not on geometric considerations.

Volume-overload patterns resulting from mitral regurgitation caused by papillary muscle dysfunction after infarction can be identified as a cause of congestive heart failure by resting gated blood pool imaging. Patients with valvular regurgitation will have an enlarged left ventricular end diastolic vol ume but a relatively preserved left ventricular ejection fraction, as long as there has not been extensive myocardial damage (see Ch. 16). Quantitative assessment of valvular regurgitation can be determined with radionuclide angiographic techniques by measuring the ratio of left ventricular stroke volume to the right ventricular stroke volume (134). In patients with no valvular regurgitation, this ratio is approximately 1.15, whereas in patients with mitral regurgitation, this ratio usually exceeds 1.30.

There are some limitations to the use of the left ventricular ejection fraction measurement by either radionuclide angiography or contrast ventriculography as a predictor of outcome in the *very early* acute phase of myocardial infarction. Some patients may demonstrate hyperkinesia of the normally perfused zone, which influences to some degree global performance. This would potentially "falsely" elevate the left ventricular ejection fraction. With diminution in this hyperkinetic function over several weeks, the true effect of infarct-related asynergy on global cardiac performance becomes evident. The ejection fraction measured 10 to 14 days after infarction, or even at 3 weeks, in patients receiving thrombolytic therapy will most truly reflect the resultant global performance and therefore be the most sensitive predictor for ultimate prognosis. The greater the uptake is of ^{201}Tl in the infarct zone in patients with acute infarction, the greater the probability is of an improvement in left ventricular ejection fraction at 3 weeks postinfarction (135).

Some investigators have recommended the use of combined ^{201}Tl scintigraphy and resting radionuclide angiography for determining prognosis in acute myocardial infarction. The Johns Hopkins group (111) examined the prognostic utility of resting ^{201}Tl imaging and resting gated blood pool imaging for separation of high-risk and low-risk patients with acute myocardial infarction (see Ch. 30). They reported that ^{201}Tl scintigraphy was more sensitive in detecting nonsurvivors than a low ejection fraction at a similar level of specificity. A ^{201}Tl defect score above 7 (according to their scoring scheme) was the best predictor of subsequent mortality, with Q waves and ejection fraction being only additive. Those patients with a high defect score that corresponded to diminished ^{201}Tl activity involving 40% of the left ventricular circumference had a 64% 6-month mortality rate. Patients with lesser defect scores had only an 8% 6-month mortality rate. Figure 11–11 summarizes some of the results of this study. Thus, with both a parameter of left ventricular function and a parameter of myocardial perfusion, postinfarction patients can be categorized into high- and low-risk groups.

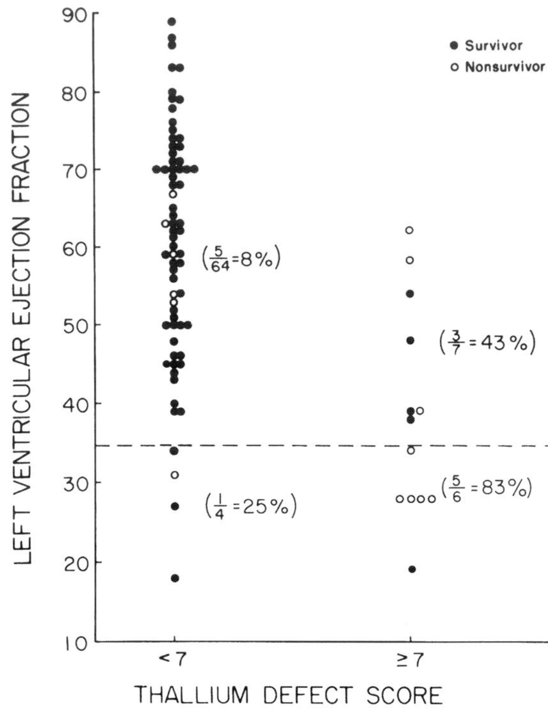

Figure 11–11. Survivors (solid circles) and nonsurvivors (open circles) following acute myocardial infarction related to the resting left ventricular ejection fraction (vertical axis) and the ^{201}Tl defect score (horizontal axis). Most of the nonsurvivors had a reduced ejection fraction and a ^{201}Tl defect score ≥7. *Reprinted from Becker et al (111), with permission.*

Thus resting radionuclide angiography may provide valuable information related to the status of global and regional left ventricular function in patients with acute myocardial infarction. The lower the ejection fraction at the time of hospital discharge, the worse the prognosis.

Infarct-Avid Imaging

Infarct-avid imaging is rarely employed clinically for either detection of acute infarction or infarct sizing. Perhaps the most useful application of the infarct-avid imaging techniques such as ^{99m}Tc pyrophosphate scintigraphy would be in the patient who presents with a clinical history compatible with acute myocardial infarction but who presents late (2 to 7 days) with a nondiagnostic electrocardiogram and negative serum enzymes. As both the ^{99m}Tc pyrophosphate scan and the ^{111}In antimyosin antibody scan remain positive for as long as 1 week after onset of symptoms, these radionuclide techniques might be helpful in identifying the presence of recent myocardial necrosis where other, more conventional diagnostic techniques may not be accurate. Discrete as opposed to diffuse myocardial uptake of these radionuclides is specific for necrosis. These techniques are less sensitive for detecting nontransmural infarction than transmural infarction (136). The extent of ^{99m}Tc pyrophosphate uptake has prognostic significance, and tomographic imaging can be employed to estimate infarct size (137).

Antimyosin antibody imaging yields a 92% sensitivity for identifying acute transmural myocardial infarction (94). Focal myocardial uptake of antimyosin corresponds to the ECG infarct location (94). Patients with inferior/posterior location have more of a "faint" uptake pattern than those with other infarct locations. Similarly, faint tracer uptake is more likely to be seen in patients with a closed-infarct vessel with absent collateral flow. The size of the antimyosin uptake pattern has shown a good correlation with computer-derived hypokinetic segment length ($r = 0.79$) and peak CK ($r = 0.90$) (92). Interestingly, when antimyosin antibody imaging was compared with technetium pyrophosphate imaging in the same patients, the pyrophosphate defect size was 1.7 times larger than antimyosin SPECT infarct size (92). Volpini et al (138) showed that previous old infarction did not take up ^{111}In antimyosin antibody; similarly, no uptake was observed in 10 healthy volunteers.

Johnson and coworkers (96) reported the value of dual-isotope ^{201}Tl and ^{111}In antimyosin SPECT imaging to identify infarct patients who might be at further risk for subsequent ischemic events. There was a significant correlation between further ischemic events and mismatching ^{201}Tl/^{111}In antimyosin activity. Thus identifying reduced perfusion in myocardial regions outside the area of actual necrosis from simultaneously recorded dual-isotope ^{111}In/^{201}Tl SPECT scans could potentially be useful for risk stratification. The results of all studies published to date show that antimyosin antibody is also safe, with no important adverse reactions noted. Despite these encouraging results, infarct-avid imaging is rarely employed for infarct localization, infarct sizing, or prognostication.

ASSESSMENT OF MYOCARDIAL VIABILITY

Table 11–2 lists the various radionuclide imaging techniques that have been utilized for detection of viable myocardium after acute myocardial infarction. Table 11–3 summarizes the criteria employed for determination of myocardial viability by these radionuclide imaging modalities. A recent review provides a comprehensive discussion of the strengths and limitations of these techniques and compares them to the echocardiographic approaches to viability assessment (138a).

Table 11–2. Detection of Myocardial Viability by Radionuclide Imaging

1. Thallium-201
   a. Stress and 3- to 4-hour redistribution imaging
   b. Stress, 3- to 4-hour redistribution, and 24-hour late imaging
   c. Stress, 3- to 4-hour redistribution, and "reinjection" imaging
   d. Early and 4-hour delayed rest imaging
2. Technetium-99*m* sestamibi
   a. Stress and rest technetium-99*m* sestamibi imaging with gating
   b. Combined first-pass radionuclide angiography and perfusion imaging
3. Positron emission tomographic imaging
   a. Imaging of perfusion with nitrogen-13 ammonia and metabolism with fluorine-18 deoxyglucose (FDG)
   b. Carbon-11 acetate imaging
   c. Serial rubidium-82 imaging
4. Imaging of radiolabeled fatty acid kinetics
   a. Iodine-123 phenylpentadecanoic acid (IPPA) rest imaging

Table 11–3. Determination of Myocardial Viability by Radionuclide Imaging in Patients With Myocardial Infarction

Resting or exercise thallium-201 scintigraphy
Normal regional thallium-201 uptake
Initial defect with delayed redistribution
Mild persistent thallium-201 defect (25% to 50% reduction in thallium-201 counts)
Resting technetium-99*m* sestamibi or tetrofosmin imaging
Regional technetium-99*m* tracer (>50% of peak) tracer uptake
Positron emission tomography
Increased regional uptake of fluorine-18, 2-deoxyglucose in zones of reduced perfusion
Preserved carbon-11 acetate kinetics
Infarct-avid imaging
Absence of technetium-99*m* pyrophosphate uptake
Absence of indium-111 antimyosin antibody uptake

Thallium-201 Scintigraphy for Assessment of Myocardial Viability

There are probably many patients with depressed left ventricular function after myocardial infarction who have viable but "stunned" or "hibernating" myocardium contributing to the heart failure syndrome. Myocardial ^{201}Tl imaging may be useful in distinguishing such patients from those with predominantly irreversible cellular injury. Patients with viable but severely asynergic myocardial regions will demonstrate significant ^{201}Tl uptake over 4 hours after intravenous administration of the radionuclide with either stress/redistribution imaging or imaging solely in the resting state. After revascularization, myocardial infarct regions showing preservation of ^{201}Tl uptake often show a significant improvement in regional wall motion postprocedure (52). This contributes to an overall enhancement of global left ventricular systolic function. For example, Yamamoto et al (139) reported that improvement in regional wall motion in the infarct zone after angioplasty was more likely to occur when mean ^{201}Tl uptake on delayed images was >50% of peak nonischemic uptake. In regions of >50% uptake in the infarct zone, mean region ejection fraction increased from 39 ± 18% before angioplasty to 47 ± 14% after angioplasty. In contrast, preangioplasty regional ejection fraction was 23 ± 9% and remained at 24 ± 12% postangioplasty in zones of ≤50% ^{201}Tl uptake on delayed images. These data are summarized in Fig. 11–12.

Certain patients may exhibit left ventricular dysfunction far in excess of infarct size, as demonstrated by ECG changes in the magnitude of CK release. In one interesting case report (140), two patients with left ventricular dysfunction demonstrated ^{201}Tl defects with delayed redistribution in myocardial regions remote from the infarct zone. Both had multivessel coronary artery disease evident on angiography and both experienced relief of symptoms and improved regional and global function after revascularization. This and other similar reports (135,139) demonstrate that viable but ischemic myocardial regions can be identified in the early or subacute postinfarction period by rest or submaximal exercise myocardial perfusion scintigraphy. Demonstration of ^{201}Tl uptake in infarct regions corresponding to severe wall motion abnormalities indicates viability (141) and predicts that improvement in function will occur after revascularization.

The clinical utility of late (18 to 72 hours) ^{201}Tl imaging as a predictor of myocardial viability has been demonstrated. In the study by Kiat et al (43),

DELAYED Tl-201 UPTAKE AND IMPROVEMENT IN WALL MOTION AFTER PTCA IN INFARCT ZONES

	Mean % Tl-201 Uptake	
	≤50%	>50%
REF-pre	23 ± 9%	39 ± 18%
REF-post	24 ± 12%	47 ± 14%*

REF = regional ejection fraction
*p < 0.05

Figure 11–12. Regional ejection fraction before angioplasty (REF-pre) and regional ejection fraction after angioplasty (REF-post) related to the mean percent ^{201}Tl uptake on delayed images acquired prior to angioplasty. Note that patients who had ≤50% regional ^{201}Tl uptake had a lower preprocedure resting ejection fraction and no significant postprocedure increase in regional ejection fraction compared with patients with >50% ^{201}Tl uptake in infarct zones. *Adapted from Yamamoto et al (139), with permission.*

85% of the myocardial segments with redistribution at 4 hours prior to coronary bypass surgery or coronary angioplasty demonstrated the expected postintervention scintigraphic improvement; 72% of the persistent defects seen at 4 hours also improved after revascularization. Ninety-five percent of the myocardial segments that showed persistent defects at 4 hours but late redistribution showed improvement in initial ^{201}Tl uptake after revascularization; however, only 37% of the 4-hour persistent defects that remained persistent at 18 to 72 hours showed improvement. In another study from this same group (44), the frequency of late redistribution was evaluated in a group of 118 patients who underwent exercise SPECT ^{201}Tl imaging. Fifty-three percent of patients showed late redistribution at 18 to 24 hours in zones that correlated with persistent defects on poststress and 4-hour redistribution images. Thirty-five percent of patients had 24-hour redistribution in at least two segments that appeared persistent on conventional redistribution imaging. Twenty-seven percent of stress defects showed reversibility at 4 hours, with an additional 16% showing reversibility at 24 hours.

The rationale for 24-hour redistribution imaging is that redistribution is an ongoing kinetic process that depends on continued uptake of ^{201}Tl in the myocardium via recirculation in regions supplied by stenotic vessels coupled with more rapid ^{201}Tl washout in normally perfused zones. It should be stated that redistribution requires some residual blood pool concentration, and such residual activity has been shown to be present for at least 24 hours following tracer injection.

The potential limitations of 24-hour redistribution images for enhancement of viability detection are suboptimal count statistics resulting in reduced image quality, the inconvenience of requiring patients to return for a second day of imaging, and inability to accurately identify in a prospective manner which patient may need to return for such 24-hour imaging. Our experience has been that most defects that exhibit late redistribution at 24 hours already demonstrate some evidence for delayed redistribution on 2.5- to 4-hour images when quantitative scan analysis is employed (142).

As mentioned previously in this chapter, another technique advocated for enhancement of detection of reversibility in poststress defects involves the injection of a second dose of ^{201}Tl at rest following acquisition of the 4-hour redistribution images. This has been referred to as the "reinjection" technique. In this protocol, 50% of the original dose that was administered during stress is reinjected at rest. Dilsizian et al (45), employing stress, redistribution, and reinjection SPECT ^{201}Tl scintigraphy in 100 patients with coronary artery disease, found that 33% of abnormal segments demonstrated nonreversible defects on conventional 4-hour redistribution images. Following reinjection of a second dose of ^{201}Tl, approximately half of these nonreversible defects demonstrated improved or normalized ^{201}Tl uptake. Figure 11–13 shows stress, redistribution, and reinjection short-axis tomograms from a representative patient in this study. Dilsizian et al (45) in this study also demonstrated that 87% of myocardial regions exhibiting enhanced ^{201}Tl reversibility after reinjection on preangioplasty images showed improved or normalized regional wall motion following balloon dilatation. Regions that

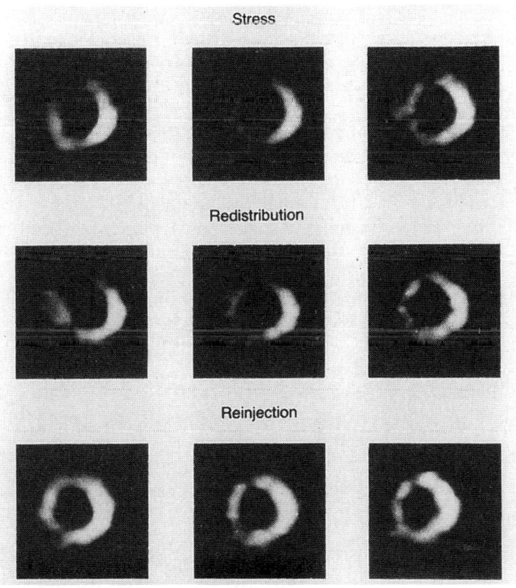

Figure 11–13. Stress (first row), redistribution (second row), and reinjection (third row) ^{201}Tl SPECT short-axis tomograms in a patient demonstrating hypoperfusion in the anteroseptal region. Note the enhanced ^{201}Tl uptake in the defect region following reinjection of a second dose of ^{201}Tl compared with redistribution and poststress tomograms. *Reprinted from Dilsizian et al (45), with permission.*

showed no enhanced ^{201}Tl uptake after reinjection preangioplasty exhibited both abnormal ^{201}Tl uptake and persistently abnormal regional wall motion after the procedure.

Tamaki and coworkers reported that reinjection ^{201}Tl imaging identified viability in 29% of patients with persistent defects and no evidence of delayed redistribution in any myocardial segment on standard 3- to 4-hour delayed imaging (143). Thus the reinjection protocol was the only way in which defect reversibility was identified in this subset of patients who solely showed persistent ^{201}Tl defects when comparing stress and conventional 4-hour redistribution images. The authors, however, did not quantitate ^{201}Tl uptake to determine if such persistent defects that demonstrated enhanced ^{201}Tl uptake after reinjection had >50% uptake compared with peak on stress and delayed 4-hour redistribution images.

Dilsizian et al (46) undertook an investigation to determine which persistent defects on ^{201}Tl redistribution imaging would most likely show enhanced ^{201}Tl uptake after reinjection. Mild to moderate (51% to 85% of normal activity) persistent defects were more likely to show an increase in absolute ^{201}Tl activity after reinjection than more severe persistent defects (<50% of normal peak uptake).

The validity of reinjection ^{201}Tl imaging for enhancing the detection of myocardial viability was further explored by Bonow and coworkers (144), who compared ^{201}Tl reinjection imaging with PET imaging employing FDG in the same patients. Uptake of FDG was observed in 94% of defects that showed complete or partial ^{201}Tl redistribution on conventional postexercise and 4-hour delayed redistribution imaging. Of the persistent defects, 51% demonstrated enhanced ^{201}Tl uptake after reinjection, and 51% demonstrated viability by FDG uptake. Detection of myocardial viability in these persistent defects by the two techniques was concordant in 88% of segments.

There are a number of alternative protocols that have been tested dealing with the timing of reinjection of ^{201}Tl after completion of the stress portion of the imaging protocol. Favaro et al (145) studied a group of patients with coronary artery disease who had at least one persistent defect on conventional 3-hour redistribution images. One protocol involved reinjection of ^{201}Tl immediately after redistribution imaging, with imaging commencing 15 minutes later. In a second protocol, patients were reinjected 48 to 96 hours later, and images were obtained at 30 and 180 minutes after reinjection. The rationale for the latter time period was to permit any possible rest redistribution of ^{201}Tl to occur in zones of resting hypoperfusion. The uptake of ^{201}Tl in irreversible defects seen at 3-hour redistribution imaging was enhanced in 35% using the protocol in which reinjection immediately followed acquisition of redistribution imaging, 43% when reinjection images were acquired 30 minutes after reinjection on a different day, and 49% when images were acquired 180 minutes after reinjection on the "different day" protocol. From this work, the authors concluded that perhaps the best protocol to differentiate irreversible from reversible myocardial injury was to give the second dose of ^{201}Tl on a different day and acquire images 3 hours later. This finding is not surprising because the 3 hour duration following a resting injection permits the process of "rest redistribution" previously demonstrated to enhance identification of viable but asynergic myocardium (53,54).

The utility of reinjection ^{201}Tl imaging performed on a separate day and followed by rest redistribution imaging was assessed in a multicenter trial comprising 402 consecutive patients with ischemic heart disease and exercise ^{201}Tl defects (146). This protocol was compared with the standard reinjection protocol in which ^{201}Tl reinjection and imaging were performed immediately after stress/redistribution imaging. Thallium-201 reinjection improved detection of reversibility in 30% of partially reversible defects and in 31% of irreversible defects during redistribution imaging. Thallium-201 reinjection was less effective in detecting reversibility in 5% of abnormal segments observed on the stress/redistribution study. The discordance between ^{201}Tl reinjection and stress/redistribution was less in this multicenter trial (146) than had been previously reported for smaller single-institution studies in which nearly 50% of defects that showed no reversibility on stress/redistribution imaging showed improved ^{201}Tl uptake after reinjection (45). Figure 11–14 shows that 31 of the 58 patients in the trial who demonstrated increased reversibility after reinjection in which only fixed de-

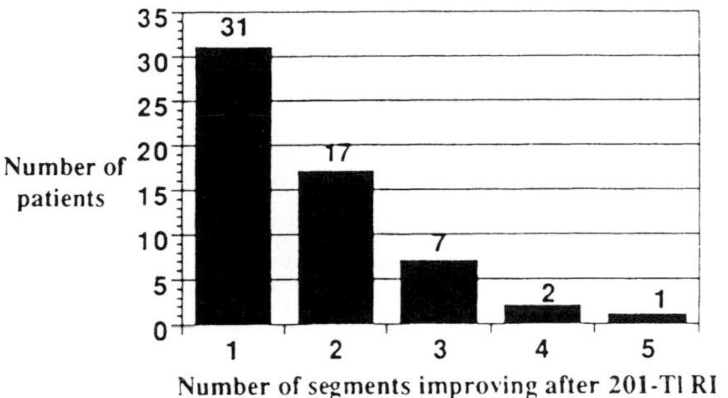

Figure 11–14. Frequency distribution of improving segments after ^{201}Tl reinjection in 58 patients with only fixed defects at redistribution and reversibility during reinjection imaging. The median number of fixed defects on redistribution imaging was 4 segments/patient. These data indicate that in 31 of the 58 patients, only one fixed defect at redistribution showed improvement in ^{201}Tl uptake after reinjection. 201-Tl RI = ^{201}Tl reinjection. *Reprinted from Inglese et al (146), with permission.*

fects were seen at redistribution had this improvement in only one myocardial segment. Only 10 of the 58 patients had three or more segments demonstrating improved ^{201}Tl uptake after reinjection.

When the only information required is whether or not an area of asynergic myocardium is viable, ^{201}Tl imaging performed entirely at rest is the procedure of choice for distinguishing reversible from irreversible injury. This technique employs an injection of ^{201}Tl at rest, with imaging performed 15 minutes and 4 hours later. Ideally, quantitative scan analysis should be performed to determine residual ^{201}Tl activity at 4 hours in infarct and noninfarct myocardial regions. Early studies by Berger and coworkers (51) and Gewirtz and colleagues (52) demonstrated that many segments showing severe asynergy at rest showed substantial ^{201}Tl uptake on rest/redistribution imaging. In the study by Berger et al (51), 80% of patients who showed rest redistribution preoperatively showed at least a 5% increase in left ventricular ejection fraction after revascularization.

Mori et al (147) studied a group of patients with regional dysfunction and prior acute myocardial infarction, all of whom underwent pre- and postoperative radionuclide angiography and preoperative rest ^{201}Tl imaging. The majority of regions showing rest ^{201}Tl redistribution exhibited improved systolic function after revascularization. Zones demonstrating a persistent severe reduction in ^{201}Tl activity on serial imaging did not demonstrate an improvement. In contrast, some mild persistent defects did show improved regional systolic function after revascularization, confirming the earlier observations of Berger et al (51).

More recently, Ragosta et al (53) performed rest ^{201}Tl scintigraphy and resting radionuclide ventriculography before and after coronary bypass surgery in a group of 21 patients with a preoperative mean left ventricular ejection fraction of 27%. All had a prior myocardial infarction. Among severely asynergic myocardial segments (severe hypokinesis or akinesis/dyskinesis), 73% showed evidence for preserved viability defined as either normal ^{201}Tl uptake, an initial resting defect with delayed redistribution at 3 hours, or a mild persistent defect showing >50% ^{201}Tl uptake compared with peak nonischemic uptake. As shown in Fig. 11–15, patients who had >7 viable asynergic segments preoperatively had a significant increase in left ventricular ejection fraction following coronary

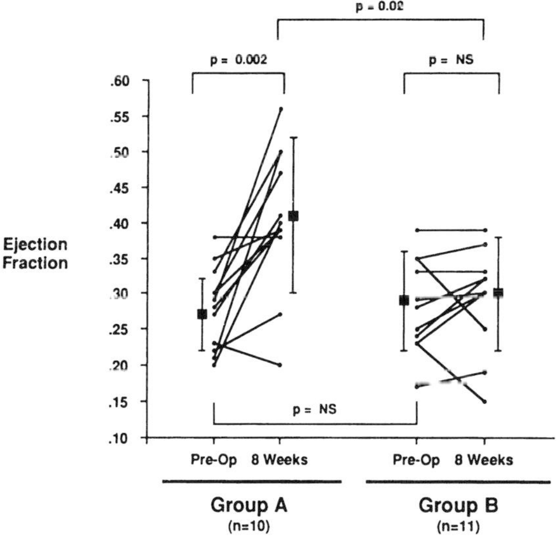

Figure 11–15. Resting left ventricular ejection fraction prior to (Pre-Op) and 8 weeks after coronary artery bypass graft surgery in 10 patients with >7 viable asynergic segments preoperatively by ^{201}Tl criteria (**group A**) and in 11 patients with ≤7 viable asynergic segments preoperatively on resting and delayed ^{201}Tl scintigraphy (**group B**). Note that the mean ejection fraction significantly increased only in group A patients who had more viable asynergic segments than group B patients, although the preoperative ejection fraction was similar in both groups. *Reprinted from Ragosta et al (53), with permission.*

revascularization. In contrast, patients with ≤7 viable asynergic segments prerevascularization on resting scintigraphy had no significant change in ejection fraction after surgery.

Lomboy et al (135) investigated the utility of early rest/redistribution ^{201}Tl imaging in detecting residual myocardial viability after acute myocardial infarction in 31 patients undergoing rest/redistribution ^{201}Tl imaging at 2 ± 1 days after admission (see Chs. 30–31). Viability was defined on the resting ^{201}Tl scan as an initial mild resting defect or any defect that demonstrated delayed redistribution. Approximately 50% of the patients were predicted to have viable myocardium in the infarct zone. These patients were more likely to have had a patent infarct-related artery, a higher initial ejection fraction, and fewer abnormal ^{201}Tl segments. In the group of patients demonstrating preserved viability in the infarct zone on early imaging, ejection fraction improved (57 ± 13% to 66 ± 10%, $p < 0.05$) in follow-up studies. In the group of patients in which predominantly nonviable myocardium was identified in the infarct zone on early imaging, ejection fraction deteriorated during follow-up (53 ± 10% to 46 ± 8%, $p < 0.05$). Figure 11–16 shows

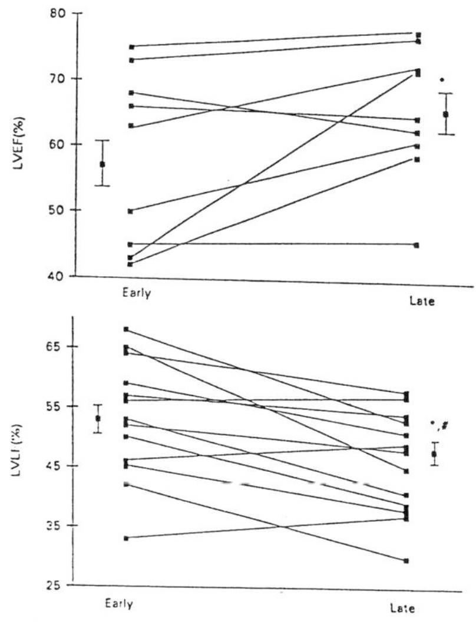

Figure 11–16. Early and late left ventricular ejection fraction (LVEF) in patients with a follow-up radionuclide angiogram (Group 1 [top], Group 2 [bottom]). Individual data and mean value ± SEM are presented (vertical bars). *p < 0.01, early versus late ejection fraction. #p < 0.0001, Group 1 versus Group 2.

the early and late left ventricular ejection fraction in patients predicted to have predominantly viable myocardium in the infarct zone on early imaging compared with patients who have predominantly nonviable myocardium by ^{201}Tl scan criteria. Thus early rest/redistribution ^{201}Tl imaging may be a useful approach for identifying residual viability in the zone of infarction, similarly to how it has already been shown useful for identifying viability in patients with remote infarction and chronic left ventricular dysfunction.

In summary, ^{201}Tl imaging performed solely in the resting state appears to have clinical utility and good positive and negative predictive value for identifying which asynergic myocardial segments will demonstrate improved regional systolic function after either angioplasty or coronary bypass surgery. Segments corresponding to resting ^{201}Tl defects that show enhanced ^{201}Tl uptake on rest redistribution imaging exhibit the greatest amount of improvement in regional wall motion after revascularization, whereas segments corresponding to severe persistent reduction in ^{201}Tl defects (>50% reduction) show the least improvement in regional contractility after revascularization. Perhaps as many as 60% of mild persistent defects (25% to 50% of peak uptake) also show substantial improvement in systolic function after revascularization. This implies that quantitation of regional ^{201}Tl activity is of great importance for enhancing the accuracy of SPECT ^{201}Tl imaging for differentiating between viable and nonviable asynergic myocardial regions.

A substantial number of patients with acute infarction have had a prior infarction and demonstrate angiographic multivessel coronary artery disease. Often such patients demonstrate symptoms and signs of congestive heart failure and may be hemodynamically unstable (see Ch. 23). Rest ^{201}Tl scintigraphy may provide important information to the surgeon pertaining to the expected improvement in function after revascularization. Those patients with substantial ^{201}Tl uptake in the zone of acute infarction, as well as in remote asynergic zones, would expect to have the greatest improvement in regional and global function after revascularization, with an associated improvement in heart failure symptoms. In contrast, patients with a low ejection fraction and predominantly nonviable myocardium would expect to have significantly less favorable outcome after revascularization, with a higher perioperative complication rate and mortality rate (147a). Further studies in a larger number of patients are warranted to validate this supposition.

Technetium-99*m* Sestamibi for Assessment of Myocardial Viability

The kinetics of ^{99m}Tc sestamibi uptake in normal, ischemic, and necrotic myocardium was discussed earlier in this chapter. As seen in the animal experiments cited previously, ^{99m}Tc sestamibi uptake can provide information comparable to that of ^{201}Tl for determination of myocardial viability. There is some controversy regarding whether or not resting ^{99m}Tc sestamibi has equal or less sensitivity than ^{201}Tl for predicting improvement in regional systolic function after revascularization. Several groups (148,149) reported that ^{99m}Tc sestamibi underestimated myocardial viability compared with ^{201}Tl scintigraphy. Maurea et al (150) found that resting ^{201}Tl uptake was higher than ^{99m}Tc sestamibi uptake in segments supplied by a totally occluded artery. Uptake of ^{201}Tl and ^{99m}Tc sestamibi, however, was comparable in segments supplied by vessels with 50% to 99% stenoses. In a subsequent study by this group (151), rest/redistribution ^{201}Tl imaging and resting ^{99m}Tc sestamibi imaging were undertaken in the same patients with coronary artery disease and regional left ventricular dysfunction (mean left ventricular ejection fraction: 35 ± 9%). When ^{201}Tl and ^{99m}Tc sestamibi uptake values were directly compared, no differences were observed in segments showing normal or hypokinetic wall motion. Technetium-99*m* sestamibi uptake was slightly but significantly lower than delayed ^{201}Tl uptake in zones demonstrating more severe reduction in systolic function (^{99m}Tc sestamibi uptake: 67 ± 14%, versus ^{201}Tl uptake: 73 ± 12%).

Several studies (54,152) employing quantitative SPECT imaging and rest/redistribution ^{201}Tl imaging and resting ^{99m}Tc sestamibi imaging found comparable worth of the two techniques for assessment of myocardial viability in predicting improvement in regional function after revascularization. Figure 11–17 demonstrates the quantitative analysis of resting ^{201}Tl activity and ^{99m}Tc sestamibi activity in perfusion defects grouped according to the mean normalized resting ^{201}Tl activity in 31 patients with chronic coronary artery disease, all of whom had a history of prior infarctions (54). Note that ^{99m}Tc sestamibi uptake was comparable to the delayed resting ^{201}Tl uptake in mild, moderate, and severe defects. In this study, concordancy in defect severity between ^{201}Tl and ^{99m}Tc sestamibi was 87%. Seventy-five percent of segments with ^{201}Tl activity of ≥60% of peak activity showed improved wall motion after revascularization. This was comparable with the segments that had ≥60% uptake of ^{99m}Tc sestamibi, 80% of which demonstrated functional recovery. No difference between the two techniques in predicting outcome after revascularization was observed.

Preliminary data from Kauffman et al (152) also demonstrate comparable ^{201}Tl and ^{99m}Tc sestamibi uptake in zones of severe regional dysfunction as categorized by preoperative resting echocardiography.

Thus, although ^{99m}Tc sestamibi does not redistribute over time after resting injection, significant uptake of the tracer occurs in asynergic myocardial

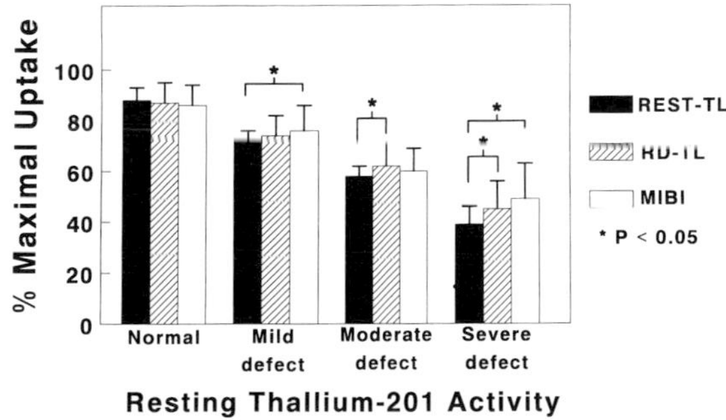

Figure 11–17. Maximal myocardial uptake of ^{201}Tl and ^{99m}Tc sestamibi in patients with chronic coronary artery disease and left ventricular dysfunction. Perfusion defects are grouped according to the mean normalized resting ^{201}Tl activity in 31 patients. Note that ^{99m}Tc sestamibi uptake (MIBI) was comparable to the delayed resting ^{201}Tl uptake (RD-TL) in mild, moderate, and severe defects. *Reprinted from Udelson et al (54), with permission.*

zones perfused by stenotic arteries. Recent studies cited above indicate that the magnitude of ^{99m}Tc sestamibi uptake in zones of hypoperfusion and regional dysfunction is comparable with the magnitude of delayed ^{201}Tl uptake (54,152). Because of better count statistics and less attenuation, ^{99m}Tc sestamibi uptake may be similar to ^{201}Tl uptake on SPECT imaging, although greater intracellular ^{201}Tl activity than ^{99m}Tc sestamibi activity can be demonstrated in vitro. The advantage of ^{201}Tl over ^{99m}Tc sestamibi in uptake kinetics (because of greater ^{201}Tl redistribution) may be lost with in vivo scintigraphy because of more ^{201}Tl attenuation.

Little data are available concerning the utility of ^{99m}Tc sestamibi SPECT imaging for evaluation of viability after acute myocardial infarction. Galli et al (152a) showed that early imaging after acute infarction with ^{99m}Tc sestamibi underestimated the extent of residual viability since a spontaneous reduction in infarct size was observed up to 8 months after the event.

Positron Emission Tomography of Myocardial Metabolic Activity

More sophisticated techniques such as positron emission computed tomography are even more sensitive than ^{201}Tl scintigraphy or radionuclide angiography in identifying zones of myocardial viability within a region of infarction. It has been shown that increased regional uptake of FDG in the ischemic zone identifies regions of myocardium that are metabolically active and thus will benefit from revascularization (153–155).

Thallium-201 and FDG were compared in an open chest canine model in which 2 hours of occlusion of the left anterior descending coronary artery were followed by 4 hours of reflow (155). Thallium-201 was injected prior to reperfusion, and FDG was administered 3 hours after reperfusion. These authors found that both normal FDG uptake and delayed ^{201}Tl redistribution reflected myocardial viability after reperfusion. Lack of redistribution and depressed FDG uptake were observed in irreversibly injured infarcted myocardial zones.

Positron emission tomography with $^{13}NH_3$ and FDG was used to assess regional perfusion and glucose uptake in 31 chronic ECG Q wave regions in 20 patients (153). Infarcted regions were identified by a matched reduction in regional $^{13}NH_3$ activity and glucose utilization, whereas regions of ischemia were identified by an enhanced FDG uptake in regions of diminished $^{13}NH_3$ activity (mismatch). Only 10 of these ECG Q wave regions (32%) truly exhibited infarction by these PET criteria. In contrast, viability was seen in 21 regions, 15 of which were normal and 6 of which revealed ischemia. Positron emission tomography revealed evidence of persistent tissue metabolism in a high proportion of regions associated with chronic ECG Q waves, thereby identifying viable regions that were not reliably detected by conventional tests. Schwaiger et al (156) performed FDG imaging studies in postinfarction patients within 72 hours of onset of symptoms. Decreased metabolic activity in the infarct zone was predictive of absence of subsequent improvement in regional systolic function. Uptake of FDG was higher in patients with patent infarct vessels than in those with an occluded infarct-related artery. Similarly, Pierard et al (157) compared FDG uptake patterns in acute infarction with subsequent outcome. Absence of metabolic activity on PET scans was associated with absence of enhanced systolic function with intravenous dobutamine. The extent of a mismatch pattern between perfusion and FDG uptake was unrelated to either presence or magnitude of collateral vessels, in a study by Di Carli and coworkers (158).

Positron emission tomographic imaging of perfusion and FDG uptake has been shown to have prognostic value. Postinfarction patients with an increase in FDG uptake demonstrated increased cardiac event rate during follow-up (159). Figure 11–18 shows the survival curves for eight uncomplicated infarction patients in this study who had an increase in FDG activity in at least one myocardial segment, compared with those without any evidence for increased FDG uptake. Note that the event-free survival rate was below 50% in patients with evidence for residual myocardial viability by PET criteria after infarction. In fact, this PET finding was the best predictor of future events among all clinical, angiographic, and ^{201}Tl scintigraphic variables.

Brunken and coworkers (154) showed that PET imaging can demonstrate evidence of preserved

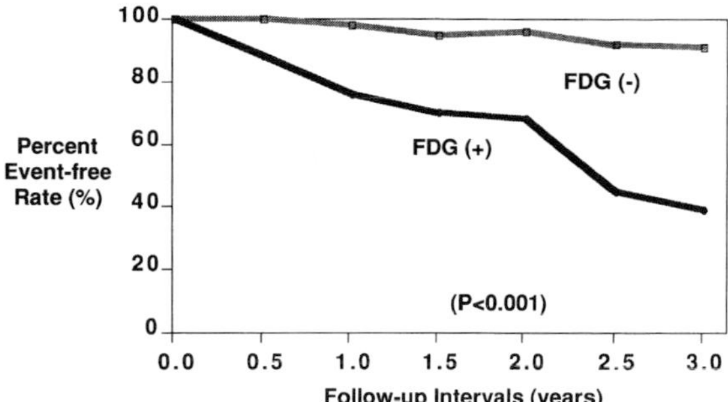

Figure 11–18. Event-free survival after acute myocardial infarction in patients who demonstrated an increase in fluorine-18 deoxyglucose (FDG) activity in at least one myocardial segment in the zone of infarction [FDG (+)], compared with those without any evidence of increased FDG uptake [FDG (−)]. *Reprinted from Tamaki et al (159), with permission.*

glucose uptake, indicating viability, in many segments with partial ^{201}Tl redistribution or persistent ^{201}Tl defects on stress/rest ^{201}Tl scintigraphy. In that study, 58% of segments showing no ^{201}Tl redistribution at 4 hours demonstrated some regional FDG uptake. These authors concluded that markers of perfusion alone may underestimate the extent of viable tissue in hypoperfused myocardial segments. It should be mentioned that late (24-hour) redistribution imaging or reinjection of a second dose of ^{201}Tl at 4 hours was not undertaken to enhance the sensitivity of the ^{201}Tl imaging procedure for distinguishing viable from nonviable myocardium.

Tillisch et al (160) monitored the functional outcome of segmental wall motion abnormalities following bypass surgery relative to preoperative metabolic findings on PET. Systolic function was enhanced in 85% of myocardial segments showing "mismatch patterns" between blood flow and metabolism, whereas no improvement was noted in 92% of patients with a flow–metabolism match (criteria for nonviability). Other studies (161) have confirmed these findings and suggest the potential clinical applicability for PET imaging of blood flow and metabolism in the pre-revascularization evaluation of patients with depressed left ventricular function with or without a recent myocardial infarction. Many of these patients have severe regional wall motion abnormalities, and myocardial viability is an important issue with respect to consideration of surgery that could be risky. In patients with ischemic cardiomyopathy, the magnitude of improvement in heart failure symptoms after revascularization is related to the preoperative extent and magnitude of viability as assessed by PET-FDG imaging (161a).

More recently, PET imaging of carbon-11 acetate has been evaluated to image myocardial oxygen consumption (84,162–164). Measurement of the oxidation of the acetate may provide an indirect measure of myocardial oxygen consumption; therefore, this approach may also be shown useful for assessing viable myocardium in areas of regional myocardial asynergy. Metabolic PET imaging with carbon-11 acetate can be employed to detect residual myocardial metabolic activity after reperfusion in acute myocardial infarction. Walsh et al (162) found that reduction in carbon-11 acetate clearance rate from the infarct zone reflected impaired oxidative metabolism. Peri-infarction zones with reduced blood flow showed only a mild decrease of carbon-11 acetate clearance.

Myocardial blood flow has been measured using oxygen-15-labeled water and PET imaging in postinfarction patients. In one study by Hanes et al (165), postinfarction patients who received t-PA were imaged by 24 hours after thrombolytic therapy, 24 to 48 hours after treatment, and before hospital discharge. These investigators found that myocardial blood flow was restored toward normal levels in most patients at the time of the first scan, without a subsequent decrement in flow. They concluded that the "no reflow" phenomenon was not observed in patients undergoing reperfusion therapy in this particular study.

Rubidium-82 imaging can also be undertaken for the assessment of myocardial viability, employing the PET technique. The rationale for the use of ^{82}Rb imaging for assessing myocardial viability is based on the concept that ischemic but viable myocardium can retain extracted ^{82}Rb, whereas nonviable myocardium exhibits back-diffusion of the tracer, yielding a faster washout rate from necrotic compared with normal myocardium. Upon delivery by coronary blood flow to myocardial tissue, ^{82}Rb is extracted by viable cells, where it equilibrates with the intracellular potassium pool. Necrotic cells cannot retain the tracer, and ^{82}Rb washes rapidly after initial redistribution. The rate of ^{82}Rb washout can be measured by rapid sequential PET imaging.

In a study reported by Gould and coworkers (83), 43 patients with evolving myocardial infarction had PET imaging using FDG and ^{82}Rb. Infarct size based on ^{82}Rb kinetics correlated closely with size and location on FDG images ($r = 0.93$), suggesting that loss of cellular mechanisms for sequestering ^{82}Rb intracellularly parallel the loss of metabolic integrity of cellular glucose extraction. In a subsequent report from the Houston group (166), the size of scar and viable myocardium by ^{82}Rb PET imaging was highly predictive of 3-year mortality in patients with a previous infarction. Infarction involving 23% or more of the left ventricle on PET imaging was associated with a 3-year mortality rate of 43%, versus 5% for those with scar comprising less than 23% of the left ventricle. Patients in this study with viable myocardium had a significantly lower mortality rate than patients with nonviable myocardium. This most likely was attributed to the fact that 75% of these patients underwent revascularization.

MYOCARDIAL PERFUSION IMAGING AFTER THROMBOLYTIC THERAPY IN ACUTE MYOCARDIAL INFARCTION

Thallium-201 Imaging

Rest ^{201}Tl scintigraphy can be utilized to assess the extent of reflow in myocardial salvage after coronary reperfusion. Several investigators administered ^{201}Tl intravenously before administration of a thrombolytic agent and obtained postthrombolysis images several hours later (167–169). These studies demonstrated that patients exhibiting successful thrombolysis had more ^{201}Tl redistribution and smaller final ^{201}Tl defect sizes compared with patients with persistently occluded infarct-related vessels. Patients who demonstrate ^{201}Tl redistribution at 4 hours after institution of thrombolytic therapy may show even further improvement in perfusion when imaging is repeated 4 days and 6 weeks later (167).

There are some significant limitations to the use of serial rest ^{201}Tl redistribution imaging in the early evaluation of patients receiving thrombolytic therapy. It may take up to 30 minutes to obtain pretreatment images, which would delay institution of thrombolytic therapy. On the other hand, if ^{201}Tl is injected for the first time immediately after reperfusion, the degree of salvage might be overestimated, because the radionuclide is taken up in proportion to the hyperemic flow and not in proportion to viable myocardial tissue.

Another approach to myocardial ^{201}Tl scintigraphy in patients undergoing thrombolytic therapy is to administer two separate intravenous ^{201}Tl injections, before and 24 hours or later after treatment (170). By delaying the second imaging procedure to 24 hours, the trapping of ^{201}Tl in the infarct region during the hyperemic flow phase that immediately follows reflow might be avoided (171). Several groups of investigators have utilized this approach. Schwartz et al (170) performed resting ^{201}Tl scintigraphy before and 24 hours after treatment in patients receiving intravenous followed by intracoronary streptokinase. The regional ejection fraction was serially measured up to 4 weeks after thrombolytic therapy. The improvement in ^{201}Tl defect size was greatest in those patients undergoing successful recanalization. Regional ejection fraction was improved only in the patients with the greatest reduction in the ^{201}Tl defect size who experienced successful reflow.

In the Western Washington Intracoronary Streptokinase in Myocardial Infarction Trial, Ritchie et al (172) performed quantitative SPECT ^{201}Tl resting imaging in 100 patients 8 weeks after infarction. They found no difference in ^{201}Tl defect size between control and streptokinase-treated patients. They also found no difference in global or regional ejection fraction between the two groups. Also in that study, there was no relation between radionuclide measures of perfusion and function and vessel patency; however, the time to vessel opening approximated 5 hours. In a subsequent intravenous thrombolytic trial, infarct size by SPECT ^{201}Tl imaging was smaller in treated patients compared with controls ($15 \pm 13\%$ versus $19 \pm 13\%$, $p = 0.03$) (173). These patients were treated sooner than patients in the intracoronary streptokinase trial conducted by the same group (172). These results emphasize that when reflow is accomplished late after the onset of infarction, significant salvage cannot be expected or, alternatively, the technique has limitations with respect to the measurement of infarct size. A long-term follow-up of this patient population showed that patients with large ^{201}Tl defects had a significantly higher 5-year mortality rate compared with those having small defects after streptokinase therapy (Fig. 11–19) (174).

Technetium-99*m* Isonitrile Imaging

A promising alternative to ^{201}Tl scintigraphy for assessment of thrombolytic therapy is the administration of ^{99m}Tc sestamibi. This agent does not redistribute; therefore, the first dose can be administered just before thrombolytic therapy, but imaging can be postponed several hours later after thrombolytic drug administration is complete, to obtain the pretreatment assessment of risk area. This way, institution of thrombolysis is not delayed as with ^{201}Tl scintigraphy. A "snapshot" of the perfusion pattern at time of admission is obtained with the first injection of ^{99m}Tc sestamibi. Even images obtained 6 hours after injection show the perfusion pattern that existed at the time of tracer administration. A second injection is given sometime after thrombolytic therapy and after the first images are obtained, to delineate the degree of improvement in flow and extent of myocardial salvage. Technetium-99*m* sestamibi imaging could become a useful technique to incorporate in clinical research trials aimed at evaluating efficacy of pharmacologic approaches for reperfusion.

Several experimental and clinical studies have been undertaken to validate this technique. Wackers et al (175) and Gibbons et al (176), with the assistance of several collaborating institutions, have successfully applied serial ^{99m}Tc sestamibi imaging in patients with acute myocardial infarction undergoing thrombolytic therapy (Fig. 11–20). Patients with a patent infarct artery had a significantly greater decrease in defect size on repeat images performed 18 to 48 hours after thrombolytic therapy than did patients with persistently occluded vessels. Wackers et al (175) found that a relative decrease of greater than 30% in the size of the ^{99m}Tc sestamibi perfusion defect predicted patency of the infarct-related artery, providing noninvasive evidence of the efficacy of treatment. This observation is important because there are few reliable nonangiographic methods to predict successful reperfusion (see Chs. 22,28).

Technetium 99*m* sestamibi defect size prior to reperfusion is significantly greater with anterior compared with inferior infarction (52 ± 9% versus 18 ± 10% of the left ventricle) (177). The final defect size after thrombolytic therapy or angioplasty was also significantly larger with anterior compared

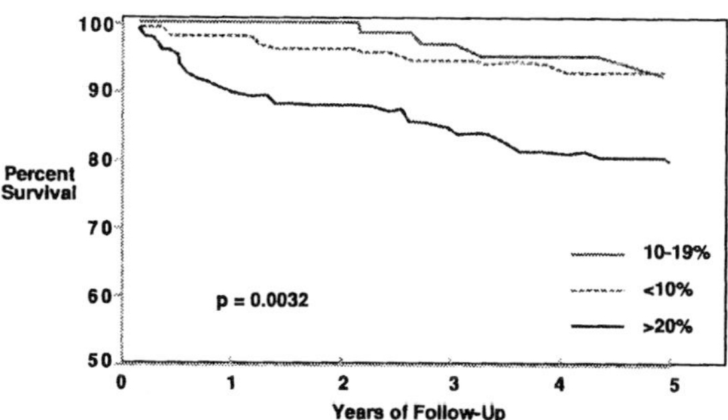

Figure 11–19. Event-free survival during five years of follow-up related to ^{201}Tl defect size after intravenous streptokinase therapy in patients with acute myocardial infarction. *Adapted from Cerqueira et al (174), with permission.*

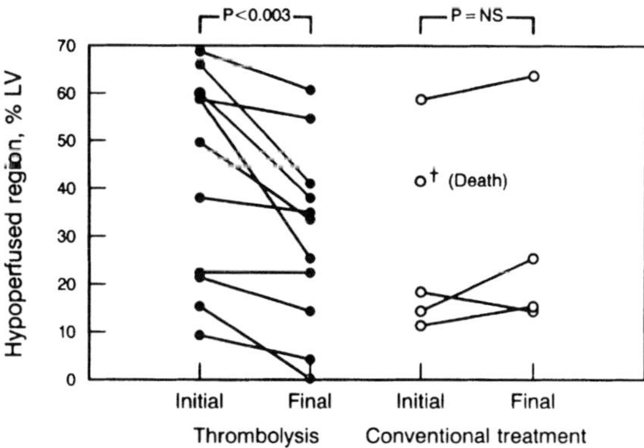

Figure 11–20. Extent of regional left ventricular (LV) hypoperfusion in the zone of acute myocardial infarction prior to (initial) and after either thrombolytic therapy or conventional treatment (final). Note a significant reduction in the hypoperfused region in the patients receiving thrombolytic therapy compared with those receiving conventional treatment. *Reprinted from Gibbons et al (176), with permission.*

with inferior infarction (30 ± 20% versus 9 ± 8%, $p < 0.01$). Nevertheless, in this study the proportion of jeopardized myocardium salvaged by reperfusion was not significantly different for patients with anterior and inferior infarction. Those patients with an occluded infarct-related artery had no change in defect size. In four patients who received ^{99m}Tc sestamibi before experiencing fatal cardiogenic shock, the extent of infarction by pathologic assessment was smaller than the ^{99m}Tc sestamibi perfusion defect (178). This observation points out that many perfusion abnormalities in patients with acute infarction represent the combination of necrosis and ischemia, particularly when such patients are imaged early.

The results of early ^{99m}Tc sestamibi imaging in patients receiving thrombolytic therapy are predictive of late functional improvement, or lack thereof, as assessed by echocardiography, radionuclide angiography, or contrast ventriculography. Santoro et al (179) found a good correlation ($r = 0.9$) between the 5-day ^{99m}Tc sestamibi scintigraphic estimate of infarct area and the enzymatic infarct size (Fig. 11–21). The reduction in defect size over time predicted late functional improvement that was demonstrated by echocardiography performed 1 month later ($r = 0.89$). Similarly, ^{99m}Tc sestamibi imaging after reperfusion therapy is predictive of the left ventricular ejection fraction at 1 year ($r = -0.78$) (180). It was also predictive of end-diastolic and end-systolic volume indices. The left ventricular ejection fraction at the time of discharge may not accurately reflect perfusion defect size because of the effects of stunning and compensatory hyperkinesia (181). The relationship between ^{99m}Tc sestamibi defect as a percentage of the left ventricle correlates well with global ejection fraction when the functional measurement is made at 6 weeks postinfarction, when compensatory hyperkinesis may abate (181). Infarct sizes of greater than 40% of the left ventricle despite acute reperfusion therapy were documented in 16 of 166 patients with acute myocardial infarction who underwent ^{99m}Tc sestamibi SPECT imaging (182). Ejection fraction by radionuclide angiography in those patients was 33% at discharge and 38% at 6 weeks. One patient who had cardiogenic shock died, but the remaining 15 patients were asymptomatic at 1 year follow-up. The authors point out that in the age of reperfusion therapy, even patients with large residual myocardial infarction can survive without heart failure.

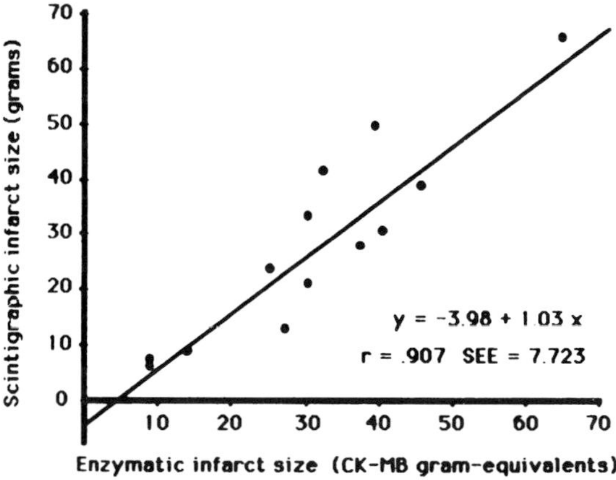

Figure 11–21. Correlation between scintigraphic infarct size determined by ^{99m}Tc sestamibi SPECT imaging at 5 days with the enzymatic infarct size determined by creatine kinase–MB (CK-MB) determinations. The correlation was good ($r = 0.907$). *Reprinted from Santoro et al (179), with permission.*

Oh et al (182a) found a good correlation (0.71) between improvement in echocardiographic wall motion score and the change in extent of ^{99m}Tc sestamibi perfusion defect in patients treated with reperfusion therapy during acute myocardial infarction. In that study, 52% of the improvement in wall motion score was achieved within 18 to 48 hours after reperfusion.

The extent of myocardial damage as assessed by ^{99m}Tc sestamibi imaging is predictive of subsequent change in left ventricular volume and function in the year after myocardial infarction (183) (see Ch. 29). In this study, the larger the infarct size is by ^{99m}Tc sestamibi activity, the greater the amount is of left ventricular remodeling after discharge. Infarct size at discharge correlated well with end-systolic volume ($r = 0.80$) and ejection fraction ($r = -0.84$) at 1 year. Interestingly, the correlation between ^{99m}Tc sestamibi infarct size and these functional parameters was not good when the correlations were made at the time of discharge. This observation may have significant relevance in that patients with extensive myocardial damage as assessed at the time of discharge by rest/stress ^{99m}Tc sestamibi imaging may benefit from angiotensin converting enzyme inhibitor therapy even though end-systolic and end-diastolic dimensions have not yet shown evidence for left ventricular remodeling.

Technetium-99*m* sestamibi imaging can be utilized to determine the efficacy of primary angioplasty in salvaging myocardium and acute infarction (184–187). Behrenbeck et al (184) found a significant reduction in defect size after primary angioplasty in patients with a first transmural infarction (Fig. 11–22). Acute ^{99m}Tc sestamibi defect size prior to angioplasty was 48 ± 17% of the left ventricle and diminished significantly to 29 ± 19% on repeat imaging undertaken 6 to 10 days following dilation of the infarct-related artery. No correlation was found between the time to therapy and the ultimate reduction in defect size. Gibbons and coworkers (186) found that myocardial salvage as assessed by measuring the percent reduction in ^{99m}Tc sestamibi defect size was similar in patients randomized to primary angioplasty than patients randomized to thrombolytic therapy. Clements et al (185) found that residual antegrade flow prior to direct angioplasty and demonstration of collateral flow were associated with a significantly smaller final ^{99m}Tc SPECT sestamibi defect size and more myocardial salvage after angioplasty.

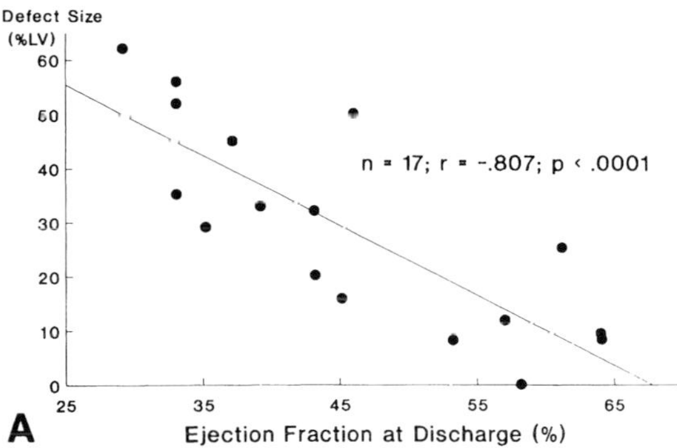

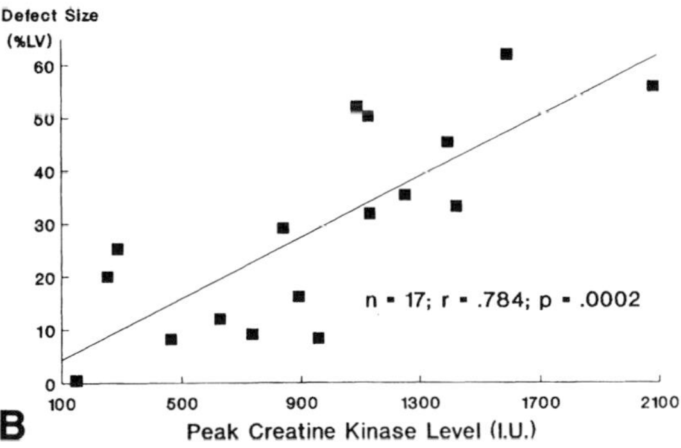

Figure 11–22. A. Correlation between late perfusion defect size by ^{99m}Tc sestamibi imaging and ejection fraction at discharge in patients undergoing primary angioplasty after myocardial infarction. **B.** Correlation between late perfusion defect size and peak creatine kinase levels in the same patients. *Reprinted from Behrenbeck et al (184), with permission.*

Christian and coworkers (188) performed exercise ^{201}Tl scintigraphy with reinjection and resting ^{99m}Tc sestamibi in a group of 20 patients, 18 of whom underwent acute reperfusion. They found that ^{99m}Tc sestamibi defect size was 12 ± 13% of the left ventricle, which was significantly smaller than the ^{201}Tl defect size as assessed by quantitative SPECT imaging using the polar map method (25 ± 17% of the left ventricle). Infarct size with ^{99m}Tc sestamibi provided a closer correlation with ejection fraction ($r = 0.81$) compared with the ^{201}Tl imaging method ($r = 0.69$). The authors concluded that ^{99m}Tc sestamibi imaging may be a more accurate technique for assessing infarct size than stress/redistribution/reinjection ^{201}Tl scintigraphy.

Serial ^{99m}Tc sestamibi imaging performed several hours apart, rather than 24 hours apart, might contribute to decision-making with respect to which patients may benefit from "rescue" angioplasty after thrombolytic therapy (see Ch. 22). If the prethrombolysis ^{99m}Tc sestamibi defect was small and the posttreatment defect remained small even if not reduced, emergent angiography would not be considered. This is because the risk area was initially minimal and even if vessel patency was not restored, prognosis would be excellent. If the pretreatment defect was large and the posttreatment defect was significantly reduced, then it could be assumed that thrombolysis had been successful in restoring nutrient blood flow. Emergent angiography would not be required since reflow was accomplished. If, however, the initial defect was large and remained large after thrombolytic therapy, then it might be assumed that the infarct-related vessel was still occluded. Such a patient would be at high risk for extensive myocardial damage. Thus emergent angiography, with a view toward rescue angioplasty (if the vessel was still occluded), would be undertaken. Further clinical research studies are required to evaluate this potential decision-making process.

PREDISCHARGE EXERCISE IMAGING FOR RISK STRATIFICATION

Exercise or Vasodilator Stress Thallium-201 Scintigraphy

Stress perfusion imaging can be utilized to separate high- and low-risk subsets of patients with uncomplicated myocardial infarction prior to hospital discharge (see Ch. 31). Table 11–4 lists the high-risk exercise radionuclide variables that can be recognized on stress perfusion scintigraphy. Detection of ischemia remote from the infarct zone, which would reflect physiologically significant multiple-vessel coronary artery disease, or residual ischemia within the infarct zone, which would suggest an "incomplete infarct," or both, should be the aim of predischarge exercise scintigraphy. Dunn and coworkers (189) showed that among 37 patients with previous myocardial infarction who had ^{201}Tl defects in more than one designated vascular region, 92% had multiple-vessel coronary disease compared with 72% of the 39 patients who had a positive exercise electrocardiogram.

Table 11–4. High-Risk Exercise Test and Imaging Variables After Acute Myocardial Infarction

Exercise electrocardiographic stress testing
Failure to reach target heart rate (120–130 beats per minute)
Failure to achieve >4 METs
Failure to increase systolic blood pressure by ≥10 mm Hg
Exercise-induced ST segment depression (>1.0 mm)
Inducible angina
Exercise or pharmacologic stress myocardial perfusion imaging
Multiple perfusion defects in more than one vascular region (for example, left anterior descending and circumflex zones)
Presence of defect reversibility
Increased lung thallium-201 uptake
Exercise-induced LV cavity dilation
Exercise radionuclide angiography
Decrease of >5% in LV ejection fraction from rest to exercise
Absolute exercise LV ejection fraction <50%
Exercise-induced increase in end-systolic volume
Rest radionuclide imaging
Resting LV ejection fraction <45%
Extensive resting thallium-201 or technetium-99*m* sestamibi or tetrofosmin defects
Large areas of technetium pyrophosphate or indium-111 antimyosin antibody uptake
Large nitrogen-13 ammonia defect with no fluorine-18, 2-deoxyglucose uptake

LV = left ventricular.

Gibson and coworkers (190) showed that approximately 50% of patients with an uncomplicated myocardial infarction who demonstrated (i) multiple ^{201}Tl defects in more than one vascular region, (ii) delayed redistribution within or remote from the infarct zone, or (iii) abnormal lung ^{201}Tl uptake on predischarge submaximal exercise imaging either suffered a cardiac death, had a nonfatal infarction, or developed class III or IV angina at a mean follow-up of 15 months. In contrast, the cardiac event rate was only 6% in those postinfarction patients who had either a normal scan or solely persistent defects and no associated redistribution. Thallium-201 scintigraphic variables separated high- and low-risk subgroups better than did exercise electrocardiographic stress test variables (Fig. 11–23). Hung et al (191) confirmed these observations and reported that the magnitude of exercise-induced ^{201}Tl defects and the extent of ^{201}Tl redistribution 3 weeks postinfarction was significantly predictive of subsequent death or nonfatal infarction.

Brown and coworkers (192) examined the prognostic implications of ischemia within the territory of a prior acute myocardial infarction versus is-

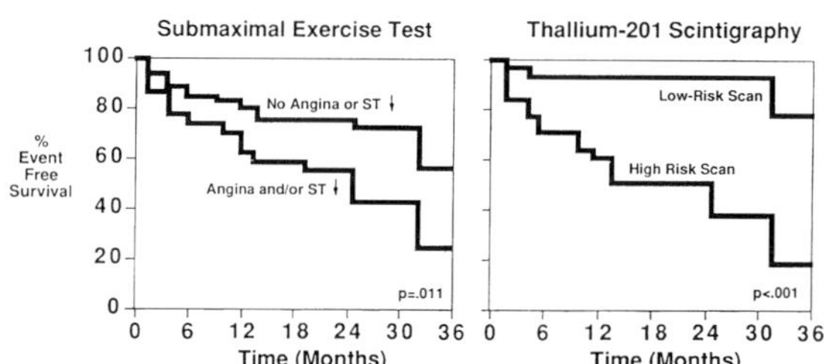

Figure 11–23. Left panel: Event-free survival in patients with a high-risk (angina and/or ST depression [↓]) or a low-risk (no angina or ST depression) submaximal exercise tests prior to hospital discharge in patients with uncomplicated acute infarction.
Right panel: Event-free survival in patients with a high-risk or low-risk planar ^{201}Tl perfusion scan obtained in conjunction with submaximal exercise testing in the same patients. Note that low- and high-risk patients were better separated by ^{201}Tl scintigraphy than by submaximal exercise testing alone. *Adapted from Gibson et al (190), with permission.*

chemia at a distance that developed late after infarction. In a group of 61 consecutive patients who underwent both exercise ^{201}Tl imaging and cardiac catheterization for evaluation of chest pain that developed after discharge from the hospital after acute infarction, 29 had ^{201}Tl redistribution confined to the infarct zone and 16 had redistribution outside the infarct zone. Stepwise multivariate logistic regression analysis revealed that both the presence of any ^{201}Tl redistribution and multivessel angiographic coronary artery disease were significant predictors of total cardiac events during a 10 ± 17-month follow-up. When, however, coronary revascularization was excluded as an endpoint, ^{201}Tl redistribution limited to the prior infarct zone was the only significant predictor of cardiac events.

High-risk non–Q wave infarct patients can also be identified by demonstration of ^{201}Tl redistribution within the zone of infarction on predischarge exercise scintigraphy (see Ch. 18) (193). In a study by Gibson (193), the prevalence and extent of ^{201}Tl redistribution within the zone of infarction were greater in patients with non–Q wave compared with those with Q wave infarction (60% versus 36%) (Fig. 11–24). Patients with non–Q wave infarction who subsequently experienced cardiac events had a higher incidence of infarct zone redistribution compared with patients whose course was event free. This is not surprising, as patients with non–Q wave infarction have less myocardial necrosis and therefore more myocardium still jeopardized in the risk area of the infarct-related vessel.

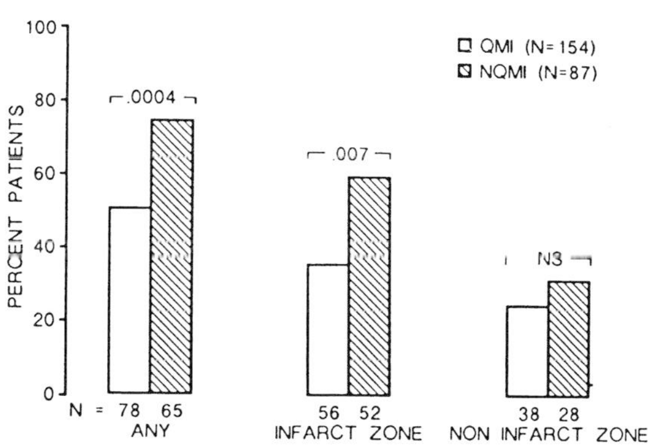

Figure 11–24. Percent of patients with Q wave myocardial infarction (open bars) and non–Q wave myocardial infarction (cross-hatched bars) with any ^{201}Tl distribution, ^{201}Tl redistribution confined to the infarct zone, and ^{201}Tl redistribution in the noninfarct zone in patients undergoing submaximal exercise testing with quantitative planar ^{201}Tl scintigraphy prior to hospital discharge. Note that the prevalence of redistribution within the infarct zone is significantly greater for non–Q wave infarction patients. *Reprinted from Gibson et al (193), with permission.*

Risk Stratification in the Era of Acute Reperfusion

Controversy exists regarding the value of exercise radionuclide perfusion imaging for risk stratification in the thrombolytic era or after primary angioplasty (194) (see Chs. 30–31). In patients who have undergone thrombolytic therapy, ^{201}Tl redistribution is still more prevalent than ST segment depression on exercise stress testing. Tilkemeier et al (195) reported a 42% prevalence of Tl-201 redistribution compared with 15% for ST segment depression in postinfarction patients who receive thrombolytic therapy. Similar findings were reported by Haber et al (196), who found a 48% prevalence of ^{201}Tl redistribution, which was significantly higher than the 14% of prevalence of ST segment depression (Fig. 11–25). Although exercise perfusion imaging remains more sensitive than exercise ECG testing alone following thrombolytic therapy, the prevalence of redistribution defects is less than seen in the prethrombolytic era in uncomplicated infarction patients undergoing

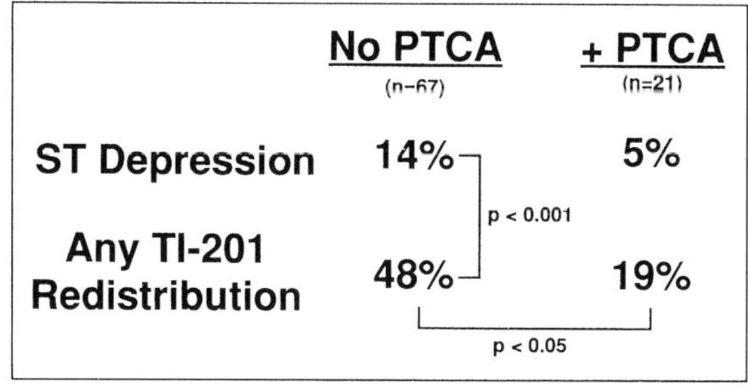

Figure 11–25. Prevalence of ST segment depression and any ^{201}Tl redistribution on predischarge exercise testing in patients with acute myocardial infarction who received thrombolytic therapy and had either no angioplasty (No PTCA; first column) or angioplasty (+ PTCA; second column) prior to testing. Note that the prevalence of ^{201}Tl redistribution was significantly greater than the prevalence of ischemic ST depression. *Reprinted from Haber et al (196), with permission.*

predischarge exercise testing. When a prethrombolytic cohort (190) was compared with a later thrombolytic cohort (196) who underwent predischarge ^{201}Tl imaging prior to hospital discharge, the prevalence of ST segment depression decreased from 32% to 14%, and the prevalence of ^{201}Tl redistribution fell from 59% to 48%.

Multivessel coronary artery disease is one of the most important prognostic variables for identifying high-risk patients who survive an acute myocardial infarction. One of the primary goals of risk assessment is to identify those patients with multivessel disease and residual myocardial ischemia who might benefit from referral for early coronary angiography and revascularization. Haber et al (196) reported that 35% of patients treated with a thrombolytic agent had underlying multivessel coronary artery disease by angiography. Twenty-two percent had two-vessel disease, and 13% had three-vessel disease. A ^{201}Tl defect identified remote from the infarct zone was observed in only 35% of these patients (Fig. 11–26). The sensitivity for detection of multivessel disease by ^{201}Tl scintigraphy (35%) was slightly, but not significantly, higher than that of exercise-induced ST segment depression (29%). If a remote ^{201}Tl defect and ST segment depression were considered as a single variable for multivessel disease detection, 58% of patients with angiographic multivessel disease had either one or the other. Using either ST segment depression or a remote ^{201}Tl defect as a single variable diminished the specificity for multivessel coronary artery disease detection from 97% to 78% (Fig. 11–26).

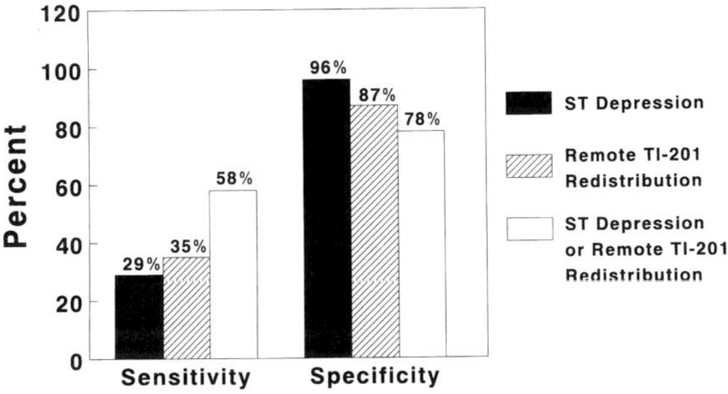

Figure 11–26. Prevalence of ischemic ST segment depression, remote ^{201}Tl redistribution, and ST depression or remote ^{201}Tl redistribution in postinfarction patients who received thrombolytic therapy and had multivessel coronary artery disease on angiography. *Reprinted from Haber et al (196), with permission.*

In the prethrombolytic era, the sensitivity for detection of multivessel coronary artery disease was higher than the 35% detection rate reported by Haber and coworkers in postinfarction patients who received thrombolytic therapy. In a series of studies collated from reports in the prethrombolytic era, which comprised a total of 508 patients, there was a 72% sensitivity of the remote ^{201}Tl defect for detecting multivessel coronary artery disease, with an 86% specificity (194). In these prior series, 59% of patients with multivessel disease have ischemic ST segment depression. The positive predictive value of a remote ^{201}Tl defect for identifying multivessel coronary artery disease was significantly higher than the positive predictive value of ST segment depression for multivessel disease identification. Possible explanations for the diminished sensitivity of exercise ^{201}Tl scintigraphy for identifying multivessel disease in cohorts of patients who received thrombolytic therapy are described below.

First, as cited previously, prethrombolytic cohorts of patients with an acute infarction had a 55% to 60% prevalence of underlying multivessel coronary artery disease compared with approximately 35% prevalence of multivessel disease in series of patients reported in the literature who are enrolled in thrombolytic trials. Such patient groups have been found to only have a 10% to 15% prevalence of three-vessel disease. For example, in the TIMI-II trial, the prevalence of three-vessel disease was 5% in the "routine catheterization" subgroup and 11% in the "selective catheterization" subgroup (123). In the GUSTO angiographic trial (125), only 14% of patients had three-vessel disease. Since a defect remote from the infarct zone is more likely to be induced by submaximal exercise in the presence of three-vessel than two-vessel disease, it is not surprising that the sensitivity of remote defects for multivessel disease identification is less than thrombolytic patient populations. Postinfarction patients with three-vessel disease would be expected to have more extensive perfusion defects remote from the infarct zone than patients with one- or two-vessel disease.

A second explanation relates to the fact that the prevalence of previous infarction is lower in patients enrolled in trials of thrombolytic therapy compared with series in the prethrombolytic era. A prior infarction at a site remote from the zone of new necrosis would be associated with a greater probability of a remote defect on ^{201}Tl scintigraphy.

A third explanation for the diminished sensitivity of ^{201}Tl scintigraphy for multivessel disease identification in postinfarction patients is that early reperfusion with attainment of TIMI grade 3 flow in the infarct-related vessel may result in minimal infarction after reperfusion. Thallium-201 uptake may be normal or minimally reduced in the risk zone perfused by the infarct-related vessel. This enhanced salvage could be associated with only one defect region being demonstrable on exercise scintigrams in a patient with angiographic multivessel disease.

A fourth explanation relates to the observation that non–Q wave infarct patients comprised a substantial percentage of postinfarction patient series reported in the prethrombolytic era, whereas patients without ST segment elevation on the admission electrocardiogram comprised a very small percentage of patients reported in thrombolytic therapy series. Patients with a non–Q wave infarction have comparable extent of angiographic coronary artery disease to patients with Q wave infarction but have a higher prevalence of stress-induced ischemia (193). With less myocardial damage in the infarct zone, patients with non–Q wave infarction can exercise to higher peak heart rates or workloads, yielding a greater probability that a defect remote from the infarct zone in the supply region of a stenotic vessel will be induced.

Thus a diminished sensitivity of ^{201}Tl scintigraphy for multivessel disease identification in the thrombolytic era could be attributed to a change in the patient population undergoing testing. Patients enrolled in thrombolytic series appear to be a lower risk population compared with patients who were evaluated in the prethrombolytic series of sequential patients.

Some observers have stated that exercise ECG testing with or without myocardial perfusion imaging is of little value for use in the risk stratification process in patients with acute myocardial infarction seen in the thrombolytic era (197,198). Krone et al (197) found that the exercise test with or without ^{201}Tl imaging added little to the overall prediction of primary cardiac events in 936 patients who recovered from myocardial infarction of unstable angina. It should be pointed out that these patients were enrolled at a mean of 2.7 months after the index event. Thirty-one percent had thrombolytic therapy, 67% underwent coronary angiography, and 39% had coronary angioplasty before enrollment. Excluded from study enrollment were those patients who underwent coronary bypass surgery after the index event (21.5% of the original eligible candidates). Also excluded were patients on digitalis or other drugs thought likely to induce false-positive or nondiagnostic ST segment changes on exercise ECG recordings. Patients who had resting ST–T wave changes were also excluded from enrollment. As expected in a patient population in which most high-risk patients were either not enrolled or underwent coronary angioplasty before enrollment, the cardiac mortality rate at 1 year in this study was only 1.2% and the rate of recurrent nonfatal infarction was only 3.4%. Interestingly, only 2% of the patients had increased lung ^{201}Tl uptake in conjunction with at least one redistribution ^{201}Tl defect. This reflects the lack of inclusion of many high-risk patients with multivessel disease and/or resting ventricular dysfunction who were medically treated. Also, consistent with the supposition that many high-risk patients were never enrolled is that 91% of the patients who were enrolled achieved exercise stage II or greater and only 3% had evidence of inducible ischemia during stage I of the exercise test protocol.

Finally, no matter how sensitive and specific a noninvasive test may be for subgrading high- and low-risk subgroups of postinfarction patients, it cannot accurately identify a subgroup with a mortality rate of only 1.2%, which was the mortality rate observed in this multicenter trial reported by Krone et al (197). If most of the high-risk patients who are prone to residual ischemia, or who have multivessel disease and left ventricular dysfunction, are either never enrolled or undergo coronary revascularization before or soon after enrollment, the only patients remaining on medical therapy and included for long-term follow-up comprise a very low-risk subgroup.

Miller et al (198a) also concluded that there was limited prognostic value of ^{201}Tl exercise testing early after myocardial infarction in patients treated with thrombolysis. Of the 210 patients in this retrospective study, 178 underwent coronary angiography prior to stress testing and 79 had angioplasty with thrombolytic therapy. Twenty-six percent of the patients underwent revascularization after the ^{201}Tl study. Those undergoing revascularization soon after ^{201}Tl perfusion imaging had more extensive and severe ischemia, indicating that the high-risk patients were referred to revascularization *on the basis* of their exercise scintigraphic findings. Another 18 patients underwent late revascularization. The 2-year survival rate for this patient cohort was 97%. Again, exercise ^{201}Tl stress testing will have "limited prognostic value" if most high-risk patients undergo either preexercise test or postexercise test revascularization, leaving only very low-risk postinfarction patients treated solely with medical therapy.

Vasodilator Stress Perfusion Imaging After Acute Myocardial Infarction

Dipyridamole ^{201}Tl imaging has been successfully employed for predischarge risk assessment in patients with an uncomplicated myocardial infarction. Leppo and coworkers (199) were the first to show that dipyridamole ^{201}Tl scintigraphy could be performed safely in uncomplicated postinfarction patients when performed 1 to 2 weeks after admission. Eleven of twelve patients who died during follow-up or sustained a recurrent infarction showed dipyridamole-induced redistribution defects at predischarge testing, as did 22 of 24 patients who were readmitted for angina. Among all clinical and ^{201}Tl scintigraphic variables tested, the presence of redistribution was the only significant predictor of these subsequent cardiac events and was more sensitive than exercise ST segment depression in predicting outcome. Dipyridamole ^{201}Tl scintigraphy can safely be performed very soon after admission for acute infarction. Brown et al (200) performed dipyridamole scintigraphy at an average of 62 ± 21 hours after hospitalization. By stepwise multivariate logistic regression analysis, the best and only statistically significant predictor of in-hospital ischemic cardiac events was the presence of dipyridamole-induced ^{201}Tl redistribution within the infarct zone. Forty-five percent of patients who demonstrated infarct zone redistribution on dipyridamole scans developed in-hospital events; this was in contrast to patients without infarct zone redistribution, of whom none had an event.

Hendel and coworkers (201) determined the utility of dipyridamole ^{201}Tl scintigraphy for predicting late cardiac death and recurrent infarction in 71 uncomplicated postinfarction patients who received thrombolytic therapy. They found that no scintigraphic variable was predictive of hard events in this patient population; however, it should be pointed out that coronary angioplasty was performed in 29 of the 71 patients before hospital discharge. There were only two deaths in this study, and most events were recurrent infarction in the 10 patients who did experience a subsequent event.

Adenosine can be substituted for dipyridamole as a vasodilator for stress perfusion imaging postinfarction patients with a comparable safety profile. Mahmarian et al (202) related adenosine SPECT defect size to future cardiac events in patients who underwent early imaging after hospitalization for uncomplicated infarction. Perfusion defect size was larger in patients who had in-hospital cardiac events (45 ± 18%) compared with those who had no events (22 ± 15%). Ninety percent of patients with events had at least a 20% perfusion defect. Perfusion defect size was 51 ± 14% in patients who either developed congestive heart failure, died, or had ventricular tachycardia. Overall sensitivity for detecting individual coronary stenoses was 87%. Sixty-three percent of patients with two-vessel disease and 91% percent of patients with three-vessel disease had a multivessel disease scan pattern.

In a follow-up report from Mahmarian et al (203), 146 patients who underwent adenosine ^{201}Tl scintigraphy during hospitalization for acute myocardial infarction were followed for more than 1 year. Excluded were 51 patients with revascularization soon after imaging. Cardiac events occurred in 33% of 92 patients over 15.7 months of follow-up. Univariate predictor events were quantified perfusion defect size ($p < 0.001$), absolute extent of left ventricular ischemia ($p < 0.000001$), and ejection fraction ($p < 0.001$). Adenosine ^{201}Tl scintigraphic variables were equally predictive in patients who underwent early reperfusion therapy compared with those who did not. Figure 11–27 shows that quantified extent of ischemia predicted risk irrespective of initial therapy during acute infarction. Other studies have also shown that vasodilator myocardial perfusion can accurately detect jeopardized myocardium after acute myocardial infarction and is useful for predicting future cardiac events (203a,203b).

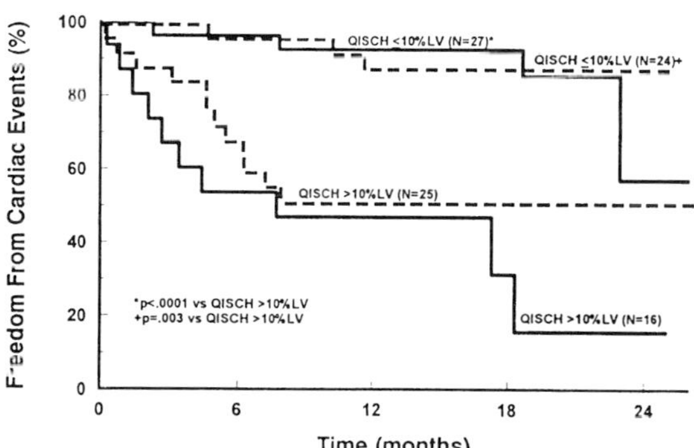

Figure 11–27. Freedom from cardiac events in 146 patients who were followed after undergoing adenosine ^{201}Tl scintigraphy during hospitalization for acute myocardial infarction. Groups are separated by the extent of ischemia of the left ventricle (QISCH) and by whether or not they received thrombolytic therapy (solid line) or no thrombolytic therapy (dotted line). Note that patients with ischemia comprising >10% of the left ventricle had significantly worse event-free survival compared with patients with >10% of the left ventricle rendered ischemic. *Reprinted from Mahmarian et al (203), with permission.*

Stress Technetium-99*m* Sestamibi Imaging After Acute Myocardial Infarction

Little data are available concerning the worth of stress ^{99m}Tc sestamibi imaging for separation of high- and low-risk subsets of patients with uncomplicated myocardial infarction. One study by Travin and coworkers (204) found that exercise ^{99m}Tc sestamibi SPECT imaging after myocardial infarction often reveals residual ischemia and is superior than the clinical information, symptoms, and stress ECG data in identifying patients with a high probability of a subsequent cardiac event. By Cox regression analysis of all variables utilized, the number of ischemic defects on SPECT ^{99m}Tc sestamibi imaging was the only significant correlate of a future cardiac event. Patients with ≥3 reversible ^{99m}Tc sestamibi defects had an event rate of 38%. Figure 11–28 shows the cardiac event rate in relation to the numbers of reversible ^{99m}Tc sestamibi defects in this study. As in the studies employing exercise ^{201}Tl scintigraphy, ischemia was detected more often with ^{99m}Tc sestamibi imaging than with exercise electrocardiography in this study. It should be pointed out that 25% of the patients in this study were referred for revascularization and comprised those with the most extensive ischemia. Thus the clinical value of ^{99m}Tc sestamibi imaging may have been more obvious had such patients been treated medically. Figure 11–29 shows exercise and rest ^{99m}Tc sestamibi SPECT images in a patient with an

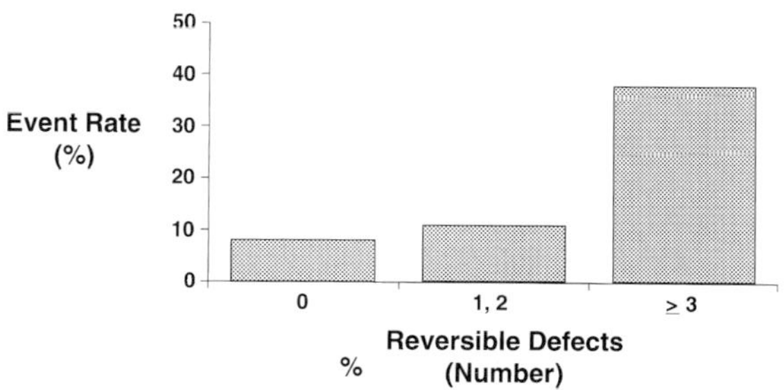

Figure 11–28. Cardiac event rate after discharge in patients who underwent exercise ^{99m}Tc sestamibi SPECT imaging after acute myocardial infarction. Patients with ≥3 reversible ^{99m}Tc sestamibi defects had an event rate of 38%. *Adapted from Travin et al (204), with permission.*

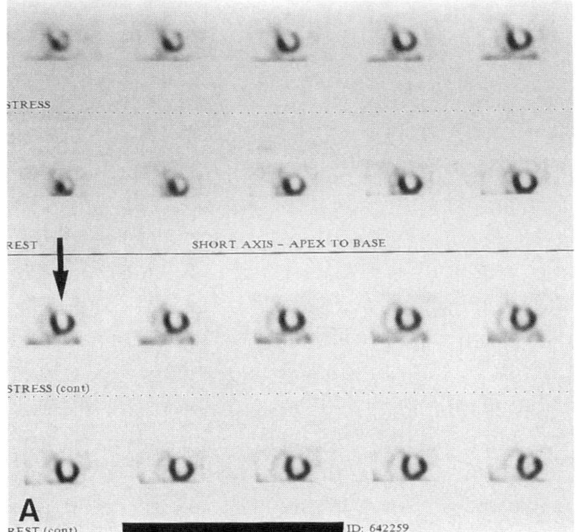

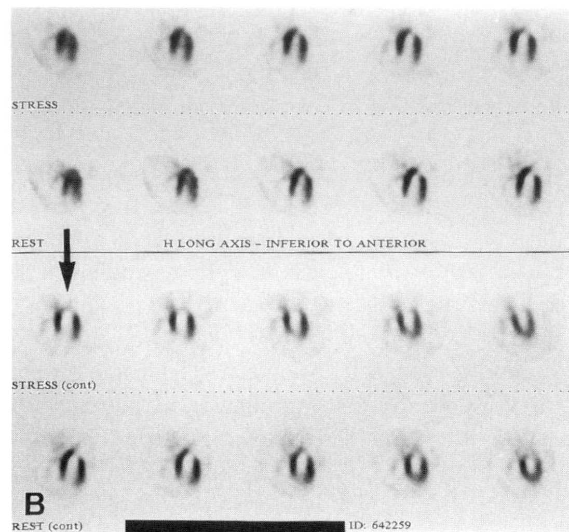

Figure 11–29. **A.** Postexercise (STRESS) and rest (REST) short-axis ^{99m}Tc sestamibi tomograms in a patient with nonreversible apical and anterior (arrow) defects. No evidence for defect reversibility is seen, and the reduction in anterior ^{99m}Tc sestamibi uptake is marked. **B.** Postexercise and resting horizontal long-axis ^{99m}Tc sestamibi tomograms in the same patient showing a nonreversible apical defect (arrow).

anterior myocardial infarction who exhibited only nonreversible apical and anterior defects. No inducible ischemia is apparent.

Heller et al (204a) from the same institution found that dipyridamole ^{99m}Tc sestamibi imaging in 512 patients provided independent prognostic information in predicting cardiac events. Patients with reversible defects had the highest event rates. The patients in this study did not all have a prior myocardial infarction.

Decision-Making Algorithm

Based on the literature cited above, as well as other reports, a decision-making algorithm might now be proposed for the prognostic evaluation of postinfarction patients (see Chs. 30–31). Patients who are clinically at high risk with congestive heart failure, prior myocardial infarction, or postinfarction angina would be candidates for direct referral for coronary angiography. However, a significant number of patients with congestive heart failure and a depressed left ventricular ejection fraction after acute infarction could benefit by a test that distinguishes viable from nonviable myocardium both within and remote from the infarct zone. For example, rest ^{201}Tl imaging or resting ^{99m}Tc sestamibi imaging could identify asynergic segments that have high probability of improving function after revascularization. Zones of asynergy that showed markedly reduced tracer activity would unlikely show improved systolic function if revascularization was performed.

Patients at intermediate risk by clinical criteria and who had an uncomplicated hospital course would be candidates for noninvasive risk assessment. Such patients may have undergone reperfusion ≥3 hours after the onset of chest pain but still had preserved left ventricular function. Stress perfusion imaging could be undertaken as early as 4 to 5 days after onset of symptoms. High-risk patients demonstrating residual ischemia or a multivessel disease scan pattern would be scheduled for coronary angiography, whereas patients exhibiting low-risk noninvasive findings would be eligible for medical therapy. Low risk would be defined as lack of inducible ischemia at completion of a submaximal exercise test protocol. Figure 11–30 demonstrates high-risk scan findings in a patient with an uncomplicated acute myocardial infarction who

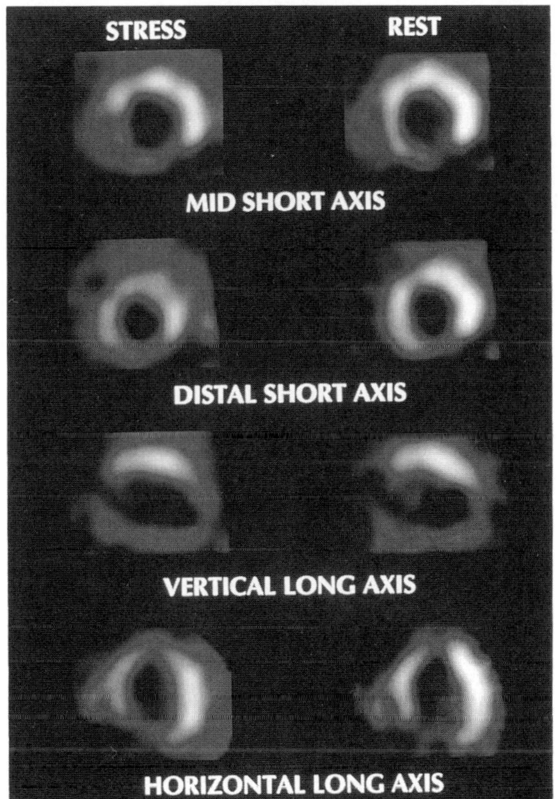

Figure 11–30. Postexercise stress (left column) and rest (right column) ^{99m}Tc sestamibi tomograms in a patient with an inferior infarction who demonstrates nonreversible inferior and apical defects and a partially reversible anteroseptal defect. This is an example of a high-risk scan demonstrating remote ischemia in the supply region of a stenotic left anterior descending coronary stenosis.

underwent predischarge submaximal exercise SPECT ^{99m}Tc sestamibi perfusion imaging. In addition to a nonreversible defect in the inferior wall, reversible defects in the anterior and septal segments can be seen consistent with a multivessel scan pattern.

Patients classified as low risk by clinical variables might first be assessed by exercise electrocardiography rather than by initially combining exercise testing with radionuclide imaging. These patients typically will have a left ventricular ejection fraction of >50%, most often have undergone reperfusion soon after onset of symptoms, and have no prior infarction and no postinfarction angina or heart failure. If the resting electrocardiogram shows persistence of ST depression or T wave abnormalities, then perfusion imaging should be performed in conjunction with testing, since additional ST segment changes during exercise might not be reflective of ischemia. If in such a low-risk patient the exercise electrocardiogram shows an ischemic ST segment response, the patient could be referred directly to coronary angiography or undergo repeat testing with a perfusion imaging agent. Patients who demonstrate no inducible chest pain or ST depression, or who are hemodynamically stable during the exercise protocol and demonstrate good exercise tolerance, could be followed medically, with repeat testing performed at maximal exercise workloads perhaps at 6 weeks to 3 months. Such low-risk patients should have a 2% or less mortality rate during follow-up.

In the United States, less than 50% of patients with acute myocardial infarction undergo early reperfusion therapy. Many are not eligible for a thrombolytic agent and do not undergo early angiography with direct angioplasty. These are the patients who were successfully risk stratified in the prethrombolytic era by a noninvasive strategy. In the thrombolytic era, such patients who are clinically stable should still be referred for a predischarge stress perfusion imaging for purposes of risk stratification. The exception might be patients who are clinically at high risk who could be referred directly to angiography. Further studies in larger clinical populations are warranted to definitively ascertain the role of a noninvasive risk assessment strategy in postinfarction patients in the thrombolytic era and age of interventional cardiology.

Exercise Radionuclide Angiography

Exercise radionuclide angiography has been performed before hospital discharge to identify high-risk and low-risk subsets after uncomplicated myocardial infarction, similar to what is undertaken with exercise ^{201}Tl scintigraphy (204–213). High-risk exercise angiographic variables are listed in Table 11–4. Patients who subsequently experience a fatal or nonfatal cardiac event have a higher prevalence of an abnormal ejection fraction or end-systolic volume response to exercise on predischarge stress testing compared with those who remain event free. Patients with inferior infarction and single-vessel right coronary artery disease tend to show an increase in left ventricular ejection fraction with exercise, whereas inferior infarction patients with multivessel disease most often show a flat response or a decline in ejection fraction with exercise (207). In the study by Hung et al (191), peak treadmill workload and the change in left ventricular ejection fraction during exercise were significant predictors of cardiac events, as assessed by multivariate analysis in men tested 3 weeks postinfarction. A peak treadmill workload of 4 METs or less, or a decrease in ejection fraction of 5% or more below the value at rest during submaximal effort, distinguished high-risk from low-risk subgroups with a 23% and 2% event rates, respectively.

Morris et al (210) reported that both rest and exercise ejection fractions were correlated inversely with subsequent mortality in 106 consecutive survivors of acute myocardial infarction (Fig. 11–31). Using the Cox regression model, they showed that as the exercise ejection fraction fell below 45%, mortality increased dramatically. The expected mortality at 2 years was 11% with an exercise ejection fraction of 50%, 29% with an exercise ejection fraction of 30%, and 56% with an exercise ejection fraction of 15%. Corbett et al (209) observed that the change in ejection fraction from rest to exercise in postinfarction patients was the most important prognostic variable in predicting the combined events of death, recurrent infarction, refractory angina, and heart failure. When the exercise ejection fraction is less than 50% compared with an ejection fraction of 50% or more, the 2-year survival rate free of medical complications is almost twice as low (212). Exercise radionuclide angiography is seldom performed today for purposes of risk stratification unless it is part of a ^{99m}Tc sestamibi or ^{99m}Tc tetrofosmin protocol where a first-pass study is performed immediately after tracer injection followed 30 minutes to 1 hour later by acquisition of SPECT tomograms for assessment of perfusion. As with stress perfusion imaging, exercise radionuclide angiography is not as predictive for identifying high-risk patients among those who receive thrombolytic therapy (213). In this study by Zaret et al (213) from the TIMI-IIB patient cohort, peak exercise ejection fraction did not provide appreciable prognostic information beyond that obtained with solely a resting ejection fraction (Fig. 11–32).

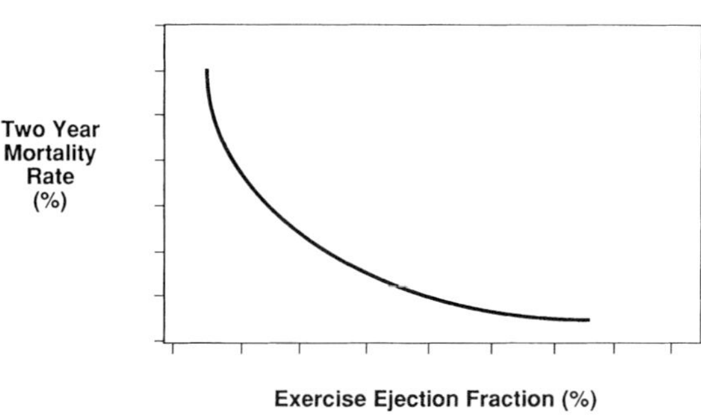

Figure 11–31. Relationship between predischarge exercise ejection fraction and 2-year mortality rate in patients with a myocardial infarction who underwent predischarge exercise radionuclide angiography. *Reprinted from Morris et al (210), with permission.*

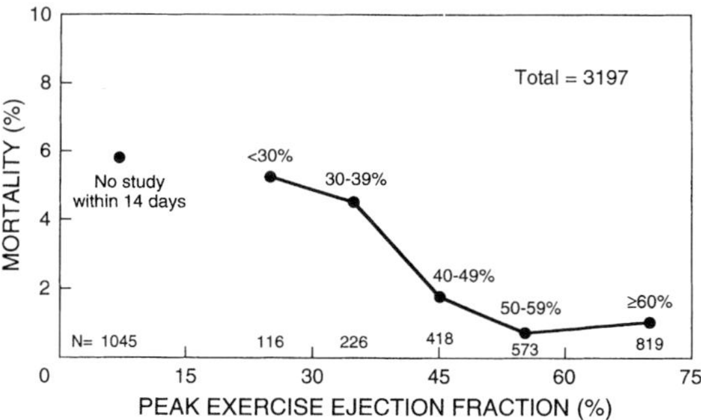

Figure 11–32. Peak exercise ejection fraction versus mortality rate in patients in the TIMI-IIB study who underwent exercise radionuclide angiography following acute myocardial infarction treated with thrombolysis. Note the increased mortality rate in patients with a peak ejection fraction below 45%. In this study, peak ejection fraction did not provide appreciable supplementary prognostic information beyond that obtained solely from a resting ejection fraction determination. *Reprinted from Zaret et al (213), with permission.*

LIMITATIONS OF NUCLEAR CARDIOLOGY PROCEDURES

Thallium-201 Scintigraphy

Thallium-201 imaging has some significant limitations. Solely visual interpretation of unprocessed scintigrams can be difficult if the clinician is not knowledgeable about image artifacts or variants of normal findings. Attenuation artifacts caused by overlying breast tissue, a high diaphragm, and an enlarged right ventricular blood pool overlying the inferior wall can cause false-positive interpretations. Exaggerated apical thinning can be misconstrued as a defect. Patients with complete left bundle branch block and normal coronary arteries may have septal ^{201}Tl defects that may be misinterpreted as anteroseptal infarction (214). Circumflex coronary lesions are less easily detected by both planar and SPECT imaging than are left anterior descending or right coronary stenoses. Branch lesions from the left anterior descending and circumflex arteries are also less well identified than stenoses that are situated in the more proximal portions of the three major coronary vessels. Even when quantitative computer-assisted scintigraphy is used, some false-positive findings can occur. Oversubtraction of background may yield defects that are not due to underlying coronary artery disease. This is most often observed when there is increased lung ^{201}Tl uptake on the initial anterior image. Isolated regional washout abnormalities without associated defects elsewhere should not be interpreted as indicative of coronary artery disease.

It has been proposed that SPECT ^{201}Tl imaging would enhance both sensitivity and specificity of the myocardial perfusion technique. Unfortunately, SPECT imaging is also associated with certain problems. With SPECT ^{201}Tl scintigraphy, artifacts caused by patient motion are more likely to occur than with planar imaging, primarily because the patient remains in an awkward position for a rather lengthy period. Patient motion is a source of artifactual defects during the tomographic reconstruction. Friedman and coworkers (215) have observed that although chest point sources inscribe a straight line on the summation image, upward motion of the area containing myocardial activity is present. They term this phenomenon *upward creep* of the heart. They show that in normal individuals, upward creep of a ≥2-pixel shift was associated with a high incidence of reversible inferior or septal perfusion defects in the absence of coronary artery disease. Friedman et al observed that upward creep occurred more often in patients who exercised longer and achieved a higher heart rate, raising the possibility that this phenomenon is related to persistent hyperventilation after exhaustive stress. Attenuation artifacts such as those produced by overlying breast tissue appear on SPECT imaging as well as on planar scintigrams. Finally, absolute quantitation of myocardial blood flow in milliliters per minute per gram of myocardium cannot be obtained with ^{201}Tl scintigraphy. This is one potential advantage of PET imaging of regional myocardial blood flow.

Radionuclide Angiography

There are some limitations to exercise radionuclide angiography for prognostication after uncomplicated myocardial infarction. Inadequate stress resulting from physical disability may be associated with a suboptimal response despite underlying residual ischemia. Patients receiving antianginal agents may also not demonstrate the expected ischemic wall motion and ejection fraction responses with exercise stress. Approximately one-third of women with chest pain and normal coronary arteries will demonstrate a decrease or a failure to increase the radionuclide ejection fraction during stress. In women who experience a myocardial infarction, therefore, the ejection fraction response may not be reflective of subsequent prognosis. Hemodynamic variables can also influence the ejection fraction response to exercise. Gibbons et al (216) showed that resting pulse pressure, adequate exercise, resting ejection fraction, changes in end-diastolic volume with exercise, positive ECG changes, and to a lesser degree, number of diseased vessels were significant independent predictors of the left ventricular ejection fraction response to exercise.

Positron Emission Tomography

There remain major questions concerning the cost-effectiveness of PET imaging in patients with coronary artery disease. The methodology employed is expensive and sophisticated and requires the existence of a nearby cyclotron for optimum utilization. No carefully undertaken comparative studies of PET and conventional perfusion imaging techniques have been undertaken to determine the added diagnostic and prognostic value of the PET approach. It certainly appears that assessment of viability using FDG imaging may be very valuable compared with perfusion or functional imaging with conventional nuclear cardiology techniques.

ACKNOWLEDGMENT

I am grateful to Mr. Jerry Curtis for his excellent editorial assistance in the revision of this chapter.

REFERENCES

1. Beller GA: Radionuclide imaging in acute myocardial infarction, in *Clinical Nuclear Cardiology.* Philadelphia, WB Saunders Co, 1995. pp 192–235.
2. Guidelines for clinical use of cardiac imaging. Report of the American College of Cardiology/American Heart Association Task Force on Assessment of Diagnostic and Therapeutic Cardiovascular Procedures (Committee on Radionuclide Imaging), developed in collaboration with the American Society of Nuclear Cardiology. *J Am Coll Cardiol* 1995;25: 521–547.
3. Pitt B: Evaluation of the postinfarct patient. *Circulation* 1995;91:1855–1860.
4. Verani MS: Exercise and pharmacologic stress testing for prognosis after acute myocardial infarction. *J Nucl Med* 1994;35:716–720.
5. Strauss HW, Harrison K, Langan JK, Lebowitz E, Pitt B: Thallium-201 for myocardial imaging: Relation of thallium-201 to regional myocardial perfusion. *Circulation* 1975;51:641–645.
6. Weich HF, Strauss HW, Pitt B: The extraction of thallium-201 by the myocardium. *Circulation* 1977; 56:188–191.
7. Okada RD, Glover D, Gaffney T, Williams S: Myocardial kinetics of technetium-99m-hexakis-2-methoxy-3-methyl-propyl-isonitrile. *Circulation* 1988; 77:491–498.
8. Beller GA, Watson DD: Physiological basis of myocardial perfusion imaging with the technetium 99m agents. *Semin Nucl Med* 1991;21:173–181.
9. Sinusas AJ, Wackers FJ: Assessing myocardial reperfusion with technetium-99m-labeled myocardial perfusion agents: Basic concepts and clinical applications. *Am J Card Imaging* 1993;7:24–38.
10. Shea MJ, Wilson RA, deLandsheere CM, et al: Use of short- and long-lived rubidium tracers for the study of transient ischemia. *J Nucl Med* 1987;28: 989–997.
11. Gould KL: PET perfusion imaging and nuclear cardiology. *J Nucl Med* 1991;32:579–606.
12. Schwaiger M: Myocardial perfusion imaging with PET. *J Nucl Med* 1994; 35:693–698.
13. Beller GA: Instrumentation in nuclear cardiology, in *Clinical Nuclear Cardiology.* Philadelphia, WB Saunders Co 1995, pp 1–36.
14. Garcia EV: Physics and instrumentation of radionuclide imaging, in Marcus M, Schelbert H, Skorton D, Wolf G (eds): *Cardiac Imaging: A Companion to Braunwald's "Heart Disease."* Philadelphia, WB Saunders Co 1991, pp 977–1005.
15. Garvin AA, Cullum J, Garcia EV: Myocardial perfusion imaging using single-photon emission computed tomography. *Am J Card Imaging* 1994;8: 189–198.
16. Faber TL: Multiheaded rotating gamma cameras in cardiac single-photon emission computed tomographic imaging. *J Nucl Cardiol* 1994;1:292–303.
17. Wallis JW, Miller TR, Koppel P: Attenuation correction in cardiac SPECT without a transmission measurement. *J Nucl Med* 1995;36:506–512.
18. Mahmarian JJ, Boyce TM, Goldberg RK, Cocanougher MK, Roberts R, Verani MS: Quantitative exercise thallium-201 single photon emission computed tomography for the enhanced diagnosis of ischemic heart disease. *J Am Coll Cardiol* 1990;15: 318–329.
19. Garcia EV, DePuey EG, Sonnemaker RE, et al: Quantification of the reversibility of stress-induced thallium-201 myocardial perfusion defects: A multicenter trial using bull's-eye polar maps and standard normal limits. *J Nucl Med* 1990; 31:1761–1765.

20. Chua T, Kiat H, Germano G, et al: Gated technetium-99m sestamibi for simultaneous assessment of stress myocardial perfusion, postexercise regional ventricular function and myocardia viability: Correlation with echocardiography and rest thallium-201 scintigraphy. *J Am Coll Cardiol* 1994;23: 1107–1114.

20a. Williams KA, Taillon LA: Reversible ischemia in severe stress technetium-99m-labeled sestamibi perfusion defects assessed from gated single-photon emission computed tomographic polar map Fourier analysis. J Nucl Cardiol 1995;2:199–206.

21. Pohost GM, Zir LM, Moore RH, McKusick KA, Guiney TE, Beller GA: Differentiation of transiently ischemic from infarcted myocardium by serial imaging after a single dose of thallium-201. *Circulation* 1977;55:294–302.

22. Nielson AT, Morris KG, Murdock R, Bruno FP, Cobb FR: Linear relationship between the distribution of thallium-201 and blood flow in ischemic and non-ischemic myocardium during exercise. *Circulation* 1980;61:797–801.

23. Melin JA, Becker LC: Quantitative relationship between global left ventricular thallium uptake and blood flow: Effects of propranolol, ouabain, dipyridamole and coronary artery occlusion. *J Nucl Med* 1986;27:641–652.

24. Glover DK, Ruiz M, Edwards NC, et al: Comparison between ^{201}Tl and ^{99m}Tc sestamibi uptake during adenosine-induced vasodilation as a function of coronary stenosis severity. *Circulation* 1995;91: 813–820.

25. Leppo JA, Macneil PB, Moring AF, Apstein CS: Separate effects of ischemia, hypoxia, and contractility on thallium-201 kinetics in rabbit myocardium. *J Nucl Med* 1986;27:66–74.

26. Moore CA, Cannon J, Watson DD, Kaul S, Beller GA: Thallium 201 kinetics in stunned myocardium characterized by severe postischemic systolic dysfunction. *Circulation* 1990;81:1622–1632.

27. Sinusas AJ, Watson DD, Cannon JM Jr, Beller GA: Effect of ischemia and postischemic dysfunction on myocardial uptake of technetium-99m-labeled methoxyisobutyl isonitrile and thallium-201. *J Am Coll Cardiol* 1989;14:1785–1793.

28. Sinusas A, Bergin JD, Edwards N, et al: Redistribution of ^{99m}Tc-sestamibi and ^{201}Tl in the presence of a severe coronary stenosis. *Circulation* 1994;89: 2332–2341.

29. Grunwald AM, Watson DD, Holzgrefe HH Jr, Irving JF, Beller GA: Myocardial thallium-201 kinetics in normal and ischemic myocardium. *Circulation* 1981;64:610–618.

30. Khaw BA, Strauss HW, Pohost GM, Fallon JT, Katus H, Haber E: Relation of immediate and delayed thallium-201 distribution to localization of iodine-125 antimyosin antibody in acute experimental myocardial infarction. *Am J Cardiol* 1983;51: 1428–1432.

31. Manyari DE, Knudtson M, Kloiber R, Roth D: Sequential thallium-201 myocardial perfusion studies after successful percutaneous transluminal coronary artery angioplasty: Delayed resolution of exercise-induced scintigraphic abnormalities. *Circulation* 1988;77:86–95.

32. Miller DD, Verani MS: Current status of myocardial perfusion imaging after percutaneous transluminal coronary angioplasty. *J Am Coll Cardiol* 1994; 24:260–266.

33. Uren NG, Crake T, Lefroy DC, de Silva R, Davies GJ, Maseri A: Delayed recovery of coronary resistive vessel function after coronary angioplasty. *J Am Coll Cardiol* 1993;21:612–621.

34. Okada RD, Jacobs ML, Daggett WM, et al: Thallium-201 kinetics in nonischemic myocardium. *Circulation* 1982;65:70–77.

35. Okada RD: Myocardial kinetics of thallium-201 after stress in normal and perfusion-reduced canine myocardium. *Am J Cardiol* 1985;56:969–973.

36. Schwartz JS, Ponto R, Carlyle P, Forstrom L, Cohn JN: Early redistribution of thallium-201 after temporary ischemia. *Circulation* 1982;57:332–335.

37. Schelbert HR, Schuler G, Ashburn WL, Covell JW: Time-course of "redistribution" of thallium-201 administered during transient ischemia. *Eur J Nucl Med* 1979;4:351–358.

38. Steingart RM, Bontemps R, Scheuer J, Yipintsoi T: Gamma camera quantitation of thallium-201 redistribution at rest in a dog model. *Circulation* 1982; 65:542–550.

39. Pohost GM, Okada RD, O'Keefe DB, et al: Thallium redistribution in dogs with severe coronary artery stenosis of fixed caliber. *Circ Res* 1981;48: 439–466.

40. Beller GA, Holzgrefe HH, Watson DD. Effects of dipyridamole-induced vasodilation on myocardial uptake and clearance kinetics of thallium-201. *Circulation* 1983;68:1328–1338.

41. Beller GA, Holzgrefe HH, Watson DD: Intrinsic washout rates of thallium-201 in normal and ischemic myocardium after dipyridamole-induced vasodilation. *Circulation* 1985;71:378–386.

42. Granato JE, Watson DD, Belardinelli L, Cannon JM, Beller GA: Effects of dipyridamole and aminophylline on hemodynamics, regional myocardial blood flow and thallium-201 washout in the setting of a critical coronary stenosis. *J Am Coll Cardiol* 1990;16:1760–1770.

43. Kiat H, Berman DS, Maddahi J, et al: Late reversibility of tomographic myocardial thallium-201 defects: An accurate marker of myocardial viability. *J Am Coll Cardiol* 1988;12:1456–1463.

44. Yang LD, Berman DS, Kiat H, et al: The frequency of late reversibility in SPECT thallium-201 stress-redistribution studies. *J Am Coll Cardiol* 1990;15: 334–340.

45. Dilsizian V, Rocco TP, Freedman NM, Leon MB, Bonow RO: Enhanced detection of ischemic but viable myocardium by the reinjection of thallium after stress-redistribution imaging. *N Engl J Med* 1990;323:141–146.

46. Dilsizian V, Freedman NM, Bacharach SL, Perrone-Filardi P, Bonow RO: Regional thallium uptake in irreversible defects. Magnitude of change in thallium activity after reinjection distinguishes viable from nonviable myocardium. *Circulation* 1992; 85:627–634.

47. Dilsizian V, Smeltzer WR, Freedman NM, Dextras R, Bonow RO: Thallium reinjection after stress-redistribution imaging. Does 24-hour delayed imaging after reinjection enhance detection of viable myocardium? *Circulation* 1991;83:1247–1255.

48. Galli M, Marcassa C: Thallium-201 redistribution after early reinjection in patients with severe stress defects and ventricular dysfunction. *Am Heart J* 1994;128:41–52.

49. Dilsizian V, Perrone-Filardi P, Arrighi JA, et al: Concordance and discordance between rest-redistribution-reinjection thallium imaging for assessing viable myocardium: Comparison with metabolic activity by positron emission tomography. *Circulation* 1993;88:941–952.

50. Kayden DS, Sigal S, Soufer R, Mattera J, Zaret BL, Wackers FJ: Thallium-201 for assessment of myocardial viability: Quantitative comparison of 24-hour redistribution imaging with imaging after reinjection at rest [published erratum appears in *J Am Coll Cardiol* 1991;19:1121]. *J Am Coll Cardiol* 1991;18:1480–1486.

51. Berger BC, Watson DD, Burwell LR, et al: Redistribution of thallium at rest in patients with stable and unstable angina and the effect of coronary artery bypass surgery. *Circulation* 1979;60:1114–1125.

52. Gewirtz H, Beller GA, Strauss HW, et al: Transient defects of resting thallium scans in patients with coronary artery disease. *Circulation* 1979;59: 707–713.

53. Ragosta M, Beller G, Watson D, Kaul S, Gimple L: Quantitative planar rest-redistribution ^{201}Tl imaging in detection of myocardial viability and prediction of improvement in left ventricular function after coronary bypass surgery in patients with severely depressed left ventricular function. *Circulation* 1993;87:1630–1641.

54. Udelson JE, Coleman PS, Metherall J, et al: Predicting recovery of severe regional ventricular dysfunction. Comparison of resting scintigraphy with ^{201}Tl and ^{99m}Tc-sestamibi. *Circulation* 1994;89: 2552–2561.

55. Galassi AR, Centamore G, Fiscella A, et al: Comparison of rest-redistribution thallium-201 imaging and reinjection after stress-redistribution for the assessment of myocardial viability in patients with left ventricular dysfunction secondary to coronary artery disease. *Am J Cardiol* 1995;75:436–442.

56. Gioia G, Powers J, Heo J, Iskandrian AS, Russell J, Cassel D: Prognostic value of rest-redistribution tomographic thallium-201 imaging in ischemic cardiomyopathy. *Am J Cardiol* 1995;75:759–762.

57. Gibson RS, Watson DD, Taylor GJ, et al: Prospective assessment of regional myocardial perfusion before and after coronary revascularization surgery by quantitative thallium-201 scintigraphy. *J Am Coll Cardiol* 1983;1:804–815.

58. Weiss AT, Maddahi J, Lew AS, et al: Reverse redistribution of thallium-201: A sign of nontransmural myocardial infarction with patency of the infarct-related coronary artery. *J Am Coll Cardiol* 1986;7:61–67.

59. Canby RC, Silber S, Pohost GM: Relations of the myocardial imaging agents ^{99m}Tc-MIBI and ^{201}Tl to myocardial blood flow in a canine model of myocardial ischemic insult. *Circulation* 1990;81: 289–296.

60. Li Q-S, Frank TL, Franceschi D, Wagner HN Jr, Becker LC: Technetium-99m methoxyisobutyl isonitrile (RP30) for quantification of myocardial

ischemia and reperfusion in dogs. *J Nucl Med* 1988; 29:1539–1548.

61. Sansoy V, Glover DK, Watson DD, et al: Comparison of thallium-201 resting redistribution with technetium-99m sestamibi uptake and functional response to dobutamine for assessment of myocardial viability. *Circulation* 1995;92:994–1004.
62. Leppo JA, Meerdink DJ: Comparison of the myocardial uptake of a technetium-labeled isonitrile analogue and thallium. *Circ Res* 1989;65:632–639.
63. Kahn JK, McGhie I, Akers MS, et al: Quantitative rotational tomography with ^{201}Tl and ^{99m}Tc 2-methoxy-isobutyl-isonitrile. A direct comparison in normal individuals and patients with coronary artery disease. *Circulation* 1989;79:1282–1293.
64. Berman DS, Kiat HS, Van Train KF, Germano G, Maddahi J, Friedman JD: Myocardial perfusion imaging with technetium-99m-sestamibi: Comparative analysis of available imaging protocols. *J Nucl Med* 1994;35:681–688.
65. Van Train KF, Garcia EV, Maddahi J, et al: Multicenter trial validation for quantitative analysis of same-day rest-stress technetium-99m-sestamibi myocardial tomograms. *J Nucl Med* 1994;35: 609–618.
66. Piwnica-Worms D, Kronauge JF, Chiu ML: Uptake and retention of hexakis (2-methoxyisobutyl isonitrile) technetium(I) in cultured chick myocardial cells. Mitochondrial and plasma membrane potential dependence. *Circulation* 1990;82:1826–1838.
67. Piwnica-Worms D, Chiu ML, Kronauge JF: Divergent kinetics of ^{201}Tl and ^{99m}Tc-sestamibi in cultured chick ventricular myocytes during ATP depletion. *Circulation* 1992;85:1531–1541.
68. Beanlands RS, Dawood F, Wen WH, et al: Are the kinetics of technetium-99m methoxyisobutyl isonitrile affected by cell metabolism and viability? *Circulation* 1990;82:1802–1814.
69. Beller GA, Glover DK, Edwards NC, Ruiz M, Simanis JP, Watson D: ^{99m}Tc-sestamibi uptake and retention during myocardial ischemia and reperfusion. *Circulation* 1993;87:2033–2042.
70. Leppo JA, Meerdink DJ: Comparative myocardial extraction of two technetium labeled BATO derivatives (SQ30217, SQ32014) and thallium. *J Nucl Med* 1990;31:67–74.
71. Di Rocco RJ, Rumsey WL, Kuczynski BL, et al: Measurement of myocardial blood flow using a co-injection technique for technetium-99m-teboroxime, technetium-96-sestamibi and thallium-201. *J Nucl Med* 1992;33:1152–1159.
72. Beanlands R, Muzik O, Nguyen N, Petry N, Schwaiger M: The relationship between myocardial retention of technetium-99m teboroxime and myocardial blood flow. *J Am Coll Cardiol* 1992;20: 712–719.
73. Gray WA, Gewirtz H: Comparison of ^{99m}Tc-teboroxime with thallium for myocardial imaging in the presence of a coronary artery stenosis. *Circulation* 1991;84:1796–1807.
74. Glover DK, Ruiz M, Bergmann EE, et al: Myocardial technetium-99m-teboroxime uptake during adenosine-induced hyperemia in dogs with either a critical or mild coronary stenosis: Comparison to thallium-201 and regional blood flow. *J Nucl Med* 1995;36:476–483.
75. Serafini AN, Topchik S, Jimenez H, Friden A, Ganz WI, Sfakianakis GN: Clinical comparison of technetium-99m-teboroxime and thallium-201 utilizing a continuous SPECT imaging protocol. *J Nucl Med* 1992;33:1304–1311.
76. Johnson LL: Myocardial perfusion imaging with technetium-99m-teboroxime. *J Nucl Med* 1994;35: 689–692.
77. Kelly JD, Forster AM, Higley B, et al: Technetium-99m-tetrofosmin as a new radiopharmaceutical for myocardial perfusion imaging. *J Nucl Med* 1993;34: 222–227.
78. Sinusas AJ, Shi QX, Saltzberg MT, et al: Technetium-99m-tetrofosmin to assess myocardial blood flow: Experimental validation in an intact canine model of ischemia. *J Nucl Med* 1994;35:664–671.
79. Zaret BL, Rigo P, Wackers FJ, et al, and the Tetrofosmin International Trial Study Group: Myocardial perfusion imaging with ^{99m}Tc tetrofosmin: Comparison to ^{201}Tl imaging and coronary angiography in a phase III multicenter trial. *Circulation* 1995;91:313–319.
80. Koplan BA, Beller GA, Ruiz M, Yang JY, Watson DD, Glover DK: Comparison between thallium-201 and technetium-99m-tetrofosmin uptake under experimental conditions of sustained low flow and profound systolic dysfunction. *J Nucl Med*, in press.

80a. Johnson G III, Allton IL, Nguyen KN, et al: Clearance of technetium 99m N-NOET in normal, ischemic-reperfused, and membrane-disrupted myocardium. *J Nucl Cardiol* 1996;3:42–54.

80b. Fagret D, Marie P-Y, Brunotte F, et al: Myocardial perfusion imaging with technetium-99m-Tc NOET: comparison with thallium-201 and coronary angiography. *J Nucl Med* 1995;36:936–943.

81. Demer LL, Gould KL, Goldstein RA, et al: Assessment of coronary artery disease severity by positron emission tomography. Comparison with quantitative arteriography in 193 patients. *Circulation* 1989;79:825–835.

82. Hutchins GD, Schwaiger M, Rosenspire KC, Krivokapich J, Schelbert H, Kuhl DE: Noninvasive quantification of regional blood flow in the human heart using N-13 ammonia and dynamic positron emission tomographic imaging. *J Am Coll Cardiol* 1990;15:1032–1042.

83. Gould KL, Yoshida K, Hess MJ, Haynie M, Mullani N, Smalling RW: Myocardial metabolism of fluorodeoxyglucose compared to cell membrane integrity for the potassium analogue rubidium-82 for assessing infarct size in man by PET. *J Nucl Med* 1991;32:1–9.

84. Bergmann SR, Herrero P, Markham J, Weinheimer CJ, Walsh MN: Noninvasive quantitation of myocardial blood flow in human subjects with oxygen-15-labeled water and positron emission tomography. *J Am Coll Cardiol* 1989;14:639–652.

85. Zaret B, Berger H: Radionuclide studies of ventricular performance in coronary artery disease, in Yu PN, Goodwin JF (eds): *Progress in Cardiology*, vol 12. Philadelphia, Lea & Febiger, 1983, pp 33–58.

86. Gal RA, Grenier RP, Port SC, Dymond DS, Schmidt DH: Left ventricular volume calculation using a count-based ratio method applied to first-pass radionuclide angiography. *J Nucl Med* 1992;33: 2124–2132.

87. Maltz DL, Treves S: Quantitative radionuclide angiocardiography: Determination of Qp:Qs in children. *Circulation* 1973;47:1049–1056.

88. Berger HJ, Davies RA, Batsford WP, Hoffer PB, Gottschalk A, Zaret BL: Beat-to-beat left ventricular performance assessed from the equilibrium cardiac blood pool using a computerized nuclear probe. *Circulation* 1981;63:133–142.

89. Tamaki N, Yasuda T, Moore RH, et al: Continuous monitoring of left ventricular function by an ambulatory radionuclide detector in patients with coronary artery disease. *J Am Coll Cardiol* 1988;12:669–679.

90. Pace L, Cuocolo A, Mangoni di Santo Stefano ML, et al: Left ventricular systolic and diastolic function measurements using an ambulatory radionuclide monitor: Effects of different time averaging on accuracy. *J Nucl Med* 1993;34:1602–1606.

91. Willerson JT, Parkey RW, Bonte FJ, Meyer SL, Atkins JM, Stokely EM: Technetium stannous pyrophosphate myocardial scintigrams in patients with chest pain of varying etiology. *Circulation* 1975;51:1046–1052.

92. Khaw BA, Gold HK, Yasuda T, et al: Scintigraphic quantification of myocardial necrosis in patients after intravenous injection of myosin-specific antibody. *Circulation* 1986;74:501–508.

93. Khaw BA, Yasuda T, Gold HK, et al: Acute myocardial infarct imaging with indium-111-labeled monoclonal antimyosin Fab. *J Nucl Med* 1987;28: 1671–1678.

94. Johnson LL, Seldin DW, Becker LC, et al: Antimyosin imaging in acute transmural myocardial infarctions: Results of a multicenter clinical trial. *J Am Coll Cardiol* 1989;13:27–35.

95. Khaw B-A, Narula J: Antibody imaging in the evaluation of cardiovascular diseases. *J Nucl Cardiol* 1994;1:457–476.

96. Johnson LL, Seldin DW, Keller AM, et al: Dual isotope thallium and indium antimyosin SPECT imaging to identify acute infarct patients at further ischemic risk. *Circulation* 1990;81:37–45.

97. Schelbert HR: Metabolic imaging to assess myocardial viability. *J Nucl Med* 1994;35(Suppl): 8S–14S.

98. Buxton DB, Nienaber CA, Luxen A, et al: Noninvasive quantitation of regional myocardial oxygen consumption in vivo with [1-^{11}C] acetate and dynamic positron emission tomography. *Circulation* 1989;79:134–142.

99. Hansen CL: Preliminary report of an ongoing phase I/II dose range, safety and efficacy study of iodine-123-phenylpentadecanoic acid for the identification of viable myocardium. *J Nucl Med* 1994;35(Suppl):38S–42S.

99a. Hansen CL, Heo J, Oliner C, Van Decker W, Iskandrian AS: Prediction of improvement in left ventricular function with iodine-123-IPPA after coronary revascularization. *J Nucl Med* 1995;36: 1987–1993.

100. van der Wieken LR, Kan G, Belfer AJ, et al: Thallium-201 scanning to decide CCU admission in patients with non-diagnostic electrocardiograms. *Int J Cardiol* 1983;4:285–295.

101. Wackers FJT, Lie KI, Liem KL, et al: Thallium-201 scintigraphy in unstable angina pectoris. *Circulation* 1978;57:738–742.

102. Parodi O, Uthurralt N, Severi S, et al: Transient reduction of regional myocardial perfusion during angina at rest with ST-segment depression or normalization of negative T waves. *Circulation* 1981;63:1238–1247.

103. Wackers FJT, Sokole EB, Samson G, et al: Value and limitations of thallium-201 scintigraphy in the acute phase of myocardial infarction. *N Engl J Med* 1976;295:1–5.

104. Tamaki S, Kambara H, Kadota K, et al: Improved detection of myocardial infarction by emission computed tomography with thallium-201. Relation to infarct size. *Br Heart J* 1984;52:621–627.

105. Ritchie JL, Williams DL, Harp G, Stratton JL, Caldwell JH: Transaxial tomography with thallium-201 for detecting remote myocardial infarction: Comparison with planar imaging. *Am J Cardiol* 1982;50:1236–1241.

106. Huey BL, Beller GA, Kaiser DL, Gibson RS: A comprehensive analysis of myocardial infarction due to left circumflex artery occlusion: Comparison with infarction due to right coronary artery and left anterior descending artery occlusion. *J Am Coll Cardiol* 1988;12:1156–1166.

107. Imamura T, Araki H, Fukuyama T, et al: Significance of collateral circulation on peri-infarct zone: Assessment with stress thallium-201 scintigraphy. *Clin Cardiol* 1986;9:137–144.

108. Gibson RS, Taylor GJ, Watson DD, et al: Prognostic significance of resting anterior thallium-201 defects in patients with inferior myocardial infarction. *J Nucl Med* 1980;21:1015–1021.

109. Hakki A-H, Nestico PF, Heo J, Unwala AA, Iskandrian AS: Relative prognostic value of rest thallium-201 imaging, radionuclide ventriculography and 24-hour ambulatory electrocardiographic monitoring after acute myocardial infarction. *J Am Coll Cardiol* 1987;10:25–32.

110. Prigent F, Maddahi J, Garcia EV, Satoh Y, Van Train K, Berman DS: Quantification of myocardial infarct size by thallium-201 single-photon emission computed tomography: Experimental validation in the dog. *Circulation* 1986;74:852–861.

111. Becker LC, Silverman KJ, Bulkley BH, Kallman CH, Mellits ED, Weisfeldt M: Comparison of early thallium-201 scintigraphy and gated blood pool imaging for predicting mortality in patients with acute myocardial infarction. *Circulation* 1983;67:1272–1282.

112. Botvinick EH, Perez-Gonzalez JF, Dunn R, Ports T, Chatterjee K, Parmley W: Late prognostic value of scintigraphic parameters of acute myocardial infarction size in complicated myocardial infarction without heart failure. *Am J Cardiol* 1983;51:1045–1051.

113. Nestico PF, Hakki A-H, Felsher J, Heo J, Iskandrian AS: Implications of abnormal right ventricular thallium uptake in acute myocardial infarction. *Am J Cardiol* 1986;58:230–234.

114. Wackers FJ, Becker AE, Samson G, et al: Location and size of acute transmural myocardial infarction estimated from thallium-201 scintiscans: A clinicopathological study. *Circulation* 1977;56:72–78.

115. Tamaki S, Nakajima H, Murakami T, et al: Estimation of infarct size by myocardial emission computed tomography with thallium-201 and its relation to creatine kinase–MB release after myocardial infarction in man. *Circulation* 1982;66:994–1001.

116. Mahmarian JJ, Pratt CM, Borges-Neto S, Cashion WR, Roberts R, Verani MS: Quantification of infarct size by ^{201}Tl single-photon emission computed tomography during acute myocardial infarction in humans: Comparison with enzymatic estimates. *Circulation* 1988;78:831–839.

117. Starling MR, Dell'Italia LJ, Chaudhuri TK, et al: First transit and equilibrium radionuclide angiography in patients with inferior transmural myocardial infarction: Criteria for the diagnosis of associated hemodynamically significant right ventricular infarction. *J Am Coll Cardiol* 1984;4:923–930.

118. The Multicenter Postinfarction Research Group: Risk stratification and survival after myocardial infarction. *N Engl J Med* 1983;309:331–336.

119. Bonow RO: Prognostic assessment in coronary artery disease: Role of radionuclide angiography. *J Nucl Cardiol* 1994;1:280–291.

120. Holmes DR, Califf RM, Topol EJ: Lessons we have learned from the GUSTO trial. *J Am Coll Cardiol* 1995;25(Suppl):10S–17S.

121. Simoons ML, Vos J, Tijssen JGB, et al: Long-term benefit of early thrombolytic therapy in patients with acute myocardial infarction: 5 year follow-up of a trial conducted by the Interuniversity Cardiology Institute of the Netherlands. *J Am Coll Cardiol* 1989;14:1609–1615.

122. Terrin ML, Williams DO, Kleiman NS, et al: Two- and three-year results of the Thrombolysis in Myocardial Infarction (TIMI) Phase II clinical trial. *J Am Coll Cardiol* 1993;22:1763–1772.

123. Rogers WJ, Bourge RC, Papapietro SE, et al, for the TIMI Investigators: Variables predictive of good functional outcome following thrombolytic therapy in the Thrombolysis in Myocardial Infarction phase II (TIMI II) pilot study. *Am J Cardiol* 1989;63:503–512.

124. White HD, Cross DB, Elliott JM, Norris RM, Yee TW: Long-term prognostic importance of patency of the infarct-related coronary artery after thrombolytic therapy for acute myocardial infarction. *Circulation* 1994;89:61–67.

125. The GUSTO Angiographic Investigators: The effects of tissue plasminogen activator, streptokinase or both on coronary-artery patency, ventricular function, and survival after acute myocardial infarction. *N Engl J Med* 1993;329:1615–1622.

126. Harrison JK, Califf RM, Woodlief LH, et al: Systolic left ventricular function after reperfusion therapy for acute myocardial infarction. Analysis of determinants of improvement. The TAMI Study Group. *Circulation* 1993;87:1531–1541.

126a. Welty FK, Mittleman MA, Lewis SM, et al: A patent infarct-related artery is associated with reduced long-term mortality after percutaneous transluminal coronary angioplasty for postinfarction ischemia and an ejection fraction <50%. *Circulation* 1996;93:1496–1501.

127. Grines CL, Browne KF, Marco J, et al, for the Primary Angioplasty in Myocardial Infarction Study Group: A comparison of immediate angioplasty with thrombolytic therapy for acute myocardial infarction. *N Engl J Med* 1993;328:673–679.

128. Ong L, Green S, Reiser P, Morrison J: Early prediction of mortality in patients with acute myocardial infarction: A prospective study of clinical and radionuclide risk factors. *Am J Cardiol* 1986;57:33–38.

129. Gibson RS, Beller GA, Gheorghiade M, et al: The prevalence and clinical significance of residual myocardial ischemia 2 weeks after uncomplicated non–Q wave infarction: A prospective natural history study. *Circulation* 1986;73:1186–1198.

130. Reduto LA, Berger HJ, Cohen LS, Gottschalk A, Zaret BL: Sequential radionuclide assessment of left and right ventricular performance after acute transmural myocardial infarction. *Ann Intern Med* 1978;89:441–447.

131. Rigo P, Murray M, Strauss HW, Pitt B: Scintiphotographic evaluation of patients with suspected left ventricular aneurysm. *Circulation* 1974;50: 985–991.

132. Botvinick EH, Shames D, Hutchinson JC, Roe BB, Fitzpatrick M: Noninvasive diagnosis of a false left ventricular aneurysm with radioisotope gated cardiac blood pool imaging: Differentiation from true aneurysm. *Am J Cardiol* 1976;37: 1089–1093.

133. Sorensen SG, Crawford MH, Richards KL, Chaudhuri TK, O'Rourke RA: Noninvasive detection of ventricular aneurysm by combined 2-dimensional echocardiography and equilibrium radionuclide angiography. *Am Heart J* 1982;104: 145–152.

134. Rigo P, Alderson PO, Robertson RM, Becker LC, Wagner HN Jr: Measurement of aortic and mitral regurgitation by gated cardiac blood pool scans. *Circulation* 1979;60:306–312.

135. Lomboy CT, Schulman DS, Grill HP, Flores AR, Orie JE, Granato JE: Rest-redistribution thallium-201 scintigraphy to determine myocardial viability early after myocardial infarction. *J Am Coll Cardiol* 1995;25:210–217.

136. Lyons KP, Olson HG, Aronow WS: Sensitivity and specificity of Tc-99m pyrophosphate myocardial scintigraphy for the detection of acute myocardial infarction. *Clin Nucl Med* 1980;5:9–12.

137. Corbett JR, Lewis SE, Wolfe CL, et al: Measurement of myocardial infarct size by technetium pyrophosphate single-photon tomography. *Am J Cardiol* 1984;54:1231–1236.

138. Volpini M, Giubbini R, Gei P, et al: Diagnosis of acute myocardial infarction by indium-111 antimyosin antibodies and correlation with the traditional techniques for the evaluation of extent and localization. *Am J Cardiol* 1989;63:7–13.

138a. Hendel RC, Chaudhry FA, Bonow RO: Myocardial viability. *Curr Probl Cardiol* 1996;21(3):145–224.

139. Yamamoto K, Asada S, Masuyama T, et al: Myocardial hibernation in the infarcted region cannot be assessed from the presence of stress-induced ischemia: Usefulness of delayed image of exercise thallium-201 scintigraphy. *Am Heart J* 1993;125:33–40.

140. Smucker ML, Beller GA, Watson DD, Kaul S: Left ventricular dysfunction in excess of the size of infarction: A possible management strategy. *Am Heart J* 1988;115:749–753.

141. Tamaki N, Yonekura Y, Yamashita K, et al: Relation of left ventricular perfusion and wall motion with metabolic activity in persistent defects on thallium-201 tomography in healed myocardial infarction. *Am J Cardiol* 1988;62:202–208.

142. Beller GA: Assessment of myocardial viability, in *Clinical Nuclear Cardiology*. Philadelphia, WB Saunders Co, 1995, pp 293–336.

143. Tamaki N, Ohtani H, Yamashita K, et al: Metabolic activity in the areas of new fill-in after thallium-201 reinjection: Comparison with positron emission tomography using fluorine-18-deoxyglucose. *J Nucl Med* 1991;32:673–678.

144. Bonow RO, Dilsizian V, Cuocolo A, Bacharach SL: Identification of viable myocardium in patients with chronic coronary artery disease and left ventricular dysfunction. Comparison of thallium scintigraphy with reinjection and PET imaging with ^{18}F-fluorodeoxyglucose. *Circulation* 1991; 83:26–37.

145. Favaro L, Masini F, Serra W, et al: Thallium 201 for detection of viable myocardium: Comparison of different reinjection protocols. *J Nucl Cardiol* 1994;1:515–521.

146. Inglese E, Brambilla M, Dondi M, et al, on behalf of the Italian Group of Nuclear Cardiology: Assessment of myocardial viability after thallium-201 reinjection or rest-redistribution imaging: A multicenter study. *J Nucl Med* 1995;36: 555–563.

147. Mori T, Minamiji K, Kurogane H, Ogawa K, Yoshida Y: Rest-injected thallium-201 imaging for assessing viability of severe asynergic regions. *J Nucl Med* 1991;32:1718–1724.

147a. Pagley PR, Beller GA, Watson DD, Gimple LW, Ragosta M: Improved early and late outcome after coronary bypass surgery in patients with ischemic cardiomyopathy and residual myocardial viability. *Circulation* (In press)

148. Cuocolo A, Pace L, Ricciardelli B, Chiariello M, Trimarco B, Salvatore M: Identification of viable myocardium in patients with chronic coronary artery disease: Comparison of thallium-201 scintigraphy with reinjection and technetium-99m-methoxyisobutyl isonitrile. *J Nucl Med* 1992; 33:505–511.

149. Marzullo P, Sambuceti G, Parodi O: The role of sestamibi scintigraphy in the radioisotopic assessment of myocardial viability. *J Nucl Med* 1992;33: 1925–1930.

150. Maurea S, Cuocolo A, Pace L, et al: Rest-injected thallium-201 redistribution and resting technetium-99m methoxyisobutylisonitrile uptake in coronary artery disease: Relation to the severity of coronary artery stenosis. *Eur J Nucl Med* 1993;20: 502–510.

151. Maurea S, Cuocolo A, Pace L, et al: Left ventricular dysfunction in coronary artery disease: Comparison between rest-redistribution thallium 201 and resting technetium 99m methoxyisobutyl isonitrile cardiac imaging. *J Nucl Cardiol* 1994;1: 65–71.

152. Kauffman GJ, Boyne TS, Watson DD, Smith WH, Beller GA: Comparison of rest thallium-201 imaging and rest technetium-99m sestamibi imaging for assessment of myocardial viability in patients with coronary artery disease and severe left ventricular dysfunction. *J Am Coll Cardiol,* in press.

152a. Galli M, Marcassa C, Bolli R, et al: Spontaneous delayed recovery of perfusion and contraction after the first 5 weeks after anterior infarction: evidence for the presence of hibernating myocardium in the infarcted area. *Circulation* 1994; 90:1386–1397.

153. Brunken R, Tillisch J, Schwaiger M, et al: Regional perfusion, glucose metabolism, and wall motion in patients with chronic electrocardiographic Q wave infarctions: Evidence for persistence of viable tissue in some infarct regions by positron emission tomography. *Circulation* 1986; 73:951–963.

154. Brunken R, Schwaiger M, Grover-McKay M, Phelps ME, Tillisch J, Schelbert HR: Positron emission tomography detects tissue metabolic activity in myocardial segments with persistent thallium perfusion defects. *J Am Coll Cardiol* 1987;10: 557–567.

155. Melin JA, Wijns W, Keyeux A, et al: Assessment of thallium-201 redistribution versus glucose uptake as predictors of viability after coronary occlusion and reperfusion. *Circulation* 1988;77:927–934.

156. Schwaiger M, Brunken R, Grover-McKay M, et al: Regional myocardial metabolism in patients with acute myocardial infarction assessed by positron emission tomography. *J Am Coll Cardiol* 1986;8:800–808.

157. Pierard LA, De Landsheere CM, Berthe C, Rigo P, Kulbertus HE: Identification of viable myocardium by echocardiography during dobutamine infusion

in patients with myocardial infarction after thrombolytic therapy: Comparison with positron emission tomography. *J Am Coll Cardiol* 1990;15: 1021–1031.

158. Di Carli M, Sherman T, Khanna S, et al: Myocardial viability in asynergic regions subtended by occluded coronary arteries: Relation to the status of collateral flow in patients with chronic coronary artery disease. *J Am Coll Cardiol* 1994;23: 860–868.

159. Tamaki N, Kawamoto M, Takahashi N, et al: Prognostic value of an increase in fluorine-18 deoxyglucose uptake in patients with myocardial infarction: Comparison with stress thallium imaging. *J Am Coll Cardiol* 1993;22:1621–1627.

160. Tillisch J, Brunken R, Marshall R, et al: Reversibility of cardiac wall motion abnormalities predicted by positron emission tomography. *N Engl J Med* 1986;314:884–888.

161. Tamaki N, Kawamoto M, Tadamura E, et al: Prediction of reversible ischemia after revascularization. Perfusion and metabolic studies with positron emission tomography. *Circulation* 1995; 91:1697–1705.

161a. Di Carli MF, Asgarzadie F, Schelbert HR, et al: Quantitative relation between myocardial viability and improvement in heart failure symptoms after revascularization in patients with ischemic cardiomyopathy. *Circulation* 1995;92:3436–3444.

162. Walsh MN, Geltman EM, Brown MA, et al: Noninvasive estimation of regional myocardial oxygen consumption by positron emission tomography with carbon-11 acetate in patients with myocardial infarction. *J Nucl Med* 1989;30:1798–1808.

163. Gropler RJ, Siegel BA, Sampathkumaran K, et al: Dependence of recovery of contractile function on maintenance of oxidative metabolism after myocardial infarction. *J Am Coll Cardiol* 1992;19:989–997.

164. Gropler RJ, Geltman EM, Sampathkumaran K, et al: Functional recovery after coronary revascularization for chronic coronary artery disease is dependent on maintenance of oxidative metabolism. *J Am Coll Cardiol* 1992;20:569–577.

165. Hanes C, Bergman S, Perez J, Sobel B, Geltman A: The time course of restoration of nutritive perfusion, myocardial oxygen consumption, and regional function after coronary thrombosis. *Cor Art Dis* 1990;1:687–696.

166. Yoshida K, Gould K: Quantitative relation of myocardial infarct size and myocardial viability by positron emission tomography to left ventricular ejection fraction and 3-year mortality with and without revascularization. *J Am Coll Cardiol* 1993; 22:984–997.

167. DeCoster PM, Melin JA, Detry JM, Brasseur LA, Beckers C, Col J: Coronary artery reperfusion in acute myocardial infarction: Assessment by pre- and postintervention thallium-201 myocardial perfusion imaging. *Am J Cardiol* 1985;55:889–895.

168. Reduto LA, Freund GC, Gaeta JM, Smalling RW, Lewis B, Gould KL: Coronary artery reperfusion in acute myocardial infarction: Beneficial effects of intracoronary streptokinase on left ventricular salvage and performance. *Am Heart J* 1981;102: 1168–1177.

169. Simoons ML, Wijns W, Balakumaran K, et al: The effect of intracoronary thrombolysis with streptokinase on myocardial thallium distribution and left ventricular function assessed by blood-pool scintigraphy. *Eur Heart J* 1982;3:433–440.

170. Schwarz F, Hofmann M, Schuler G, von Olshausen K, Zimmermann R, Kübler W: Thrombolysis in acute myocardial infarction: Effect of intravenous followed by intracoronary streptokinase application on estimates of infarct size. *Am J Cardiol* 1984;53:1505–1510.

171. Granato JE, Watson DD, Flanagan TL, Gascho JA, Beller GA: Myocardial thallium-201 kinetics during coronary occlusion and reperfusion: Influence of method of reflow and timing of thallium-201 administration. *Circulation* 1986;73:150–160.

172. Ritchie JL, Davis KB, Williams DL, Caldwell J, Kennedy JW: Global and regional left ventricular function and tomographic radionuclide perfusion: The Western Washington Intracoronary Streptokinase in Myocardial Infarction Trial. *Circulation* 1984;70:867–875.

173. Ritchie JL, Cerqueira M, Maynard C, Davis K, Kennedy JW: Ventricular function and infarct size: The Western Washington Intravenous Streptokinase in Myocardial Infarction Trial. *J Am Coll Cardiol* 1988;11:689–697.

174. Cerqueira MD, Maynard C, Ritchie JL, Davis KB, Kennedy JW: Long-term survival in 618 patients from the Western Washington Streptokinase in Myocardial Infarction trials. *J Am Coll Cardiol* 1992;20:1452–1459.

175. Wackers FJ, Gibbons RJ, Verani MS, et al: Serial quantitative planar technetium-99m isonitrile imaging in acute myocardial infarction: Efficacy for noninvasive assessment of thrombolytic therapy. *J Am Coll Cardiol* 1989;14:861–873.

176. Gibbons RJ, Verani MS, Behrenbeck T, et al: Feasibility of tomographic ^{99m}Tc-hexakis-2-methoxy-2-methylpropyl-isonitrile imaging for the assessment of myocardial area at risk and the effect of treatment in acute myocardial infarction. *Circulation* 1989;80:1277–1286.

177. Christian TF, Gibbons RJ, Gersh BJ: Effect of infarct location on myocardial salvage assessed by technetium-99m isonitrile. *J Am Coll Cardiol* 1991; 17:1303–1308.

178. Hvid-Jacobsen K, Møller JT, Kjøller E, et al: Myocardial perfusion at fatal infarction: Location and size of scintigraphic defects. *J Nucl Med* 1992; 33:251–253.

179. Santoro GM, Bisi G, Sciagrà R, Leoncini M, Fazzini PF, Meldolesi U: Single photon emission computed tomography with technetium-99m hexakis 2-methoxyisobutyl isonitrile in acute myocardial infarction before and after thrombolytic treatment: Assessment of salvaged myocardium and prediction of late functional recovery. *J Am Coll Cardiol* 1990;15:301–314.

180. Christian TF, Behrenbeck T, Gersh BJ, Gibbons RJ: Relation of left ventricular volume and function over one year after acute myocardial infarction to infarct size determined by technetium-99m sestamibi. *Am J Cardiol* 1991;68:21–26.

181. Christian TF, Behrenbeck T, Pellikka PA, Huber KC, Chesebro JH, Gibbons RJ: Mismatch of left ventricular function and infarct size demonstrated by technetium-99m isonitrile imaging after reperfusion therapy for acute myocardial infarction: Identification of myocardial stunning and hyperkinesia. *J Am Coll Cardiol* 1990;16:1632–1638.

182. McCallister BD, Christian TF, Gersh B, Gibbons RJ: Prognosis of myocardial infarctions involving more than 40% of the left ventricle after acute reperfusion therapy. *Circulation* 1993;88: 1470–1475.

182a. Oh JK, Gibbons RJ, Christian TF, et al: Correlation of regional wall motion abnormalities detected by two-dimensional echocardiography with perfusion defect determined by technetium 99m sestamibi imaging in patients treated with reperfusion therapy during acute myocardial infarction. *Am Heart J* 1996;131:32–37.

183. Chareonthaitawee P, Christian TF, Hirose K, Gibbons RJ, Rumberger JA: Relation of initial infarct size to extent of left ventricular remodeling in the year after acute myocardial infarction. *J Am Coll Cardiol* 1995;25:567–573.

184. Behrenbeck T, Pellikka PA, Huber KC, Bresnahan JF, Gersh BJ, Gibbons RJ: Primary angioplasty in myocardial infarction: Assessment of improved myocardial perfusion with technetium-99m isonitrile. *J Am Coll Cardiol* 1991;17:365–372.

185. Clements IP, Christian TF, Higano ST, Gibbons RJ, Gersh BJ: Residual flow to the infarct zone as a determinant of infarct size after direct angioplasty. *Circulation* 1993;88:1527–1533.

186. Gibbons RJ, Holmes DR, Reeder GS, Bailey KR, Hopfenspirger MR, Gersh BJ, for the Mayo Coronary Care Unit and Catheterization Laboratory Groups: Immediate angioplasty compared with the administration of a thrombolytic agent followed by conservative treatment for myocardial infarction. *N Engl J Med* 1993;328:685–691.

187. O'Keefe JH Jr, Grines CL, DeWood MA, Bateman TM, Christian TF, Gibbons RJ: Factors influencing myocardial salvage with primary angioplasty. *J Nucl Cardiol* 1995;2:35–41.

188. Christian TF, O'Connor MK, Hopfenspirger MR, Gibbons RJ: Comparison of reinjection thallium 201 and resting technetium 99m sestamibi tomographic images for the quantification of infarct size after acute myocardial infarction. *J Nucl Cardiol* 1994;1:17–28.

189. Dunn RF, Freedman B, Bailey IK, Uren R, Kelly DT: Noninvasive prediction of multivessel disease after myocardial infarction. *Circulation* 1980;62: 726–734.

190. Gibson RS, Watson DD, Craddock GB, et al: Prediction of cardiac events after uncomplicated myocardial infarction: A prospective study comparing predischarge exercise thallium-201 scintigraphy and coronary angiography. *Circulation* 1983;68: 321–336.

191. Hung J, Goris ML, Nash E, et al: Comparative value of maximal treadmill testing, exercise thallium myocardial perfusion scintigraphy and exercise radionuclide ventriculography for distinguishing high- and low-risk patients soon after acute myocardial infarction. *Am J Cardiol* 1984;53: 1221–1227.

192. Brown KA, Weiss RM, Clements JP, Wackers FJ: Usefulness of residual ischemic myocardium within prior infarct zone for identifying patients at high risk late after acute myocardial infarction. *Am J Cardiol* 1987;60:15–19.

193. Gibson RS: Clinical, functional, and angiographic distinctions between Q wave and non–Q wave myocardial infarction: Evidence of spontaneous

reperfusion and implications for intervention trials. *Circulation* 1987;75(Suppl V): V-128–V-138.

194. Gimple LW, Beller GA: Assessing prognosis after acute myocardial infarction in the thrombolytic era. *J Nucl Cardiol* 1994;1:198–209.

195. Tilkemeier PL, Guiney TE, LaRaia PJ, Boucher CA: Prognostic value of predischarge low-level exercise thallium testing after thrombolytic treatment of acute myocardial infarction. *Am J Cardiol* 1990;66:1203–1207.

196. Haber HL, Beller GA, Watson DD, Gimple LW: Exercise thallium-201 scintigraphy after thrombolytic therapy with or without angioplasty for acute myocardial infarction. *Am J Cardiol* 1993;71:1257–1261.

197. Krone RJ, Gregory JJ, Freedland KE, et al, for the Multicenter Myocardial Ischemia Research Group: Limited usefulness of exercise testing and thallium scintigraphy in evaluation of ambulatory patients several months after recovery from an acute coronary event: Implications for management of stable coronary heart disease. *J Am Coll Cardiol* 1994;24:1274–1281.

198. Moss AJ, Goldstein RE, Hall WJ, et al, for the Multicenter Myocardial Ischemia Research Group: Detection and significance of myocardial ischemia in stable patients after recovery from an acute coronary event. *JAMA* 1993;269:2379–2385.

198a. Miller TD, Gersh BJ, Christian TF, Bailey KR, Gibbons RJ: Limited prognostic value of thallium-201 exercise treadmill testing early after myocardial infarction in patients treated with thrombolysis. *Am Heart J* 1995;130:259–266.

199. Leppo JA, O'Brien J, Rothendler JA, Getchell JD, Lee VW: Dipyridamole–thallium-201 scintigraphy in the prediction of future cardiac event after acute myocardial infarction. *N Engl J Med* 1984;310:1014–1018.

200. Brown KA, O'Meara J, Chambers CE, Plante DA: Ability of dipyridamole–thallium-201 imaging one to four days after acute myocardial infarction to predict in-hospital and late recurrent myocardial ischemic events. *Am J Cardiol* 1990;65:160–167.

201. Hendel RC, Gore JM, Alpert JS, Leppo JA: Prognosis following interventional therapy for acute myocardial infarction: Utility of dipyridamole thallium scintigraphy. *Cardiology* 1991;79:73–80.

202. Mahmarian JJ, Pratt CM, Nishimura S, Abreu A, Verani MS: Quantitative adenosine ^{201}Tl single-photon emission computed tomography for the early assessment of patients surviving acute myocardial infarction. *Circulation* 1993;87:1197–1210.

203. Mahmarian JJ, Mahmarian AC, Marks GF, Pratt CM, Verani MS: Role of adenosine thallium-201 tomography for defining long-term risk in patients after acute myocardial infarction. *J Am Coll Cardiol* 1995;25:1333–1340.

203a. Bosch X, Magriñá J, March R, et al: Prediction of in-hospital cardiac events using dipyridamole-thallium scintigraphy performed very early after acute myocardial infarction. *Clin Cardiol* 1996;19:189–196.

203b. Claeys MJ, Vrints CJ, Krug B, et al: Adenosine technetium-99m sestamibi (SPECT) for the early assessment of jeopardized myocardium after acute myocardial infarction. *Eur Heart J* 1995;16:1186–1194.

204. Travin MI, Dessouki A, Cameron T, Heller GV: Use of exercise technetium-99m sestamibi SPECT imaging to detect residual ischemia and for risk stratification after acute myocardial infarction. *Am J Cardiol* 1995;75:665–669.

204a. Heller GV, Herman SD, Travin MI, Baron JI, Santos-Ocampo C, McClellan JR. Independent prognostic value of intravenous dipyridamole with technetium-99m sestamibi tomographic imaging in predicting cardiac events and cardiac-related hospital admissions. *J Am Coll Cardiol* 1995;26:1202–1208.

205. Corbett JR, Dehmer GJ, Lewis SE, et al: The prognostic value of submaximal exercise testing with radionuclide ventriculography before hospital discharge in patients with recent myocardial infarction. *Circulation* 1981;64:535–544.

206. Borer JS, Miller D, Schreiber T, Charash B, Gerling B: Radionuclide cineangiography in acute myocardial infarction: Role in prognostication. *Semin Nucl Med* 1987;17:89–94.

207. Wasserman AG, Katz RJ, Cleary P, Varma VM, Reba RC, Ross AM: Noninvasive detection of multivessel disease after myocardial infarction by exercise radionuclide ventriculography. *Am J Cardiol* 1982;50:1242–1247.

208. Nicod P, Corbett JR, Firth BG, et al: Prognostic value of resting and submaximal exercise radionuclide ventriculography after acute myocardial infarction in high-risk patients with single and multivessel disease. *Am J Cardiol* 1983;52:30–36.

209. Corbett JR, Nicod P, Lewis SE, Rude RE, Willerson JT: Prognostic value of submaximal exercise

radionuclide ventriculography after myocardial infarction. *Am J Cardiol* 1983;52:82A–91A.

210. Morris KG, Palmeri ST, Califf RM, et al: Value of radionuclide angiography for predicting specific cardiac events after acute myocardial infarction. *Am J Cardiol* 1985;55:318–324.

211. Kuchar DL, Freund J, Yeates M, Sammel N: Enhanced prediction of major cardiac events after myocardial infarction using exercise radionuclide ventriculography. *Aus NZ J Med* 1987;17:228–233.

212. Abraham RD, Harris PJ, Roubin GS, et al: Usefulness of ejection fraction response to exercise one month after acute myocardial infarction in predicting coronary anatomy and prognosis. *Am J Cardiol* 1987;60:225–230.

213. Zaret BL, Wackers FJ, Terrin ML, et al, for the TIMI Study Group: Value of radionuclide rest and exercise left ventricular ejection fraction in assessing survival of patients after thrombolytic therapy for acute myocardial infarction: Results of Thrombolysis in Myocardial Infarction (TIMI) phase II study. *J Am Coll Cardiol* 1995;26:73–79.

214. Rothbart RM, Beller GA, Watson DD, Nygaard TW, Gibson RS: Diagnostic accuracy and prognostic significance of quantitative thallium-201 scintigraphy in patients with left bundle branch block. *Am J Noninvas Cardiol* 1987;1:197–205.

215. Friedman J, Van Train K, Maddahi J, et al: "Upward creep" of the heart: A frequent source of false-positive reversible defects during thallium-201 stress-redistribution SPECT. *J Nucl Med* 1989; 30:1718–1722.

216. Gibbons RJ, Lee KL, Cobb F, Jones RH: Ejection fraction response to exercise in patients with chest pain and normal coronary artery arteriograms. *Circulation* 1981;64:952–957.

PART III

Acute Management

12

Pharmacologic Management of Acute Myocardial Infarction

J. Wayne Warnica, MD, FRCPC

The goals of pharmacologic therapy of acute myocardial infarction are to minimize short-term and long-term morbidity and mortality and to alleviate symptoms. As the major determinant of prognosis both in the short-term and in the long-term is the size of the infarct (1–3), the primary objective of therapy is to interrupt or limit the extent of necrosis. In this context, measures aimed at diminishing myocardial oxygen demand have become standard therapy. As discussed in Chapters 19 to 22, limiting the extent of necrosis or salvaging myocardium at risk can be significantly addressed only by restoring blood flow. All patients presenting with an acute infarct must therefore be *considered* for reperfusion therapy. Certain subsets of patients, including those presenting late after the onset of symptoms, and those patients with ST segment depression on the initial electrocardiogram, do not appear to benefit from such an approach (4–6). In patients undergoing short-term reperfusion therapy, many of the pharmacologic agents and principles discussed in this chapter play an important adjunctive role (see later in this chapter). Unfortunately, only about 25% of patients with acute myocardial infarction are reported to be eligible for a thrombolytic therapy (following currently accepted criteria) (7). A recent Canadian multicenter study, however, has reported the use of thrombolytic therapy in 43% of *all* patients presenting with acute myocardial infarction (8). In the remainder, namely, those for whom thrombolytic therapy or mechanical reperfusion therapy (primary PTCA, or a coronary arterial bypass grafting) is not possible, other pharmacologic agents alone must suffice. This chapter addresses the general pharmacologic management of acute myocardial infarction, with a particular emphasis on the management of those patients who do not receive thrombolytic therapy. The principles to be applied are, however, important for all patients with acute evolving infarction: to evaluate and treat promptly, to treat aggressively but carefully, and to individualize therapy. The objectives are to relieve pain and anxiety, to limit the extent of necrosis, and to prevent complications.

OXYGEN

Dyspnea is one of the most common symptoms of patients with acute myocardial infarction (see Ch. 24). Although oxygen administration has been routinely applied to patients with acute myocardial infarction for many years, this approach has been questioned (9). Several earlier studies have, however, shown that significant arterial hypoxemia occurs commonly in acute myocardial infarction, even in patients without primary lung disease or apparent pulmonary congestion (10–12). Correction of hypoxemia would therefore be expected to reduce the symptoms of dyspnea in these patients and to have a beneficial impact on oxygen delivery to the myocardium. Dyspnea is frequent even among patients without measurable hypoxemia, possibly related to a transient decrease in pulmonary compliance resulting from increased interstitial fluid (see Ch. 26). Regardless of the mechanisms causing dyspnea, clinicians have noted the almost immediate relief of breathlessness, anxiety, and often pain after the administration of oxygen. A placebo effect may be involved; nonetheless, with the absence of evidence for any deleterious effect of low-dose oxygen and the presence of evidence suggesting that it may improve myocardial function (13) as well as decrease anterior ST segment elevation (14), the evident relief of anxiety and pain after the administration of oxygen justifies routine use in acute myocardial infarction.

ANALGESICS

Chest pain is the most frequent presenting complaint in acute myocardial infarction. The pain, distress, and anxiety associated with acute infarction may induce significant circulatory effects, at least in part by triggering sympathetic overactivity leading to sinus tachycardia, hypertension, and increased cardiac output. It is likely that pain and anxiety are important contributors to the "hyperdynamic state" described in a proportion of patients with acute evolving infarction (15), and relief of these symptoms would be expected to aid in decreasing oxygen demands.

The mechanisms of pain production are not well defined, nor is it possible to differentiate between pain arising from irreversible necrosis and pain caused by reversible ischemia. Relief of pain in acute infarction has traditionally been achieved by the liberal use of narcotics, and they are effective. It should, however, be emphasized that the reduction in myocardial ischemia, whether by reperfusion or by diminishing myocardial oxygen demands, may have markedly beneficial effects on pain relief as well (16–18). Nitrates have a primary role, and the use of sublingual nitroglycerin followed by intravenous nitroglycerin may be extremely effective in relieving pain, as well as in meeting the other hemodynamic objectives of such therapy. When pain persists, especially in patients in a "hyperdynamic state," intravenous beta-blockade is a extremely useful (16) (see later).

Narcotic analgesics should be administered in the absence of a prompt response to nitrates. Morphine given intravenously in repeated boluses of 2 to 5 mg remains the agent of choice. Intramuscular injections (which may complicate enzyme analyses and thrombolytic therapy) should be avoided. The optimal dose of morphine is unclear, but it appears that doses greater than 10 to 15 mg per 70 kg of body weight do not produce greater degrees of analgesia. The duration of pain and the need for narcotic analgesia vary considerably. The highest use of morphine may be predicted by the extent of infarction, the initial degree of the suspicion for myocardial infarction, and male sex (19). The excessive use of morphine should be avoided in the face of potential side effects such as nausea, vomiting, hypotension, and respiratory depression. One should remain alert to the features of persistent ischemia that might necessitate a change of therapy, despite the apparent absence of pain, which may be masked by excessive doses of narcotics.

Meperidine (Demerol) has been recommended as an alternative to morphine, especially in the setting of acute inferior wall myocardial infarction with increased vagal tone. As significant adverse effects, such as hypotension, bradycardia, and tachycardia, occur in only 2% to 8% of those treated with morphine (20), the hemodynamic advantages of switching to meperidine in this setting are relatively small.

Diamorphine (heroin) and nitrous oxide are both used more frequently in Europe. Neither has been extensively used in North America. Nitrous oxide in portable containers (Entonox) has been used to good effect by paramedical personnel, i.e., ambulances, in the United Kingdom.

Nalbuphine (Nubain) is a narcotic analgesic related to the opioid oxymorphine and the narcotic antagonist naloxone. It has been shown to be useful in the management of acute myocardial infarction (21) with few adverse hemodynamic effects. Although respiratory depression does occur with this drug, there appears to be a ceiling at higher doses, which may increase the safety of its use (22).

NITRATES

Mechanisms of Action

The fundamental action of nitrates is direct vasodilation by smooth muscle relaxation. Nitrates act as an exogenous source of nitric oxide (the apparent EDRF). Thus they are nonselective vasodilators affecting veins, arteries, and arterioles. The smooth muscle of the venous system appears to be the most sensitive, with maximum dilation of venous capacitance vessels occurring even at low doses, leading to a consequent reduction of both left and right ventricular preload (23). As the dose of nitrates is increased, large conductance arteries dilate, decreasing arterial pressure and resistance (afterload). With further increases in dosage, arteriolar resistance falls with a further reduction in both peripheral vascular and coronary vascular resistance. A significant anti-ischemic effect of nitrates is mediated by decreases in preload and afterload, and the consequential fall in both left ventricular pressure and volume reduces ventricular wall tension, one of the major determinants of myocardial oxygen demand. A second mechanism by which nitrates decrease ischemia is by direct coronary artery dilation, leading to improved myocardial oxygen supply. Endothelial function over an atherosclerotic plaque is markedly altered, with diminished or absent production of EDRF (nitric oxide) (24). This not only increases vascular tone due to unopposed vasoconstrictor forces, but the lack of nitric oxide may also foster platelet aggregation and adhesion (25,26). Nitroglycerin, which is converted to nitric oxide, corrects or replaces this deficiency in EDRF production in the diseased endothelium, and the diseased artery dilates in response to nitrates. Nitroglycerin also in this way inhibits thrombin-induced release of endothelin and platelet aggregation (27–29). The major effects of nitrates are listed in Table 12–1.

Table 12–1. Major Effects of Nitrates in Ischemic Heart Disease

Anti-ischemic effects
—Coronary vasodilation
—Preload reduction
—Afterload reduction
—Redistribution of transmural coronary blood flow
—Inhibition of thrombin induced release of endothelin
—Relief of coronary vasospasm
Antiplatelet effects
—Inhibition of platelet aggregation

Clinically, nitroglycerin, given both sublingually and intravenously, has been shown to decrease regional ischemia, increase subendocardial oxygen delivery, and improve coronary collateral flow by dilation of collateral vessels (30). Nitrates dilate smaller coronary vessels to a greater degree than larger vessels (31). Nitrates also appear to redistribute flow preferentially to underperfused areas of myocardium, thereby diminishing localized ischemia (31).

In summary, nitrates have both systemic and coronary vascular effects, resulting in an improvement in the balance between myocardial oxygen supply and demand, with potentially salutary effects on the extent of necrosis, pain relief, hypertension, and heart failure that may arise secondary to ischemic or necrotic left ventricular dysfunction.

Effects on Hemodynamics and Clinical Outcome

Both sublingual nitroglycerin and intravenous nitroglycerin have been shown to decrease the duration and severity of the pain of acute myocardial infarction (32,33) and the frequency of recurrent ischemic pain during the first 24 to 48 hours. Because of the potential for nitrates to cause hypotension and either reflex tachycardia or reflex bradycardia (the latter is often a manifestation of excessive preload reduction and hypovolemia) (34), intravenous nitroglycerin has become the preferred method of administration. This allows a more accurate titration of both dose and effect. Cutaneous nitroglycerin preparations have been used clinically, but in the setting of acute myocardial infarction with enhanced sympathetic stimulation of the peripheral vasculature, the absorption of cutaneous agents is variable and provides a less reliable route for nitrate delivery.

Transient hypertension occurs in up to 40% of patients with acute infarction and is persistent in a significant proportion of others with preexisting hypertension. Hypertension has adverse effects on the extent of ischemia and infarct size and is associated with an increased frequency of complications, including congestive heart failure, infarct extension and expansion, and cardiac rupture (see Ch. 16). Reducing the blood pressure in the first few hours of therapy has been shown to decrease infarct size and reduce the incidence and severity of complications (35). Intravenous nitrates reduce blood pressure by causing a decrease in cardiac output and systemic vascular resistance. Both intravenous nitroglycerin and intravenous sodium nitroprusside have been used effectively and safely to control blood pressure in acute myocardial infarction, but intravenous nitroglycerin has become the agent of choice, primarily because of familiarity with its use and evidence to indicate a "coronary steal" syndrome with sodium nitroprusside. If hypertension does not respond promptly to intravenous nitroglycerin, sodium nitroprusside should be the next line of therapy.

Congestive heart failure occurring in the first few hours of acute myocardial infarction is related primarily to diminished left ventricular compliance, rather than to volume overload. Nitrates, by promoting rapid dilation of the capacitance bed, produce what is, in effect, a medical or internal phlebotomy, decreasing both pulmonary congestion and preload of the left and right ventricles. As the venodilating effect of the nitrates occurs at low doses, congestion may be relieved without an excessive decrease in systemic vascular resistance (36). A study has been reported comparing the effects of intravenous isosorbide dinitrate with a diurete in patients with congestive heart failure early after acute myocardial infarction (37). The diuretic decreased left ventricular filling pressure, decreased cardiac output, and transiently raised systemic blood pressure, whereas nitrates caused a decrease in systemic blood pressure and a decrease in peripheral vascular resistance with no reduction in cardiac output, despite a large fall in pulmonary vascular and left ventricular filling pressures. This suggests that the alleviation of pulmonary congestion by venodilation is hemodynamically superior to that produced by diuresis, in that the former approach reduces myocardial oxygen demand and maintains peripheral perfusion. Furthermore, the short duration of action allows careful titration to diminish pulmonary congestion without a sustained decrease in blood volume as effected by the use of diuretics. Hypertension and congestive heart failure complicating acute myocardial infarction are clear indications for intravenous nitroglycerin therapy.

Clinical and experimental studies imply that the beneficial effect of nitrates on the limitation of infarct size depends on the duration of symptoms prior to the initiation of therapy, the dose used, and possibly the site of infarction. In at least one laboratory study, low-dose intravenous nitroglycerin initiated during the first 6 hours after coronary ligation reduced the size of both inferior and anterior infarctions (38). These beneficial effects were completely abolished, however, when hypotension (mean blood pressure below 80 mm Hg) was induced by larger doses of nitroglycerin (39). A number of relatively small clinical studies have demonstrated beneficial effects of nitrates in acute myocardial infarction. These include a reduction in left ventricular filling pressure, improved global left ventricular function, decreased electrocardiographic ST segment elevation, reduced infarct size (as measured by creatine kinase release), a persistent reduction in the endocardial surface area of left ventricular asymmetry on echocardiography, and improved perfusion and defect scores on thallium scintigraphy (33,40,41). These clinical trials have further suggested that nitrate therapy is most effective when initiated early (probably within 4 hours of the onset of symptoms) and should be continued for 24 to 48 hours. More recent trials in "the modern era" appear to question this benefit of early versus late nitrate therapy (42,43). The most effective regimens utilize a dose titrated to produce a mean decrease in systolic blood pressure or mean blood pressure of approximately 10%. In *no* case should the mean blood pressure be lowered below 80 mm Hg, as reductions below this level have been associated with an increase in infarct size and complications (Fig. 12–1) (41). Using these guidelines, a trial reported by Jugdutt and Warnica demonstrated a reduction in infarct size and a clear reduction in major infarct-related complications, such as infarct expansion, infarct extension, cardiogenic shock, and in-hospital mortality (41). Echocardiographic data documented a decrease in expansion and thinning of the infarct zone in patients treated with intravenous nitroglycerin (see Ch. 29). Clinically recognized infarct *expansion* (defined as a second acute clinical event with hypotension; left ventricular failure; evidence of left ventricular dilation without electrocardiographic or enzyme evidence of new injury or necrosis; and echocardiographic evidence of regional diastolic stretching, thinning, and dilation of the infarct segment) was 87% less frequent in the nitroglycerin treated patients than in controls (41). Clinical evidence of infarct *extension* (with electrocardiographic or enzyme evidence of recurrent injury) was reduced by 50% (11% versus 23%, $p < 0.025$). Cardiogenic shock was 67% less frequent in the treated group (5% versus 15%, $p < 0.005$), and in-hospital mortality was reduced by 46%. (14% versus 26%, $p < 0.01$) (Fig. 12–2) (41). Furthermore, these beneficial effects appear to be maintained over the long term. In one study, immediate therapy with intravenous nitroglycerin followed by buccal nitroglycerin for 6 weeks led to sustained evidence of functional improvement at 1 year, as shown by diminished left ventricular volumes at rest and at exercise (44). Very recently, the use of intravenous isosorbide dinitrate in acute myocardial infarction has been reported (43). In contrast to the previously described studies, no benefit was observed with the administration of nitrates in the treatment groups as a whole for either acute or subacute infarction. Some subgroups appeared to derive more benefit than others, but the studies are too small to allow firm conclusions to be drawn. Patients with anterior infarctions appeared to benefit more than those with inferior myocardial infarctions, and those with non-Q infarction also appeared to benefit. Interestingly, a heterogeneity of nitrate effect was observed: there was a clear benefit of isosorbide dinitrate in patients with moderate ST segment elevation, and a trend toward a deleterious effect in patients with marked ST segment elevation. The mechanism for this is not clear, but it does suggest a need for caution in the use of intravenous nitrates in patients with very large infarctions. There are a number of differences between this trial, and the earlier one reported by Jugdutt and Warnica (41). In this recent trial, 97% of patients received thrombolytic therapy, whereas the earlier trial was primarily carried out in the "prethrombolytic era." In addition, patients with hypertension, or evidence of failure for which intravenous nitroglycerin was clearly indicated, were not included in the trial, so that potential beneficial

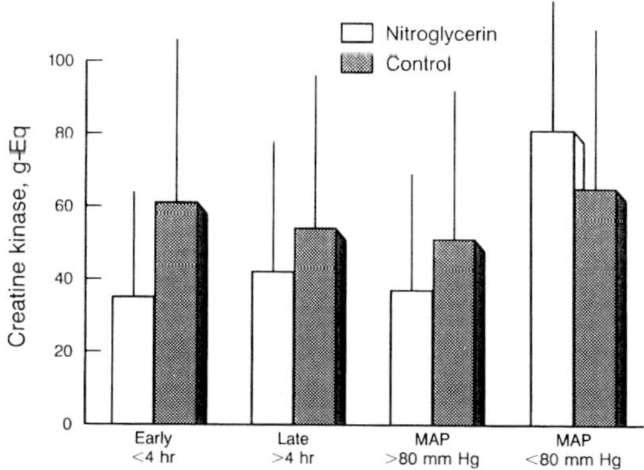

Figure 12–1. Relationship between cardiac creatine phosphate kinase enzyme release and therapy with intravenous nitroglycerin according to duration of symptoms and mean arterial blood pressure. *Adapted from Jugdutt and Warnica, (41), with permission.*

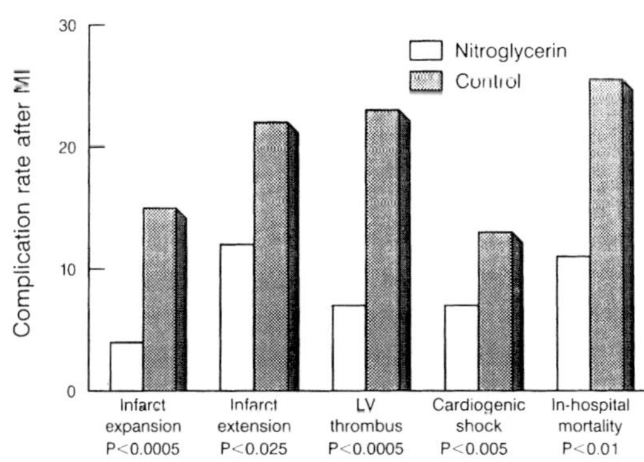

Figure 12–2. Effect of intravenous nitroglycerin on in-hospital complications of acute myocardial infarction. *Adapted from Jugdutt and Warnica (41), with permission.*

effects in this group would not have been measured. This most recent trial, however, does continue to suggest a potential role for nitrates in selected patients who have received thrombolytic therapy.

It must be emphasized that the foregoing trials are relatively small with broad confidence limits. Two "mega-trials," GISSI-3 and ISIS-IV, involving use of nitrates in acute myocardial infarction have now been reported (42,45). In GISSI-3, 19,394 patients with an acute myocardial infarction were randomized in a factorial design to receive 6 weeks of oral lisinopril or control drug, as well as nitroglycerin (IV for the first 24 hours, and then transdermal glyceryl trinitrate) (45). In this very large open-label study, systematic use of intravenous followed by transdermal nitrates did not show any independent effects on mortality or combined mortality and severe left ventricular dysfunction. It did yield a slightly lower rate of postinfarction angina, a lower frequency of cardiogenic shock ($2p = 0.009$), and a slight increase of stroke ($2p = 0.027$). However, more than half (57%) of control patients received nitrates, and 47% of these received intravenous nitroglycerin in the first 24 hours. In addition, 65% of patients in GISSI-3 started nitrate therapy after more than 6 hours from the onset of pain, and 40% started nitrate therapy after more than 12 hours from the onset of pain, so that little beneficial effect on left ventricular function or complications might be expected if early initiation of therapy plays a significant role. While a 6-week echocardiogram was part of the study protocol, no information on these results is yet available. Unfortunately, there is no information provided as to the type of infarction (Q wave versus non-Q wave, or anterior myocardial infarction versus other types of myocardial infarction), which may, by helping to define risk groups, be important in assessing the effects of nitrate therapy.

In the ISIS-IV trial, in 58,050 patients (described in more detail in the following section), there was no significant reduction in 5-week mortality, either overall (7.34% mononitrates vs. 7.54 placebo) or in any subgroup examined. No late survival advantage was apparent (42). Oral mononitrate therapy was not associated with reduction of postinfarction angina (surprising since that is the effect for which most nitrates are prescribed). Other clinical events, including congestive heart failure and cardiogenic shock, were also not affected by nitrate therapy. Again in this study, 60% of patients received their first oral dose of nitrate at more than 6 hours from the onset of symptoms, and approximately 60% of control patients received either intravenous (54%) or other forms of nitrate therapy. The investigators report (but do not provide data) that those patients receiving early nitrate therapy did not benefit more than those receiving late therapy. Little information as to the hemodynamic and clinical effects of nitrate therapy in the various types or sites of infarction is given.

Effects on Mortality

The most stringent criterion of therapeutic efficacy is a reduction in mortality. The initial clinical trials of nitrate therapy in acute myocardial infarction were each too small to satisfactorily answer the question of mortality reduction. However, the meta-analysis of 10 small trials (involving a total of 2,000 patients) of intravenous nitroglycerin and/or sodium nitroprusside in acute myocardial infarction showed that both agents were associated with a reduction in mortality (over a 13- to 18-month period), with a nonsignificant trend favoring nitroglycerin (Fig. 12–3) (46). Nitrate therapy was associated with a 35% reduction in short-term mortality (5.5% in treated patients versus 9.6% in controls), with the major benefit evident during the first 7

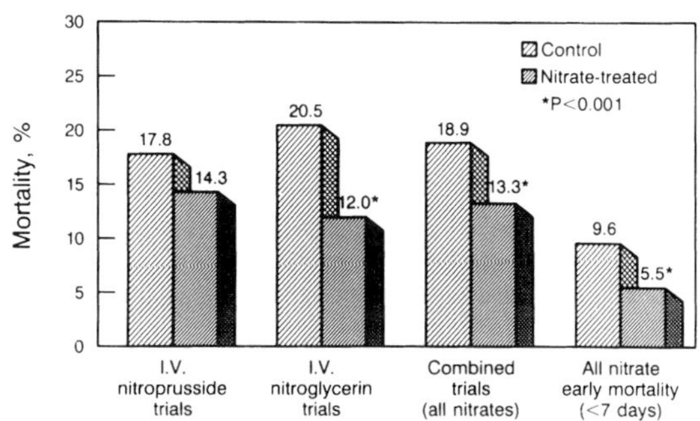

Figure 12–3. Effect on mortality, both early and total, of intravenous nitrate and introvenous nitroprusside in acute myocardial infarction.

days of follow-up (46). Persistence of the early beneficial effect was, however, maintained with a further (albeit minor) reduction in mortality thereafter. The role of nitrates on mortality in acute myocardial infarction has been addressed very carefully by the ISIS-IV and GISSI-3 trials (42,45). GISSI-3, in almost 20,000 patients, demonstrated that intravenous nitroglycerin followed by transdermal nitrates in all patients presenting with acute myocardial infarction had no independent effect on mortality, or on the combined endpoint of mortality plus severe congestive heart failure (45). The combination of lisinopril and nitrates did, however, reveal a significant reduction in overall mortality [odds ratio 0.83 (0.7–0.97)] and in combined mortality plus severe congestive heart failure [0.85 (0.76–0.941)].

ISIS-IV, in 58,050 unselected patients with acute myocardial infarction, demonstrated no significant reduction in 5-week mortality by the use of early oral mononitrate therapy (42). There was also no significant interaction (either positive or negative) with either captopril or magnesium therapies. Both trials did demonstrate conclusively the safety of nitrate use in this very broadly defined patient group.

An intriguing small study addressing a potential additional mechanism whereby nitrates might alter prognosis in acute infarction arises from a report that intravenous nitroglycerin reduced the frequency of complex ventricular ectopy (47). In the large ISIS-IV trial, nitrates as prescribed had no effect on either ventricular fibrillation or other cardiac arrests (42).

Despite widespread acceptance of acute reperfusion as the initial treatment of choice in myocardial infarction, there is a paucity of data on the role of nitrates as adjuncts to thrombolytic agents. One small study showed a prompt and persistent improvement in left ventricular function with a combination of reperfusion therapy (streptokinase and/or angioplasty) and intravenous nitroglycerin (48). A concern has recently been raised about a possible negative interaction between intravenous nitroglycerin and thrombolytic therapy with r-tPA (49). This small study suggests that intravenous nitroglycerin inhibits the lytic effects of r-tPA. Further information to clarify this important concern is obviously critical. In both the GISSI-3 and ISIS-IV trials, thrombolytic therapy was given in 71% and 70%, respectively, of all study patients. Streptokinase was the thrombolytic agent used in the great majority of patients. While no adverse interaction between streptokinase and intravenous or oral nitrate therapy was reported, neither was there any apparent benefit to adding nitrates to lytic therapy in this rather broadly defined group of patients with acute myocardial infarction (42,45).

What, then, is the role of nitrate therapy in acute myocardial infarction? Intravenous nitroglycerin has been clearly shown to be effective in treating patients with acute myocardial infarction complicated by hypertension, congestive heart failure, and ongoing or recurrent ischemic pain. The mega-trials did not support a beneficial effect of routine nitrate therapy on mortality with acute myocardial infarction. However, the populations in these studies represent the broad spectrum of acute myocardial infarction patients, including Q wave and non Q wave infarction, infarcts of all areas of the myocardium, and of varying sizes, and therapy was begun quite late. They do not exclude and, indeed, may have obscured possible benefits in both mortality and left ventricular function in selected groups of patients either treated with or without thrombolytic therapy. Moreover the widespread use of nitrates in patients in the placebo arms of both ISIS-4 and GISSI-3 trials introduces a bias and dilutes the overall potentially beneficial effect of treatment. What these data do suggest however is that although nitrates need not be routinely used in all patients, their clinical use is frequent and therapy in this broad group of patients is safe. We can therefore continue to be confident in the use intravenous nitroglycerin for ongoing ischemia, hypertension, and acute congestive heart failure complicating acute myocardial infarction as clinically indicated. In patients who are hemodynamically fragile, or with apparent large infarctions, intravenous nitroglycerin is a useful adjunct to therapy, at least until such patients can be stabilized and therapy with an angiotensin converting enzyme inhibitor is well established.

Methods of Administration

There is evidence that, at least in selected patients, intravenous nitrates can have a beneficial effect on both morbidity and mortality from acute myocardial infarction. It is interesting to reflect that at one time nitrates were considered to be contraindicated in the management of acute myocardial infarction (50). The ISIS-IV and GISSI-3 trials have at least clearly demonstrated the safety of nitrates in acute myocardial infarction (42,45). We can thus be reassured about using these medications for acute myocardial infarction where clinically indicated. The earlier recommendation to avoid the use of nitrates in acute myocardial infarction was based primarily on the potential of nitrates to induce hypotension and tachycardia, or hypotension with marked reflex bradycardia (34). Sublingual nitroglycerin, particularly the initial dose, may result in a vasovagal response with marked hypotension and bradycardia in approximately 9% of patients (34). This is likely the consequence of excessive preload reduction, especially in "relatively" hypovolemic patients or in elderly patients, and the hemodynamic sequelae are probably a manifestation of an activation of the Von Bezold–Jarisch reflex (34). The hypotension and bradycardia are, however, transient and invariably respond to increasing venous return to the heart by leg raising, fluid administration, and occasionally, atropine administration. The likelihood of such a response can be diminished by starting with intravenous nitroglycerin at low doses (5 μg/min).

From a practical standpoint, it should be emphasized that invasive pulmonary artery or systemic blood pressure monitoring is unnecessary during the routine administration of intravenous nitroglycerin, but patients need to be carefully observed, particularly during the initiation of therapy. Any decision to subsequently use hemodynamic monitoring should be based on the standard clinical indications. As the response to nitroglycerin is highly variable, the desired hemodynamic objectives rather than a preset dose should be used as therapeutic endpoints. After therapy is initiated at 5 to 10 μg per minute, the dose is increased by 10 μg every 5 to 10 minutes until mean blood pressure is reduced by 10%, but not below 80 mm Hg, in normotensive patients. In chronically hypertensive patients, the aim is to reduce blood pressure by approximately 30% but to maintain the pressure no lower than 140/90 mm Hg.

The most common complications of intravenous nitroglycerin are headache, with occasional dizziness, nausea, and vomiting. As most nitroglycerin is suspended in an alcohol-based solution, there have been occasional anecdotal reports of patients becoming intoxicated after receiving large doses over a prolonged period.

In patients with inferior wall infarctions, which may be complicated by right ventricular infarction, the administration of nitrates mandates extreme caution (see Ch. 17) (51). Such patients are often extremely "volume sensitive," and a reduction in venous pressure caused by diuretics, nitrates, or even dehydration may cause hypotension and a marked fall in cardiac output.

BETA BLOCKERS

Mechanisms of Action

Beta-adrenergic receptor blockers (beta blockers) are now considered as proven effective therapy for myocardial infarction. As such, they have been described as indicated for most patients with myocardial infarction who do not demonstrate overt congestive heart failure or shock at admission (52). To use them most effectively, we need to understand their mechanism of action.

Beta blockers were developed primarily to inhibit the cardiac effects of the sympathoadrenal system in patients with asymptomatic coronary heart disease. By decreasing heart rate, blood pressure, and the force of contraction, these agents decrease overall myocardial oxygen demand and are thus potent anti-ischemic agents (53). With an acute myocardial infarction, marked increases in the level of catecholamines (norepinephrine and epinephrine) occur rapidly, primarily due to pain and fear. Anesthetized animals with experimental infarction, however, show a similar response, suggesting that factors other than simply pain and fear are involved. In animal studies, ischemic myocardium exposed to high levels of catecholamines has been shown to have increased numbers of beta-adrenergic receptors (54). This increased number of functional receptors has the potential of further increasing oxygen demand in the ischemic area in response to increased catecholamine concentration (55). Beta blockers may directly reduce myocardial oxygen demand in this setting by inhibiting the adverse beta-receptor stimulation by the high levels of catecholamines. Because of this anti-ischemic effect, the beta blockers were among the first drugs to be tested in an attempt to limit the development or the extent of myocardial infarction. Animal experiments in 1971 showed that propranolol decreased ST segment elevation and creatine kinase enzyme release and, by implication, infarct size (56). Nonetheless, more recent studies in dogs using the concept of a "risk zone" (defined by the extent of infarction normalized as a percentage of the extent of the original zone of underperfusion) have questioned whether beta blockers can, in fact, reduce infarct size (57–60).

In humans, after coronary arterial occlusion, the progression from ischemia to infarction is usually quite rapid. Irreversible necrosis of muscle begins about 20 minutes after a coronary artery is occluded, beginning at the endocardial surface and spreading out in a wavefront-like phenomenon from the endocardium to the epicardium. Most of the damage occurs within the first 3 to 4 hours, and the infarct is essentially completed in 4 to 6 hours (61,62). This animal evidence may not apply directly to humans, in whom there may be extensive collaterals. The extent of collaterals and variations in myocardial oxygen demand may influence the rate and the extent of irreversible damage (63). This may explain why damage, as assessed by electrocardiography, appears to be only 50% complete in 4 to 6 hours, and 75% complete in 12 hours (64). Regardless of the method by which the amount of damage is assessed, it is clear that for any intervention to be successful in limiting infarct size, it must be promptly administered within the first few hours of the onset of symptoms. Late reperfusion may impart additional long-term benefits (65); however, time *is* of the essence, and any therapeutic intervention aimed at salvaging myocardium exerts its major impact when administered early during the evolving phase of infarction. Beta blockers, when given orally, produce a maximum reduction in heart rate and blood pressure after approximately 10 to 12 hours, whereas the same effect appears after approximately 15 minutes when the drug is given intravenously (66–68). Table 12–2 lists the potential mechanisms by which beta blockers could immediately reduce infarct size with a consequent impact on both early and late morbidity and mortality. Table 12–3 lists some contraindications for the use of beta blockers in myocardial infarction.

Table 12–2. Potential Beneficial Short-Term Effects of Beta Blockers on Infarct Size in Acute Evolving Myocardial Infarction

Reduction in oxygen demands as a result of decreased heart rate, blood pressure, and possibly contractility (53,56)
Counteraction of the direct cardiotoxic effects of excessive catecholamines (69)
Counteraction of indirect effects of high levels of catecholamines (prevention of increase in free fatty acids and in uptake of excess free fatty acids) (69–71)
Redistribution of blood from epicardial areas to more ischemic subendocardial tissue (72,73)
Reduction in the frequency of complex ventricular arrhythmias and possibly an elevation in ventricular fibrillation thresholds (74,75)
Reduction in the incidence of cardiac rupture (76)
Reduction in the frequency of recurrent ischemia and infarct extension (77,78)

Table 12–3. Contraindications to Beta Blocker Therapy in Acute Myocardial Infarction

Atrioventricular block
Systolic pressure less than 100 mm Hg
Congestive heart failure (crackles in greater than one-third of the posterior thorax)
Bradycardia less than 50 to 55 per minute
History of bronchial asthma

Results of Clinical Trials

Clinical trials involving the use of beta blocking agents in acute myocardial infarction should be considered as two groups: those including therapy with thrombolytic agents, and those without thrombolytic agents. The largest numbers of trials on the early administration of a variety of beta blocking agents in acute myocardial infarction occurred in the prethrombolytic era. Most of these studies have used mortality and infarct size as endpoints (Fig. 12–4). For details of individual trial designs and results, see Chapter 32. Estimates of infarct size have generally been based on the extent and patterns of enzyme release (primarily creatine kinase). The first bar in Figure 12–4 shows the pooled results from nine trials in which the drug was given within 12 hours of the onset of symptoms (79,80). In each individual trial there was a statistically significant reduction in enzyme release. An absence of any significant difference in enzyme release was noted in several other studies, all of which had a "wide window" for entry (patients were included up to 24 hours after the onset of symptoms). When all the trials are combined, the average reduction in enzyme release approximates 25%. The pivotal importance of the *early* administration of beta blockers on infarct development and both early and late outcomes was emphasized in a review by Herlitz and Hjalmarson (81).

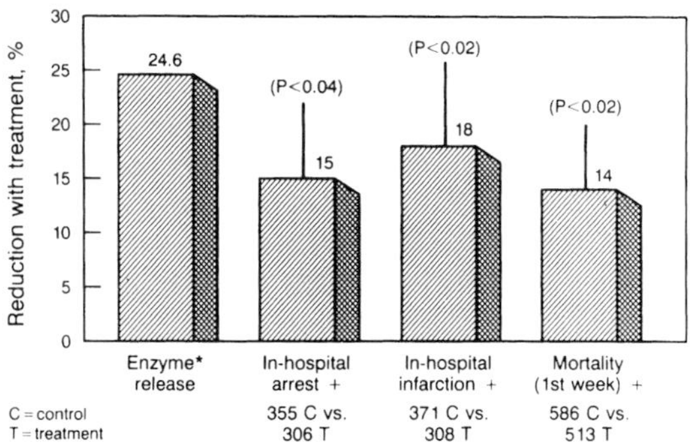

Figure 12–4. Effects of early administration of intravenous beta blockers on acute myocardial infarction, shown as a percentage reduction from controls with treatment. The reduction in enzyme release is taken from an average of nine trials in which treatment was given within 12 hours (77,79,80,82–87). The reductions shown for in-hospital arrests, in-hospital infarction, and early mortality (first week) are taken from the data pooled from 27,486 patients in 28 randomized trials. *Adapted from the ISIS-I Collaborative Group (88), with permission.*

Despite impressive evidence from numerous trials substantiating a favorable effect of beta blockers on enzyme release and presumably on infarct size, corroborative evidence as documented by an improvement in global left ventricular function has been lacking. In part this could reflect the imprecision of current techniques of assessing left ventricular function to reflect small changes in infarct size. Alternatively, changes in enzyme release may not be an accurate reflection of any preservation of viable contractile myocardium. Furthermore, the concept that beta blockers could limit infarct size, and the role of the latter in mortality, has been questioned (60,89). Nonetheless, the massive evidence accumulated from numerous randomized trials has shown that beta blockers exert a favorable and impressive effect on morbidity and mortality from acute myocardial infarction (see Fig. 12–4). Figure 12–4 also illustrates graphically the pooled results of early intravenous beta blocker therapy on early mortality, in-hospital reinfarction, and nonfatal cardiac arrests in more than 27,000 patients studied in 28 randomized controlled clinical trials (88). Mortality in the first week was reduced by 14% ($p < 0.02$), with almost all of the benefit occurring within the first 48 hours. It should be emphasized that the benefits apparent early persisted during late follow-up even after the discontinuation of beta blocker.

Although a reduction in mortality is undisputed, the mechanisms are less clearly defined. In-hospital reinfarction and nonfatal cardiac arrest were reduced by 18% and 15%, respectively (see Fig. 12–4), which could certainly account for some of the reduction in early mortality. Fitzgerald, in questioning both the existence and the importance of a reduction in infarct size with beta-blockade, has raised the intriguing possibility that beta blockers may exert their beneficial effects in infarct survivors primarily by reducing the "trigger event" leading to sudden death or reinfarction (90). This is, in most cases, due to plaque rupture with subsequent thrombosis. Beta blockers (via a reduction in heart rate and blood pressure) could reduce the wall stress of coronary vessels containing fragile plaques and thus decrease the incidence of plaque rupture (see Chs. 4 and 32). This mechanism could account for a reduction in mortality on the basis of a reduced frequently of subsequent ischemic events (both in-hospital and after discharge) independent of any effect on infarct size (see Tables 12–2 and 12–3). In this regard, several clinical trials have correlated the extent of the reduction in mortality with the magnitude of the change in heart rate (91), in concert with a lack of benefit associated with beta blocking agents that have intrinsic sympathomimetic effects and with calcium channel blockers (92,93).

A surprising and intriguing finding from the ISIS-I study was evidence to suggest that the major benefit of intravenous atenolol was due to a reduction in cardiac rupture (76) (see Ch. 16). This is understandable given the reduction in both the rate and force of contraction following beta-blockade, with a consequent impact on the stress on acutely necrotic myocardium. The information is particularly timely in the thrombolytic era, noting that in the large multicenter GISSI trial of intravenous streptokinase and placebo in acute myocardial infarction, the mortality on the first day following symptoms was actually higher in patients treated with streptokinase (94). Only the subsequent marked reduction in mortality from day 2 to discharge explained the overall improvement in mortality with streptokinase. Preliminary data from this and other studies imply that the excess *early* mortality of thrombolytic therapy may be due to cardiac rupture and possibly reperfusion injury; further validation of these hypotheses are needed, however, particularly among patients treated relatively late after the onset of symptoms. A recent retrospective autopsy review reported that the rupture rate (4%) in patients admitted for acute MI has remained constant for the past 16 years, despite the advent of thrombolytic therapy (95). However very recent data from a large national registry of myocardial infarction suggests that thrombolytic therapy accelerates the timing of cardiac rupture, typically to within 24 to 48 hours of treatment. (95a). This may be extremely important as we consider the timing of adjunctive therapies such as beta blocker therapy or ACE inhibitor therapy (see below) in an attempt to limit complications such as myocardial rupture. As mortality rates have progressively declined, the relative importance of rupture as a cause of death increases.

Most randomized trials of beta blocker therapy in acute myocardial infarction have excluded patients with moderate to severe clinical signs of acute left ventricular dysfunction. Several of the larger trials did, however, include high-risk patients who had a history of compensated heart failure or with symptoms and signs suggesting at least mild left ventricular dysfunction. In these trials, beta blocker treatment was surprisingly well tolerated by patients with left ventricular dysfunction, and mortality in this group was reduced by 20% to 30% when compared with the placebo group. Because of the high mortality in these high-risk patients, the absolute gain in number of lives saved per 100 patients treated with beta blockers is larger than in those patients without left ventricular dysfunction (96). It appears likely that all patients with left ventricular dysfunction who can tolerate beta blocker therapy will benefit from it. A strategy that includes a trial of an ultra–short acting beta blocker, esmolol, in patients with left ventricular dysfunction may be effective in increasing the numbers of patients ultimately treated with beta-blockade (97).

Benefits for Diabetics

A subgroup of patients with acute myocardial infarction who may benefit most from early therapy with beta blockers has recently been described (98). Patients with diabetes and acute myocardial infarction have a high risk of early mortality that continues over long-term follow-up (98,99). The risk is highest in the period immediately following the acute infarction. In a retrospective review of two trials of intravenous metoprolol (98), the diabetic group appeared to receive the most benefit. Both early mortality and reinfarction (up to 15 days) were reduced. For example, in patients with confirmed acute myocardial infarction in the Metoprolol in Acute Myocardial Infarction (MIAMI) trial, mortality in the entire group was not really altered with metoprolol (6.5% versus 5.9% in the treated group). In diabetics however, mortality decreased from 15.2% to 7.8% in the treated group. The numbers from neither trial were sufficient to reach significance, but the trend is highly suggestive of benefit and is certainly in agreement with the findings from other trials that suggest that patients with the poorest prognosis who are nonetheless able to tolerate the treatment benefit the most from intravenous beta-blockade (84,100). Possible explanations for the apparently greater magnitude of benefit from treatment in the diabetic population are interesting. In both studies, the mean heart rate before randomization was higher among diabetics. Moreover, the extent of beta blocker–induced heart rate reduction has been shown to correlate strongly with the decrease in postinfarction mortality (91). With this in mind, the higher initial heart rate in diabetics could explain the apparently improved prognosis with beta-blockade in this patient subset. Enhanced vagal activity and subsequent increased heart rate variability has been suggested as an alternative explanation for the preventative effects of beta blockers on sudden cardiac death (101). This may be particularly relevant in diabetics. Furthermore, diabetics have a decreased capability to produce or utilize insulin, and they may be especially susceptible to the toxic effects of the increased free fatty acids and catecholamine levels of acute myocardial infarction. Beta blockers reduce free fatty acid concentrations and also shift substrate utilization toward glucose (70,71).

Concomitant Thrombolytic Therapy

Thrombolytic therapy is now considered the standard of care for acute myocardial infarction, and its use must be *considered* in all patients with acute transmural myocardial infarction. Despite the very large numbers of patients evaluated in the mega-trials of thrombolytic therapy, there are relatively very few patients in whom the effects of combined beta blocker and thrombolytic therapy have been studied carefully. Only one clinical trial of thrombolytic therapy specifically addressed the role of beta blocking agents as adjunctive therapy: In the TIMI-II trial (78), a subgroup of patients were randomized to receive either immediate (intravenous) or delayed (at day 6) metoprolol. Immediate beta-blockade lowered the incidence of nonfatal reinfarction and recurrent ischemic events during hospitalization but did not affect mortality or affect left ventricular ejection fraction. Intravenous metoprolol appeared to be particularly beneficial in two prespecified subgroups: patients treated within 2 hours of the onset of symptoms and patients in the "low-risk" group. The results of the TIMI-II trial substantiated the theoretical hypotheses that pointed toward the utility of association of beta blocking agents with thrombolytic therapy. Further support for a possible survival benefit from the combined use of intravenous beta blocker therapy and reperfusion therapy came from a retrospective analysis by Ellis et al in 1990 (102). The TEAHAT trial also reported that reperfusion with r-tPA was most effective in reducing infarct size and improving left ventricular function when it was combined with early intravenous metoprolol therapy (103). Several other small trials have shown that intravenous beta blocker therapy when combined with thrombolytic therapy is safe, does not produce significant added hypotension, and may improve survival over the use of chronic oral beta blocker therapy in this setting (104–107). Interestingly, several of these trials have shown no effect of intravenous beta blocker therapy on major arrhythmias, either ventricular or atrial, in the early phase of acute myocardial infarction when combined with thrombolytic therapy (105–107). In patients receiving thrombolytic therapy, and with relative contraindications to beta blocker therapy, intravenous esmolol has been shown to be safe. When adverse events occur, they are short-lived. The ability to tolerate higher maintenance doses of esmolol predicted subsequent tolerance to oral beta blocker therapy (97).

Despite the relative lack of good solid evidence in support of the role of intravenous beta blocker therapy combined with thrombolytic therapy, there is evidence for increasing use of this combination in acute myocardial infarction (108). This is clearly based on the body of theoretical and clinical evidence suggesting an important potential role for this combination in improving outcome and the smaller clinical trials demonstrating the safety of this combination.

In addition to the Canadian study showing increasing use of beta blockers and thrombolytic therapy (108), more recent studies have reported on trends in the use of these therapies in acute myocardial infarction. The current use of thrombolytic therapy remains lower than expected, but beta blocker use is increasing in the United States, and calcium channel blocker use is decreasing (109). Even when beta blockers are prescribed, it appears that the doses used are considerably lower than those proven to be effective after myocardial infarction (110). Neither of these recent reviews have commented on the frequency with which combined beta blocker and thrombolytic therapy is being prescribed in the United States. The beneficial effects of such therapy reported in clinical trials clearly take an inordinate amount of time to be translated into clinical practice.

CALCIUM CHANNEL BLOCKERS

The calcium channel blockers are a heterogeneous group of organic compounds that inhibit calcium entry into smooth muscle and myocardial cells. The available agents differ primarily in their electrical effects. Only verapamil and diltiazem have significant dromotropic and chronotropic effects. All calcium channel blockers lower blood pressure by peripheral arterial dilation, and they reduce myocardial contractility to varying degrees (111). By relieving an element of coronary vasoconstriction and dilating atherosclerotic arteries, these agents may improve myocardial oxygen supply (112,113). In addition, animal research has shown that calcium channel blockers can prevent or delay calcium overload in ischemically injured myocardial cells, thus decreasing ischemic damage and potential reperfusion injury (114–116) (see Ch. 21). The property of "cardioprotection," combined with anti-ischemic effects, is theoretically appealing with respect to the potential of calcium entry blocking agents to reduce the extent of cellular damage and infarct size (see Table 32–4).

Several clinical trials of the efficacy of calcium channel blockers in acute myocardial infarction have been carried out, and the overall results are disappointing (Fig. 12–5) (see Table 32–5). For details of the design and results of individual trials, see Chapter 32. Most of the trials to date have been too small to detect minor or even modest beneficial or harmful events (namely, a difference of approximately 10% to 15%), although several of the trials have been large enough to exclude, with some confidence, a difference, whether beneficial or harmful, of approximately 30% to 40%. In view of these limitations, a recent meta-analysis of 22 randomized controlled trials of calcium channel blockers in acute myocardial infarction is helpful (see Fig. 12–5) (93).

The analysis comprised 17 studies in which treatment was begun within hours of the onset of symptoms but discontinued after hospital discharge; two studies in which calcium channel blockers were started early but were continued after discharge; and three studies that were primarily trials

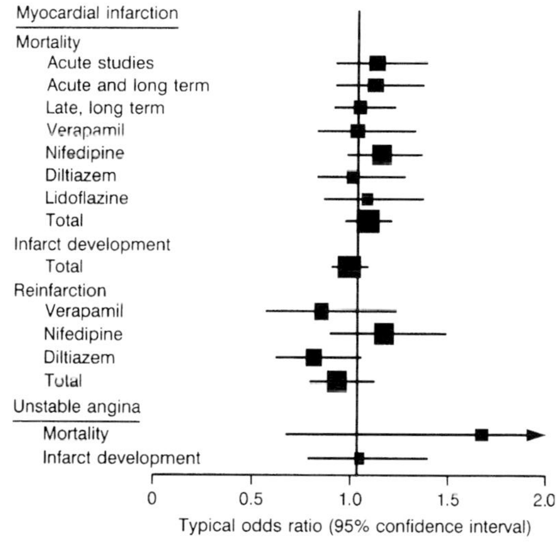

Figure 12–5. Therapy with calcium channel blockers in myocardial infarction and unstable angina. Typical odds of death, infarct development, and reinfarction by disease, types of trials, and drug used. Areas of squares are proportional to number of patients. Bars indicate 95% confidence intervals. Portions to the left of the vertical line (corresponding to odds ratio less than 1) indicate reduced risk with treatment; portions to the right of the vertical line indicate increased risk with treatment. Upper 95% confidence limit for effect on mortality in unstable angina = 6.2. Note that treatment does not seem to reduce risk of any event. *Reproduced from Held et al (96), with permission.*

of the efficacy of calcium channel blockers in secondary prevention. In only six trials were the calcium channel blockers given intravenously. The primary conclusions from this overview (93) were that calcium channel blocking agents, irrespective of the timing of their administration, have no beneficial effect on the mortality of acute myocardial infarction in patients with a suspected acute myocardial infarction: 61.3% of treated patients developed a myocardial infarction as opposed to 61.9% of controls (overall odds reduction of −3%, with 95% confidence intervals ranging from −10% to 6%).

In five of the trials, infarct size as measured by enzyme release was lower in the treated than in the control group. In seven of the trials, however, enzyme release was higher in the treated than in the control groups, and in one trial there was no difference between treated and control patients. Similarly, nonfatal reinfarction occurred in 4.2% of the treated patients and in 4.6% of the control patients.

When all of these trials were reviewed with respect to the endpoints of mortality, infarct size, and nonfatal reinfarction relative to the specific drug used, there appeared to be a trend toward a slight increase in these endpoints when nifedipine was used alone. These are shown in Fig. 12–5.

This review has subsequently been updated on several occasions (117–119) to include the results of newer trials of calcium channel blockers after acute myocardial infarction. The largest of these trials was DAVIT-II (120), the Danish Post-Infarction Verapamil Trial. The trials reviewed were primarily postinfarction studies of calcium channel blockers and will be discussed in detail in a later chapter. Based on this review, however, the overall conclusions remain the same: the routine use of calcium channel blockers for acute myocardial infarction cannot be supported by evidence of benefit.

Based on the theoretical evidence suggesting the potential of calcium channel blockers to reduce reperfusion injury (see Ch. 21), several trials of calcium channel blockers used in conjunction with thrombolysis have recently been reported. Ellis et al in 1990 reported a survival benefit with beta blockers, but no survival benefit from calcium antagonist therapy during reperfusion therapy (102). A small observational study of intravenous verapamil suggested that the potential adverse effects of verapamil could be mediated by cautious intravenous doses, the use of thrombolytic therapy for large infarctions, and potential synergistic cardioprotective effects of verapamil and nitroglycerin (121). Obviously, the potential benefits from such therapies would require a large controlled trial. Beneficial effects of combining intravenous diltiazem with reperfusion have been demonstrated only in animal studies. In one study, intravenous diltiazem reduced myocardial infarction size by 42% over that treatment with streptokinase alone (122). No clinical trials of intravenous diltiazem and thrombolytic therapy have yet been reported. More recently, a very small clinical trial using an intravenous dihydropyridine, nisoldipine, in acute myocardial infarction has been reported (123). It suggests that this more vascular-selective calcium channel blocker may improve global and regional left ventricular function in patients with acute myocardial infarction when given within the first 24 hours. In this study, two-thirds of the patients were given intravenous streptokinase, suggesting the possibility at least that the improved regional function was due to the limitations by nesoldipine of reperfusion damage or stunning. Again, such potential benefits require a large placebo-controlled trial to demonstrate clinical efficacy.

In summary, the clinical utility of calcium channel blockers when used for acute myocardial infarction, either alone or with thrombolytic agents, has not been demonstrated. Some studies have suggested a potential role for the rate-limiting calcium channel blocking agents in non-Q myocardial infarction, and as secondary prophylaxis for small, low-risk myocardial infarctions. These studies will be discussed in detail in later chapters.

ANGIOTENSIN CONVERTING ENZYME INHIBITORS

With acute myocardial infarction, the major determinant of mortality is the extent of necrosis–infarct size (1,2). Another major determinant of prognosis after acute myocardial infarction is left ventricular dilation or remodeling. Larger infarctions are more prone to subsequent left ventricular dilation, with increased development of congestive heart failure, left ventricular aneurysm, ventricular rupture, and death. The major cause of left ventricular dilation early after acute myocardial infarction (first few days) appears to be expansion of the infarct area secondary to increased wall stress. The later progressive dilation (over the first two months) results from increased wall stress as well, and subsequent remodeling of the infarcted and noninfarcted areas. For a detailed discussion of left ventricular remodeling post–myocardial infarction, please see Chapter 29. Experimental studies demonstrated that the early infarct expansion is increased with increasing wall stress, and that both angiotensin converting enzyme inhibitors and nitrates decrease wall stress.

The investigation of the role of angiotensin converting enzyme (ACE) inhibitors in acute myocardial infarction has followed a classical path, but it has progressed surprisingly rapidly from basic animal research to multicenter mega-trials in the clinical sphere. The initial studies of the effects of captopril therapy on experimental myocardial infarction (124,125) were quickly followed by small clinical trials that demonstrated both the safety and beneficial effects of captopril on left ventricular function after acute myocardial infarction (126,127). The early enthusiasm for early ACE inhibitor therapy for acute myocardial infarction was dampened by the report of the CONSENSUS II trial (128). In this trial, 6,090 patients with acute myocardial infarction were enrolled and randomized to enalapril or placebo therapy within the first 24 hours. Active therapy consisted of intravenous enalaprilat (1 mg over 2 hours) followed by oral enalapril in increasing doses. This trial was stopped by the Safety and Data Monitoring Committee after one year of recruitment. At that time it was concluded that enalapril therapy begun in the first 24 hours after acute myocardial infarction did not improve survival over the next 6 months. A subsequent echocardiographic substudy in these patients has, however, demonstrated that enalapril therapy initiated within the first 24 hours and continued for 6 months can attenuate left ventricular dilation during the first month and result in smaller left ventricular volumes after both 1 and 6 months (129). Subsequent clinical trials delayed the initiation of ACE inhibitor therapy until after the early phase of the acute myocardial infarction. The SAVE trial studied 2,231 patients with ejection fractions less than 40% and without overt congestive heart failure or ischemic symptoms (130). Therapy with oral captopril or placebo was initiated 3 to 16 days post–myocardial infarction (mean 10.6 days). Those patients treated with captopril had a 19% decrease in risk of all cause mortality, 21% reduction in risk of fatal and nonfatal major cardiovascular events, a 37% reduction in risk of development of severe congestive heart failure, and a 25% reduction in recurrent myocardial infarctions.

The AIRE trial of ramapril on mortality and morbidity of survivors of acute myocardial infarction moved the initiation time of therapy with an ACE inhibitor closer to the time of the acute myocardial infarction (131). Randomization occurred between 3 and 10 days (mean 5.4 days), at which time oral ramapril (2.5 mg BID) or placebo was started. Ramapril therapy was increased to 5 mg BID if tolerated after two days. Mortality from all causes was significantly lower in the ramapril treated group than in the placebo treated group (17% vs. 23%), with an observed risk reduction of 27%.

The most recent study assesses benefits of angiotensin converting enzyme inhibitor therapy with trandolapril in selected patients with left ventricular dysfunction after a myocardial infarction (Ref. 131a). In this study patients were selected according to an echocardiographic index of left ventricular function. Twenty-five percent of more than 6,000 consecutive patients screened were enrolled in the study. Long-term therapy with trandolapril in patients with reduced ventricular function (defined by a wall motion index less than 1.2) (131b) reduced the risk of overall mortality, cardiovascular mortality, sudden death and the development of severe heart failure. The relative reduction of risk of death (0.78) was very comparable to both the AIRE, and the SAVE Trials. The TRACE Study is the only trial of ACE inhibition after myocardial infarction to date that has shown a significant reduction in sudden death.

It must be emphasized that the SAVE trial (130) AIRE (131), and TRACE (131a) did not encompass exactly the same patient population. Patients enrolled in SAVE were asymptomatic but had left ventricular ejection fractions of less than 40%. All those patients enrolled in AIRE had clinical evidence for pulmonary congestion. In the TRACE Study, patients with evidence of left ventricular systolic dysfunction, with or without clinical congestive heart failure, were enrolled. Patients with overt heart failure were included in this study whereas they were excluded from the SAVE Trial. In the AIRE Trial, a significant proportion of patients with symptoms of pulmonary congestion had normal left ventricular function (131c) so that the TRACE Study enrolled a population at higher risk for events after myocardial infarction. Despite these differences in study design, the benefits of ACE inhibition in patients with left ventricular dysfunction early after an acute myocardial infarction are quite consistent. It appears clear that at least some patients with increased risk (both mortality and morbidity) post–myocardial infarction will be missed when selected by simple clinical criteria alone. Clinicians using both clinical acumen and some other assessment of left ventricular function will identify those most likely to benefit from ACE inhibitor therapy post–myocardial infarction (Table 12–4) (132).

Another approach to ACE inhibitor therapy post–myocardial infarction would be to treat everyone with an acute myocardial infarction without clear contraindication to such therapy (much is as currently recommended for beta blocker therapy post–myocardial infarction). Three recent trials (GISSI-3, ISIS-IV, and the Chinese captopril study) tested the safety and efficacy of treating unselected patients with acute myocardial infarction, and of initiating such therapy acutely (42,45,134). GISSI-3 was an open-labeled randomized trial of the effects of lisinopril and transdermal glyceryltrinitrate, singly and together, on 6-week mortality and ventricular function after acute myocardial infarction (45). In this trial 1,394 patients were randomized within 24 hours of symptom onset. The survival curves of the lisinopril treated patients and controls separated early and continued to diverge throughout the entire 6 weeks. Patients allocated lisinopril had an 11% lower rate of death at six weeks than controls (6.3 vs. 7.1%, $2p = 0.003$). There was also a reduction in the combined outcome measures of death and severe left ventricular dysfunction. In addition, the combined administration of lisinopril and nitrates produced significant reductions in mortality (6.2 vs. 7.2%, $2p = 0.21$) and combined endpoints (14.8 vs. 17.0%, $2p = 0.078$). Unfortunately, more than one-half of the control group also received some form of nitrate therapy in the acute phase, potentially blunting the measured benefit of combined angiotensin converting enzyme inhibitor and nitrate treatment in acute myocardial infarction.

No excess of unfavorable clinically relevant events in the treated group were noted, highlighting the safety of early (day 1) administration of lisinopril after acute myocardial infarction. The authors thus recommend that we treat all hemodynamically stable patients who have had an acute myocardial infarction within the past 24 hours. Some patients at higher risk (the elderly, females) seemed to benefit from lisinopril alone, and from the combined treatment of lisinopril with nitrates. Further support for very early initiation of therapy with lisinopril comes from a detailed six month analysis of the GISSI-III data (134a). The trend to early mortality reduction was consistent in all subgroups, with the greatest absolute benefit in subgroups at highest risk (for example Killip Class II and III). Interestingly, inferior wall infarctions appeared to benefit equally with anterior myocardial infarctions by such therapy. In all groups, the greatest relative reduction in cause of cardiac death was in cardiac rupture. The early initiation of lisinopril therapy then maybe particularly important to help avoid the early cardiac rupture associated with thrombolytic therapy (95a).

The ISIS-IV trial (previously described) investigates the effect of early oral captopril in suspected acute myocardial infarction in 58,050 patients on mortality and morbidity over 5 weeks (42). There was a small but statistically significant reduction in 5-week mortality in the captopril treated group (7.19% vs. 7.69%). This corresponds to an absolute

Table 12–4. Assessment of Risk After Myocardial Infarction by Clinical Signs and Left Ventricular Ejection Fraction

Clinical Findings	*Relative Risk* (95% confidence intervals)
Rates > bibasilar	3.3 (2.1 to 5.2)
EF ≤ 40%	2.4 (1.5 to 3.7)
Both	7.9

Adapted from Ball and Hall (133).

reduction of 4.9 deaths for 100,000 patients treated for 1 month. This survival advantage appears to be maintained over the next 12 months (5.4 fewer deaths per 1,000 in the treated group). Certain high-risk groups appear to have derived more benefit, approximately 10 fewer deaths per 1,000 treated patients with previous myocardial infarction or heart failure. Moreover the benefit on mortality was noted almost entirely in the minority of patients who presented with anterior ST-segment elevation. Captopril therapy did not produced any excessive deaths in day 0–1, even among those with low blood pressure on entry. There was, however, an increase of 52 patients per 1,000 in hypotension severe enough to terminate the study treatment, and an increase of 5 per 1,000 in reported cardiogenic shock, and 5 per 1,000 in some degree of renal insufficiency. Importantly, there appeared to be no significant interaction, either positive or negative, between captopril and the other study drugs— mononitrate and magnesium.

The Chinese captopril study (134) in itself did not demonstrate benefit from captopril started within 36 hours of suspected onset of acute myocardial infarction. When ISIS-IV and the Chinese captopril study are taken together, they demonstrate clearly that initiating ACE inhibitor therapy early in the acute phase of myocardial infarction is safe and well tolerated. Whether the modest reduction in early and late mortality in this group as a whole justifies treatment of all patients with acute myocardial infarction with an ACE inhibitor in the first 24 hours remains the subject of debate. For example, in the ISIS-IV trial, no benefit whatsoever can be seen in treating more than 20,000 patients with acute inferior wall infarction. While the confidence intervals are such that a slight increase in risk of treatment in these patients cannot be demonstrated, no benefit can be expected. Other subgroups without obvious benefit are too small to allow conclusions to be drawn.

More recently, the Survival of Myocardial Infarction Long-Term Evaluation (SMILE) investigators reported on the study of 1,556 patients with acute anterior myocardial infarction who were randomized to treatment with zofinopril or placebo for 6 weeks (135). The combined reduction of death or severe heart failure at 6 weeks was 34% (95% confidence interval 8–54%; $p = 0.018$—i.e., 7.1% in the zofinopril treated group vs. 10.6% in the placebo treated group). The reduction in risk of death was 25%, but the confidence intervals are wide (95% confidence interval −11–60%, $p = 0.19$). However, the risk reduction for severe congestive heart failure was 46% (95% confidence interval 11–71%; $p = 0.018$). Even though ACE inhibitor therapy by protocol was only for 6 weeks, survival at 1 year was greater in the zofinopril treated group, 10.0% vs. 14.1% (risk reduction 29%, $p = 0.011$). This SMILE study is consistent with GISSI-III and ISIS-IV data in demonstrating a substantial reduction in mortality within the first several days of treatment. This new demonstration of survival benefit with ACE inhibitors indicates that therapy should be started soon after the infarction.

An important difference between the SMILE study and the ISIS-IV and GISSI-3 trials was in patient selection. In SMILE, only patients with anterior myocardial infarction, already higher risk, and who were ineligible for thrombolytic therapy (putting them in the highest risk category), were randomized to zofinopril or placebo therapy. In the ISIS and GISSI trials, all suspected acute myocardial infarctions were eligible, and a high proportion (approximately 70%) received thrombolytic therapy. The apparently large effect of early zofinopril therapy may have been magnified by the selection of relatively high-risk patients, whereas the lower benefit in ISIS-IV and GISSI-3 may be related to the inclusion of lower-risk patients and patients receiving thrombolysis. Does thrombolytic therapy in itself lower the risk and thus diminish the benefit from ACE inhibitors, or is there some other interaction?

Several small trials have investigated the effect of angiotensin converting enzyme inhibitor therapy before, or in combination with, thrombolysis in acute myocardial infarction and in combination with other adjunctive therapy such as nitrates and beta blockers (136–139). These confirm the safety of ACE inhibitor therapy with thrombolysis, and when used in combination with beta blockers or nitrate therapy. Each trial was too small to allow definitive conclusions to be drawn about the efficacy of such combinations.

Recommendations for Use

Data from the mega-trials (ISIS-IV and GISSI-3) support the use of ACE inhibitors in the broad group of patients with acute myocardial infarction and systolic blood pressures over 100 mm Hg. Within this broad group, there may be subgroups of patients who benefit greatly (repeat infarctions, anterior infarctions, etc.) and subgroups with apparently little or no benefit (for example, inferior wall infarctions in ISIS-IV). It is difficult to justify treating all patients when significant subgroups have little potential benefit and thus dilute the overall benefit of such a strategy. Patients with clinical left ventricular dysfunction should have therapy initiated early and continued over the long term. The most practical approach would seem to be one that is tailored to fit individual circumstances. Because of the potential for significant hypotension, ACE inhibitor therapy should be begun in a monitored setting. Hemodynamically unstable patients with hypertension or significant left ventricular failure in the first hours after a myocardial infarction may be best treated with intravenous nitroglycerin for the first 24 hours or until stability is achieved. Then ACE inhibitor therapy should be initiated. For the asymptomatic, hemodynamically stable patient with acute myocardial infarction, some evidence of left ventricular dysfunction should be sought (echocardiography or radionuclide ventriculography) and ACE inhibitor therapy initiated for evidence of left ventricular dysfunction. If one were to calculate the lives saved using a more selective strategy (perhaps by combining enrollment criteria from SAVE and from the AIRE study), the total number would equal those saved by treating all eligible patients as in the ISIS-IV study. The selective approach appears the safest and most cost-effective over the long term (139a).

Which ACE inhibitor should be prescribed? The trial data to date supports ACE inhibition as a class effect. Only one trial has compared enalapril versus captopril directly (140). No significant difference was found in the benefit achieved from either ACE inhibitor. It is most important to become familiar with one or more of the various ACE inhibitors currently available, and to prescribe them at doses demonstrated to be effective in the large clinical trials. The physician should have a working knowledge of the proper initiation dose for these agents and the correct manner of titration to achieve the best effects at least risk.

MAGNESIUM

Magnesium is the second most common intracellular cation, with only 1% of the total body stores found in the extracellular compartment. It functions as a cofactor for various enzymes of cellular metabolism and appears to be essential in maintaining resting membrane potential (through activation of Na- K- ATPase). It also plays an important role in the modification of vascular tone (141). A number of animal and human studies (in vitro and in vivo) have described the effects of the administration of magnesium to supraphysiological levels that may have beneficial cardiovascular effects during acute myocardial injury. These potential beneficial effects are summarized in Table 12–5. In addition, a direct protective effect of magnesium pretreatment on myocardial cells during ischemia and reperfusion has been reported (142).

Based on these studies suggesting potential beneficial effects of magnesium on the ischemic injured

Table 12–5. Potential Beneficial Cardiovascular Effects of Increased Serum Magnesium Levels in Acute Myocardial Infarction

Site of Action	Effect
Myocardium	—Preservation of high-energy phosphates (143,144) —Protection of mitochondrial function by preventing Ca^{2+} overload (145,146) —Suppression of arrhythmias during ischemia and reperfusion (147–150)
Vascular Smooth Muscle	—Coronary vasodilation (151–154) —Reduced peripheral vascular resistance (141,155)
Platelet Function	—Inhibition of aggregation, disaggregation of platelet thrombi (156,157)

Modified from Yusuf et al (158).

myocardial cell, and some epidemiological studies linking low magnesium levels in drinking water with increased ischemic heart disease and myocardial infarction (159), clinical trials of magnesium in acute myocardial infarction were initiated. Several small trials were reported (150,160) and suggested benefit in terms of mortality and arrhythmia suppression. These were largely ignored until the present decade. Two meta-analyses were published, both indicating a substantial reduction in mortality from magnesium therapy in acute myocardial infarction (161,162). In addition, in an era of ever increasing costs and diminishing added benefit of new interventions to reduce mortality in acute myocardial infarction, magnesium therapy appeared to be very attractive. It is cheap, relatively easy and safe to administer, and can be utilized in every coronary care unit treating acute myocardial infarctions, not just in the tertiary care centers.

In the first meta-analysis (161), mortality in the magnesium treated group, 3.8%, was substantially less than in the placebo group 8.2% ($p < 0.001$). They also reported a reduction in deaths due to heart failure in the magnesium treated group (6.7% vs. 9.0% in controls), but this was not significant. In the second report (162), Horner reviewed eight randomized control trials of magnesium therapy in acute myocardial infarction totaling 930 patients. A 54% reduction in mortality in the magnesium treated group was apparent (95% confidence interval −27% to −72%). In addition, cardiac arrest was reduced by 58%, and ventricular tachycardia and fibrillation were reduced by 49%. Not surprisingly, the conclusion from both reports was that intravenous magnesium is a safe, effective treatment for acute myocardial infarction to reduce mortality and ventricular arrhythmias.

These two reports were followed by a large single-center randomized placebo-controlled trial of intravenous magnesium in acute myocardial infarction—LIMIT-2 (163). Among 2,316 patients with suspected acute myocardial infarction and randomized to intravenous magnesium or placebo therapy, the magnesium treated group (8 mmol/5 minutes followed by 65 mmol/24 hours, and initiated before thrombolytic therapy) had a 7.8% all cause mortality vs. 10.3% in the control group ($2p = 0.04$), a relative reduction of 24%. Acute left ventricular failure was also reduced by 25% in the magnesium treated group ($2p = 0.009$). Interestingly, no effects were seen on the incidence of heart block, severe ventricular arrhythmias (164), or the development of myocardial infarction in those presenting with unstable angina. Nor was there any apparent interaction of magnesium therapy with thrombolysis, aspirin, or previous treatment with beta blockers, calcium channel blockers, or diuretics.

When these patients were followed out to 1 year, improved long-term survival in the magnesium treated group was apparent (165). Mortality from ischemic heart disease was reduced by 21% ($p = 0.01$) and all cause mortality was reduced by 16% ($p = 0.003$) in the magnesium treated group.

The third arm of the giant ISIS-IV trial (42), previously described in detail, included acute therapy with intravenous magnesium in the same doses as those used in LIMIT-2. Surprisingly, and to many a great disappointment, intravenous magnesium in this mega-trial did not appear to confer any benefit on mortality. Indeed, there was no significant reduction in 5-week mortality, either overall (7.64% in magnesium treated patients vs. 7.24% in controls) or in any subgroup examined such as early or late therapy, or in the presence or absence of thrombolytic therapy. There was a significant excess of 12 per 1,000 patients in heart failure and 5 per 1,000 in reported cardiogenic shock in magnesium treated patients. Magnesium treatment also caused more hypotension (11 per 1,000 treated patients) and bradycardia (3 per 1,000). There was no net adverse effect on mortality in days 0–1. The likelihood of a significant benefit being missed in this trial was very small. There were, however, some potentially significant differences between LIMIT-2 and ISIS-IV. In the latter trial, magnesium infusions were started substantially later (median 8 hours vs. 3 hours in LIMIT-2) and after 12 hours (median time) for the 30% of patients not receiving thrombolytic therapy. That the timing of magnesium may be crucial in patients undergoing reperfusion is suggested by a powerful body of experimental data which would suggest that *early* treatment with magnesium may modify infarct size and perhaps reperfusion injury. In order to achieve cardioprotective effects with magnesium, the blood level must be elevated either before or within a short interval after reperfusion, whether spontaneous or drug-induced. (194–197) The lack of therapeutic effect of magnesium in ISIS-IV may reflect the absence of this medication at the time of reperfusion. In ISIS-IV, however, a very large number of patients received intravenous magnesium within the time limits defined by LIMIT-2, without any apparent added benefit of this early treatment.

Two recent smaller trials have further contributed to this discussion. In 109 patients with acute myocardial infarction randomized to intravenous magnesium therapy or placebo, 63% of all patients received intravenous thrombolytic therapy. In this trial, a small but significant reduction in mortality and heart failure was reported for those patients not receiving thrombolytic therapy (167). No such benefit was apparent in the thrombolytic treated group, nor was there added benefit in terms of arrhythmias, reinfarction, or heart failure (167). In the second, more recent, study, intravenous magnesium or placebo was administered to 194 patients with acute myocardial infarction who were considered ineligible for thrombolytic therapy. The magnesium treated group had decreased incidences of arrhythmias (27% vs. 40%, $p < 0.04$), congestive heart failure (18% vs. 23%, $p = 0.27$) and conduction disturbances (10% vs. 15%, $p = 0.21$) (166). In-hospital mortality and left ventricular function (early, and 1 to 2 months later) were both improved in the magnesium treated group (166).

What is the clinician to conclude about magnesium therapy for acute myocardial infarction? Despite the large numbers of treated patients studied, the jury must still be considered to be out. At the present time, the great weight of the evidence is that there is no substantiated role for the routine use of intravenous magnesium in acute myocardial infarction, especially in those receiving thrombolytic therapy. There is a suggestion of benefit for those patients who are ineligible for thrombolysis and for whom emergency revascularization is not possible. Intravenous magnesium therapy continues to be indicated in those clinical situations where it has demonstrated benefit—torsades des pointes (168) and digitalis intoxication (169). It is also commonly used as part of therapy for refractory or difficult to control ventricular arrhythmias, either in the setting of acute myocardial infarction or congestive heart failure.

In view of the potential benefits in terms of efficacy and cost, a large trial satisfying all of the above concerns about the use of intravenous magnesium therapy in acute myocardial infarction would appear to be justified. Numerous clinical trials have shown the mortality reduction with magnesium is greatest in patients with the highest baseline risk and there appears to be a correlation between the benefit from magnesium therapy over control with increasing mortalities in the control population. In this respect, patients in the ISIS trail were at low risk in comparison to the patients studied by Schecter et al, all of whom were not candidates for thrombolytic therapy. (196, 197) It would be logical therefore for such a trial to be confined to higher risk patients (aged < 65 yrs) receiving reperfusion therapy in addition to patients who are not candidates for thrombolytic therapy.(198)

ANTIARRHYTHMIC DRUGS

In the pre–coronary care unit era and among patients who do not survive to reach hospital, primary ventricular arrhythmias were and are the main cause of death. As such, the critical role of antiarrhythmic therapy in the management of acute myocardial infarctions is undisputed and discussed in detail in Chapter 14. The controversy over the prophylactic use of lidocaine has, however, persisted through two decades, and the popularity of this approach has fluctuated. Three recent large meta-analyses of several trials are helpful in placing the issue in perspective (170–172). Indisputably, it is preferable to prevent primary ventricular fibrillation, even though successful resuscitation is nearly always achieved in a carefully monitored environment. Nonetheless, the event itself may, via a number of hemodynamic mechanisms, adversely affect long-term outcome, probably by increasing infarct size. The crucial issue is whether prophylactic lidocaine actually reduces the incidence of primary ventricular fibrillation and, if so, whether this is achieved at the expense of other unwanted side effects.

Review of the trials to date would suggest that the incidence of primary ventricular fibrillation is relatively low (1.4%) and fatal asystole occurs even less commonly (0.2%) (170,171). The low incidence of ventricular fibrillation may reflect the fact that most of these studies were begun several hours after the onset of the acute infarction, beyond the most critical period for primary ventricular arrhythmias. Overall, prophylactic treatment with lidocaine reduced the risk of ventricular fibrillation by 36% (1.4% to 0.9%). The incidence for fatal asystole, however, doubled (although the difference was not statistically significant), and it is certainly possible that this could offset the small decrease in mortality associated with prophylactic lidocaine for ventricular fibrillation. A meta analysis of six prehospital trials of lidocaine revealed no difference in mortality, but in six to eight hospital-phase trials in which 24–48 hour mortality information was provided, there appeared to be an increase in mortality with lidocaine (172). The pendulum that has oscillated over the years has currently swung against the routine "prophylactic" use of lidocaine in acute myocardial infarction; however, there may exist a subset of patients at high risk from very large infarctions with frequent ventricular arrhythmias early in the hospital course in whom lidocaine may decrease the incidence of ventricular fibrillation and improve mortality. A recent review of antiarrhythmic prophylaxis after acute myocardial infarction does not substantially alter these recommendations (173). Nattel and Arenal conclude that lidocaine prophylaxis does not alter prognosis but may be reasonable in high-risk patients, namely, younger patients (<65 years) with acute transmural infarction, if they are less than 6 hours from the onset of symptoms. In all others, including those >70 years of age, prophylactic treatment with lidocaine is not warranted. They do recommend intramuscular lidocaine administration for probable myocardial infarction occurring in isolated locations and where transport to a location providing prompt arrhythmia detection and treatment is warranted. A potential concern would be the risk for subsequent thrombolytic therapy in these patients. Intramuscular injections should in general be avoided if thrombolytic therapy may be given in the next few hours.

Prophylactic lidocaine is no longer commonly used as an adjunct to thrombolytic therapy. Accelerated idioventricular rhythms are very common and often herald reperfusion. No treatment is recommended as a routine. Lidocaine may actually lower the fibrillation threshold. Other ventricular tachyarrhythmias are treated with lidocaine or procainamide as necessary. Intravenous magnesium is often used for difficult to control arrhythmias as well.

Bradyarrhythmias also may complicate an acute myocardial infarction. Inferior wall infarctions in particular are frequently complicated by the early appearance of varying degrees of transient (usually) A-V block that may be hemodynamically significant. There is substantial laboratory and clinical evidence that endogenous adenosine may play a mechanistic role in the bradyarrhythmias associated with myocardial ischemia or infarction (173a, 173b, 173c). The role of adenosine in mediating the early A-V block with acute myocardial infarction is further supported by a recent clinical study that also has significant therapeutic potential. In this very small study, theophylline (up to 250 mg intravenously) rapidly restored normal conduction in 11 of 11 patients (173d). Because of the small size however, more work must be done in this area before this can be accepted as standard therapy.

Patients who have survived the acute myocardial infarction continue to be at risk for premature death. The degree of risk is highly variable and depends upon a number of factors including the presence of recurrent or on-going myocardial ischemia, the extent of necrosis, and the presence and complexity of ventricular ectopy. The detection of left ventricular systolic dysfunction or of frequent or complex ventricular ectopy early after an acute myocardial infarction identifies patients at higher risk for early mortality. Unfortunately, clinical trials aimed at treating ventricular ectopy in this population have not been successful in preventing death. Indeed, increased mortality in the treated group was seen in trials of Class I antiarrhythmic agents (CAST) (173e). In early 1996 however two trials of the use of amiodarone in survivors of acute myocardial infarction were reported. EMIAT (European Myocardial Infarct Amiodarone Trial) included 1,486 patients 5–21 days post myocardial infarction with ejection fractions ≤ to 40% (173f). After a mean follow up of twenty months, the group randomized to amiodarone had reduced arrhythmic death by 35% (P = 0.053). Nevertheless, the risk reduction in arrhythmic death was not reflected in a reduction in all-cause mortality. CAMIAT (Canadian Amiodarone Myocardial Infarction Arrhythmia Trial) studied 1,202 patients 6–45 days post myocardial infarction with frequent (≥ to 10 VPD's per hour) or complex ventricular ectopy (173g). At 24 months, amiodarone reduced the incidence of arrhythmic death or resuscitated cardiac arrests from 6% to 3.3% (RR = 48%, P = 0.016).

Neither study showed evidence for pro-arrhythmic effects with Amiodarone in these patients with structural heart disease, or for increased mortality from any cause. Unfortunately, 35 and 42.3% of patients were withdrawn from EMIAT and CAMIAT respectively due to side effects of amiodarone.

Patients who are at the highest risk for early mortality after an acute myocardial infarction can safely be treated with amiodarone with a reasonable expectation of reduced risk for premature arrhythmic death. A number of questions remain to be answered however. Should all patients post myocardial infarction be treated with amiodarone? Unlikely. Should all patients with left ventricular dysfunction and/or complex ventricular ectopy post myocardial infarction be treated with amiodarone? Possibly. Would all such patients at high risk be better served with an implantable defibrillator device rather than medical therapy with its potential side effects? Possibly. The definitive answer to these questions must await further clinical trials.

OTHER PHARMACOLOGICAL AGENTS FOR POTENTIAL MYOCARDIAL SALVAGE

Aspirin

Aspirin, as primary therapy or as adjunct to thrombolytic therapy, should be prescribed for every patient with acute myocardial infarction for whom no absolute contraindication exists. The routine use of heparin in this setting is more controversial. For a detailed discussion of antiplatelet agents and anticoagulants, see Chapters 20 and 32.

Hyaluronidase

The enzyme hyaluronidase depolymerizes mucopolysaccharides. Its apparent ability to retard edema in infarcted areas and to dilate lymphatic channels in the myocardium suggested a potential for enhanced myocardial salvage (174,175). In the large prospective Multicenter Investigation for the Limitation of Infarct Size (MILIS) trial, propranolol and hyaluronidase were compared with placebo in patients with acute infarction admitted within 18 hours of the onset of symptoms. Hyaluronidase (500 IU/kg given every 6 hours for 48 hours) had no effect on mortality or infarct size in the overall population; however, in patients with early-peaking plasma creatine kinase MB or those with nontransmural ischemic changes (suggesting possibly early spontaneous reperfusion), hyaluronidase did appear to have a significant benefit on cardiac mortality overall and at 4 years (176). Despite these apparent benefits, interest in hyaluronidase has been superseded by the introduction of acute thrombolytic therapy, although its role as an adjunct to such an approach has not been discounted.

Glucose–Insulin–Potassium

Solutions containing glucose, regular insulin, and potassium chloride have been shown to result in increases in plasma and free fatty acid concentrations, improved left ventricular function, and, in animals, a reduction in the extent of myocardial necrosis (177–179). In a prospective randomized study of acute infarction in patients admitted within 12 hours of symptoms, a trend toward lower hospital mortality was seen with glucose–insulin–potassium infusions, although there was no long-term difference in survival between treated and control groups (180). In a 1987 study of 17 patients with anterior myocardial infarctions receiving streptokinase, glucose–insulin–potassium improved ventricular function and reduced the size of segmental wall motion abnormalities in comparison with placebo (181).

Anti-inflammatory Agents

A case for the use of corticosteroids was based on experimental evidence showing a reduction in the inflammatory response to injury and infarct size with both corticosteroids (182) and ibuprofen (183). On the other hand, an impairment of healing with increased scar thinning, infarct expansion, and reduced left ventricular function has been reported with corticosteroids (184,185), ibuprofen, and indomethacin in animals (186,187). These data, in conjunction with clinical evidence that corticosteroid therapy appears to increase the incidence of complications, strongly imply that its use should be avoided in acute infarction (188). In patients with acute pericarditis, indomethacin is effective in relieving symptoms, but it should be used sparingly and only until the symptoms are relieved. These recommendations are based on experimental data suggesting that indomethacin may interfere with scar healing, as well as on a loose clinical association between indomethacin administration and cardiac rupture (189,190).

POTENTIAL NEW DIRECTIONS OF THERAPY

Inotropic Therapy

Acute congestive heart failure remains a significant complication of acute myocardial infarction. Dopamine and dobutamine represent the most common of the inotropic therapies in this setting (190a). The phosphodiesterase inhibitors milrinone and amrinone, both potent inotropic agents, are also available for short-term intravenous use. In congestive heart failure not related to acute myocardial infarction, both milrinone and dobutamine, both potent inotropic agents, are also available for short-term intravenous use. In congestive heart failure not related to acute myocardial infarction, both milrinone and dobutamine produced comparable beneficial hemodynamic effects (190a, 190b). Because of milrinone's combined vasodilating and positive inotropic characteristics, it has potential advantages in the post-infarction setting. In a study of patients with acute congestive heart failure within twelve hours to five days after acute myocardial infarction, short-term intravenous milrinone compared very favorably with dobutamine in the setting of congestive heart failure following acute myocardial infarction (190c). Despite the small numbers in the study, milrinone appeared to have advantages in rapid reduction of pulmonary congestion without alterations of the double product. It thus appears to be a reasonable alternative to dobutamine therapy in this setting. A small study comparing intravenous enoximone with dobutamine reports that enoximone is better tolerated with fewer side effects than dobutamine in acute myocardial infarction when inotropic therapy is indicated (191). Similar increases in cardiac output occurred with both agents, but dobutamine produced more increased heart rate and more runs of superventricular and ventricular tachycardia. Ibopamine has also been demonstrated to have beneficial effects in acute myocardial infarction (192). In this animal study, ibopamine and captopril both attenuated ventricular dilation (possibly by reducing plasma norepinephrine levels), but only ibopamine reduced infarct size and preserved myocardial function.

An interesting new direction is the use of free radical scavengers and antioxidants to limit the damage and improve the prognosis for patients with acute myocardial infarction receiving thrombolytic therapy. The European Myocardial Infarction Project—Free Radicals Pilot Study reported on the early use of trimetazidine in patients with acute myocardial infarction receiving thrombolytic therapy (193). Trimetazidine has potent antioxidant properties without any direct hemodynamic effects, and it appears to prevent or limit the deleterious effects of free radicals on the myocardium. It also has been used for several years in patients suffering from chronic angina and is well tolerated. In this pilot trial, no significant differences between the treatment groups was observed for either major or minor adverse events. A large-scale mortality and morbidity trial was initiated in October 1992. The results are pending.

CONCLUSION

What is the currently recommended "cocktail" for the pharmacological management of acute myocardial infarction? Patients presenting with a history compatible with acute myocardial infarction should be placed in bed, nasal oxygen administered, an intravenous line established, and an electrocardiogram recorded. While the electrocardiogram is being interpreted, sublingual nitroglycerin should be administered providing pain persists and hypotension is not present. Analgesia in the form of intravenous morphine should be considered and administered in repeated doses to render the patient comfortable but not comatose. All patients with acute impending or developing transmural myocardial infarction should be considered for thrombolytic therapy, and this should be administered with a minimum of delay. All patients should be given aspirin (crushed or chewed, and swallowed) and probably intravenous heparin depending primarily on the thrombolytic agent chosen. If thrombolysis is contraindicated, or in hemodynamically unstable patients with exceptionally high risk, consider primary revascularization. Selected patients should be administered intravenous nitroglycerin (including those with hypertension, acute congestive heart failure, ongoing ischemic chest pain, and probably, acute transmural anterior infarctions), being careful to avoid hypotension. Intravenous beta blockers should be considered and administered where no contraindications exist, and oral beta blocker therapy should follow unless complications arise. Calcium channel blockers should be avoided in the acute myocardial infarction setting. If evidence for pulmonary congestion or significant left ventricular dysfunction is present, continue with intravenous nitroglycerin for the first 18 to 24 hours and then begin ACE inhibitor therapy. In the absence of indications for intravenous nitroglycerin, and in the absence of clinical evidence of left ventricular dysfunction, some measure of left ventricular function should be obtained early (either echocardiography or radionuclide ventriculography) and ACE inhibitor therapy initiated only for those with evidence of left ventricular dysfunction (ejection fraction less than 40%) and blood pressure greater than 100 mm Hg. By tailoring our therapeutic regimen to best fit individual risk groups, we are most likely to achieve the best balance of cost, effectiveness, and risk.

REFERENCES

1. Sobel BE, Bresnahan JF, Shell WE: Estimations of infarct size and its relation to prognosis. *Circulation* 1972;46:640–648.
2. Thanavaro S, Krone RJ, Kleiger RE: In-hospital prognosis of patients with first nontransmural infarction. *Circulation* 1980;61:29–33.
3. Herlitz J, Karlson BW, Hjalmarson A: Ten year mortality in relation to original size of myocardial infarct: Results from the Gothenburg metoprolol study. *Br Heart J* 1994;7:238–241.
4. Gruppo Italiano per lo Studio Dell Streptrochinasi Nell'Infarto Miocardio (GISSI): Effectiveness of intravenous thrombolytic treatment in acute myocardial infarction. *Lancet* 1986;1:397–401.
5. ISIS-2 Collaborative Group: Randomized trial of intravenous streptokinase, oral aspirin, both or neither among 17,187 cases of suspected acute myocardial infarction. *Lancet* 1988;2:349.
6. The TIMI IIIB Investigators: Effects of tissue plasminogen activator and a comparison of early invasive and conservative strategies in unstable angina and non-Q-wave myocardial infarction. *Circulation* 1989;89:1545–1556.
7. Lee TH, Weisberg MD, Brand DA: Candidates for thrombolysis among emergency patients with acute chest pain. Potential true- and false-positive rates. *Ann Intern Med* 1989;110:957–962.
8. Rouleau JL, Talajic M, Sussex B, et al: Myocardial infarction patients in the Nineties, their risk factors, stratification and survival in Canada: The Canadian Assessment of Myocardial Infarction (CAMI) Study. Submitted for publication, 1995.
9. Conti CR: Conventional drug therapy of patients with acute myocardial infarction. *Cardiovasc Clin* 1989;20:259–281.
10. Valencia A, Burgess JH: Arterial hypoxemia following acute myocardial infarction. *Circulation* 1969;40: 641–652.
11. Fillmore SJ, Guimaraes AC, Scheidt SS: Blood gas changes and pulmonary hemodynamics following acute myocardial infarction. *Circulation* 1972;45: 583–591.
12. Warnica JW, White AVM, Burgess JH: Cardiorespiratory function and extravascular lung water following acute myocardial infarction. *Am Heart J* 1997;97:469–476.
13. Maroko PR, Fadvany P, Branuwald E: Reduction of infarct size by oxygen inhalation following acute coronary occlusion. *Circulation* 1975;52: 360–368.
14. Madias JE, Hood WB: Reduction of precordial ST segment elevation in patients with anterior myocardial infarction by oxygen breathing. *Circulation* 1976;53(Suppl I): I-198–I-200.

15. Forrester JH, Diamond GA, Chatterjee K: Medical therapy of acute myocardial infarction by application of hemodynamic subsets. *N Engl J Med* 1975; 295:1356–1362.

16. Herlitz J, Hjalmarson A, Holmberg S: Effect of metoprolol on chest pain in acute myocardial infarction. *Br Heart J* 1984;51:438–444.

17. The MIAMI Trial Research Group: Narcotic analgesics and other anti-anginal drugs. *Am J Cardiol* 1985;56:30G–34G.

18. Anderson JL, Marshall HW, Askins JC: A randomized trial of intravenous and intracoronary streptokinase in patients with acute myocardial infarction. *Circulation* 1984;70:606–618.

19. Karlson BW, Sjolin M, Herlitz J: Clinical factors associated with pain in acute myocardial infarction. *Cardiology* 1993;83:107–117.

20. Semekovitch CFG, Jaffe AS: Adverse effects due to morphine sulfate—challenge to previous clinical doctrine. *Am J Med* 1985;79:325–330.

21. Lee G, Low RI: Hemodynamic effects of morphine and nalbuphine in acute myocardial infarction. *Clin Pharmacol Ther* 1981;29:576–581.

22. Romagnoli A, Keats A: Comparative hemodynamics effects of nalbuphine and morphine in patients with coronary artery disease. *Cardiovasc Dis Bull* 1978;5:19–24.

23. Loos D, Schneider R, Schorner W: Changes in regional body blood volume caused by nitroglycerin. *Z Kardiol* 1983;72:29–34.

24. Mehta JL: Endothelium, coronary vasodilation, and organic nitrates. *Am Heart J* 1995;129:382–391.

25. Schafer AT, Alexander RW, Handin RI: Inhibition of platelet function by organic nitrate vasodilators. *Blood* 1980;55:649–654.

26. DeCaterina R, Giannessi R, Crea F: Inhibition of platelet function by infectable isosorbide dinitrate. *Am J Cardiol* 1984;53:1683–1687.

27. Mellion BT, Ignarro LJ, Ohlstein EG: Evidence for the inhibitory role of guanosine 3′,5′ monophosphate in ADP-induced human platelet aggregation in the presence of nitric oxide and related vasodilators. *Blood* 1981;57:946–955.

28. Folts JD, Stamler J, Loscalzo J: Intravenous nitroglycerin infusion inhibits cyclic blood flow response caused by periodic platelet thrombus formation in steonsed coronary arteries. *Circulation* 1991;83: 2122–2127.

29. Diodati J, Theroux P, Latour JG: Effects of nitroglycerin at therapeutic doses on platelet aggregation in unstable angina pectoris and acute myocardial infarction. *Am J Cardiol* 1990;66:683–687.

30. Mehta JL, Pepine CJ: Effect of sublingual nitroglycerin on regional flow. *Circulation* 1978;58: 803–807.

31. Brown BG, Bolson E, Petersen RB: The mechanisms of nitroglycerin: Stenosis vasodilation as a major component of the drug response. *Circulation* 1981;64:1089–1097.

32. Kim YI, Williams JF: Large dose sublingual nitroglycerin in acute myocardial infarction: Relief of chest pain and reduction of Q-wave evolution. *Am J Cardiol* 1982;49:842–848.

33. Bussman WD, Passek D, Seidel W: Reduction of CK and CK MB indexes of infarct size by intravenous nitroglycerin. *Circulation* 1981;63:615–622.

34. Come PC, Pitt B: Nitroglycerin-induced severe hypotension and bradycardia in patients with acute myocardial infarction. *Circulation* 1976;54: 624–628.

35. Shell WE, Sobel BE: Protection of jeopardized ischemic myocardium by reduction of ventricular afterload. *N Engl J Med* 1974;291:481–486.

36. Abrams J: Hemodynamics effects of nitroglycerin and long-acting nitrates. *Am Heart J* 1985;110: 216–224.

37. Nelson GIC, Ahuja RC, Silke B: Hemodynamic advantages of isosorbide dinitrate over frusemide in acute heart failure following myocardial infarction. *Lancet* 1983;1:730–732.

38. Jugdutt BI, Becker LC, Hutchins GM: Effect of intravenous nitroglycerin on collateral blood flow and infarct size in the conscious dog. *Circulation* 1981;63: 17–28.

39. Jugdutt BI: Myocardial salvage by intravenous nitroglycerin in conscious dogs: Loss of beneficial effect with marked nitroglycerin-induced hypotension. *Circulation* 1983;68:673–684.

40. Jugdutt BI, Sussex BA, Warnica JW: Persistent reduction in left ventricular asynergy in patients with acute myocardial infarction by intravenous infusion of nitroglycerin. *Circulation* 1983;68: 1264–1273.

41. Jugdutt BI, Warnica JW: Intravenous nitroglycerin therapy to limit myocardial infarction infarct size, expansion, and its complications: Effect of timing, dosage, and infarct location. *Circulation* 1988;78: 906–919.

42. ISIS-IV Collaborative Group: ISIS-4: A randomised factorial trial assessing early oral captopril, oral mononitrate, and intravenous magnesium

sulphate in 58,050 patients with suspected acute myocardial infarction. *Lancet* 1995;345:669–685.

43. Morris JL, Zaman AG, Smyllie JH, Cowan JC: Nitrates in myocardial infarction: Influence on infarct size, reperfusion, and ventricular remodelling. *Br Heart J* 1995;73:310–319.

44. Humen DP, McCormick L, Jugdutt BI: Chronic reduction of left ventricular volumes at rest and exercise in patients with nitroglycerin following anterior MI (abstract). *J Am Coll Cardiol* 1989;13:25A.

45. GISSI-3 Gruppo Italiano per to Studio della Soprawivenza nell'Infarcto Miocardicoo: GISSI-3: Effects of lisinopril and transdermal glyceryl trinitrate singly and together on 6-week mortality and ventricular function after acute myocardial infarction. *Lancet* 1994;343:1115–1122.

46. Yusuf S, Collins R, MacMahon S: Effect of intravenous nitrates on mortality in acute myocardial infarction: An overview of the randomized trials. *Lancet* 1988;1:1088–1092.

47. Bussman WD, Neumann K, Kaltenbach M: Effects of intravenous nitroglycerin on ventricular ectopic beats in acute myocardial infarction. *Am Heart J* 1984;107:940–944.

48. Tymchak WJ, Michorowski BL, Burton JR: Preservation of left ventricular function and topography with combined reperfusion and intravenous nitroglycerin in acute myocardial infarction (abstract). *J Am Coll Cardiol* 1988;2:90A.

49. Nicolini FA, Ferrini D, Ottani F, et al: Concurrent nitroglycerin therapy impairs tissue-type plasminogen activator-induced thrombolysis in patients with acute myocardial infarction. *Am J Cardiol* 1994;74:662–666.

50. Friedberg CK: *Acute Coronary Occlusion and Myocardial Infarction.* Philadelphia, 1966, pp 913–914.

51. Ferguson JJ, Diver DJ, Boldt M: Significance of nitroglycerin-induced hypotension with inferior wall acute myocardial infarction. *Am J Cardiol* 1989;64:311–314.

52. Reeder GS, Gersh BJ: Modern management of acute myocardial infarction. *Curr Prob Cardiol* 1993;XV11:

53. Mueller H: Propranolol in acute myocardial infarction in man: Effects of hemodynamics and myocardial oxygenation. *Acta Med Scan* 1976;587:177–183.

54. Mukherjee A, Bush LR, McCoy KE, et al: Relationship between beta-adrenergic receptor numbers and physiological responses during experimental canine myocardial ischemia. *Circ Res* 1982;50:735–741.

55. Muntz KH, Hagler HK, Boulas HJ, Willerson JT, Buja LM: Redistribution of catecholamines in the ischemic zone of the dog heart. *Am J Path* 1984;114:64–78.

56. Maroko PR, Kjekshus JK, Sobel BE: Factors influencing infarct size following experimental coronary artery occlusion. *Circulation* 1971;43:67–82.

57. Jennings RB, Reimer KA: *Modulation of Sympathetic Tone in the Treatment of Cardiovascular Disease.* Berne, Hans, Huber, 1979, pp 103–114.

58. Kudoh Y, Maxwell MP, Hearse DJ: Failure of metoprolol to limit infarct size during 24 hour of coronary artery occlusion in a closed chest dog. *J Cardiovasc Pharmacol* 1984;6:1201–1209.

59. Lange R, Nieminen MS, Kloner RA: Failure of pindolol and metoprolol to reduce the size of non-reperfused infarcts in dogs using area at risk techniques. *Cardiovasc Res* 1984;18:37–43.

60. Hearse DJ, Yellon DM, Downey JM: Can beta blockers limit myocardial infarct size? *Eur Heart J* 1986;7:925–930.

61. Reimer KA, Lowe J,E., Rasmussen MM, Jennings RB: The wavefront phenomenon of ischemic cell death: 1. Myocardial infarct size vs duration of coronary occlusion in dogs. *Circulation* 1977;56:786–794.

62. Reimer KA, Jennings RB: The "wavefront phenomenon" of myocardial ischemic cell death: II. Transmural progression of necrosis within the framework of ischemic bed size (myocardium at risk) and collateral flow. *Lab Invest* 1979;40:633–644.

63. Schaper W, Binz K, Sass S, Winkler B: Influence of collateral blood flow and of variations in MV02 on tissue ATP content in ischemia and infarcted myocardium. *J Mol Cell Cardiol* 1987;19:19–37.

64. Yusuf S, Lopez R, Maddison A: Variability of electrocardiographic and enzyme evolution of myocardial infarction. *Br Heart J* 1981;45:271–280.

65. Rentrop KP, Feit F, Sherman W, et al: Late thrombolytic therapy preserves left ventricular function in patients with collaterlized total coronary occlusion: Primary end point findings of the second Mount Sinai–New York University reperfusion trial. *J Am Coll Cardiol* 1989;1:58–64.

66. Yusuf S: Early intravenous beta blockade in acute myocardial infarction, special report. *Postgrad Med J* 1988;90–95.

67. Held PH, Corbeij HMA, Dunselman P: Hemodynamic effects of metoprolol in acute myocardial infarction: A randomized, placebo-controlled multicenter study. *Am J Cardiol* 1985;56:47G–54G.

68. Murray DP, Murray RG, Rafigi E: Beta-adrenergic blockade in acute myocardial infarction: A haemodynamic radionuclide study. *Eur Heart J* 1987;8: 845–854.

69. Mueller HS, Ayres SM: Propranolol decreases sympathetic nervjous system activity reflected by plasmic catecholamines during evolution of myocardial infarction in man. *J Clin Invest* 1980;65:338–346

70. Fitzgerald JD: *Handbook of Hypertension, Vol. 3, Pharmacology of Anti-hypertensive Drugs.* Amsterdam, Elsevier, 1984, pp 249–306.

71. Opie LH, Thomas M: Propranolol and experimental myocardial infarction: Substrate effects. *Postgrad Med J* 1976;52:124–132.

72. Pitt B, Craven P: Effect of propranolol on regional myocardial blood flow in acute ischemia. *Cardiovasc Res* 1970;4:176 179.

73. Vanter SF, Baig H, Manders TW: Effects of propranolol on regional myocardial function electrocardiograms and blood flow on conscious dogs with my ocardial ischemia. *J Clin Invest* 1977;60:353–360.

74. Jewitt DE, Singh BN: The role of beta adrenergic blockade in myocardial infarction. *Prog Cardiovasc Dis* 1974;16:421–438.

75. Ryden L, Ariniego R, Arnman K: A double-blind trial of metoprolol in acute myocardial infarction: Effects on ventricular tachyarrhythmias. *N Engl J Med* 1983;308:614–618.

76. ISIS-1 Collaborative Group: Mechanisms for the early mortality reduction produced by beta-blockade started early in acute myocardial infarction. *Lancet* 1989;1:921–923.

77. Herlitz J, Elmfeldt D, Hjalmarson A: Effect of metoprolol on indirect signs of the size and severity of acute myocardial infarction. *Am J Cardiol* 1983; 51:1282–1288.

78. The TIMI Study Group: Comparison of invasive and conservative strategies after treatment with intravenous tissue plasminogen activity in acute myocardial infarction: Results of the thrombolysis in myocardial infarction (TIMI) phase II trial. *N Engl J Med* 1989;320:618–627.

79. Jurgensen JH, Frederiksen J, Hansen DA: Limitation of myocardial infarct size in patients less than 66 years treated with alprenolol. *Br Heart J* 1981;45: 583–588.

80. Rogue R, for the TIARA Group Investigators: Limitation of infarct size and reduction of late ventricular arrhythmias with early administered timolol in acute myocardial infarction: A one-month follow-up study (abstract). *J Am Coll Cardiol* 1986;7:67A.

81. Herlitz J, Hjalmarson A: The role of beta blockade in the limitation of infarct development. *Eur Heart J* 1986;7:916–924.

82. Yusuf S, Sleight P, Rossi P: Reduction in infarct size, arrhythmias and chest pain by early intravenous beta blockade in suspected acute myocardial infarction. *Circulation* 1983;67:32–41.

83. Salathia KS, Barber JM, McIlmoyle EL: Very early intervention with metoprolol in suspected acute myocardial infarction. *Eur Heart J* 1985;6: 190–198.

84. MIAMI Trial Research Group: Metoprolol in acute myocardial infarction (MIAMI): A randomized placebo controlled international trial. *Eur Heart J* 1985;6:199–226.

85. Peter T, Norris RM, Clarke ED: Reduction of enzyme levels by propranolol after acute myocardial infarction. *Circulation* 1978;57:1091–1095.

86. Norris RM, Clarke ED, Sammel NL: Protective effect of propranolol in threatened myocardial infarction. *Lancet* 1978;2:907–909.

87. The International Collaborative Study Group: Reduction of infarct size with early use of timolol in acute myocardial infarction. *N Engl J Med* 1984; 310:9–15.

88. ISIS-1 Collaborative Group: Randomized trial of intravenous atenolol among 16,027 cases of suspected acute myocardial infarction. *Lancet* 1986;2: 57–66.

89. Fitzgerald JD: By what means might beta blockers prolong life after acute myocardial infarction? *Eur Heart J* 1987;8:945–951.

90. Rytter L, Troelsen S, Beck-Nielsen H: Prevalence and mortality of acute myocardial infarction patients with diabetes mellitus. *Diabetes Care* 1985;8: 230–234.

91. Kjerkshus J: Heart rate reduction, a mechanism of benefit. *Eur Heart J* 1985;6:29–30.

92. Sleight P: Adrenoceptor blockade in the treatment of coronary heart disease. *Eur Heart J* 1986;6. 81–91.

93. Held PH, Yusuf S, Furgerg CO: Calcium channel blockers in acute myocardial infarction and unstable angina. *Br Med J* 1989;299:1187–1189.

94. Mauri F, DeBiase AM, Franzosi MG: GISSI: Analisi della cause di morte intraospedaliera. *G Ital Cardiol* 1987;17:37–44.

95. Pollak H, Nobis H, Miczoch H: Frequency of left ventricular free wall rupture complicating acute myocardial infarction since the advent of thrombolysis. *Am J Cardiol* 1994;74:184–186.

95a. Becker RC, Gore JM, Lambrew C, et al: A Composite View of Cardiac Rupture in the United States National Registry of Myocardial Infarction. *J Am Coll Cardiol* 1996; 27:1321–1326.

96. Held P: Effects of beta blockers on ventricular dysfunction after myocardial infarction: Tolerability and survival effects. *Am J Cardiol* 1993;71: 39C–44C.

97. Moss AN, Hillerman DE, Mohiudin SM, Hunter CB: Safety of esmolol in patients with acute myocardial infarction treated with thrombolytic therapy who had relative contraindications to beta-blocker therapy. *Ann Pharmacother* 1994;28: 701–703.

98. Malmberg K, Herlitz J, Hjalmarson A: The effects of metoprolol mortality and late infarction in diabetics with suspected acute myocardial infarction: Retrospective data from two large studies. *Eur Heart J* 1989;10:423–428.

99. Malmberg K, Ryden L: Myocardial infarction in patients with dibetes mellitus. *Eur Heart J* 1988;9: 259–264.

100. Beta Blocker Heart Attack Trial Research Group: A randomized trial of propranolol in patients with acute myocardial infarction: Mortality results. *JAMA* 1982;247:1707–1714.

101. Molgaard H, Mickley H, Pless P, Bjerregaard P, Moller M: Effects of metoprolol on heart rate variability in survivors of acute myocardial infarction. *Am J Cardiol* 1993;71:1357–1359.

102. Ellis SC, Muller DW, Topol EJ: Possible survival benefit from concomitant beta but not calcium-antagonist therapy during reperfusion for acute myocardial infarction. *Am J Cardiol* 1990;66: 125–128.

103. Risenfars M, Herlizt J, Berg C-H, et al: Early treatment with thrombolysis and beta-blockade in suspected acute myocardial infarction: Results from the TEAHAT Study. *J Intern Med* 1991;229: 35–42.

104. Green BKW, Gordon GD, Horak AR, Millar RNS, Commerford PJ: Safety of combined intravenous beta-adrenergic blockade (atenolol or metroprolol) and thrombolytic therapy in acute myocardial infarction. *Am J Cardiol* 1992;69: 1389–1392.

105. Van de Werf F, Janssens L, Brzostek T, et al: Short-term effects of early intravenous treatment with a beta-adrenergic blocking agent or a specific bradycardiac agent in patients with acute myocardial infarction receiving thrombolytic therapy. *J Am Coll Cardiol* 1993;22:407–416.

106. Heidbuchel H, Tack J, Vanneste L, Ballet A, Ector H, Van de Werf F: Significance of arrhythmias during the first 24 hours of acute myocardial infarction treated with altplase and effect of early administration of a beta blocker or a bradycardiac agent on their incidence. *Circulation* 1994;89: 1051–1059.

107. Hohnloser SH, Zabel M, Olschewski M, Kasper W, Just H: Arrhythmias during the acute phase of reperfusion therapy for acute myocardial infarction: Effects of beta-adrenergic blockade. *Am Heart J* 1992;123:1530–1535.

108. Montague TJ, Roger YW, Burton JR, Kyung SB, Catellier DJ, Koon KT: Changes in acute myocardial infarction risk and patterns of practice for patients older and younger than 70 years, 1987–90. *Can J Cardiol* 1992;8:596–600.

109. Pashos CL, Normand ST, Garfinkle JB, Newhouse JP, Epstein AM, McNeil BJ: Trends in the use of drug therapies in patients with acute myocardial infarction: 1988 to 1992. *J Am Coll Cardiol* 1994;23:1023–1030.

110. Viskin S, Kitzis I, Lev E, et al: Treatment with beta-adrenergic blocking agents after myocardial infarction: From randomized trials to clinical practice. *J Am Coll Cardiol* 1995;25:1327–1332.

111. Singh BN, G Ellrodt, K Nademanee: *Clinical Essays on the Heart.* New York, McGraw-Hill, 1984, pp 65–98.

112. Brown BG, Bolson EL, Dodge HT: Dynamic mechanisms in human coronary stenosis. *Circulation* 1984;70:917–922.

113. Waters DD, Theroux P, Szlachic J: Effects of calcium antagonists on infarcting myocardium. *Am J Cardiol* 1981;48:123–130.

114. Kloner RA, Braunwald E: Effects of calcium antagonists on infarcting myocardium. *Am J Cardiol* 1987;59:84B–94B.

115. Nayler WG, Grau A, Slade A: A protective effect of verapamil on hypoxic heart muscle. *Cardiovasc Res* 1976;10:650–662.

116. Nayler WG: Calcium antagonists at the ischemic myocardium. *Int J Cardiol* 1987;15:267–285.

117. Yusuf S, Held P, Furberg C: Update of effects of calcium antagonists in myocardial infarction or angina in light of the Second Danish Verapamil Infarction Trial (DAVIT-II) and other recent studies. *Am J Cardiol* 1991;67:1295–1297.

118. Held PH, Yusuf S: Effects of beta blockers and calcium channel blockers in acute myocardial infarction. *Eur Heart J* 1993;14:18–25.

119. Held P, Yusuf S: Calcium antagonists in the treatment of ischemic heart disease: Myocardial infarction. *Cor Art Dis* 1994;5:21–26.

120. The Danish Study Group on Verapamil in Myocardial Infarction: Effect of verapamil on mortality and major events after acute myocardial infarction (the Danish Verapamil Infarction Trial II—DAVIT II). *Am J Cardiol* 1990;66: 779–785.

121. Arstall MA, Beltrame JF, Mohan P, Wuttke RD, Esterman AJ, Horowitz JD: Incidence of adverse events during treatment with verapamil for suspected acute myocardial infarction. *Am J Cardiol* 1992;70:1611–1612.

122. Knabb RM, Rosamond TL, Fox KAA, Sobel BE, Bergmann SR: Salvage of reperfused ischemic myocardium myocardium by diltiazem. *J Am Coll Cardiol* 1986;8:861–871.

123. van der Wall EE, Cats VM, Chin JC, Pauwels JK, Bruschke VG: Acute effects of intravenous nisoldipine on left ventricular function after acute myocardial infarction. *Cardiovasc Drugs Ther* 1994;8: 345–351.

124. Pfeffer JM, Pfeffer MA, Braunwald E: Influence of chronic captopril therapy on the infarcted left ventricle of the rat. *Circ Res* 1985;57:84–95.

125. Pfeffer M, Pfeffer J, Steinberg C, Finn P: Survival after an experimental myocardial infarction: Beneficial effects of long-term therapy with captopril. *Circulation* 1985;72:406–412.

126. Pfeffer M, Lamas G, Vaughan D: Effect of captopril on progressive ventricular dilatation after anterior myocardial infarction. *N Engl J Med* 1988; 319:80–86.

127. Sharpe N, Murphy J, Smith H, Hannan S: Treatment of patients with symptomless left ventricular dysfunction after myocardial infarction. *Lancet* 1988;1:255–259.

128. Swedberg K, Held P, Kjekshus J: Effects of the early administration of enalapril on mortality in patients with acute myocardial infarction. *N Engl J Med* 1992;327:678–684.

129. Bonarjee VVS, Carstensen S, Caidahl K, Nilsen DWT, Edner M, Berning J: Attenuation of left ventricular dilatation after acute myocardial infarction by early initiation of enalapril therapy. *Am J Cardiol* 1993;72:1004–1009.

130. Pfeffer MA, Braunwald E, Moye LA: Effect of captopril on mortality and morbidity in patients with left ventricular dysfunction after myocardial infarction. *N Engl J Med* 1992;327:669–677.

131. The Acute Infarction Ramipril Efficacy (AIRE) Study Investigators: Effect of ramipril on mortality and morbidity of survivors of acute myocardial infarction with clinical evidence of heart failure. *Lancet* 1993;343:821–828.

131a. Kober L, Torp-Pedersen C, Carlsen JE, et al for the Trandolapril Cardiac Evaluation (TRACE) Study Group: A Clinical Trial of the Angiotensin Converting Enzyme Inhibitor Trandolapril in Patients With Left Ventricular Dysfunction After Myocardial Infarction. *NEJM* 1995;33:1670–1676.

131b. The TRACE Study Group: The TRAndolapril Cardiac Evaluation (TRACE) Study: Rationale, Design and Baseline Characteristics of the Screened Population. *Am J Cardiol* 1994;73: 44C–50C.

131c. Ball SG, Hall AS, Murray GD: Angiotensin-Converting Inhibitors After Myocardial Infarction: Indications and Timing. *J Am Coll Cardiol* 1995;25:Suppl:42S–46S.

132. Multicentre Postinfarction Research Group: Risk stratification and survival after acute myocardial infarction. *N Engl J Med* 1983;309:331–336.

133. Ball SG, Hall AS: What to expect from ACE inhibitors after myocardial infarction. *Br Heart J* 1994;72:70–74.

134. Chinese Cardiac Study Collaborative Group: Oral captopril versus placebo among 13 634 patients with suspected acute myocardial infarction: Interim report from the Chinese Cardiac Study (CCS-1). *Lancet* 1995;345:686–687.

134a. Pizzetti F, Maggioni AP, Santoro E, et al for the GISSI-3 Investigators: Effects of Lisinopril Treatment on Early Mortality in Patients with Acute Myocardial Infarction at Different Risk Profile: data from the GISSI-3 Study. *J Am Coll Cardiol* 1996;27:(Suppl A):82A (Abstract).

135. Ambrosioni E, Borghi C, Magnani B: The effect of the angiotensin-converting-enzyme inhibitor

zofenopril on mortality and morbidity after anterior myocardial infarction. *N Engl J Med* 1995;332: 80–85.

136. Kingma JH, van Gilst WH, Peels CH, Dambrink J-H, Verheugt FWA, Wielenga RP: Acute intervention with captopril during thrombolysis in patients with first anterior myocardial infarction. *Eur Heart J* 1994;15:898–907.

137. Tohmo H, Karanko M, Korpilahti K: Haemodynamic effects of enalaprilat and preload in acute severe heart failure complicating myocardial infarction. *Eur Heart J* 1994;15:523–527.

138. Pasquale PD, Paterna S, Bucca V, Maringhini G, Magatti M: Effects of the administration of captopril, metoprolol and of the captopril–metoprolol combination as adjuvant therapy during thrombolysis in acute myocardial infarction. *Int J Cardiol* 1994;46:107–112.

139. Tranchesi B Jr, Santos RD, Caramelli B, et al: Early administration of captopril and nitroglycerin in combination after acute myocardial infarction: An invasive haemodynamic study. *Eur Heart J* 1993;14:90–95.

139a. Walsh JT, Gray D, Keating NA, et al: ACE for Whom? Implications for Clinical Practice of Post-Infarct Trials. *Br Heart J* 1995;73:470–474.

140. Foy SG, Crozier IG, Turner JG, et al: Comparison of enalapril versus captopril on left ventricular function and survival three months after acute mycocardial infarction (the "PRACTICAL" study). *Am J Cardiol* 1994;73:1180–1186.

141. Mroczek WJ, Lee WR, Davidov ME: Effect of magnesium sulfate on cardiovascular hemodynamics. *Angiology* 1977;28:720–724.

142. Hearse DJ, Stewart DA, Braimbridge MV: Myocardial protection during ischemic cardiac arrest: The importance of magnesium in cardioplegic solutions. *J Thorac Cardiovasc Surg* 1978;75: 877–855.

143. Hearse DJ: Reperfusion of the ischemic myocardium. *J Mol Cell Cardiol* 1977;9:605–616.

144. Borchgrevink PC, Bergan AS, Bakoy O, Jynge P: Magnesium and reperfusion of ischemic rat heart as assessed by 31P-NMR. *Am J Physiol* 1986;18: 487–498.

145. Favaron M, Bernardi P: Tissue-specific modulation of the mitochondrial calcium uniporter by magnesium ions. *FEBS Lett* 1985;183:260–264.

146. Ferrari R, Albertini A, Curello S, et al: Myocardial recovery during post-ischemic reperfusion: Effects of nifedipine, calcium and magnesium. *J Mol Cell Cardiol* 1986;18:487–498.

147. Barros LFM, Da-Luz PL, Silveria MC, Chagas ACP, Pileggi F: Ventricular fibrillation in acute experimental myocardial ischemia: Protection by magnesium sulfate. *Braz J Med Biol Res* 1988;21: 791–799.

148. Crampton RS, Clark CW: Varying extracellular (Mg_2) alters ischemic and reperfusion tachyarrhythmias (abstract). *Circulation* 1983;68 (Suppl III):III-146.

149. Haverkamp W, Hindricks G, Keteller T, Allberty D, Wiethold D, Gulker H: Prophylactic antiarrhythmic and antifibrillatory effects of intravenous magnesium sulphate during acute myocardial ischemia (abstract). *Eur Heart J* 1988;9:288.

150. Ceremuzynski L, Jurgiel R, Kulakowski P, Gebalska J: Threatening arrhythmias in acute myocardial infarction are prevented by intravenous magnesium sulfate. *Am Heart J* 1989;118: 1333–1334.

151. Kimura T, Yasue H, Sakaino N, Rokutanda M, Jougasaki M, Araki H: Effects of magnesium on the tone of isolated human coronary arteries. *Circulation* 1989;79:1118–1124.

152. Altura BN, Altura BT, Carella A, Gerbrewold A, Murakawa T, Nishio A: Mg^{2+}–Ca^{2+} interaction in contractility of vascular smooth muscle: Mg^{2+} versus organic calcium channel blockers on myogenic tone and agonist-induced responsiveness of blood vessels. *Can J Physiol Pharmacol* 1987;65: 729–745.

153. Vigorito C, Giordano A, Ferraro P, et al: Hemodynamic effects of magnesium sulfate on the normal human heart. *Am J Cardiol* 1991;67:1435–1437.

154. Kugiyama K, Yasue H, Okumura K, et al: Suppression of exercise-induced angina by magnesium sulphate in patients with variant angina. *J Am Coll Cardiol* 1988;12:1177–1183.

155. Nadler JL, Goodson R, Rude R: Evidence that prostacyclin mediates the vascular action of magnesium in humans. *Hypertension* 1987;9:379–383.

156. Adams JH, Mitchell JRA: The effects of agents which modify platelet behavior and of magnesium ions on thrombus formation in vivo. *Thromb Haemost* 1979;42:603–610.

157. Watson KV, Moldow CF, Ogburn PL, Jacob HS: Magnesium sulfate: Rationale for its use in preeclampsia. *Proc Natl Acad Sci USA* 1986;83: 1075–1078.

158. Yusuf S, Teo K, Woods K: Intravenous magnesium in acute myocardial infarction. *Circulation* 1993;87:2043–2046.
159. Luoma H, Aromaa A, Helminen S, et al: Risk of myocardial infarction in Finnish men in relation to fluoride, magnesium and calcium concentration in drinking water. *Acta Med Scand* 1983;213: 171–176.
160. Ghani MF, Rabah M: Effect of magnesium chloride on electrical stability of the heart. *Am Heart J* 1977;94:600–602.
161. Teo KK, Yusuf S, Collins R, Held PH, Peto R: Effect of intravenous magnesium in suspected acute myocardial infarction: Overview of randomized trials. *Br Med J* 1991;303:1499–1503.
162. Horner SM: Efficacy of intravenous magnesium in acute myocardial infarction in reducing arrhythmias and mortality. *Circulation* 1992;86: 774–779.
163. Woods KL, Fletcher S, Roffe C, Haider Y: Intravenous magnesium sulphate in suspected acute myocardial infarction: Results of the second Leicester Intravenous Magnesium Intervention Trial (LIMIT-2). *Lancet* 1992;339:1553–1558.
164. Roffe C, Fletcher S, Woods KL: Investigation of the effects of intravenous magnesium sulphate on cardiac rhythm in acute myocardial infarction. *Br Heart J* 1994;71:141–145.
165. Woods KL, Fletcher S: Long-term outcome after intravenous magnesium sulphate in suspected acute myocardial infarction: The second Leicester Intravenous Magnesium Intervention Trial (LIMIT-2). *Lancet* 1994;343:816–819.
166. Shechter M, Hod H, Chouraqui P, Kaplinsky E, Rabinowitz B: Magnesium therapy in acute myocardial infarction when patients are not candidates for thrombolytic therapy. *Am J Cardiol* 1995; 75:321–323.
167. Thogersen AM, Johnson O, Wester PO: Effects of magnesium infusion on thrombolytic and non-thrombolytic treated patients with acute myocardial infarction. *Int J Cardiol* 1993;39: 13–22.
168. Tzivoni D, Banai S, Schuger C, et al: Treatment of torsade de pointes with magnesium sulfate. *Circulation* 1988;77:392–397.
169. Beller GA, Hood WB Jr, Smith TW, Abelmann WH, Wacker WAC: Correlation of serum magnesium levels and cardiac digitalis intoxication. *Am J Cardiol* 1974;33:225–229.
170. McMahon S, Collins R, Peto K: Effects of prophylactic lidocaine in suspected acute myocardial infarction: An overview of results from the randomized controlled trials. *JAMA* 1988;260: 1910–1916.
171. Yusuf S, Wittes J, Friedman L: Overview of results of randomized clinical trials in heart disease. *JAMA* 1988;260:2088–2093.
172. Hine LK, Laird N, Hewitt P: Meta-analytic acute myocardial infarction. *Arch Intern Med* 1989;149: 2694–2698.
173. Nattel S, Arenal A: Antiarrhythmic prophylaxis after acute myocardial infarction. *Drugs* 1993;45: 9–14.

173a. Belardinelli L., West GA, Clemo SH. Regulation of Atrioventricular Node Function by Adenosine. In: Gerlach E, Belker BF, eds. Topics and Perspectives in Adenosine Research: Proceedings of the 3rd International Symposium on Adenosine, Munich, June 1986. New York: Springer-Verlag; 1987:346–353.

173b. Wesley RC Jr, Lerman BB, DiMarco JP, Berne RM, Belardinelli L: Mechanism of Atropine-Resistant Atrioventricular Block During Inferior Myocardial Infarction: Possible Role of Adenosine. *J Am Coll Cardiol* 1986;8: 1232–1234.

173c. Shah PK, Nalos P, Peter T: Atropine Resistant Post Infarction Complete AV Block: Possible Role of Adenosine and Improvement With Aminophylline. *Am Heart J* 1986;113:194–195.

173d. Bertolet BD, McMurtrie EB, Hill JA, Belardinelli L: Theophylline for the Treatment of Atrial Ventricular Block after Myocardial Infarction. *Ann Intern Med* 1995;123:509–511.

173e. The Cardiac Arrhythmic Suppression Trial (CAST) Investigators Preliminary Report: Effect of Encainide and Flecainide on Mortality in a Randomized Trial of Arrhythmia Suppression After Myocardial Infarction. *N Engl J Med* 1989;321:406–412.

173f. The European Myocardial Infarct Amiodarone Trial (EMIAT) presented at the 45th Annual Scienfitic Session of the American College of Cardiology, Orlando, Florida, March 26, 1996.

173g. The Canadian Amiodarone Myocardial Infarction Arrhythmia Trial (CAMIAT) presented at the 45th Annual Scientific Session of the American College of Cardiology, Orlando, Florida, March 26, 1996.

174. Szlavy L, Adams DF, Hollenberg NK: Cardiac lymph and lymphatics in normal and infarcted myocardium. *Am Heart J* 1980;100:323–331.

175. Wolf RA, Chaung LY, Muller JE: Intravenous bovine testicular hyaluronidase depolymerizes myocardial hyaluronic acid in dogs with coronary artery occlusion. *Circ Res* 1981;48:88–95.

176. Roberts R, Braunwald E, Muller JE: Effect of hyaulronidase on mortality and morbidity in patients with early peaking of plasma creatinine kinase MB and non-transmural ischemia. *Br Heart J* 1988;60:290–298.

177. Rogers WJ, Russel RO, McDaniel HJ: Acute effects of glucose–insulin–potassium infusion on myocardial substrates, coronary blood flow, and oxygen consumption in man. *Am J Cardiol* 1977; 40:421–428.

178. Rogers WJ, Segall PH, McDaniel HJ: Prospective randomized trial of glucose–insulin–potassium in acute myocardial infarction: Effects on myocardial hemodynamics, substrates, and rhythm. *Am J Cardiol* 1979;43:801–809.

179. Maroko PR, Libby P, Sobel BE: Effective glucose–insulin–potassium infusion and myocardial infarction following experimental coronary artery occlusion. *Circulation* 1972;45:1160–1175.

180. Rogers WJ, McDaniel HJ, Mantle: Prospective randomized trial of glucose–insulin–potassium in acute myocardial infarction: Effects on hemodynamics, short- and long-term survival (abstract). *J Am Coll Cardiol* 1983;1:628.

181. Satler LF, Green CE, Kent KM: Metabolic support during coronary reperfusion. *Am Heart J* 1987;114:54–58.

182. Spath JA, Lane DL, Lefer AM: Protective action of methylprednisolone on the myocardium during experimental ischemia in the cat. *Circ Res* 1974;35:44–51.

183. Jugdutt BI, Hutchins GM, Bulkley BH: Salvage of ischemic myocardium by ibuprofen during infarction in the conscious dog. *Am J Cardiol* 1980;46: 74–82.

184. Kloner RA, Fishbein MC, Lew H: Mummification of the infarcted myocardium by high dose corticosteroids. *Circulation* 1978;57:56–63.

185. Hammerman H, Kloner RA, Hele S: Dose-dependent effects of short-term methylprednisolone and myocardial infarct extent, scar formation, and ventricular function. *Circulation* 1983; 68:446–452.

186. Brown EJ, Kloner RA, Schoen FJ: Scar thinning due to ibuprofen administration after experimental myocardial infarction. *Am J Cardiol* 1983;51: 877–833.

187. Hammerman H, Schoen FJ, Braunwald E: Drug-induced expansion of infarct: Morphologic and functional correlation. *Circulation* 1984; 69:611–617.

188. Siever SJ, Johansson BW, Nilsson SE: Corticosteroid therapy in acute myocardial infarction. IVth World Congress of Cardiology, Mexico City 1963;4-B:222–225.

189. Hammerman H, Kloner RA, Schoen FJ: Indomethacin-induced scar thinning after experimental myocardial infarction. *Circulation* 1983;67: 1290–1295.

190. Silverman HS, Pfeifer MP: Relation between use of anti-inflammatory agents and left ventricular free wall rupture during acute myocardial infarction. *Am J Cardiol* 1987;59:363–364.

190a. Maikawa K, Liang CS, Hood WB: Comparison of Dobutamine and Dopamine in Acute Myocardial Infarction. *Circulation* 1983;67:750–758.

190b. Biddle TL, Benotti JR, Creager MA, et al: Comparison of Intravenous Milrinone and Dobutamine for Congestive Heart Failure Secondary to Either Ischemic or Dilated Cardiomyopathy. *Am J Cardiol* 1987;59:1345–1350.

190c. Karlsberg RP, De Wood MA, De Maria AN, et al: Comparitive Efficacy of Short-Term Intravenous Infusions of Milrinone and Dobutamine in Acute Congestive Heart Failure Following Acute Myocardial Infarction. *Clin Cardiol* 1996; 19:21–30.

191. Caldicott LD, Hawley K, Heppell PA, Woodmansey PA, Channer KS: Intravenous enoximone or dobutamine for severe heart failure after acute myocardial infarction: A randomized double-blind trial. *Eur Heart J* 1995;14:696–700.

192. van Gilst WH, van Veldhuisen DJ, Hegeman H, et al: Effect of ibopamine on ventricular remodeling after experimental myocardial infarction: A comparison with captopril. *J Cardiovasc Pharmacol* 1994;24:171–174.

193. EMIP-FR Pilot Study Group: Free radicals, reperfusion and myocardial infarction therapy: European Myocardial Infarction Project—free radicals pilot study. *Eur Heart J* 1993;14:48–51.

194. du Toit EF, Opie LH. Modulation of severity of reperfusion and stunning in the isolated rat heart

by agents altering calcium flux at reperfusion. *Circulation Research* 1992;70:960–967.

195. Herzog WR, Scholssberg ML, MacMurdy KS, et al. Timing of magnesium therapy affects experimental infarct size. *Circulation* 1995;92:2622–2626.

196. Christensen CW, Reeder MA, Silverstein EL, et al. Magnesium sulfate reduces myocardial infarct size when administered prior to but not after coronary reperfusion in a canine model. *Circulation* 1995;92:2617–2621.

197. Antman EM. Magnesium and acute MI. Timing is critical. *Circulation* 1995;92:2367–2372 (editorial).

198. Antman E. Randomized trials of magnesium for acute myocardial infarction; Big numbers do not tell the whole story. *Am J Cardiol* 1995;75:391–393.

13

Pathophysiology and Management of Cardiogenic Shock Due to Primary Pump Failure

John Webb, MD, and Judith S. Hochman, MD

INTRODUCTION

Cardiogenic shock remains the most frequent mode of death for patients who are hospitalized with acute myocardial infarction (MI) (1). The reported incidence of cardiogenic shock complicating acute MI ranges from 5% to 15%, and the associated mortality ranges from 70% to 80% (2–10). Despite rapid advances in the medical management of acute MI during the prethrombolytic era, neither the frequency nor the outcome of cardiogenic shock were significantly affected (2). The high early mortality associated with cardiogenic shock has been compounded by a high late mortality, with reported 1-, 2-, and 3-year mortality rates of 18%, 25%, and 28% respectively (11).

Definition

Cardiogenic shock can be defined as a state of severe tissue hypoperfusion resulting from underlying cardiac dysfunction. This usually manifests itself as persistent systemic arterial hypotension unresponsive to fluid resuscitation combined with evidence of hypoperfusion, such as cool skin, altered mental status, and markedly diminished urine output. The diagnosis of shock usually requires hemodynamic confirmation as evidenced by sustained systemic hypotension (systolic arterial pressure (<90 mm Hg or mean arterial pressure >30 mm Hg below basal levels) in the absence of vasopressor agents, combined with evidence of adequate left ventricular filling pressures (pulmonary artery wedge pressure [PAWP] >15 mm Hg) and a reduced cardiac output (cardiac index <2.2 L/min/m^2).

There is wide variability in the criteria used for cardiogenic shock in different published studies. Pulmonary congestion need not necessarily be present for the diagnosis of cardiogenic shock, and all manifestations of end organ hypoperfusion may not be present (4). However, reliance on hypotension alone in the absence of hemodynamic confirmation of adequate left ventricular filling pressure and reduced cardiac output has led to inclusion of some relatively low-risk patients not in true shock in some clinical series.

The above definition of classic cardiogenic shock defines those patients with the most profound hemodynamic abnormality and the worst prognosis. These are the patients referred to by the AHA/ACC Task Force on the management of myocardial infarction as subset 2 (1). In this classification subset 1 included patients without frank hypotension, but with low cardiac output (<2.5 L/min/m^2) and PAWP >15 mm Hg. These two subsets are included in Forrester hemodynamic subset 4, in which mortality was demonstrated to be related to the degree of hemodynamic abnormality as shown in Fig. 13–1 (12). It should be appreciated that systemic arterial pressure may be well maintained at the expense of a very high systemic vascular resistance (SVR); however, the low output state will lead to tissue ischemia and lactate production and initiate the vicious spiral leading to further LV dysfunction. This early shock or "preshock" must be recognized for earlier intervention. Some studies have defined hypotension to be a mean arterial pressure 30 mm Hg lower than baseline; it is clear that these patients are also at high risk, even if absolute systolic blood pressure remains within the "normal range."

Cardiogenic shock may be due to either severe left or right ventricular dysfunction, or mechanical causes such as acute mitral insufficiency, ventricular septal rupture, free wall rupture, or tamponade. To some extent the ability of an individual patient to tolerate poor tissue perfusion depends on the suddenness of the reduction; some patients with chronic congestive heart failure due to dilated cardiomyopathy may have chronic low output and degrees of LV dysfunction similar to those in shock, but remain functional (13). We will restrict our discussion to acute dysfunction of the left ventricular myocardium or "primary pump failure" complicating acute myocardial infarction.

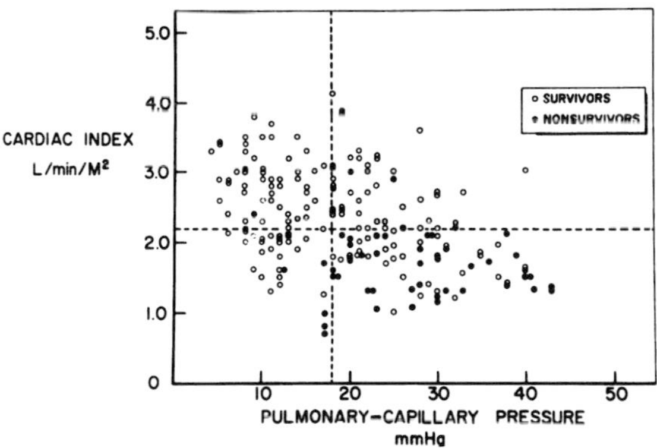

Figure 13–1. Survival in acute myocardial infarction is related to the severity of the hemodynamic abnormality. Four subsets (quadrants) are defined by Cardiac Index less than or greater than 2.2 L/min/m^2 and PCWP less than 18 mm Hg (upper left is subset 1, upper right is subset 2, lower left is subset 3, and lower right is subset 4). *From Forrester et al (12), with permission.*

PATHOPHYSIOLOGY

The Timing of Shock

From 1% to 5% of patients with acute MI present to hospital in cardiogenic shock, while another 5% to 7% develop shock during their hospitalization (2–5,8,14–16). In the recent SHOCK Registry, cardiogenic shock was not present at the time of hospital admission in the majority of acute MI patients who were ultimately diagnosed with shock (17). However, in this large multicenter prospective series, the median interval from MI onset to shock diagnosis was only 8 hours. In the GUSTO trial, where all participants were candidates for thrombolysis, only 0.8% presented in shock and 6.5% developed it (14). Overall, approximately one-half of shock patients develop shock early (<24 hours); of these, one-third are in shock at the time of hospital arrival (2–5,8,14–16).

Mechanisms of Development of Shock

Cardiogenic shock that develops soon after the onset of myocardial infarction is due to extensive myocardial damage. Typically, this results from occlusion of a coronary artery that supplies a large region of myocardium at risk with no appreciable collateral flow. Massive infarction may result in a sudden precipitous fall in cardiac output and systemic pressure and very rapid death. A small to moderate infarct may precipitate shock when there has been extensive prior damage. The downward spiral leading to irreversible cardiogenic shock is multifactorial (Fig. 13–2) (13). The pathogenesis of shock occurring later in the course of myocardial infarction is more complex. Important factors include infarct expansion, infarct extension, reduced coronary perfusion pressure, and increased myocardial oxygen demands as well as metabolic abnormalities.

Infarct extension is the most clearly documented process whereby late cardiogenic shock may develop after initial presentation. Progressive myocardial necrosis is suggested by persistently elevated cardiac enzyme levels consistent with ongoing or recurrent infarction (5,18–20). Pathologic

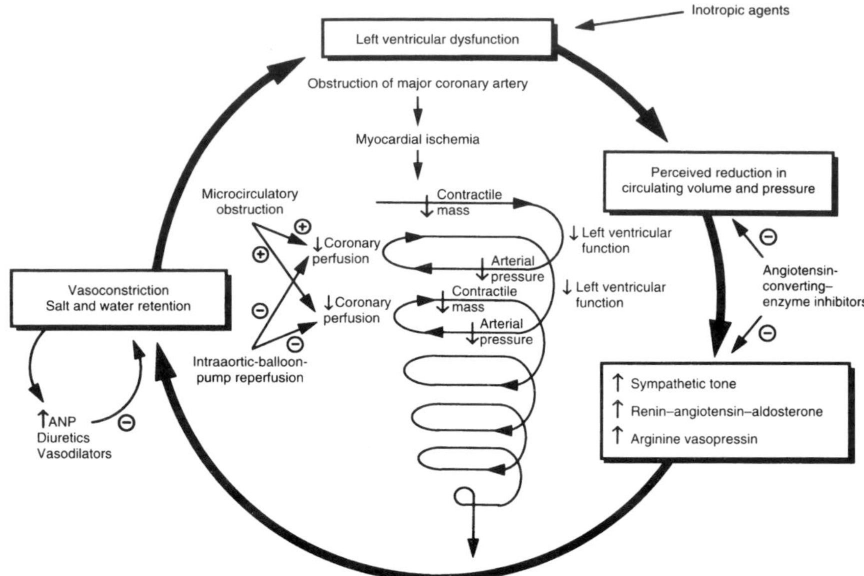

Figure 13–2. The vicious cycle of mechanical and neurohormonal events that lead from coronary obstruction to death in patients with cardiogenic shock. (See text for discussion of abnormalities in the infarct and remote, uninfarcted myocardium that result in LV dysfunction.) *From Califf and Bengston (13), with permission.*

examination frequently reveals myocardium in varying stages of infarction, suggesting stepwise extension of necrosis as demonstrated in Fig. 13–3 (18,19,21–23). The MILIS study group conservatively estimated that late (>48 hours after the onset of infarction) reinfarction or infarct extension occurred in 23% of 60 patients who developed shock while in hospital, in contrast to 7% in those without shock ($p < 0.0001$) (5). Similarly the GUSTO study found reinfarction or recurrent ischemia to be more frequent in patients who later developed cardiogenic shock than those who did not (29.3% vs. 6.1%, $p < 0.05$) (14).

Infarct extension may occur by several mechanisms. Reocclusion of a patent infarct-related artery is probably the most common mechanism. Such reocclusion may occur regardless of whether initial coronary reperfusion occurred spontaneously (24), with thrombolysis (25), or with percutaneous transluminal coronary angioplasty (PTCA) (26). Infarct extension may occur due to propagation of thrombus retrograde so as to occlude more proximal coronary branches or due to embolization into more distal branches. Infarction may also occur in a territory distant from the myocardium initially at risk, perhaps due to thrombosis of a critical coronary lesion in the setting of low coronary blood flow and a hypercoaguable state. Finally, infarct extension adjacent to the infarct territory or remote from it may occur due to increased myocardial oxygen demands secondary to left ventricular dilation, tachycardia, and inotropes in combination with reduced coronary perfusion pressure and flow.

In the normal heart, coronary blood flow is determined primarily by changes in coronary vascular resistance. Coronary perfusion pressure is of secondary importance. The ability of the microvasculature to dilate may allow normal coronary blood flow even in the presence of marked systemic arterial hypotension and aortic pressures as low as 50 mm Hg. However, in patients with critical coronary stenoses the microvasculature may already be fully dilated and vasodilator reserve exhausted (27). At this point further reductions in aortic pressure may lead to directly proportional reductions in coronary blood flow. Increased left ventricular diastolic pressures further serve to reduce coronary perfusion pressure (Fig. 13–4) (28). Since the normal heart ex-

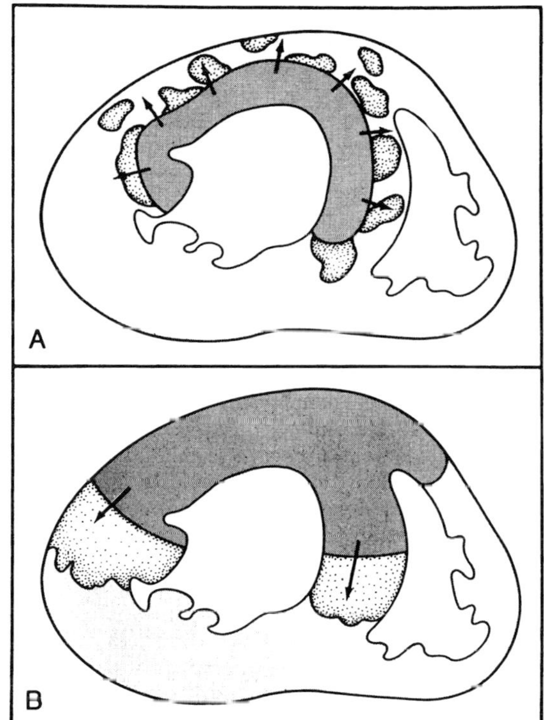

Figure 13–3. Patients in cardiogenic shock consistently demonstrate marginal extension at autopsy, which can involve the subepicardial region (**A**) or lateral margins (**B**). *From Pasternak et al (18) and Alonso et al (19), with permission.*

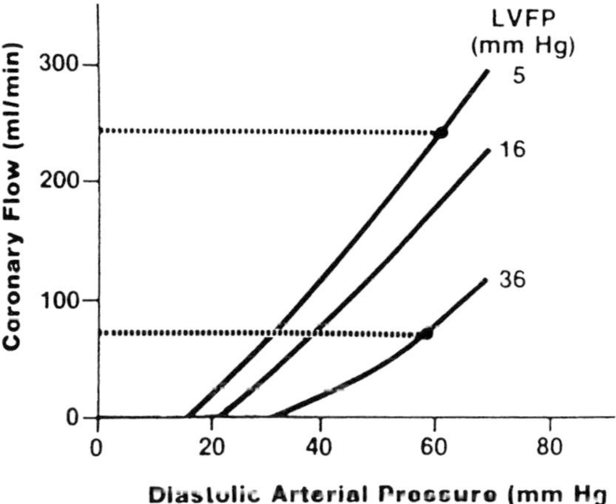

Figure 13–4. Effect of diastolic arterial pressure and left ventricular filling pressure (LVFP) on coronary blood flow. Coronary blood flow may be enhanced by interventions that increase diastolic pressure within the aorta and reduce diastolic left ventricular filling pressures. *From McGhie and Goldstein (28), with permission.*

tracts approximately 65% of the oxygen present in coronary blood, there is little room for further oxygen extraction; ischemia and anaerobic metabolism ensue. If reduced coronary perfusion persists, the resultant lactic acidosis and reduced levels of high-energy phosphates may further impair the contractility of the remaining viable myocardium (29,30).

Infarct expansion may also contribute to the late development of cardiogenic shock (5). Expansion occurs as a result of remodeling of the structurally weakened infarct zone, which thins and dilates, often leading to functional aneurysm formation (31,32). As infarct expansion occurs, left ventricular function further deteriorates due to reduced mechanical efficiency (33,34). Infarct expansion is particularly notable after large anterior infarctions involving the left ventricular apex (34–36).

Anatomic Features

Although occlusion of a single major coronary artery may result in cardiogenic shock, most often there is involvement of all three major coronary arteries with predominant involvement of the left anterior descending artery (19,21,37–42). One postmortem study found significant stenosis of the left anterior descending artery in 80% and triple-vessel disease in 68% of patients dying of cardiogenic shock (43). The absence of collaterals to the infarct artery distal to the site of occlusion markedly increases the likelihood of cardiogenic shock. The incidence of prior MI has been reported as approximately 40% (2,5).

Autopsy studies of patients dying from cardiogenic shock have typically shown that at least 40% of the left ventricular mass is affected (19,21). However, at times, cardiogenic shock may occur in patients without this degree of aggregate necrosis (22,23). In patients with extensive prior myocardial compromise, even a small infarction may lead to decompensation and shock (44). Infarction of one area of myocardium supplied by an occluded coronary artery is usually associated with compensatory hyperkinesis of the remaining myocardium.

Echocardiographic studies have shown that failure to develop this hypercontractility of remote myocardial segments may predispose to shock in patients who suffer smaller infarctions (44–46). The high incidence of multivessel disease in these patients suggests that ischemia remote to the infarct region compromises the potential for compensation and predisposes to the development of cardiogenic shock (47).

Physiologic Features

In patients with cardiogenic shock, major systemic compensatory mechanisms include activation of the sympathetic nervous system, altered renal and neurohormonal regulation, and local vasoregulation (Fig. 13–2). Sympathetic nervous system activation is triggered by baroreceptors in the aortic arch, carotid sinus, splanchnic bed, and heart, leading to an increase in heart rate, contractility, and both arterial and venous vasoconstriction. The renin–angiotensin system is activated by decreased renal perfusion and by increased sympathetic tone. Angiotensin II levels rise, resulting in peripheral vasoconstriction and synthesis of aldosterone. In turn, aldosterone leads to increased renal sodium and water resorption and increased blood volume. Atrial distension results in increased levels of atrial natriuretic peptide, which leads to renal sodium and water excretion while reducing the formation of renin and counteracting the effects of angiotensin II. Hypotension triggers increased levels of antidiuretic hormone, leading to increased renal water resorption. Vasoactive metabolites may initially result in vasodilatation of the tissue microvasculature; however, vascular autoregulation favors redistribution of blood to the heart, brain, and kidneys at the expense of the skin, skeletal muscle, and intestines.

Impairment of myocardial function in segments remote from the site of infarction may occur in the presence of only minimally decreased or normal coronary perfusion (48,49). Metabolic changes include preferential use of glucose rather than fatty acids for energy production, diminished ATP production and utilization, and other abnormalities (50–58). These disturbances may lead to a lack of compensatory hyperkinesis or frank hypokinesis of

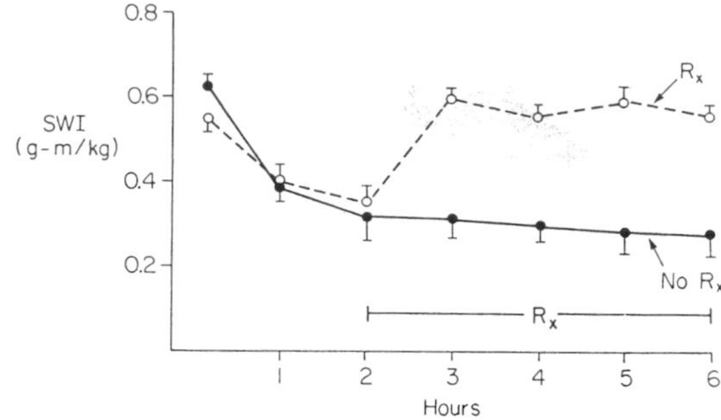

Figure 13–5. Response of left ventricular stroke work index (SWI) after left anterior descending artery occlusion in dogs that have a mild (50%) circumflex stenosis. SWI falls rapidly but is restored to normal in the group that received the metabolic support solution, which contains glutamate, aspartate, glucose–potassium–insulin, and coenzyme Q. Ultrasonic studies (not shown) demonstrate progressive impairment of contraction in the uninfarcted myocardium (circumflex distribution) and normalized contraction with the metabolic support solution. *From Beyersdorf et al (44), with permission.*

noninfarcted segments (44,54,55). It has been suggested that reduced substrate delivery may adversely affect this process, and preliminary studies suggest that intravenous substrate infusions can favorably influence contractility of remote myocardial segments (44) (Fig. 13–5). Since metabolic compromise and myocardial energy depletion may be progressive, this may predispose to the late development of pump failure, even in the setting of single-vessel disease with a large infarction.

As cardiogenic shock becomes more prolonged, tissue hypoperfusion leads to microvascular injury, myocardial depression, and multisystem failure. In the absence of supportive therapy, progressive deterioration is usual.

CLINICAL FEATURES

Patient Profile

The multicenter SHOCK Registry profiled 251 consecutive patients presenting with cardiogenic shock complicating acute MI prospectively identified in 19 international centers, as shown in Fig. 13–6 (17). The mean age was 67.5 ± 11.7 years. Although the majority (57%) were male, females were

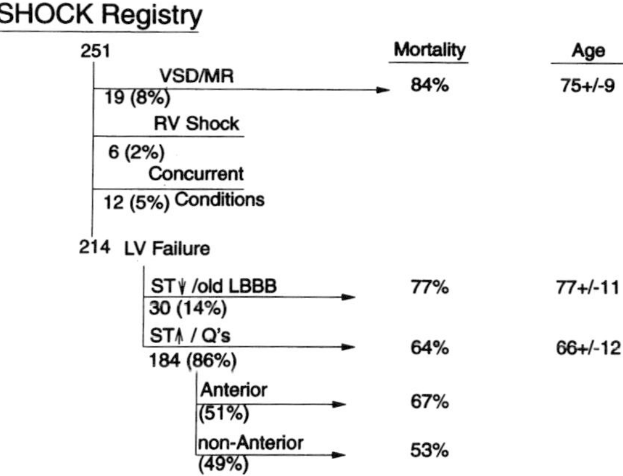

Figure 13–6. The multicenter SHOCK Registry profiled 251 consecutive patients with cardiogenic shock complicating acute MI prospectively identified in 19 centers (17). The heterogeneous nature of patients with shock complicating acute MI is demonstrated. Acute ventricular septal defect (VSD) or acute severe mitral regurgitation (MR) caused shock in 8% of cases and were associated with the highest in-hospital mortality rate (84%) and advanced age (75 ± 9 years).

disproportionately represented in this registry compared with the typical MI study representation rates of 20–25% (5,16,25,59). Women were significantly older than men (69.5 ± 11.2 vs. 65.9 ± 11.8 years, $p = 0.014$). Shock was due to mechanical causes, that is, ventricular septal rupture or mitral insufficiency, in 8%, isolated right ventricular failure in 2%, and concurrent medical illness in 5%. Primary left ventricular pump failure accounted for shock in 214 patients (85%) (Fig. 13–6). Age was highly associated with mortality. Patients discharged alive had a mean age of 63.8 ± 11.2 years, while nonsurvivors were on average 68.4 ± 11.5 years old ($p = 0.006$). Age was the strongest predictor of mortality in patients with cardiogenic shock receiving thrombolytic therapy in the GUSTO trial (60). Other variables significantly associated with mortality were nonsmoker status, Killip class 3 or 4 on hospital arrival, anterior MI, prior MI, diabetes, and hemodynamic variables.

Predictors of the development of cardiogenic shock in nonthrombolysed patients include age >65, female sex, prior infarction, diabetes, MB-CK > 160 IU/L, elevated blood lactate, ejection fraction less than 35%, persistent occlusion of the infarct-related artery, and the absence of hyperkinesis of the nonacutely infarcted segments of the left ventricular wall (2,4,5,8,46,47,61–63).

Clinical Assessment

In evaluating acute MI patients with hypotension, it is important to exclude noncardiogenic causes of shock. Confusion can arise in patients presenting with acute MI and volume depletion, sepsis, aortic dissection or rupture, pulmonary embolism, and pericardial tamponade. Mechanical causes of cardiogenic shock such as ventricular septal rupture or acute severe mitral regurgitation must be considered. A brief history and physical examination, an electrocardiogram (ECG), and a blood gas analysis should be obtained immediately. A chest film will aid in the assessment of pulmonary congestion, infection, tamponade, and aortic dissection.

Electrocardiogram

In the SHOCK Registry the majority (86%) of 214 patients with primary pump failure had ECG findings of acute transmural infarction: ST elevations, new Q waves, or new LBBB (Fig. 13–6). Half (51%) of all infarcts were anterior, 38% inferior, 11% posterior, and 24% lateral (patients had multiple infarct sites). Within this group, 67% of patients with anterior infarction died and 53% of patients with inferior infarction died ($p = 0.097$) (17). This relatively large proportion of inferior infarcts is consistent with other recent series (11,64) but is contrary to prior series that demonstrated a marked anterior predominance (5).

The Worcester study reported that 30% of all patients with shock did not have evidence of a Q wave infarction (2). Similarly, 14% of patients with primary pump failure in the SHOCK Registry did not have ECG findings of acute transmural infarction (17). These patients had findings of subendocardial infarction/ischemia, i.e., ST depression, nonspecific ST changes, or old left bundle branch block. They were significantly older (70.7 ± 10.5 vs. 66.1 ± 11.7 years, $p = 0.012$) and had a nonsignificantly higher mortality (77% vs. 64%, $p = 0.215$) compared with the group with ECG criteria for transmural infarction.

Echocardiogram and Doppler Flow Study

A transthoracic echocardiogram should be considered routine in the initial investigation of cardiogenic shock. Pump dysfunction can be readily confirmed, and other causes of low output excluded (65,66). This can be particularly helpful when the electrocardiogram does not allow the diagnosis of acute infarction, as may be the case in patients with prior infarction, nontransmural infarction, conduction block, or pacemakers. Right ventricular function, pericardial effusions, and tamponade can be assessed. Doppler imaging allows assessment of valvular function and shunts, and estimation of pulmonary arterial pressure.

Transesophageal echocardiography can be safely performed in patients with cardiogenic shock and may be invaluable in selected patients in whom routine transthoracic studies do not provide adequate information (67). Mechanically ventilated, critically ill patients may be particularly difficult to assess by transthoracic means, but they can be readily assessed by esophageal intubation. Transesophageal echocardiography may be particularly useful in the diagnosis of aortic dissection, mitral regurgitation (MR), and ventricular septal rupture. We have noted several cases in the ongoing SHOCK trial Registry where only moderate MR was diagnosed on a technically limited transthoracic echocardiogram, but a flail mitral leaflet and severe MR were seen on transesophageal echo. These patients had a first inferior infarction and no regurgitation murmur appreciated. A mechanical cause of LV shock should be suspected in the setting of a first inferior infarct.

MANAGEMENT OF SEVERE PUMP DYSFUNCTION

General Measures

Once cardiogenic shock is suspected, a fluid challenge is warranted in patients without pulmonary congestion. Insertion of an arterial cannula allows accurate determination of blood pressure and its response to interventions while facilitating frequent blood sampling. Catheterization of the bladder is advisable to assess urine output. Central venous access should be obtained. In patients who have recently received thrombolytic drugs, use of a compressible site such as the basilic vein, femoral vein below the inguinal ligament, or posterior approach internal jugular may be safer than the more commonly used medial or anterior approach jugular or subclavian sites.

Endotracheal intubation and mechanical ventilation should be considered early in the management of cardiogenic shock. In the patient who is obtunded, hypoxemic, acidotic, and hypoperfused, prompt intubation with ventilatory support may improve oxygen delivery, reduce the work of breathing, and improve cardiac output as well as protect the airway. Attention to cardiac rhythm is important. Even moderate bradycardia and atrioventricular dissociation may suggest potential benefit from atropine or pacing, as cardiac output is directly related to heart rate. New onset atrial fibrillation should be cardioverted.

Aspirin reduces mortality and reinfarction in acute infarction (59). Although not specifically tested in cardiogenic shock, it should be administered routinely to facilitate reperfusion and reduce the likelihood of reinfarction. Full anticoagulation with heparin is indicated to reduce the risk of reinfarction, left ventricular mural thrombus, and deep vein thrombosis.

Hemodynamic Monitoring

Right heart catheterization is indicated to confirm the diagnosis of cardiogenic shock and to exclude other possible causes of hypotension. Intravascular volume depletion or excessive venodilation may be diagnosed if low right atrial and/or pulmonary wedge pressures are recorded. Inappropriate vasodilation may be detected by an unexpectedly low systemic vascular resistance. Right ventricular infarction may be suggested by an inappropriately elevated right heart filling pressure (e.g., right atrial pressure/pulmonary wedge pressure > 0.7) (68). Ventricular septal rupture can be diagnosed by finding a step-up in oxygen saturation from right atrium to right ventricle (69). Mitral insufficiency may be suggested, but not proven, by large V waves in the pulmonary wedge tracing (70,71). Equalization of diastolic pressures suggests tamponade.

Cardiogenic shock is characterized hemodynamically by low systemic arterial pressure (systolic blood pressure < 90 mm Hg), high left ventricular filling pressure (mean pulmonary arterial wedge pressure > 18 mm Hg), low cardiac index (<2.2 L/min/m^2), low stroke volume index (<20 ml/m^2), and elevated systemic vascular resistance >1200 dynes-sec/m^2). Mixed venous oxygen saturation is low, reflecting reduced tissue oxygen delivery (72–75) and increased extraction.

PHARMACOLOGIC SUPPORT

Sympathomimetic Inotropic and Vasopressor Agents

Dopamine is the drug of first choice in the setting of cardiogenic shock with marked hypotension (28). The effects of dopamine are dose dependent. At low doses (1 to 3 μg/kg/min), dopaminergic renal vasodilatation occurs; at intermediate doses (5 to 10 μg/kg/min), beta-1 adrenergic increased cardiac contractility is evident; at high doses (>15 μg/kg/min), alpha-1 arterial vasoconstriction predominates. High-dose dopamine typically results in increased systemic and pulmonary vascular pressures.

Dobutamine is the drug of first choice in the setting of cardiogenic shock without severe hypotension (28). Dobutamine acts mainly as a beta-1 agonist increasing cardiac contractility, with beta-2 vasodilation. Typically, cardiac output increases with a decrease in systemic vascular resistance. Diastolic coronary blood flow increases with the increase in cardiac output and reduction in LV end-diastolic pressure. Systemic pressure may rise slightly due to the increase in cardiac output.

Norepinephrine is a powerful vasopressor agent and is used mainly as a last resort to maintain an adequate systemic and coronary perfusion pressure when high-dose dopamine is inadequate. Epinephrine is a powerful inotropic agent. Its propensity to cause tachycardia, arrhythmias, and ischemia limit its use in the setting of cardiogenic shock.

The lowest doses of these agents necessary to maintain adequate systemic perfusion and blood pressure should be used. Doses that are higher than necessary may have an adverse effect on heart rate, arrhythmias, myocardial oxygen consumption, coronary arterial tone, disparity in myocardial regional blood flow, and renal and peripheral perfusion.

Cardiac Glycosides

Digoxin is a weak inotropic agent with a delayed onset of action and with no clear role in the routine management of the shock patient. Acute administration is associated with alpha-adrenergically mediated coronary and systemic vasoconstriction (76). Metabolic abnormalities in the setting of shock may increase the risk of arrhythmias.

Phosphodiesterase Inhibitors

Amrinone and milrinone are agents in this class and are available for intravenous administration. These drugs inhibit cAMP-specific phosphodiesterase activity, indirectly increasing intracellular cAMP, which in turn increases myocardial contractility. These effects are additive to those of beta agonists. Unlike beta agonists, these effects are not altered by receptor density. There is greater vasodilatation with these agents than with dobutamine, with the associated risk of hypotension. The longer half-life makes dosing somewhat more complex than dobutamine, and there is a higher incidence of side effects including thrombocytopenia, fever, and gastrointestinal upset. Milrinone has a shorter half-life and causes less thrombocytopenia than amrinone.

Vasodilators

Arterial vasodilation lowers afterload, thereby reducing myocardial work and oxygen consumption while increasing cardiac output. Venous dilation lowers preload, thereby reducing pulmonary and systemic venous congestion while reducing left ventricular wall stress and thus myocardial oxygen consumption. Nitroprusside acts on both the arterial and venous circulation. It may be particularly useful when systemic vascular resistance and filling pressures are elevated and/or when mitral insufficiency is present. Nitroglycerin has a greater effect on the venous circulation and is beneficial when filling pressures are high and/or ischemia is present. Angiotensin converting enzyme (ACE) inhibitors are not generally used in this setting in the acute phase due to their prolonged duration of action. While the utility of vasodilators is proven in patients with heart failure, reduced systemic and coronary perfusion pressures limit their utility in the setting of cardiogenic shock. There is a clear role for long-term ACE inhibitor use for survivors of cardiogenic shock, as they have demonstrated survival benefit for patients with depressed LV function (77).

General Pharmacologic Approach

A common approach to the patient with an inadequate systemic arterial pressure is to initiate treatment with dopamine and increase the dose as needed to obtain an adequate systemic arterial pressure. Dobutamine may be added and titrated to achieve adequate systemic perfusion as determined by peripheral perfusion, mentation, and increase in cardiac output and urine output. If arterial pressure can be stabilized, then the dopamine dose may be reduced. Low-dose dopamine may be continued to maximize renal blood flow. However, if blood pressure remains inadequate despite high-dose dopamine, then norepinephrine may be added. Similarly, if cardiac output remains inadequate despite high-dose dobutamine, then epinephrine or milrinone may be added. If the cardiac output is low but blood pressure is maintained by a high systemic vascular resistance, careful addition of nitroglycerin or nitroprusside is indicated. Intravenous diuretics or volume should be administered as needed to maintain an optimal pulmonary arterial wedge pressure. An optimal pulmonary artery wedge pressure is the point on Starling's curve where the plateau is reached, and no further increase in cardiac output results from increasing the filling pressure. Furthermore, cardiac output must be maximized without compromising ventilation. For most patients with acute left ventricular dysfunction, this optimal pulmonary artery wedge pressure is in the range of 15–18 mm Hg.

There are special considerations for vigorously maintaining coronary perfusion pressure during reperfusion, which are discussed below.

MECHANICAL CIRCULATORY SUPPORT

Temporary circulatory support by mechanical means may play an important role in the management of cardiogenic shock (78). There are several options for circulatory support currently available. They vary in their ability to provide systemic circulatory support, coronary perfusion, left ventricular unloading, and oxygenation. In general, however, they only provide temporary support and should be used in the setting of an underlying condition amenable to correction (i.e., reperfusion with thrombolysis, PTCA, or coronary artery bypass grafting CABG) or the possibility of long-term support (i.e., bridge to transplantation).

Intraaortic Balloon Pump Counterpulsation

Synchronized intraaortic balloon counterpulsation (IABP) has become a standard component of therapy for cardiogenic shock at tertiary care centers. However, data from the GUSTO study reflect low overall rates of utilization for shock (22%) (14). Based on its proven efficacy for initial stabilization (79), it should be considered *early* in the management of any patient requiring temporary support of systemic or coronary perfusion (29,80). The ability to augment diastolic coronary blood flow while simultaneously decreasing left ventricular afterload without increasing myocardial oxygen consumption makes it superior to vasopressors. Improved coronary blood flow (Fig. 13–7) is greatest in patients with the most compromised hemodynamic status (that is, lowest basal systolic pressures) (81). The improved diastolic coronary flow and reduced left ventricular wall stress may result in reduced myocardial oxygen requirements and improved myocardial lactate extraction, effects not seen with inotropic or vasopressor therapy (29,30,79,80,82).

Early nonrandomized studies suggested that IABP reduced mortality compared with historical controls (83,84). A large cooperative study found that the majority of patients with shock that was *refractory* to pharmacologic support demonstrated clinical improvement with IABP (Table 13–1), although in this prethrombolytic study mortality re-

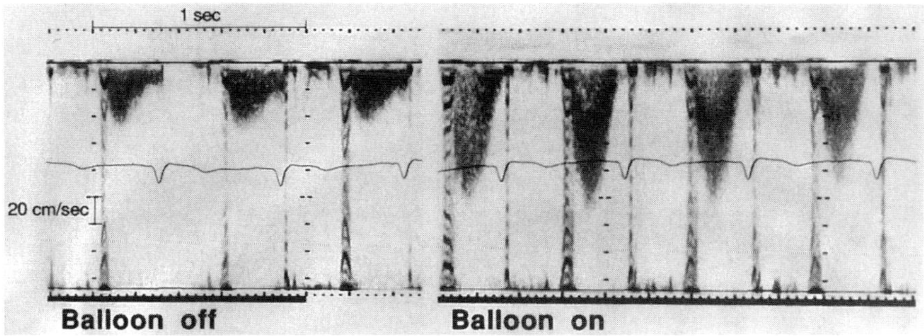

Figure 13–7. Coronary flow velocity measured in the left main coronary artery by transesophageal Doppler echocardiography in a patient with and without intraaortic balloon counterpulsation. Peak flow velocity was 45 cm/s with the intraaortic balloon pump off (**left**), and increased to 95 cm/s with intraaortic balloon pump on (**right**). Similar findings were confirmed with intracoronary Doppler measurement. *From Kern et al (81), with permission.*

mained high (79). One small randomized trial in the prethrombolytic era found no reduction in mortality (85). A recent report demonstrated an increased survival in shock patients admitted to a unit in which IABP was used frequently compared with an otherwise identical unit in which IABP was not available (38% vs. 46%, $p < 0.001$) (86). More than 40% of those patients received thrombolysis, and in recognition of the delayed recovery of stunned myocardium, counterpulsation was continued for longer periods than previous studies. The multicenter SHOCK Registry found a significantly lower mortality with the use of IABP (17). However, selection bias was evident, as patients receiving IABP support were significantly younger and more likely to be selected to undergo cardiac catheterization, which correlated strongly with survival.

Table 13–1. Intraaortic Balloon Counterpulsation (IABP) in Cardiogenic Shock: Report of a Cooperative Clinical Trial.

IABP Cooperative Trial - Refractory Shock (n = 87).

Response to IABP		
Abnormality before IABP	(n)	Improvement to Normal with IABP (%)
Oliguria (<20 ml/hr)	(46)	70%
Acidemia (pH < 7.35)	(32)	69%
Arrhythmia	(34)	68%
Abnormal Mental Status	(57)	44%

This trial assessed IABP for patients with shock that was *refractory* to vasopressors. In spite of persistent hypotension and hypoperfusion on norepinephrine, IABP temporarily normalized systemic perfusion in many cases, as demonstrated in this table. (*n*) represents the number of patients with the abnormality, and the right-hand column represents the percent of those patients that responded to IABP with normalization of the abnormality. *From Scheidt et al (79), with permission.*

Scheidt et al NEJM 1973

Despite initial enthusiasm, current data suggests that, despite the marked efficacy for initial stabilization, IABP does not improve survival in the absence of reperfusion therapy, i.e., thrombolysis, PTCA, or CABG. Conversely, data does suggest that IABP may improve outcome in patients undergoing reperfusion therapy in the setting of cardiogenic shock. Although proximal coronary flow may be enhanced by IABP, blood flow distal to subtotal coronary occlusions may not be improved (81,87,87a,87b). Recently Ohman et al demonstrated improved angiographic patency in patients randomized to routine IABP following infarct vessel PTCA in patients without shock (88). At follow-up there was a significant reduction in reocclusion (8% vs. 21%, $P < 0.03$) and in the composite clinical endpoint (death, stroke, reinfarction, revascularization, or ischemia) (13% vs. 24%, $p < 0.04$). In addition, canine studies have shown that improving coronary perfusion pressure with IABP significantly increases the rate and extent of thrombolysis (Fig. 13–8) (89), and small nonrandomized studies suggest an improved outcome in patients receiving IABP support in conjunction with thrombolytic administration (90,91). In contrast, recent preliminary data from the randomized PAMI-2 study did not demonstrate significant clinical benefit in relatively stable

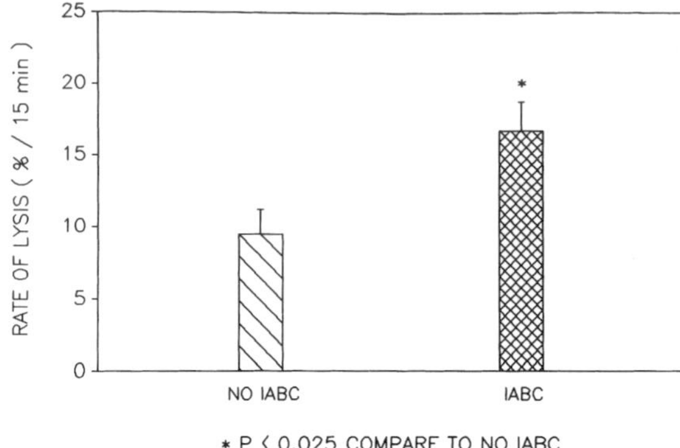

Figure 13–8. The effect of intraaortic balloon counterpulsation (IABC) on the rate of coronary thrombolysis. Dogs with a left anterior descending artery occlusion by thrombus were made hypotensive by phlebotomy. Rates of thrombolysis (% per 15 minutes) were depressed by hypotension (no IABC) and restored with IABC * ($p<0.025$). Values expressed as mean value ± SE. *From Prewitt et al (89), with permission.*

patients from routine IABP use after PTCA for acute myocardial infarction (91b) without shock.

Although bleeding and vascular complications have been relatively frequent in the past, the use of newer lower profile devices, sheathless insertion, and increased expertise has reduced these risks (80,88,90,92,93). Ohman et al (88) reported that IABP in the setting of direct PTCA for acute MI was associated with a slightly increased risk of severe bleeding (2% vs. 1%) and vascular repair or thrombectomy (5% vs. 2%).

Hemopump

The Hemopump (Medtronic) is a motor-driven turbine catheter that is advanced retrograde across the aortic valve into the left ventricle (Fig. 13–9). The device aspirates blood from the left ventricle and ejects it into the aorta, thereby decompressing the left ventricle while maintaining cardiac output (94). Flows of up to 4 L/min can be achieved with the larger device inserted by femoral cutdown, while the more recently developed, smaller percutaneous device produces lower flows. The device may be superior to IABP in terms of left ventricular unloading and circulatory support (95). Hemopump support of the systemic circulation can be maintained for prolonged periods, which is an advantage

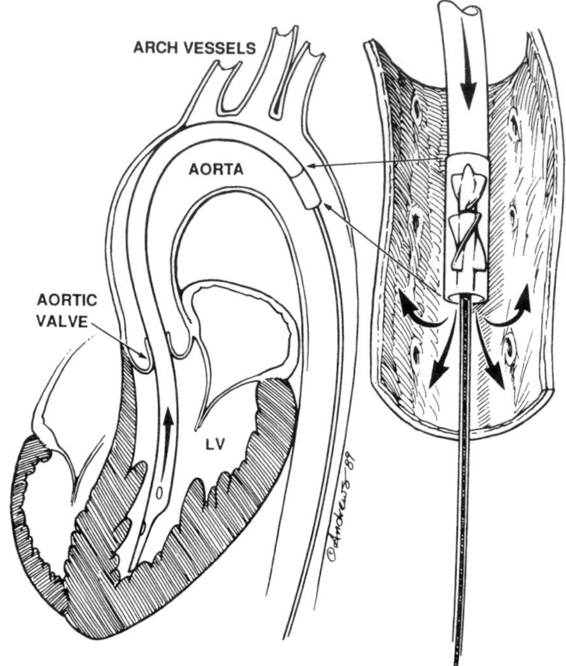

Figure 13–9. Hemopump. The device is advanced from the femoral artery retrograde to the left ventricle. A rotating turbine aspirates left ventricular blood and ejects it into the aorta using the principle of Archimedes screw. *From Duncan et al (94a), with permission.*

over cardiopulmonary bypass. Smalling et al demonstrated significant hemodynamic and functional improvement in 11 patients with cardiogenic shock complicating MI, although mortality remained high (64%) (96).

Percutaneous Cardiopulmonary Support

Cardiopulmonary support (CPS) is accomplished by percutaneous or cutdown cannulation of the femoral artery and vein with large 18F to 20F catheters. Blood is withdrawn from the right atrium through a centrifugal pump, oxygenator, and heat exchanger. Oxygenated, warmed blood passes into the femoral artery. Percutaneous cardiopulmonary support can provide up to 3 to 6 L/min of systemic blood flow even in the absence of cardiac function. Circuits mounted on mobile carts allow the institution of total circulatory support in the intensive care unit or catheterization laboratory (97–103).

Grambow et al reported a survival rate of 20% in 30 patients receiving percutaneous cardiopulmonary support following cardiac arrest or shock due to a cardiac catheterization laboratory complication (102). Overlie et al reported a registry survival rate of 48% in patients placed on percutaneous bypass within 15 minutes of circulatory collapse (103). Hill et al (100) and Phillips (101) have reported favorable results in shock patients treated with percutaneous cardiopulmonary bypass as a bridge to further therapies.

There are limitations to this modality. Although nonpulsatile coronary perfusion is maintained, as with other systemic support systems, myocardial ischemia in the territory of a severely stenotic or occluded coronary artery may not be relieved. Significant ventricular unloading is not achieved with CPS. The risks, including peripheral vascular injury and blood loss, are significant. Importantly, specialized expertise is required, and the limited duration of support possible (hours) makes it applicable only for patients in whom temporary support is required to facilitate emergency interventions such as PTCA or surgery.

Ventricular Assist Devices

Ventricular assist devices consist of prosthetic pumps that are connected in series to the heart and great vessels by cannulas, often through a sternotomy. Both pulsatile and nonpulsatile, univentricular and biventricular systems have been utilized. Left ventricular assist devices of various designs have been used in a relatively small number of patients with cardiogenic shock complicating acute infarction. Survival rates as high as 45% to 76% have been reported when used as a bridge to transplantation (104–106). The availability of donor hearts severely limits this approach.

MYOCARDIAL REPERFUSION

Spontaneous Reperfusion

Although spontaneous reperfusion of an infarct related artery is a common occurrence in MI, this occurs less often in patients with cardiogenic shock (37,107). In the Mayo Clinic series (37), subtotal or total occlusion of the infarct-related artery was demonstrated in 44/45 (98%) of patients undergoing PTCA for cardiogenic shock at varying times after complicating acute MI. In a study by Bengtson et al, 65% (50/85) of patients in shock who underwent cardiac catheterization and had not received thrombolytics had a totally occluded infarct artery (11).

Thrombolysis

Early thrombolytic treatment of acute MI has been shown unequivocally to reduce mortality and improve myocardial function (16,25,59). Late reperfusion may also exert beneficial effects on left ventricular remodeling and electrical stability. In placebo-controlled trials, the incidence of shock development was significantly reduced by thrombolytics, as is shown in Table 13–2 (9,10). In the APSAC Multicenter trial (9) thrombolysis reduced the incidence of shock within the first 24 hours from 7.1% to 6.0% (not significant) and the onset of late shock after 24 hours from 9.5% to 3.2% (p = 0.031). In the ASSET study (10) t-PA reduced the incidence of shock from 5.1% to 3.8% ($p < 0.05$). Nevertheless, patients presenting in cardiogenic shock with acute MI are less likely to receive thrombolytic therapy than other patients, and most trials of thrombolytic therapy have specifically excluded patients in cardiogenic shock (108).

The only large placebo-controlled thrombolytic study that specifically examined patients presenting with cardiogenic shock was GISSI 1 (16), which used streptokinase (SK) without adjunctive aspirin or heparin, and this study found no benefit. However, the small number—280—of shock patients leaves wide confidence limits that substantially overlap the 20% mortality reduction seen in the overall study population. Subgroup analyses initially suggested a lack of benefit in GISSI-1 in all patients with MI who had nonanterior infarction, age > 65 years, and treatment > 6 hours after symptom onset. These subset analyses have been refuted by larger studies, leaving any conclusions based on subgroup analyses questionable (108).

Other data suggest, but do not prove, a potential benefit of thrombolysis in shock patients. The ISIS-2 study reported a lower mortality rate in SK

Table 13–2. Effect of Thrombolysis on the Incidence of Subsequent Development of Cardiogenic Shock.

	Thrombolytic agent	Incidence of Shock: Thrombolysis (%)	Incidence of Shock: Heparin alone (%)	*p* value
APSAC Multicenter Trial (9)				
Shock onset <24 hours	APSAC	6.0	7.4	NS
Shock onset >24 hours	APSAC	3.2	9.5	0.031
ASSET Study (10)	t-PA	3.8	5.1	<0.05

A reduction of the incidence of subsequent development of in-hospital cardiogenic shock has been demonstrated in two randomized placebo-controlled trials comparing APSAC (anisoylated plasminogen streptokinase activator complex) and tissue plasminogen activator with heparin alone.

treated patients presenting with a systolic blood pressure under 100 mm Hg than with placebo, although many of these patients may not have met criteria for cardiogenic shock (58). In a pooled analysis of patients with a systolic blood pressure < 100 mm Hg by the Fibrinolytic Therapy Trialists, thrombolysis reduced 35-day mortality from 35% to 29% ($p < 0.01$) as shown in figure 10 (109). In the subgroup of 276 patients with hypotension and heart rate > 100, thrombolytic therapy reduced mortality from 61% to 54%. However, due to the small number of patients, these differences were not statistically significant. Although the mortality rate remained high for the thrombolytic administered group, the potential of 7 lives saved for every 100 patients treated constitutes a large absolute benefit.

In cardiogenic shock, thrombolytic administration is associated with lower rates of reperfusion and higher rates of reocclusion than in nonshock patients (110). Kennedy et al documented a lower rate of reperfusion with intracoronary streptokinase (SK) in patients with shock than for those not in shock (43% vs. 71%, $p < 0.0001$) (111). However, patients in whom reperfusion was successful had a lower mortality rate than those with persistent coronary occlusion (42% vs. 84%), with rates similar to the more recent reports of PTCA for shock (see below). There are dramatic case reports of successful intravenous thrombolysis for acute MI with left main disease (113,114). Bengtson et al (11) demonstrated a patent infarct-related artery in 33/69 (48%) patients who received thrombolysis before cardiac catheterization, and the in-hospital mortality rate was only 30% for these patients. This mortality rate was comparable with that of other modalities that resulted in a patient infarct-related artery.

Noncontrolled studies provide additional support for thrombolysis in shock (Table 13–3). The TIMI-2B trial, which used tissue plasminogen activator (t-PA) and an aggressive heparin regimen, had a 6-week mortality of 51% in shock patients (15). The GUSTO study reported a 30-day mortality of 55% in shock patients receiving thrombolysis and aggressive heparinization (14). These mortality outcomes are similar to those reported from pooled PTCA data (115) and are superior to those reported in nonthrombolysed patients (2).

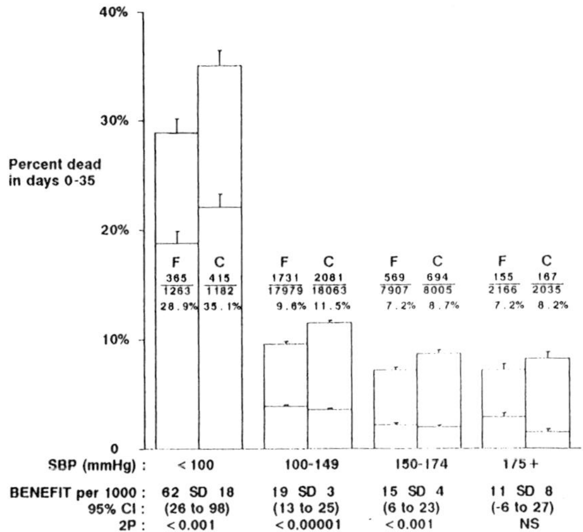

Figure 13–10. Effect of fibrinolysis on mortality in patients as a function of blood pressure at the time of treatment. This meta-analysis of all large randomized trials of fibrinolysis (F) versus control (C) found that the absolute reduction in mortality by fibrinolysis was greatest among patients with hypotension. A similar mortality reduction was demonstrated for patients with hypotension and tachycardia. (see text) *From the Fibrinolytic Therapy Trialists Group (109), with permission.*

Table 13–3. Thrombolysis and Mortality in Cardiogenic Shock.

		Mortality	
1. Society for Cardiac Angiography Registry		*Intracoronary Streptokinase (SK)*	
		Successful reperfusion	*Unsuccessful Reperfusion*
	n = 45	42%	84%
		(43% successful reperf.)	
			$p < 0.0001$
2. GISSI		*I.V. SK*	*Placebo*
	n = 281	69%	70%
		(no ASA, no Heparin, ST ↑ and ST ↓ MIs)	
3. FTT Collaborative Group		*Thrombolytic*	*Control*
	n = 276	54%	61%
		(patients with HR > 100 and BP < 100 on presentation) (ST ↑ and ST ↓ MIs)	
4. TIMI 2		*t-PA*	
	n = 193	51%	
		(ASA and heparin) (ST ↑ only)	
5. GUSTO		*t-PA or SK or t-PA/SK*	
	n = 2500	55%	
		(ASA and heparin) (ST ↑ only)	

The 4- to 6-week mortality rates are shown for thrombolytic trials. The types of MIs included in the trial, as well as selected other features of treatment, are shown. See text for full discussion of each study.

It has been suggested that low coronary perfusion pressure may slow the rate of thrombolysis in shock patients. Possible mechanisms include a reduction in pressure-dependent diffusion of thrombolytic drugs into thrombus (116,117), reduced coronary blood flow velocity, and reduced mechanical distension and diameter of collapsible coronary arteries (118,119). Studies have shown that improving coronary perfusion pressure in hypotensive dogs with either norepinephrine or IABP significantly increases the rate and extent of thrombolysis (89,120). IABP also increases the rate of thrombolysis in normotensive dogs (121). One small nonrandomized series suggests that rapid, moderate increases in low aortic pressure achieved with pressor agents or IABP combined with rapid t-PA administration may increase thrombolytic efficacy in hypotensive patients (91). A retrospective community study of patients with cardiogenic shock found a survival of 23% with thrombolysis alone, 28% with IABP alone, and 68% in patients who received both ($p < 0.005$)(90). Of interest, these authors found a lower mortality rate for shock patients who were transferred to a tertiary care center compared with those who remained at a community hospital (69% vs. 7%, $p < 0.001$) (90). Many of the former subsequently underwent PTCA or CABG at a mean of 84 hours after shock onset. Case selection confounds these data, with patients who die very rapidly not being transferred.

Adjunctive therapy has been shown to be important in improving the efficacy of thrombolysis. Aspirin has been shown to reduce reinfarction and mortality in patients given thrombolytics (59). Heparinization, when combined with t-PA, may increase sustained arterial patency (25). Recent studies suggest that newer antithrombin agents such as hirudin may result in further improvements in sustained arterial patency (122). Antiplatelet and antithrombin agents should probably be considered routine in the management of cardiogenic shock, particularly when thrombolysis is utilized.

There are few data with which to compare the relative efficacy of SK and t-PA. The ISIS-3 trial compared SK, t-PA, and streptokinase plasminogen activator complex (APSAC) and found that the rates of development of cardiogenic shock were similar (7). Subsequently, the GUSTO trial compared a more rapidly administered, front-loaded t-PA regimen with SK and found a lower incidence of the subsequent development of cardiogenic shock with t-PA (5.1% vs. 6.6%, $p < 0.05$). In contrast, GISSI-2 (123) and GUSTO (25) both found that SK was associated with a lower mortality (55% vs. 63% and 65% vs. 78%, respectively) when administered to patients presenting with cardiogenic shock. Unfortunately, all of these studies are limited by the very small number of shock patients and resultant wide confidence intervals.

Based on current evidence it is difficult to recommend one thrombolytic drug over another in the setting of cardiogenic shock. Streptokinase has potential disadvantages in that (i) hypotension may limit the rate of drug administration, (ii) prior administration may reduce the effectiveness of SK, (iii) there is a small risk of allergic reactions, and (iv) a prolonged fibrinolytic state may be of concern in the patient who may undergo PTCA or surgery. t-PA has potential advantages in that reperfusion is more rapid, and improved outcome has been demonstrated in larger patient groups with MI (25). However, the short half-life and fibrin specificity may be disadvantageous in shock, and the current data suggest a trend toward a lower mortality rate with the less fibrin-specific agent that lowers blood viscosity (streptokinase) in the setting of shock. With any agent, thrombolysis should be combined with vigorous and rapid measures to support the blood pressure and thereby facilitate reperfusion.

Although definite evidence of efficacy is lacking in the subgroup of MI patients presenting with shock, thrombolysis should be the initial reperfusion strategy, particularly in the absence of facilities for direct PTCA. Patients presenting in cardiogenic shock with acute MI should *not* be considered "ineligible" for thrombolysis.

Percutaneous Transluminal Coronary Angioplasty

Recently there has been increasing interest in the role of mechanical reperfusion for acute MI. Early (<90 minutes), complete (TIMI 3 flow grade), and sustained infarct artery reperfusion correlates highly with a lower mortality rate and improved left ventricular function (112). The importance of a patent infarct artery in determining outcome in cardiogenic shock (regardless of how patency is established) is demonstrated by Fig. 13–11 (11).

Primary PTCA for acute MI within 6–12 hours of symptoms has been demonstrated to achieve higher early TIMI 3 flow rates (80% to over 90%) than thrombolysis (26,124,125). A meta-analysis of 1,145 patients undergoing primary PTCA for acute MI reported encouraging 6-week mortality rates of 3.7% compared with 6.4% for thrombolysis (126). However, patients with shock have either been excluded or insufficiently represented in randomized PTCA trials, and the results of primary PTCA for acute MI may not be directly applicable to patients with cardiogenic shock. The PTCA success rate in shock is lower, and risks of complications are higher. PTCA is often not performed early after MI onset for cardiogenic shock, as shock most often de-

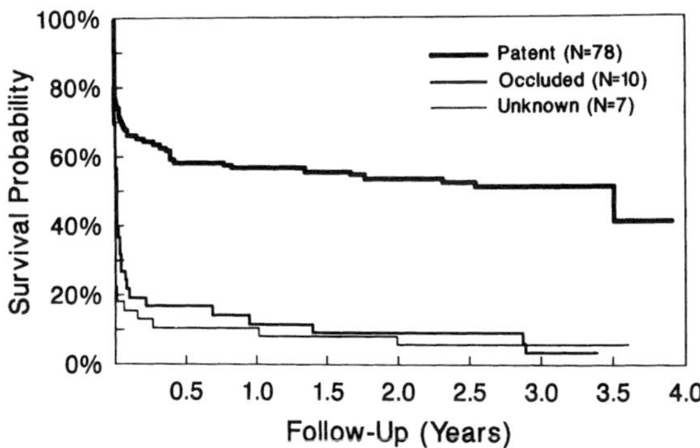

Figure 13–11. Late survival in cardiogenic shock patients discharged alive from hospital whose infarct related arteries were patent, occluded, or of unknown status. Respective mortality rates were 33%, 75%, and 84% at hospital discharge and 43%, 88%, and 88% after one year. Infarct-related artery patency was the strongest predictor of survival, regardless of the means by which patency was established, namely, spontaneous thrombolysis (47% in-hospital mortality), thrombolytic therapy (30% in-hospital mortality), PTCA (45% in-hospital mortality), or CABG (12% in-hospital mortality). *From Bengston et al (11), with permission.*

velops relatively late after MI onset. In an unselected population with shock, multivessel disease is most often present, and results of infarct artery PTCA are disappointing in this setting (see below).

Several uncontrolled, retrospective series have specifically examined the role of PTCA in shock patients. Pooled data shown in Table 13–4 (6,38–41,64,78,127–137) suggest an improved outcome with PTCA for cardiogenic shock. These series consistently demonstrated that shock patients who undergo PTCA have a lower mortality rate (i) than historical controls (38–41,64,125–135), (ii) than nonrandomized shock patients who do not undergo PTCA (38,41), (iii) if PTCA is successful than if it is not successful (38,40,64,134), and (iv) are more likely to have a patent infarct artery than thrombolysed or nonthrombolysed patients (64).

O'Neill reviewed available series and found that successful PTCA, compared with failed PTCA, is associated with a markedly improved survival rate of 73% vs. 22% (64). A multicenter registry found that the improved survival seen at 30 days in patients undergoing PTCA for cardiogenic shock was maintained at 2-year follow-up (39). The long-term survival was 54% in patients who had undergone immediate, successful PTCA and only 11% in patients in whom PTCA had been unsuccessful.

Patency of the infarct artery seems to be the critical factor associated with outcome after PTCA. A review of the Duke database found that infarct artery patency was among the most important predictors of survival, as is demonstrated in Fig. 13–11 (11). Mortality was 33% in shock patients with patent infarct arteries, regardless of how patency was achieved, versus 75% in patients with an occluded artery. Other studies have reported 1-year mortality rates of 4% to 20% in patients who underwent successful PTCA and survived to hospital discharge (38,40,41,78).

Verna et al documented that successful PTCA may lead to an immediate improvement in left ventricular function (132). These investigators reported

Table 13–4. Coronary Angioplasty for Cardiogenic Shock Complicating Acute Myocardial Infarction.

			Mortality rate (%)		
Study	# of patients	PTCA Success Rate (%)	Total (%)	Successful PTCA (%)	Unsuccessful PTCA (%)
O'Neill (64)	27	88	30	25	67
Shani (127)	9	67	33	N/A	N/A
Heuser (128)	10	60	30	17	75
Brown (129)	38	61	57	42	82
Laramee (130)	39	86	41	N/A	N/A
Lee (39)	24	54	50	23	82
Lee (40)	69	71	45	31	80
Gacioch (78)	25	72	44	22	100
Disler (131)	7	71	57	40	100
Verna (132)	7	100	14	14	0
Meyer (133)	25	88	47	41	100
Hibbard (38)	45	62	44	29	71
Moosvi (41)	38	76	47	38	78
Eltchaninoff (134)	33	76	36	24	75
Yamamoto (135)	26	62	62	44	90
Seydoux (136)	21	85	43	33	100
Himbert (6)	18	89	78	81	50
Total (%)	100	74	46	34	81
Total (n=)	451	332	207	99/293	89/110

Modified from Bates and Topol (110) and O'Neill et al (64).

Pooled data on 451 patients with cardiogenic shock who underwent PTCA during hospitalization for myocardial infarction are shown. The timing of the PTCA in relation to MI and shock onset was highly variable, ranging from less than an hour to several days.

an immediate rise in ejection fraction from 27% to 41%, a fall in left ventricular filling pressure from 26 to 18 mm Hg, and a rise in systolic pressure from 86 to 126 mm Hg. Yamamoto et al reported a similar rise in cardiac index over a 24-hour period after successful PTCA (1.9 ± 0.3 to 2.2 ± 0.6 L/min/m^2) and no improvement in those with a failed PTCA (135). Seydoux et al reported rapid improvement in hemodynamic status in 18 patients undergoing successful PTCA with continued improvement over the following day (136). Reports of resolution of ischemic mitral insufficiency following successful angioplasty indicate that this occasionally may be a reversible problem (139,140). More often, PTCA for mitral regurgitation with acute MI yields disappointing results.

It seems reasonable to expect that early reperfusion (<6 hours) would be most beneficial (141). However, Lee found no clear relationship between the timing of PTCA reperfusion and outcome. This may be a function of patient selection, with those who survive the acute phase of shock being selected to undergo cardiac catheterization and PTCA (39). Benefit was reported for PTCA performed 20 ± 32 hours after shock, and shock had developed 28 ± 30 hours after MI onset. In contrast, Moosvi et al demonstrated that early revascularization (<24 hours) after shock resulted in improved outcome compared with late revascularization (>24 hours) (41). PTCA was performed 12.4 ± 16 hours in survivors compared with 58 ± 93 hours in nonsurvivors. Since the majority of patients developing cardiogenic shock do so many hours to days after the onset of infarction (2,5,8,14–17), it is possible that many patients may have limited potential for reduction in infarct size with late reperfusion strategies. Nevertheless, recent data suggesting benefit with late thrombolysis (142) supports a potential role for late reperfusion in selected shock patients. Even delayed reperfusion without myocardial salvage may be beneficial by reducing ischemia in the peri-infarct zone or in other regions, preventing infarct extension (64,121,141), and reducing infarct expansion (142–146). Late reperfusion may be particularly beneficial after right ventricular infarction (146a–146c).

Most authorities recommend PTCA only of the infarct artery culprit lesion in patients with acute MI, with consideration given to dilation of other vessels at a later time once the patient has been stabilized. Patients with shock most often have multivessel disease, and a more aggressive approach may be appropriate for selected patients. Lee et al reported a disappointing 83% mortality in shock with multivessel disease, despite successful PTCA of the infarct artery (40). Conversely, other small series have reported favorable results in multivessel disease (38,98). Shawl and colleagues (99) attributed their favorable results in part to the relatively complete revascularization achieved with multivessel PTCA. Ellis et al suggested that early (<6 hours) and more complete reperfusion may be particularly important in multivessel disease (141). Since ischemia at a distance from the infarct zone may play an important role in cardiogenic shock (44,46,47), single-stage multivessel PTCA for more complete revascularization is an approach that is being examined as an alternative to coronary artery bypass graft surgery. The frequency of multivessel disease in shock patients limits the applicability of PTCA for cardiogenic shock.

Although encouraging, it is possible that the superior outcome described in nonrandomized reports of patients undergoing revascularization for cardiogenic shock may, in part, be related to patient selection. In general, patients undergoing PTCA in these nonrandomized series tend to be younger, be less critically ill, and have less prior myocardial damage and comorbidity (41), and are more likely to receive IABP support than controls (64). Survival data may be biased by inclusion of early deaths in the medical arm, while including only those patients who survived long enough to undergo cardiac catheterization in the revascularization arm (6,13,17). Furthermore, PTCA series only include patients whose coronary anatomy is suitable for PTCA. In the multicenter SHOCK Registry, nonrandomized patients who were selected by their physicians for cardiac catheterization were significantly younger, more often had ST elevation MI, as opposed to subendocardial, infarction (non ST elevation MI), and had a lower mortality rate than patients not selected for catheterization, even if revascularization was not accomplished. Typically, the most critically ill patients may not be taken to the cardiac catheterization laboratory, and the most unstable patients may not survive long enough to have this option. Consequently, caution must be used in interpreting the results of these noncontrolled studies. The significance of these selection biases in the prior studies is highlighted by the results of the first study of consecutive, unselected patients with cardiogenic shock early after MI onset all treated with an aggressive strategy of cardiac catheterization followed by PTCA in most (18/25) or CABG (5/25) (6). The patient characteristics in this consecutive series were representative of an unselected shock population, with 60% undergoing CPR prior to cardiac catheterization and 69% with three-vessel and 13% left main coronary disease. The in-hospital mortality was a disappointing 72%, with 13/16 (81%) of patients with successful PTCA dying.

The reported success rates of PTCA in shock patients (mean 74%, Table 13–4) are substantially lower than those reported in nonshock patients, presumably due to the combination of multivessel disease, thrombus, unstable plaque, and unstable patients with coronary hypoperfusion (38–41,64,78, 127–136). Failed PTCA may be associated with a higher mortality (147). Furthermore, extensive infarction present in shock patients is associated with loss of capillary integrity and microvascular platelet plugging, which prevent the reestablishment of normal flow (e.g., no reflow). The well-described phenomenon of no reflow may occur more often in shock. Radiographic contrast dye may induce arrhythmias, hypotension, pulmonary congestion, ischemia, and renal failure. Transient bradycardia and hypotension may complicate reperfusion of an acutely occluded right coronary artery. Embolization of coronary thrombus, reperfusion arrhythmias, and bleeding complications may occur. All of these potential complications are more serious in the patient already compromised by cardiogenic shock. In general, PTCA in the shock patient demands a high degree of technical expertise and support. Favorable results reported in the literature come primarily from high-volume centers with highly skilled operators. It is reasonable to assume that results will be less favorable in lower-volume centers with less skilled operators.

The potential for rapid, complete, and sustained reperfusion with PTCA is very appealing, and the data from nonrandomized studies suggest that PTCA is promising for reducing mortality in cardiogenic shock. Definitive data on whether there is a mortality reduction with PTCA, and if so, its magnitude, and the optimal timing of PTCA in shock, is the subject of two ongoing randomized trials, SHOCK (SHould we *emergently* revascularize Occluded Coronaries for cardiogenic shocK: an international randomized trial of emergency PTCA/CABG.) and SMASH (Swiss Multicenter evaluation of early Angioplasty for SHock following myocardial infarction). Pending the results of these trials, individual judgments should be made regarding emergency angiography soon after shock onset. Based on the coronary anatomy and the skills of the staff, individual decisions should be made on the mode of revascularization, namely, PTCA or CABG.

Increasing experience as well as newer modalities (148) and adjunctive therapies may improve the outcome associated with interventional management. Coronary stents were thought to be contraindicated in acute myocardial infarction and cardiogenic shock. However, recent information suggests that they may be an important adjunct to balloon angioplasty in selected patients (148,148a,148b). We have recently reported the initial favorable experience with the care of coronary stents in cardiogenic shock (148). Newer stent designs may incorporate antithrombotic and antiplatelet properties (148c). Recent data suggest an important role and markedly improved outcome with the use of platelet glycoprotein IIb/IIIa antagonists following angioplasty in the presence of unstable ischemic syndromes (148d).

Coronary Artery Bypass Surgery

In 1980 DeWood et al. (149) reported their favorable experience with coronary artery bypass surgery for cardiogenic shock. Although there was no overall difference in survival with surgery in this nonrandomized series, those patients who underwent surgery within 16 hours of MI onset had a lower late mortality rate than those who did not undergo surgery (25% vs. 71%, $p < 0.03$). Additional nonrandomized surgical series have reported similar favorable results compared with historical controls (11,150–157), while other series have not been so encouraging (158,159). As with the currently available noncontrolled, nonrandomized PTCA series, substantial patient selection bias is likely present. The patient who is sufficiently stable to undergo diagnostic catheterization and subsequent surgery is highly selected. Nevertheless, the available pooled data on surgery for cardiogenic shock due to pump failure (Table 13–5) (11,13,149–153, 155–169) are encouraging, particularly for the large cohort with triple-vessel disease discussed above.

Left main stenosis is generally considered an indication for coronary artery bypass surgery. Quigley reported clinical outcome in patients presenting to Duke University with "left main shock syndrome" (169). Mortality was a disappointing 94% in 16 patients who underwent salvage PTCA or CABG and 100% in 7 patients treated medically. The authors attributed these disappointing results in part to the relatively late presentation to this referral center. Others have reported a more favorable outcome in limited numbers of patients with left main disease treated with CABG and PTCA, suggesting that this condition may be amenable to revascularization if achieved promptly (170,171). While PTCA of an occluded left main coronary artery may be appropriate as a temporizing measure (Fig. 13–12), currently a patent but stenotic left main coronary is generally more appropriately dealt with by immediate surgery.

An area of considerable interest has been the use of newer cardioplegic solutions that may improve myocardial salvage and reduce the potential for reperfusion injury. Improved surgical outcome has been reported with the use of "controlled reperfusion" using amino acid–enriched warm whole blood cardioplegic solution on total vented bypass (172). These investigators reported an incredible 6% mortality in 66 patients who were in cardiogenic shock preoperatively (168). Controlled reperfusion may be

Table 13–5. Coronary Artery Bypass Surgery for Cardiogenic Shock Complicating Acute Myocardial Infarction.

			Mortality	
First author	Year	Pts.	No.	%
Dunkman (160)	1972	15	6	40
Mundth (161)	1973	33	20	61
Miller (159)	1974	12	7	58
Willerson	1975	3	2	67
Johnson (162)	1977	5	3	60
Ehrich (163)	1977	3	2	67
Bardet (164)	1977	4	2	50
O'Rourke (165)	1979	6	4	67
Subramanian (150)	1980	20	6	45
DeWood (149)	1980	19	8	42
Berg (151)	1981	19	1	5
Rosenkranz (152)	1983	23	19	83
Kirklin (153)	1985	4	0	0
Phillips (166)	1986	34	8	24
Laks (155)	1986	50	15	30
Guyton (156)	1987	9	2	22
Bolooki (157)	1989	7	3	43
Beyersdorf (167)	1990	11	6	55
Bengston (11)	1992	17	2	12
Allen (168)	1993	66	6	9
Quigley (169)**	1993	5	4	80
Himbert (6)	1994	5	2	40
Total		370	128	35%*

Modified from Bates and Topol (110).

Pooled data for 370 patients with cardiogenic shock who underwent CABG during hospitalization for myocardial infarction are shown. The timing of CABG in relation to MI and shock onset was highly variable.

*The mean reported mortality in this series is 44%.

(**Left main Stenoses only.)

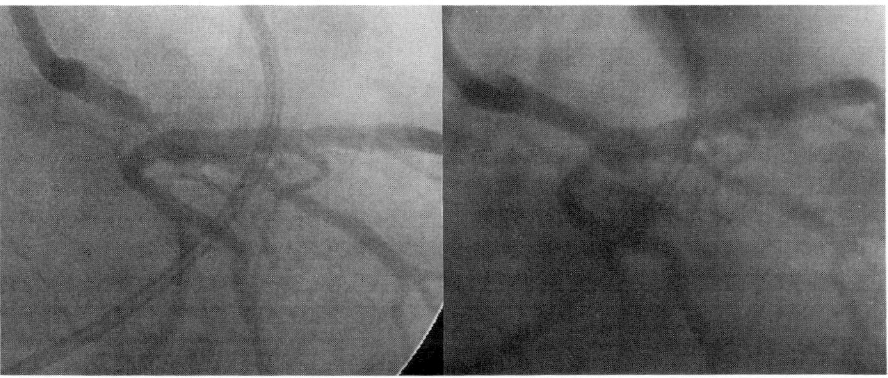

Figure 13–12. **A.**Critical stenosis of the left main coronary artery in a patient who refused surgery. **B.** With percutaneous femoral arteriovenous cardiopulmonary support, left main angioplasty and stenting was well tolerated, following which the left main artery is widely patent.

a potential advantage of surgical revascularization compared with PTCA. An additional advantage of surgical revascularization is the potential to revascularize myocardium in areas remote from the site of infarction, which may be important in the development of shock. Nevertheless, the inherent delays, high operative mortality rates, and high degree of surgical expertise required pose limitations for this therapy. Whether *emergency* CABG (or *emergency* PTCA) reduces mortality when shock complicates MI is being evaluated in the SHOCK trial.

METABOLIC SUPPORT

The importance of metabolic abnormalities in the remote, uninfarcted myocardial segments as well as within the ischemic/injured risk region have been discussed in the pathophysiology section. Experimentally, glutamate and aspartate enriched solutions with glucose, potassium, insulin, coenzyme Q, and a sulfhydryl donor have been demonstrated to improve contractility in the myocardium remote from the infarct zone (44) (Fig. 13 5). Studies of nonrandomized patients using this metabolic support solution for "controlled reperfusion" with coronary artery bypass graft surgery have demonstrated promising results.

Prior studies of glucose–insulin–potassium (G–I–K) infusions for patients with acute MI failed to show improved outcome (57). However, there are no studies combining this metabolic support with reperfusion and/or mechanical circulatory support for patients with pump failure. Ongoing work in the rabbit model of cardiogenic shock is encouraging for the potential adjunctive role of G–I–K (173).

Administration of L-carnitine results in restoration of adenine nucleotide translocase activity, which increases high-energy phosphate levels. In one favorable noncontrolled trial, an infusion administered to 27 patients with cardiogenic shock was associated with a 78% survival rate (21/27) at 10 days (174).

Although reperfusion injury does not appear to play a significant role clinically in patients with acute MI who are reperfused (175), the role of these agents, for example, free radical scavengers and inhibitors of leukocytes, has not been systematically investigated in reperfusion for cardiogenic shock complicating acute MI.

The role of agents that metabolically support ischemic tissue in the risk region and remote myocardial segments, and of agents that limit reperfusion injury in cardiogenic shock need further investigation.

FUTURE DIRECTIONS

The mortality associated with cardiogenic shock remains exceedingly high. Rapid diagnosis and initial medical stabilization are important. Patients must be identified in the early phase of left ventricular failure (preshock or early-phase shock), before frank hypotension develops. Current evidence suggests that early reperfusion is critical if outcome is to be improved. One recent study found a lower mortality in shock patients who were transferred to a tertiary care center compared with those who remained at a community hospital (7% vs. 69%, $p <$ 0.001) (90). Hospitals without special expertise or facilities for intraaortic balloon pumping, high-risk PTCA, or cardiac surgery should initiate supportive measures and simultaneously make a rapid decision regarding the appropriateness of transfer to a tertiary care facility. A decision with regard to transfer should be based on the physician's estimate of the possibility of survival coupled with patient and family wishes and expectations.

Two multicenter randomized trials are currently under way to determine whether a strategy of *emergency* early revascularization can reduce mortality associated with postinfarction cardiogenic shock. In the SHOCK trial, eligible patients are those that develop cardiogenic shock within 36 hours of infarction with less than 12 hours duration of shock. Patients are randomized to one of two strategies: (i) initial medical stabilization followed by revascularization as clinically determined, or (ii) *emergency early* revascularization. All patients receive aggressive medical management including thrombolysis (if no direct PTCA), pulmonary artery pressure monitoring, pharmacologic support, IABP, and assisted ventilation when appropriate. Patients randomized to emergency early revascularization undergo prompt diagnostic catheterization. On the basis of the angiographic findings, emergency PTCA or CABG is performed. The SMASH trial is similarly designed, with predominantly PTCA being assessed.

As cardiogenic shock complicating acute myocardial infarction is associated with extensive myocardial damage, future efforts must focus on limitation of infarct size and testing of early intervention strategies for those at risk for development of shock. In addition to the defined high-risk baseline characteristics (age, prior MI, anterior MI, and large infarction), those with lack of hyperkinesis of the remote myocardium are at risk for development of shock and may benefit from early complete revascularization.

In light of the relatively high mortality rate associated with the most favorable PTCA and CABG reports, and the even less favorable mortality rates with successful reperfusion reported in the Himbert series (6), adjunctive modalities for the treatment of cardiogenic shock must be aggressively pursued. Metabolic support the myocardium supplied by the infarct-related artery *and* the nonculprit vessels, with agents such as glucose–potassium–insulin and carnitine, are being investigated. Agents that limit reperfusion injury and prevent the no reflow phenomenon may have their greatest potential in patients with cardiogenic shock. Recent developments in coronary stenting and newer anticoagulants hold significant promise.

SUMMARY

Initial management of the patient with postinfarction shock requires rapid confirmation of the diagnosis of pump failure and exclusion of other potentially correctable conditions with a systematic, organized approach. The general approach to cardiogenic shock is shown in Table 13–6. Pulmonary artery catheterization and echocardiography should be considered routine. Initial stabilization should include prompt and aggressive respiratory support and pharmacologic hemodynamic support, most often with dopamine for hypotension. Most patients are potential candidates for intraaortic balloon counterpulsation, which should be instituted rapidly. Options for reperfusion should be rapidly assessed. Thrombolysis with IABP or direct PTCA or CABG are potential options, based on availability and individual judgment. The dismal prognosis expected with medical therapy alone suggests that patients with a reasonable possibility of survival should be considered for prompt transfer to a center with capabilities for intraaortic balloon support and coronary interventions.

ACKNOWLEDGMENTS

We thank Ann Eagan for her expert secretarial assistance, Jennifer Webb for her editing, Mark Gelernt, MD, for his assistance in review of the literature, and Angela Palazzo, MD, and Richard Fuchs, MD, for their review of the manuscript.

REFERENCES

1. ACC/AHA Task Force Report: Guidelines for the early management of patients with acute myocardial infarction. *J Am Coll Cardiol* 1990;16:249–292.
2. Goldberg R, Gore J, Alpert J, et al: Cardiogenic shock after acute myocardial infarction. Incidence and mortality from a community wide perspective, 1975–1988. *N Engl J Med* 1991;325:1117–1122.

Table 13–6. Diagnostic and Therapeutic Approach to Cardiogenic Shock.

General measures		*Diagnostic testing*
Support ventilation		ECG, CXR
Optimize intravascular volume		Pulmonary artery catheter
Aspirin, heparin		2D echo and Doppler
		Consider transesophageal echo
		Consider early cardiac catheterization
Pharmacologic support	*Mechanical support*	*Reperfusion/revascularization*
Inotropes	IABP	Thrombolysis
Vasopressors	Newer devices	PTCA
(vasodilators)		CABG

3. Killip T III, Kimball JT: Treatment of myocardial infarction in a coronary care unit: A two year experience with 250 patients. *Am J Cardiol* 1967;20: 457–464.
4. Scheidt S, Ascheim R, Killip T III: Shock after acute myocardial infarction: A clinical and hemodynamic profile. *Am J Cardiol* 1970;26:556–564.
5. Hands ME, Rutherford JD, Muller JE, et al: The in-hospital development of cardiogenic shock after myocardial infarction: Incidence, predictors of occurrence, outcome and prognostic factors. *J Am Coll Cardiol* 1989;14:40–46.
6. Himbert D, Juliard J, Steg PG, Karrillon GJ, Aumont M, Gourgon R: Limits of reperfusion therapy for immediate cardiogenic shock complicating acute myocardial infarction. *Am J Cardiol* 1994;4: 492–494.
7. ISIS-3 (Third International Study of Infarct Survival) Collaborative Group: ISIS-3: a randomised comparison of streptokinase vs tissue plasminogen activator vs anistreplsae and of aspirin plus heparin vs aspirin alone among 41 299 cases of suspected acute myocardial infarction. *Lancet* 1992; 339:753–770.
8. Leor J, Godbourt U, Reicher-Reiss H, Kaplinsky E, Behar S, and the SPRINT Study Group: Cardiogenic shock complicating acute myocardial infarction in patients without heart failure on admission: Incidence, risk factors, and outcome. *Am J Med* 1993;94:265–273.
9. Meinertz T, Kasper W, Schumacher M, Just H, for the APSAC Multicenter Trial Group: The German multicenter trial of anisoylated plasminogen streptokinase activator complex versus heparin for acute myocardial infarction. *Am J Cardiol* 1988;62: 347–351.
10. Wilcox RG, Von Der Lippe G, Olsson CG, et al, for the ASSET Study Group: Trial of tissue plasminogen activator for mortality reduction in acute myocardial infarction. *Lancet* 1988;2:525–530.
11. Bengtson JR, Kaplan AJ, Pieper KS, et al: Prognosis in cardiogenic shock after acute myocardial infarction in the interventional era. *J Am Coll Cardiol* 1992;20:1482 1429.
12. Forrester JS, Diamond G, Chatterjee K, Swan HJC: Medical therapy of acute myocardial infarction by application of hemodynamic subsets. *N Engl J Med* 1976;295:1356–1362.
13. Califf RM, Bengston JR: Cardiogenic shock. *N Engl J Med* 1994;330:1724–1730.
14. Holmes DR, Bates E, for the GUSTO investigators: Cardiogenic shock during myocardial infarction. The GUSTO experience with thrombolytic therapy (abstract). *Circulation* 1993;88:I-25.
15. Garrahy PJ, Hazlowa MJ, Forman S, Rogers WJ: Has thrombolysis improved survival from cardiogenic shock? Thrombolysis in myocardial infarction (TIMI II) results. *Circulation* 1989;80;(Suppl II):II-623.
16. Gruppo Italiano per lo Sudio della Streptochinasi nell'Infarto Miocardico (GISSI): Effectiveness of intravenous thrombolytic treatment in acute myocardial infarction. *Lancet* 1986;1:397–401.
17. Hochman JS, Boland J, Sleeper LA, et al, and the SHOCK Registry Investigators: Current spectrum of cardiogenic shock and effect of early revascularization on mortality: Results of an international registry. *Circulation* 1995;91:873–881.
18. Pasternak RC, Braunwald E, Sobel, BE: Acute myocardial infarction. In: *Heart Dis* Ed: Braunwald E., W.B. Saunders 1992;2:1228.
19. Alonso DR, Scheidt S, Post M, Killip T: Pathophysiology of cardiogenic shock: Quantitation of myocardial necrosis, clinical, pathologic and electrocardiographic correlations. *Circulation* 1973;48: 588–596.
20. Gutovitz AL, Sobel BE, Roberts R: Progessive nature of myocardial injury in selected patients with cardiogenic shock. *J Am Coll Cardiol* 1978;41(3): 469–475.
21. Page DL, Caulfield JB, Kastor JA, DeSanctis RW, Sanders CA: Myocardial changes associated with cardiogenic shock. *N Engl J Med* 1971;285: 133–137.
22. Ong L, Green S, Reiser P, Morrison J: Early prediction of mortality in patients with acute myocardial infarction: A prospective study of clinical and radionuclide risk factors. *Am J Cardiol* 1986;57: 33–38.
23. Shah PK, Maddahi J, Staniloff HM, et al: Variable spectrum and prognostic implications of left and right ventricular ejection fractions in patients with and without heart failure after acute myocardial infarction. *Am J Cardiol* 1986;58:387–393.
24. DeWood MA, Spores J, Notske R: Prevalence of total coronary occlusion during the early hours of transmural myocardial infarction. *N Engl J Med* 1980;303:897–902.
25. The GUSTO Investigators: An international randomized trial comparing four thrombolytic strategies

for acute myocardial infarction. *N Engl J Med* 1993; 329:673–682.

26. Grines CL, Browne KF, Marco J, et al: A comparison of immediate angioplasty with thrombolytic therapy for acute myocardial infarction. *N Engl J Med* 1993;328:673–679.
27. Fuchs RM, Brinker JA, Maughan WL, Weisfeldt ML, Lin FC: Coronary flow limitation during the development of ischemia. Effect of atrial pacing in patients with left anterior descending coronary artery disease. *Am J Cardiol* 1981;48:1029–1036.
28. McGhie AI, Goldstein RA: Pathogenesis and management of acute heart failure and cardiogenic shock: Role of intropic therapy. *Chest* 1992;102: 626S–632S.
29. Mueller H, Ayres SM, Giannelli S, Conklin EF, Mazzara JT, Grace WJ: Effect of isoproterenol, 1-norepinephrine, and intraaortic balloon counterpulsation on hemodynamics and myocardial metabolism in shock following acute myocardial infarction. *Circulation* 1972;45:335–351.
30. Mueller HS, Ayres SM, Gregory JJ, Giannelli S, Grace WJ: Hemodynamics, coronary blood flow and myocardial metabolism in cardiogenic shock; response to 1-norepinephrine and isoproterenol. *J Clin Invest* 1970;49:1885–1902.
31. Hochman JS, Bulkley BH: Expansion of acute myocardial infarction: An experimental study. *Circulation* 1982;65:1446–1450.
32. Hochman JS, Bulkley BH: The pathogenesis of left ventricular aneurysms: An experimental study in the rat model. *Am J Cardiol* 1982;50:83–88.
33. Erlebacher JA, Weiss JL, Eaton LW, Kallman C, Weisfeldt ML, Bulkley BH: Late effects of acute infarct dilatation on heart size: A two-dimensional echocardiographic study. *Am J Cardiol* 1982;49: 1120–1126.
34. Grossman W, Jones D, McLaurin LD: Wall stress and patterns of hypertrophy in the human left ventricle. *J Clin Invest* 1975;56:56–64.
35. Pirolo JS, Hutchins GM, Moore GW: Infarct expansion versus extension: Two different complications of acute myocardial infarction. *Am J Cardiol* 1976;37:345–351.
36. Picard MH, Wilkins GT, Gilliam LD, Thomas JD, Weyman AE: Immediate regional endocardial surface expansion following coronary occlusion in the canine left ventricle: Disproportionate effects of anterior versus inferior ischemia. *Am Heart J* 1991; 121:753–762.
37. Blumgart H, Schlesinger M, Davis D: Studies on the relation of the clinical manifestations of angina pectoris, coronary thrombosis and myocardial infarction to the pathologic findings. *Am Heart J* 1940;19:1–91.
38. Hibbard MD, Holmes DR Jr, Bailey KR, Reeder GS, Bresnahan JF, Gersh BJ: Percutaneous transluminal coronary angioplasty in patients with cardiogenic shock. *J Am Coll Cardiol* 1992;19:639–646.
39. Lee L, Bates ER, Pitt B, Walton JA, Laufer N, O'Neill WW: Percutaneous transluminal coronary angioplasty improves survival in acute myocardial infarction complicated by cardiogenic shock. *Circulation* 1988;78:1345–1351.
40. Lee L, Erbel R, Brown TM, Laufer N, Meyer J, O'Neill WW: Multicenter registry of angioplasty therapy of cardiogenic shock: Initial and long-term survival. *J Am Coll Cardiol* 1991;17:599–603.
41. Moosvi AR, Khaja F, Villanueva L, Gheorghiade M, Douthat L, Goldstein S: Early revascularization improves survival in cardiogenic shock complicating acute myocardial infarction. *J Am Coll Cardiol* 1992;19:907–914.
42. Swan HJC, Forrester JS, Diamond GA, Chatterjee K, Parmley WW: Hemodynamic spectrum of myocardial infarction and cardiogenic shock. A conceptual model. *Circulation* 1972;45:1097–1110.
43. Wackers F, Lie K, Becker A, Durrer D, Wellers H: Coronary artery disease in patients dying from cardiogenic shock or congestive heart failure in the setting of acute myocardial infarction. *Br Heart J* 1976;38:906–910.
44. Beyersdorf F, Acar C, Buchberg GD, et al: Studies on prolonged acute regional ischemia: III. Early natural history of simulated single and multivessel disease with emphasis of remote myocardium. *J Thorac Cardiovasc Surg* 1989;98:368–380.
45. Beyersdorf F, Buckberg GD, Acar C, et al: Cardiogenic shock after acute coronary occlusion: Pathogenesis, early diagnosis and treatment. *Thorac Cardiovasc Surg* 1989;37:28–36.
46. Widimsky P, Gregor P, Cervenka V, et al: Severe diffuse hypokinesis of the remote myocardium—the main cause of cardiogenic shock? An echocardiographic study of 75 patients with extremely large myocardial infarctions. *Cor Vasa* 1988;30: 27–34.
47. Berning J, Steensgard-Hansen F: Early estimation of risk by echocardiographic determination of wall motion index in an unselected population with

acute myocardial infarction. *Am J Cardiol* 1990;65: 567–576.

48. Kerber RE, Marcus ML, Ehrhardt J, Wilson R, Abboud FM: Correlation between echocardiographically demonstrated segmental dyskinesis and regional myocardial perfusion. *Am Heart J* 1984; 107:458–464.

49. Lie KI, Liem KL, Schuilenburg RM, David GK, Durrer D: Early identification of patients developing late in-hospital ventricular fibrillation after discharge from the coronary care unit. *Am J Cardiol* 1978;41:674–677.

50. Liedtke AJ, Nellis SH, Whitesell LF: Effects of regional ischemia on metabolic function in adjacent aerobic myocardium. *J Mol Cell Cardiol* 1982;1: 195–205.

51. Mudge GH, Mills RM, Taegtmeyer H, Gorlin R, Lesch M: Alterations of myocardial amino acid metabolism in chronic ischemic heart disease. *J Clin Invest* 1976;58:1185–1192.

52. Schwaiger M, Schelbert HR, Ellison D, et al: Sustained regional abnormalities in cardiac metabolism after transient ischemia in the chronic dog model. *J Am Coll Cardiol* 1985;6:336–347.

53. Folkers K, Watanabe T, Kaji M: Critique of coenzyme Q10 in biomedical research and in 10 years of clinical research on cardiovascular disease. *J Mol Med* 1977;2:431–460.

54. Theroux P, Franklin D, Ross J, Kemper WS: Regional myocardial function during acute coronary artery occlusion and its modification by pharmacologic agents in the dog. *Circ Res* 1974;35:896–908.

55. Guth BD, White FC, Gallagher KP, Bloor CM: Decreased systolic wall thickening in myocardium adjacent to ischemic zones in conscious swine during brief coronary artery occlusion. *Am Heart J* 1984; 107:458–464.

56. Sodi-Pallares D, Testelli MD, Fisleder BL, Bisteni A, Friedland C: Effects of an intravenous infusion of a potassium–glucose–insulin solution on the electrocardiographic signs of myocardial infarction. *Am J Cardiol* 1965;9:166–181.

57. Rogers WJ, Segall PH, McDaniel HG, Mantle JA, Russell RO, Rackley CE: Prospective randomized trial of glucose–insulin–potassium in acute myocardial infarction. Effects on myocardial hemodynamics, substrates and rhythm. *Am J Cardiol* 1979; 21:537–545.

58. Pissarek M, Goos H, Nohring J, et al: Beneficial effect of combined glucose–insulin–potassium and mechanical support in acute myocardial ischemia. *Biomed Biochem Acta* 1986;45:629–636.

59. ISIS-2 (Second International Study of Infarct Survival) Collaborative Group: Randomized trial of intravenous streptokinase, oral aspirin, both or neither among 17 187 cases of suspected acute myocardial infarction: ISIS-2. *Lancet* 1988;2:349–360.

60. Holmes DR, Berger PB, Bates E, et al, and the GUSTO Investigators: Predictors of mortality in cardiogenic shock: The GUSTO experience. *J Am Coll Cardiol* (Suppl) 1995;87A:715–1.

61. Sharps DS, Onde C, Cameron B, et al: Resting peripheral blood lactate elevation in survivors of prehospital cardiac arrest: Correlation with hemodynamic, electrophysiologic and oxyhemoglobin dissociation indexes. *Am J Cardiol* 1979;44: 1276–1282.

62. Kessler KM, Kozlovskis P, Trohman RG, Myerburg RJ: Serum lactate: Prognostic marker for recurrent cardiac arrest? *Am Heart J* 1987;113:1540–1544.

63. Mavric Z, Zaputovic L, Zagar D, Matana A, Smokvina D: Usefulness of blood lactate as a predictor of shock development in acute myocardial infarction. *Am J Cardiol* 1991;67:565–568.

64. O'Neill WW, Erbel R, Laufer N: Coronary angioplasty therapy of cardiogenic shock complicating acute myocardial infarction. *Circulation* 1985; 72(suppl III):III-309.

65. Nishimura RA, Schaff HV, Shub C, Gersh BJ, Edwards WD, Tajik AJ: Papillary muscle rupture complicating acute myocardial infarction: Analysis of 17 patients. *Am J Cardiol* 1983;51:373–377.

66. Nishimura RA, Tajik AJ, Shub C, Miller FA, Ilstrup DM, Harison CE: Role of two-dimensional echocardiography in the prediction of in-hospital complications after acute myocardial infarction. *J Am Coll Cardiol* 1984;4:1080–1087.

67. Oh JK, Sinak LJ, Freeman WK, et al: Transesophageal echocardiography in patients with shock syndrome. *Circulation* 1991;78(Suppl II):II-127.

68. Dell'Italia LJ, Starling MR, Crawford MH, Boros BL, Chaudhuri TK, O'Rourke RA: Right ventricular infarction: Identification by hemodynamic measurements before and after volume loading and correlation with non-invasive techniques. *J Am Coll Cardiol* 1984;4:931–939.

69. Meister SG, Helfant RH: Rapid bedside differentiation of ruptured intraventricular septum from acute mitral insufficiency. *N Engl J Med* 1972;287: 1024–1025.

70. Morrow AG, Cohen LS, Roberts WC, Braunwald NS, Braunwald E: Severe mitral regurgitation following acute myocardial infarction and ruptured papillary muscle: Hemodynamic findings and results of operative treatment in four patients. *Circulation* 1968;37(Suppl II):II-124–II-132.

71. Fuchs RM, Heuser RR, Yin FC, Brinker JA: Limitations of pulmonary wedge V waves in diagnosing mitral regurgitation. *Am J Cardiol* 1982;49: 849–854.

72. Scheinman MN, Brown MA, Rapaport E: Critical assessment of use of central venous oxygen saturation as a mirror of mixed venous oxygen in severely ill cardiac patients. *Circulation* 1969;40:165–172.

73. Kasnitz P, Druger GL, Yorra F, Simmons DH: Mixed venous oxygen tension and hyperlactemia: Survival in severe cardiopulmonary disease. *JAMA* 1976;236:570–574.

74. da Luz PL, Cavanilles JM, Michaels C, Weil MH, Shubin H: Oxygen delivery, anoxic metabolism and hemoglobin–oxygen affinity (P_{50}) in patients with acute myocardial infarction and shock. *Am J Cardiol* 1975;36:148–154.

75. Yang SC, Puri VK, Raheja R: Oxygen delivery and consumption and P_{50} in patients with acute myocardial infarction. *Circulation* 1986;73:1183–1185.

76. Hamlin NP, Willerson JT, Garan H, Powell WR Jr: The neurogenic vasoconstrictor effect of digitalis on coronary vascular resistance. *J Clin Invest* 1974; 53:288–296.

77. Pfeffer MA, Braunwald E, Moye LA: Effect of captopril on mortality and morbidity in patients with left ventricular dysfunction after myocardial infarction—results of the Survival and Ventricular Enlargement Trial. *N Engl J Med* 1992;327:669–676.

78. Gacioch GM, Ellis SG, Lee L, et al: Cardiogenic shock complicating acute myocardial infarction: The use of coronary angioplasty and the integration of the new support devices into patients management. *J Am Coll Cardiol* 1992;19:647–653.

79. Scheidt S, Wilner G, Mueller H, et al: Intra-aortic balloon counterpulsation in cardiogenic shock: Report of a cooperative clinical trial. *N Engl J Med* 1973;288:979–984.

80. Nanas JN, Moulopoulos SD: Counterpulsation: Historical background, technical improvements, hemodynamic and metabolic effects. *Cardiology* 1994;84:156–167.

81. Kern MJ, Aguirre FV, Tatineni S, et al: Enhanced coronary blood flow velocity during intraaortic balloon counterpulsation in critically ill patients. *J Am Coll Cardiol* 1993;21:359–368.

82. Mueller H, Ayres SM, Conklin EF, et al: The effects of intra-aortic balloon counterpulsation on cardiac performance and metabolism in shock associated with acute myocardial infarction. *J Clin Invest* 1971;50:1885–1900.

83. Kantrowitz A, Tjonneland S, Krakauer JS, Phillips SJ, Freed PS, Butner AN: Mechanical intra-aortic cardiac assistance in cardiogenic shock: Hemodynamic effects. *Arch Surg* 1968;97:100–104.

84. O'Rourke M, Chang H, Windsor H, et al: Acute severe cardiac failure complicating myocardial infarction. Experience with 100 patients referred for consideration of mechanical left ventricular assistance. *Br Heart J* 1975;37:169–181.

85. O'Rourke MF, Norris RM, Campbell TJ, Chang VP, Sammel NL: Randomized controlled trial of intraaortic balloon counterpulsation in early myocardial infarction with acute heart failure. *Am J Cardiol* 1981;47:815–820.

86. Waksman R, Weiss AT, Gotsman MS, Hasin Y: Intra-aortic balloon counterpulsation improves survival in cardiogenic shock complicating acute myocardial infarction. *Eur Heart J* 1993;14:71–74.

87. Hutchinson SJ, Thaker KB, Chandraratna PA: Effects of balloon counterpulsation on flow velocity in stenotic left main coronary arteries from transesophageal echocardiography. *Am J Cardiol* 1994; 74:1063–1065.

87a. Kimura A, Toyota E, Songfang L, Goto M, Yada T, Chiba Y, Ebata J, Tachibana H, Ogasawara Y, Tsujioka K, Kajiya F: Effects of intraaortic balloon pumping on the septal arterial blood flow velocity waveform during severe left main coronary artery stenosis. *J Am Coll Cardiol* 1996;27:810–816.

87b. Williams DO: Intraaortic balloon counterpulsation: deciphering its effects on coronary flow. *J Am Coll Cardiol* 1996;27:817–818.

88. Ohman EM, George BS, White CJ, et al: Use of aortic counterpulsation to improve sustained coronary artery patency during acute myocardial infarction. Results of a randomized trial. The Randomized IABP Study Group. *Circulation* 1994;90:792–799.

89. Prewitt RM, Gu S, Schick U, Ducas J: Intraaortic balloon counterpulsation enhances coronary thrombolysis induced by intravenous administration of a thrombolytic agent. *J Am Coll Cardiol* 1994;23:794–798.

90. Stomel RJ, Rasak M, Bates ER: Treatment strategies for acute myocardial infarction complicated by cardiogenic shock in a community hospital. *Chest* 1994;105:997–1002.

91. Garber PJ, Mathieson AL, Ducas J, Patton JN, Geddes JS, Prewitt RM: Thrombolytic therapy in cardiogenic shock: Effect of increased aortic pressure and rapid tPA administration. *Can J Cardiol* 1995;1(1):30–36.

91a. Griffin J, Grines C, Marsalese D, et al: A prospective randomized trial evaluating early the prophylactic use of balloon pumping in high risk patients with myocardial infarction: PAMI-2. *J Am Coll Cardiol* 1995;Feb:86A.

92. Mueller HS: Role of intra-aortic counterpulsation in cardiogenic shock and acute myocardial infarction. *Cardiology* 1994;84:168–174.

93. Silverman AJ, Williams AM, Wetmore WR, Stomel RJ: Complications of intra-aortic balloon pump counterpulsation in patients receiving thrombolytic therapy for acute myocardial infarction. *J Intervent Cardiol* 1991;4:49–52.

94. Wampler RK, Baker BA, Wright WM: Circulatory support of cardiac interventional procedures with the Hemopump cardiac assist system. *Cardiology* 1994;84:194–201.

94a. Duncan JM, Frazier OH, Radovancevic B, Velebit V: Implantation techniques for the Hemopump. *Ann Thorac Surg* 1989;48:733–735.

95. Smalling RW, Cassidy DB, Barrett R, Lachterman B, Felli P, Amirian J: Improved regional myocardial blood flow, left ventricular unloading and infarct salvage using an axial flow, transvalvular left ventricular assist device: A comparison with intra-aortic balloon counterpulsation and reperfusion alone in a canine infarction model. *Circulation* 1992;85:1152–1159.

96. Smalling RW, Sweeney M, Lachterman B, et al: Transvalvular left ventricular assistance in cardiogenic shock secondary to acute myocardial infarction. *J Am Coll Cardiol* 1994;23:637–644.

97. Tomaso CL: Use of percutaneously inserted cardiopulmonary bypass in the cardiac catheterization laboratory. *Cathet Cardiovasc Diagn* 1990;20:32–38.

98. Shawl F, Domanski M, Hernandez T, Punja S: Emergency percutaneous cardiopulmonary bypass support in cardiogenic shock from acutemyocardial infarction. *Am J Cardiol* 1989;64:967–980.

99. Vogel R, Shawl F, Tommanso CL, et al: Initial report of the national registry of elective cardiopulmonary bypass supported coronary angioplasty. *J Am Coll Cardiol* 1990;15:23–29.

100. Hill JG, Bruhn PS, Cohen SE, et al: Emergent applications of cardiopulmonary support: A multi-institutional experience. *Ann Thorac Surg* 1992;54: 699–704.

101. Phillips SJ: Resuscitation from cardiogenic shock with extracorporeal membrane oxygen systems. *Sem Thorac Cardiovasc Surg* 1994;6:131–135.

102. Grambow DW, Deeb GM, Pavlides GS, Margulis A, O'Neill WW, Bates ER: Emergent percutaneous cardiopulmonary bypass in patients having cardiovascular collapse in the cardiac catheterization laboratory. *Am J Cardiol* 1994;73:872–875.

103. Overlie PA, Walter PD, Hurd HP II, et al: Emergency cardiopulmonary support with cardiopulmonary support devices. *Cardiology* 1994;84: 231–237.

103a. Harrington JC, Teirstein PS: Cardiopulmonary support for complex angioplasty. *J Interven Cardiol* 1995;8:249–255.

103b. Overlie PA. Emergency use of cardiopulmonary bypass. *J Interven Cardiol* 1995;8:239–247.

104. Farrar DJ, Lawson JH, Litwak P, Cederwall G: Thoratec VAD system as a bridge to heart transplantation. *J Heart Transplant* 1990;9:415–423.

105. Miller CA, Pae WE, Pierce WS: Combined registry for the clinical use of mechanical ventricular assist devices. Postcardiotomy cardiogenic shock. *Trans Am Soc Artif Intern Organs* 1990;34:43–46.

106. Moritz A, Wolner E: Circulatory support with shock due to acute myocardial infarction. *Ann Thorac Surg* 1993;55:238–244.

106a. Macris MP, Frazier OH: Progress in the development of mechanical circulatory support devices. *ACC Curr J Review* 1995;4:47–50.

107. Becker RC: Hemodynamic, mechanical, and metabolic determinants of thrombolytic efficacy; a theoretic framework for assessing the limitations of thrombolysis in patients with cardiogenic shock. *Am Heart J* 1993;125:919–929.

108. Col N, Gurwitz J, Alpert J, Goldberg R: Frequency of inclusion of patients with cardiogenic shock in trials of thrombolytic therapy. *Am J Cardiol* 1994;73:149–157.

109. Fibrinolytic Therapy Trialists (FTT) Group: Indications for fibrinolytic therapy in suspected acute myocardial infarction: Collaborative overview of early mortality and major morbidity results from

all randomized trials of more than 1000 patients. *Lancet* 1994;343:311–322.

110. Bates E, Topol E: Limitations of thrombolytic therapy for acute myocardial infarction complicated by congestive heart failure and cardiogenic shock. *J Am Coll Cardiol* 1991;18:1077–1084.

111. Kennedy JW, Gensini GG, Timmis GC, Maynar C: Acute myocardial infarction treated with intracoronary streptokinase: A report of the Society for Cardiac Angiography. *Am J Cardiol* 1985;55: 871–877.

112. Fajadet J, Brunel P, Jordan C, Cassagneau B, Maro J: Is stenting of left main coronary artery a reasonable procedure? *Circulation* 1995;92: I–74.

113. Lew AS, Weiss AT, Shah PK, Fishbein MC, Berman DS, Maddahi J: Extensive myocardial salvage and reversal of cardiogenic shock after reperfusion of the left main coronary artery by intravenous streptokinase. *Am J Cardiol* 1984;54: 450–452.

114. Ajosilla CE, Bell WW, Ferree J, Torre ADL: Thrombolytic therapy during acute myocardial infarction due to sudden occlusion of the left main coronary artery. *J Am Coll Cardiol* 1985;5: 1253–1236.

115. O'Neill WW: Angioplasty therapy of cardiogenic shock: Are randomized trials necessary? *J Am Coll Cardiol* 1992;19:915–917.

116. Blinc A, Planinsic G, Keber D, et al: Dependence of blood clot lysis on the mode of transport of urokinase into the clot: A magnetic resonance imaging study in vitro. *Thromb Haemost* 1991;65: 549–552.

117. Zidansek A, Blinc A: The influence of transport parameters and enzyme kinetics of the fibrinolytic system on thrombolysis: Mathematical modeling of two idealized cases. *Thromb Haemost* 1991;65:553–552.

118. Li KS, Sanatamore WP, Morley DL, Tulenko TN: Stenotic amplification vasoconstriction responses. *Am J Physiol* 1989;256:H1044–H1051.

119. Freedman B, Richmond DR, Kelly DT: Pathophysiology of coronary artery spasm. *Circulation* 1982;66:705–709.

120. Prewitt RM, Gu S, Garger PJ, Ducas J: Marked systemic hypotension depresses coronary thrombolysis induced by intracoronary administration of recombinant tissue-type plasminogen activator. *J Am Coll Cardiol* 1992;20:1626–1633.

121. Gurbel PA, Anderson RD, MacCord CS, et al: Arterial diastolic pressure augmentation by intraaortic balloon counterpulsation enhances the onset of coronary artery reperfusion by thrombolytic therapy. *Circulation* 1994;89:361–365.

122. Cannon CP, McCabe CH, Henry TD, et al: A pilot trial of recombinant desulfatohirudin compared to heparin in conjunction with tissue plasminogen activator and aspirin for acute myocardial infarction: Results of the Thrombolysis in Myocardial Infarction (TIMI) 5 trial. *J Am Coll Cardiol* 1994;23:993–1003.

123. Gruppo Italiano per lo Studio della Sopravvivenza nell'Infarto Miocardico: GISSI-2: A factorial randomised trial of alteplase versus streptokinase and heparin versus no heparin among 12 490 patients with acute myocardial infarction. *Lancet* 1990;336:65–71.

124. Zijlstra F, de Boer MJ, Hoorntje JCA, Reiffers S, Reiber JHC, Suryapranata H: A comparison of immediate coronary angioplasty with intravenous streptokinase in acute myocardial infarction. *N Engl J Med* 1993;328:680–684.

125. Gibbons RJ, Holmes DR, Reeder GS, Bailey KR, Hopfenspirger MR, Gersh BJ: Immediate angioplasty compared with the administration of a thrombolytic agent followed by conservative treatment for myocardial infarction. *N Engl J Med* 1993;328:685–691.

126. Michels KB, Yusuf S: Does PTCA in acute myocardial infarction affect mortality and reinfarction rates? A quantitative overview (meta-analysis) of the randomized clinical trials. *Circulation* 1995;91(2):476–485.

127. Shani J, Rivera M, Greengart A: Percutaneous transluminal coronary angioplasty in cardiogenic shock. *J Am Coll Cardiol* 1986;7:219A.

128. Heuser RR, Maddoux GL, Goss JE: Coronary angioplasty in the treatment of cardiogenic shock: The therapy of choice. *J Am Coll Cardiol* 1986;7: 219A.

129. Brown TM, Iannone LA, Gordon DF: Percutaneous myocardial reperfusion reduces mortality in acute myocardial infarction complicated by cardiogenic shock. *Circulation* 1985;72(Suppl III): III-309.

130. Laramee LA, Rutherford BD, Ligon RW, McConahay DR, Hartzler GO: Coronary angioplasty for cardiogenic shock following myocardial infarction. *Circulation* 1988;78(Suppl II):II-634.

131. Disler L, Haitas B, Benjamin J, Steingo L, McKibbin J: Cardiogenic shock in evolving myocardial infarction: Treatment by angioplasty and streptokinase. *Heart Lung* 1987;16:649–652.
132. Verna E, Repetoo S, Boscarina M, Ghezzi I, Binaghi G: Emergency coronary angioplasty in patients with severe left ventricular dysfunction of cardiogenic shock after acute myocardial infarction. *Eur Heart J* 1989;10:958–966.
133. Meyer P, Blanc P, Badouy M, Morand P: Treatment de choc cardiogenique primaire par angioplastie transluminale coronarienne à la phase aigüe de l'infarctus. *Arch Mal Coeur Vaiss* 1990;83: 329–334.
134. Eltchaninoff H, Simpendorfer C, Whitlow PL: Coronary angioplasty improves both early and 1-year survival in acute myocardial infarction complicated by cardiogenic shock. *J Am Coll Cardiol* 1991;17:167A.
135. Yamamoto H, Hayashi Y, Oka Y, et al: Efficacy of percutaneous transluminal coronary angioplasty in patients with acute myocardial infarction complicated by cardiogenic shock. *Jpn Circ J* 1992;56: 815–821.
136. Seydoux C, Goy JJ, Beuret P, et al: Effectiveness of percutaneous transluminal coronary angioplasty in cardiogenic shock during acute myocardial infarction. *Am J Cardiol* 1992;69:968–969.
137. Rothbaum DA, Linnemeir TJ, Landin RJ, et al: Emergency percutaneous transluminal angioplasty in acute myocardial infarction: A 3 year experience. *J Am Coll Cardiol* 1987;10:264–272.
138. Stack RS, O'Connor CM, Mark DB, et al: Coronary perfusion during acute myocardial with a combined therapy of coronary angioplasty and high-dose intravenous streptokinase. *Circulation* 1988;77:151–161.
139. Heuser RR, Maddoux GL, Goss JE, Ramo BW, Raff GL, Shadoff N: Coronary angioplasty for acute mitral regurgitation due to myocardial infarction. *Ann Intern Med* 1987;107:852–855.
140. Shawl F, Forman M, Punja S, Goldbaum T: Emergent coronary angioplasty in the treatment of acute ischemic mitral regurgitation: Long-term results in five cases. *J Am Coll Cardiol* 1989;14: 986–991.
141. Ellis SG, O'Neill WW, Bates ER, et al: Implications for triage from survival and left ventricular functional recovery analyses in 1500 patients treated with coronary angioplasty for acute myocardial infarction. *J Am Coll Cardiol* 1989;13: 1251–1259.
142. LATE Study Group: Late assessment of thrombolytic efficacy (LATE) study with alteplase 6–24 hours after onset of acute myocardial infarction. *Lancet* 1993;342:759–766.
143. Hochman JS, Choo H: Limitation of myocardial infarct expansion by reperfusion independent of myocardial salvage. *Circulation* 1987;75:299–306.
144. Brown EJ, Swinford RD, Gadde P, Lillis O: Acute effects of delayed reperfusion on myocardial infarct shape and left ventricular volume: A potential mechanism of additional benefits from thrombolysis therapy. *J Am Coll Cardiol* 1991;17: 1641–1650.
145. Hahn R, Brown R, Mogtader A, et al: Early benefits of late coronary reperfusion on reducing myocardial infarct expansion; echo findings and ultrastructural basis. *J Am Coll Cardiol* 1993;21: 301A.
146. Kemper FT, Leavitt M, Parisi AF: Acute reduction in functional infarct expansion with late coronary reperfusion: Assessment with quantitative two-dimensional echocardiography. *J Am Coll Cardiol* 1988;11:192–200.
146a. Laster S, Shelton T, Barzilai B, Goldstein J: Determinants of the recovery of right ventricular performance following experimental chronic right coronary artery occlusion. *Circulation* 1993;88: 696–708.
146b. Laster S, Ohnishi Y, Saffitz G, Goldstein J. Effects of reperfusion on ischemic right ventricular dysfunction. *Circulation* 1994;90:1398–409.
146c. Kinn GW, Ajluni SC, Samyn JG, Bates ER, Grines CL, O'Neill W. Rapid hemodynamic improvement after reperfusion during right ventricular infarction. *J Am Coll Cardiol* 1995;26:1230–4.
147. Abbotsmith CW, Topol EJ, George BS, et al: Fate of patients with acute myocardial infarction with patency of the infarct-related vessel achieved with successful thrombolysis versus rescue angioplasty. *J Am Coll Cardiol* 1990;16:770–778.
148. Ahmad T, Webb J, Carere R, Dodek A: Stenting for acute myocardial infarction. *Am J Cardiol* 1995;76:77–80.
148a. Garcia-Cantu E, Spaulding C, Corcos T, Ben Hamda K, Roussel L, Favereau X, Guerin Y, Chalet Y, Souffrant G, Guerin F. Stent implantation in acute myocardial infarction. *Am J Cardiol* 1996;77:451–454.

148b. Webb JG, Carere RG, Hilton JD, Buller E, Rabinowitz A, Dodek AA. Coronary stenting for cardiogenic shock. (in press).

148c. Williams DO. Dressing up the Palmaz-Schatz stent. *Circulation* 1996;93:400–402.

148d. Ferguson JJ. EPILOG and CAPTURE trials halted because of positive interim results. *Circulation* 1996;93:637.

149. DeWood M, Notske R, Hensley G, et al: Intraaortic balloon counterpulsation with and without reperfusion for myocardial infarction shock. *Circulation* 1980;61:1105–1112.

150. Subramanian VA, Roberts AJ, Zema MJ, et al: Cardiogenic shock following acute myocardial infarction: Late functional results after emergency cardiac surgery. *NY State J Med* 1980;80: 947–952.

151. Berg R, Selinger S, Leonard J, Grunwald R, O'-Grady W: Immediate coronary artery bypass surgery for acute evolving myocardial infarction. *J Thorac Cardiovasc Surg* 1981;81:493–497.

152. Rosenkranz ER, Buckberg GD, Laks H, Mulder DG: Warm induction of cardioplegia with glutamate-enriched blood in coronary patients who are dependent on inotropic drugs and intra-aortic balloon support. *J Thorac Cardiovasc Surg* 1983;86: 507–518.

153. Kirklin JK, Blackstone EH, Zorn GL, et al: Intermediate-term results of coronary artery bypass grafting for acute myocardial infarction. *Circulation* 1985;72(Suppl II):II-175–II-178.

154. Phillips S, Kongtahvam C, Slanner J, Zeff M: Emergency coronary artery reperfusion: A choice for evolving myocardial infarction: Results in 339 patients. *J Thorac Cardiovasc Surg* 1983;86: 679–688.

155. Laks H, Rosenkranz E, Buckerg GD: Surgical treatment of cardiogenic shock after myocardial infarction. *Circulation* 1986;74:(Suppl III):III-11–III-16.

156. Guyton RA, Arcidi JM, Langford DA, Morris DC, Liberman HA, Hatcher CR: Emergency coronary artery bypass for cardiogenic shock. *Circulation* 1987;76(Suppl V):V-22–V-27.

157. Bolooki H: Emergency cardiac procedures in patients in cardiogenic shock due to complications of coronary artery disease. *Circulation* 1989; 79(Suppl I):I-137–I-148.

158. Willerson JT, Curry GC, Watson JT, et al: Intraaortic balloon counterpulsation in patients in cardiogenic shock, medically refractory left ventricular failure and/or recurrent ventricular tachycardia. *Am J Med* 1975;58:183–191.

159. Miller MG, Hedley-Whyte J, Weintraub RM, Restall DS, Alexander M: Surgery for cardiogenic shock. *Lancet* 1974;1:1342–1345.

160. Dunkman W, Leinbach R, Buckley M, et al: Clinical and hemodynamic results of intra-aortic balloon pumping and surgery for cardiogenic shock. *Circulation* 1972;46:465–477.

161. Mundth ED, Buckley MJ, Leinbach RC, Gold HK, Daggett WM, Austen WG: Surgical intervention for the complications of acute myocardial ischemia. *Ann Surg* 1973;178:379–388.

162. Johnson S, Scanlon P, Loeb H, Moran J, Pifarre R, Gunnar R: Treatment of cardiogenic shock in myocardial infarction by intra-aortic counterpulsation and surgery. *Am J Med* 1977;62: 687–692.

163. Ehrich DA, Biddle TL, Kronenberg MW, Yu PN: The hemodynamic response to intra-aortic balloon counterpulsation in patients with cardiogenic shock complicating acute myocardial infarction. *Am Heart J* 1977;93:274–279.

164. Bardet J, Masquet C, Khan J-C, et al: Clinical and hemodynamic results of intra-aortic balloon counterpulsation and surgery for cardiogenic shock. *Am Heart J* 1977;93:598–604.

165. O'Rourke MF, Sammel N, Chang VP: Arterial counterpulsation in severe refractory heart failure complicating acute myocardial infarction. *Br Heart J* 1979;41:308–316.

166. Phillips SJ, Zeff RH, Skinner JR, Toon RS, Grignon A, Kongtahworn C: Reperfusion protocol and results in 738 patients with evolving myocardial infarction. *Ann Thorac Surg* 1986;41: 119–125.

167. Beyersdorf F, Sarai K, Wendt T, Eckel L, Schneider M, Kubitzky W: Prolonged abnormalities of LV regional wall motion after normal reperfusion of patients with preoperative cardiogenic shock. *J Thorac Cardiovasc Surg* 1990;38:165–174.

168. Allen BS, Buckberg GD, Fontan FM, et al: Superiority of controlled surgical reperfusion versus percutaneous transluminal coronary angioplasty in acute coronary occlusion. *J Thorac Cardiovasc Surg* 1993;105:864–883.

169. Quigley RL, Milano CA, Smith R, White WD, Rankin JS, Glower DD: Prognosis and management of anterolateral myocardial infarction in patients with severe left main disease and cardio-

genic shock. The left main shock syndrome. *Circulation* 1993;88(Pt 2):65–70.

170. Lijoi A, Della Rovere F, Passerone GC, et al: Emergency surgical treatment for total left main coronary artery occlusion. A report of 2 cases. *Texas Heart J* 1993;20:58–59.

171. Spiecher M, Erbel R, Rupprecht HJ, Meyer J: Emergency angioplasty of totally occluded left main coronary artery in acute myocardial infarction and unstable angina pectoris—institutional experience and literature review. *Eur Heart J* 1994;15:602–607.

172. Beyersdorf F, Acar C, Buckberg GD, et al: Studies on prolonged acute regional ischemia: V. Metabolic support of remote myocardium during left ventricular power failure. *J Thorac Cardiovasc Surg* 1989;98:567–579.

173. Coven DL, Suter TM, Eberli FR, Apstein CS: Dobutamine and glucose–insulin–potassium (GIK) improve cardiac function and survival in a randomized trial of experimental cardiogenic shock. *Circulation* 1994;90(Suppl I):I-480.

174. Kloner RA: Does reperfusion injury exist in humans? *J Am Coll Cardiol* 1993;21:537–545.

175. Corbucci GG, Loche F: L-carnitine in cardiogenic shock therapy: Pharmacodynamic aspects and clinical data. *Int J Clin Pharm Res* 1993;13(2): 87–91.

14

Tachyarrhythmias During Acute Myocardial Infarction

Alan Woelfel, MD, and Leonard S. Gettes, MD

BASIC ELECTROPHYSIOLOGY OF ACUTE ISCHEMIA

Acute myocardial ischemia consists of three components: (i) the acute interruption of coronary arterial blood flow, which leads to anaerobic metabolism and depletion of the high-energy phosphates—creatine phosphate and ATP; (ii) the absence of venous washout, which leads to accumulation of the end products of anaerobic metabolism—lactate, phosphate, potassium, carbon dioxide, adenosine, and lysophosphoglycerides; and (iii) the local release of sympathetic and parasympathetic neurotransmitters, which leads to accumulation of sympathetic amines within the ischemic zone. These events produce alterations in myocardial electrophysiologic properties capable of causing single ectopic beats as well as sustained tachyarrhythmias in response to each of the recognized mechanisms of arrhythmogenesis: reentry, abnormal automaticity, and triggered activity.

In this section, we will discuss the various local consequences of acute myocardial ischemia, explain how these alter electrical properties of the myocardium, and relate these alterations to the different mechanisms responsible for tachyarrhythmias. The intent is not to describe in detail the many studies that have contributed to our current level of understanding. The interested reader is referred to recent reviews for this information (1–4). Rather, the intent is to provide a conceptual framework that we hope will aid in understanding the electrical events that result in cardiac arrhythmias when a portion of the heart is acutely deprived of its arterial blood supply.

Ionic and Metabolic Consequences of Acute Ischemia

The arrhythmogenicity of acute coronary occlusion can be attributed in large part to the intracellular and extracellular changes that result from the hydrolysis and depletion of high-energy phosphates induced by anoxia and lack of metabolic substrate, and the accumulation of the end products of anaerobic metabolism in the extracellular space. These changes are listed in Table 14–1, and their time course is shown in Fig. 14–1. Examination of Fig. 14–1 reveals that creatine phosphate falls rapidly and ATP decreases more slowly, with 50% of the total ATP pool depleted by 10 minutes (3). Intracellular pH (pH_i) falls monotonically (5,6) and is paralleled by the fall in extracellular pH (pH_e) (1) and the rise in pCO_2 (not shown). Intracellular cal-

Table 14–1. Ionic and Metabolic Consequences of Acute Myocardial Ischemia

Intracellular Changes	Extracellular Changes
↓ Creatine phosphate	↑ Potassium
↓ ATP	↓ pH
↓ pH	↑ Lactate, carbon dioxide
↑ Calcium	↑ Lysophosphoglycerides
	↑ Catecholamines
	↑ Adenosine

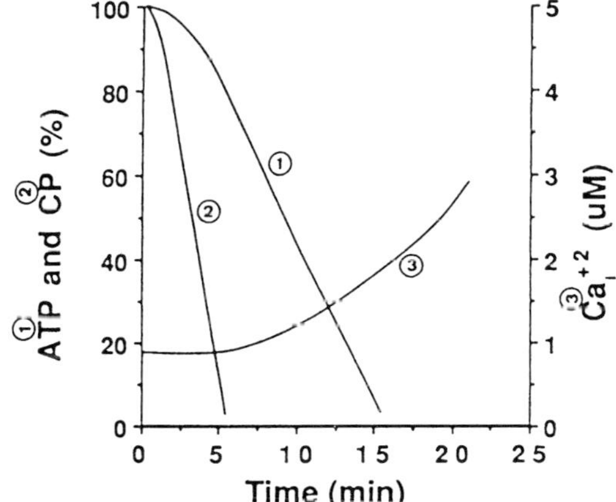

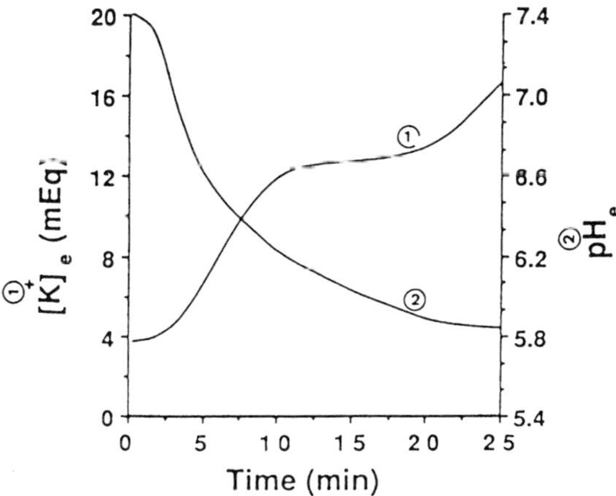

Figure 14–1. Top, Changes in ATP (1), creatine phosphate (2), and intracellular calcium, Ca_I^{2+} (3) that occur within minutes of coronary occlusion. **Bottom,** Changes in extracellular potassium (1) and pH (2) occurring over the same time interval.

cium (Ca_i) as determined by NMR spectroscopy rises over 10 to 20 minutes (7,8,8a) although information obtained using fluorescent dye techniques (9,10) suggests that the changes may occur more rapidly. The changes in extracellular potassium are triphasic (11). Potassium rises within seconds of the acute occlusion and reaches levels in excess of 10 mM within 5 to 10 minutes. A plateau phase lasting approximately 15 to 20 minutes follows, which corresponds to and may be associated with the rise in catecholamines in the extracellular space (12). In the third phase, potassium rises again as a result of cell death and loss of membrane integrity when extracellular and intracellular pH have fallen to approximately 6.0.

Myocardial Electrical Properties and Arrhythmogenesis in Acute Ischemia

The ionic and metabolic changes just described produce alterations in the electrophysiologic properties of individual myocardial fibers, which are shown in Table 14–2. Slowing in intraventricular conduction associated with acute ischemia is due to a decrease in the maximum rate of rise of the upstroke of the action potential (V_{max}) and depression of cell-to-cell transmission of the action potential, termed *cellular uncoupling*. The decrease in V_{max} occurs primarily as a result of the decrease in resting

Table 14–2. Effects of Ionic and Metabolic Changes on Electrophysiologic Properties

↑ Potassium	↓ RMP; ↓ $\dot{V}_{max}$ and prolonged recovery of $\dot{V}_{max}$; ↓ APD
↓ pO_2	↓ APD; accentuates effects of ↑ potassium on $\dot{V}_{max}$ and recovery of $\dot{V}_{max}$; cellular uncoupling
↓ pH	Accentuates effects of ↑ potassium on RMP, $\dot{V}_{max}$, and recovery of $\dot{V}_{max}$; cellular uncoupling
↑ Calcium	Cellular uncoupling; contributes to APD shortening; after potentials
↓ ATP	Contributes to ↑ potassium and to APD shortening
↑ Catecholamines	Contributes to APD shortening and to triggered activity

APD = action potential duration, RMP = resting membrane potential.

membrane potential induced by the rise in extracellular potassium (13,14). Cellular uncoupling is due primarily to intracellular acidosis and the increase in intracellular calcium (15–17); however, decreases in pO_2 and extracellular pH and the accumulation of lysophosphoglycerides also contribute to the decrease in V_{max} and promote cellular uncoupling (1,18–21). Thus the slowing of conduction is greater than would be expected from the increase in extracellular potassium alone (11,22). Slowing of conduction also becomes more pronounced as the heart rate increases (Fig. 14–2) (23,24). This rate dependence of the conduction slowing is independent of any further increase in extracellular K and more likely relates to rate-dependent changes in intracellular sodium (25) and calcium (26), and to rate-dependent increases in coupling resistance (27). This rate-dependent component of the conduction slowing is an important factor contributing to the development of reentry.

The initial change in refractoriness is a shortening of the refractory period within the ischemic zone due to shortening of the action potential duration. This shortening reflects an increase in potassium currents induced by hypoxia (28,29), increased extracellular potassium (30), and decreased intracellular ATP (31). Within minutes, the refractory period lengthens in spite of the shortening of the action potential duration. This is referred to as time-dependent refractoriness, and it is attributed primarily to prolongation of the time required for V_{max} to regain its steady-state value after a preceding depolarization (14). The fall in extracellular pH and pO_2 (20) and the decrease in resting potential induced by the rise in extracellular potassium (14) also contribute to this effect.

The changes in conduction and refractoriness produced by acute coronary occlusion are not uniform throughout the area of involved myocardium. Figure 14–3 shows inhomogeneities in extracellular

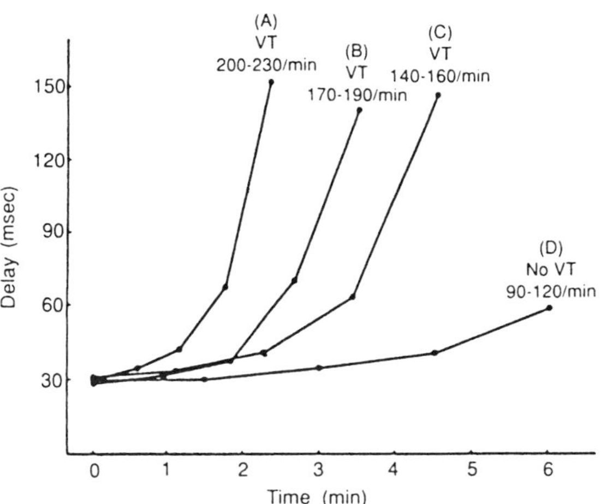

Figure 14–2. Activation delay in the center of the ischemic zone recorded at four different paced rates after coronary occlusion in the dog. The activation delay occurs earlier and is of greater magnitude as the rate is increased. The onset of ventricular tachycardia (VT) is associated with a critical activation delay of approximately 150 milliseconds. *Reproduced from Hope et al. (23), with permission.*

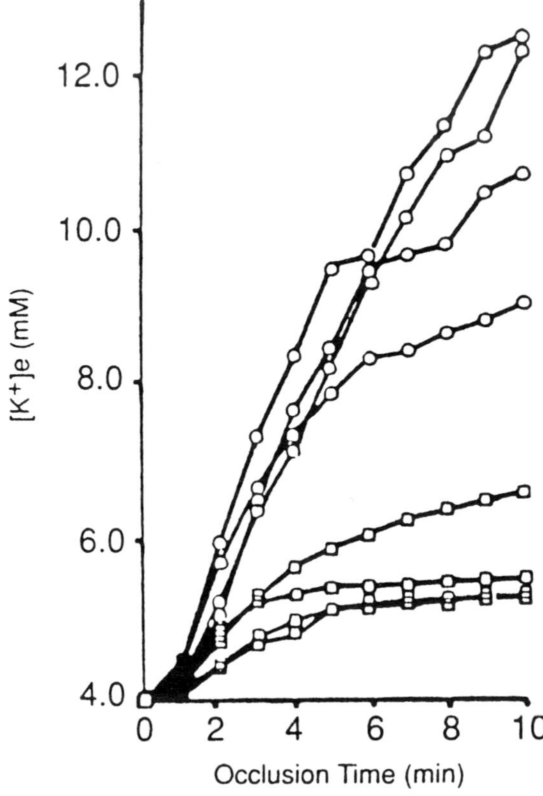

Figure 14–3. Changes in interstitial extracellular potassium recorded simultaneously by four closely spaced potassium-sensitive electrodes positioned in the mid-myocardium of the center of the ischemic zone (upper tracings) and four closely spaced potassium-sensitive electrodes positioned in the lateral border zone (lower tracings). The figure illustrates the inhomogeneities in extracellular potassium that occur within the first 10 minutes of coronary occlusion.

potassium recorded in the center and at the margin of the ischemic zone (11). Similar observations have been made with respect to changes in pH (1). These inhomogeneities probably result from different rates of ATP hydrolysis within the ischemic zone (3) and from variable diffusion of the end products of anaerobic metabolism—particularly potassium and carbon dioxide—across the borders of the ischemic zone (32). The inhomogeneities illustrated in Fig. 14–3 produce differences in resting membrane potential, V_{max}, and action potential duration within the ischemic zone. These, in turn, result in inhomogeneities in conduction and refractoriness that are important to arrhythmogenesis.

The electrophysiologic alterations discussed thus far are fundamental to the development of reentrant arrhythmias, which require a critical balance of refractoriness and conduction slowing to become manifest. It is also important that these alterations be inhomogeneous, to create areas of unidirectional conduction block that are crucial to the formation of reentry circuits (2,32). Spontaneous reentry has been documented at the lateral and subendocardial margins and within the center of the ischemic zone (1,33). Of particular importance in this regard is the finding that areas exist along the ischemic margins where, because of differences in diffusion, potassium is increased but pH has not changed significantly (34,35). This combination of ionic changes facilitates the development of very slow conduction mediated by the slow calcium-dependent inward current (36) and may be critical to the development of reentry at ischemic margins.

Inhomogeneities may also may be a cause of arrhythmias resulting from abnormal automaticity. The inhomogeneous changes in resting potential associated with the local variability in extracellular potassium generate electrical currents termed *injury currents,* which account for the ST segment changes seen on the body surface electrocardiogram (37). These currents are capable of raising the resting membrane potential in pacemaker cells to their threshold for activation, thereby inducing a spontaneous propagated response. Injury currents may also induce pacemaker activity in nonpacemaker cells (38,39).

Triggered activity is a consequence primarily of alterations in myocardial calcium. The increase in intracellular calcium that results from acute coronary occlusion (7–10) induces an oscillatory inward current known as the transient inward current. This current is capable of causing decreases in membrane potential, termed *afterdepolarizations* (40), which follow spontaneous action potentials. If these afterdepolarizations reach threshold potential, they "trigger" one or more additional action potentials, thus generating a spontaneous premature beat or more sustained tachyarrhythmia. Catecholamines increase the amplitude of afterdepolarizations, and thus they enhance the likelihood of triggered activity occurring in the ischemic zone. Afterdepolarizations may be of particular importance in the setting of myocardial hypertrophy, a situation that by itself is known to be arrhythmogenic (41) and that when combined with ischemia is even more arrhythmogenic than ischemia alone (42). It has been shown that hypertrophy causes alterations in intracellular calcium and changes in potassium conductance that lead to lengthening of action potential duration, and that these changes facilitate the induction of both early and late afterdepolarizations (43,44).

Other Aspects of Arrhythmogenesis

Abnormal spontaneous ectopic activity during ischemia may also occur as a result of myocardial fiber stretch (45), perhaps involving abnormal automaticity as well as triggered activity (Fig. 14–4). The importance of this mechanism in the genesis of the spontaneous beats and rhythms that follow acute myocardial infarction has not been delineated, but the concept that ventricular dilation in itself may be arrhythmogenic is worthy of mention.

The transformation of single spontaneously occurring premature beats into sustained arrhythmias, ventricular fibrillation in particular, is facilitated by the alterations described earlier. The propensity for ventricular arrhythmias follows a distinctive time course. Harris (46) demonstrated in an animal model that the occurrence of ventricular arrhythmias had a triphasic pattern: frequent for the first 10 to 30 minutes after coronary occlusion, rare for the next 6 to 8 hours, and then again more frequent. It

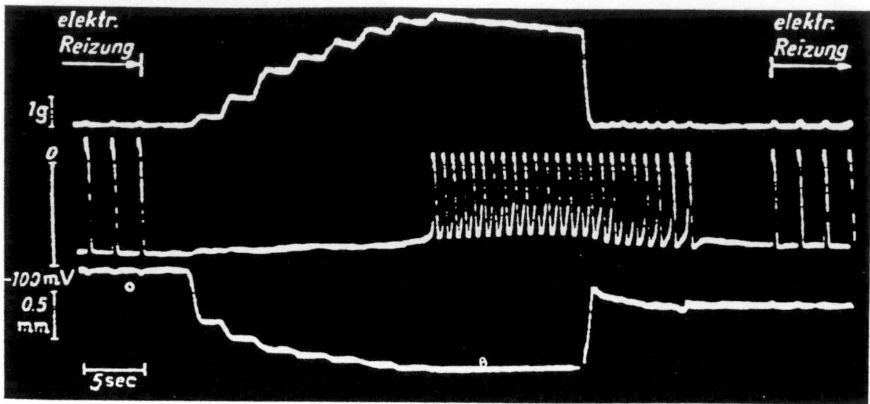

Figure 14–4. Development of spontaneous activity in monkey papillary muscle in response to stretch. Top, Stretching force in grams (g). Middle, Action potential recordings. Bottom, Changes in length of the muscle fiber. *Reproduced from Kaufman and Theophile (45), with permission.*

has been suggested that the initial arrhythmias are due to reentry and those occurring later are a manifestation of enhanced automaticity (47), but direct evidence demonstrating this mechanistic difference is lacking. Kaplinsky et al (48) subsequently showed that the first phase of arrhythmogenicity described by Harris was itself triphasic, with arrhythmias occurring frequently in the first 5 to 10 minutes after occlusion and again 10 minutes later, with a relatively quiescent period between. The precise cause of these various phases, particularly those described by Kaplinsky et al (48), is uncertain, but it is of interest that these phases correspond to the triphasic nature of the change in extracellular potassium (11), and that the 1b phase described by Kaplinsky et al (48), may relate to the onset of cellular uncoupling (49).

Sympathetic stimulation also contributes to arrhythmias after coronary occlusion. The ease of inducing ventricular fibrillation as determined by measurement of the fibrillation threshold is enhanced by sympathetic stimulation and reduced by sympathetic ablation (50). Sympathetic stimulation increases the dispersion, that is, inhomogeneity, of refractoriness (51), and the time course of this change parallels the time course of the change in the ventricular fibrillation threshold. The mechanism responsible for the inhomogeneity has not been fully determined. It is, however, known that sympathetic neurons are not distributed uniformly throughout the myocardium (52).

Coronary Reperfusion

The electrophysiologic mechanisms underlying the arrhythmias associated with coronary reperfusion are incompletely understood (53–55). It is known that these arrhythmias, which may include ventricular fibrillation, occur during a very brief period, usually within seconds of the abrupt reestablishment of coronary flow. It has been shown in experimental animals that reperfusion arrhythmias are critically related to the duration of the occlusion, rarely occurring if the occlusion lasts less than 10 minutes or longer than 30 minutes (56). The lack of response to antiarrhythmic agents that suppress ischemia-related arrhythmias (57) indicates that the electrophysiology of reperfusion differs significantly from that of occlusion. As detailed in other chapters in this volume, calcium overload and the production of oxygen free radicals occur after reperfusion (1,53) and may contribute significantly to the electrical changes responsible for these arrhythmias. There are also ionic and electrical inhomogeneities during the brief period required for them to return to their normal values after the reestablishment of coronary flow (11), which may play a role in these arrhythmias.

Subacute Arrhythmias from Myocardial Ischemia

Recurrent ischemia within the first week of infarction may cause the same sequence of events as described earlier; however, the bases for other mechanisms of arrhythmogenesis during this time period are less well understood. It has been shown that the subendocardial Purkinje fibers and several layers of endocardial muscle fibers often survive the acute ischemic event (58). The action potentials in these fibers are, however, abnormal, characterized by decreased resting potentials, slowed upstrokes, shortened plateaus, and prolonged terminal repolarization phases (58–60). In addition, there are significant anatomic and electrophysiologic inhomogeneities within the area of infarction that clearly provide the substrate for reentrant arrhythmias (59,61). The loss of sympathetic and parasympathetic fibers within and distal to the infarcted region contributes to the alterations in electrophysiologic properties (62). Thus it is clear that the recently infarcted myocardium provides an ongoing substrate capable of initiating and maintaining a variety of ventricular tachyarrhythmias, although their precise mechanisms may not be obvious.

The preceding discussion illustrates how the short-term interruption of coronary flow induces a series of metabolic, ionic, and neurohormonal changes that cause profoundly arrhythmogenic alterations in the electrophysiology of the cardiac fibers within the ischemic zone. Abrupt reperfusion reverses the ischemia-induced abnormalities, causing a separate series of changes that are also arrhythmogenic. The question remains as to why only some patients develop life-threatening arrhythmias or die suddenly, and others with ischemic insults seemingly identical with respect to size, location, and hemodynamic consequences do not. One possible explanation is that the patients are actually not identical, and that subtle differences exist that are crucial to the genesis of ventricular fibrillation. It is also possible that ventricular fibrillation is largely a random event and depends on the interaction between inhomogeneities of the ischemic myocardium and the location and timing of premature beats, being such that a premature beat travels a pathway leading to fractionation and creation of one or more reentry circuits. Because spontaneous premature beats and the substrate for reentry likely coexist in most patients with acute ischemia, the development of ventricular fibrillation may not be predictable. For example, site specificity for the induction of reentry has been observed in animal models (63–65). It is therefore possible to visualize a scenario in which the timing and site of origin of premature beats determine whether ventricular fibrillation will occur; that is, a premature beat arising from one location may not encounter an environment conducive to reentry and therefore will be benign, whereas in the same patient, a second spontaneous beat arising with the same coupling interval but from a slightly different focus will encounter local conditions that lead to ventricular tachycardia or fibrillation. Similarly, because the electrophysiologic changes that occur in the first few minutes after a coronary event are dynamic and continuously changing, it is possible that a premature beat of fixed origin and coupling interval will not initiate a sustained arrhythmia if it arises at one particular point in time, but may do so if it occurs even seconds earlier or later. Clearly, further studies are necessary to identify those patients destined to die suddenly after an acute ischemic event.

SPECIFIC TACHYARRHYTHMIAS AND THEIR MANAGEMENT

Sinus Tachycardia

Sinus tachycardia frequently accompanies acute myocardial infarction and is secondary to pain, anxiety, fever, or abnormal hemodynamics rather than any electrophysiologic consequence of acute ischemia. It is undesirable in acute infarction because it increases myocardial oxygen demands and compromises coronary perfusion by abbreviating diastole; and it will exaggerate conduction slowing within the ischemic zone. However, treatment is most appropriately directed at the underlying cause rather than the tachycardia itself. Adequate analgesia and sedation often are all that is required to restore the heart rate to normal. Sinus tachycardia that persists after these measures is usually the result of extensive infarction, and it is thus associated with a poor prognosis (66). Invasive hemodynamic monitoring should be employed in these circumstances to optimize cardiac output and filling pressures. In the absence of other indications for beta-blockade (for example, hypertension or possibly limitation of infarct size), administration of a beta-adrenergic blocking agent to reduce the heart rate should be considered only after the previously mentioned factors have been addressed. Hemodynamic monitoring is not needed routinely in the absence of features suggesting cardiac failure or severe left ventricular dysfunction. In patients with cardiogenic shock, sinus tachycardia may be an unavoidable consequence of endogenous compensatory mechanisms and/or exogenous adrenergic agents required to treat this complication.

Atrial Premature Beats

Atrial premature beats are frequently detected in patients with acute myocardial infarction; however, they are also common in the general population and therefore may be unrelated to the infarction itself. Atrial premature beats may initiate atrial tachyarrhythmias in the presence of an appropriate substrate, but they are of no consequence in themselves and do not warrant suppressive therapy.

Atrial Fibrillation and Flutter

Atrial fibrillation occurs in approximately 10% to 15% of patients with acute myocardial infarction. Episodes within the first 24 hours of inferior infarction are associated with atrial ischemia from coronary occlusions proximal to both the atrioventricular nodal artery and the atrial circumflex branch of the left circumflex artery (67). The majority of episodes occur later in the course of infarction and are associated with increasing patient age and elevation of pulmonary capillary wedge pressure, accounting for the relatively high mortality observed in patients with atrial fibrillation (68). Atrial flutter is much less common in acute infarction than atrial fibrillation, but its pathophysiology and significance are probably similar to those of the latter arrhythmia. Atrial fibrillation and flutter are particularly detrimental when they occur in acute myocardial infarction and therefore, in general, are managed more aggressively in this setting than in the absence of acute infarction. Exacerbation of ischemia by the rapid heart rate increases the urgency of slowing the ventricular response, and impairment of cardiac output by the loss of organized and appropriately timed atrial contraction in the setting of ventricular systolic dysfunction and increased diastolic stiffness from acute infarction may make restoration of sinus rhythm preferable to simply slowing the ventricular response.

In the individual patient with atrial fibrillation, selection among therapeutic alternatives depends on the patient's clinical status. Patients who are asymptomatic with a moderate ventricular response resulting from intrinsic conduction disease require little or no therapy; those with severe hemodynamic compromise from an exceptionally rapid response require prompt electrical countershock. Moderately symptomatic patients should be treated initially with one or more atrioventricular nodal blocking agents. Of the available drugs, digoxin has the advantage of not having negative inotropic action, but it does not reach peak effect for 8 to 12 hours. In addition, its principal mechanism of action, enhancement of parasympathetic tone with resultant prolongation of atrioventricular nodal refractoriness (69), is easily overridden by the adrenergic conditions that often accompany acute infarction. Beta-adrenergic blocking agents and the calcium channel blocking agents verapamil and diltiazem are generally more effective and act more rapidly than digoxin. But both classes of drugs possess important negative inotropic potential. For this reason, careful observation is essential to ascertain that the net hemodynamic effect of drug administration is beneficial. When atrioventricular nodal blocking agents produce inadequate rate control or are not tolerated in required dosages, restoration of sinus rhythm by electrical or other pharmacologic means is indicated. Direct current cardioversion is most expeditious and is usually effective, but adequate anesthesia must be provided. A pharmacologic alternative is intravenous procainamide (70), up to 20 mg/kg infused over at least 30 minutes to avoid excessive hypotension from vasodilation. The oral administration of class 1a, class 1c, and class 3 antiarrhythmic drugs may be employed on a short-term basis to maintain sinus rhythm after chemical or electrical cardioversion. However, regardless of the drug chosen, careful observation is mandatory because of their potential negative inotropic effect and because of the risk of proarrhythmic effects, particularly the polymorphic ventricular tachycardia termed torsade de pointes (71).

These management principles generally apply to atrial flutter as well as atrial fibrillation. The relatively well-organized nature of atrial electrical activity in flutter decreases the energy requirement for electrical cardioversion, while making the ventricular response more difficult to control with drugs. In addition, attempted pharmacologic conversion of atrial flutter with procainamide or quinidine must be accompanied by administration of an atrioventricular nodal blocking agent to prevent a paradoxical increase in ventricular rate from 1:1 atrioventricular conduction of the slower atrial rate produced by these drugs.

Supraventricular Tachycardia

There is little reliable information on paroxysmal supraventricular tachycardias in acute myocardial infarction other than atrial fibrillation and flutter. Reports of "paroxysmal atrial tachycardia" in 2% to 7% of infarction patients (72,73) predate modern terminology based on a more complete understanding of the mechanisms of atrial tachyarrhythmias. The term *junctional reciprocating tachycardia*, which encompasses most arrhythmias formerly designated "paroxysmal atrial tachycardia," refers to reentrant tachyarrhythmias involving either an accessory atrioventricular connection or dual conduction pathways within the atrioventricular node. These abnormalities are congenital and cannot be acquired from myocardial infarction. It is possible that in patients with one of these substrates, atrial or ventricular ectopy or autonomic disturbances from acute infarction might potentiate reciprocating tachycardia, but a past history of paroxysmal tachycardia would be expected. The term *ectopic atrial tachycardia* refers to a heterogeneous group of atrial arrhythmias resulting from abnormal automaticity, triggered activity, and reentry. Nonsustained ectopic atrial tachycardia is common in the general population, so that its relationship to acute myocardial infarction is uncertain if detected in this setting. Sustained ectopic atrial tachycardia may be a manifestation of digitalis toxicity, especially if associated with atrioventricular block. It is also possible for atrial flutter to go unrecognized and be labeled instead as apparent supraventricular tachycardia. Given these considerations, it should be unusual for acute myocardial infarction to be directly responsible for clinically important, true paroxysmal supraventricular tachycardia.

There is similar confusion surrounding the terms *paroxysmal* and *nonparoxysmal junctional tachycardia*. Most instances of paroxysmal junctional tachycardia represent junctional reciprocating tachycardia as described earlier. Tachycardia greater than 120 beats per minute that arises from the atrioventricular junction and that is not due to reentry is very rare, with or without acute infarction. The more appropriate term for nonparoxysmal junctional tachycardia is *accelerated junctional rhythm*, which refers to junctional rates of 60 to 120 beats per minute that exceed the sinus rate. This rhythm may be detected in up to 10% of continuously monitored patients (74), usually within the first 48 hours of infarction, and is most likely a consequence of enhanced automaticity of the junctional pacemaker from ischemia or autonomic factors. It tends to occur in brief, self-limited episodes, the occurrence of which is potentiated by sinus bradycardia. Despite the consequent loss of atrioventricular synchrony, accelerated junctional rhythm generally does not produce hemodynamic compromise and is not associated with an adverse prognosis.

Ventricular Premature Beats

Ventricular premature beats, like several of the arrhythmias previously discussed, are so common in the general population that their relationship to acute myocardial infarction in a given patient is uncertain. They are not of any hemodynamic or electrical importance in themselves, but historically they have been considered to represent "warning arrhythmias" for ventricular fibrillation, especially when they are frequent, multiform, or occur early in the cardiac cycle ("R on T" phenomenon) (72). Studies, however, have shown that warning arrhythmias are absent in as many as half of patients who develop ventricular fibrillation during the acute phase of myocardial infarction, and that they are as frequent in patients who do not develop ventricular fibrillation as in those who do (75,76). Because ventricular premature beats are not accurate predictors of ventricular fibrillation, they do not constitute a sufficient indication for administration of prophylactic antiarrhythmic therapy. They are also of no use in determining the efficacy of therapy for more clinically important sustained ventricular tachyarrhythmias: persistence of ventricular premature beats does not necessarily imply inadequacy of therapy for the sustained tachyarrhythmia, and conversely, suppression of ventricular premature beats does not guarantee effectiveness of that therapy.

Accelerated Ventricular Rhythm

Accelerated ventricular rhythm, or "idioventricular rhythm" as it is sometimes labeled, refers to consecutive beats of ventricular origin at a rate of less than 100 to 120 beats per minute. In the prethrombolytic era, it was detected in up to 40% of continuously monitored patients, and it did not appear to adversely affect prognosis (77). Like accelerated junctional rhythm, it generally occurs in brief, self-limited episodes, is more likely to become manifest when there is underlying sinus bradycardia, and produces no hemodynamic compromise despite the loss of atrioventricular synchrony. Rarely, this arrhythmia may result from exit block from the focus of origin of a more rapid ventricular tachycardia (77,78). In these cases, tachycardia rates that are multiples of the apparent "accelerated ventricular" rate may occur intermittently, and suppressive therapy is indicated.

Studies of thrombolytic therapy is acute myocardial infarction suggest that accelerated ventricular rhythm is usually a consequence of myocardial reperfusion after acute coronary occlusion. In studies combining serial coronary angiography and continuous electrocardiographic monitoring, this arrhythmia has been observed to be a reasonably sensitive and specific marker of restoration of antegrade coronary flow (79,80), although this is disputed by others (81). Thus its occurrence in the absence of thrombolytic therapy may well signify spontaneous reperfusion.

Ventricular Tachycardia

It is difficult to interpret much of the historical literature concerning ventricular tachycardia in acute myocardial infarction, because the term has been used nonspecifically to encompass a wide variety of tachyarrhythmias—from those that are brief, asymptomatic, and relatively slow and occur early in infarction, on one extreme, to those that are sustained, are sufficiently rapid to produce cardiovascular collapse, and occur several days after infarction, on the other. Because the pathophysiology, clinical implications, and appropriate therapy of these diverse forms of ventricular tachycardia may be quite different, it is crucial to address specifically the duration, rate, appearance (monomorphic or polymorphic), and timing with respect to infarction of the arrhythmias to which this term may be applied.

The transient local ionic and metabolic derangements that occur in the early hours after coronary occlusion tend to produce ventricular tachycardia that is polymorphic. Episodes of this arrhythmia often terminate spontaneously, but on occasion continue into ventricular fibrillation. When rapid (>200 beats per minute) polymorphic ventricular tachycardia is observed, continuous electrocardiographic monitoring and immediate availability of defibrillation are mandatory to ensure prompt detection and treatment of ventricular fibrillation should it occur. Intravenous lidocaine should be administered in an attempt to avert this complication, and measures undertaken to relieve myocardial ischemia. In most patients, polymorphic ventricular tachycardia subsides within 24 to 48 hours of infarction as the electrophysiologic environment stabilizes. Long-term therapy is unnecessary, and prognosis is not adversely affected.

In contrast, residual alterations in myocardial structure and electrical properties after myocardial infarction may constitute a substrate capable of supporting sustained monomorphic ventricular tachycardia. This substrate is most likely to evolve in patients with extensive infarctions that tend to be accompanied by congestive heart failure or new myocardial conduction disturbances. It is also relatively persistent, so that sustained monomorphic ventricular tachycardia may recur over a longer period than polymorphic ventricular tachycardia. It is possible for arrhythmia susceptibility to eventually disappear because of continued structural and electrical evolution of the infarcted area over ensuing weeks to months, but this cannot be reliably predicted in individual patients. Patients with sustained monomorphic ventricular tachycardia should therefore receive chronic antiarrhythmic therapy assessed by a reliable endpoint. If the arrhythmia is frequent before treatment, elimination of spontaneous recurrences as determined by ambulatory electrocardiographic monitoring may be adequate (82), but in the absence of such frequent spontaneous events, electrophysiologic testing is advisable to determine the effect of a given therapy on arrhythmia susceptibility. Mortality is very high in patients with sustained ventricular tachycardia, because of both ventricular dysfunction and recurrent arrhythmia.

In our experience, sustained monomorphic ventricular tachycardia is unusual before the second or third day following infarction, probably reflecting the time necessary for the requisite substrate to evolve. In patients who initially present with sustained ventricular tachycardia and develop elevated myocardial creatine kinase levels, the arrhythmia is probably the cause rather than the consequence of acute ischemia (83). This conclusion is supported by the presence of a preexisting substrate for ventricular tachycardia in the form of old myocardial infarction in such patients, the predominance of tachyarrhythmic symptoms in the clinical presentation rather than chest pain, and the absence of electrocardiographic changes diagnostic of acute infarction. The enzyme elevations detected in this setting are relatively modest, and they probably reflect myocardial injury resulting from prolonged tachyarrhythmia. In contrast to patients with polymorphic ventricular tachycardia or ventricular fibrillation (see later) early after clear-cut myocardial infarction, whose susceptibility to arrhythmia is usually transient, these patients with sustained monomorphic ventricular tachycardia and acute myocardial injury remain chronically susceptible to recurrent arrhythmia, and therefore require long-term antiarrhythmic therapy.

The short-term treatment of sustained ventricular tachycardia depends on the clinical status of the individual patient. Tachycardia at moderate rates may be stable and hemodynamically well tolerated, allowing time for intravenous administration of one or more drugs in an attempt to restore sinus rhythm. Lidocaine is easiest to administer most quickly; procainamide also can be given in the manner detailed previously for atrial fibrillation. If drugs are ineffective, or if ventricular tachycardia produces myocardial ischemia, hypotension, or pulmonary congestion, electrical cardioversion should be performed promptly. Adequate anesthesia must, however, be administered before this procedure in patients who remain conscious during their arrhythmia. There is never any justification for subjecting an awake patient to the extreme discomfort of external countershock (84). Monomorphic ventricular tachycardia may be converted with energies below 10 joules, but because unsuccessful low-energy shocks may produce ventricular fibrillation on occasion, it is our practice to use energies of at least 60 joules. When syncope and hemodynamic collapse result from rapid ventricular tachycardia or its degeneration into ventricular fibrillation, immediate high-energy countershock is mandatory.

Patients with recent infarction and sustained ventricular tachycardia refractory to conventional drug therapy rarely survived in the past (85), but recent advances have substantially improved their prognosis. Intravenous administration of amiodarone may be capable of salvaging patients who otherwise appear destined to die from refractory recurrent ventricular tachyarrhythmias. In one study (86), one or more 300-mg boluses of amiodarone sustained sinus rhythm after cardioversion in the majority of patients who previously had only brief periods of normal rhythm between recurrences of ventricular tachycardia and fibrillation. The use of antitachycardia and automatic defibrillating devices that can be inserted without thoracotomy provides an important addition to the therapeutic options available in this often desperate situation (87). Acute coronary angioplasty or bypass surgery to open an occluded vessel or to relieve acute ischemia may still be considered in appropriate patients. In patients with ventricular aneurysms who require bypass surgery, aneurysmectomy, with map-guided endocardial resection, may still be a reasonable option (88,89).

Ventricular Fibrillation

Ventricular fibrillation is both the most devastating and most potentially treatable complication of acute myocardial infarction. Its incidence peaks in the early hours of infarction and subsequently declines as the cellular electrophysiologic environment stabilizes. It occurs most commonly in patients with large Q wave infarctions, and in this situation, excess in-hospital mortality is related to left ventricular failure. However, patients with ventricular fibrillation who survive the hospital discharge exhibit a long-term mortality no different from that of patients without ventricular fibrillation (90,91). The short-term derangements responsible for this arrhythmia have generally resolved by this point, so that in the absence of a new ischemic insult, ventricular fibrillation is unlikely and long-term antiarrhythmic therapy is unnecessary. Prior to 1990, the incidence of ventricular fibrillation was reported to be 7% to 8% (90,91), not including patients who died from ventricular fibrillation prior to receiving medical assistance (92,93). As a result, there was modest enthusiasm for the prophylactic administration of lidocaine to all patients with suspected or proven myocardial infarctions (94,95). More recent reports indicate that the incidence of primary ventricular fibrillation, i.e., that occurring in the absence of hypotension or cardiac failure, has fallen to less than 1% (96).

The cause of this decline is not known with certainty. Several possible explanations have been suggested (96). These include greater CCU bed availability, the administration of beta-adrenergic blocking agents, more aggressive use of potassium and possibly magnesium, the use of antiplatelet and thrombolytic agents, and more effective sedation. Regardless of cause, the declining incidence has lessened enthusiasm for the routine prophylactic use of intravenous lidocaine to prevent ventricular fibrillation (96,97), particularly since ventricular fibrillation, when it occurs in those who reach medical attention, is rarely fatal because of prompt defibrillation and continuous electrocardiographic monitoring.

Other prophylactic measures, particularly the use of intravenous magnesium and the intravenous administration of beta-adrenergic blocking agents, are also viewed less enthusiastically now than in the past. In spite of suggestions that the use of IV magnesium might be safe, inexpensive, and effective in preventing life-threatening arrhythmias (98–100), more recent results obtained in the ISIS-4 trial (101) failed to substantiate any significant improvement in mortality in the magnesium treated patients. However, recent data obtained in patients who do not receive thrombolytic therapy (102), when combined with the previous randomized trials (99), suggest that there may be a subset of patients in whom intravenous magnesium therapy is a useful and effective strategy (103). The routine use of IV beta-blockers has also been advocated as an effective means for reducing the incidence of ventricular fibrillation (104,105). However, two large multicenter trials, Metoprolol in Acute Myocardial Infarction, MIAMI (106), and the ISIS-1 trial (107), failed to demonstrate any significant reduction in the incidence of ventricular fibrillation in patients treated with intravenous beta-blockers. When the results from all randomized trials of early interventions of beta-blockers in acute infarction are pooled, only small, albeit significant, differences in the incidence of ventricular fibrillation in treated patients are observed (2.2% vs. 2.6%) (107). Recent studies considering the use of beta-adrenergic blocking agents with thrombolytic agents, particularly the TIMI-2 trial (108), suggest that the use of beta-blockers may lessen the incidence of ventricular rupture and reinfarction following thrombolytic therapy. However, insufficient data is available at this time to demonstrate this effect in a statistically significant fashion (109).

In summary, acute myocardial infarction causes a variety of ionic, metabolic, and neurohumoral events that lead to electrophysiologic abnormalities entirely consistent with the ventricular arrhythmias observed in the clinical setting. The recent decline in the incidence of lethal arrhythmias that occur in this setting, while not completely understood, is obviously a welcome observation. However, sudden cardiac death occurring in the setting of acute myocardial ischemia and infarction and following infarction remains a major cause of death in the United States (110). Thus continued investigation into the causes of these arrhythmias and the continued search for agents that prevent infarction, protect the ischemic myocardium, and affect the electrical abnormalities and clinical arrhythmias detailed in this chapter remain as vital now as in the past.

REFFRENCES

1. Gettes LS: Effects of ischemia on cardiac electrophysiology, in Fozzard HNA, Haber E, Jennings RB, et al (eds): *The Heart and Cardiovascular System, Scientific Foundations,* 2nd ed. New York, Raven Press, 1991, pp 2021–2054.
2. Janse MJ, Opthof T: Mechanisms of ischemia-induced arrhythmias, in Zipes DP, Jalife J (eds): *Cardiac Electrophysiology: From Cell to Bedside,* 2nd ed. Philadelphia, WB Saunders, 1995, pp 489–496.
3. Reimer KA, Jennings RB: Myocardial ischemia, hypoxia and infarction, in Fozzard HNA, Haber E, Jennings RB, et al (eds): *The Heart and Cardiovascular System, Scientific Foundations,* 2nd ed. New York, Raven Press, 1991, pp 1875–1973.
4. Fozzard HA, Makielski JC: The electrophysiology of acute myocardial ischemia. *Ann Rev Med* 1985;36: 275–284.
5. Pieper GM, Todd GL, Wu ST, et al: Attenuation of myocardial acidosis by propranolol during ischemic arrest and reperfusion: Evidence with 31P nuclear magnetic resonance. *Cardiovasc Res* 1980;14:646–653.
6. Garlick PB, Radde GK, Seeley PJ: Studies of acidosis in the ischemic heart by phosphorous magnetic resonance. *Biochem J* 1979;184:547–554.
7. Steenbergen C, Murphy E, Levy L, London RE: Elevation in cytostolic free calcium concentration early in myocardial ischemia in perfused rat heart. *Circ Res* 1987;60:700–707.
8. Marban E, Kitakaze M, Kusuoka H, et al: Intracellular free calcium concentration measured with 19F NMR spectroscopy in intact ferret hearts. *Proc Natl Acad Sci USA* 1987;84:6005–6009.

8a. Owens LM, Fraliz TA, Murphy E, Cascio WE, Gettes LS: Correlation of ischemia induced extracellular and intracellular ion changes to cell-to-cell electrical uncoupling in isolated blood-perfused rabbit hearts. *Circulation* (in press).

9. Lee HC, Smith N, Mohabir R, Clusin WT: Cytosolic calcium transients from the beating mammalian heart. *Proc Natl Acad Sci USA* 1987;84:7793–7797.
10. Kihara Y, Grossman W, Morgan JE: Direct measurement of changes in intracellular calcium transients during hypoxia, ischemia and reperfusion in intact mammalian heart. *Circ Res* 1989;65: 1029–1044.
11. Hill JL, Gettes LS: Effect of acute coronary artery occlusion on local myocardial K^+ activity in swine. *Circulation* 1980;61:768–778.
12. Lathers CM, Kelliher GJ, Roberts J, Beasly AB: Nonuniform cardiac sympathetic nerve discharge. Mechanism for coronary artery occlusion and digitalis-induced arrhythmias. *Circulation* 1978;57: 1058–1065.
13. Weidmann S: The effect of the cardiac membrane potential on the rapid availability of the sodium carrying system. *J Physiol* 1955;127:213–224.
14. Gettes LS, Reuter H: Slow recovery from inactivation of inward currents in mammalian myocardial fibers. *J Physiol* 1974;240:703–724.
15. DeMello WC: Modulation of junctional permeability. *Fed Proc* 1984;43:2692–2696.
16. Pressler ML: Effects of Ca_i and pH_i on cell-to-cell coupling. *Experientia* 1987;43:1084–1091.
17. Spray DC, Stern JH, Harris AL, Bettett MVL: Gap junctional conductance: Comparison of sensitivities to H and Ca ions. *Proc Natl Acad Sci USA* 1982; 79:441–445.
18. Kagiyama Y, Hill JK, Gettes LS: Interaction of acidosis and increased extracellular potassium on action potential characteristics and conduction in guinea pig ventricular muscle. *Circ Res* 1982;51: 614–623.
19. Morena H, Janse MJ, Fiolet JWT, et al: Comparison of the effects of regional ischemia, hypoxia, hyperkalemia, and acidosis on intracellular and extracellular potentials and metabolism in the isolated porcine heart. *Circ Res* 1980;46:634–646.
20. Kodama L, Wilde AAM, Janse MJ, et al: Combined effects of hypoxia, hyperkalemia and acidosis on membrane action potential and excitability of guinea-pig ventricular muscle. *J Mol Cell Cardiol* 1984;16:247–259.
21. Corr PB, Dobmeyer DJ: Amphipathic lipid metabolites and arrhythmogenesis: A perspective, in Rosen MR, Palti Y (eds): *Lethal Arrhythmias Resulting*

from Myocardial Ischemia and Infarction. Boston, Dordrecht, Lancaster, Kluwer Academic Publishers, 1989, pp 91–104.

22. Kleber AG, Janse MJ, Wilms-Schopman FJG, et al: Changes in conduction velocity during acute ischemia in ventricular myocardium of the isolated porcine heart. *Circulation* 1986;73:189–198.
23. Hope RR, Williams DO, El-Sherif N, et al: The efficacy of antiarrhythmic agents during acute myocardial ischemia and the role of heart rate. *Circulation* 1974;50:507–514.
24. Harper JR Jr, Johnson TA, Engle CL, Martin DG, Fleet W, Gettes LS: Effect of rate on changes in conduction velocity and extracellular potassium concentration during acute ischemia in the in situ pig heart. *J Cardiovasc Electrophysiol* 1993;4:661–671.
25. Cohen CJ, Fozzard HA, Sheu SS: Increase in intracellular sodium ion activity during stimulation in mammalian cardiac muscle. *Circ Res* 1982;50: 651–662.
26. Lado MG, Sheu SS, Fozzard HA: Changes in intracellular Ca^{2+} activity with stimulation in sheep cardiac Purkinje strands. *Am J Physiol* 1982;243:133–137.
27. Hiramatsu Y, Buchanan JW, Knisley SB, et al: Influence of rate-dependent cellular uncoupling on conduction change during simulated ischemia in guinea pig papillary muscles: Effects of verapamil. *Circ Res* 1989;65:95–102.
28. Vleugels A, Vereecke J, Carmeliet E: Ionic currents during hypoxia in voltage clamped ventricular muscle. *Circ Res* 1980;47:501–508.
29. Carmeliet E: Cardiac transmembrane potentials and metabolism. *Circ Res* 1978;42:577–587.
30. Weidmann S: Shortening of the action potential due to brief injections of KCI following the onset of activity. *J Physiol* 1956;132:156–163.
31. Noma A: ATP-regulated K^+ channels in cardiac muscle. *Nature* 1983;305:147–148.
32. Coronel R, Fiolet JWT, Wilms-Schopman FJG, et al: Distribution of extracellular potassium and its relation to electrophysiologic changes during acute myocardial ischemia in the isolated perfused porcine heart. *Circulation* 1988;77:1125–1138.
33. Pogwizd SM, Corr PB: Reentrant and nonreentrant mechanisms contribute to arrhythmogenesi during early myocardial ischemia: Results using three dimensional mapping. *Circ Res* 1987;61:352–371.
34. Wilensky RL, Tranum-Jensen J, Coronel R, Wilde AAM, Fiolet, Janse MJ: The subendocardial border zone during acute ischemia of the rabbit heart: An electrophysiologic, metabolic and morphologic correlative study. *Circulation* 1986;74:1137–1146.
35. Fleet WF, Johnson TA, Engle CL, et al: $[K+]_e$–pH_e combinations at the ischemic margin in the pig. *Circulation* 1993;88(Pt II):I7.
36. Fleet WF, Johnson TA, Cascio WE, et al: Marked activation delay caused by ischemia initiated after regional K^+ elevation in in situ pig hearts. *Circulation* 1994;90:3009–3017.
37. Holland R, Brooks H: The QRS complex during myocardial ischemia: An experimental analysis in the porcine heart. *J Clin Invest* 1976;57:541–550.
38. Antoni H, Toppler J, Krause H: Polarization effects of sinusoidal 50-cycle alternating current on membrane potential of mammalian cardiac fibers. *Pflugers Arch Ges Physiot* 1970;314:274–291.
39. Katzung BG, Morgenstern JA: The effects of extracellular potassium on ventricular automaticity and evidence for a pacemaker current in mammalian ventricular myocardium. *Circ Res* 1977;40:105–111.
40. Wit AL, Rosen MR: After depolarizations and triggered activity: Distinction from automaticity as an arrhythmogenic mechanism, in Fozzard HA, Haber E, Jennings RB, et al (eds): *The Heart and Cardiovascular System, Scientific Foundations, Second Edition,* New York, Raven Press, 1991, pp 2113–2163.
41. Rials SJ, Wu Y, Ford N, Pauletto FJ, et al: Effect of left ventricular hypertrophy and its regression on ventricular electrophysiology and vulnerability to inducible arrhythmias in the feline heart. *Circulation* 1995;91:426–430.
42. Kohya T, Kimura S, Myerburg RJ, Bassett AL: Susceptibility of hypertrophied rat hearts to ventricular fibrillation during acute ischemia. *J Mol Cell Cardiol* 1988;20:159–168.
43. Hart G: Cellular electrophysiology and cardiac hypertrophy and failure. *Cardiovasc Res* 1994;28: 933–946.
44. Aronson RS: Mechanisms of arrhythmias in ventricular hypertrophy. *J Cardiovasc Electrophysiol* 1991; 32:249–261.
45. Kaufman R, Theophile U: Automatie-fordernde Dehnungseffekte an Purkinje-Faden, Papillarmuskein und Vorhoftrabekeln von Rhesus-Affen. *Pflugers Arch Ges Physiol* 1967;297:174–189.
46. Harris AS: Delayed development of ventricular ectopic rhythms following experimental coronary occlusion. *Circulation* 1950;1:1318–1325.
47. Bigger JT, Dresdale RF, Heissenbuttel RH, et al: Ventricular arrhythmias in ischemic heart disease:

Mechanisms, prevalence, significance and management. *Proc Cardiovasc Dis* 1977;19:255–277.

48. Kaplinsky E, Ogawa S, Balke W, Dreifus LS: Two periods of early ventricular arrhythmia in the canine acute myocardial infarction model. *Circulation* 1979;60:397–403.
49. Smith WT IV, Fleet WF, Johnson TA, Engle CL, Cascio WE, and the Experimental Cardiology Group: The I-b phase of ventricular arrhythmias in ischemic in situ porcine heart is related to changes in cell-to-cell electrical coupling. *Circulation* 1995;92:3051–3060.
50. Kliks BR, Burgess MJ, Abildskov JA: Influence of sympathetic tone on ventricular fibrillation threshold during experimental coronary occlusion. *Am J Cardiol* 1975;36:45–51.
51. Han J, Garcia de Jalon PD, Moe GK: Adrenergic effects on ventricular vulnerability. *Circ Res* 1964; 14:516–524.
52. Lathers CM, Levin RM, Spivey WH: Regional distribution of myocardial β-adrenoceptors in the cat. *Eur J Pharmacol* 1986;130:111–117.
53. Manning AS, Hearse DJ. Reperfusion induced arrhythmias: Mechanisms and prevention. *J Mol Cell Cardiol* 1984;16:497–518.
54. Opie LH: Reperfusion injury and its pharmacologic modification. *Circulation* 1989;80:1049–1062.
55. Bolli R, Patel B: Factors that determine the occurrence of reperfusion arrhythmias. *Am Heart J* 1988; 115:20–29.
56. Balke CW, Kaplinsky E, Michelson EL, et al: Reperfusion ventricular tachyarrhythmias: Correlation with antecedent coronary artery occlusion tachyarrhythmias and duration of myocardial ischemia. *Am Heart J* 1981;101:449–456.
57. Naito M, Michelson EL, Kmetzo JJ, et al: Failure of antiarrhythmic drugs to prevent experimental reperfusion ventricular fibrillation. *Circulation* 1981; 63:70–79.
58. Friedman PL, Fenoglio JJ, Wit AL: Time course for reversal of electrophysiological and ultrastructural abnormalities in subendocardial Purkinje fibers surviving extensive myocardial infarction in dogs. *Circ Res* 1975;36:127–144.
59. Spear JF, Horowitz LN, Hodess AB, et al: Cellular electrophysiology of human myocardial infarction. *Circulation* 1979;59:247–256.
60. Lazzara R, Scherlag BJ: Role of the slow current in the generation of arrhythmias in ischemic myocardium, in Zipes DP, Bailey JC, Elharrar V (eds): *The Slow Inward Current and Cardiac Arrhythmias.* The Hague, Martinus Nijhoff, 1980, pp 399–416.
61. Michelson EL, Spear JM, Moore EN: Electrophysiologic and anatomic correlates of sustained ventricular tachyarrhythmias in a model of chronic myocardial infarction. *Am J Cardiol* 1980;45:583–590.
62. Barber MJ, Mueller TM, Henry DP, et al: Transmural myocardial infarction in the dog produces sympathectomy in noninfarcted myocardium. *Circulation* 1983;67:787–796.
63. Wallace AG, Mignone RJ: Physiologic evidence concerning the re-entry hypothesis for ectopic beats. *Am Heart J* 1966;72:60.
64. Burgess MJ, Williams D, Ershler P: Influence of test site on ventricular fibrillation threshold. *Am Heart J* 1977;94:55–61.
65. Kuo CS, Munakata K, Reddy CP, Surawicz B: Characteristics and possible mechanism of ventricular arrhythmias dependent on the dispersion of action potential duration. *Circulation* 1983;67: 1356–1367.
66. Lown B, Klein MD, Hershberg P: Coronary and precoronary care. *Am J Med* 1969;46:705.
67. Hod H, Lew AS, Keltai M, et al. Early atrial fibrillation during evolving myocardial infarction: A consequence of impaired left atrial perfusion. *Circulation* 1987;75:146–150.
68. Sugiura T, Iwasaka T, Ogawa A, et al: Atrial fibrillation in acute myocardial infarction. *Am J Cardiol* 1985;56:27–29.
69. Simpson RJ Jr, Foster JR, Woelfel AK, Gettes LS: Management of atrial fibrillation and flutter: A reappraisal of digitalis therapy. *Postgrad Med* 1986;8: 241–253.
70. Halpern SW, Ellrodt G, Singh BN, Mandel WJ: Efficacy of intravenous procainamide infusion in converting atrial fibrillation to sinus rhythm: Relation to left atrial size. *Br Heart J* 1980;44:1247.
71. Jackman WM, Friday KJ, Anderson JL, Aliot EM, Clark M, Lazzara R: The long QT syndromes: A critical review, new clinical observations and a unifying hypothesis. *Prog Cardiovasc Dis* 1988;31: 115–172.
72. DeSanctis RW, Block P, Hutter AM: Symposium: Myocardial infarction 1972: Tachyarrhythmias in myocardial infarction. *Circulation* 1972;155:681–702.
73. Jewitt DE, Balcon R, Raferty EB, Oram S: Incidence and management of supraventricular arrhythmias after acute myocardial infarction. *Lancet* 1967;2:734–738.

74. Konecke LL, Knoebel SB: Nonparoxysmal junctional tachycardia complicating acute myocardial infarction. *Circulation* 1972;155:367–374.

75. Lie KI, Wellens HJJ, Downar E, Durrer D: Observations on patients with primary ventricular fibrillation complicating acute myocardial infarction. *Circulation* 1975;52:755–759.

76. Lawrie DM, Higgins MR, Godman MJ, et al: Ventricular fibrillation complicating acute myocardial infarction. *Lancet* 1968;2:523.

77. Lichstein E, Ribas-Meneclier C, Gupta PK, Chadda KD: Incidence and description of accelerated ventricular rhythm complicating acute myocardial infarction. *Am J Med* 1975;58:192–198.

78. de Soyza N, Bissett JK, Kane JJ, et al: Association of accelerated idioventricular rhythm and paroxysmal ventricular tachycardia in acute myocardial infarction. *Am J Cardiol* 1974;34:667–670.

79. Goldberg S, Greenspon AJ, Urban PL, et al: Reperfusion arrhythmia: A marker of restoration of antegrade flow during intracoronary thrombolysis for acute myocardial infarction. *Am Heart J* 1983; 105:26–32.

80. Ganz W, Geft L, Shah PK, et al: Intravenous streptokinase in evolving myocardial infarction. *Am J Cardiol* 1984;53:1209–1216.

81. Califf RM, O'Neill W, Stack RS, et al: Failure of simple clinical measurements to predict perfusion status after intravenous thrombolysis. *Ann Intern Med* 1988;108:658–662.

82. Mason JW, for the Electrophysiologic Study Versus Electrocardiographic Monitoring Investigators: A comparison of electrophysiologic testing with Holter monitoring to predict antiarrhythmic-drug efficacy for ventricular tachyarrhythmias. *N Engl J Med* 1993;329:445–451.

83. Woelfel A, Wohns DHW, Foster JR: Implications of sustained monomorphic ventricular tachycardia associated with myocardial injury. *Ann Intern Med* 1990;112:141–143.

84. Kowey PR: The calamity of cardioversion of conscious patients. *Am J Cardiol* 1988;61:1106–1107.

85. Wellens HJJ, Bar FW, Vanast EJ, Brugada P: Medical treatment of ventricular tachycardia: Considerations in the selection of patients for surgical treatment. *Am J Cardiol* 1982;49:186–193.

86. Williams ML, Woelfel A, Cascio W, et al: Intravenous amiodarone during prolonged resuscitation from cardiac arrest. *Ann Intern Med* 1988;110: 839–842.

87. Mitrani RD, Klein LS, Reardon DP, Zipes DP, Miles WM: Current trends in the implantable cardioverter-defibrillator, in *Cardiac Electrophysiology: From Cell to Bedside,* 2nd ed. Zipes DP, Jalife J (eds): Philadelphia, WB Saunders, 1995.

88. Haines DE, Lerman BB, Kron IL, DiMarco JP: Surgical ablation of ventricular tachycardia with sequential map-guided subendocardial resection: Electrophysiologic assessment and long-term follow-up. *Circulation* 1988;77:131–141.

89. Kleiman RB, Miller JM, Buxton AE, et al: Prognosis following sustained ventricular tachycardia occurring early after myocardial infarction. *Am J Cardiol* 1988;62:528–533.

90. Nicod P, Gilpin E, Dittrich H, et al: Late clinical outcome in patients with early ventricular fibrillation after myocardial infarction. *J Am Coll Cardiol* 1988;11:464–470.

91. Tofler GH, Stone PH, Muller JE, and the MILIS Study Group: Prognosis after cardiac arrest due to ventricular tachycardia of ventricular fibrillation associated with acute myocardial infarction (MILIS study). *Am J Cardiol* 1987;60:755–761.

92. Davies MJ, Thomas A: Thrombosis and acute coronary-artery lesions in sudden cardiac ischemic death. *N Engl J Med* 1984;18:1137–1140.

93. Cobb LA, Baum RS, Alvarez H III, Schaffer WA: Resuscitation from out-of-hospital ventricular fibrillation: 4 years follow-up. *Circulation* 1975; 5152(Suppl III):III-223–III-228.

94. Dunn HM, McComb JM, Kinney CD, et al: Prophylactic lidocaine in the early phase of suspected myocardial infarction. *Am Heart J* 1985;110: 353–362.

95. Lie KI: Lidocaine and prevention of ventricular fibrillation complicating acute myocardial infarction. *Int J Cardiol* 1985;7:321–325.

96. Antman EM, Berlin JA: Declining incidence of ventricular fibrillation in myocardial infarction. *Circulation* 1992;86:764–773.

97. Singh BN: Routine prophylactic lidocaine administration in acute myocardial infarction. *Circulation* 1992;86:1033–1035.

98. Horner, SM: Efficacy of intravenous magnesium in acute myocardial infarction in reducing arrhythmias and mortality. Meta-analysis of magnesium in acute myocardial infarction. *Circulation* 1992;86: 774–779.

99. Teo KK, Yusuf S, Collins R, Held PH, Peto R: Effects of intravenous magnesium in suspected acute

myocardial infarction: Overview of randomized trials. *Br Med J* 1991;303:1499–1503.

100. Yusuf S, Teo K, Woods K: Intravenous magnesium in acute myocardial infarction. An effective, safe, simple, and inexpensive intervention (editorial). *Circulation* 1993;87:2043–2046.

101. ISIS-4 (Fourth International Study of Infarct Survival) Collaborative Group: ISIS-4: A randomized factorial trial assessing early oral captopril, oral mononitrate, and intravenous magnesium sulfate in 58,050 patients with suspected acute myocardial infarction. *Lancet* 1995;345:669–685.

102. Shechter M, Hod H, Chouraqui P, Kaplinsky E, Rabonowitz: Magnesium therapy in acute myocardial infarction when patients are not candidates for thrombolytic therapy. *Am J Cardiol* 1995; 75:321–323.

103. Antman EM: Randomized trials of magnesium in acute myocardial infarction: Big numbers do not tell the whole story. *Am J Cardiol* 1995;75: 391–393.

104. Yusuf S, Ramsdale D, Rossi P, et al: Reduction in infarct size, arrhythmias and chest pain by early intravenous beta blockade in suspected acute myocardial infarction. *J Am Coll Cardiol* 1983; 1:676.

105. Norris RM, Brown MA, Clarke ED, et al: Prevention of ventricular fibrillation during myocardial infarction by intravenous propranolol. *Lancet* 1984; 2:883–886.

106. The MIAMI Trial Research Group: Metroprolol in acute myocardial infarction (MIAMI). A randomized placebo-controlled international trial. *Eur Heart J* 1985;6:199–226.

107. ISIS-1 (First International Study of Infarct Survival) Collaborative Group: Randomized trial of intravenous atenolol among 16,027 cases of suspected myocardial infarction: ISIS-1. *Lancet* 1986; 2:57–66.

108. Roberts R, Rogers WL, Mueller HS, et al: Immediate versus deferred β blockade following thrombolytic therapy in patients with acute myocardial infarction. *Circulation* 1991;83:422–437.

109. Borzak S, Gheorghiade M: Early intravenous β-blocker combined with thrombolytic therapy for acute myocardial infarction: The thrombolysis in myocardial infarction (TIMI-2) trial. *Prog Cardiovasc Dis* 1993;36:261–266.

110. Poole JE, Bardy GH: Sudden cardiac death, in Zipes DP, Jalife J (eds): *Cardiac Electrophysiology: From Cell to Bedside*, 2nd ed. Philadelphia, WB Saunders, 1995.

15

Conduction Disturbances: Temporary and Permanent Pacing in Patients with Acute Myocardial Infarction

Joseph S. Alpert, MD

Disorders of rhythm and electrical conduction were among the first complications of acute myocardial infarction described. Although conduction disturbances are clearly less common in patients treated with thrombolytic agents, they remain a continuing source of concern for the physician who is caring for a patient with acute myocardial infarction (MI). Moreover, uncertainty about the short-term and long-term prognosis of conduction disturbances in acute myocardial infarction has led to contradictory recommendations concerning temporary and permanent pacing in these patients. This chapter reviews what is known about the pathophysiology and prognosis of conduction disturbances in the setting of acute MI. With this information as background material, recommendations for temporary and permanent pacing therapy are made.

ANATOMY AND BLOOD SUPPLY OF THE CONDUCTION SYSTEM

The sinus node is located at the junction of the superior vena cava and the high right atrium (Fig. 15–1). It is connected to the atrioventricular (AV) node by a series of interatrial conduction tracts. Blood is supplied to the sinus node by a separate sinus node artery originating from the proximal right coronary artery in 53% of patients, from the circumflex coronary artery in 35% of individuals, and from both arteries (dual supply) in 11% of patients (1). The interatrial conduction system connecting the sinus and AV nodes has a dual blood supply: the sinus node artery and the AV node artery. The sinus node is extensively innervated by branches of both the sympathetic and parasympathetic nervous systems.

The AV node is located in the posteromedial region of the right atrium just anterior to the coronary sinus. This node consists of interlacing whorls of fibers organized into three histologic/electrophysiologic zones: (i) a region of transition from working atrial muscle to AV nodal cells, (ii) a compact central zone, and (iii) a second transitional zone between AV nodal cells and His bundle cells (2–5). Arterial blood is supplied to the AV node via the AV node artery, which is a branch of the right coronary artery in 84% of patients, a branch of the left circumflex coronary artery in 8% of individuals, and two arteries (one from the right and one from the left circumflex) in 8% of cases (1). Collateral circulation to the AV node is often supplied by

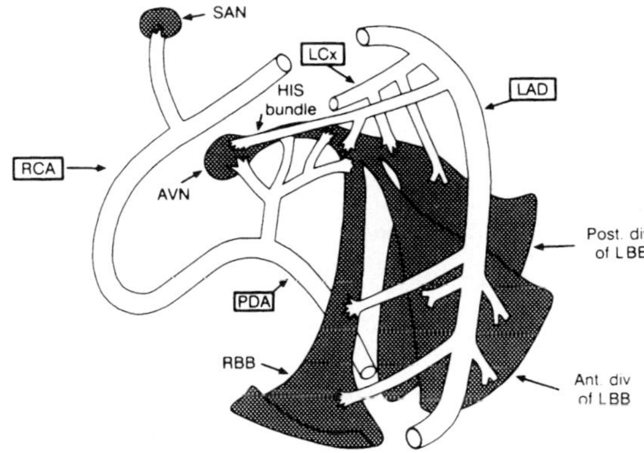

Figure 15–1. Diagram of the conduction system and its blood supply. SAN = sinoatrial node, AVN = atrioventricular node, LCx = left circumflex coronary artery, LAD = left anterior descending coronary artery, RBB = right bundle branch block, LBB = left bundle branch block, PDA = posterior descending coronary artery. *Modified from DeGuzman et al (53), with permission.*

the left anterior descending coronary artery. The AV node is also richly innervated by the sympathetic and parasympathetic nervous systems.

The AV node is connected to the bundle of His, which, in turn, gives rise to the left and right bundle branches. The left bundle separates into two divisions: an anterior (or superior) division and a posterior (or inferior) division. The His bundle passes through the fibrous atrioventricular ring near the central fibrous body, the membranous septum, and the noncoronary cusp of the aortic valve (6). Usually, the His bundle lies on the left side of the interventricular septum. It has a dual blood supply from branches of the AV node artery and left anterior descending septal perforator arteries.

The right bundle branch is often considered the continuation of the His bundle following the branching of the left bundle branch in the region of the membranous septum (6). The right bundle branch arises distal to the septal leaflet of the tricuspid valve, coursing anteriorly past the membranous septum, within the interventricular septum and subendocardium toward the base of the anterior papillary muscle of the right ventricle (7). The blood supply of the right bundle branch is also dual, arising from branches of the AV node artery and left anterior descending septal perforator arteries.

The left bundle branch is a less discrete structure compared with the right bundle branch. The left bundle branch is a fanlike structure radiating from the left side of the interventricular septum. It originates near the right and noncoronary cusps of the aortic valve and gives rise to two branches, the anterior and posterior subdivisions. These two subdivisions are quite variable in morphology from individual to individual (6). In general, the broader posterior branch passes posteriorly and inferiorly from the subaortic region into the interventricular septum toward the posterior left ventricular papillary muscle (6). Thereafter, it branches into the peripheral Purkinje network. The thinner anterior branch of the left bundle courses across the left ventricular outflow tract toward the anterior papillary muscle of the left ventricle. The blood supply of the anterior fascicle of the left bundle branch is derived from branches of the septal perforator arteries of the left anterior descending coronary artery. The posterior fascicle is usually supplied by branches derived from both the anterior and the posterior descending coronary arteries. The bundle branches have relatively little autonomic nervous innervation.

PATHOPHYSIOLOGY OF CONDUCTION DISTURBANCES IN ACUTE MYOCARDIAL INFARCTION

Two different mechanisms account for the abnormalities of conduction observed in patients with acute MI: (i) reversible or irreversible ischemic injury to the conduction system, and (ii) abnormal autonomic reflexes precipitated by myocardial ischemia.

In patients with inferoposterior MI, conduction system abnormalities may result from ischemia and/or necrosis involving part or all of the sinoatrial node and/or the AV node. Injury to the sinoatrial node can result in sinus exit block with loss of P waves from the electrocardiogram. Sinus exit block may be complicated by atrial arrhythmias (for example, atrial fibrillation, atrial flutter) if atrial infarction or left ventricular failure is present; however, most conduction disturbances following inferoposterior MI are the result of injury or abnormal autonomic activity involving the AV node.

The right coronary artery supplies the inferoposterior aspect of the left ventricle, most of the right ventricle, and the AV node in most individuals. Obstruction of the right coronary artery often produces ischemic dysfunction of the AV node without necrosis (8,9). Apparently, irreversible damage to the AV node is very unusual in this setting; however, Bilbao and associates noted that patients with fatal inferoposterior MI and AV block had necrosis of prenodal atrial myocardial fibers (10). It is of interest that patients without AV block had no such prenodal atrial necrosis. Bassan and associates (11) observed a marked increase in high-grade AV block in patients with inferoposterior MI and obstruction of the left anterior descending coronary artery. This latter finding emphasizes the importance of collateral blood flow to the AV node from the left anterior descending coronary artery in preventing ischemic injury/dysfunction of the AV node in patients with inferoposterior MI. Increased vagal tone is also a common cause of AV nodal dysfunction in patients with inferoposterior MI. Such vagal dysfunction may be mediated by abnormal function of cholinergic ganglia, which lie in the proximity of the AV node. Stimulation of these ganglia may be the human counterpart of the Von Bezold–Jarisch reflex noted in experimental MI in dogs (12). Another possible mechanism of AV nodal dysfunction in patients with inferoposterior MI is local AV nodal hyperkalemia. Cohen and associates observed increased potassium concentrations in lymph draining from the infarcted inferoposterior wall of dogs after right coronary artery occlusion producing experimental MI (13). Lymph with increased potassium concentration was present in lymphatic channels that passed in close proximity to the AV node (13).

Adenosine is an ischemic metabolite which depresses the sino-atrial activity and has negative effects on atrio-ventricular conduction. It has been postulated that transient hypoxia at the AV node may cause the release of adenosine (62). Atropine-resistant AV block occurring in the early phase of inferior myocardial infarction has been shown to be promptly reversed with intravenous aminophylline in a small series (63). The suggested mechanism is via competitive antagonism of adenosine.

Anterior and anteroseptal myocardial infarctions occur secondary to left anterior descending coronary arterial obstruction. Bundle branch and AV block in this setting is almost always the result of extensive septal necrosis, with concomitant destruction of the His bundle and bundle branches. The AV node is usually spared.

Acute right bundle branch block following anterior myocardial infarction may transiently disappear during electrical stimulation of the distal His bundle area in some patients. Cortadellas and coworkers performed electrophysiologic studies in nine such patients. They observed normal HV intervals in all these individuals. Ventricular tachycardia or fibrillation and a high mortality rate were associated with this form of conduction disturbance. The right bundle branch block rarely reverted spontaneously (14).

Prognosis of Bundle Branch Block and/or High-Grade Atrioventricular Block

The serious prognostic implications of bundle branch block and high-grade atrioventricular (AV) block were recognized more than 25 years ago by investigators working in early coronary care units (15–18). Mortality rates of 40–50% or higher were often associated with the development of complete left or right bundle branch block or complete (third-degree) AV block. Third-degree AV block was noted to be associated with a worse prognosis in patients with anterior as compared with inferior infarction. The prognosis for patients with these conduction disturbances has improved markedly during recent years in large part secondary to early thrombolytic therapy.

Among 2215 consecutive patients with an acute inferior Q-wave myocardial infarction hospitalized in Israel between 1981 and 1983, bundle branch block was present in 4.9%. Bundle branch block was a harbinger of hospital complications, irrespective of the site and time of the appearance of block, and these included atrial fibrillation, complete atrial ventricular block and congestive heart failure. Both in hospital and five year mortality were higher in patients with block, (22%, 33%) than those without it (13% and 23% respectively). New right bundle branch block emerged as an independent predictor of death and for the development of complete atrial ventricular block. Twenty-three of the 108 patients had left bundle branch block, but from a practical standpoint this should also be considered an adverse predictor of early and late prognosis (64). This and other studies (41) and to date, the widespread use of thrombolytic therapy in primary angioplasty, and there is a general impression that the frequency of bundle branch block has declined in such patients. Nonetheless, from a practical standpoint, one would assume that even in patients treated with acute re-perfusion therapy, new, persistent bundle branch block is an adverse prognostic factor.

SPECIFIC CONDUCTION DISTURBANCES IN ACUTE MYOCARDIAL INFARCTION

Sinus Node Dysfunction

The diagnosis of sinus node dysfunction is made by observing marked sinus bradycardia or loss of atrial activity on the electrocardiogram. Sinoatrial exit block is diagnosed when a pause is noted that is a multiple of the spontaneous sinus cycle length. A pause that is not a multiple of the spontaneous sinus cycle length is referred to as a *sinus pause.* A prolonged sinus pause is termed a *sinus arrest.* The asystolic period (rarely longer than 5 to 10 seconds) terminates with restoration of atrial activity or with a junctional escape rhythm. Most patients who demonstrate this rhythm abnormality have sick sinus syndrome that either predates the onset of the acute MI or is the result of sinus node ischemia and/or infarction. Abnormally increased vagal stimulation in the setting of inferoposterior MI can also produce these rhythm disturbances.

A blow to the lower sternum often restores normal sinus node activity. Alternatively, intravenous atropine (0.5 to 1.0 mg) may be administered. Atropine is only of use if sinus node dysfunction is the result of increased vagal tone. More aggressive therapy of this rhythm disturbance includes intravenous isoproterenol and temporary external or transvenous pacing; however, this arrhythmia is often benign, occurring rather infrequently and usually in the setting of inferoposterior myocardial infarction (15). It is therefore prudent not to treat this arrhythmia unless it is clearly the cause of decreased cardiac output or ventricular escape rhythms.

First-Degree Atrioventricular Block

First-degree AV block that develops during acute MI may be the result of increased vagal tone (inferoposterior MI), AV nodal ischemia/necrosis (inferoposterior MI), or more extensive necrosis of the His-Purkinje system (anterior/anteroseptal MI). First-degree AV block occurs in 4% to 13% of patients with acute MI (16,17). Most patients with first-degree AV block have had an inferoposterior MI, and hence vagatonia or AV nodal ischemia/infarction are the usual mechanisms. First-degree AV block is usually a benign rhythm disturbance in the setting of acute MI. It rarely, if ever, requires therapy. The patient with anterior myocardial infarction and first-degree AV block has often sustained a significant injury to the His-Purkinje system. Higher-degree AV block may develop, and such patients require careful monitoring (18). Patients with inferoposterior MI and first-degree AV block may also progress to higher-grade AV block, although such progression is not as ominous as in patients with anterior MI.

Type I Second-Degree Atrioventricular Block

Type I second-degree AV block (Wenckebach or Mobitz type I) is usually the result of vagally induced AV nodal dysfunction. Consequently, it is usually seen in patients with inferoposterior MI. This rhythm disturbance is the result of increased vagal stimulation or ischemia/necrosis of the AV node. Often, patients with inferoposterior MI develop progressive AV block, starting with first-degree and progressing to type I second-degree AV block. Further progression to higher degrees of AV block can also occur. Patients with type I second-degree AV block usually demonstrate a narrow QRS complex on the electrocardiogram, and the ventricular rate is sufficient to maintain an adequate cardiac output. His bundle recordings demonstrate prolongation of the AH interval, confirming the location of the block at or above the AV node. Type I second-degree AV block usually occurs early (within the first 72 hours) after inferoposterior MI (18,19). It seldom lasts for more than 7 days, and is almost invariably benign requiring no therapy (18,19). Of course, such patients should be carefully monitored.

Type I second-degree AV block is unusual in patients with anterior/anteroseptal MI. When it occurs, it reflects extensive septal injury with necrosis of the His-Purkinje system. Higher degrees of AV block may develop suddenly, and the patient should be monitored very closely. Some cardiologists favor prophylactic placement of a transvenous demand right ventricular pacing system. Others would employ close observation and external pacing followed by transvenous pacing if higher-grade AV block developed.

Type II Second-Degree Atrioventricular Block

Type II second-degree AV block is usually the result of injury to the conduction system at or *below* the AV node. Patients with this form of block and a narrow QRS complex usually have the conduction block located within the AV node. This is typically seen in patients with inferoposterior MI. His bundle recordings demonstrate AH prolongation, confirming the nodal or supranodal location of the block.

Patients with type II second-degree AV block and a wide QRS complex usually have the conduction block below the AV node. This is most often seen in patients with anterior or anteroseptal MI with extensive injury to the His-Purkinje system. His bundle electrocardiography demonstrates HV (infranodal) prolongation of conduction. The prognosis for type II second-degree AV block in anterior or anteroseptal MI is much worse than in individuals with inferoposterior MI. Patients with this conduction disturbance and anterior/anteroseptal MI may suddenly develop third-degree (complete) AV block with a slow (20 to 40 beats per minute) ventricular escape rhythm and hypotension.

Observation of the QRS width in type II second-degree AV block is not a completely reliable method of predicting whether the conduction disturbance is infranodal and hence more dangerous. For example, a patient may have a preexisting ventricular conduction defect, that is, right or left bundle branch block, making QRS width an unreliable predictor of conduction disturbance location. Conversely, type I second-degree AV block may, on occasion, result from block below the AV node (20). If doubt exists concerning the location of the conduction disturbance and its prognosis. His bundle electrocardiography is indicated.

Type I and II second-degree AV blocks usually develop during the first 24 hours of the patient's stay in the cardiac care unit. Rarely does the patient present with these rhythm disturbances. Progression to third-degree AV block occurs in approximately one third of individuals with type II second-degree AV block (16,18). The duration of the block is usually short, rarely lasting more than 72 hours (21).

The majority of patients with type II second-degree AV block have inferoposterior MI. As noted earlier, in this setting, the prognosis is much better than in anterior/anteroseptal MI. Approximately 20% of patients with inferoposterior MI, treated in the prethrombolytic era, manifested second-degree AV block (19). This incidence has been greatly reduced by thrombolytic therapy.

Type II second-degree AV block in the setting of inferoposterior MI usually requires no therapy as long as the heart rate exceeds 45 to 50 beats per minute. If clinical deterioration (hypotension, congestive heart failure, ventricular arrhythmias) is observed, therapy with intravenous atropine, isoproterenol, or temporary pacing may be undertaken. Patients with anterior/anteroseptal MI and type II second-degree AV block may suddenly develop third-degree AV block with a slow ventricular escape rhythm. A prophylactic temporary transvenous pacing wire is therefore often inserted in such individuals in anticipation of third-degree AV block. Alternatively, external pacing electrodes might be placed on such a patient, and a transvenous pacing wire may be inserted only if third-degree AV block occurs. Nonconducted atrial premature beats may superficially resemble the onset of second-degree AV block. In the setting of anterior/anteroapical MI, such nonconducted atrial premature beats should be carefully distinguished from second-degree AV block (22).

Third-Degree (Complete) Atrioventricular Block

Third-degree or complete AV block has been reported in 3% to 19% of patients with acute MI managed without thrombolytic therapy (18,23,24). Patients with inferoposterior MI usually develop third-degree AV block after progression through first-degree and second-degree AV block (Table 15–1). The QRS complex is often narrow and the block is located at or above the AV node. His bundle electrocardiography demonstrates *related* AH spikes and unrelated V spikes, confirming the nodal or supranodal location of the conduction disturbance. In the setting of inferoposterior. MI, third-degree AV block is usually the result of marked vagatonia or AV nodal is ischemia/infarction (see Table 15–1). The prognosis is good, and most patients recover normal AV conduction after 3 to 7 days. An occasional patient will manifest third-degree AV block for 2 weeks or more. Two-thirds of patients with third-degree AV block have had an inferoposterior MI (25).

Most patients with inferoposterior MI and third-degree AV block do not require therapy as they have a nodal escape rhythm with a rate of 50 to 60 beats per minute. Hemodynamic compromise is usually not present (see Table 15–1). An occasional patient may demonstrate clinical signs of inadequate cardiac output (hypotension, oliguria) or increasing ventricular ectopy. Intravenous atropine, isoproterenol, or pacing should be considered for these patients. Atropine is administered in doses of 0.5 mg up to a total of 2.0 mg. Isoproterenol is initiated as a constant infusion beginning with 1 μg/min and titrating upward to achieve a heart rate of 60 to 80 beats per minute. Isoproterenol must be used with great care as ventricular arrhythmias may increase markedly during beta stimulation.

Patients with inferoposterior MI, third-degree AV block, and heart rates exceeding 50 beats per minute often respond poorly to further increases in heart rate, presumably because of more extensive left ventricular dysfunction (26). Third-degree AV block that develops in the first 6 hours after the onset of inferoposterior MI is probably the result of increased vagal activity. Complete heart block that develops after this period appears to be the result of AV nodal ischemia and/or infarction (27).

The presence of complete AV block in patients with acute inferior wall infarction worsens the in-hospital prognosis even after statistical adjustment for factors such as age, gender, infarct size, and left ventricular dysfunction (28,29). Interestingly, long-term (1 year or greater) prognosis is *not* influenced by the development of complete AV block during the acute phase of the inferior infarction (27–29).

Table 15–1. Features of Third-Degree Atrioventricular Block in Inferoposterior and Anterior/Anteroseptal Myocardial Infarction

	Anterior/Anteroseptal	Inferoposterior
Pathophysiology	Extensive infarction of the septum with widespread injury to the His-Purkinje system; infranodal location of block	Less extensive infarction of the septum with associated edema and/or modest injury to the AV node; nodal or supranodal location of block
Prognosis	High mortality	Much lower mortality
Timing	Sudden onset after type II second-degree AV block	Gradual onset after first- and second-degree AV block
QRS width	Wide	Narrow
Ventricular escape rate	20–40 beats per minute	40–60 beats per minute
Hemodynamic compromise	Present	Often absent
Treatment	Pacing	No therapy or atropine; occasional patient is paced for clinical deterioration

In thrombolysed patients, the incidence of complete AV block complicating inferior wall myocardial infarction ranges from 5–13%, perhaps slightly higher than in the prethrombolytic era (27–32). However, the mortality rate associated with this complication is substantially less with reperfusion therapy than without that intervention.

In contrast to inferoposterior MI, third-degree AV block that occurs in patients with anterior/anteroseptal MI carries a poor prognosis (see Table 15–1). These latter patients have extensive septal necrosis with widespread infarction of the His-Purkinje system. The block is infranodal in location, develops suddenly, and is usually associated with a slow ventricular escape rhythm and hemodynamic compromise (see Table 15–1). Temporary (and possibly permanent) pacing is indicated; however, these patients have a poor prognosis despite pacing therapy because of their extensive infarction.

Bundle Branch Block

Fascicular Block

Left anterior hemiblock is the most common type of intraventricular conduction abnormality seen in patients with acute MI, occurring in approximately 5% of these individuals (33). Left anterior hemiblock is defined as a QRS axis of $-30°$ to $-90°$ in the absence of an inferoposterior MI. Patients with unifascicular block generally have a good prognosis with a low incidence of progression to high-grade AV block. In one series, only 3 of 75 patients with left anterior hemiblock progressed to high-grade AV block (33). It is likely that the left anterior fascicle is more often involved than the posterior branch because of its smaller size and more tenuous blood supply (6). Left anterior hemiblock occurs almost exclusively in patients with anterior/anteroseptal MI secondary to obstruction of the left anterior descending coronary artery. Sugiura and coworkers examined a variety of variables in 131 patients with Q wave anterior MI and fascicular block to clarify the genesis and prognosis of fascicular block (34). Fourteen (11%) patients developed isolated left anterior hemiblock. Only 16% of these patients developed high-grade AV block. Mortality was 36% in patients who developed high-grade AV block, but no death was judged to be the result of AV block per se (34). Patients with fascicular block had slightly higher pulmonary capillary wedge pressures, heart rates, and serum potassium levels. The authors suggest that these variables, in addition to blood supply and infarct size, may relate to the genesis of left anterior hemiblock.

In conclusion, it seems likely that patients who develop left anterior hemiblock in the setting of acute anterior MI are at modestly increased risk for complications and mortality. They should be observed closely. Prophylactic pacing is *not* indicated.

Left Posterior Hemiblock

New left posterior hemiblock (frontal ECG axis greater than 120° in the absence of lateral MI) is quite uncommon in patients with acute MI. No patient developed this conduction disturbance in the series of Sugiura et al (34). Mullins and Atkins found only 14 patients with isolated left posterior hemiblock, none of whom progressed to high-grade AV block (33). Lewin et al noted that 0.4% of 3,160 patients with acute MI developed left posterior hemiblock (35); however, isolated left posterior hemiblock was noted in only 0.1% of these patients. Morbidity and mortality were increased in these patients compared with a group of patients who did not develop this conduction disturbance. The control group had a lower incidence of previous MI, however, and consequently might have had better left ventricular function. Moreover, most of the patients also had concomitant right bundle branch block (35). None of these patients developed complete heart block. The recommendations given earlier for patients with isolated left anterior hemiblock, that is, close observation without prophylactic pacing, are also appropriate for patients with isolated left posterior hemiblock.

Complete Right and Left Bundle Branch Block

Ten to fifteen percent of patients with acute MI demonstrate complete bundle branch block (16,36–38). Two-thirds of these individuals have right bundle branch block (RBBB), and one-third have left bundle branch block (LBBB). Many of the patients with RBBB have associated left anterior or left posterior hemiblock. Only 10% of patients with conduction disturbances after acute MI demonstrate isolated RBBB (139). Approximately two-thirds of these patients have the conduction disturbance on admission, although it is often difficult to judge if the bundle branch block is new or old because the patient has not had a recent ECG taken. RBBB is more common than LBBB probably because the right bundle is a more slender structure that is more vulnerable to injury, even from an infarct of modest dimensions.

Patients with complete RBBB and LBBB are usually older and, more frequently, women. They have larger infarcts and suffer higher morbidity and mortality than are observed in patients without bundle branch block. Transient bundle branch block carries the same increased risk as permanent block (40). High-grade AV block develops more commonly in patients with new-onset bundle branch block (39).

Extensive septal necrosis is found in the vast majority of patients with complete bundle branch block (17,37). Most of these patients have an occlusion of the left anterior descending coronary artery with an associated anterior MI; however, some patients with inferior MI develop complete RBBB because the right coronary artery often supplies the proximal portion of the right bundle branch. The extensive nature of the associated infarct accounts for the high mortality rate in these patients. The cause of death is usually pump failure secondary to extensive myocardial necrosis.

In the thrombolytic era, the occurrence of bundle branch block complicating acute myocardial infarction has diminished, as has the associated mortality (41). Thus, in the prethrombolytic era, complete bundle branch block was often associated with an in-hospital mortality rate of 40% or greater. In a series of 1,634 patients with acute inferior wall Q wave infarction collected between 1979 and 1989, right bundle branch block was observed in approximately 7% of patients (41). Fifteen percent of these patients with right bundle branch block developed complete heart block. In-hospital and 1-year mortality rates for these patients were 11% and 14%, respectively, considerably lower than that observed in earlier, prethrombolytic series. However, in-hospital and long-term mortality rates were higher for patients with than for those without right bundle branch block, probably as a result of more extensive coronary artery disease, larger infarct size, and older age (41).

Whereas the presence of bundle branch block on the admission electrocardiogram during acute myocardial infarction has long been recognized as a powerful prognostic factor, there is little information on the outcome of such patients in the thrombolytic era. Among North American patients in the GUSTO-I trial, 420 or 0.17% had bundle branch block on admission. One hundred and thirty-one patients presented with left bundle branch block, and 289 patients presented with right bundle branch block, which was isolated in 133 patients, associated with left anterior hemiblock in 145 patients, and with left posterior hemiblock in 11 patients. These patients were matched for age and Killip class on admission. Patients admitted with bundle branch block had higher event rates with 30 day mortality, 22% versus 10%, P = .003, asystole during hospitalization (18% versus 8%, P less than .001) and need for pacing 22% versus 13%, P = .006, and their matched control. After adjusting for all additional baseline prognostic variables, bundle branch block remained an independent predictor for 30 day mortality, P = .036, ration 1.5895, same confidence intervals, 1.023–2.43.

Electrocardiographic criteria for the recognition of acute myocardial infarction in the presence of left bundle branch block have been described utilizing the GUSTO database (41a).

Bifascicular Bundle Branch Block

Left bundle branch block, discussed in the preceding section, is one form of bifascicular block. Right bundle branch block, combined with left anterior or left posterior hemiblock, represents the other form of bifascicular block. Hindman and coworkers, in a large multicenter study, demonstrated that patients with bifascicular block were at particularly high risk for developing complete heart block during the short term phase of their infarction (39). Mortality rates in these patients are high because of extensive infarction. Most of these patients have left anterior descending coronary arterial occlusion and extensive septal necrosis.

THERAPY OF CONDUCTION DEFECTS COMPLICATING ACUTE MYOCARDIAL INFARCTION

As the prognosis is often worse for patients with conduction defects and acute MI, and because some of these patients develop clinically important bradyarrhythmias and/or asystole, temporary pacing therapy has been recommended in this setting for more than two decades. Unfortunately, the results of such therapy have been disappointing because of the extensive nature of the associated myocardial necrosis. Most of these patients die of left, and occasionally right, ventricular pump failure rather than primary electrical failure (17,37–57).

Until recently, pacing has been the only therapeutic modality suggested for patients with conduction abnormalities that develop following acute myocardial infarction. Bertolet and coworkers evaluated intravenous aminophylline therapy in 18 patients with acute inferior wall myocardial infarction and second or third degree atrioventricular block (57a) within 4 hours of the onset of infarction. Theophylline was administered at 100mg/min to a maximum dose of 250 mg. Normal 1:1 atrioventricular conduction was restored in all patients within 3 minutes of initiating intravenous aminophylline therapy. All patients remained free of arrhythmias for 24 hours or more following this intervention. The authors concluded that adenosine released by ischemic myocardium was an important factor in the development of atrioventricular block in these patients since it responded to the adenosine antagonist, aminophylline following unsuccessful attempts to restore sinus rhythm with intravenous atropine.

Temporary Pacing

Considerable controversy still exists as to which group of infarct patients, if any, requires temporary and/or permanent pacing. Hindman et al retrospectively examined the outcome for 494 patients with acute MI and bundle branch block 39,42. They excluded 62 patients with cardiogenic shock and, hence, a very poor prognosis regardless of therapy. The remaining 432 patients had a high in-hospital mortality (28%), which, not unexpectedly, correlated with the severity of left ventricular dysfunction. High-grade AV block occurred in 22% of these patients and also correlated with in-hospital case fatality rates. These investigators identified three factors that correlated with the development of high-grade AV block: (i) first-degree AV block, (ii) new or indeterminate time of onset of bundle branch block, and (iii) bilateral bundle branch block (that is, bifascicular block or alternating RBBB and LBBB). The presence of any two of these factors was associated with an increased risk of developing high-grade AV block (Fig. 15–2). The authors recommend temporary, prophylactic pacemaker placement in patients with two of these three risk factors (39,42).

Lamas and coworkers examined the MILIS (Multicenter Investigation of the Limitation of Infarct Size) data bank to identify patients who were at high risk for developing complete heart block. As in the study of Hindman et al cited earlier, complete AV block tended to occur in patients with extensive infarction and poor left ventricular function (43). Thirty-eight patients (5.4%) developed complete AV block. These investigators were able to identify patients with a high likelihood (up to a 36% chance) of developing complete AV block. Risk fac-

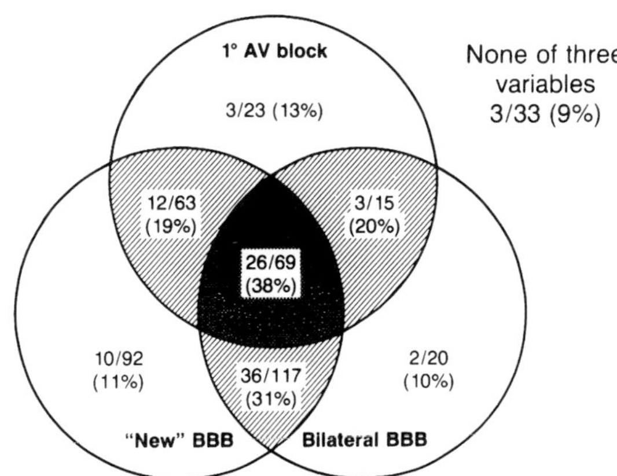

Figure 15–2. Representation of 432 patients with acute myocardial infarction and bundle branch block, excluding 62 patients with cardiogenic shock. The circles represent patient populations with one of the three risk factors and areas that represent patients with two or three variables. The denominator of each fraction indicates the total number of patients in that subgroup, and the numerator indicates the number of patients who developed high-degree AV block. *Adapted from Hindman et al (42), with permission.*

tors examined included first-degree AV block, type I second-degree AV block, type II second-degree AV block, left anterior hemiblock, left posterior hemiblock, complete RBBB, and complete LBBB (Fig. 15–3). Patients with any two of these risk factors had a 25% chance of developing complete heart block; patients with three risk factors had a 36% chance of developing third-degree AV block (43). Neither Hindman et al nor Lamas et al separated patients with anterior MI from those with inferior MI. As patients with anterior MI usually have a worse prognosis as compared with individuals with inferoposterior MI, these two retrospective studies present some difficulties for the clinician who must decide about temporary pacer therapy in a patient with inferoposterior MI.

It is worth noting that some smaller series of patients, including one prospective trial, have failed to demonstrate benefit from prophylactic pacing therapy in patients with bundle branch block (38,53). Most of the patients in these series had anterior MI with marked left ventricular dysfunction. Mortality was generally due to pump failure or late sudden death (presumably ventricular fibrillation), neither of which were prevented by temporary pacing. Despite these discouraging results, many cardiologists continue to recommend temporary prophylactic pacing in patients with extensive infarction and complete bundle branch block in the hope of salvaging an occasional individual in whom sudden high-grade AV block develops. Of course, temporary pacing is also indicated in patients with symptomatic high-grade AV block after inferoposterior MI. A summary of reasonable, *suggested,* indications for temporary pacing is found in Table 15–2.

Zoll and coworkers have called attention to the use of temporary external ventricular pacing for patients with high-grade AV block (58). This simple, safe, and effective method of temporary pacing enables the clinician to maintain an adequate heart rate and hence blood pressure while an intravenous pacing wire is inserted. Thus an alternative strategy to prophylactic intravenous pacing (see Table 15–2) for bundle branch block and acute MI is close monitoring of such patients with support via external pacing if high-grade AV block develops. Intravenous pacing wires are inserted only into patients who develop high-grade AV block. The external pacing modality should be tested when the patient is asymptomatic to ensure that it *can* capture the ventricles if required.

For most patients who develop high-grade AV block, ventricular pacing is sufficient to restore arterial blood pressure and circulatory compensation. It is, however, important to note that some patients for example, individuals with right ventricular infarction or markedly decreased left ventricular compliance should receive AV sequential pacing (59,60). Ventricular pacing alone does not restore blood pressure and circulatory homeostasis in these patients.

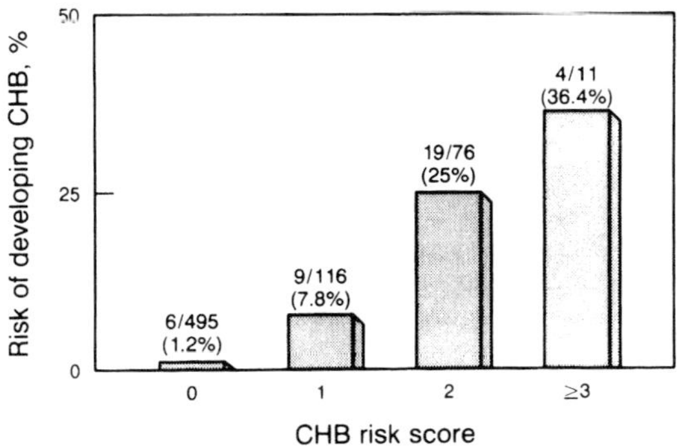

Figure 15–3. Risk of developing complete heart block based on the number of "risk factors" examined (see text). Data from the Multicenter investigation of the Limitation of Infarct Size. *Adapted from Lamas et al (43), with permission.*

Table 15–2. Possible Indications for Intravenous Pacing Therapy

Symptomatic Atrioventricular Block
- Complete heart block with slow ventricular response and wide QRS complex (usually anterior MI)
- Complete heart block with slow ventricular response and narrow QRS complex (usually inferoposterior MI) (Right ventricular infarction may require AV pacing.)
- Marked sinus bradycardia or sinus arrest unresponsive to atropine

Prophylactic Pacing
- Second-degree AV block with anterior MI
- Alternating bundle branch block
- RBBB with either left anterior or left posterior hemiblock
- LBBB and first-degree AV block
- ? New RBBB

Permanent Pacing

Some investigators have suggested that selected patients with bundle branch block who develop high-grade AV block in the setting of acute MI should have permanent pacing therapy (39,42, 44,46,48,52–55). For example, Hindman et al noted that a number of patients who developed bundle branch block and transient third-degree AV block in the setting of acute MI redeveloped high-grade AV block later in the clinical course (39). Some of these patients were still in-hospital although no longer monitored. Many of these investigators advise that patients who develop transient third-degree AV block with a wide QRS complex and persistent RBBB or LBBB should be continuously monitored during their hospitalization and undergo placement of a permanent pacemaker before discharge. In contradistinction to these authors, Watson et al found no benefit from permanent pacing in these patients (156). This trial randomized 50 patients with RBBB with or without concomitant fascicular block to permanent pacing or usual medical care. Patients with symptomatic or persistent AV block were excluded. There was no difference in mortality or sudden death rates during a 5-year follow-up between the paced group and the control group; however, it should be noted that the authors fail to specify how many of these patients experienced transient third-degree AV block. Probably, many of these patients did *not* develop transient complete heart block and consequently were at lower risk for subsequent development of high-grade AV block. Although recommendations for these patients remain tentative, many cardiologists favor implantation of permanent pacemakers (Table 15–3).

Table 15–3. Reasonable Indications for Permanent Pacing Therapy in Patients with Acute Myocardial Infarction

Persistent high-grade AV block after acute MI
Bifascicular bundle branch block that persists in a patient who demonstrated transient complete heart block after acute MI
Alternating bundle branch blocks (RBBB and LBBB) after acute MI with persistence of RBBB or LBBB

Role of Electrophysiologic Study in Selecting Patients for Pacing Therapy

Intracardiac electrophysiologic study is a useful technique for evaluating infarct patients with conduction defects in whom permanent pacing is being considered. A markedly prolonged HV interval implies extensive damage to the His-Purkinje system and such patients should receive a permanent pacemaker. Most infarct patients with conduction abnormalities, however, have only mild or moderate prolongation of the HV interval, implying an intermediate risk for developing complete heart block. Consequently, the decision for or against permanent pacing is usually made on clinical grounds (see Table 15–3) in these letter individuals.

POTENTIAL PROBLEMS FOR PATIENTS WITH POSTINFARCTION CONDUCTION ABNORMALITIES

Most patients with conduction abnormalities after myocardial infarction have had an extensive infarct with resultant left ventricular dysfunction. These patients are at high risk for malignant ventricular arrhythmias and sudden death. Their clinical course may be complicated by atrial arrhythmias and/or unstable angina pectoris. Consequently, the clinician may consider therapy with antiarrhythmic agents, beta blockers, and/or calcium antagonists. All of these agents can slow cardiac electrical conduction with resultant worsening of the preexisting conduction abnormality. Great care and meticulous ECG monitoring should be employed when such pharmacologic agents are employed in patients with post-infarct conduction abnormalities. Intracardiac electrophysiologic study may be required.

REFERENCES

1. Vieweg WVR, Alpert JS, Hagan AD: Origin of the sinoatrial and atrioventricular node arteries in right, mixed, and left inferior emphasis systems. *Cathet Cardiovasc Diag* 1975;1:361.

2. Becker AE, Anderson RH: Morphology of the human atrioventricular junctional area, in Wellens HJJ, Lie KI, Janse MJ (eds): *The Conduction System of the Heart.* Philadelphia, Lea & Febiger, 1976, pp 263–286.
3. Anderson RH, Janse MJ, van Capelle JL, et al: A combined morphological and electrophysiological study of the atrioventricular node of the rabbit heart. *Circ Res* 1974;35:909.
4. Paes de Carvalho A, de Almeide DF: Spread of activity through the atrioventricular node. *Circ Res* 1960;8:801.
5. Truex RC: Anatomical considerations of the human atrioventricular function, in Dreifus LS, Likoff W (eds): *Mechanisms and Therapy of Cardiac Arrhythmias.* New York, Grune & Stratton, 1966, pp 333–340.
6. Massing GK, James TN: Anatomic configuration of the His bundle and proximal bundle branches in the human heart. *Circulation* 1971;44(Suppl II): II-I–II-64.
7. James TN, Sherf L, Urthaler F: Fine structure of the bundle branches. *Br Heart J* 1974;36:1.
8. Sutton R, Davies M: The conduction system in acute myocardial infarction complicated by heart block. *Circulation* 1968;38:987.
9. Blondeau M, Rizzon P, Lenegre J: Les trouble de la conduction auriculoventriculaire dans l'infarctus myocardique recent: II, Etude anatomique. *Arch Mal Coeur* 1961;54:1104.
10. Bilbao FJ, Zabalza IE, Vilanova JR, Froufe J: Atrioventricular block in posterior acute myocardial infarction: A clinicopathologic correlation. *Circulation* 1987;75:733.
11. Bassan R, Maia IG, Bozza A, et al: Atrioventricular block in acute inferior wall myocardial infarction: Harbinger of associated obstruction of the left anterior descending artery. *J Am Coll Cardiol* 1986;8: 773–778.
12. Paes de Carvalho A: Excitation of the atrioventricular node during normal rhythm. Effects of acetylcholine, in Dreifus LS, Likoff W (eds): *Mechanisms and Therapy of Cardiac Arrhythmias.* New York, Grune & Stratton, 1966, pp 341–352.
13. Cohen HC, Gozo EG Jr, Pick A: The nature and type of arrhythmias in acute experimental hyperkalemia in the intact dog. *Am Heart J* 1971;82:777.
14. Cortadellas J, Cinca J, Moya A, et al: Clinical and electrophysiologic findings in acute ischemic intraHisian bundle branch block. *Am Heart J* 1990; 119:23–29.
15. Bouvrain Y, Slama R, Temkine J: Le Bloc sino-auriculaire et les "maladies du sinus." Reflexions a propos de 63 observations. *Arch Mal Coeur* 1967; 60:753.
16. Julian DG, Valentine PA, Miller GG: Disturbances of rate, rhythm and conduction in acute myocardial infarction. A prospective study of 100 consecutive unselected patients with the aid of electrocardiographic monitoring. *Am J Med* 1964; 37:915.
17. Fauchier J-P, Raynaud PH, Brochier M, et al: Le bloc auriculo-ventriculaire a la phase aigue de l'infarctus du myocarde. A propos de 46 cas. *Sem Hop Paris* 1969;45:101.
18. Brown RW, Hunt D, Sloman JG. The natural history of atrioventricular conduction defects in acute myocardial infarction. *Am Heart J* 1969;78:460.
19. Rotman M, Wagner GS, Wallace AG: Bradyarrhythmias in acute myocardial infarction. *Circulation* 1972;45:703.
20. Strasberg B, Sclarovsky S, Agmon J: Wenckebach block in the distal conduction system complicating a non-Q wave acute myocardial infarction. *Chest* 1987;92:745.
21. Pentecost BL, Mayne NMC: Results of a general hospital coronary care service. *Br Med J* 1968; 1:830.
22. Massie B, Scheinman MM, Peters R, et al: Clinical and electrophysiologic findings in patients with paroxysmal slowing of the sinus rate and apparent Mobitz type II AV block. *Circulation* 1978;58:305.
23. Paulk EA Jr, Hurst JW: Complete heart block in acute myocardial infarction. A clinical evaluation of the intracardiac bipolar catheter pacemaker. *Am J Cardiol* 1966;17:695.
24. Friedberg CK, Cohen H, Donoso E: Advanced heart block as a complication of acute myocardial infarction: Role of pacemaker therapy. *Progr Cardiovasc Dis* 1968;10:466.
25. Johansson BW: Complete heart block. A clinical, hemodynamic and pharmacological study in patients with and without an artificial pacemaker. *Acta Med Scand* 1966;180(suppl):451.
26. Tans AC, Lie KI, Durrer D: Clinical setting and prognostic significance of high degree atrioventricular block in acute inferior myocardial infarction. *Am Heart J* 1980;99:4.

27. Feigl D, Ashkenazy J, Kishon Y: Early and late atrioventricular block in acute inferior myocardial infarction. *J Am Coll Cardiol* 1984;4:35.

28. Behar S, Zissman E, Zion M, et al: Complete atrioventricular block complicating inferior wall myocardial infarction: Short and long-term prognosis. *Am Heart J* 1993;125:1622–1627.

29. Goldberg RJ, Zevallos JC, Yarzebski J, et al: Prognosis of acute myocardial infarction complicated by complete heart block (The Worcester Heart Attack Study). *Am J Cardiol* 1992;69:1135–1141.

30. Nicod P, Gilpin E, Dittrich H, et al: Long-term outcome in patients with inferior myocardial infarction and complete atrioventricular block. *J Am Coll Cardiol* 1988;12:589–594.

31. Clemmensen P, Bates ER, Califf RM, et al: Complete atrioventricular block complicating inferior wall acute myocardial infarction treated with reperfusion therapy. *Am J Cardiol* 1991;67:225–230.

32. Berger PB, Ruocco NA, Ryan TJ, et al: Incidence and prognostic implications of heart block complicating inferior myocardial infarction treated with thrombolytic therapy. Results from TIMI II. *J Am Coll Cardiol* 1992;20:533–540.

33. Mullins CB, Atkins JM: Prognosis and management of ventricular conduction blocks in acute myocardial infarction. *Mod Concepts Cardiovasc Dis* 1976;45:129.

34. Sugiura T, Iwasaka T, Takayama Y, et al: The factors associated with fascicular block in acute anteroseptal infarction. *Arch Intern Med* 1988;148:529.

35. Lewin RF, Sclarovsky S, Strasberg B, et al: Right axis deviation in acute myocardial infarction: Clinical significance, hospital evolution, and long-term follow-up. *Chest* 1984;85:489.

36. Restieaux N, Bray C, Bullard H, et al: 150 patients with cardiac infarction treated in a coronary unit. *Lancet* 1967;1:1285.

37. Hunt D, Sloman G: Bundle branch block in acute myocardial infarction. *Br Med J* 1969;1:85.

38. Godman MJ, Lassers BW, Julian DG: Complete bundle branch block complicating acute myocardial infarction. *N Engl J Med* 1970;282:237.

39. Hindman MC, Wagner GS, Jaro M, et al: The clinical significance of bundle branch block complicating acute myocardial infarction: I, Clinical characteristics, hospital mortality, and one-year follow-up. *Circulation* 1978;4:679.

40. Dubois C, Pierard LA, Smeets JP, et al: Short and long-term prognostic importance of complete bundle branch block complicating acute myocardial infarction. *Clin Cardiol* 1988;11:292.

41. Ricou F, Nicod P, Gilpin E, et al: Influence of right bundle branch block on short and long-term survival after inferior wall Q-wave myocardial infarction. *Am J Cardiol* 1991;67:1143–1146.

41a. Sgarbossa, EB, Pinski, SL, Barbagelata, A, et al: Electrocardiographic diagnosis of evolving acute myocardial infarction in the presence of left bundle-branch block. *N Engl J Med* 1996;334:481–487.

42. Hindman MC, Wagner GS, Jaro M, et al: The clinical significance of bundle branch block complicating acute myocardial infarction: 2, Indications for temporary and permanent pacemaker insertion. *Circulation* 1978;4:689.

43. Lamas GA, Muller JE, Turi ZG, et al: A simplified method to predict occurrence of complete heart block during acute myocardial infarction. *Am J Cardiol* 1986;57:1213.

44. Dominghetti G, Perret C: Intraventricular conduction disturbances in acute myocardial infarction: Short- and long-term prognosis. *Eur J Cardiol* 1980; 11:51.

45. Hollander G, Nadiminti V, Lichstein E, et al: Bundle branch block in acute myocardial infarction. *Am Heart J* 1983;105:738.

46. Waugh RA, Wagner GS, Haney TL, et al: Immediate and remote prognostic significance of fascicular block during acute myocardial infarction. *Circulation* 1973;47:765.

47. Scanlon PJ, Pryor R, Blount SG: Right bundle branch block associated with acute myocardial infarction. *Circulation* 1970;42:135.

48. Atkins JM, Leshin SJ, Blomquist G, Mullins CB: Ventricular conduction blocks and sudden death in acute myocardial infarction: Potential indications for pacing. *N Engl J Med* 1973;288:281.

49. Nimetz AA, Shubrooks SJ, Hutter AM, DeSanctis RW: The significance of bundle branch block during acute myocardial infarction. *Am Heart J* 1975; 90:439.

50. Godman MJ, Alpert BA, Julian DG: Bilateral bundle branch block complicating acute myocardial infarction. *Circulation* 1972;46:753.

51. Lichstein E, Gupta PK, Chadda KD, et al: Findings of prognostic value in patients with incomplete bilateral bundle branch block complicating acute myocardial infarction. *Am J Cardiol* 1973;32:913.

52. Waters DD, Mizgala HF: Long-term prognosis of patients with incomplete bilateral bundle branch

block complicating acute myocardial infarction: Role of cardiac pacing. *Am J Cardiol* 1974;34:1.

53. Hauer RNW, Lie KI, Liem KL, Durrer D: Long-term prognosis in patients with bundle branch block complicating acute anteroseptal infarction. *Am J Cardiol* 1982;49:1581.

54. Ginks WR, Sutton R, Oh W, Leatham A: Long-term prognosis after acute anterior infarction with atrioventricular block. *Br Heart J* 1977;39:186.

55. Ritter WA, Atkins JM, Blomquist CG, Mullins CB: Permanent pacing in patients with transient trifascicular block during acute myocardial infarction. *Am J Cardiol* 1976;38:205.

56. Watson RSD, Glover DR, Page AJF, et al: The Birmingham trial of permanent pacing in patients with intraventricular conduction disorders after myocardial infarction. *Am Heart J* 1984;108:496.

57. Pagnoni F, Finzia A, Valentini R, et al: Long-term prognostic significance and electrophysiological evaluation of intraventricular conduction disturbances complicating acute myocardial infarction. *PACE* 1986;9:91.

57a. Bertolet, BD, McMurtrie, EB, Hill, JA, et al: Theophylline for the treatment of atrioventricular block after myocardial infarction. *Ann Intern Med* 1995; 123:509–511.

58. Zoll PM, Zoll RH, Falk RH, et al: External noninvasive temporary cardiac pacing: Clinical trials. *Circulation* 1985;71:937.

59. Chamberlain D, Leinbach R: Electrical pacing in heart block complicating acute myocardial infarction. *Br Heart J* 1970;32:2.

60. Love JC, Haffajee CI, Gore JM, et al: Reversibility of hypotension or shock by atrial or AV sequential pacing in patients with right ventricular infarction. *Am Heart J* 1984;108:5.

61. DeGuzman M, Rahimtoola SH: What is the role of pacemakers in patients with coronary artery disease and conduction abnormalities? *Cardiovasc Clin* 1983;13:191–207.

62. Belardinelli L, Linden J, Burne RM. The cardiac effects of adenosine. *Progress in Cardiovascular Diseases* 1987;32:783–797.

63. Goodfellow J and Walker PR. Reversal of atropine-resistant atrio-ventricular block with intravenous aminophylline in the early phase of inferior wall myocardial infarction following treatment with streptokinase. *Eur H J* 1995;16:862–865.

64. Hod H, Goldbur TU, Beh RS, et al: Bundle Branch Block in Acute Q-Wave Inferior Wall Myocardial Infarction, A High Risk Subgroup of Inferior Myocardial Infarction Patients. *Eur J Cardiol* 1991;67: 1143–1146.

65. Sgarbossa EB, Pinski SL, Gates KB, et al: Outcome of Patients with Acute Myocardial Infarction and Bundle Branch Block in the Thrombolytic Era; Observations from GUSTO. *J Am Coll Cardiol* 1995, (suppl):Abstract 59A.

16

Pathophysiology, Diagnosis, and Management of Mechanical Complications

Carole A. Warnes, MD, MRCP, FACC,
and Bernard J. Gersh, MB, ChB, DPhil, FRCP

As the prognosis of cardiogenic shock resulting from primary pump failure is so poor in the absence of short-term successful early reperfusion (see Ch. 13), it is essential to exclude other potentially reversible causes, for example, hypovolemia, anaphylaxis, sepsis, vasodilation secondary to drugs, pulmonary embolus, and arrhythmias. In addition, other major mechanical complications of myocardial infarction, including severe mitral regurgitation secondary to papillary muscle rupture, ventricular septal defect, and cardiac rupture, must also be excluded before cardiogenic shock secondary to global impairment of left ventricular function can be confirmed. These catastrophic complications must be excluded because the majority require urgent operative intervention. Each of these complications is reviewed in this chapter.

ACUTE MITRAL REGURGITATION

Mitral regurgitation is common in the early phase of acute myocardial infarction and is present on auscultation in up to 80% of all patients (1). It is usually transient, however, and does not cause hemodynamic compromise. There exists a subset of patients who develop hemodynamically significant mitral regurgitation from a number of causes, including dilation of the mitral annulus from left ventricular enlargement, papillary muscle dysfunction, and papillary muscle rupture. This discussion focuses on papillary muscle rupture and not the other causes of mitral regurgitation following acute myocardial infarction.

Although recognized from autopsy specimens as far back as 1803, the first antemortem diagnosis of papillary muscle rupture was made by Davison in 1948 (2). Since that time, more than 200 cases have been reported in the literature (3–12). Rupture of the papillary muscle is less common than rupture of the ventricular septum, occurring in 0.9% to 5% of all patients dying from myocardial infarction (4). When it occurs, papillary muscle rupture is usually fatal, with more than 50% of patients dying within the first 24 hours and 80% within the first 2 weeks (5). Immediate and accurate diagnosis is essential, as prompt surgical intervention may be lifesaving.

Pathology and Pathophysiology

The mitral valve apparatus is composed of the mitral valve leaflets, the chordae tendineae, the mitral annulus, and the papillary muscles (13,14) (see also Ch. 2). The papillary muscles occupy the middle third of the left ventricle and arise from the trabeculae carnae of the anterolateral and posteromedial free wall. The papillary muscles themselves may be multiple separate muscle bundles or may consist of one large muscle bundle with multiple heads. Usually, the anterolateral muscle is single and the posteromedial muscle has multiple heads. The papillary muscles prevent retroversion of the mitral valve leaflets into the left atrium during systole by maintaining tension on the chordal apparatus (15,16). When partial rupture of one of the papillary muscles occurs, there is loss of support of several chordae tendineae, and severe mitral regurgitation results (17). In the presence of complete rupture of the entire trunk of a papillary muscle, there is massive regurgitation, with the left atrium and left ventricle becoming essentially a single chamber.

The arterial supply to the papillary muscles consists of small coronary vessels derived from the large epicardial arteries, which in turn traverse the entire thickness of the left ventricular wall and the papillary muscles themselves (18,19). The excessive length of the arteries and their subendocardial location may account for the susceptibility to ischemia (2,11). Because of the single blood supply to the posteromedial papillary muscle from the posterior descending artery, this muscle has a greater propensity to rupture than the anterolateral muscle and is involved with ruptures 6 to 12 times more frequently than the anterolateral muscle, which has a dual blood supply from the left anterior descending artery and left circumflex arteries (3–5,7,11).

The degree of involvement of the myocardium by infarction is usually small in patients with papillary muscle rupture (4,7). More than half of postmortem examinations show the infarction is limited to the subendocardium and is frequently smaller than 6 cm^2 (7). There is often a limited extent of coronary artery disease, as half of the patients have either single-vessel disease or no significant coronary disease in which the occlusion resulted from a thrombus alone (7). This results in hyperdynamic function of the noninfarcted regions. It is conceivable that the patients with the smaller infarctions are prone to rupture, as their relatively good ventricular function may result in a greater "shearing" force at the site of the potential rupture (7,12).

Clinical Presentation and Diagnosis

The clinical course of a patient with papillary muscle rupture is characterized by the acute onset of pulmonary edema or hypotension (or both), usually 2 to 7 days after an acute myocardial infarction (7,12). Although a new murmur is said to be common, the murmur may be soft or even absent because of the hemodynamics of severe mitral regurgitation and the resultant pressure equalization between the left atrium and left ventricle (12). Because of the single blood supply to the posteromedial papillary muscle from the posterior descending artery, papillary muscle rupture occurs most commonly in the setting of an inferior myocardial infarction (7,12). In contrast to an infarction producing a ventricular septal defect, there need not be pathologic Q waves on the electrocardiogram, and many of these ruptures occur with a non-Q wave infarction.

In the setting of acute hemodynamic deterioration, the differential diagnosis rests between papillary muscle rupture, acute rupture of the interventricular septum, and free wall rupture with pericardial tamponade. The physical examination is often nondiagnostic in this setting (7,20), as a murmur may not be audible. The advent of two-dimensional echocardiography has provided an immediate noninvasive method for diagnosis (9,20–25) (see Figs. 10–4, 10–5, and 10–6; Color Plates 3 and 5). Partial rupture of the papillary muscle has been visualized directly by two-dimensional echocardiography (26). Complete rupture of the papillary muscle is diagnosed when a freely mobile mass is attached to the mitral valve chordae, representing the head of the muscle itself (20) (see Ch. 10). When the papillary muscle cannot be visualized, the diagnosis can be made by the appearance of a flail mitral leaflet, indicating loss of support structure apparatus (27).

Color flow imaging has provided a method for semiquantitation of the degree of mitral regurgitation (28); and this combined with two-dimensional imaging has been shown to be sensitive for the detection of isolated mitral regurgitation (29), but it may underestimate the degree of mitral regurgitation. In many critically ill patients, the use of color flow imaging may be limited by the lack of adequate resolution. The striking finding in most patients with papillary muscle rupture is that ventricular function appears hyperdynamic or fairly well preserved in the presence of hemodynamic deterioration. In this instance, even if the papillary muscle or mitral valve cannot be visualized, the diagnosis of some type of mechanical complication must be entertained, and further diagnostic tests are required. The importance of a high index of clinical suspicion cannot be overemphasized.

Transesophageal echocardiography has provided a new window to the heart, especially in the critically ill patient in whom a precordial echo may not provide optimal imaging (30) (see Color Plates 3 and 5). If available, transesophageal echocardiography should facilitate the diagnosis of papillary muscle rupture as it enables direct visualization of the papillary muscle. Thus the need for left ventricular angiography may be obviated. Cineangiography can be used to confirm severe mitral regurgitation if transesophageal echocardiography is not available and the diagnosis is still in doubt.

Because a major cause of morbidity and mortality in the postoperative period arises from decreased ventricular function and recurrent myocardial infarction (31), it is recommended that coronary angiography be performed before surgical intervention if the hemodynamic condition permits (32). In the hemodynamically unstable patient, however, there should not be a delay; the patient should proceed directly to operation after the diagnosis has been made.

Management

The prognosis of a patient with papillary muscle rupture is poor. Thirty-three percent die immediately, 50% die within 24 hours, and more than 80% die within 2 weeks (5). Aggressive medical management with afterload reduction and vasodilator therapy has been advocated for stabilization, as these interventions can potentially reduce the degree of regurgitation (33). The degree of success with medical therapy alone is, however, limited in these patients whose hemodynamic deterioration is due to mechanical causes.

Intraaortic balloon pump counterpulsation may be used in the hemodynamically unstable patient, often resulting in adequate clinical improvement (34). It must, however, be emphasized that this procedure is temporary and should be used only as a stabilization maneuver before definitive repair (20,34).

Because of the dismal natural history of these complications, surgical intervention has been advocated (10,11,34–44). The first report of successful valve replacement for papillary muscle rupture was by Austen et al in 1965 (35). With a satisfactorily functioning left ventricle, patients have survived rupture of the entire trunk of the papillary muscle with surgical intervention (36). In certain situations, valve repair has been successful (37), particularly when the mitral regurgitation is due to rupture of a single papillary muscle head and the surrounding muscle is not extensively infarcted (38).

It must be emphasized that most patients with papillary muscle rupture have maintained excellent ventricular function due to the small amount of myocardium involved by infarction (4,7). In addition, the extent of coronary artery disease is limited (4,7). Therefore, the hemodynamic deterioration is due to a mechanical process. These factors portend a good prognosis if the hemodynamic abnormality itself can be corrected.

Although it is generally accepted that all patients with myocardial rupture will require an operation at some time, the precise timing of operation has been controversial. Earlier retrospective reports noted that the lowest operative mortality occurred in patients operated on more than 6 weeks after their myocardial infarction (41–43). These observations, combined with the work of Mallory et al (45), who described a 3- to 6-month interval for healing of the myocardium after an infarct, led to the recommendation that operation be delayed as long as possible (41–43). If operation is delayed for more than 3 months after myocardial infarction, operative mortality is reported to be lowered from 35–50% to 15–25% (39,40). This treatment strategy, however, may be the result of a selection process whereby patients with good ventricular function and less severe mitral regurgitation will be those who survive the waiting period.

Figure 16–1 illustrates the outcomes of 17 patients who had papillary muscle rupture at the Mayo Clinic from 1939 to 1981 (7). Of 11 patients who presented with pulmonary congestion alone, 6 remained stable and had subsequent mitral valve operation at a delayed date. Five patients who initially stabilized with medical therapy suddenly deteriorated after a variable period (1 to 60 days) and thereafter died. Of the 6 patients who presented with shock, 4 were treated medically and died. One of the two who underwent urgent surgical intervention survived. Thus the delayed surgical strategy may result in excellent surgical survival; however, 50% of patients who are stable may die suddenly while awaiting surgery. Almost all patients with cardiogenic shock succumb with medical therapy. It is felt that the overall outcome of patients with acute papillary muscle rupture might be improved by proceeding with operation early after the diagnosis is made, even in those patients whose symptoms are well controlled (7,20). This may increase the early surgical mortality but should improve overall patient salvage. This concept has recently been supported by several papers on acute rupture that have shown excellent results after early operation, approaching 100% perioperative survival and 90% 1-year survival (20,46,47).

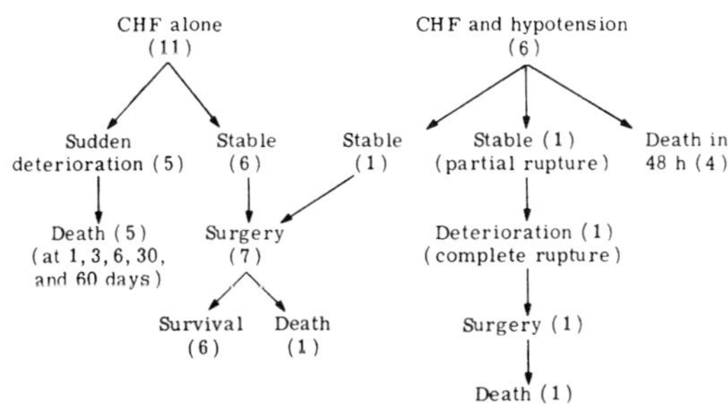

Figure 16–1. Clinical course of 17 patients with papillary muscle rupture. *Reproduced from Nishimura et al (7), with permission.*

Long-term follow-up of a small group of such patients estimated a 64% 7-year survival rate for patients who survived the operation (48). The concomitant performance of coronary artery bypass grafting was the only factor identified that improved both immediate and long-term survival. While revascularization may be a desirable objective, however, the potential benefit must be balanced in each case against the consequences of prolonging the surgical procedure. Despite the limitations of nonrandomized series and the small number of patients, therefore, these results reinforce the need for urgent recognition and referral for surgical repair in these patients with severe but potentially reversible heart failure and shock after myocardial infarction.

FREE WALL RUPTURE

Incidence and Timing

Free wall rupture is a catastrophic and usually unexpected complication of acute myocardial infarction; after arrhythmias and cardiogenic shock, it is the most common cause of death following myocardial infarction (see Ch. 2). Free wall rupture is estimated to cause 25,000 fatalities the United States (49), although its true incidence is unknown.

The generally accepted incidence rate of cardiac rupture in hospitalized patients who die of acute myocardial infarction is approximately 10% (46), with a range of 4% to 24% (50–53). The incidence rate is higher in large epidemiologic studies and in coroners' cases (54), which may reflect the higher autopsy rates in these communities. Because such cases involve little selection bias, this higher rate may represent the true incidence in the population at large. High incidence rates have also been reported from mental institutions (55,56), suggesting that continued activity after undetected myocardial infarction may be implicated in the etiology of rupture, but this may also reflect the higher autopsy rates in these patients and has not been supported by other studies (57,58).

More than 50% of ruptures occur within the first 5 days of infarction (49,58), and some investigators using both histologic (23) and clinical criteria (32,52,59) have reported that more than 22% may occur within the first 24 hours. Precise timing is difficult, however, as there may be discrepancies between the onset of clinical symptoms of acute myocardial infarction and the histologic age of the myocardial infarction at necropsy (50), suggesting that "silent myocardial infarction" may also be implicated or that there may be confusion between initial and recurrent infarctions. Bates et al (49) reported that 87% of ruptures occurred within 14 days of myocardial infarction, and ruptures occurring later probably represent recurrent infarct, infarct extension (60), or rupture through a false aneurysm (61,62).

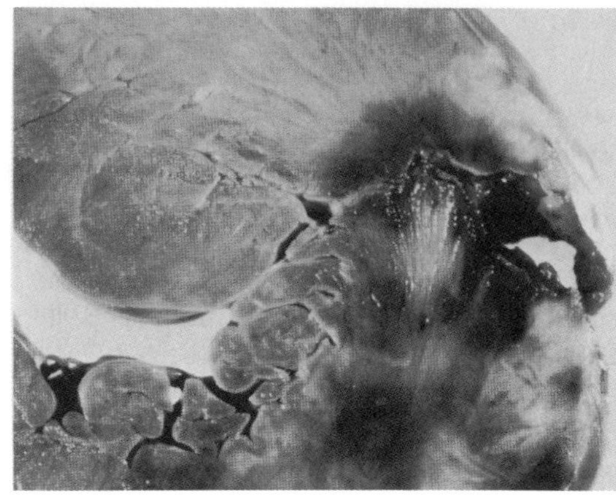

Figure 16–2. Rupture of the lateral wall of the left ventricle in association with acute myocardial infarction. The rupture takes a circuitous path from endocardium to epicardium.

Pathology and Pathophysiology

Rupture of the myocardial free wall occurs much more commonly in the left than the right ventricle (49) and infrequently may occur in the atria (63). Although "blowout" ruptures may occur (64), more commonly a ragged dissecting hematoma takes a circuitous route through the necrotic myocardium (Fig. 16–2). The size of the epicardial tear varies from several millimeters to several centimeters (59,65) and is frequently larger than the endocardial component. The tear is usually located within the area of infarction, but in an eccentric position rather than in the center of the infarct (59) (see Ch. 2).

Controversy exists regarding the location of infarction leading to rupture. Many reports suggest that the most common site of rupture is the anterior wall, involving the area of the terminal distribution of the left anterior descending coronary artery (59,66), but others have reported an equal distribution between anterior, posterior, and lateral walls (51,67,166).

The infarction associated with rupture is usually transmural (67), but the size of the infarction is variable, and it has been suggested that of patients dying with acute transmural infarction, those with cardiac rupture have the smallest infarcts (68). Previous myocardial infarction is present in less than 25% of patients (69–72,82f), and evidence of significant congestive heart failure is also uncommon (32,58–65,67), the implication being that those hearts with large areas of infarction or fibrosis have a decreased force of contraction and do not generate sufficient tensile stress to produce rupture. Similarly, it has been held that myocardial rupture is associated with coronary artery disease less severe than that found in cases of nonruptured myocardial infarction. The protective effect attributed to more severe coronary artery disease has been related to the development of a collateral circulation and fibrosis, offering resistance to rupture (59,65,73). Those patients at highest risk of free wall rupture appear to be women older than 60 years (32,59, 65,66); in one study, rupture was responsible for 30.3% of deaths among women aged 60 to 69 admitted to hospitals with acute myocardial infarction (70).

Preexisting hypertension has also been implicated by several authors as an important contributing factor to myocardial rupture (51,52,59,74). The presence of sustained on initial systemic hypertension after acute infarction may be more important (32,82f), as rupture may be the consequence of mechanical stress placed on infarcted tissue by the forcible contraction of surrounding normal tissue

(75) or by the increased intramural pressure transmitted from high intraventricular pressures during systole (74). Both of these mechanisms could be affected by systolic hypertension (76). One large prospective study (76) did demonstrate that systemic hypertension after acute infarction is accompanied by an increased incidence of myocardial rupture, but only among men. Systolic hypertension may not be a major factor leading to rupture, as in one large series (70) only one-third of patients developing rupture suffered from systemic hypertension. Dellborg et al (32) suggested that after acute myocardial infarction, sustained hypertension may be regarded as a sign of preserved left ventricular function and, hence, a good prognostic sign. Notwithstanding, hypertension after acute myocardial infarction should be treated promptly.

Concern has been expressed that anticoagulants may predispose patients to cardiac rupture by potentiating bleeding at the site of infarction and producing intramural hematoma and eventual rupture (77,78). These reports, however, have been refuted by others (52,58,66). Recent reports, particularly the GISSI trial, have also implicated thrombolytic agents and have suggested that their use, particularly if given late after the onset of symptoms, may increase the risk of cardiac rupture within the first 24 hours (79–82).

Honan et al (80) reported a meta-analysis of the effects of streptokinase on cardiac rupture. While the loading dose, total dose, and duration of the infusion differed, the odds ratio of cardiac rupture increased significantly ($p = 0.013$) with delay in the mean time to treatment. On the other hand, a number of studies have shown that thrombolytic therapy early after myocardial infarction improves survival and decreases the risk of cardiac rupture (82a,82b). The TIMI investigators examined the hearts of 61 patients who died a median of three days after a fatal first acute myocardial infarction (82a). The frequency of myocardial rupture of the left ventricular free wall or septum was lower in those who received thrombolytic therapy in comparison with patients who did not (22% versus 46%). Initial suggestions that the late administration of thrombolytic therapy might increase the risk of cardiac rupture were not substantiated by data from the Late Assessment of Thrombolytic Efficacy (LATE) Trial in which patients were randomized to receive tissue-type plasminogen activator or placebo, 6 to 24 hours after the onset of symptoms. Late thrombolysis did not increase the risk of cardiac rupture but it did appear however to accelerate the time of onset of rupture and the majority of ruptures in patients treated with thrombolytics occurred within 24 hours of therapy (82b). Becker et al (82c) reviewed 350,755 patients enrolled in the United States National Registry of Myocardial Infarction, of whom 122,243 received thrombolytic therapy. In-hospital mortality for those not treated with thrombolysis ($n = 228{,}512$) and those given thrombolytics was 12.9% and 5.9%, respectively ($p < 0.001$). The incidence of cardiac rupture was low (<1%) but was responsible for 6.1% and 12.1%, respectively, of in-hospital deaths. Death from rupture occurred earlier in patients given thrombolytic therapy, with a clustering of events within 24 hours of drug administration. Most patients received thrombolytic therapy within 6 hours of symptom onset; thus, thrombolysis appeared to accelerate cardiac rupture in this study. Other studies, including patients treated with PTCA suggest that persistent occlusion or ineffective reperfusion in patients with a "no-reflow phenomenon" after the procedure was more common in patients with rupture (82d,82e).

Corticosteroid therapy has also been held responsible for defective healing and scar formation predisposing to cardiac rupture (32,83,84). Methylprednisolone (85), indomethacin (86), and ibuprofen (87) induced scar thinning and infarct expansion in the setting of experimental infarction, and an apparent association between the use of these drugs and increased incidence of myocardial rupture has been demonstrated in humans (88).

Data showing a beneficial effect of drugs on the incidence of free wall rupture are scarce and contradictory. The ISIS-I trial suggested that early administration of beta blockers might reduce the incidence of rupture in the first two days following infarction (89). The Metoprolol in Acute Myocardial Infarction Trial (MIAMI) in contrast, showed a similar incidence of rupture in the placebo and metoprolol group (90).

It has been suggested that nitrates may reduce the risk of free wall rupture by approximately 30%, perhaps by reducing infarct expansion (91).

Schuster and Bulkley (92) emphasized the importance of infarct expansion in the pathophysiology of rupture and observed on necropsy that 54 (49%) of 110 patients who died of acute myocardial infarction showed some degree of myocardial expansion. Of those, 23 (43%) sustained cardiac rupture. Of the 56 patients without infarct expansion, only 1 (2%) had rupture. Other authors have suggested that the degree of polymorphonuclear infiltrate in the area of myocardial infarction correlates with the incidence of rupture (93), and eosinophils in particular, rich in proteolytic enzymes, might further weaken the necrotic myocardium (71). These reports are not confirmed by others (59), and some have suggested that intramyocardial blood vessels are stretched and torn when the infarct bulges during systole, causing the hematoma formation (94).

An incomplete rupture may become sealed by mural thrombus formation and, together with the pericardium, prevent the formation of hemopericardium. A left ventricular diverticulum may form at the site that communicates with the left ventricular lumen by a small orifice but produces no perceptible bulge in the cardiac outline (95). When rupture is prevented by adherent pericardium, there may occur formation of a false left ventricular aneurysm with a narrow neck opening into a large cavity, the wall of which is composed of fibrous tissue containing no myocardial cells. Contrast this with a true left ventricular aneurysm, the wall of which always contains myocardial elements.

Clinical Presentation and Diagnosis

The course of rupture is commonly catastrophic, with an acute "blowout" leading to immediate death, or with profound shock and tamponade causing complete cardiovascular collapse and death within a few minutes. Occasionally, however, the interval between onset of rupture and collapse is longer, possibly permitting surgical intervention. The concept of "subacute" rupture was first reported by O'Rourke (96) in 1973 when he described patients who developed shock later with signs of right as well as left ventricular failure. He suggested that minor episodes of bleeding occur, producing hemopericardium before terminal massive rupture.

Recently, Oliva et al (97) reported a characteristic symptom complex associated with cardiac rupture. On review of 70 patients with rupture, they observed a significantly greater incidence of pericarditis, repetitive emesis, restlessness, and agitation than in patients without rupture. More than 80% of patients with rupture had two or more symptoms compared with 3% of patients without rupture ($p < 0.002$). An abrupt transient episode of hypotension and bradycardia (probably due to the initial tearing with a resultant small hemopericardium) was observed in 21% of patients with rupture. In addition, a deviation from the expected evolutionary T wave pattern occurred in 94% of patients with rupture and 34% of control patients ($p < 0.02$). Patients displaying these symptoms, signs, and electrocardiographic changes should have an urgent bedside echocardiogram.

When cardiovascular collapse occurs secondary to rupture, it is imperative to make the correct diagnosis promptly, stabilize the hemodynamics, and repair the rupture site as quickly as possible. Frequently, electromechanical dissociation accompanies rupture but is not pathognomonic. Other bradyarrhythmias, including sinus bradycardia and junctional and idioventricular escape rhythm, are common (66,98).

Immediate pericardiocentesis may facilitate accurate diagnosis and, much more importantly, temporarily stabilize the hemodynamics by relieving tamponade (99). Volume loading and inotropes may also help to improve the hemodynamics (100). If time permits, diagnosis may be confirmed by two-dimensional echocardiography (101,102), and stabilization may be achieved by the prompt insertion of an intraaortic balloon pump (98,103). Achieving hemodynamic stability is imperative, and management has to be swift and aggressive. Intraaortic balloon pump counterpulsation may allow coronary angiography to be performed, but the majority of patients are too tenuous for this. Some have suggested that it is unnecessary and wastes valuable time before surgical repair (96). Most commonly, the patients are transferred to the operating room while undergoing cardiopulmonary resuscitation (99). The management strategy must be determined by the clinical stability of the patient, the most important imperative being repair of the rupture site. It has been suggested that in patients without previous angiography, "blind" left anterior descending and left coronary artery bypass grafting should be done if lesions are palpable proximally in these major coronary arteries (99). Because many myocardial free wall ruptures occur in association with small or modest-sized infarctions, the potential exists for successful surgical repair and as a result good myocardial function. Indeed, long-term survival after successful surgical repair has been reported (105).

Different surgical approaches have been employed to achieve successful repair: cardiopulmonary bypass (96,106), partial cardiopulmonary bypass and hypothermia (107), or partial bypass alone (108,109). Cardiopulmonary bypass appears to be the preferred approach because more of the heart is accessible, facilitating a more careful repair (110). Surgical options include infarctectomy with closure of viable ventricular muscle (95,110, 111), or covering the tear and surrounding infarcted myocardium with a Teflon (112) or Dacron (113,114) patch. Closing the rupture with Teflon-reinforced sutures may not be ideal, because the sutures are placed into necrotic myocardium, which is likely to tear.

Left Ventricular False Aneurysm

Although left ventricular false aneurysm is an uncommon consequence of free wall rupture (67,114), the diagnosis and management are important because of the tendency of these aneurysms to rupture (115). They may occur at any site in the ventricular wall in contrast to true left ventricular aneurysms, which are more commonly anterior (115). Examination of the mouth of the aneurysm reveals a sudden interruption of continuity of myocardial cells, the wall of the aneurysm being lined by fibrous tissue without parietal pericardium adherent to the outer surface (67) (see Color Plate 4 and Ch. 10).

In view of the propensity for false aneurysms to rupture irrespective of size or chronicity (115), their identification is crucial. Clinical features may be indistinguishable from a true left ventricular aneurysm, although flow through the narrow neck may produce a to-and-fro murmur (116) or an apical systolic murmur (117) sometimes associated with a pericardial friction rub. Frequently, they may also produce left ventricular failure (114,117). The chest x-ray may reveal a "bulge" in the lateral or posterior wall of the left ventricle, which, if seen early after acute myocardial infarction, may progressively enlarge (117). Onik et al (118) reported that of 87 patients with false aneurysms, only 5 had normal chest radiographs.

Two-dimensional echocardiography is a valuable diagnostic tool in this setting and can usually distinguish true and false aneurysms because of the narrow neck of the latter (119,120). The diagnosis has also been made by radionuclide angiography (121,122), although difficulty may be encountered localizing the narrow neck by this technique. Left ventricular angiography may also facilitate the diagnosis if contrast is seen traversing the narrow neck into the cavity of the false aneurysm during systole (117), but orientation may limit visualization, and if the narrow neck is not demonstrated, it may be difficult to distinguish a true from a false aneurysm.

Management

Once the diagnosis of false aneurysm is established, surgical therapy is the only option regardless of the temporal proximity to the acute infarction. Successful resection of the false aneurysm has been accomplished both early and late after infarction (123,124) and may be combined with coronary artery bypass grafting (125). The aggressive surgical approach appears justified not only because of the propensity of these lesions to rupture, but also because of the improvement in functional capacity and long-term survival that patients may achieve (67,117,124).

ACUTE INTERVENTRICULAR SEPTAL RUPTURE

Acute interventricular septal rupture is another catastrophic complication of acute myocardial infarction and usually occurs within the first week after the infarction (126) (see Color Plate 2). It is estimated to complicate 1% to 3% of acute myocardial infarctions and to cause approximately 5% of peri-infarction deaths (127). The pathologic substrate is invariably a transmural infarction, frequently the first infarction (47,128), and more commonly in an anterior or anterolateral location than an inferior or inferolateral location (3). Septal rupture may coexist with rupture at other sites including the free wall of the left and right ventricles (60). The perforation may be a direct hole or may be irregular and serpiginous and described as "complex" (128) (see Color Plate 2 and Ch. 2). These "complex" ruptures are more likely to be associated with rupture at other sites such as the papillary muscles and free wall of the left ventricle (128). Rupture may occur in patients who have single-vessel coronary artery disease (47,129), although some authors have reported that multivessel coronary artery disease is more commonly associated (47). Some authors have proposed that many patients with septal rupture have a paucity of septal collateral vessels, suggesting that an abrupt cessation in flow such as that produced by thrombosis is responsible for the infarction that leads to rupture (47).

Like free wall rupture, hypertension has been implicated in the pathogenesis of free wall rupture (74,130), but the association, if it exists, is not a close one (47). Thrombolysis has also been implicated in the pathogenesis (131).

Clinical Presentation and Diagnosis

The diagnosis is usually suggested by the development of acute and severe right-sided heart failure associated with shock and commonly a new, loud pansystolic murmur. A thrill is present in up to 50% of cases (132). The major differential diagnosis is mitral regurgitation secondary to papillary muscle dysfunction or rupture, and bedside differential diagnosis can be difficult. The electrocardiogram is not specific for the diagnosis of septal rupture and may demonstrate heart block, bradyarrhythmia, tachyarrhythmia, or marked elevation of the ST segments (115,133).

The diagnosis may be made most rapidly and safely with two-dimensional echocardiography and Doppler techniques (see Ch. 10). These allow direct visualization of the defect as well as assessment of ventricular function (134–139), and differentiation from mitral regurgitation is usually possible (see Color Plate 6).

If urgent access to echocardiography is not available, Swan–Ganz catheterization will facilitate diagnosis by demonstrating a "step-up" in the oxygen saturation of the right ventricle or pulmonary artery. Careful attention needs to be paid to sampling sites, however, as patients with severe acute mitral regurgitation may produce a step-up in oxygen in the right or left pulmonary artery or their branches because of the transmission of large V waves (140).

Emergency cardiac catheterization with left ventriculography also helps to define the rupture site, but more importantly coronary angiography is necessary if bypass grafting is being considered. The decision to proceed with angiography is determined by the patient's hemodynamic stability.

Management

Management must be swift and aggressive and, if hemodynamic stability is not rapidly achieved with diuretics, inotropes, and the judicious use of vasodilators, an intraaortic balloon pump should be inserted. Subsequent stabilization, however, may only be temporary, but sufficient to allow safe conduct of cardiac catheterization and perioperative hemodynamic support (44). Even patients who appear hemodynamically stable may experience sudden and unexpected hemodynamic deterioration and death (141), and indeed with medical therapy alone, most patients die within 6 weeks. In one series, all 13 unoperated patients died within 3 months (47).

Although an operation for repair of ventricular septal rupture has been available for more than 30 years (142), there has been considerable debate regarding the optimum timing for surgical intervention. Early reports (143–145) suggested that surgery should be delayed to allow sufficient time for healing of the infarcted area, so that sutures would not be inserted into friable necrotic tissue that would easily tear. Following this recommendation, a lower operative mortality was reported in patients who were operated on 8 weeks after septal rupture compared with those operated on less than 3 weeks after the event (146). In one series, operative mortality in those patients operated on less than 3 weeks was 40% but fell to 6% when operation was deferred for more than 3 weeks (145). An alternative interpretation of the data, however, might suggest that those patients who survived more than 3 weeks were "selected" by the fact they were less ill with smaller infarcts and perhaps smaller shunts and hence were able to survive and subsequently have a lower operative mortality.

More recently, the trend has been toward early surgical repair (20), although many studies still show a high perioperative mortality in these patients. In one series, the operative mortality of patients operated on within 48 hours of rupture was 71%, compared with 26% in those operated on 2 days or more after rupture (147). The implication is that these patients needed urgent surgery because they were in cardiogenic shock and were generally more hemodynamically unstable, and thus they were a "sicker" group of patients in whom high operative mortality might be anticipated (148). One critical deciding factor appears to be the presence or absence of cardiogenic shock (47,149), as the prognosis for shock with medical therapy with or without an intraaortic balloon pump is abysmal (47), and many patients suffer sudden and unpredictable deterioration and death while awaiting surgery. In a recent study of 77 patients, no patient with cardiogenic shock survived without surgery (150). Radford et al (47) reported that perioperative survival was much higher in patients who were not in shock preoperatively (14/27, 52%) than in those who were (3/11, 27%), and that neither the magnitude of the shunt nor left ventricular ejection fraction correlated well with perioperative survival. Others have suggested that those with a QP/QS > 3:1 and/or refractory congestive heart failure should have early surgery (151,152), but most authors agree that the degree of shunt has poor predictive value.

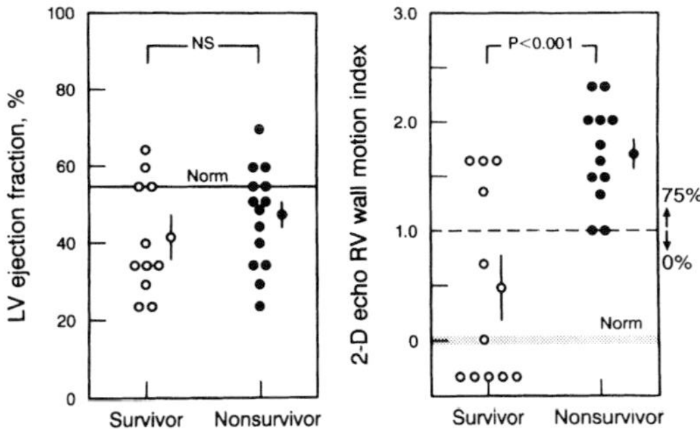

Figure 16–3. Left ventricular (LV) and right ventricular (RV) function parameters in 25 patients, survivors and nonsurvivors, with postinfarction ventricular septal rupture. Compared with survivors, the nonsurvivors had greater impairment of RV function as determined by a higher two-dimensional echocardiographically derived RV wall motion index. Percentages represent the overall mortality rate based on the presence or absence of significant RV dysfunction. *Adapted from Moore et al (154), with permission.*

Several reports have suggested that patients with inferior infarction also have a worse prognosis (47,153,154), the explanation being that they are usually associated with more extensive right ventricular dysfunction and the already damaged right ventricle cannot cope with the added volume load of the shunt (Fig. 16–3). In one necropsy study of patients with a postinfarction septal rupture, the incidence of right ventricular infarction was 100% (155) (Fig. 16–4).

In summary, therefore, acute septal rupture carries a grave prognosis, particularly when associated with cardiogenic shock and inferior infarction.

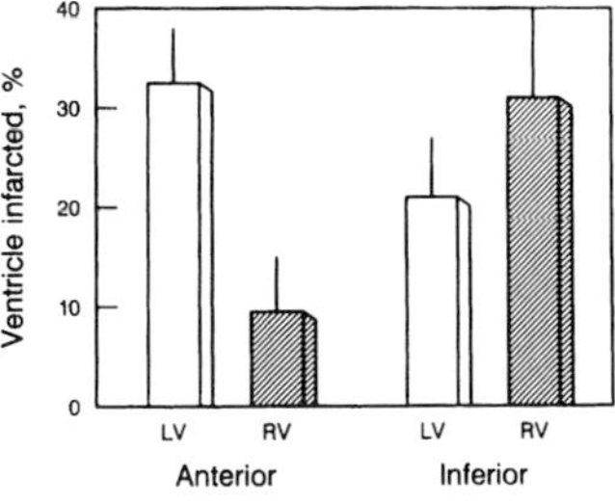

Figure 16–4. Percentages of left and right ventricles infarcted in anterior and inferior locations in patients with postinfarction ventricular septal defect. The amount of right ventricular infarction in anterior locations was notable, but inferior infarctions were associated with more extensive right ventricular infarction. *Adapted from Cummings et al (155), with permission.*

Aggressive medical management aimed at achieving hemodynamic stability should be followed by rapid diagnosis and surgical repair. Coronary angiography is appropriate if time permits. Early operative repair is indicated even though it may carry a high mortality; the long-term outlook appears better with this approach. If patients are not in cardiogenic shock, deferment of surgery for 3 weeks or more may be a reasonable option provided they are carefully managed with the knowledge that unpredictable deterioration may occur.

Several technical advances in the repair of septal rupture have been made in recent years, and the current preferred approach is to place the ventriculotomy in the left ventricular infarction and perform an infarctectomy. This approach permits better visualization of the septal defect and avoids disruption of noninfarcted myocardium (49). The defect may be closed with buttressed sutures or prosthetic patch material, the latter being more common for posterior defects, to prevent reopening of the defect or dehiscence of the ventriculotomy (49,156). Mitral valve replacement or coronary artery bypass grafting may be performed at the time of septal repair, although the benefits of the latter have not been proven absolutely (44). Muehrcke et al reported that coronary artery bypass grafting did not affect hospital mortality but significantly increased long-term survival when compared with that of patients with unbypassed coronary artery disease (157).

The surgical mortality for septal rupture remains high despite early intervention and is currently approximately 25% and probably slightly higher in those with preoperative shock and inferior infarcts (155). Cautious optimism for the long-term follow-up, however, appears appropriate with good functional capacity in the survivors and a low incidence of late death (20,47,153,158–160). Comparable survival has even been demonstrated in patients over the age of 70 (161).

ACKNOWLEDGMENT

The authors acknowledge the contribution of Dr. R. A. Nishimura in the discussion of papillary muscle rupture.

REFERENCES

1. Heikkila J: Myocardial infarction as complication of acute myocardial infarction. *Acta Med Scand* 1967 (Suppl);475:1–139.
2. Davison S: Spontaneous rupture of a papillary muscle. *J Mount Sinai Hosp* 1948;14:941–953.
3. Vlodaver Z, Edwards JE: Rupture of ventricular septum or papillary muscle complicating myocardial inJarction. *Circulation* 1971;55:815–822.
4. Wei JY, Hutchins GM, Bulkley BH: Papillary muscle rupture in fatal acute myocardial infarction: A potentially treatable form of cardiogenic shock. *Ann Intern Med* 1979;90:149–152.
5. Sanders RJ, Neubuerger KT, Ravin A: Rupture of papillary muscles: Occurrence of rupture of the posterior muscle in posterior myocardial infarction. *Dis Chest* 1957;31:316–323.
6. DeBusk RF: The clinical spectrum of papillary muscle disease. *N Engl J Med* 1969;281:1458–1467.
7. Nishimura RA, Schaff HV, Shub C, et al: Papillary muscle rupture complicating acute myocardial infarction: Analysis of 17 patients. *Am J Cardiol* 1983; 51:373–377.
8. Cederqvist L, Soderstrom J: Papillary muscle rupture in myocardial infarction: A study based upon an autopsy material. *Acta Med Scand* 1964;176:287.
9. Mintz GS, Victor MF, Kotler MN, et al: Two-dimensional echocardiographic identification of surgically correctable complications of acute myocardial infarction. *Circulation* 1981;64:91–96.
10. Morrow AG, Cohen LS, Roberts WC, et al: Severe mitral regurgitation following acute myocardial infarction and ruptured papillary muscle: Hemodynamic findings and results of operative treatment in four patients. *Circulation* 1968;37 (suppl II):II-124–II-132.
11. Fox AC, Glassman E, Osom OW: Surgically remediable complications of myocardial infarction. *Prog Cardiovasc Dis* 1979;21:461–484.
12. Roberts WC, Perloff JK: Mitral valvular disease: A clinicopathologic survey of the conditions causing the mitral valve to function abnormally. *Ann Intern Med* 1972;77:939–975.
13. Rusted IE: Studies of the mitral valve. *Circulation* 1952;6:825–831.
14. Roberts WC: Left ventricular papillary muscles. *Circulation* 1972;46:138–154.

15. Burch GE: Clinical manifestations of papillary muscle dysfunction. *Arch Int Med* 1963;112:112–117.
16. Burch GE: The syndrome of papillary muscle dysfunction. *Am Heart J* 1968;75:399–415.
17. Barbour DJ, Roberts WC: Rupture of a left ventricular papillary muscle during acute myocardial infarction: Analysis of 17 patients. *J Am Coll Cardiol* 1986;8:558–565.
18. Estes EH: The anatomy and blood supply of the papillary muscles of the left ventricle. *Am Heart J* 1966;71:356–362.
19. James TN: Blood supply of the human interventricular septum. *Circulation* 1958;17:391–396.
20. Nishimura RA, Schaff HV, Gersh BJ, et al: Early repair of mechanical complications after acute myocardial infarction. *JAMA* 1986;256:47–50.
21. Bishop HL, Gibson RS, Stamm RB, et al: Role of two-dimensional echocardiography in the evaluation of patients with ventricular septal rupture postmyocardial infarction. *Am Heart J* 1981;102: 965–971.
22. Scanlan JG, Seward JB, Tajik AJ: Visualization of ventricular septal rupture utilizing wide-angle two-dimensional echocardiography. *Mayo Clin Proc* 1979;54:381–384.
23. Farcot JC, Bolsante L, Rigaud M, et al: Two-dimensional echocardiographic visualization of ventricular septal rupture after acute anterior myocardial infarction. *Am J Cardiol* 1980;45:370–377.
24. Ahmad S, Kleiger RE, Connors J, Krone R: The echocardiographic diagnosis of rupture of a papillary muscle. *Chest* 1978;73:232–243.
25. Erbel R, Schweizer P, Bardos P, Meyer J: Two-dimensional echocardiographic diagnosis of papillary muscle rupture. *Chest* 1981;79:595–598.
26. Nishimura RA, Shub C, Tajik AJ: Two-dimensional echocardiographic diagnosis of partial papillary muscle rupture. *Br Heart J* 1982;48:598–600.
27. Godley RW, Weyman AE, Feigenbaum H, et al: Patterns of mitral leaflet motion in patients with probable papillary muscle dysfunction (abstract). *Am J Cardiol* 1979;43:411.
28. Helmcke F, Nanda NC, Hsuing MC, et al: Color Doppler assessment of mitral regurgitation with orthogonal planes. *Circulation* 1987;75:175–183.
29. Smyllie JH, Sutherland GR, Geuskens R, et al: Doppler color flow mapping in the diagnosis of ventricular septal rupture and acute mitral regurgitation after myocardial infarction. *J Am Coll Cardiol* 1990;15:1449–1455.
30. Seward JB, Khandheria BK, Oh JK, et al: Transesophageal echocardiography technique, anatomic correlations, implementation, and clinical applications. *Mayo Clin Proc* 1988;63:649–680.
31. Merin G, Giuliani ER, Pluth JR, et al: Surgery for mitral valve incompetence after myocardial infarction. *Am J Cardiol* 1973;32:322–324.
32. Dellborg M, Held P, Swedberg K, Vedin A: Rupture of the myocardium: Occurrence and risk factors. *Br Heart J* 1985;54:11–16.
33. Chatterjee K, Parmley WW, Swan HJC, et al: Beneficial effects of vasodilator agents in severe mitral regurgitation due to dysfunction of subvalvular apparatus. *Circulation* 1973;48:684–690.
34. Gold HK, Leinbach RC, Sanders CA, et al: Intraaortic balloon pumping for ventricular septal defect or mitral regurgitation complicating acute myocardial infarction. *Circulation* 1973;47:1191–1196.
35. Austen WG, Sanders CA, Averill JH, Friedlich AL: Ruptured papillary muscle: Report of a case with successful mitral valve replacement. *Circulation* 1965;32:597–601.
36. DeBusk RF, Kleiger RE, Ebnother CL, et al: Successful early operation for papillary muscle rupture. *Chest* 1970;58:175–178.
37. Gula G, Yacoub MH: Surgical correction of complete rupture of the anterior papillary muscle. *Ann Thorac Surg* 1981;32:88–91.
38. David TE: Techniques and results of mitral valve repair for ischemic mitral regurgitation. *J Card Surg* 1994;9(Suppl):274–277.
39. Kouchoukos NT: Surgical treatment of acute complications of myocardial infarction. *Cardiovasc Clin* 1981;11(3):141–149.
40. Buckley MJ, Mundth ED, Daggett WM, et al: Surgical management of ventricular septal defects and mitral regurgitation complicating acute myocardial infarction. *Ann Thorac Surg* 1973;16:598–607.
41. Mary DA, Pakrashi BC, Ionescu MI: Papillary muscle rupture following myocardial infarction: Successful treatment by resection of akinetic left ventricular area, mitral valve replacement, and aorta to coronary artery bypass graft. *Thorax* 1973;28:390–393.
42. Giuliani ER, Danielson GK, Pluth JR et al: Postinfarction ventricular septal rupture: Surgical considerations and results. *Circulation* 1974;49:455–459.

43. Merin G, Giuliani ER, Pluth JR, et al: Surgery for mitral valve incompetence after myocardial infarction. *Am J Cardiol* 1973;32:322–324.
44. Daggett WM, Guyton RA, Mundth ED: Surgery for post–myocardial infarct ventricular septal defect. *Ann Surg* 1977;186:260–270.
45. Mallory GK, Whie PD, Salcedo-Salgar J: The speed of healing of myocardial infarction: A study of pathologic anatomy in 72 cases. *Am Heart J* 1939;18:647–671.
46. Montoya A, McKeever L, Scanlon P, et al: Early repair of ventricular septal rupture after infarction. *Am J Cardiol* 1980;45:345–348.
47. Radford MJ, Johnson RA, Daggett WM Jr, et al: Ventricular septal rupture: A review of clinical and physiologic features and an analysis of survival. *Circulation* 1981;64:545–553.
48. Kishon Y, Oh JK, Schaff HV, et al: Mitral valve operation in post infarction rupture of a papillary muscle: Immediate results and long-term follow-up of 22 patients. *Mayo Clin Proc* 1992;67:1023–1030.
49. Bates RJ, Beutler S, Resnekov L, et al: Cardiac rupture: Challenge in diagnosis and management. *Am J Cardiol* 1977;40:429–437.
50. Oblath RW, Levenson DC, Griffith GC: Factors influencing rupture of the heart after myocardial infarction. *JAMA* 1952;149:1276–1281.
51. Naeim F, De la Maza LM, Robbins SL: Cardiac rupture during myocardial infarction: A review of 44 cases. *Circulation* 1972;45:1231–1239.
52. Griffith GC, Hedge B, Oblath RW: Factors in myocardial rupture. An analysis of 204 cases at Los Angeles County Hospital between 1924 and 1957. *Am J Cardiol* 1961;8:792–798.
53. Spiekerman RE, Brandenberg JT, Achor RWP, Edwards JE: The spectrum of coronary heart disease in a community of 30,000: A clinicopathologic study. *Circulation* 1962;25:57–65.
54. Crawford MD, Morris JN: Ruptured ventricle: Incidence in population of London, 1957–1958. *Br Med J* 1960;2:1624–1626.
55. Jetter WW, White PD: Rupture of the heart in patients in mental institutions. *Ann Intern Med* 1944;21:783–802.
56. Mundth ED: Rupture of the heart complicating myocardial infarction. *Circulation* 1972;46:427–429.
57. Kavelman DA: Myocardial rupture: A study of nonpsychotic and psychotic patients. *Can Med Assoc J* 1960;82:1105–1107.
58. Maher JF, Mallory GK, Laurend GA: Rupture of the heart after myocardial infarction. *N Engl J Med* 1956;255:1–10.
59. Lewis AJ, Burchell HB, Titus JL: Clinical and pathologic features of postinfarction cardiac rupture. *Am J Cardiol* 1960;23:43–53.
60. Meurs AAH, Vos AK, Verhey JB, Gerbrandy J: Electrocardiogram during cardiac rupture by myocardial infarction. *Br Heart J* 1970;32:232–235.
61. Ersek RA, Chesler E, Korns ME, Edwards JE: Spontaneous rupture of a false left ventricular aneurysm following myocardial infarction. *Am Heart J* 1969;77:677–680.
62. Rasmussen S, Leth A, Kjoller E, Pedersen A: Cardiac rupture in acute myocardial infarction: A review of 72 consecutive cases. *Acta Med Scand* 1979; 205:11–16.
63. Lowe TE, Wartman WB: Myocardial infarction. *Br Heart J* 1944;6:115–128.
64. McMullan MH, Kilgore TJ, Dear D, Hindman SH: Sudden blow-out rupture of the myocardium after infarction: Urgent management. *J Thorac Cardiovasc Surg* 1985;89:259–263.
65. Wessler S, Zoll PM, Schlesinger MJ: The pathogenesis of spontaneous cardiac rupture. *Circulation* 1952;6:334–351.
66. London RE, London SB: Rupture of the heart: A critical analysis of 47 consecutive autopsy cases. *Circulation* 1965;31:202–208.
67. vanTassel RA, Edwards JE: Rupture of the heart complicating myocardial infarction: Analysis of 40 cases including nine examples of left ventricular false aneurysm. *Chest* 1972;61:104–116.
68. Saffitz JE, Fredrickson RC, Roberts WC: Relation of size of transmural acute myocardial infarct to mode of death, interval between infarction and death and frequency of coronary arterial thrombus. *Am J Cardiol* 1986;57:1249–1254.
69. Herlitz J, Samuelson SO, Richter A, Hjalmarson A: Prediction of rupture in acute myocardial infarction. *Clin Cardiol* 1988;11:63–69.
70. Shapira I, Isakov A, Burke M, Almog C: Cardiac rupture in patients with acute myocardial infarction. *Chest* 1987;92:219–223.
71. Atkinson JB, Robinowitz M, McAllister HA, Virmani R: Association of eosinophils with cardiac rupture. *Hum Pathol* 1985;16:562–568.
72. Mann JM, Roberts WC: Rupture of the left ventricular free wall during acute myocardial infarc-

tion: Analysis of 138 necropsy patients and comparison with 50 necropsy patients with acute myocardial infarction without rupture. *Am J Cardiol* 1988;62:847–860.

73. Mann JM, Roberts WC: Fatal rupture of both left ventricular free wall and ventricular septum (double rupture) during acute myocardial infarction: Analysis of seven patients studied at necropsy. *Am J Cardiol* 1987;60:722–724.

74. Edmondson HA, Hoxie HJ: Hypertension and cardiac rupture: A clinical and pathologic study of 72 cases, in 13 of which rupture of the interventricular septum occurred. *Am Heart J* 1942;24:719–723.

75. Levene E: Spontaneous rupture of the heart. *Br Heart J* 1960;22:660–670.

76. Christensen DJ, Ford M, Reading J, Castle CH: Effect of hypertension on myocardial rupture after acute myocardial infarction. *Chest* 1977;72:618–622.

77. Waldron BR, Fennell RH Jr, Castleman B, Bland EF: Myocardial rupture and hemopericardium associated with anticoagulant therapy: A postmortem study. *N Engl J Med* 1954;251:892–894.

78. Capeci NE, Levy RL: The influence of anticoagulant therapy on the incidence of thromboembolism, hemorrhage and cardiac rupture in acute myocardial infarction. *Am J Med* 1959;26:76–80.

79. Honan MB, Harrell FE, Reimer KA, et al: Cardiac rupture and timing of thrombolytic therapy: A meta analysis. *Circulation* 1988;78(Suppl II):II-503 (abstract).

80. Honan MB, Harrell FE, Reimer KA, et al: Cardiac rupture, mortality, and the timing of thrombolytic therapy: A meta-analysis. *J Am Coll Cardiol* 1990;16: 359–367.

81. Lonkinen KL, O'Neill W, Laufer N, et al: Myocardial rupture complicating tissue plasminogen activator therapy of acute myocardial infarction (abstract). *J Am Coll Cardiol* 1989;13:94A.

82. Mauri F, DeBiase AM, Franzosi MG, et al: GISSI: Analisi delle cause di morte intraospedaliera. *G Ital Cardiol* 1987;17:37–44.

82a. Gertz SD, Kragel AH, Kalan JM, et al: Comparison of Coronary and Myocardial Morphologic Findings in Patients With and Without Thrombolytic Therapy During Fatal First Acute Myocardial Infarction. The TIMI Investigators, *Amer J Cardiol* 1990;66:904.

82b. Becker RC, Charlesworth A, Wilcox RG, et al: Cardiac Rupture Associated with Thrombolytic Therapy: Impact of Time to Treatment in the Late Assessment of Thrombolytic Efficacy (LATE) Study. *J Am Coll Cardiol* 1995;5:1063.

82c. Becker RC, Gore JM, Lambrew C et al: A composite view of cardiac rupture in the United States National Registry of Myocardial Infarction *J Am Coll Cardiol* 1996;6:1321–1326.

82d. Morishima I, Sone T, Mokuno S, et al: Clinical Significance of No-Reflow Phenomenon Observed on Angiography After Successful Treatment of Acute Myocardial Infarction with Percutaneous Transluminal Coronary Angioplasty, *Amer Heart J* 1995; 130:239.

82e. Cheriex EC, de Swart H, Dijkman LW, et al: Myocardial Rupture After Myocardial Infarction is Related to the Perfusion Status of the Infarct-Related Coronary Artery, *Amer Heart J* 1995; 129:644.

82f. Figueras J, Curos A, Cortadellas J et al., Relevance of Electrocardiographic Findings, Heart Failure and Infarct Site in Assessing Risk and Timing of Left Ventricular Free Wall Rupture During Acute Myocardial Infarction. *Amer J Cardiol* 1995;76: 543–547.

83. Bulkley BH, Roberts WC: Steroid therapy during acute myocardial infarction: A cause of delayed healing and of ventricular aneurysm. *Am J Med* 1974;56:244–250.

84. Roberts R, DeMello V, Sobel BE: Deleterious effects of methylprednisolone in patients with myocardial infarction. *Circulation* 1976;53(Suppl I): I-204–I-206.

85. Hammerman H, Kloner RA, Hale F, et al: Dose-dependent effects of short-term methylprednisolone on myocardial infarct extent, scar formation and ventricular function. *Circulation* 1983;68: 446–453.

86. Hammerman H, Cloner RA, Schoen FJ, et al: Indomethacin-induced scar thinning after experimental myocardial infarction. *Circulation* 1983;67: 1290–1295.

87. Brown EJ Jr, Kloner RA, Schoen FJ, et al: Scar thinning due to ibuprofen administration after experimental myocardial infarction. *Am J Cardiol* 1983;51:877–883.

88. Silverman HF, Pfeifer MP: Relation between use of anti-inflammatory agents in left ventricular free wall rupture during acute myocardial infarction. *Am J Cardiol* 1987;59:363–364.

89. ISIS-1 Collaborative Group: Mechanisms for the early mortality reduction produced by beta blockade started early in acute myocardial infarction: ISIS-1. *Lancet* 1988;1:921–923.
90. The MIAMI Trial Research Group: Mortality. *Am J Cardiol* 1985;56:15G–22G.
91. Pollak H, Miczoch J: Effect of nitrates on the frequency of left ventricular free wall rupture complicating acute myocardial infarction: A case-controlled study. *Am Heart J* 1994;128: 466–471.
92. Schuster EH, Bulkley BH: Expansion of transmural myocardial infarction: A pathophysiologic factor in cardiac rupture. *Circulation* 1975;60: 1532–1538.
93. Ross RM, Young JA: Clinical and necropsy findings in rupture of the myocardium: A review of forty-three cases. *Scott Med J* 1963;8:222–226.
94. Kamil M, Miller M, Messelolf CR, Lepow HI: Cardiac rupture in myocardial infarction. *NY State J Med* 1962;62:2327–2335.
95. Datta BN, Bowes VF, Silver MD: Incomplete rupture of the heart with diverticulum formation. *Pathology* 1975;7:179–185.
96. O'Rourke MF: Subacute heart rupture following myocardial infarction: Clinical features of a correctable condition. *Lancet* 1973;2:124–126.
97. Oliva PB, Hammill SC, Edwards WD: Cardiac rupture, a clinically predictable complication of acute myocardial infarction: Report of 70 cases with clinicopathologic correlations. *J Am Coll Cardiol* 1993;22:720–726.
98. Friedman HF, Kuhn LA, Katz AM: Clinical and electrocardiographic features of cardiac rupture following acute myocardial infarction. *Am J Med* 1971;50:709–720.
99. Cohn LH: Surgical management of acute and chronic cardiac mechanical complications due to myocardial infarction. *Am Heart J* 1981;102: 1049–1060.
100. Coma-Canella I, Lopez-Sendon J, Garcia AG: Hemodynamic effect of dextran, dobutamine, and pericardiocentesis in cardiac tamponade secondary to subacute heart rupture. *Am Heart J* 1987;114:78–84.
101. Desoutter P, Halphen C, Haiat R: Two-dimensional echographic visualization of free ventricular wall rupture in acute anterior myocardial infarction. *Am Heart J* 1984;108:1360–1361.
102. Hagemeijer F, Verbaan CJ, Sonke PC, de Rooij CH: Echocardiography and rupture of the heart. *Br Heart J* 1980;43:45–46.
103. Hochreiter C, Goldstein J, Borer JS, et al: Myocardial free-wall rupture after acute infarction: Survival aided by percutaneous intraaortic balloon counterpulsation. *Circulation* 1982;65:1279–1282.
104. Feneley MP, Chang VP, O'Rourke MF: Myocardial rupture after acute myocardial infarction: Ten year review. *Br Heart J* 1983;49:550–556.
105. Cobbs BW Jr, Hatcher CR Jr, Robinson PH: Cardiac rupture: Three operations with two long-term survivals. *JAMA* 1973;223:532–535.
106. Anagnostopoulos E, Beutler S, Levett JM, et al: Myocardial rupture: Major left ventricular infarct rupture treated by infarctectomy. *JAMA* 1977; 238:2715–2716.
107. Lillehei CW, Todd DB Jr, Levy MJ, Ellis RJ: Partial cardiopulmonary bypass, hypothermia, and total circulatory arrest. *J Thorac Cardiovasc Surg* 1969;58:530–544.
108. FitzGibbon GM, Hooper GD, Heggtveit HA: Successful surgical treatment of postinfarction external cardiac rupture. *J Thorac Cardiovasc Surg* 1972;63:622–630.
109. Parr GVS, Pae WE Jr, Pierce WS, Zelis R: Cardiogenic shock due to ventricular rupture: A surgical approach. *J Thorac Cardiovasc Surg* 1981;82: 889–891.
110. Kendall RW, DeWood MA: Postinfarction cardiac rupture: Surgical success and review of the literature. *Ann Thorac Surg* 1978;25:311–315.
111. Pifarre R, Sullivan HJ, Grieco J, et al: Management of left ventricular rupture complicating myocardial infarction. *J Thorac Cardiovasc Surg* 1983;86: 441–443.
112. Nunez L, de la Llana R, Lopez-Sendon J, et al: Diagnosis and treatment of subacute free wall ventricular rupture after infarction. *Ann Thorac Surg* 983;35:525–529.
113. Calick A, Kerth W, Barbour D, Cohn K: Successful surgical therapy of ruptured myocardium. *Chest* 1974;66:188.
114. Chesler E, Korns ME, Semba T, Edwards JE: False aneurysms of the left ventricle following myocardial infarction. *Am J Cardiol* 1969;23:76–82.
115. Vlodaver Z, Coe JI, Edwards JE: True and false left ventricular aneurysms: Propensity for the latter to rupture. *Circulation* 1975;51:567–572.

116. Cone RB, Hawley RL: Pseudoaneurysm of the heart following infarction. *Arch Pathol* 1964;77:166–171.

117. Gueron M, Wanderman KL, Hirsch M, Borman J: Pseudoaneurysm of the left ventricle after myocardial infarction: A curable form of myocardial rupture. *J Thorac Cardiovasc Surg* 1975;69:736–742.

118. Onik G, Recht L, Edwards JE, et al: False left ventricular aneurysm: Diagnosis by noninvasive means. *J Nucl Med* 1980;21:177–182.

119. Reeder GS, Seward JB, Tajik AJ: The role of two-dimensional echocardiography in coronary artery disease: A critical appraisal. *Mayo Clin Proc* 1982; 57:247–258.

120. Gatewood RP Jr, Nanda NC: Differentiation of left ventricular pseudoaneurysm from true aneurysm with two dimensional echocardiography. *Am J Cardiol* 1980;46:869–878.

121. Van Mechelen R, Van Hemel M, Van Rijk PP: Noninvasive diagnosis of pseudoaneurysm of left ventricle. *Br Heart J* 1978;40:812–816.

122. Winzelberg GC, Miller SW, Okada RD, et al: Scintigraphic assessment of false left ventricular aneurysms. *Am J Radiol* 1980;135:569–574.

123. Stewart S, Huddle R, Stuard I, et al: False aneurysm and pseudo-false aneurysm of the left ventricle: Etiology, pathology, diagnosis, and operative management. *Ann Thorac Surg* 1981;31:259–265.

124. Rittenhouse EA, Sauvage LR, Mansfield PB, et al: False aneurysm of the left ventricle: Report of four cases and review of surgical management. *Ann Surg* 1979;189:409–415.

125. Buehler DL, Stinson EB, Oyer PE, Shumway NE: Surgical treatment of aneurysms of the inferior left ventricular wall. *J Thorac Cardiovasc Surg* 1979; 78:74–78.

126. Sanders RJ, Kern WH, Blount SG: Perforation of the interventricular septum complicating myocardial infarction. *Am Heart J* 1956;51:736–748.

127. Hutchins GM: Rupture of the interventricular septum complicating myocardial infarction: Pathological analysis of 10 patients with clinically diagnosed perforations. *Am Heart J* 1979;97:165–173.

128. Edwards BS, Edwards WD, Edwards JE: Ventricular septal rupture complicating acute myocardial infarction: Identification of simple and complex types in 53 autopsied hearts. *Am J Cardiol* 1984;54:1201–1205.

129. Hill JD, Lary D, Kerth WJ, Gerbode F: Acquired ventricular septal defects: Evolution of an operation, surgical technique, and results. *J Thorac Cardiovasc Surg* 1975;70:440–449.

130. Roberts WC, Ronan JA Jr, Harvey WP: Rupture of the left ventricular free wall (LVFW) or ventricular septum (VS) secondary to acute myocardial infarction (AMI): An occurrence virtually limited to the first transmural AMI in a hypertensive individual (abstract). *Am J Cardiol* 1975;35:166.

131. Westaby S, Parry A, Ormerod O, et al: Thrombolysis and post infarction ventricular septal rupture. *J Thorac Cardiovasc Surg* 1992;104:1506–1509.

132. Perloff JK, Talano JV, Ronan JA Jr: Noninvasive techniques in acute myocardial infarction. *Prog Cardiovasc Dis* 1971;13:437–464.

133. James TN: De subitaneis mortibus XXIV: Ruptured interventricular septum and heart block. *Circulation* 1977;55:934–946.

134. Scanlan JG, Seward JB, Tajik AJ: Visualization of ventricular septal rupture utilizing wide-angle two-dimensional echocardiography. *Mayo Clin Proc* 1979;54:381–384.

135. Bishop HL, Gibson RS, Stamm RB, et al: Role of two-dimensional echocardiography in the evaluation of patients with ventricular septal rupture postmyocardial infarction. *Am Heart J* 1981;102:965–971.

136. Drobac M, Gilbert B, Howard R, et al: Ventricular septal defect after myocardial infarction: Diagnosis by two-dimensional contrast echocardiography. *Circulation* 1981;67:335–341.

137. Recusani F, Raisaro A, Sgalambro A, et al: Ventricular septal rupture after myocardial infarction: Diagnosis by two-dimensional and pulsed Doppler echocardiography. *Am J Cardiol* 1984;54:277–281.

138. Miyatake K, Okamoto M, Kinoshito N, et al: Doppler echocardiographic features of ventricular septal rupture in myocardial infarction. *J Am Coll Cardiol* 1985;5:182–187.

139. Smith G, Endresen K, Sivertssen E, Semb G: Ventricular septal rupture diagnosed by simultaneous cross-sectional echocardiography and Doppler ultrasound. *Eur Heart J* 1985;6:631–636.

140. Tatooles CJ, Gault JH, Mason DT, Ross J Jr: Reflux of oxygenated blood into the pulmonary artery in severe mitral regurgitation. *Am Heart J* 1968;5:102–106.

141. Montoya A, McKeever L, Scanlon P, et al: Early repair of ventricular septal rupture after infarction. *Am J Cardiol* 1980;45:345–348.
142. Cooley DA, Belmonte BA, Zeis LB, Schnur S: Surgical repair of ruptured interventricular septum following acute myocardial infarction. *Surgery* 1957;41:930–937.
143. Kitamura S, Mendez A, Kay JH: Ventricular septal defect following myocardial infarction: Experience with surgical repair through a left ventriculotomy and review of the literature. *J Thorac Cardiovasc Surg* 1971;61:186–199.
144. Giuliani ER, Danielson GK, Pluth JR, et al: Postinfarction ventricular septal rupture. *Circulation* 1974;49:455–459.
145. Brandt B, Wright CB, Ehrenhaft JL: Ventricular septal defect following myocardial infarction. *Ann Thorac Surg* 1979;27:580–589.
146. Austen WC, Sokol DM, DeSanctis RW, Sanders CA: Surgical treatment of papillary muscle rupture complicating myocardial infarction. *N Engl J Med* 1968;278:1137–1141.
147. Parry G, Goudevenos J, Adams PC, et al: Septal rupture after myocardial infarction: Is very early surgery really worthwhile? *Eur Heart J* 1992;13: 373–382.
148. Windsor HM, Chang VP Shanahan MX: Postinfarction cardiac rupture. *J Thorac Cardiovasc Surg* 1982;84:755–761.
149. Killen DA, Reed WA, Wathanacharoen S, et al: Postinfarction rupture of the interventricular septum. *J Cardiovasc Surg* 1981;22:113–126.
150. Lemery R, Smith HC, Gersh BJ, et al: Prognosis in rupture of the ventricular septum after acute myocardial infarction: Role of early surgical intervention. *Am J Cardiol* 1992;70:147–151.
151. Mundth ED, Buckley MJ, Daggett WM, et al: Surgery for complications of acute myocardial infarction. *Circulation* 1972;45:1279–1291.
152. Khan MM, Patterson GC, O'Kane HO, Adgey AAJ: Management of ventricular septal rupture in acute myocardial infarction. *Br Heart J* 1980; 44:570–576.
153. Gaudiani VA, Miller C, Stinson EB, et al: Post infarction ventricular septal defect: An argument for early operation. *Surgery* 1981;89:43–54.
154. Moore CA, Nygaard TW, Kaiser DL, et al: Postinfarction ventricular septal rupture: The importance of location of infarction and right ventricular function in determining survival. *Circulation* 1986;74:45–55.
155. Cummings RG, Reimer KA, Califf R, et al: Quantitative analysis of right and left ventricular infarction in the presence of postinfarction ventricular septal defect. *Circulation* 1988;77:33–42.
156. Dagget WM: Surgical technique for early repair of posterior ventricular septal rupture. *J Thorac Cardiovasc Surg* 1982;84:306–312.
157. Muehrcke DD, Daggett WM, Buckley MJ, et al: Postinfarct ventricular septal defect repair: Effect of coronary artery bypass grafting. *Ann Thorac Surg* 1992;54:876–883.
158. Jones MT, Schofield PM, Dark JF, et al: Surgical technique for early repair of acquired ventricular septal defect. *J Thorac Cardiovasc Surg* 1987;93: 680–686.
159. Matsui K, Kay JH, Mendez M, et al: Ventricular septal rupture secondary to myocardial infarction: Clinical approach and surgical results. *JAMA* 1981;245:1537–1539.
160. Davies RH, Dawkins KD, Skillington PD, et al: Late functional results after surgical closure of acquired ventricular septal defect. *J Thorac Cardiovasc Surg* 1993;106:592–598.
161. Muehrcke DD, Blank S, Daggett WM: Survival after repair of postinfarction ventricular septal defects in patients over the age of 70. *J Cardiac Surg* 1992;7:290–300.

17

Right Ventricular Myocardial Infarction

L. J. Dell'Italia, MD, and R. A. O'Rourke, MD

Right ventricular myocardial infarction (RVMI) usually occurs after occlusion of a dominant right coronary artery in the clinical setting of an inferior or diaphragmatic myocardial infarction. When predominant infarction of the right ventricle is present, the patient may present with a unique combination of clinical findings that include hypotension, an elevated jugular venous pressure, and clear lung fields. This clinical syndrome requires a unique form of therapy clearly distinct from that of hypotension associated with predominant infarction of the left ventricle. Since it was first described in the early 1970s, there has been great interest in the function of the right ventricle in acute myocardial infarction, and this has resulted in a number of studies describing various methods for diagnosis of RVMI. These studies have led to some confusion with respect to the incidence of RVMI in acute inferior myocardial infarction because hemodynamic monitoring and various noninvasive diagnostic methods report an incidence of RVMI ranging between 10% to 50% in patients who present with acute inferior myocardial infarction. Nevertheless, it is clear that this clinical syndrome has a better acute and long-term prognosis than that associated with predominant infarction of the left ventricle. In this chapter the unique anatomic and physiologic features of the right ventricle will be related to the clinical presentation of RVMI in order to provide a clear understanding of its incidence, treatment, and acute and long-term prognosis.

ANATOMY AND POSTMORTEM STUDIES

The right coronary artery provides blood supply to the right ventricular outflow tract via the conus artery, to the right ventricular free wall via the right ventricular free wall branches, and to the right ventricular lateral and posterior walls via the right ventricular marginal branches (see Chs. 2 and 15). In addition, the right coronary artery provides blood supply to the posterior one-third of the interventricular septum and variable blood supply to the posterior wall of the left ventricle depending on the dominance of the right coronary artery. The left coronary artery provides very little blood supply to the right ventricle in the form of small arterial branches to the right ventricular anterior wall from the left anterior descending artery. Accordingly, right ventricular ischemia or infarction occurs in the majority of cases after occlusion of a dominant right coronary artery resulting in various grades of right ventricular ischemia and/or necrosis, which can be summarized as follows (1) (Fig. 17–1):

Grade I: Necrosis of less than 50% of the right ventricular posterior wall

Grade II: Necrosis limited to but not involving more than 50% of the posterior wall

Grade III: Necrosis of the posterior wall and less than 50% of the anterolateral wall

Grade IV: Necrosis of the right ventricular posterior wall and more than 50% of the anterolateral wall

From this anatomic scheme of resultant right ventricular necrosis, one can appreciate the spectrum of hemodynamic and noninvasive findings in this condition. Furthermore, it is clear that necrosis of the right ventricle is usually associated with a small amount of left ventricular posterior necrosis. Consequently, RVMI generally produces predominant right ventricular dysfunction with relative preservation of overall left ventricular systolic function.

Not all right coronary artery occlusions result in significant right ventricular necrosis and dysfunction. This is quite different from the situation encountered in left coronary artery occlusion and resultant left ventricular necrosis and may be related to the different anatomy and physiology of the right ventricle. A rich system of thebesian veins may directly supply the thin right ventricular myocardium with venous oxygenated blood, and the low-pressure system in the right heart may decrease right ventricular myocardial oxygen demands during acute right coronary artery occlusion. Postmortem studies by Isner (1) and Ratliff (2) reported that three-fourths of all heart specimens with right ventricular necrosis had a greater than 75% stenosis of the left anterior descending artery, suggesting that impaired left-to-right collateral blood flow may be important in the pathogenesis of RVMI. Nonetheless, RVMI does occur in the absence of significant disease of the left coronary artery system and, consequently, may depend upon interindividual differ-

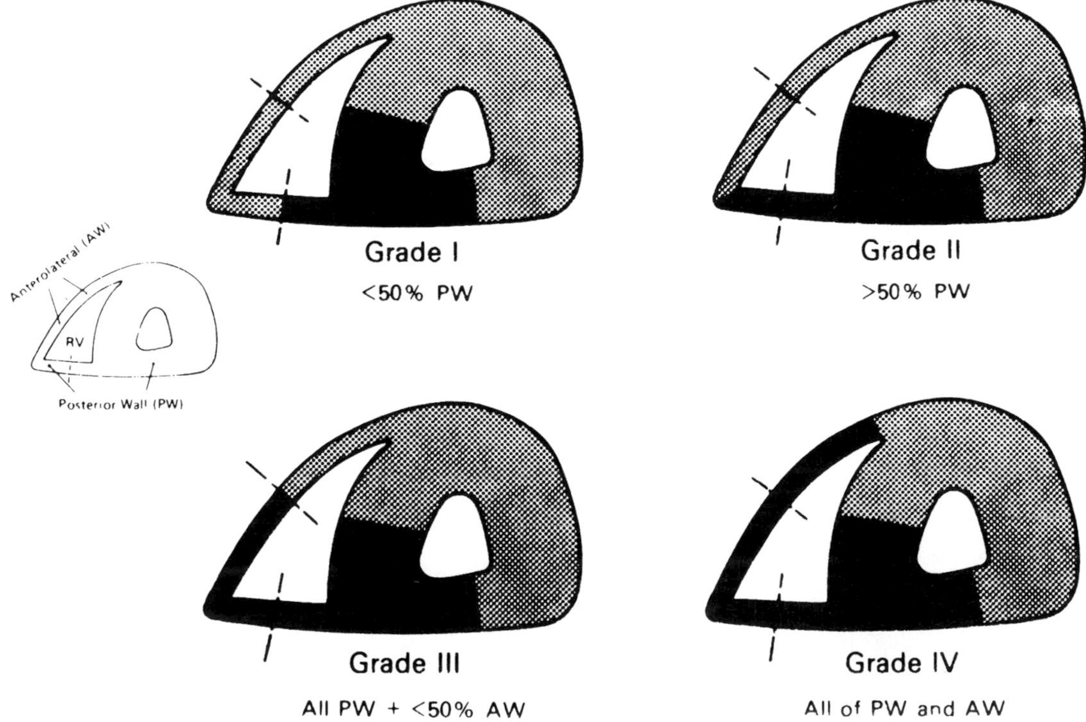

Figure 17–1. Schematic diagram of transverse slices of the right and left ventricles illustrating the scheme for grading the extent of right ventricular myocardial infarction (RVMI). PW = posterior wall; AW = anterolateral wall. *Reproduced by permission of the American Journal of Cardiology.*

ences in the rate of collateral vessel development. Other human postmortem studies and animal models have demonstrated that RVMI occurs more frequently or exclusively in the presence of preexisting right ventricular hypertrophy because this condition may increase right ventricular myocardial oxygen demands and enhance ischemic injury during acute right coronary artery occlusion (2–6). However, there are numerous documented cases of RVMI in the absence of significant right ventricular hypertrophy (1,7). Thus the pathogenesis of RVMI may be multifactorial, resulting in a yet unpredictable presence or absence of necrosis with acute right coronary artery occlusion.

PHYSICAL EXAMINATION

Prompt clinical recognition of acute RVMI in patients is extremely important because appropriate therapy for hypotension and shock oftentimes must be started before performance of invasive hemodynamic monitoring or noninvasive tests. Therefore, the physical examination must provide an important initial guide for appropriate therapy to achieve circulatory stability. Any patient with an acute inferior wall myocardial infarction should be suspected of having right ventricular dysfunction. However, less than 10% of these patients will suffer from hypotension and shock. In contrast, for patients who do not present in shock, one must also recognize the potential presence of right ventricular dysfunction in order to avoid therapy that will further lower right heart filling pressures (e.g., nitrates, diuretics, morphine) and produce hypotension.

Cohn and coworkers were the first to describe the triad of hypotension, elevated jugular venous pressure, and clear lung fields as physical examination markers of RVMI in acute inferior myocardial infarction (8). Other studies have reported the presence of Kussmaul's sign and various clinical findings associated with RVMI, all of which result from systolic and diastolic dysfunction of the right ventricle (9–14). However, a systematic and prospective approach is necessary to determine the accuracy of these physical examination findings for identifying significant right ventricular dysfunction in those patients who present with and without shock in the setting of acute inferior wall myocardial infarction.

In 53 consecutive patients with acute inferior myocardial infarction evaluated within 36 hours of the onset of symptoms, we identified 8 patients with hemodynamic findings consistent with RVMI (right atrial pressure [RAP] ≥ 10 mm Hg and RAP : pulmonary arterial wedge pressure [PAWP] ratio ≥ 0.8) (15). The physical examination findings of both an elevated jugular venous pressure (≥8 cm H_2O) and Kussmaul's sign were the most sensitive (88%) and specific (100%) markers for hemodynamically important RVMI. The classic triad of hypotension, elevated jugular venous pressure, and clear lung fields was only 25% sensitive but 96% specific, whereas an elevated jugular venous pressure alone was more sensitive (88%) but less specific (69%) for RVMI. Therefore, careful physical examination of the neck veins provides a rapid diagnostic screen so that appropriate therapy may be initiated for treatment of hypotension and, treatment with nitroglycerin and morphine may be administered with caution in order to avoid system arterial hypotension resulting from a deleterious decrease in right heart filling pressures.

Table 17–1 lists other physical examination findings that may be present in patients presenting with acute RVMI. Because right ventricular chamber dilation frequently accompanies RVMI, tricuspid regurgitation may be identified by a systolic murmur aucultated at the lower left sternal border that increases with inspiration. This finding must be distinguished from the murmurs of papillary muscle dysfunction and ventricular septal defect that may result from acute inferior wall myocardial infarction. Other physical examination features of right

Table 17–1. Clinical Findings Associated with Right Ventricular Infarction.

Hypotension
Elevated jugular venous pressure
Kussmaul's sign
Abnormal jugular venous pressure pattern (Y ≥ X descent)
Tricuspid regurgitation
Right-sided S_3 and S_4
Pulsus paradoxus
High-grade atrioventricular block

ventricular diastolic dysfunction include atrial and ventricular gallops and an abnormal waveform of the jugular venous pressure. In addition to elevation of the jugular venous pressure, its pattern may demonstrate an abnormal pressure wave form manifested by an A wave and V wave that are equal in magnitude and a Y descent greater than or equal to the X descent. These findings reflect a poorly compliant or stiff right ventricle, which may become more apparent during inspiration or hepatojugular reflux maneuver. Careful recording of the blood pressure by cuff sphygmomanometer may demonstrate a pulsus paradox. Finally, high-grade atrioventricular (AV) block can occur, resulting from AV nodal ischemia, and loss of atrial/ventricular synchrony can exacerbate hypotension and shock when severe right ventricular dysfunction is present. It has been reported that the incidence of high-grade AV block is two to four times as high in patients with acute inferior wall myocardial infarction than those with anterior wall infarction, and this finding may be associated with a poor prognosis (14).

In summary, all of the potential physical examination findings that may be associated with RVMI depend on the amount of right ventricular necrosis present. Of all the previously mentioned features, elevation of the jugular venous pressure and Kussmaul's sign provide the most accurate clinical markers of significant right ventricular ischemia and/or necrosis (15). The syndrome of hypotension, poor peripheral perfusion and/or shock in the *absence* of pulmonary edema should alert one to the existence of right ventricular infarction, particularly in a patient with an inferior myocardial infarction.

HEMODYNAMIC FUNCTION

Invasive hemodynamic monitoring identifies RVMI by a combination of findings that suggest systolic and diastolic dysfunction of the right ventricle—e.g., low cardiac output and a disproportionate elevation of the right atrial pressure (RAP) compared with the pulmonary arterial wedge pressure (PAWP) (16–22). Decreased right ventricular systolic function results in low cardiac output and hypotension. Decreased compliance of the right ventricle produces an elevated right atrial pressure, Kussmaul's sign, and a poorly compliant right atrial pressure waveform manifested by A and V waves which are equal in amplitude and the Y descent greater than or equal to the X descent (Fig. 17–2). These diastolic abnormalities represent the decreased compliance of the right atrial and ventricular myocardium, which produces a rise in right atrial pressure during inspiration (Kussmaul's sign) and a prominent V wave and Y descent during rapid diastolic filling of the right ventricular cavity.

The currently accepted hemodynamic criteria of RVMI come from a combined autopsy/hemodynamic study performed by Lopez-Sendon and coworkers (21). These investigators report 60 patients dying of acute myocardial infarction who underwent hemodynamic monitoring before death

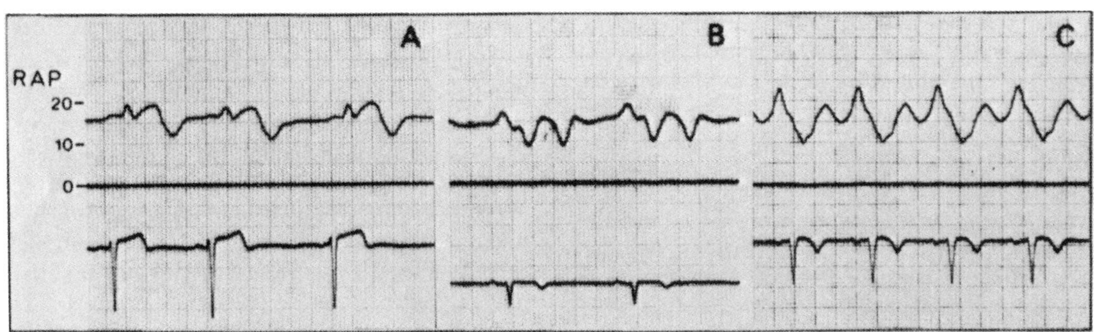

Figure 17–2. Right atrial pressure (RAP, mm Hg) waveforms with Y > X descent (**A**), Y = X descent (**B**), and X > Y descent (**C**). **A** and **B** represent severe and mild forms of the poorly compliant pattern of the right atrial pressure waveform, while a normal pattern is demonstrated in **C.** *Reproduced with permission of the American Heart Journal.*

and subsequent postmortem examination. Autopsy-proven right ventricular necrosis in 22 of 60 heart specimens correlated with a RAP ≥ 10 mm Hg and a RAP : PAWP ratio of >0.86. If these conditions were met, along with a poorly compliant pattern of the right atrial pressure waveform (Y descent greater than or equal to X descent), the sensitivity and specificity for detecting RVMI by hemodynamic monitoring were 82% and 97%, respectively. However, in 18% of cases these hemodynamic criteria were not fulfilled despite well-documented right ventricular necrosis. Careful inspection of the data demonstrates that 15 patients had a PAWP greater than 20 mm Hg, which precluded volume administration, and 10 of these 15 patients had acute or healed necrosis of the left ventricular anterior wall. Consequently, a close relation between the right atrial pressure and pulmonary arterial wedge pressure was not observed in these patients because there was concomitant significant left ventricular dysfunction, and this accounted for the reduced sensitivity. However, when this latter situation exists, right atrial pressure is often persistently elevated after appropriate diuresis or treatment with other agents aimed at unloading the left ventricle.

The importance of this study and other studies evaluating hemodynamic function in the setting of acute inferior myocardial infarction demonstrates that patients with RVMI may present with a spectrum of hemodynamic findings that are best summarized as follows:

1. RAP ≥ 10 mm Hg, RAP : PAWP ratio > 0.86, and systolic arterial pressure (SAP) less than 100 mm Hg
2. RAP ≥ 10 mm Hg, RAP : PAWP > 0.86, and SAP greater than 100 mm Hg
3. RAP ≥ 10 mm Hg and RAP : PAWP > 0.86 only after volume loading, with or without SAP greater than 100 mm Hg
4. RAP ≥ 10 mm Hg and RAP : PAWP < 0.86 due to marked elevation of the PAWP and greater amount of left ventricular damage

Clinical studies by Bairgre (16) and Coma-Canella (17) have demonstrated that volume loading may increase the yield of RVMI hemodynamics in patients presenting with acute inferior myocardial infarction. In our study of 53 consecutive patients with acute inferior myocardial infarction, we found that 8 patients had hemodynamic criteria consistent with RVMI at rest (RAP ≥ 10 mm Hg and RAP : PAWP ratio ≥ 0.8) and an additional 6 patients developed RVMI hemodynamics after volume loading with normal saline ($p < 0.05$) (22). Thus the *majority* of patients with acute inferior myocardial infarction present hemodynamically stable without evidence of significant right ventricular dysfunction. However, a small percentage of patients may present with elevation of both right- and left-sided filling pressures because of concomitant significant left ventricular myocardial infarction.

Other cardiac conditions can produce an elevation and equalization of right and left heart pressures along with an abnormal right atrial pressure waveform. These cardiac problems can be subdivided into pathophysiologic conditions affecting predominantly right ventricular diastolic and/or systolic dysfunction. Those conditions predominantly affecting diastolic function include cardiac tamponade, constrictive pericarditis, and restrictive or infiltrative cardiomyopathy, all of which may be associated with normal or near-normal right ventricular systolic function. In contrast, severe right ventricular systolic dysfunction may result from pulmonary hypertension secondary to acute pulmonary embolism or severe chronic obstructive lung disease. In addition, severe, chronic right and left heart failure may result in both elevation and equalization of right and left heart filling pressures in some instances. In most cases, a careful history and physical examination coupled with an electrocardiogram and two-dimensional echocardiography may rule out these potential cardiac problems that may mimic RVMI hemodynamics.

NONINVASIVE DIAGNOSIS OF RVMI

The most commonly used noninvasive methods for identifying RVMI in the setting of acute inferior wall myocardial infarction include electrocardiography, two-dimensional echocardiography, radionuclide ventriculography, and technetium pyrophosphate myocardial scintigraphy. Using these techniques the incidence of RVMI has been reported to range between 25% and 50%. This variability is related to the inherent limitations of each technique and to the interstudy variability in criteria for the diagnosis of RVMI. Nevertheless, electrocardiography may provide a rapid diagnosis of RVMI, and radionuclide angiography and echocardiography may provide important complementary information to invasive hemodynamic monitoring for complete treatment of patients in the coronary care units.

Electrocardiography

The electrocardiographic manifestation of acute right ventricular injury has been reported using the V_{4R} lead placed in the fifth intercostal space in the right mid-clavicular line. Erhardt (23) reported that ST segment elevation of more than 1 mm in lead V_{4R} was a highly specific finding for subsequent postmortem documentation of right ventricular necrosis in 18 of 92 patients with acute inferior myocardial infarction (Fig. 17–3). Sixteen of the seventy-two surviving patients also had ST segment elevation in V_{4R}, and these patients had a higher incidence of hypotension ($p < 0.05$) and right heart failure ($p < 0.01$) than the remaining 58 survivors. Subsequently, Chou and coworkers reported transient ST segment elevation in precordial lead V_1 in 8 of 11 patients presenting with acute inferior myocardial infarction (24). Right ventricular infarction was documented by autopsy in 5 patients and by hemodynamic monitoring in 6. In a prospective analysis of 110 consecutive patients with acute inferior transmural myocardial infarction, Klein and coworkers demonstrated greater than 0.5 mm ST elevation in lead V_{4R} in 48 of 58 patients with hemodynamic or noninvasive evidence of RVMI (83% sensitivity) and 12 of the remaining 52 patients without evidence of RVMI (77% specificity) (25). Subsequent studies over the past 15 years have demonstrated a similar sensitivity and specificity for detecting either hemodynamic or noninvasive evidence of RVMI when ST segment elevation greater than 1 mm was used as the criteria for right ventricular necrosis in lead V_{4R} (26–30). However, all of these studies have documented that this finding may be present for only 24 to 48 hours after the onset of chest pain, thereby limiting the sensitivity of this electrocardiographic finding. Furthermore, cardiac problems other than RVMI may produce ST segment elevation in lead V_{4R}, including acute pulmonary embolism, left ventricular hypertrophy, acute anterior septal myocardial infarction, pericarditis, and previous anterior myocardial infarction with aneurysm formation.

Geft and coworkers have described five patients with acute inferior myocardial infarction who pre-

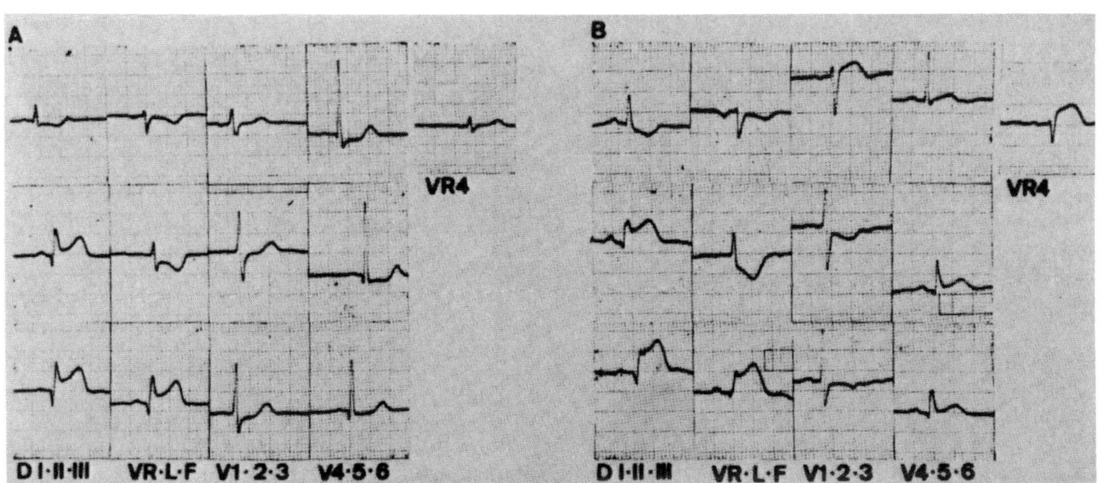

Figure 17–3. Electrocardiogram demonstrating acute inferior myocardial infarction in two patients with a normal ST segment in V_{4R} (**A**) and with >1 mm ST segment elevation in V_{4R} (**B**) consistent with RVMI. *Reproduced by permission of the American Heart Journal.*

sented with significant ST segment elevation in leads V_1–V_5 without Q waves and minimal ST segment elevation in the inferior leads (31). Subsequent cardiac catheterization within 4 hours of the onset of chest pain demonstrated proximal right coronary artery obstruction without significant left coronary artery disease. These five patients also had technetium-99*m* pyrophosphate myocardial scintigraphy and radionuclide angiographic evidence of RVMI. Thus these electrocardiographic findings represent a manifestation of predominant right ventricular injury early in the course of myocardial infarction. These investigators produced infarction of the right ventricle in a dog model and demonstrated ST segment elevation in V_{4R} to V_{6R} in this model, where the right coronary artery supplies the right ventricular free wall and no blood supply to the left ventricular posterior wall. However, when an occlusion of the right coronary artery was followed by occlusion of the left circumflex coronary artery, ST segment elevation in the right precordial leads that overlie the right ventricle were suppressed. Thus, in this animal model and most likely in man, left ventricular necrosis appears to cancel the ST segment elevation associated with right ventricular injury and may account for the infrequent occurrence in early left precordial leads (V_1–V_3) and its transient nature in the right precordial leads (V_{4R}), especially when right ventricular necrosis is not extensive. Thus the finding of ST segment elevation in the right precordial or early transitional precordial leads is a very specific marker for right ventricular necrosis (Fig. 17–3); however, the sensitivity of this finding is limited by its transient appearance, which may be related to the relative proportion of right ventricular compared with left ventricular necrosis.

In spite of the foregoing limitations, recent studies have suggested that ST segment elevation in right-sided precordial leads is a strong, independent predictor of major complications and in-hospital mortality (32–36). In a prospective study of 200 consecutive patients with acute inferior myocardial infarction, Zehender and associates (32) demonstrated that the presence of ST segment elevations of ≥1 mm in lead V_{4R} identified subgroups of patients with increased hospital mortality ($p < 0.001$) and major complications ($p < 0.001$) including cardiogenic shock, ventricular fibrillation, third-degree block, and the need for temporary pacing. The in-hospital mortality after inferior myocardial infarction was 19% for the group. However, two-thirds of the patients with inferior myocardial infarction had contraindications to thrombolytic therapy, and these patients accounted for a substantial proportion of the high overall in-hospital mortality. Among the 36% who were suitable for thrombolytic therapy, the in-hospital mortality was 7%. Moreover, it is likely that some of the patients with electrocardiographic signs of right ventricular dysfunction had concomitant severe left ventricular dysfunction as well (37). Since isolated inferior wall myocardial infarction without complication is generally associated with a favorable prognosis, the early detection of right ventricular infarction by recording lead V_{4R} has been recommended by some for quickly stratifying patients into low- and high-risk subgroups (36). As emphasized above, the diagnostic usefulness of right precordial ST segment elevation is greatest during the first 10 hours post–acute inferior infarction. A complete electrocardiographic assessment should be obtained on all patients with inferior infarctions as soon after presentation as possible. In many hospitals, right-sided precordial leads are obtained routinely in all patients with inferior wall myocardial infarctions.

Echocardiography

Two-dimensional echocardiography offers a technique for assessing global right ventricular size and performance, segmental wall motion, valvular structures, and left ventricular size and performance (16,22,38,39) (see Ch. 10). Lopez-Sendon and coworkers studied 63 consecutive patients with inferior myocardial infarction with two-dimensional echocardiography and acute hemodynamic monitoring within 4 days of the onset of symptoms (39). The lateral right ventricular free wall and interventricular septum were evaluated in multiple views for evidence of akinesis or dyskinesis. There was a significant relation between the number of asynergic right ventricular wall segments and the severity of the hemodynamic pattern encountered. A total of 32 patients manifested hemodynamic criteria of RVMI, while the remaining 31 patients never demonstrated hemodynamics consistent with RVMI during their clinical observation period. A total of 11 patients had abnormal two-dimensional echocardiographic evaluation with normal hemodynamic function. In our study of 53 consecutive patients with inferior myocardial infarction, two-dimensional echocardiography was a highly sensitive technique for documenting the presence of hemodynamically important RVMI using echocardiographic wall motion abnormalities of akinesis or dyskinesis of right ventricular wall segments (22). However, this technique identified right ventricular wall motion abnormalities in patients who never developed hemodynamic criteria consistent with RVMI. The reduced specificity of echocardiographic manifestations of right ventricular wall motion abnormalities may reflect the superior sensitivity of a good-quality two-dimensional echocardiogram for detecting right ventricular ischemia and/or infarction. However, because of the difficulty in assessing wall motion abnormalities of the thin-walled right ventricle by this technique, it is important to include right ventricular dilation in addition to akinesis of dyskinesis in order to document hemodynamically important RVMI with a high degree of accuracy (Fig. 17–4).

The addition of color Doppler increases the diagnostic utility of this technique because tricuspid and mitral valvular function and shunt flow across a patent foramen ovale or ventricular septal defect may also be evaluated at bedside.

Radionuclide Angiography

Assessment of right ventricular performance is problematic because its complex structure does not conform to simple geometric assumptions and makes accurate right ventricular volumes and ejection fraction difficult to ascertain. Radionuclide angiography offers a significant advantage because it is based on count density and, therefore, can be used to access right ventricular performance independent of geometry. Using either the first-pass technique or equilibrium studies, right ventricular dysfunction has been reported to occur in approximately 40% to 50% of patients with acute inferior myocardial infarction (40–45), manifested by right ventricular enlargement or an ejection fraction value of less than 45% as markers for RVMI. However, these studies lack a systematic evaluation of right ventricular wall motion, which is an important feature in identifying right ventricular dysfunction secondary to RVMI

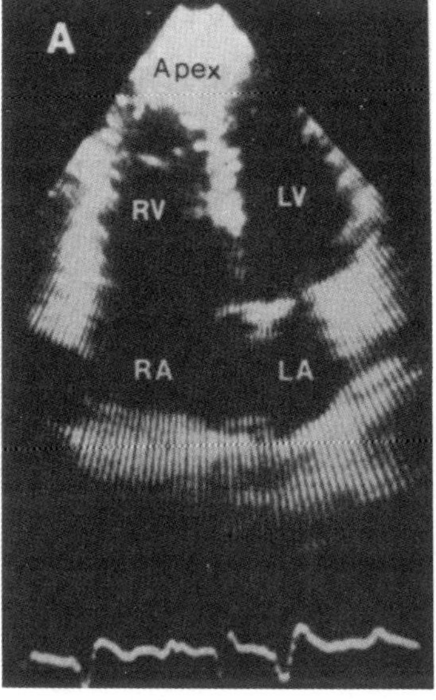

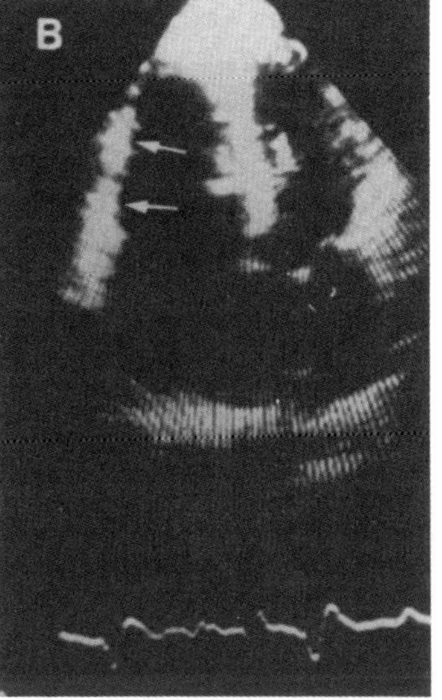

Figure 17–4. Two-dimensional echocardiogram demonstrating end-diastolic (**A**) and end-systolic (**B**) images of an apical four-chamber view that demonstrates right ventricular (RV) dilatation and akinesis of the RV lateral wall (arrows). RA = right atrium; LA = left atrium; LV = left ventricle. *Reproduced by permission of the Journal American College of Cardiology.*

because the normal right ventricular ejection fraction may range between 35% and 75%. This wide range of normal values may be attributed to factors other than ischemia that may decrease right ventricular systolic performance. The most frequently encountered conditions are chronic obstructive lung disease, pulmonary emboli, valvular heart disease, and left ventricular failure.

In a prospective evaluation of 53 consecutive patients with acute inferior myocardial infarction, we identified 14 patients with hemodynamic evidence of RVMI (RAP $\geq$ 10 mm Hg and RAP : PAWP ratio $\geq$ 0.8) (22). Radionuclide ventriculography was 92% sensitive and 82% specific for identifying hemodynamically important RVMI when both the right ventricular ejection fraction value of less than 40% and segmental wall motion abnormalities of akinesis or dyskinesis were used as radionuclide angiographic criteria for RVMI. Thus, by using both a global depression of right ventricular performance and wall motion abnormalities of akinesis or dyskinesis, acute diagnosis of hemodynamically important RVMI can be made with a high degree of accuracy because akinesis or dyskinesis is highly specific for ischemia or infarction.

Right ventricular systolic function may be depressed in the setting of acute anterior myocardial infarction. Marmor and coworkers have reported that low right ventricular ejection fraction values are associated with symmetric depression in the lateral, inferior, and apical wall segments in patients with anterior infarction (45). In contrast, in patients with inferior infarction, inferior and lateral segments were most severely depressed. In addition, there was a linear correlation between right ventricular ejection fraction and left ventricular ejection fraction in patients with anterior myocardial infarction. Therefore, these data suggest that an increased afterload may have been responsible for the acutely depressed right ventricular performance in the group of patients who present with anterior myocardial infarction. These findings are consistent with the insignificant blood supply to the anterior wall of the right ventricle by the left anterior descending artery and underscore the importance of right ventricular segmental wall motion abnormalities in addition to a reduction in systolic performance for accurate diagnosis of RVMI by radionuclide angiography (Fig. 17–5).

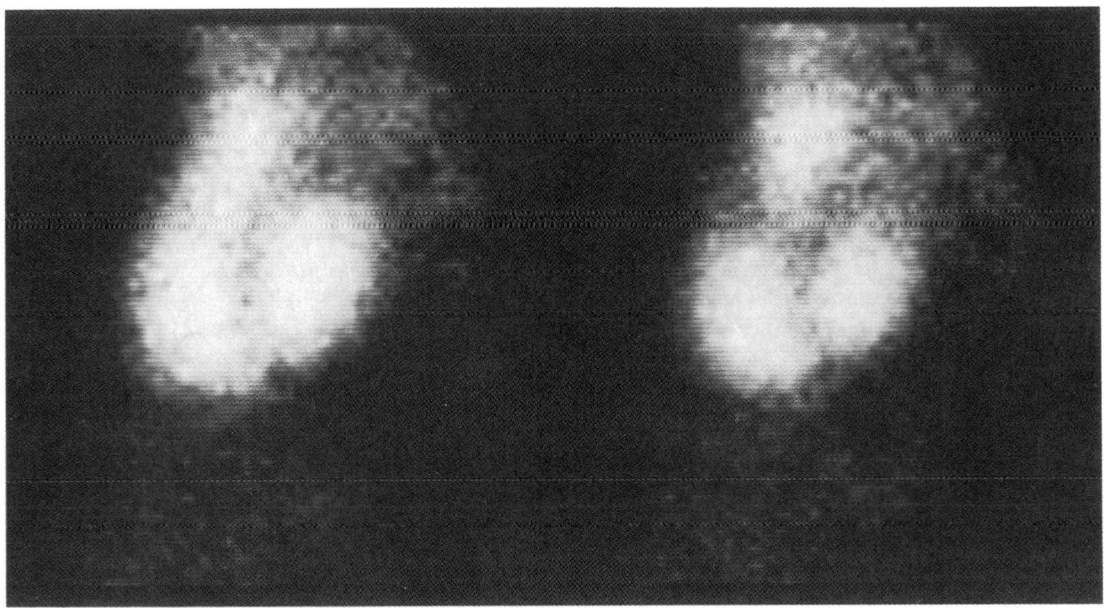

Figure 17–5. Radionuclide angiogram demonstrating end-diastolic (left) and end-systolic (right) images of the right and left ventricles. In this example of RVMI, the apex and lateral wall are akinetic, with the high outflow tract demonstrating normal contractility. Right ventricular ejection fraction is 25%.

Technetium-99*m* Pyrophosphate Myocardial Scintigraphy

Technetium-99*m* myocardial scintigraphy is a highly sensitive and specific marker for detecting left ventricular myocardial infarction. However, application of this technique in the acute setting is limited because diagnostic scans cannot be obtained until 72 hours after the onset of infarction. Documentation of RVMI has been reported to occur in approximately 40% of patients with acute inferior myocardial infarction in one study (46). However, other investigations have reported a much lower incidence in patients with inferior myocardial infarction, even when unequivocal hemodynamic evidence of RVMI is documented (16). This discrepancy demonstrates the potential problem in the performance of this technique, the proper timing of the study after the onset of infarction, and interpretation of the images because of uptake of radionuclide in noncardiac structures (chest wall, bone, and cartilage) that overlie the right ventricle.

PATHOPHYSIOLOGY AND TREATMENT

The hemodynamic consequences of predominant right ventricular damage were first described by Starr and coworkers in 1943. In this animal model the heart was suspended in a pericardial cradle, and there was no appreciable increase in venous pressure or decrease in cardiac output after cauterization of the right ventricular lateral wall (47). Other open pericardial dog models reported similar findings and demonstrated adequate ventricular performance as long as pulmonary vascular resistance remained normal (48–50). Therefore, these reports led to the belief that right ventricular function was not essential to maintain circulatory stability, and that the pressure pulse that developed in the right ventricular cavity after extensive destruction of the lateral wall of the right ventricle might be generated by the left ventricle.

Subsequent to the description of the clinical syndrome of RVMI in 1974, Guiha and coworkers demonstrated a mild increase in right heart filling pressures associated with a decrease in cardiac output after extensive cauterization of the right ventricular lateral wall using a similar open pericardial canine model (51). Progressive volume loading produced a greater increase in right heart filling pressures over left heart filling pressures, as well as an increase in systolic arterial pressure and cardiac output. The result of this study provided the rationale behind volume administration in the treatment of RVMI, which achieves maximal benefit from the Frank–Starling mechanism by maintaining an adequate right ventricular preload. However, data from clinical studies demonstrate that volume infusion does not uniformly produce an increase in cardiac output when given to patients who present with hemodynamic criteria of RVMI (52–54). In 36 patients with acute RVMI (RAP $\geq$ 10 mm Hg and not 5 mm Hg below the PAWP), volume was infused until the PAWP increased more than 5 mm Hg. The response was highly variable, and there was no significant increase in cardiac index in the 36 study patients, in those patients who presented with a cardiac index less than 2.2 L/min/m^2, or in those patients who presented with a cardiac index greater than 2.2 L/min/m^2.

In a study of 13 patients with hemodynamic and radionuclide ventriculographic evidence of RVMI, we demonstrated that progressive volume loading significantly increased RAP (11 $\pm$ 2 to 15 $\pm$ 2 mm Hg, $p < 0.001$) and PAWP (10 $\pm$ 4 to 15 $\pm$ 2 mm Hg, $p < 0.001$), but produced no significant change in cardiac index (1.9 $\pm$ 0.5 to 2.1 $\pm$ 0.4 L/min/m^2) (54). Thus, despite an increase in right heart and left heart filling pressures, cardiac index did not improve. Simultaneously acquired radionuclide angiographic studies demonstrated an increase in right ventricular end-diastolic volume as left ventricular end-diastolic volume remained unchanged. Therefore, the PAWP did not accurately reflect true preload or end-diastolic volume of the left ventricle. Furthermore, by increasing right ventricular cavity size, volume loading may limit the left ventricular filling through a mechanism of ventricular interaction.

This physiologic mechanism is nicely demonstrated in closed pericardial animal models of RVMI in the dog where the right coronary artery supplies blood solely to the right ventricular myocardium

(55,56). After right coronary artery occlusion, Goldstein and coworkers demonstrated typical RVMI hemodynamics:

1. Elevation and equalization of right- and left-sided filling pressures
2. Increase in right ventricular cavity size and decrease in left ventricular end-diastolic size
3. Decrease in cardiac output

Subsequent volume loading increased the left ventricular end-diastolic pressure from 7 to 12 mm Hg with minimal change in left ventricular cavity size, and there was a small but significant increase in cardiac output. However, after the pericardium was removed, equalization of right and left heart diastolic pressures resolved, left ventricular end-diastolic pressure decreased to 11 mm Hg as diastolic cavity size increased, and cardiac output increased significantly over the post–volume load values when the pericardium was intact. Thus, despite a significant increase in left ventricular end-diastolic pressure after volume loading, the true distending pressure or transmural pressure of the left ventricle was diminished because of an increased intrapericardial pressure. In another closed chest canine model of RVMI, the right coronary artery was embolized with mercury through a catheter inserted into the femoral artery and positioned at the orifice of the right coronary artery (57). After embolization, the transeptal pressure gradient reversed from 3 ± 1 to −1 ± 1 mm Hg ($p < 0.001$) (left ventricular minus right ventricular end-diastolic pressure). In addition, the shape of the interventricular septum was flattened at end-diastole in the short-axis cross-sectional two-dimensional echocardiographic view (see Fig. 17–6). Thus, despite a significant increase in left ventricular end-diastolic pressure in both animal models, left ventricular end-diastolic dimension decreased or did not change due to acute distention of the right ventricle in the intact pericardial sac. Therefore, it would seem that the right ventricle must also be unloaded by a primary or secondary mechanism in order to allow for better filling of the left ventricle.

To determine the relative efficacy of inotropic therapy or afterload reduction as adjunctive therapy to volume infusion, we studied the effects of dobutamine and nitroprusside randomly infused in nine patients with RVMI after volume loading with normal saline (54). Dobutamine produced a statistically significant increase in cardiac index, stroke volume index, and right ventricular ejection fraction when compared with nitroprusside. From this study we concluded that nitroprusside deleteriously decreased preload in patients with RVMI to the extent that right ventricular stroke volume was unchanged, while dobutamine maintained preload and augmented systolic performance and stroke output. Therefore, this study suggests that if an initial volume infusion raises right and left heart filling pressures without a significant improvement in cardiac output, copious amounts of volume are unlikely to improve cardiac output, and dobutamine should be administered to improve right ventricular systolic performance (19).

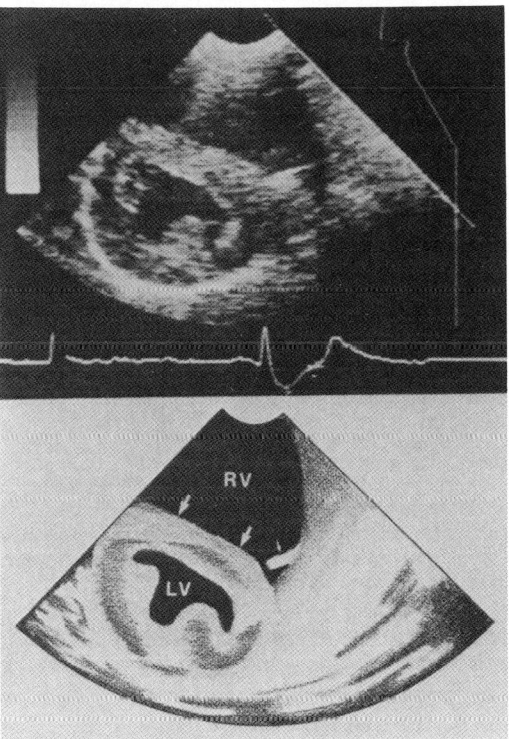

Figure 17–6. Still-frame echocardiographic image after embolization of the right coronary artery in the closed chest dog model, demonstrating an enlarged right ventricle and a ventricular septum that has shifted toward the left ventricle, resulting in decreased left ventricular cavity size. *Reproduced by permission of the American Heart Journal.*

The apparent discrepancy between these recent studies and earlier series that documented an impressive response to fluid loading can be reconciled (8,19). It is likely that many of the earlier patients were "hypovolemic" right ventricular infarcts, in part a function of an initial misdiagnosis and treatment of the low-output syndrome with diuretics.

Other studies have reported improvement in cardiac index and mean arterial pressure after AV sequential pacing in patients with acute RVMI (58). These studies demonstrate the salutary effect of atrial contraction on both ventricular filling and stroke volume in the setting of acute myocardial infarction. This form of therapy may be beneficial in those patients who manifest persistent hypotension and high-grade AV block despite maximal therapy with inotropic agents and volume infusion.

The benefits of acute reperfusion achieved by primary angioplasty in 27 patients with acute inferior myocardial infarction and right ventricular involvement by electrocardiographic and hemodynamic criteria have been demonstrated (59). Patients with successful reperfusion demonstrated an improved right atrial pressure, pulmonary capillary wedge pressure and right atrial/pulmonary capillary wedge pressure ratio as early as 8 hours after reperfusion, with the greatest improvement noted in right atrial pressure (See Fig. 17–7). Persistent elevation of the latter was associated with increased mortality.

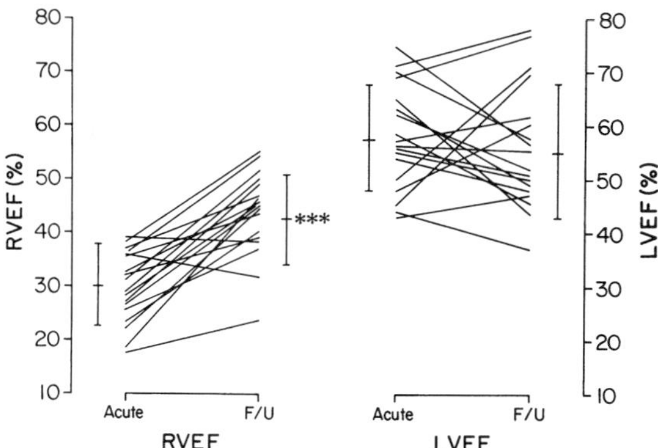

Figure 17–7. Right atrial (RA) pressure during right ventricular infarction with and without reperfusion. Open circles = successful reperfusion after coronary angioplasty (n = 17); solid circles = non-reperfusion (n = 10); * $p < .05$, significant difference versus baseline measurements; $p < .05$, significant difference versus time-matched control subjects. *Reproduced by permission of the Journal American College of Cardiology.*

COMPLICATIONS OF RVMI

Complications of RVMI may adversely affect acute prognosis. Numerous case reports have described severe hypoxemia and arterial desaturation resulting from right-to-left shunting across an atrial septal defect or patent foramen ovale (60,61). This is an interesting and not uncommon complication of RVMI, which may be diagnosed at bedside using current echo Doppler techniques. Because these patients present with hypoxemia, the differential diagnosis includes acute pulmonary embolism, because right ventricular thrombus is a potential source for pulmonary emboli (62). Perfusion scanning of the lung with macroaggregated albumin is a very sensitive technique for detecting intracardiac shunting manifested by uptake of radionuclide in the brain, thyroid, and kidneys. Rupture of the interventricular septum may occur in the setting of acute inferior myocardial infarction, and several surgical series have reported that acute and perioperative mortality may be determined by the severity of right ventricular dysfunction (63–65).

SHORT-TERM PROGNOSIS

The acute outcome of patients with RVMI is primarily determined by the amount of accompanying left ventricular necrosis. In 27 patients presenting with both hemodynamic and radionuclide ventriculographic criteria for RVMI, extensive postmortem infarction of the right and left ventricles was found in all three patients who died within 72 hours of presentation (66). All three had ≥10 mm of summed ST segment depression leads V_1–V_4 that was disproportionate to the extent of ST segment elevation in the inferior leads and therefore likely not due to reciprocal changes. Such electrocardiographic changes most likely represent extensive left ventricular posterior and lateral wall ischemia. This report and data from other series (67–69) indicate that the early mortality of RVMI is not due principally to the severity of right ventricular dysfunction, but rather to the presence of extensive left ventricular and/or mechanical or electrical complications of myocardial infarction. Studies have demonstrated that patency of the right coronary artery achieved by acute thrombolytic therapy (70) or primary percutaneous transluminal angioplasty (59) results in improved survival compared to those patients with occluded right coronary arteries. Right ventricular necrosis assessed by technetium-99 m pyrophosphate was significantly lower in patients who achieved successful early reperfusion with thrombolytic therapy than in those who did not (27% versus 64%, $p < 0.01$) (71). In another study, however, right ventricular systolic function improved in spite of positive uptake of technetium-99 m pyrophosphate in the right ventricle (72). Thus, these data and the data from the prethrombolytic era (66) indicate that right ventricular dysfunction commonly associated with acute inferior wall infarction is often transient, and improvement is the rule, irrespective of early recanalization of the infarct vessel. Whether reduction in early mortality in patients with inferior myocardial infarction is related to preservation of right ventricular or left ventricular myocardium is an open question.

Although the acute prognosis of RVMI is directly related to the amount of coexisting left ventricular damage, occasional patients die with hemodynamically important RVMI who have a normal left coronary artery and normal left ventricular systolic function. Other factors determining the hemodynamic status of patients with acute RVMI have been delineated. Goldstein et al (73) evaluated 16 patients with hemodynamically important RVMI confirmed by right-heart catheterization and two-dimensional echocardiography. The right atrial waveform had two characteristic patterns, depending on the amplitude of the "a" wave. These two distinct right atrial waveforms were associated with disparate clinical courses. Eight patients had prominent "a" waves, and the remaining eight had depressed "a" waves. Those with augmented "a" waves had a higher average right ventricular systolic pressure, a better mean cardiac output, and a more favorable response to volume and inotropic therapy, and less frequently required emergency revascularization for refractory shock. All differences were statistically significant. Coronary artery stenoses proximal to the major right atrial branches of the right or circumflex coronary artery were demonstrated in all six patients with diminished "a" waves and who had coronary arteriography.

Interestingly, global left ventricular function was near normal or normal in all but 2 of the 16 patients, and assessment of the interventricular septum echocardiographically revealed diastolic septal flattening in 10 and frank reversal of septal curvature during diastole in the remaining 6 patients. Definite systolic paradoxical septal motion was present in 14 of 16 patients and difficult to assess in the remaining 2 due to technical limitations. Thus all 16 patients had both hemodynamic and echocardiographic evidence of severe RVMI, and in 8 the loss of enhanced atrial transport contributed to a low cardiac output. The finding of a diminished "a" wave on the right atrial pressure waveform in patients with hemodynamically important RVMI may be an important acute prognostic indicator, even in the presence of well-preserved left ventricular systolic function.

LONG-TERM PROGNOSIS

It has been well documented that right ventricular ejection fraction increases significantly in the recovery period in survivors after acute RVMI (66,72,74) (Fig. 17–8). Dell'Italia and associates (66) demonstrated that the response of the right ventricular ejection fraction to exercise is also well preserved in patient 1–3 years after RVMI. This remarkable capacity of the right ventricle to regain systolic function after myocardial infarction most likely explains the finding of Haines and associates (75), who reported the myocardial infarction predominantly affecting the right ventricle was associated with excellent short- and long-term prognoses. They demonstrated that exercise tolerance as assessed by treadmill time, blood pressure–heart rate product, and peak workload in metabolic equivalents (METs) was comparable among 47 patients who had normal right ventricular function, 12 patients with moderate dysfunction, and 50 patients with severe right ventricular dysfunction as determined by

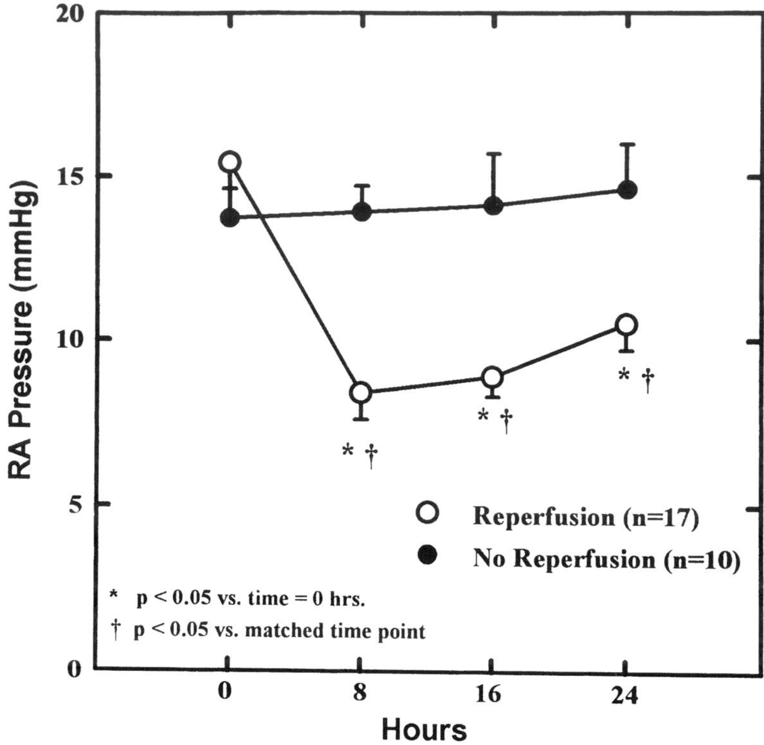

Figure 17–8. Short-term and follow-up (F/U) resting, supine right ventricular ejection fraction (RVEF), and left ventricular ejection fraction (LVEF) determinations in 18 survivors. ***$p < 0.001$. *Reproduced by permission of Circulation.*

radionuclide ventriculography before hospital discharge.

To elucidate further the factors affecting exercise capacity in patients with well-documented right ventricular infarction, Dell'Italia and coworkers (66) evaluated the response in the radionuclide right and left ventriculographic ejection fraction and the respiratory gas exchange analysis in patients 1–3 years after hemodynamically important RVMIs. The onset of anaerobic threshold during exercise correlated significantly with peak exercise, right ventricular ejection fraction ($r = 0.82$, $p < 0.02$), but not with left ventricular ejection fraction. Importantly, both the baseline and exercise left ventricular function were well preserved or normal in most of these patients. During upright exercise the right ventricular ejection fraction increased significantly, from 41 ± 10% to 47 ± 12%. In this study, the direction and extent of change in right ventricular ejection fraction correlated well with the change in left ventricular ejection fraction ($r = 0.82$, $p < 0.02$). Deviations from this good correlation occurred only in patients who had a decreased 1-second force expiratory volume and an abnormal ventilatory reserve during exercise as measured by respiratory gas exchange analysis. Thus, in the recovery phase after RVMI, the right ventricular ejection fraction often improves and the right ventricular functional reserve usually is preserved during exercise in patients who are not limited by angina, pulmonary disease, or left ventricular failure.

These studies indicate that hemodynamic evidence of RVMI usually is associated with excellent short- and long-term prognoses. Although hemodynamic compromise and death can occur in the presence of RVMI alone, the prognosis is most cases is excellent as long as severe left ventricular dysfunction is absent. This favorable prognosis is even more impressive considering that these prognostic studies were conducted before thrombolytic therapy and early direct coronary angioplasty were widely utilized. They affirm the remarkable resistance of the right ventricle to necrosis in acute right coronary artery occlusion. However, the right ventricle often may develop transient ischemic injury that sometimes produces reversible severe arterial hypotension. Accordingly, prompt recognition by physical examination of the V_{4R} electrogram, appropriate treatment with judicious volume loading, and early inotropic therapy when needed are important in maintaining circulatory stability. A careful clinical evaluation including risk stratification, noninvasive testing, and coronary arteriography as appropriate to rule out important left coronary artery disease, recurrent myocardial ischemia, and severe left ventricular dysfunction prior to discharge results in an excellent long-term survival.

REFERENCES

1. Isner J, Roberts WC: Right ventricular infarction complicating left ventricular infarction secondary to coronary heart disease. *Am J Cardiol* 1978;42:885.
2. Ratliff NB, Hackel DB: Combined right and left ventricular infarction: Pathogenesis and clinicopathologic correlations. *Am J Cardiol* 1980;45:217.
3. Wade WG: The pathogenesis of infarction of the right ventricle. *Br Heart J* 1959;21:545.
4. Ratliff NB, Peter RH, Ramo BW, et al: A model for the production of right ventricular infarction. *Am J Pathol* 1970;58:471.
5. Ramo BW, Peter RH, Ratliff N, et al: The natural history of right coronary arterial occlusion in the pig. *Am J Cardiol* 1970;26:156.
6. Peter RH, Ramo BW, Ratliff N, et al: Collateral vessel development after right ventricular infarction in the pig. *Am J Cardiol* 1972;29:56.
7. Erhardt LR: Clinical and pathological observations in different types of acute myocardial infarction: A study of 84 patients deceased after treatment in a coronary care unit. *Acta Med Scand* 1974;26 (Suppl):7.
8. Cohn JN, Guiha NH, Broder MI, et al: Right ventricular infarction. *Am J Cardiol* 1974;33:209.
9. Cintron GB, Hernandez E, Linares E, et al: Bedside recognition, incidence and clinical course of right ventricular infarction. *Am J Cardiol* 1981;47:224.
10. Lorell B, Leinbach RC, Pohost GM, et al: Right ventricular infarction. Clinical diagnosis and differentiation from cardiac tamponade and pericardial constriction. *Am J Cardiol* 1979;43:465.
11. Eisenberg S, Suyemoto J: Rupture of a papillary muscle of the tricuspid valve following acute myocardial infarction. *Circulation* 1964;30:588.
12. McAllister RG, Friesinger GC, Sinclair-Smith BC: Tricuspid regurgitation following inferior myocardial infarction. *Arch Intern Med* 1976;136:95.
13. Zone DD, Botti RE: Right ventricular infarction with tricuspid insufficiency and chronic right heart failure. *Am J Cardiol* 1976;37:445.
14. Braat SH, de Zwann C, Brugada P, et al: Right ventricular involvement with acute inferior wall myocardial infarction identifies high risk of developing atrioventricular nodal conduction disturbances. *Am Heart J* 1984;107:1181.
15. Dell'Italia LJ, Starling MR, O'Rourke RA: Physical examination for exclusion of hemodynamically important right ventricular infarction. *Ann Intern Med* 1983;99:608.
16. Baigre RS, Hag A, Morgan CD, et al: The spectrum of right ventricular involvement in inferior wall myocardial infarction: A clinical, hemodynamic and noninvasive study. *J Am Coll Cardiol* 1983;1:1396.
17. Coma-Cannella I, Lopez-Sendon J: Ventricular compliance in ischemic right ventricular dysfunction. *Am J Cardiol* 1980;45:555.
18. Coma-Canella I, Lopez-Sendon J, Gamallo C: Low output syndrome in right ventricular infarction. *Am Heart J* 1979;98:613.
19. Lloyd EA, Gersh BJ, Kennelly BM: Hemodynamic spectrum of "dominant" right ventricular infarction in 19 patients. *Am J Cardiol* 1981;48:1016.
20. Jensen DP, Goolsby JP, Oliva PB: Hemodynamic pattern resembling pericardial constriction after acute inferior myocardial infarction with right ventricular infarction. *Am J Cardiol* 1978;42:858.
21. Lopez-Sendon J, Coma-Cannella I, Gamallo C: Sensitivity and specificity of hemodynamic criteria in the diagnosis of acute right ventricular infarction. *Circulation* 1981;64:515.
22. Dell'Italia LJ, Starling MR, Crawford MH, et al: Right ventricular infarction: Identification by hemodynamic measurements before and after volume loading and correlation with noninvasive techniques. *J Am Coll Cardiol* 1984;4:931.

23. Erhardt LR, Sjogem A, Wahlberg I: Single right-sided precordial lead in the diagnosis of right ventricular involvement in inferior myocardial infarction myocardial infarction. *Am Heart J* 1976;91:571.
24. Chou T, Van Der Bel-Kahn J, Allen J, et al: Electrocardiographic diagnosis of right ventricular infarction. *Am J Med* 1981;70(6):1175.
25. Klein HO, Tordjman T, Ninio R, et al: The early recognition of right ventricular infarction: Diagnostic accuracy of the electrocardiographic V_{4R} lead. *Circulation* 1983;67:558.
26. Croft CH, Nicod P, Corbett JR, et al: Detection of acute right ventricular infarction by right precordial electrocardiography. *Am J Cardiol* 1982;50:421.
27. Bratt SH, Brugada P, De Zwaan C, et al: Value of electrocardiogram in diagnosing right ventricular involvement in patients with an acute inferior wall myocardial infarction. *Br Heart J* 1983;49:368.
28. Candell-Riera J, Figueras J, Valle V, et al: Right ventricular infarction: Relationships between ST segment elevation in V_{4R} and hemodynamic, scintigraphic, and echocardiographic findings in patients with acute inferior myocardial infarction. *Am Heart J* 1981;101:281.
29. Morgera T, Alberti E, Silvestri F, et al: Right precordial ST and QRS changes in the diagnosis of right ventricular infarction. *Am Heart J* 1984;108:13.
30. Lopez-Sendon J, Coma-Canella I, Alcasena S, et al: Electrocardiographic findings in acute right ventricular infarction: Sensitivity and specificity of electrocardiographic alterations in right precordial leads V_{4R}, V_{3R}, V_1, V_2, and V_3. *J Am Coll Cardiol* 1984;6:1273.
31. Geft LL, Shah PK, Rodriguez L, et al: ST elevations in leads V_1 to V_5 may be caused by right coronary artery occlusion and acute right ventricular infarction. *Am J Cardiol* 1984;53:991.
32. Zehender M, Kasper W, Kauder E, et al: Right ventricular infarction as an independent predictor of prognosis after acute inferior myocardial infarction. *N Engl J Med* 1993;328:981.
33. Wellens HJJ: Right ventricular infarction. *N Engl J Med* 1993;328:1036.
34. Rodrigues EA, Dewhurst NG, Smart LM, Hannan WJ, Muir AL: Diagnosis and prognosis of right ventricular infarction. *Br Heart J* 1986;56:19.
35. Anderson HR, Nielson D, Lung O, Falk E: Prognostic significance of right ventricular infarction diagnosed by ST elevation in right chest leads V_{3R} to V_{7R}. *Int J Cardiol* 1988;23:349.
36. Berger PB, Ryan TJ: Inferior myocardial infarction high-risk subgroups. *Circulation* 1990;81(2):401–411.
37. Shah PK. Right ventricular infarction. *N Engl J Med* 1993;329:1043.
38. D'Arcy B, Nanda NC: Two-dimensional echocardiographic features of right ventricular infarction. *Circulation* 1982;65:167.
39. Lopez-Sendon J, Garcia-Fernandez MA, Coma-Canella I, et al: Segmental right ventricular function after acute myocardial infarction: Two-dimensional echocardiographic study in 63 patients. *Am J Cardiol* 1983;51:390.
40. Rigo P, Murray M, Taylor DR: Right ventricular dysfunction detected by gated scintiphotography in patients with acute inferior myocardial infarction. *Circulation* 1975;52:268.
41. Sharpe DN, Botvinick EH, Shames DM, et al: The noninvasive diagnosis of right ventricular infarction. *Circulation* 1978;57:483.
42. Tobinick E, Schelbert HR, Henning H, et al: Right ventricular ejection fraction in patients with acute anterior and inferior myocardial infarction assessed by radionuclide angiography. *Circulation* 1978;57:1078.
43. Reduto LA, Berger HJ, Cohen LS, et al: Sequential radionuclide assessment of left and right ventricular performance after acute transmural myocardial infarction. *Ann Intern Med* 1978;89:441.
44. Starling M, Dell'Italia LJ, O'Rourke RA, et al: First transit and equilibrium radionuclide angiography in inferior transmural myocardial infarction patients: Criteria for the diagnosis of associated hemodynamically significant right ventricular infarction. *J Am Coll Cardiol* 1984;9:15.
45. Marmor A, Geltman EM, Biello DR, et al: Functional response of the right ventricle to myocardial infarction: Dependence on the site of left ventricular infarction. *Circulation* 1981;64:1005.
46. Wackers FJT, Lie KI, Sokole EB, et al: Prevalence of right ventricular involvement in inferior wall infarction assessed with myocardial imaging with thallium-201 and technetium-99m pyrophosphate. *Am J Cardiol* 1978;42:358.
47. Starr I, Jeffers WA, Meade RH: The absence of conspicuous increments of venous pressure after severe damage to the right ventricle of the dog, with a discussion of the relation between clinical

congestive failure and heart disease. *Am Heart J* 1943;26:291.

48. Bakos ACP: The question of the function of the right ventricular myocardium: An experimental study. *Circulation* 1950;1:724.
49. Kagan A: Dynamic responses of the right ventricle following extensive damage by cauterization. *Circulation* 1952;5:816.
50. Donald DE, Essex HE: Pressure studies after inactivation of the major portion of the canine right ventricle. *Am J Physiol* 1954;176:155.
51. Guiha NH, Limas CJ, Cohn JN: Predominant right ventricular dysfunction after right ventricular destruction in the dog. *Am J Cardiol* 1974;33:254.
52. Lopez-Sendon J, Coma-Canella I, Adanez JV: Volume loading in patients with ischemic right ventricular dysfunction. *Eur Heart J* 1981;2:329.
53. Shah PK, Maddahi J, Berman DS, et al: Scintigraphically detected predominant right ventricular dysfunction in acute myocardial infarction: Clinical and hemodynamic correlates and implications for therapy and prognosis. *J Am Coll Cardiol* 1985;6:1264.
54. Dell'Italia LJ, Starling MR, Blumhardt R, et al: Comparative effects of volume loading, dobutamine and nitroprusside in patients with predominant right ventricular infarction. *Circulation* 1985; 72:1327.
55. Goldstein JA, Vlahakes GJ, Verrier ED, et al: Volume loading improves low cardiac output in experimental right ventricular infarction. *J Am Coll Cardiol* 1983;2:270.
56. Goldstein JA, Vlahakes GJ, Verrier ED, et al: The role of right ventricular systolic dysfunction and elevated intrapericardial pressure in the genesis of low output in experimental right ventricular infarction. *Circulation* 1982;65:513.
57. Sharkey SW, Shelley W, Carlyle PF, et al: M-mode and two-dimensional echocardiographic analysis of the septum in experimental right ventricular infarction: Correlation with hemodynamic alterations. *Am Heart J* 1985;110:1210.
58. Topol EJ, Goldschlager N, Ports TA, et al: Hemodynamic benefit of atrial pacing in right ventricular myocardial infarction. *Ann Intern Med* 1982;96:594.
59. Kinn JW, Ajluni SC, Samyn JG, et al: Rapid hemodynamic improvement after reperfusion during right ventricular infarction. *J Am Coll Cardiol* 1995; 26:1230.
60. Rietveld AP, Merrman L, Essed CE, et al: Right to left shunt, with severe hypoxemia, at the atrial level in a patient with hemodynamically important right ventricular infarction. *J Am Coll Cardiol* 1983;2:776.
61. Manno BV, Bhennis CE, Carver J, et al: Right ventricular infarction complicated by right to left shunt. *J Am Coll Cardiol* 1983;2:554.
62. Stowers SA, Leiboff RH, Wasserman AG, et al: Right ventricular thrombus formation in association with acute myocardial infarction: Diagnosis by two-dimensional echocardiography. *Am J Cardiol* 1983;52:912.
63. Radford MJ, Johnson RA, Daggett WM, et al: Ventricular septal rupture: A review of clinical and physiologic features and an analysis of survival. *Circulation* 1981;64:545.
64. Fananapazir L, Bray CL, Dark JR, et al: Right ventricular dysfunction and surgical outcome in postinfarction ventricular septal defect. *Eur Heart J* 1983;4:157.
65. Grose R, Spindola-Franco H: Right ventricular dysfunction in acute ventricular septal defect. *Am Heart J* 1981;101:67.
66. Dell'Italia LJ, Lembo NJ, Starling MR, et al: Hemodynamically important right ventricular infarction: Follow-up evaluation of right ventricular systolic function at rest and during exercise with radionuclide ventriculography and respiratory gas exchange. *Circulation* 1987;75:996.
67. Jugdutt BI, Sussex BA, Sivaram CA, Rossall RE: Right ventricular infarction: Two-dimensional echocardiographic evaluation. *Am Heart J* 1984;107: 505.
68. Legrand V, Rigo P, Demoulin JC, et al: Right ventricular myocardial infarction diagnosed by 99m pyrophosphate scintigraphy: clinical course and follow-up. *Eur Heart J* 1983;4:9.
69. Shah PK, Maddahi J, Staniloff HM, et al: Variable spectrum and prognostic implications of left and right ventricular ejection fractions in patients with and without heart failure after acute myocardial infarction. *Am J Cardiol* 1986;58:387.
70. Schuler G, Hofmann M, Schwarz, et al: Effect of successful thrombolytic therapy on right ventricular function in acute inferior wall myocardial infarction. *Am J Cardiol* 1984;54:951.
71. Asano H, Sone T, Tsuboi H, et al: Diagnosis of right ventricular infarction by overlap images of simultaneous dual emission computed tomography

using technetium-99m pyrophosphate and thallium-201. *Am J Cardiol* 1993;71:902.

72. Verrani MS, Tortoledo FE, Batty JW, Raizner AE: Effect of coronary artery recanalization on right ventricular function patients with acute myocardial infarction. *J Am Coll Cardiol* 1985;5:1029.

73. Goldstein JA, Barzilai B, Rosamond TL, et al: Determinants of hemodynamic compromise with severe right ventricular infarction. *Circulation* 1990;82:359.

74. Steele P, Kirch D, Ellis J, et al: Prompt return to normal of depressed right ventricular ejection fraction in acute inferior infarction. *Br Heart J* 1977;39:1319.

75. Haines DE, Beller GA, Watson DD, et al: A prospective clinical, scintigraphic, angiographic and functional evaluation of patients after inferior myocardial infarction with and without right ventricular dysfunction. *J Am Coll Cardiol* 1985;6:995.

18

Non-Q Wave Myocardial Infarction: Prognosis, Changing Incidence, and Management

Robert S. Gibson, MD

Historically, two types of myocardial infarction (MI) have been described: the "transmural" infarction and the "nontransmural" infarction, also called the subendocardial or intramural infarction. In clinical practice, this distinction is made on the basis of the occurrence of abnormal Q waves on the surface electrocardiogram (ECG); for example, infarcts that alter the sequence of ventricular depolarization in such a way that Q waves are produced, are designated transmural. If the QRS complex is unchanged and only ST–T wave changes occur, the infarct is considered nontransmural or subendocardial.

Because the traditional classification scheme involves the use of pathologic nomenclature to describe a clinical entity, Spodick and others in 1983 (1,2) suggested that the terms *transmural* and *nontransmural* be eliminated when referring to the ECG pattern of myocardial infarction, and that the more appropriate terms *Q wave* and *non-Q wave infarction* be used instead. The validity of this recommendation, which has been widely accepted, is obvious because to distinguish with certitude between transmural and subendocardial infarction on the basis of ECG data alone does not seem possible (3–10). Moreover, available evidence suggests that the differences between Q wave and non-Q wave infarction, particularly in prognosis and changing incidence, have important clinical implications that make their understanding imperative to the practicing physician (11).

CLINICAL COURSE AND PROGNOSIS OF NON-Q WAVE INFARCTION

Since 1962, there have been at least 45 reports in the literature comparing the clinical outcome of patients with Q wave infarction with that of patients with non-Q wave infarction (12–56). Each of these reports essentially asked the same question, namely, Do patients with non-Q wave infarction enjoy a more favorable prognosis than their Q wave counterparts? To answer this question, investigators used three somewhat different epidemiologic approaches. The first approach examined group-specific mortality (usually all cause) as the primary indicator of prognosis. Of the 45 reports, 43 evaluated this outcome measure. A second approach was to assess incident morbidity rates (that is, the issue of the quality of life) by tabulating data on reinfarction ($n = 15$) and/or postinfarction angina ($n = 6$). The third approach was to differentiate between the short-term and the long-term prognosis of the two infarct groups. Of the 45 reports, 16 compared only short-term mortality (12–27), 9 compared only long-term mortality (28–36), and 18 compared both short-term and long-term mortality (37–54).

Short-Term Mortality Comparisons

Of the 34 studies that reported mortality results, 32 (94%) found a lower case-fatality rate among patients with non-Q wave infarction. As Figure 18–1 shows, when data from all 34 studies are pooled, the short-term mortality rate for patients with Q wave infarction averages 18.3% versus 9.3% for patients with non-Q wave infarction ($p < 0.0001$). Not surprisingly, the mortality differences between the Q wave and the non-Q wave groups are greatest in the studies that excluded patients with prior infarctions (15.1% versus 5.5%, respectively, $p < 0.0001$).

Relationship Between Short-Term Prognosis and Infarct Size

Many studies have shown that non-Q wave infarction is associated with less myocardial necrosis than Q wave infarction. Indeed, this has been demonstrated in no fewer than 47 studies with a wide variety of techniques (11) including serial creatine kinase (CK) measurements, technetium-99*m* inorganic pyrophosphate infarct-avid scintigraphy, thallium-201 perfusion imaging, two-dimensional echocardiography, radionuclide and contrast ventriculography, and, in two studies, positron emission tomography (57,58). In view of the well-documented relationship between infarct size, left ventricular ejection fraction, and major cardiovascular morbidity and mortality, it is not surprising that patients with non-Q wave MI, in general, have a lower frequency of congestive heart failure and life-threatening arrhythmias, and a better short-term survival than their Q wave counterparts.

Long-Term Mortality Comparisons

As non-Q wave infarction is usually associated with less extensive injury and better left ventricular function, it is logical to expect long-term follow-up studies to show lower mortality among patients with non-Q wave infarcts. In reviewing the literature, however, the case-fatality rate for non-Q wave infarction is similar to or higher than that for Q wave infarction. When data from all 27 long-term studies are pooled, the aggregate postdischarge mortality rate averages 23.7% for Q wave infarcts

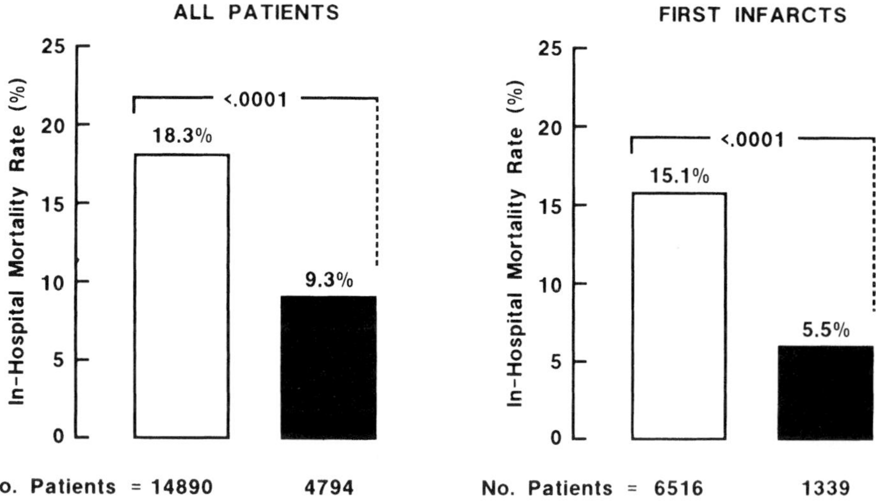

Figure 18–1. In-hospital mortality rate for patients with Q wave (open bars) and non-Q wave (solid bars) infarction.

versus 28.6% for non-Q wave infarcts ($p < 0.001$). Furthermore, in the 18 studies that report both short-term and long-term data, it has been shown by multiple investigators that patients with non-Q wave infarcts have a higher postdischarge mortality, despite a significantly lower in-hospital or 30-day mortality (Fig. 18–2). These results have led to the conclusion that the early survival advantage of the non-Q wave infarct group is lost in the first 6 to 12 months after hospital discharge.

Comparison of Incident Morbidity Rates

As Figure 18–3 illustrates, patients with non-Q wave MI are two to three times more likely to experience recurrent ischemia and infarction than their Q wave counterparts. Also, the frequency of coronary artery bypass surgery and/or percutaneous transluminal coronary angioplasty for angina relief is significantly greater after non-Q wave infarction (34,54). These findings suggest that the amount of viable but hypoperfused myocardium that remains at risk for recurrent ischemia and infarction is substantial and significantly greater after non-Q wave than Q wave MI.

Value and Limitations of Observational Studies

Examination of the 45 studies published between 1962 and 1989 identifies a pattern of consistent clinically important findings that support the dichotomous classification of infarcts as either Q wave or non-Q wave. Although this ECG classification scheme does not accommodate the heterogeneity that clearly exists within the non-Q wave group (see later), it does seem to represent a prognostically meaningful distinction (11).

It is important to recognize that observational data and epidemiologic associations cannot provide a scientific explanation for the smaller infarct size with non-Q wave infarction. Also, the pathophysiologic basis that accounts for the greater clinical instability after non-Q wave infarction and the reason that these patients lose their initial prognostic advantage are not clearly evident nor fully explained by the 45 clinical outcome studies. In part, this is because very few of the studies were specifically designed to examine directly the issue of ischemic jeopardy or delineate the exact nature of the underlying coronary atherosclerotic process. In the sections that follow, information relevant to these

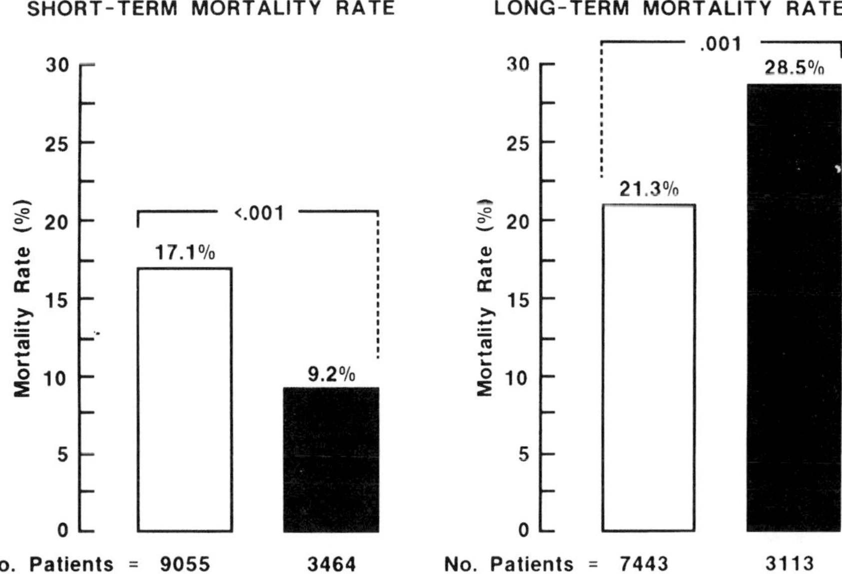

Figure 18–2. Comparison of short-term (left) and long-term (right) mortality rates for patients with Q wave (open bars) and non-Q wave (solid bars) infarction.

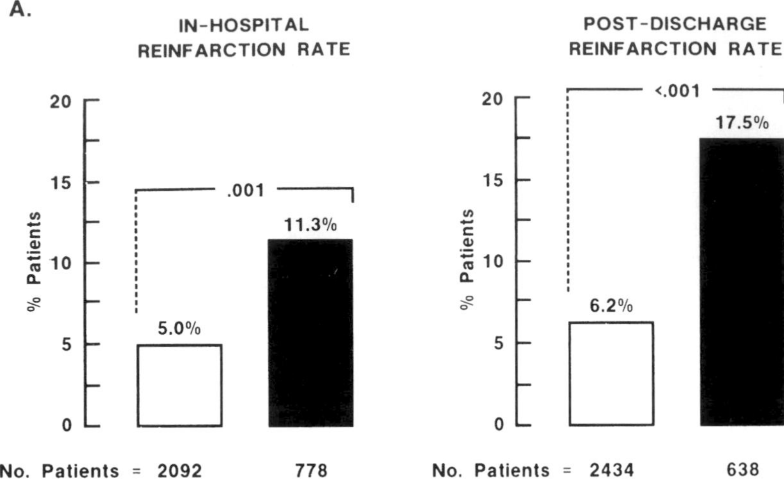

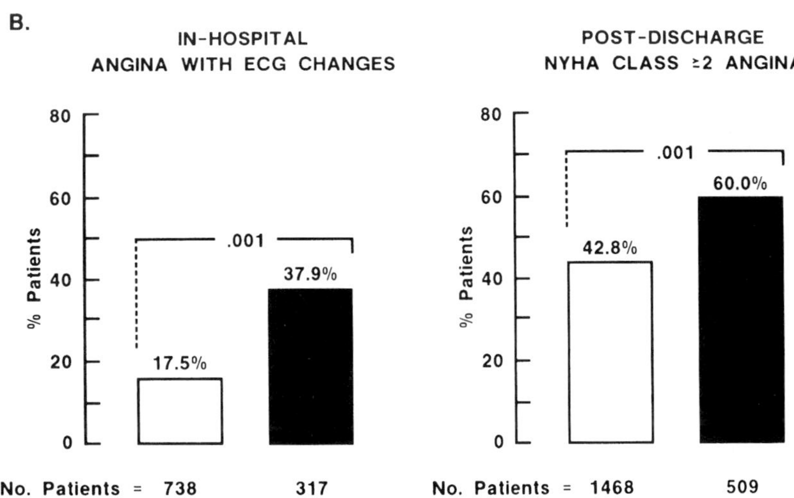

Figure 18–3. Pooled data from 19 studies showing a higher incidence of recurrent ischemia and infarction after non-Q wave infarction (solid bars) compared with Q wave infarction (open bars).

areas as well as the pathogenesis of non-Q wave infarction is presented.

CORONARY PATHOANATOMY AFTER NON-Q WAVE INFARCTION

Several natural history studies performed in the early 1970s suggested that the prognosis of patients with coronary artery disease (CAD) is best correlated with a degree of coronary stenosis and the number of vessels involved as documented by angiography, rather than the clinical manifestations of coronary disease such as angina pectoris or acute MI (see also Ch. 2). If this is true, the unexpectedly poor long-term prognosis of patients with non-Q wave infarction may simply indicate that these patients have more advanced coronary atherosclerosis than patients with Q wave infarctions.

Extent of Coronary Artery Disease

As Table 18–1 illustrates, only 2 of the 14 published studies found significant between-group differences in the extent of atherosclerotic CAD (11). In both instances, the angiographic findings could be attributed either to a "referral bias" or to important differences in baseline clinical characteristics between the two infarct groups. For example, in the study by Ogawa et al (24), the prevalence of multivessel disease was 73% in the non-Q wave group versus 51% in the Q wave group ($p < 0.01$). This finding of more extensive disease in the non-Q wave group is understandable, as more patients with non-Q wave infarcts had early postinfarction angina with ECG changes (55% versus 21% in the Q wave group, $p < 0.01$), and angiography typically shows severe multivessel disease in such patients (11). In the study by Coll et al (46), only 34% of patients with non-Q wave MI had multivessel disease compared with 58% of patients with Q wave MI ($p < 0.05$). This finding of less extensive disease in the non-Q wave group may reflect the fact that patients with non-Q wave MI were significantly younger (mean age 46 ± 10 years) and had significantly fewer risk factors than patients with Q wave MI.

Infarct Vessel Patency

Although most studies have shown that the extent and severity of CAD are equivalent in the two infarct groups, one angiographic difference exists that consistently stands out in both pathologic and clinical studies (11) (see Ch. 4). As Fig. 18–4 shows, patients with non-Q wave infarction are two to four times more likely to have an open infarct-related vessel than patients with Q wave infarction. In each of the 12 studies, the between-group difference in vessel patency was statistically significant at a level of 0.007 or less. This finding raises several interesting possibilities relevant to the pathogenesis of non-Q wave infarction. One possibility is that a flow-limiting stenosis caused by atherosclerosis was present, but that the infarct-related vessel was never occluded. In this situation, non-Q wave infarction may simply represent an imbalance between supply and demand in the presence of a patent but severely narrowed coronary artery. An alternative hypothesis, which seems more likely (11), is one that allows for a transient reduction in flow sufficient to cause subendocardial necrosis but not enough to compromise subepicardial viability. As DeWood et al (59) point out, this could occur as a result of complete thrombotic coronary occlusion with subsequent

Table 18–1. Prevalence of Multivessel Coronary Artery Disease in 3,252 Patients with Q Wave and Non-Q Wave Myocardial Infarction

		Q Wave MI		Non-Q Wave MI	
Study	Stenosis Criteria %	N	2–3VD %	N	2–3VD %
Fuster (1975)	50	73	62	63	58
Schulze (1978)	50	31	a68	17	65
Turner (1980)	70	94	76	23	74
Taylor (1980)	50	64	72	42	76
DeWood (1981)	50	440	71	261	82
Roubin (1983)	70	148	38	48	32
Coll (1983)	50	378	58	24	34*
Zema (1985)	50	25	64	12	67
Ogawa (1985)	75	199	51	70	73*
Kouvaras (1985)	70	258	73	42	67
Gibson (1986)	50	154	60	87	54
Theroux (1986)	70	291	54	157	62
L'Abbate (1986)	50	29	66	42	60
Huey (1987)	50	115	58	35	51
Pooled data		2,299	62	923	61

N = number of patients, 2–3VD = two- or three-vessel disease.

* $p < 0.05$ compared with Q wave group.

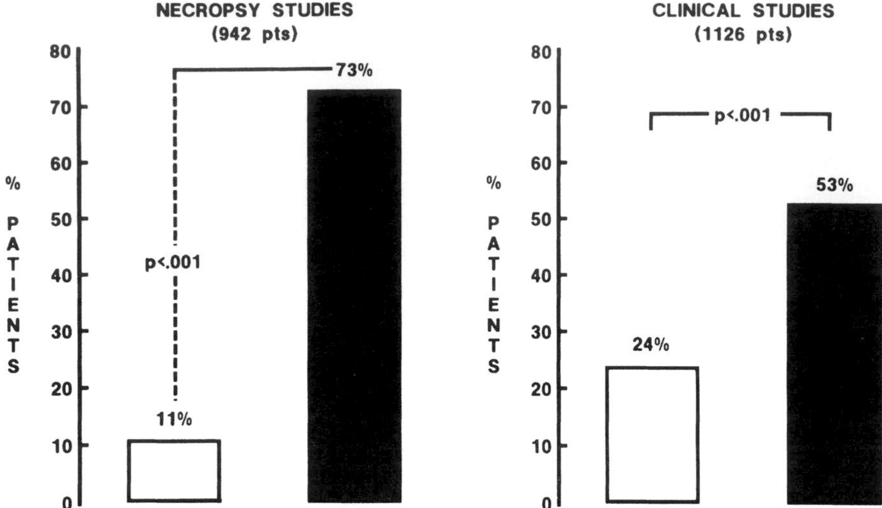

Figure 18–4. Patency rates of infarct-related artery after Q wave (open bars) and non-Q wave (solid bars) infarction. See text. *Reprinted from Gibson RS: Non-Q wave myocardial infarction: Pathophysiology, prognosis, and therapeutic strategy. Ann Rev Med 1989;40:395–410, with permission.*

spontaneous thrombolysis, severe coronary spasm with or without coronary thrombosis, or severe atherosclerotic obstruction with a variable component of coronary vasoconstriction.

On the basis of available data, it is reasonable to postulate that in many patients, residual antegrade flow beyond the coronary obstruction is responsible for the preservation of viable myocardium. The open but severely stenotic coronary artery allows for viable but potentially ischemic myocardium to survive and, because of the instability of the obstructive lesion (60), places the patient at risk for future events. Those patients with a completely occluded artery who have myocardial salvage because of adequate collaterals may have a more stable situation and less danger of sudden acute changes resulting in reinfarction. These patients, especially the subset with "nonjeopardized" collaterals (that is, collateral vessels arising from a nonstenotic coronary artery), may be at lesser risk of future events.

MYOCARDIAL PERFUSION AND TISSUE VIABILITY STUDIES

In a recent series of studies published by our group (34,61,62), we found that the proportion of patients with thallium-201 redistribution (that is, ischemia) within the perfusion zone of the infarct-related vessel was greater in the non-Q wave group as compared with the Q wave group (60% versus 36%, $p = 0.007$) (see Ch. 11). We also found that the number of scan segments showing peri-infarction ischemia was greater among patients with non-Q wave than Q wave infarction ($p = 0.0003$). This observation, which has been confirmed by others (63), provides strong evidence that patients with non-Q wave infarction have a larger residual mass of viable but jeopardized myocardium than patients with Q wave infarction. Because ischemic tissue remains, the heart is understandably more prone to recurrent ischemia and infarction. One might actually view the non-Q wave infarction as an incomplete or aborted Q wave infarction, possibly because early spontaneous reperfusion occurred in the first hour or two after onset of symptoms.

Geltman et al (57), using positron emission tomography (PET) and metabolic imaging with ^{11}C-palmitate, have reported substantial morphologic differences in the tomographic appearance of Q wave and non-Q wave infarctions. Patients with Q wave infarcts were found to have large confluent regions of homogeneously diminished tissue metabolism extending from the subendocardial to the subepicardial surface. In contrast, PET reconstructions from patients with non-Q wave infarction showed less regional depression but greater spatial heterogeneity in metabolism, suggesting the presence of ischemic, infarcted, and normal myocardium interspersed with one another. This situation may, in some patients, provide the substrate for reentrant ventricular arrhythmias, and help explain the findings of Cannom et al (38) and others (30,34,64), who showed that a significant number of the deaths in patients with non-Q wave MI are sudden.

In a recent study of 22 patients using the ^{18}F-deoxyglucose PET technique, Hashimoto and colleagues (58) demonstrated preserved metabolic integrity (that is, residual tissue viability as evidenced by regional ^{18}F-deoxyglucose accumulation) in 10 of 11 areas (91%) with non-Q wave MI. In contrast, residual tissue viability was found in only 4 of 11 areas (36%) with Q wave infarction. These results and the earlier observations of Brunken et al (65) provide further support that the mass of viable but jeopardized tissue within the perfusion zone of the infarct-related artery is greater after non-Q wave than Q wave infarction.

CHANGING INCIDENCE OF NON-Q WAVE INFARCTION

Perhaps of equal importance to recent knowledge defining the prognosis and pathophysiologic features of non-Q wave infarction is the epidemiologic evidence that the incidence of the syndrome may be increasing, both naturally and iatrogenically, relative to a decade ago (11). In almost all of the studies published between 1969 and 1980, the ratio of Q wave to non-Q wave infarction ranged from 4:1 to 6:1. As Fig. 18–5 illustrates, results from a recently published community-wide survey show a substantial increase in the incidence of non-Q wave infarction (52). In this study, Goldberg and associates found that the age-adjusted hospital attack rate (per 100,000) for non-Q wave infarction increased from 46 in 1975 to 89 in 1981, a relative increase of 93% ($p < 0.001$). The authors concluded that their findings indicated a significant change in either the occurrence or the recognition rates of non-Q wave myocardial infarction.

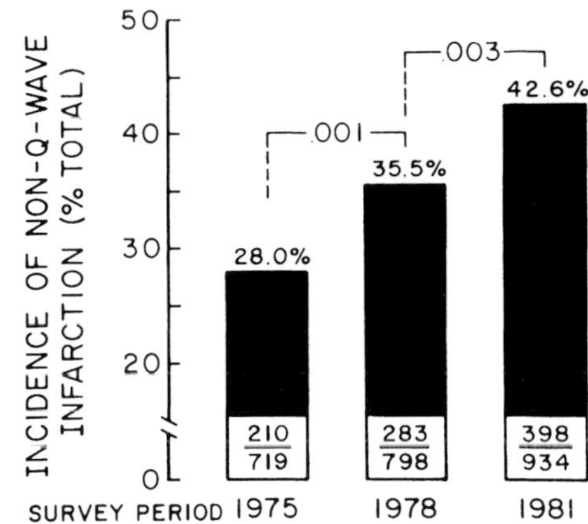

Figure 18–5. Change in incidence of non-Q wave myocardial infarction between 1975 and 1981. See text. *Adapted from Goldberg et al (52), with permission.*

The apparent increased incidence of non-Q wave infarction may be related to the recent widespread adoption of antiplatelet, anticoagulant, and other aggressive therapies for the management of the acute intermediate ischemic syndromes (that is, unstable angina, coronary insufficiency, threatened infarction). Certainly, patients with these syndromes appear to have coronary anatomy, morbidity, and mortality risks similar to those of patients with non-Q wave infarction (60,66). It seems reasonable to speculate that successful therapy, although possibly avoiding transmural infarction and death, may predispose patients to repetitive ischemic events including subsequent non-Q wave infarction.

Similarly, if one accepts the concept that the underlying coronary artery defect in acute non-Q wave MI is the critically compromised lumen of the infarct-related artery, it seems appropriate to speculate that patients who have received successful thrombolytic therapy for acute Q wave MI have similar pathophysiologic features. Angiography in such patients performed soon after thrombolytic therapy often reveals a patent but severely narrowed infarct-related vessel. Moreover, there appears to be a significant risk of recurrent ischemia (~35%) and infarction (8% to 15%) in these patients (67). A recent meta-analysis by Yusef et al of the pooled data of 27 intravenous and 9 intracoronary thrombolytic therapy studies revealed that the relative risk of reinfarction in the treated group was 57% higher in the intravenous studies and 100%

higher in the intracoronary studies. Obviously, the rapidly increasing use of such therapy and other acute interventions to effect reperfusion in the early phase of infarction may, in minimizing the mural extent of myocardial damage (68), modify the course of evolving MI with a resultant increased likelihood of aborted Q wave infarctions whose postlytic infarct-related coronary anatomy and risk of reinfarction are similar to those of patients with naturally occurring non-Q wave infarction.

PREDICTORS OF POOR PROGNOSIS AFTER NON-Q WAVE INFARCTION

Examination of data from the 45 cohort studies of non-Q wave infarction reveals considerable variation in mortality and incident morbidity rates (Table 18–2). The degree of difference in reported outcomes suggests that patients with non-Q wave MI have highly heterogeneous risk profiles, and that the identification of prognostically relevant variables that effectively stratify patients into low-risk, intermediate-risk, and high-risk subgroups is vitally important to our understanding and management of individual patients.

Admission Electrocardiographic Findings

Several studies have shown that patients with insignificant or no ECG changes at the onset of infarction have a very low mortality risk and incident morbidity rate compared with patients with frankly abnormal findings (48,64,69–71). Among patients with a definitely abnormal ECG on admission, it seems clear that classification of non-Q wave infarcts according to the predominant waveform change (for example, ST depression, ST elevation, or T wave inversion without significant ST deviation) provides valuable information about short-term and long-term prognosis, extent of underlying CAD, and the status of left ventricular function (13,48,72–78). As Table 18–3 illustrates, pooled data from multiple studies show a significantly higher cardiac event rate in patients who present with ST segment depression versus those with ST segment elevation or T wave inversion.

Table 18–2. Event Rate Variability in 45 Clinical Outcome Studies of Non-Q Wave Myocardial Infarction[a]

	Reported Range of Event Rates (%)	
Outcome Measure	In-hospital	Postdischarge[b]
Mortality	0–23	6–48
Reinfarction	7–43	0–32
Recurrent ischemia	13–55	36–66

[a] Data on 4794 patients.

[b] Length of follow-up varies from 6 to 96 months.

Persistent ST Segment Depression

Many investigators have reported that ST segment depression on the discharge ECG is an independent predictor of prognosis (64,79–81). Only one study, however, has examined the prognostic value of both the admission ECG and the discharge ECG in patients with MBCK-confirmed acute non-Q wave MI (64,81). In this study by Schechtman et al, "persistent" ST segment depression (that is, ST depression on admission and at discharge) was found to be the single most powerful predictor of 1-year mortality ($p = 0.0009$) and late reinfarction ($p = 0.0058$) (64). As Figure 18–6 demonstrates, both outcomes were significantly more likely in patients with persistent ST depression compared with those with transient or no ST depression. Of particular note is the fact that highly significant differences in mortality between the three groups emerged very early in follow-up; at 3 months, mortality was 0.5% (1 of 199) for patients with no ST depression, 5.0% (7 of 139) for patients with transient ST depression, and 13.7% (16 of 117) for patients with persistent ST depression. These data indicate that the relative risk of death within 3 months of hospital discharge is increased by a factor of 9.5 with transient ST segment depression and by a factor of 27.2 with persistent ST segment depression.

Anterior Infarct Location

The results of two recent studies suggest that location of infarction, as determined by ECG, may

Table 18–3. Comparison of Outcomes of Patients with Non-Q Wave Myocardial Infarction According to Admission ECG-Determined Infarct Subtype[a]

	ST Depression		ST Elevation		T Wave Inversion	
	N	Rate	N	Rate	N	Rate
In-hospital events[b]						
Death	304	77(25)*	248	14(5.6)	143	5(3.4)
Infarct extension	97	24(25)*	207	19(9.2)	0	NA
Recurrent ischemia	97	50(52)*	207	58(28)	0	NA
Heart failure	113	49(43)*	41	6(15)	168	33(20)
Postdischarge events[b]						
Death	147	33(23)*	95	11(12)	162	23(14)
Infarct extension	104	12(12)	195	6(3.1)	114	28(25)
Angina pectoris	22	9(41)	0	NA	114	38(33)
Heart failure	65	20(31)	175	31(18)	0	NA

N = number of patients. NA = not available; event rate not calculated because of no data or too few patients in sample.

[a] Event rates represent average values from pooled data (13,48,72–78).

[b] Percentages given in parentheses.

* $p < 0.05$ compared with group with ST segment elevation or T wave inversion.

be an extremely important discriminator of risk (82,83). In both studies, investigators observed significantly higher mortality and incident morbidity rates in patients with anterior versus inferior or lateral non-Q wave MI. Importantly, Cox regression analysis showed that anterior infarct location retained its independent prognostic significance even after adjusting for baseline between-group differences in clinical variables, size of infarction, and indices of heart failure (Fig. 18–7). These findings appear to support previous observations (61,84,85) that anterior non-Q wave MI is a largely incomplete event associated with a large amount of viable but hypoperfused myocardium that predisposes patients to a higher incidence of morbid cardiac events. Inferior and lateral or nonlocalizable non-Q wave infarcts may, on the other hand, represent either completed events or aborted initial infarctions, but with a relatively small amount of remaining jeopardized myocardium.

Left Ventricular Hypertrophy

Since 1961, there have been numerous reports showing that left ventricular hypertrophy (LVH), whether detected by standard ECG criteria or by echocardiography, is an independent predictor of increased cardiovascular morbidity and mortality (86–94). Only one study, however, has evaluated the prognostic importance of LVH in patients with non-Q wave myocardial infarction. In this study (94), Boden and coworkers found that 126 of 544 patients (23%) exhibited LVH using standard ECG voltage criteria. Compared with patients without LVH, those with LVH were significantly older (65 versus 60 years, $p < 0.0001$) and had smaller peak adjusted CK levels (490 ± 376 IU/L versus 666 ± 726 IU/L, $p < 0.001$). Although in-hospital clinical outcome was similar in the two groups, patients with LVH were more likely to die (19% versus 9%, $p = 0.044$) or suffer reinfarction (24% versus 12%, $p < 0.005$) during the first year of follow-up. Multivariate regression analysis revealed that the relative risk of death and reinfarction during the initial year after non-Q wave MI was increased by factors of 1.7 and 2.1 among patients with LVH, respectively.

Early Recurrent Ischemia

Historically, the occurrence of early postinfarction angina has indicated a poor prognosis, as extension of infarction, serious ventricular arrhythmias, or even death may follow (95–99). In recent years, however, some investigators have begun to question whether all patients with recurrent angina

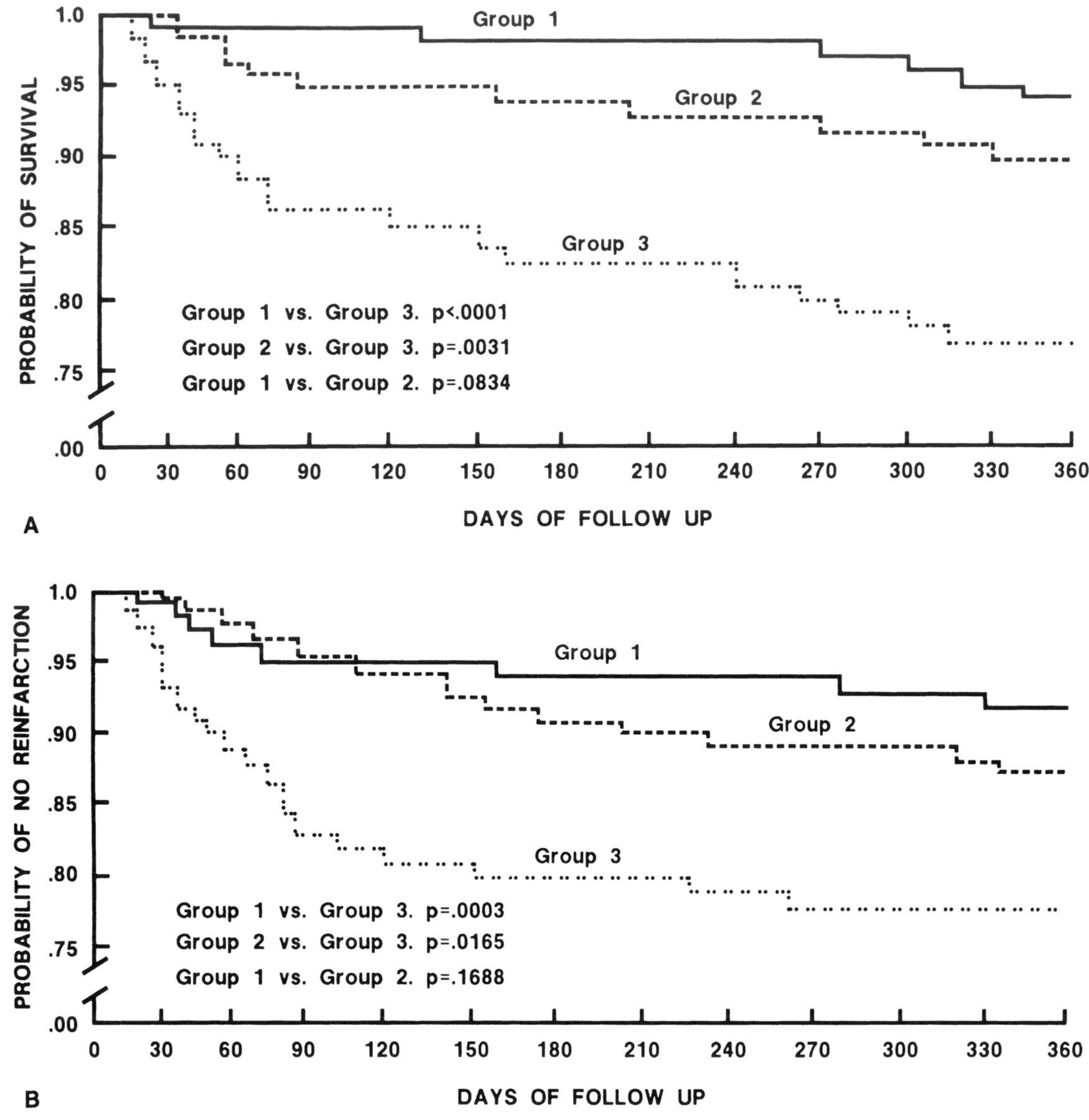

Figure 18–6. A. Kaplan–Meier survival curves for patients with no ST segment depression (group 1), ST segment depression at baseline or discharge (group 2), and ST segment depression at baseline and discharge (group 3). Mortality at 1 year was 5.5% in group 1 (n = 199), 10.1% in group 2 (n = 168), and 22.2% in group 3 (n = 117). **B.** Kaplan–Meier curves for cumulative incidence of late reinfarction for patients with no ST segment depression (group 1), ST segment depression at baseline or discharge (group 2), and ST segment depression at baseline and discharge (group 3). Reinfarction rates at 1 year were 7.8% in group 1, 12.3% in group 2, and 21.4% in group 3. *Reprinted from Schechtman et al (64), with permission.*

have the same risk. Results from two different studies of patients with early postinfarction angina have now shown that the short-term and long-term risk of reinfarction and/or death is confined predominantly to the patients who show transient ECG changes during their anginal episodes (100–102). This seems especially true for patients with early angina after non-Q wave infarction. In one study of 246 such patients, the likelihood of subsequent reinfarction, death, or either event was significantly

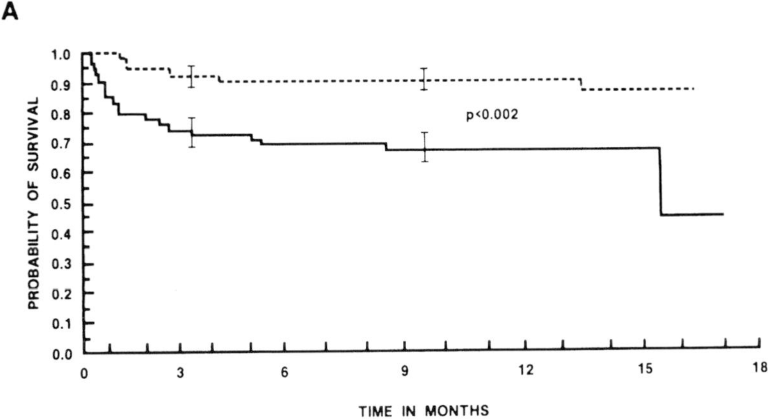

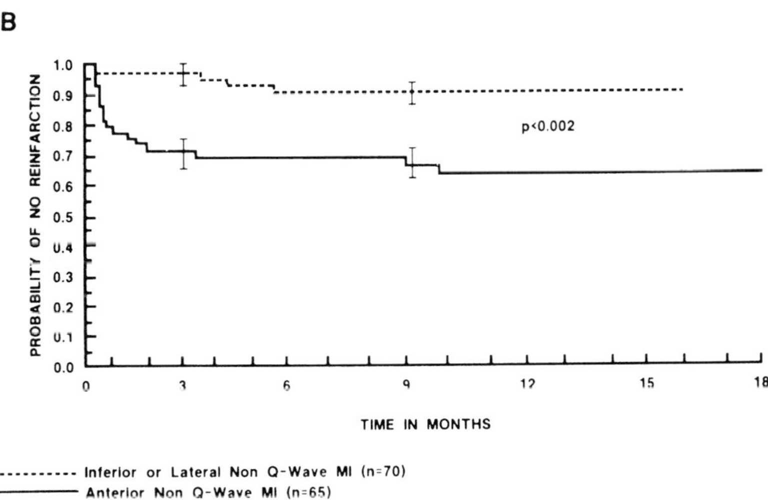

Figure 18–7. Kaplan Meier probabilities of survival (**A**) and of no reinfarction (**B**) in patients with anterior non-Q wave MI (solid line) and with inferior and/or lateral non-Q wave MI (dotted line). *Reprinted from Kao et al (83), with permission.*

higher if transient ST–T wave changes accompanied the episode of angina. Compared with patients with angina alone, those with angina and associated ECG changes were 3.9 times more likely to suffer reinfarction or death during hospitalization (6.8% versus 27%, $p < 0.001$) (101). Also, patients with angina and ECG changes had higher peak MBCK levels with reinfarction than those with angina alone (91 ± 76 IU/L versus 37 ± 19 IU/L, $p = 0.059$ [Wilcoxon rank sum test]). These observations combined with the results illustrated in Figure 18–8 demonstrate the importance of obtaining an ECG during episodes of early postinfarction angina; whereas patients with ST–T wave changes have a very poor outlook (that is, a 27% probability of death and/or reinfarction during 14 days of follow-up), those with angina alone exhibit a prognosis similar to that of patients with no angina at all.

Early Recurrent Infarction

In 1981, Marmor and associates (43) reported that reinfarction in patients recovering from an initial non-Q wave infarction has a highly deleterious effect on left ventricular function and survival.

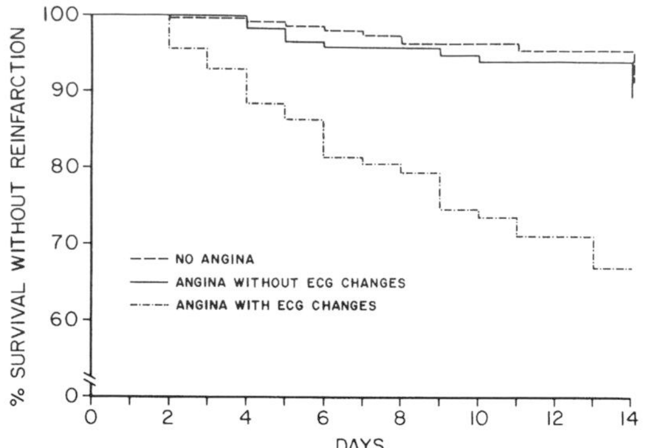

Figure 18–8. Kaplan–Meier survival curves for patients with no angina ($n = 330$), patients with angina alone ($n = 131$), and patients with angina associated with transient ST–T changes ($n = 115$) after MBCK-confirmed acute non-Q wave infarction. At 14 days, the survival rates without reinfarction were 92%, 90%, and 63% for the three groups, respectively ($p < 0.0001$). *Reprinted from Gibson et al (101), with permission.*

Subsequently, a comprehensive analysis of two large databases established conclusively the independent prognostic significance of recurrent myocardial infarction (47,64,80). On the basis of available data, it is therefore clear that reinfarction events, whether occurring in-hospital or later, significantly change the mortality risk (by a factor of 4.5) of patients with an initial non-Q wave infarction (Fig. 18–9).

Inability to Perform a Low-Level Exercise Test

Between 15% and 25% of patients with non-Q wave MI are deemed ineligible for predischarge exercise stress testing. In most instances, this is because of ongoing ischemia. Other less common contraindications include signs of persistent heart failure on physical examination, poorly controlled arrhythmias, or musculoskeletal handicap. Studies have shown that these patients, compared with those who are tested, have a higher frequency of multivessel CAD (81% versus 58%, $p < 0.01$) and lower left ventricular ejection fractions (49 ± 11% versus 43 ± 12%, $p < 0.01$) (34). As such, it is not surprising that the incidence of death and reinfarction in the several years subsequent to the index MI is significantly higher in patients deemed ineligible for testing (24% versus 11% for patients who are tested, $p < 0.05$) (103).

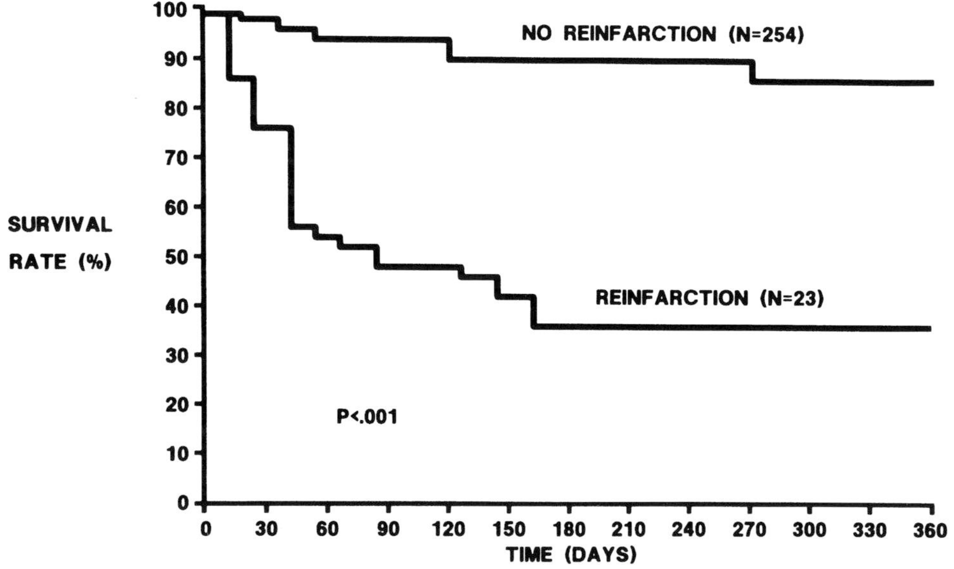

Figure 18–9. Effect of reinfarction on 1-year survival after acute non-Q wave MI. *Reprinted from Maisel et al (47), with permission.*

Predictive Value of Thallium-201 Scintigraphy

A considerable amount of data indicate that exercise electrocardiography has limited value in the predischarge risk assessment of asymptomatic patients recovering from acute non-Q wave MI (103–105). Because of this and the well-recognized advantages of thallium-201 stress-redistribution scintigraphy (106), there appears to be a strong rationale for recommending exercise or dipyridamole perfusion imaging, rather than exercise ECG testing alone, as the preferred noninvasive method for evaluating mortality and morbidity risks after acute MI. This recommendation seems justified given that the presence and extent of inducible ischemia have been shown to be a key predictor of future cardiac events in postinfarction patients with uncomplicated hospital courses (11); thallium-201 scintigraphy is more reliable (that is, more sensitive and specific than exercise testing) in detecting and quantifying ischemic jeopardy (the amount of viable myocardium "jeopardized" by atherosclerotic coronary lesions) (106–108); thallium-201 scintigraphy, unlike the exercise ECG, can localize ischemia to a specific area or areas subtended by a specific coronary artery (that is, it can identify the ischemia-producing or "culprit" vessel) (109); and thallium-201 scintigraphy has been shown to be more accurate in risk stratification of individual patients than exercise testing alone (105,110–112). The more optimal prognostic efficiency of thallium-201 scintigraphy is due, in part, to the fact that the error rate in falsely classifying patients as low-risk is substantially and significantly smaller with thallium-201 scintigraphy than with stress echocardiography (Fig. 18–10).

Several laboratories have independently demonstrated the value of stress-redistribution thallium-201 imaging for determining prognosis in patients with CAD (106), including those recovering from acute Q wave and non Q wave infarction (108). In addition to indicating simply the positive or negative nature of the test, these studies have defined a number of key prognostic indicators, including the number of vascular beds involved (105,110–113), relative size of the defect and reversibility of hypoperfusion (105,110 114), abnormally increased lung uptake (110,115,116), and ischemic left ventricular dilation (117). These factors can be identified qualitatively as well as quantitatively, and the prognostic window can be modulated according to the combination of criteria employed.

At the present time, only one study (105) has compared the ability of predischarge exercise ECG testing and thallium-201 stress-redistribution

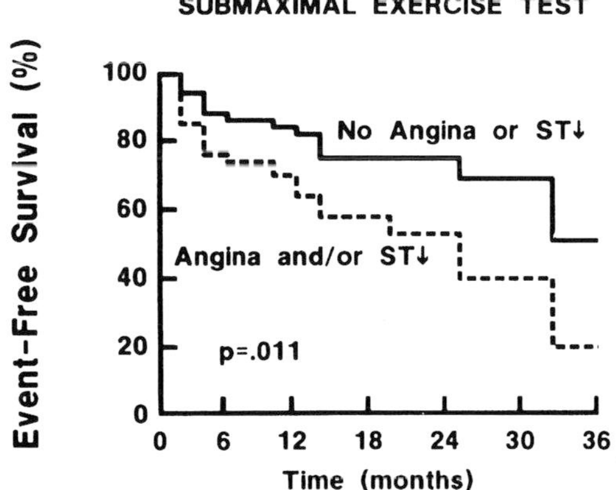

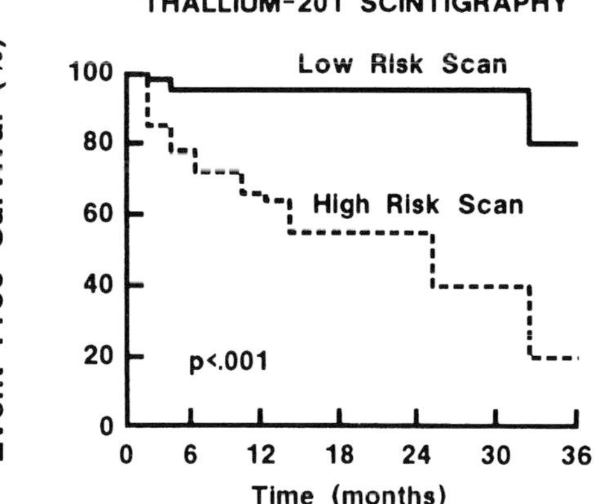

Figure 18–10. Cumulative probability of event-free survival for four different subgroups of postinfarction patients formed by the submaximal exercise test results (**left**) and thallium-201 scintigraphic findings (**right**). Because thallium-201 scintigraphy correctly identified 94% of patients with events during follow-up (versus only 56% for exercise ECG test, $p < 0.01$), the error rate in falsely classifying patients as low-risk was substantially less with thallium-201 scintigraphy than with exercise ECG. *Reprinted from Gibson et al (108), with permission.*

scintigraphy to predict prognosis after non-Q wave MI. In this study, 87 asymptomatic patients with uncomplicated hospital courses underwent testing 10 ± 3 days after onset of MI. During 23 ± 18 months of follow-up, 8 patients (9.2%) died, 16 (18.4%) experienced reinfarction, and 21 patients (24%) had unstable angina pectoris necessitating readmission and myocardial revascularization. As shown in Table 18–4, there was no exercise test variable that discriminated patient outcome. In contrast, the number of scintiscan segments showing numerically significant defects, the number of hypoperfused vascular regions, and the presence of thallium-201 redistribution in scan segments remote from the zone of MI (that is, multivessel disease pattern) were all significant univariate predictors ($p < 0.05$) of postdischarge cardiac events. Moreover, multivariate analysis of 67 clinical, historical, exercise test, and thallium-201 variables identified only three independent predictors of patient outcome: (i) number of risk factors ($p < 0.01$), (ii) angina preceding the index infarction ($p < 0.02$), and (iii) number of hypoperfused vascular regions by thallium-201 criteria ($p < 0.02$). The results of this study indicate that in contrast to submaximal exercise ECG testing, stress-redistribution thallium-201 scintigraphy is useful in the predischarge risk assessment of patients recovering from acute non-Q wave MI.

Multivessel Disease

Several studies have shown that postinfarction patients with single-vessel CAD have a negligible mortality rate (≤1% to 2% per year) and a very low cumulative risk of recurrent infarction (~5%) during the first several years after hospital discharge (111,118,119). As it has also been demonstrated that the vast majority of postdischarge deaths (85% to 100%) and most reinfarctions (70% to 85%) occur in patients with two-vessel or three-vessel disease, it appears that the presence of multivessel dis-

Table 18–4. Results of Submaximal Treadmill Testing in 87 Patients with Uncomplicated Acute Non-Q Wave Myocardial Infarction[a]

Exercise Test Variable	Event Group (N = 34)	Nonevent Group (N = 53)	*p*
Exercise duration (minutes)	6.7 ± 4.7	7.5 ± 4.6	NS
Peak heart rate (beats per minute)	107 ± 13	108 ± 18	NS
Workload achieved (METS)	4.4 ± 2.8	4.2 ± 1.8	NS
Peak systolic blood pressure (mm Hg)	144 ± 25	144 ± 29	NS
Peak rate-pressure product (× 10^3)	15.7 ± 3.5	15.7 ± 4.3	NS
Test endpoints			
Limiting angina	7(21)[b]	10(19)	NS
Dyspnea or fatigue	11(32)	19(36)	NS
Achieved heart rate/workload target[a]	5(15)	12(23)	NS
Other	11(32)	11(12)	NS
Abnormal systolic blood pressure response	1(3)	1(2)	NS
Exercise-induced VEA+[c]	5(15)	5(10)	NS
Any angina	12(35)	14(26)	NS
ST segment response			
Number of patients with ≥ 0.1 mV ST ↓	15(45)	17(31)	NS
Leads with ≥ 0.1 mV ST ↓	2.0 ± 0.4	1.4 ± 0.3	NS
Total ST ↓ score (mm)	2.7 ± 0.6	1.9 ± 0.5	NS

[a] Naughton protocol with heart rate and workload targets of 130 beats per minutes and 5 METS.

[b] Percentages given in parentheses.

[c] VEA = ventricular ectopic activity (≥ 5 premature ventricular contractions [PVCs] per minute, multifocal or paired PVCs, or ventricular tachycardia/ventricular fibrillation).

ease is an extremely important covariate of risk (34,118,119). Indeed, Varma and Gibson (120) have recently shown that the presence of multivessel disease, but not infarct-vessel patency or percentage residual stenosis, is one of the most powerful independent predictors of adverse clinical outcome after non-Q wave infarction.

Some investigators have speculated that multivessel disease, especially severe three-vessel disease, is a marker of risk because of its effect on physiologic "autorevascularization" of the infarct zone. Experimental and clinical data have shown that there is a gradual increase in collateral flow during the first 7 to 14 days after myocardial infarction that often restores flow to normal values in previously ischemic "border-zone" regions (59,121,122). In the presence of multivessel disease, collateralized flow to the partially viable infarct zone may be severely compromised, resulting in a larger lateral and transmural dimension of noninfarcted myocardium at risk, and thus predisposing patients to recurrent infarction and death.

MANAGEMENT OF NON-Q WAVE INFARCTION

It is now well documented that patients with non-Q wave infarction have less extensive injury but a high propensity for recurrent ischemia and infarction. Studies have also shown that the non-Q wave infarction represents an incomplete infarction and that the increased risk of additional ischemic injury is due to the presence of a large residual mass of viable but jeopardized myocardium within the perfusion zone of the infarct-related vessel. As extensive damage from reinfarction has a significant deleterious effect on left ventricular function and long-term survival, patients with non-Q wave infarction would be expected to benefit from an intervention that prevents reinfarction. Indeed, this subset of patients appears to offer a unique opportunity to modify favorably the natural history of ischemic heart disease.

During the past 20 years, a large number of randomized, placebo-controlled clinical trials have been performed in patients recovering from acute MI. Most of these studies have evaluated the effect of experimental therapy on mortality, and some also assess evidence of other benefits such as reduction in reinfarction and early recurrent ischemia. Unfortunately, many of these placebo-controlled studies evaluated therapeutic efficacy in large, undifferentiated populations; i.e., the trials did not specify an a priori test of drug efficacy based on the presence or absence of electrocardiographic Q waves. Because of this, there is a relative paucity of data collected prospectively that addresses the specific problem of secondary prevention after acute non-Q wave infarction.

Effect of Antiplatelet Agents

The RISC investigators were the first to prospectively show that in non-Q wave MI, as well as unstable angina, aspirin therapy (75 mg/day) significantly reduces the incidence of subsequent MI or death from the levels associated with administration of placebo (123). In a later analysis, the RISC group also observed that aspirin therapy effectively reduced the incidence of severe postinfarction angina requiring revascularization (124). At least four other clinical trials of patients with unstable CAD have shown a beneficial treatment-related effect with either aspirin or ticlopidine on mortality and nonfatal MI (125–128). In all of these trials, the effect attributable to antiplatelet therapy on these endpoints was impressive and highly significant (e.g., a 50% reduction in risk compared to placebo, $p < 0.005$).

A strong argument can also be made for aspirin treatment in the chronic phase of acute MI. The Part 2 analysis of the Persatine/Aspirin Reinfarction Study (PARIS-2) (129) is particularly informative in this regard. At the end of 1 year of follow-up, there was a 48% reduction in mortality and reinfarction among patients with non-Q wave MI who received active treatment. By comparison, the combined mortality and recurrent MI rate was reduced only 7% in the Q wave group.

Effect of Combined Antithrombotic Therapy

Therapeutic intravenous heparin has been found to be of benefit in unstable angina (125), and since a common pathophysiology has been proposed for unstable angina and non-Q wave MI (130,131), some investigators have advocated the use of heparin on presentation and for several days after non-Q wave MI. Heparin may be even more appealing with the knowledge that most infarct-related vessels are patent at angiography and that most reinfarctions occur in the same vascular bed as the original injury. Also, it has been demonstrated that among patients presenting with ST segment elevation who undergo successful thrombolysis, the combination of heparin and aspirin is superior to heparin or aspirin alone in maintaining patency of the infarct-related artery (132–135). Findings indicate that combination antithrombotic therapy (aspirin plus heparin versus aspirin alone) significantly reduced the incidence of ischemic events (death, reinfarction, or recurrent angina associated with ECG changes) at 14 days; analysis by intention to treat showed that 26.6% of patients assigned to aspirin experienced an ischemic event versus only 10.5% of patients assigned to combination therapy (a 63% reduction in risk $p = 0.004$). When the results from all available studies are pooled, the relative risk for death or MI with combination antithrombotic therapy compared with aspirin alone is 0.44 (95% confidence interval, 0.21–0.93, $p < 0.001$) (123, 135–138).

It is important to emphasize that heparin has a beneficial effect in patients with unstable CAD provided that it is started early and adequate control of anticoagulation is ensured. The protective effect appears to apply to patients with unstable angina and non-Q wave MI, as well as patients with and without ischemic ECG changes on presentation. As such, there is now general agreement that the treatment of patients with unstable angina or non-Q wave MI should include antithrombotic therapy with an antithrombin (presently heparin) and an antiplatelet agent (presently aspirin).

Effect of Thrombolytic Therapy

Theoretically, thrombolytic therapy for non-Q wave myocardial infarction and the closely related syndrome of unstable angina, particularly if it is administered early, would be expected to reduce the severity of obstruction of the culprit coronary lesion or the tendency of the subtotally occluded vessel to progress and thereby improve the clinical outcome. However, when the results of two large-scale trials were examined (post hoc), the effect of thrombolytic therapy on patients with ST segment depression were disappointing. In the GISSI trial, 451 patients had ST segment depression. Patients treated with intravenous streptokinase had a 20.5% mortality rate at 21 days, compared with 16.3% in patients receiving standard care (138). In ISIS-2, 1,137 patients were found to have ST segment depression at study entry (139). Five-week vascular mortality rates in these patients were not influenced by treatment with streptokinase, low-dose aspirin, or a combination of the two.

During the past year, the results of the TIMI-3 study were reported (140,141). Pertinent findings from this trial which included 1,779 analyzable patients with unstable angina ($n = 1,205$) or non-Q wave MI ($n = 574$) included (i) t-PA was more effective than placebo in achieving measurable improvement in the "culprit" coronary lesion of patients with non-Q wave MI (33% versus 8%, $p = 0.003$); (ii) the occurrence of any event making up the "unfavorable outcome" endpoint (death, MI, or objective evidence of recurrent ischemia) was similar in the two treatment groups (t-PA or placebo) by the time of the 6-week visit; (iii) the effect of t-PA on the incidence of fatal and nonfatal acute MI by 6 weeks appeared to be different in patients with unstable angina versus those with non-Q wave MI. Patients with unstable angina exhibited a higher occurrence of MI if treated with t-PA than if treated with placebo (8.3% versus 4.6%, $p = 0.01$), whereas in patients with a diagnosis of non-Q wave MI, the rates for reinfarction were similar (5.6% versus 5.4%, p = NS); and (iv) intracranial hemorrhage, confirmed by computerized tomography, was more common in t-PA versus placebo treated patients ($p = 0.06$). Not surprisingly, the intracranial hemorrhage rate was higher in patients over the age of 75 years than it was in patients aged 75 years or younger (6.7% versus 0.2%, $p = 0.01$). These disappointing results for the TIMI-3 study, particularly when combined with findings from other trials (142–146), lead to the inevitable conclusion that thrombolytic therapy offers no clinically important advantage compared with intravenous heparin, oral aspirin, and vigorous use of pharmacologic anti-ischemic therapy.

The reasons for this lack of benefit of thrombolytic therapy are not clear, but several possibilities have been considered. In an excellent discussion of this issue (140,141), the TIMI-3 investigators point out that the balance between the clot-dissolving and procoagulant actions of thrombolytic agents might well differ in patients with non-Q wave MI versus those with Q wave MI. The thrombi in patients with unstable angina and non-Q wave MI appear to be composed predominantly of platelets rather than erythrocytes, and it has been demonstrated that the former are considerably more resistant to lysis by t-PA than the latter (147–149). In addition, the subtotal occlusion characteristic of unstable angina and non-Q wave MI provide continued access of procoagulant substances to the thrombus. As such, it has been postulated that the balance between the two opposing actions of thrombolytic agents leads to a less favorable effect with patients with unstable angina and non-Q wave MI who have subtotal coronary occlusions and platelet-rich thrombi than in patients with evolving Q wave and total occlusion due to erythrocyte-rich thrombi.

Effect of Intravenous Nitroglycerin

Intravenous nitroglycerin has found growing support for its potential role in limiting infarct size and reducing mortality in patients with Q wave or unspecified infarction (150,151). However, no study has addressed the non-Q wave MI population, and current recommendations of the American College of Cardiology/American Heart Association do not support the routine use of intravenous nitroglycerin in all patients with infarction (152). Nitroglycerin is well established for relieving ischemic symptoms, and it may improve collateral flow to jeopardized myocardium. However, in the absence of a well-designed and properly executed clinical trial, a firm new recommendation cannot be made.

Effect of Beta Blockers

A beneficial effect of long-term administration of beta blockers has been demonstrated in numerous controlled trials, ranging in size from 100 to more than 4,000 patients (153). In evaluating these trials, it is useful to divide beta blockers into those with intrinsic sympathonometic activity (ISA), such as alprenolol, practolol, pindolol, and oxyprenolol, and those without ISA, such as atenolol, metoprolol, propranolol, and timolol. Pooled data for beta blockers with ISA indicate a minimal (usually less than 5–10%) reduction in mortality. Studies of beta blockers without ISA have shown significantly greater benefit. In the two largest trials, the Norwegian Timolol Trial and the β-Blocker Heart Attack Trial (βHAT), the results are statistically significant (154,155). Pooled analysis of data from all trials using beta blockers without ISA shows a 30% reduction in all cause mortality and an approximately 25% reduction in cumulative incidence of nonfatal reinfarction.

Although retrospective subgroup analysis should always be interpreted with caution (156), it is interesting that three of the largest beta blocker trials observed little or no benefit with treatment in patients with non Q wave MI. The βHAT, for example, demonstrated reduced mortality and a lower reinfarction rate with propranolol compared with placebo in patients with Q wave MI, but showed no effect on either endpoint in patients with non Q wave MI (157). Similarly, the Metoprolol in Acute Myocardial Infarction (MIAMI) trial found no reduction in mortality or reinfarction among the non-Q wave group (158). By comparison, the Norwegian Timolol Trial showed prolonged survival in timolol treated patients regardless of infarct type; however, the incidence of reinfarction during long-term follow-up was reduced only in patients with Q wave MI (159). In light of these findings, the routine use of prophylactic beta-adrenergic blockade does not seem justified for all patients recovering from acute non-Q wave MI.

Effect of Calcium Channel Blockers

Currently, the Diltiazem Reinfarction Study (DRS) is the only study that has prospectively addressed the issue of secondary prevention after non-Q wave infarction (101,160). In this trial involving 576 patients, the cumulative incidence of reinfarction within 14 days of randomization was 12.9% in the placebo group and 6.1% in the diltiazem group ($p = 0.029$, Fig. 18–11). Diltiazem also reduced the frequency of refractory postinfarction angina by 49.7% ($p = 0.035$) and the incidence of angina associated with transient ST–T wave changes by 28% ($p = 0.005$). As diltiazem proved to be safe and well tolerated, the investigators recommended prophylactic diltiazem as a valuable addition to the early in-hospital management of cases of non-Q wave MI. This certainly seems reasonable, given the consistency of the reductions in the three prognostically important endpoints (reinfarction, angina refractory therapy, and angina-associated transient ECG changes) and the fact that treatment with other drugs (e.g., beta blocker, nifedipine and verapamil) is largely unproven in this subset of patients.

In 1988, the results of the Multicenter Diltiazem Postinfarction Trial (MDPIT) were published (161). This study, in contrast to the DRS, evaluated the long-term effect of diltiazem on mortality and reinfarction in a mixed clinical population of 2,466 patients with Q wave and non-Q wave MI. When the subset of 634 patients with non-Q wave MI were analyzed (post hoc), the cumulative 1-year cardiac event rate (death and/or nonfatal reinfarction) was found to be 14.8% in placebo treated patients and 8.4% in diltiazem treated patients (162). Thus MDPIT showed an overall 34% reduction among non-Q wave MI patients who received diltiazem ($p = 0.03$). Because the propensity for late reinfarction and death after an index non-Q wave MI is appreciable, the long-term results of the MDPIT subset analysis provide a convincing therapeutic rationale for recommending diltiazem as effective pharmacotherapy to prevent both early and late ischemic sequelae in these patients without congestive heart failure (Fig. 18–12) (152).

Other studies of calcium channel blockers cannot be directly compared with the DRS or the subset analysis of the MDPIT, as a prior distinction was not made between Q wave and non-Q wave MI (Table 18–5). When the results of these studies are reviewed, however, the published findings are generally disappointing (163). For example, none of the 13 trials of nifedipine, comprising a total of 9,990 patients, showed a salutary effect on mortality, reinfarction, or the incidence of early recurrent ischemia, and several studies actually suggest an increased risk of death or reinfarction among patients given nifedipine versus placebo. Only one of the six verapamil trials have reported (post hoc) a beneficial effect of treatment among patients with non-Q wave MI (164).

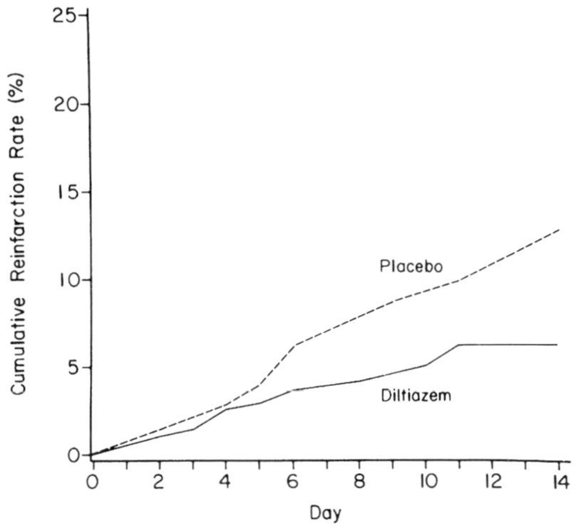

Figure 18–11. Cumulative life-table incidence of reinfarction according to treatment group assignment. At 14 days, the reinfarction rate was 51.2% lower in the diltiazem treated group. *Reprinted from Gibson (130), with permission.*

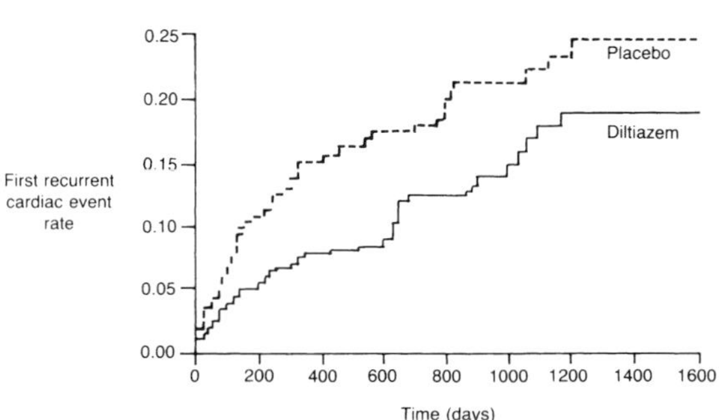

Figure 18–12.

Table 18–5. Clinical Trials of Calcium Channel Blockers in Patients with Threatened or Confirmed Acute Myocardial Infarction

Study	Total Number of Patients (% with MI)	Criteria for MI Diagnosis[a]	Trial Endpoint				
			Progression to Q Wave MI	Infarct Size	Mortality Rate	Reinfarction Rate	Angina Pectoris
Nifedipine							
NAMIS (1984)	171(84)	A	+	+	+	0	0
Norwegian (1984)	222(71)	A	0	+	+	0	0
Loogna et al (1985)	57(100)	B	0	+	0	0	0
Eisenberg et al (1985)	50(100)	A	0	0	0	+	+
TRENT (1986)	4,491(64)	B	0	0	+	+	0
SPRINT-1 (1986)	2,276(100)	C	0	0	+	+	+
HINT (1986)[b]	515(18)	B	+	0	0	+	+
Branagan et al (1986)	98(52)	A	+	+	+	0	0
Jaffe et al (1987)	22(100)	A	0	+	0	0	0
Gottlieb et al (1988)	22(100)	C	+	+	+	+	+
Walker et al (1988)	434(68)	A	+	+	+	+	0
Erbel et al (1988)[b]	149(100)	A	0	+	+	+	0
SPRINT-II (1988)	1,373(85)	C	0	0	+	+	0
Versapsmil							
Hansen et al (1980)[c]	61(100)	B	0	0	+	+	0
Thuesen et al (1983)	100(100)	B	0	+	0	0	0
Danish-I (1984)	1,436(100)	B	0	0	+	+	+
Bussmann et al (1984)[c]	54(100)	A	0	+	0	0	0
Crea et al (1985)[c]	15(100)	A	0	0	0	+	+
Danish-II (1990)[c]	1,775(100)	B	0	0	+	+	0
Diltiazem							
DRS (1986)	576(100)	A	0	0	+	+	+
Zannad et al (1988)	32(100)	A	0	+	0	0	0
MDPIT (1988)	2,466(100)	B	0	0	+	+	0

[a] A = New Q waves and/or diagnostic rise and fall of MB CK; B = Elevated enzymes required but diagnosis of MI not confirmed in all patients by MB CK levels; C = WHO "2 of 3" criteria (that is, chest pain, ECG changes, and elevated enzymes).

[b] Evaluated effect(s) of trial medication as adjunctive therapy in combination with beta blocker or streptokinase.

[c] Single-blind or open-label study.

Effect of Angiotensin Converting Enzyme Inhibitors

Preliminary data suggests that treatment with an angiotensin converting enzyme (ACE) inhibitor may be therapeutic when used in the chronic phase of non-Q wave infarction. In a recently published placebo-controlled trial, Søgarrd and colleagues showed a significant anti-ischemic effect of captopril on the duration of ambulatory ST segment depression during 180 days of treatment (165). Of interest, the anti-ischemic effect was independent of changes in ventricular volume, assessed by serial echocardiography. Based on earlier observations, it was postulated that the reduction in ambient ischemia was due to favorable effects on platelet function and/or vascular remodeling, a decrease in myocardial oxygen demand, or prevention of diastolic dysfunction (165–168). If these results can be confirmed by others and linked to improved prognosis, it may be appropriate to use ACE inhibitors more widely after non-Q wave MI.

Effect of Angioplasty on Clinical Outcome

Percutaneous transluminal coronary angioplasty (PTCA) has assumed an important role in the general treatment of acute MI (52). However, its routine use after MI, and in particular its role after non-Q wave MI, is still being evaluated. Use of PTCA after non-Q wave MI is fortified by the high rates of reinfarction and recurrent angina in these patients. Recent studies have shown that PTCA for angina after non-Q wave MI has a high initial success rate, a low incidence of subsequent death or infarction, and may improve regional myocardial dysfunction (Table 18–6) (169–170). Although these findings are encouraging, caution should be exercised before touting PTCA as an effective treatment strategy for abolishing ischemia, preventing reinfarction, and prolonging life in the first several years after non-Q wave MI. The reasons for this include the following.

1. All of the studies listed in Table 18–6 are observational in nature, and lack a randomized control group.
2. The study cohorts appear to be heavily biased toward a relatively young population of patients with first infarcts, well-preserved left ventricular function, and single-vessel disease—i.e., patients who in general have a relatively good prognosis (111,119,177).
3. The results apply only to a very specific anatomic subset of patients—i.e., patients with discrete lesions of the infarct-related artery "amenable to PTCA."
4. The indications for PTCA were highly variable, and many of the patients included in the studies did not have angina at rest associated with transient ECG changes and/or repetitive episodes of angina resistant to medical therapy.
5. No attempt was made to quantitate the amount of residual ischemia after PTCA; for example, none of the studies employed stress-redistribution thallium-201 scintigraphy in the follow-up assessment.
6. The clinical restenosis rate and need for subsequent interventions (repeat PTCA or bypass surgery) was uniformly high in each of the seven studies.
7. In most of the studies, PTCA was performed relatively late after onset of non-Q wave infarction, thus hindering assessment of the safety of performing angioplasty in immediate postinfarction period.

Given these limitations and the enormous gaps that they create in our knowledge, it seems prudent to conclude that we lack definitive data on the safety and efficacy of PTCA, especially in patients with multivessel disease and/or reduced left ventricular function.

Table 18–6. Results of PTCA in Patients with Angina After Non-Q Wave Infarction

			Outcome Data (%)[a]				
Study (year)	Total No. (% with NQMI)	% Success	Death	MI	AP	Repeat PTCA	CABG
Defeyter (1986) (169)	53(66)	89	1(2)	6(11)	13(28)	3(6)	10(4)
Safian (1987) (170)	68(100)	87	1(1)	3(4)	24(41)	17(25)	5(7)
Gottlieb (1987) (171)	47(70)	91	1(2)	3(6)	17(40)	6(13)	3(6)
Holt (1988) (172)	70(54)	80	2(3)	5(7)	15(27)	7(10)	16(23)
Suryapranta (1988) (173)	114(100)	86	0(0)	11(10)	31(32)	18(16)	19(17)
Bellamy (1989) (174)	52(100)	100	0(0)	3(6)	13(25)	9(17)	4(8)
Alfonso (1990) (175)	33(100)	91	0(0)	0(0)	10(30)	5(15)	0(0)
Pooled Data	437(85)	**91%**	**1.1%**	**7.1%**	**28%**	**15%**	**13%**

[a] Data represents number of patients with an event (inclusive of procedure-related events) during average follow-up of 18 months (range 6 to 27 months). AP = angina recurrence rate in patients with initially successful PTCA.

Safety and Efficacy of Predischarge Bypass Graft Surgery

As previously discussed, the prognosis of patients with early recurrent ischemia defined as rest angina associated either with ECG changes or as repetitive episodes refractory to medical therapy, is very poor (56, 97, 101, 102, 178). Because most studies show that 80–90% of these patients have severe multivessel CAD and 10–20% have left mainstem stenosis (58, 179–190), it has been suggested that complete surgical revascularization, rather than PTCA of the presumed culprit lesion, may be the best long-term therapeutic intervention for these patients (191). Unfortunately, at the present time, there are no prospective data from randomized clinical trials that clearly favor one approach over the other (192,193). Nevertheless, it is noteworthy that a relatively large experience from 10 different institutions (Table 18–7) indicates that early surgery for unstable postinfarction angina is highly effective in relieving ischemic symptoms and can be accomplished with a remarkably low operative mortality (e.g., <2% among patients with non-Q wave MI). Published reports have also shown a favorable effect on left ventricular function and excellent long-term outlook with respect to survival without reinfarction (180–190).

Compared with the published experience with single-vessel PTCA, the literature on CABG surgery offers more compelling evidence, albeit indirect, that revascularization may improve the prognosis of patients with recurrent angina after non-Q wave infarction. This is because the surgical experience has focused on high-risk patients with significant ongoing ischemia and severe multivessel CAD. Thus, although data from controlled clinical trials that compare alternative treatments are not available, the results with CABG surgery appear to be superior to results observed with noninterventional treatment for similar patients with unstable postinfarction angina.

Value of Routine Early Cardiac Catheterization

In many hospitals, it has become standard practice to perform predischarge coronary arteriography in patients convalescing from uncomplicated acute myocardial infarction (194). The rationale for routine catheterization is that (i) it provides detailed information about the coronary anatomy responsible for the infarction, the location and extent of atherosclerotic disease, the extent of left ventricular dysfunction, and the presence and severity of coexisting cardiac disorders such as valvular or congenital lesions; (ii) it offers the potential to prevent

Table 18–7. Results of Coronary Artery Bypass Graft Surgery in Postinfarction Patients with Early Recurrent Ischemia[a]

		Extent of CAD			Mortality %		Reinfarction %		Recurrent
Study (year)	Total No. of Patients (% with NQMI)	2–3VD	Grafts/ Patients	Follow-up (Months)	Early	Late	Early	Late	Angina[a] (%)
Madigan (1977) (180)	28(100)	64	2.1	16	3.6	0	10.7	0	24
Jones (1981) (181)	116(28)	72	2.6	14	0	4.3	5.0	—	29
Roberts (1983) (182)	20(60)	100	2.8	12	0	0	15.0	—	—
Nunley (1983) (183)	80(39)	83	2.2	35	5.0	9.0	2.5	—	—
Williams (1983) (184)	103(82)	91	3.1	15	1.9	0	1.0	—	4
Breyer (1985) (185)	75(61)	97	3.1	13	8.0[a]	0	—	—	17
Singh (1985) (186)	108(45)	96	2.7	35	1.8	7.5	4.6	3.8	27
Kouchoukos (1985) (187)	240(93)	96	4.0	—	3.3	—	3.3	—	—
Gardner (1989) (188)	300(46)	—	3.5	23	5.0[a]	5.5	—	—	—
Kennedy (1989) (189)	793(63)	—	3.5		5.7[a]			—	—
Sintek (1994) (190)	530(38)	—	2.9	1	1.7[a]	—	1.9	—	—
Pooled Data	2393(54)	**90**	**3.0**	**18**	**3.3**	**4.4**	**3.5**	**3.1**	**20**

[a]Operative early (or 30-day) mortality was lower in patients with non-Q wave MI.

reinfarction and premature death by identifying for subsequent mechanical revascularization subsets of patients with "high-risk" coronary anatomy, such as those with left main-stem or three-vessel CAD, or large zones of viable myocardium jeopardized by critically narrowed coronary arteries; (iii) the knowledge of coronary anatomy may allow more prompt institution of appropriately tailored therapy, and a shortened hospitalization and subsequent convalescence; and (iv) it may prevent new admissions and reduce health care costs.

When considering the issue of predischarge coronary arteriography, the primary care physician should keep in mind several important points:

1. Coronary arteriography does not directly benefit patient outcome, and its value as a diagnostic test derives from its ability to estimate risk for future cardiac events in order to select the most appropriate long-term management strategy.
2. The pathophysiological basis that accounts for the greater clinical instability after non-Q wave infarction is related to the amount of hypoperfused but viable myocardium that remains at risk for recurrent ischemia and infarction.
3. Careful clinical assessment and exercise stress testing techniques, particularly myocardial perfusion scintigraphy, can identify most patients with prognostically important residual ischemia.
4. In asymptomatic patients recovering from an uncomplicated acute MI, the absence of an ischemic result on predischarge exercise radionuclide imaging is predictive of an excellent 1-year prognosis (34,195–197). Moreover, Ellis et al have observed that medical management of these patients is probably superior to prophylactic PTCA (197).
5. Coronary arteriography, when used alone to determine the need for myocardial revascularization, has several important limitations (most notably, the risk that routine catheterization may lead to many unnecessary, and potentially harmful, revascularization procedures).
6. Patients with non-Q wave MI constitute a highly heterogeneous group. Although some will have what is termed an "incomplete infarction" and exhibit residual preinfarction ischemia, others will not. These latter patients, who constitute between 30% and 50% of the total population, have a very low nonfatal cardiac event rate during the subsequent year, with a mortality rate of only 1–2%.

Should all patients with non-Q wave MI undergo coronary arteriography for risk stratification? Presently, there is no evidence that routine, as compared with selective, catheterization is of any benefit when applied without evidence of exercise-induced or spontaneous ischemia. Data from 10 studies indicate that a conservative approach, with catheterization reserved for selected patients at increased risk, is as effective in reducing subsequent acute cardiac events as is a routine catheterization approach (197–204). On the basis of available data concerning the indication for and the timing of coronary arteriography after non-Q wave MI, the inevitable conclusion is that conservative instead of aggressive management is appropriate for the 30–50% of patients at low risk who do not have spontaneous myocardial ischemia or myocardial ischemia provoked during predischarge exercise testing.

RECOMMENDATIONS

On the basis of our current understanding and the available data, the following guidelines for the management of non-Q wave infarction can be recommended: (i) combination antithrombotic therapy with heparin and aspirin, along with diltiazem, should be administered to all patients with non-Q wave MI, unless contraindications exist; (ii) patients with early recurrent ischemia—i.e., angina with associated ECG changes or persistent angina despite maximal medical therapy—should undergo prompt cardiac catheterization and myocardial revascularization; and (iii) patients with entirely uncomplicated hospital courses who are asymptomatic should undergo exercise stress testing, preferably in conjunction with stress-redistribution thallium-201 scintigraphy, before hospital discharge. Only those with evidence of significant residual ischemia need cardiac catheterization and myocardial revascularization.

CONCLUDING REMARKS

From this review, it should be readily apparent that the current ECG classification scheme for acute myocardial infarction represents a meaningful clinical and prognostic distinction. Non-Q wave MI differs from Q wave MI in three important respects: (i) smaller infarct size, which possibly is due to early reperfusion as a result of spontaneous thrombolysis, relief of spasm, or both; (ii) more frequent patency of the infarct-related artery; and (iii) a larger residual mass of viable but jeopardized myocardium within the perfusion zone of the infarct-related vessel. Left ventricular function, unless impaired by previous MI, is generally better. The prognosis is worse after the acute phase, when residual ischemia is present, and reinfarction rates during hospitalization and in the subsequent year of follow-up are higher. Obviously, as myocardial ischemia is potentially reversible, its presence should be energetically sought in all patients with recognized non-Q wave MI.

Non-Q wave MI should be considered an unstable ischemic syndrome. If significant residual ischemia is documented either clinically or by exercise stress testing techniques, coronary arteriography should be performed before hospital discharge in search of significant atherosclerotic lesions that might be amenable to PTCA or coronary artery bypass graft surgery.

REFERENCES

1. Spodick DH: Q wave infarction versus S–T infarction: Nonspecificity of electrocardiographic criteria for differentiating transmural and nontransmural lesions. *Am J Cardiol* 1983;51:913–915.
2. Phibbs B: Transmural versus subendocardial myocardial infarction: An electrocardiographic myth. *J Am Coll Cardiol* 1984;1:561–564.
3. Cook RW, Edwards JE, Pruitt RD: Electrocardiographic changes in acute subendocardial infarction: I, Large subendocardial and large nontransmural infarcts. *Circulation* 1958;18:603–611.
4. Cook RW, Edwards JE, Pruitt RD: Electrocardiographic changes in acute subendocardial infarction: II, Small subendocardial infarcts. *Circulation* 1958;18:613–622.
5. Durrer D, Vanlier AAW, Buller J: Epicardial and intramural excitation in chronic myocardial infarction. *Am Heart J* 1964;68:765–775.
6. Savage RM, Wagner GS, Ideker RE, et al: Correlation of postmortem anatomic findings with electrocardiographic changes in patients with myocardial infarction. *Circulation* 1977;55:279–285.
7. Raunio H, Rissanen V, Romppanen T, et al: Changes in the QRS complex and ST segment in transmural and subendocardial myocardial infarction: A clinicopathologic study. *Am Heart J* 1979;98:176–184.
8. Freifeld AG, Schuster EH, Bulkley BH: Nontransmural versus transmural myocardial infarction: A morphologic study. *Am J Med* 1983;75:423–432.
9. Mirvis DM, Ingram L, Holly MK, et al: Electrocardiographic effects of experimental nontransmural myocardial infarction. *Circulation* 1985;71:1206–1214.
10. Antaloczy Z, Barcsak J, Magyar E: Correlation of electrocardiologic and pathologic findings in 100 cases of Q wave and non-Q wave myocardial infarction. *J Electrocardiol* 1988;21:331–335.
11. Gibson RS: Non-Q wave myocardial infarction: Diagnosis, prognosis and management. *Curr Probl Cardiol* 1988;13:9–72.
12. Peel AA, Semple T, Wang I, et al: A coronary prognostic index for grading the severity of infarction. *Br Heart J* 1962;24:745–755.
13. Lown B, Vassaux C, Hood WB, et al: Unresolved problems in coronary care. *Am J Med* 1967;20:494–508.
14. Norris RM, Brandt PWT, Caughey DE, et al: A new coronary prognostic index. *Lancet* 1969;1:274–278.
15. Venkatachalapathy D, Kuhn L, Waxman H: Clinical features, early and later prognosis of acute subendocardial infarction: Comparison with transmural infarction. *Circulation* 1973;48(Suppl IV):IV-226.
16. Scheinman MM, Abbott JA: Clinical significance of transmural versus nontransmural electrocardiographic changes in patients with acute myocardial infarction. *Am J Med* 1973;55:602–607.
17. Madias JE, Chahine RA, Gorlin A, et al: A comparison of transmural and nontransmural acute myocardial infarction. *Circulation* 1974;49:498–507.

18. Schor S, Shani M, Modan B: Factors affecting immediate mortality of patients with acute myocardial infarction: A nationwide study. *Chest* 1975;68: 217–221.
19. Strauss H, Sobel BE, Roberts R: Acute and long-term prognosis in patients with transmural versus subendocardial infarction. *Circulation* 1978;58 (Suppl II):II-193.
20. Schroter H, Schulte KL, Beck OA, et al: Transmuraler und nichttransmuraler myokardinfarkt. *Herz* 1978;3:185–190.
21. Connolly DC, Elveback LR: Comparison of hospital and post-hospital course of patients with transmural and subendocardial myocardial infarction. *Am J Cardiol* 1979;43:370.
22. Ahmed SS, Brancato RR: Transmural versus nontransmural myocardial infarction: Influence of location on clinical features and mortality. *Angiology* 1979;30:240–248.
23. Thanavaro S, Krone RJ, Kleiger RE, et al: In-hospital prognosis of patients with first nontransmural and transmural infarction. *Circulation* 1980; 61:29–33.
24. Ogawa H, Hiramori K, Haze K, et al: Comparison of clinical features of non-Q wave and Q wave myocardial infarction. *Am Heart J* 1986;11:513–518.
25. L'Abbate A, Carpeggiani C, Testa R, et al: In-hospital myocardial infarction: Preinfarction features and their correlation with short-term prognosis. *Eur Heart J* 1986;7(Suppl A):53-61.
26. Bourke S, Conroy RM, Mulcahy R, Robinson K: Etiological and prognostic correlates of site of myocardial infarction. *Eur Heart J* 1988;9:734–739.
27. Fesmire FM, Percy RF, Wears RL, MacMath TL: Initial ECG in Q wave and non-Q wave myocardial infarction. *Ann Emerg Med* 1989;18:741–746.
28. Norris RM, Caughey DE, Deeming LW, et al: Coronary prognostic index for predicting survival after recovery from acute myocardial infarction. *Lancet* 1970;1:485–488.
29. Norris RM, Caughey DE, Mercer CJ, et al: Prognosis after myocardial infarction: Six year follow-up. *Br Heart J* 1974;36:786–790.
30. Fabricius-Bjerre N, Munkvad M, Knudsen JB: Subendocardial and transmural myocardial infarction: A five year survival study. *Am J Med* 1979;66:986–990.
31. Pohjola A, Siltanen P, Romo M: Five year survival of 728 patients after myocardial infarction: A community study. *Br Heart J* 1980;43:176–183.
32. Lekakis J, Katsoyanni K, Trichopoulos D, et al: Q wave versus non-Q wave myocardial infarction: Clinical characteristics and 6 month prognosis. *Clin Cardiol* 1984;7:283–288.
33. Krone RJ, Friedman E, Thanavaro S, et al: Long-term prognosis after first Q wave (transmural) or non-Q wave (nontransmural) myocardial infarction: Analysis of 583 patients. *Am J Cardiol* 1983; 52:234–239.
34. Gibson RS, Beller GA, Gheorghiade M, et al: The prevalence and clinical significance of residual myocardial ischemia two weeks after uncomplicated non-Q wave infarction: A prospective natural history study. *Circulation* 1986;73:1186–1198.
35. Theroux P, Kouz S, Bosch X, et al: Clinical and angiographic features of non-Q wave and Q wave myocardial infarction. *Circulation* 1986;74:303.
36. Smeets JP, Legrand V, Rigo P, et al: Subendocardial myocardial infarction: A follow-up study of 55 cases. *Eur Heart J* 1981;2:57–63.
37. Rigo P, Murray M, Taylor DR, et al: Hemodynamic and prognostic findings in patients with transmural and nontransmural infarction. *Circulation* 1975;51:1064–1070.
38. Cannom D, Levy W, Cohen L: The short- and long-term prognosis of patients with transmural and nontransmural infarction. *Am J Med* 1976;61: 452–458.
39. Szklo M, Goldberg R, Kennedy HL, et al: Survival of patients with nontransmural myocardial infarction: A population based study. *Am J Cardiol* 1978;42:648–652.
40. Boxall J, Saltups A: A comparison of nontransmural and transmural myocardial infarction. *Aust NZ J Med* 1980;10:176–179.
41. Mahony C, Hindman MC, Aronin N, et al: Prognostic differences in subgroups of patients with electrocardiographic evidence of subendocardial or transmural myocardial infarction: The favorable outlook for patients with an initially normal QRS complex. *Am J Med* 1980;69:183–186.
42. Hutter AM, DeSanctis RW, Flynn T, et al: Nontransmural myocardial infarction: A comparison of hospital and late clinical course of patients with that of matched patients with transmural anterior and transmural inferior myocardial infarction. *Am J Cardiol* 1981;48:595–602.
43. Marmor A, Sobel BE, Roberts R: Factors presaging early recurrent myocardial infarction (extension). *Am J Cardiol* 1981;48:603–610.

44. Bayley N, Hunt D, Penington C, et al: Subendocardial myocardial infarction. *Aust NZ J Med* 1982;12:166–169.

45. Marmor A, Geltman EM, Schechtman K, et al: Recurrent myocardial infarction: Clinical predictors and prognostic implications. *Circulation* 1982; 66:415–421.

46. Coll S, Castaner A, Sanz G, et al: Prevalence and prognosis after first nontransmural myocardial infarction. *Am J Cardiol* 1983;51:1584–1588.

47. Maisel AS, Ahnve S, Gilpin E, et al: Prognosis after extension of myocardial infarction: The role of Q wave or non-Q wave infarction. *Circulation* 1985;71:211–217.

48. Zema MJ: Q wave, ST segment and T wave myocardial infarction: Useful clinical distinction. *Am J Med* 1985;78:391–398.

49. VanRensburg CJ, Przybojewski JZ, Soolman J: Clinical characteristics of and prognosis in acute transmural anterior, transmural inferior and nontransmural myocardial: A comparative retrospective study. *S Afr Med J* 1985;67:487–495.

50. Connolly DC, Elveback LR: Coronary heart disease in residents of Rochester, Minnesota: Hospital and post-hospital course of patients with transmural and subendocardial myocardial infarction. *Mayo Clin Proc* 1985;60:375–381.

51. Herlitz J, Hjalmarson A, Bengtsson A, Sillfors L: Long-term prognosis in relation to ECG findings in acute myocardial infarction. *Cardiologica* 1987; 42:79–89.

52. Goldberg RJ, Gore JM, Alpert JS, et al: Non-Q wave myocardial infarction: Recent changes in occurrence and prognosis—a community wide perspective. *Am Heart J* 1987;113:273–279.

53. Nicod P, Gilpin E, DiHrich H, et al: Short- and long-term clinical outcome after Q wave and non-Q wave myocardial infarction in a large patient population. *Circulation* 1989;79:528–536.

54. Stone PH, Raabe DS, Jaffe AS, et al: Prognostic significance of location and type of myocardial infarction: Independent adverse outcome associated with anterior location. *J Am Coll Cardiol* 1988;11:453–463.

55. McQuay NW, Edwards JE, Burchell HB: Types of death in acute myocardial infarction. *Arch Intern Med* 1955;96:1–10.

56. Bosch X, Theroux P, Waters DD, et al: Early postinfarction ischemia: Clinical, angiographic and prognostic significance. *Circulation* 1987;75:988–995.

57. Geltman EM, Biello D, Welch MJ, et al: Characterization of nontransmural myocardial infarction by positron: Emission tomography. *Circulation* 1982;65:747–755.

58. Hashimoto T, Kambara H, Fudo T, et al: Non-Q wave versus Q wave myocardial infarction: Regional myocardial metabolism and blood flow assessed by positron emission tomography. *J Am Coll Cardiol* 1988;12:88–93.

59. DeWood MA, Stifter WF, Simpson CS, et al: Coronary arteriographic findings soon after non Q wave myocardial infarction. *N Engl J Med* 1986; 315:417–423.

60. Ambrose JA, Hjemdahl-Monsen CE, Borrico S, et al: Angiographic demonstration of a common link between unstable angina pectoris and non-Q wave acute myocardial infarction. *Am J Cardiol* 1986;61:244–247.

61. Gibson RS: Clinical, functional and angiographic distinctions between Q wave and non-Q wave myocardial infarction: Evidence of spontaneous reperfusion and implications for intervention trials. *Circulation* 1987;75(Suppl V):V-128–V138.

62. Hucy BL, Ghcorghiadc M, Crampton RS, et al: Acute non-Q wave myocardial infarction associated with early ST segment elevation: Evidence for spontaneous reperfusion and implications for thrombolytic trials. *J Am Coll Cardiol* 1987;9:18–25.

63. Bissett JK, Matts J, Sharma B, et al: Residual myocardial jeopardy in patients with Q wave and non-Q wave infarctions. *Br Hart J* 1987;58:460–464.

64. Schechtman KB, Capone RJ, Kleiger RE, et al: Risk stratification of patients with non-Q wave myocardial infarction: The critical role of ST segment depression. *Circulation* 1989;80:1148–1158.

65. Brunken R, Tillisch J, Schwaiger M, et al. Regional perfusion, glucose metabolism, and wallmotion in patients with chronic electrocardiographic Q wave infarction: Evidence for persistence of viable tissue in some infarct regions by positron emission tomography. *Circulation* 1986;73:951–963.

66. Conti CR, Hill JA, Mayfield WR: Unstable angina pectoris: Pathogenesis and management. *Curr Probl Cardiol* 1989;14:551–623.

67. Schaer DH, Ross AM, Wasserman AG: Reinfarction, recurrent angina and reocclusion after thrombolytic therapy. *Circulation* 1987;76(Suppl II):II-57–II-62.

68. Reimer KA, Lowe JE, Rasmussen MM, Jennings AB: The wave front phenomenon of ischemic cell

death: Myocardial infarct size versus duration of coronary occlusion in dogs. *Circulation* 1977;56: 786–794.

69. Brush JE, Brand DA, Acamporci D, et al: Use of the initial electrocardiogram to predict in-hospital complications of acute myocardial infarction. *N Engl J Med* 1985;312:1137–1141.
70. Slater DK, Hlatky MA, Mark DB, et al: Outcome in suspected acute myocardial infarction with normal or minimally abnormal admission electrocardiographic findings. *Am J Cardiol* 1987; 60:766–770.
71. Boden WE, Kleiger RE, Gibson RS, et al: Favourable long term prognosis in patients with non-Q wave acute myocardial infarction not associated with specific electrocardiographic changes. *Br Heart J* 1989;61:396–402.
72. Abbott JA, Scheinman MM: Nondiagnostic electrocardiogram in patients with acute myocardial infarction: Clinical and anatomic correlations. *Am J Med* 1973;55:608–613.
73. Poehlman JH, Silverman ME: Clinical characteristics, electrocardiographic and enzyme correlations, and long-term prognosis of patients with chest pain associated with ST depression or T wave inversion. *Am Heart J* 1980;99:173–180.
74. Hollander G, Ozick H, Greengart A, et al: High mortality early reinfarction with first nontransmural myocardial infarction. *Am Heart J* 1984; 108:1412–1416.
75. Verat MA: Nontransmural infarction: Clinical distinction between patients with ST depression and those with T wave inversion. *J Electrocardiol* 1985;18:15–20.
76. Ogawa H, Hiramori K, Haze K, et al: Classification of non-Q wave myocardial infarction according to electrocardiographic changes. *Br Heart J* 1985;54:473–478.
77. Willich SN, Stone PH, Muller JE, et al: High-risk subgroups of patients with non-Q wave myocardial infarction based on direction and severity of ST segment deviation. *Am Heart J* 1987;114: 1110–1119.
78. Herlitz J, Hjalmarson A: Appearance of T wave inversions without raised serum enzyme activity in suspected acute myocardial infarction: Clinical outcome in relation to subendocardial infarction. *Clin Cardiol* 1986;9:209–214.
79. The Coronary Drug Project Research Group: The prognostic importance of the electrocardiogram after myocardial infarction. *Ann Intern Med* 1972;77:672–680.
80. Siltanen P, Pohjola-Sintonen S, Haapakoski J, et al: The mortality predictive power of discharge electrocardiogram after first acute myocardial infarction. *Am Heart J* 1985;109:1231–1237.
81. Schechtman KB, Capone RJ, Kleiger RE, et al: Differential risk patterns associated with three-month as compared to three to 12 month mortality and reinfarction following non-Q wave myocardial infarction. *J Am Coll Cardiol* 1990;15:940–948.
82. Stone PH, Raabe DS, Jaffe AS, et al: Prognostic significance of location and type of myocardial infarction: Independent adverse outcome associated with anterior location. *J Am Coll Cardiol* 1988;11:453–463.
83. Kao W, Khaja F, Goldstein S, Gheorghiade M: Cardiac event rate after non-Q wave acute myocardial infarction and the significance of its anterior location. *Am J Cardiol* 1989;64:1236–1242.
84. Boden WE, Bough EW, Benham I, Shulman RS: Unstable angina with episodic ST segment elevation and minimal creatinine kinase release culminating in extensive, recurrent infarction. *J Am Coll Cardiol* 1983;2:11–20.
85. Hands ME, Lloyd BL, Robinson JS, et al: Prognostic significance of electrocardiographic site of infarction after correction for enzymatic size of infarction. *Circulation* 1986;73:885–891.
86. Kannel WB, Dawber TR, Kaga A, et al: Factors of risk in the development of coronary heart disease—six year follow-up experience: The Framingham Study. *Ann Intern Med* 1961;55:33–50.
87. Kannel WB, Gordon T, Offutt D: Left ventricular hypertrophy by electrocardiogram: Prevalence, incidence, and mortality in the Framingham Study. *Ann Intern Med* 1969;71:89–105.
88. Kannel WB, Gordon T, Castelli WP, Margolis JR: Electrocardiographic left ventricular hypertrophy and risk of coronary artery disease: The Framingham Study. *Ann Intern Med* 1970;72:813–822.
89. Coronary Drug Project Research Group: Left ventricular hypertrophy patterns and prognosis. *Circulation* 1974;49:862–871.
90. Borhani NO, Blaufox D, Oberman A, et al: Incidence of coronary heart disease and left ventricular hypertrophy in the HDFP. *Prog Cardiovasc Dis* 1986;29:55–62.
91. Casale PN, Devereux RB, Milner M, et al: Value of echocardiographic measurement of left ven-

tricular mass in predicting cardiovascular morbid events in hypertensive men. *Ann Intern Med* 1986; 105:173–178.

92. Levy P, Anderson KM, Savage DD, et al: Echocardiographically detected left ventricular hypertrophy: Prevalence and risk factors: The Framingham Heart Study. *Ann Intern Med* 1988; 108:7–13.

93. MacMahon S, Collins G, Rautaharju P, et al: Electrocardiographic left ventricular hypertrophy and effects of antihypertensive drug therapy in hypertensive participants in the Multiple Risk Factor Intervention Trial. *Am J Cardiol* 1989;63: 202–210.

94. Boden WE, Kleiger RE, Schechtman KB, et al and the Diltiazem Reinfarction Study Research Group: Clinical significance and prognostic importance of left ventricular hypertrophy in non-Q wave acute myocardial infarction. *Am J Cardiol* 1988;62:1000–1004.

95. Chaturvedi NC, Walsh MJ, Evans A, et al: Selection of patients for early discharge after acute myocardial infarction. *Br Heart J* 1974;36:533–535.

96. Lofmark R: T wave changes and postinfarction angina pectoris is predictive of recurrent myocardial infarction. *Br Heart J* 1981;45:512–516.

97. Schuster EH, Bulkley BH: Early postinfarction angina: Ischemia at a distance and ischemia in the infarct zone. *N Engl J Med* 1981;205:1101–1105.

98. Figueras J, Cinca J, Valle V: Prognostic implications of early spontaneous angina after acute transmural myocardial infarction. *Int J Cardiol* 1983;4:264–272.

99. Sellier P, Plat F, Corona P, et al: Prognostic significance of angina pectoris recurring soon after myocardial infarction. *Eur Heart J* 1988;9:447–452.

100. Bosch X, Theroux P, Waters DD, et al: Early postinfarction ischemia: Clinical, angiographic and prognostic significance. *Circulation* 1987;75: 988–995.

101. Gibson RS, Young PM, Boden WE, et al: Prognostic significance and beneficial effect of diltiazem on the incidence of early recurrent ischemia after non-Q wave myocardial infarction: Results from the multicenter Diltiazem Reinfarction Study. *Am J Cardiol* 1987;60:203–209.

102. Boden WE, Gibson RS, Kleiger RE, et al: Importance of early recurrent ischemia on one-year survival after non-Q wave myocardial infarction. *Am J Cardiol* 1989;64:799–801.

103. Krone RJ, Dwyer EM, Greenberg H, et al: Risk stratification in patients with first non-Q wave infarction: Limited value of the early low level exercise test after uncomplicated infarcts. *J Am Coll Cardiol* 1989;14:31–37.

104. Levy WS, Katz RJ, Ross AM: Limited prognostic value of submaximal exercise testing following non-Q wave MI. *Circulation* 1987;76(Suppl IV): IV-170.

105. Varma SK, Gibson RS: Predischarge exercise ECG versus thallium-201 scintigraphy in predicting prognosis after non-Q wave infarction. *Circulation* 1987;76(Suppl IV):IV-157.

106. Gibson RS: A comparative analysis of the diagnostic and prognostic value of exercise ECG and thallium-201 scintigraphic markers of myocardial ischemia in asymptomatic and symptomatic patients. *Cardiol Clin* 1989;7(3):565–575.

107. Gibson RS, Beller GA, Kaiser DL: Prevalence and clinical significance of painless ST segment depression during early postinfarction exercise testing. *Circulation* 1987;75(Suppl II):II-36–II-39.

108. Gibson RS: The role of predischarge thallium-201 imaging in risk stratification of patients recovering from acute myocardial infarction. *Circulation* 1990 (in press).

109. Gibson RS: The prognostic value of predischarge exercise thallium 201 scintigraphy after acute myocardial infarction. *J Cardiovasc Rehab* 1985;5:28–39.

110. Gibson RS, Watson DD, Craddock GB, et al: Prediction of cardiac events after uncomplicated myocardial infarction: A prospective study comparing predischarge exercise thallium 201 scintigraphy and coronary angiography. *Circulation* 1983;68: 321–336.

111. Wilison WW, Gibson RS, Nygaard TW, et al. Acute myocardial infarction associated with single vessel coronary artery disease: An analysis of clinical outcome and the prognostic importance of vessel patency and residual ischemic myocardium. *J Am Coll Cardiol* 1988;11:223–234.

112. Reed DC, Kaiser DL, Gibson RS: The prognostic significance of left anterior descending disease in asymptomatic patients after acute uncomplicated inferior myocardial infarction. *J Am Coll Cardiol* 1988;11(Suppl 2):194.

113. Brown KA, Boucher CA, Okada RD, et al: Prognostic value of exercise thallium-201 imaging in patients presenting for evaluation of chest pain. *J Am Coll Cardiol* 1983;1:994–1001.

114. Ladenheim ML, Pollock BH, Rozanski A, et al: Extent and severity of myocardial hypoperfusion as predictors of prognosis in patients with suspected coronary artery disease. *J Am Coll Cardiol* 1986;7:464–471.

115. Gibson RS, Watson DD, Carabello BA, et al: Clinical implications of increased lung uptake of thallium-201 during exercise scintigraphy 2 weeks after myocardial infarction. *Am J Cardiol* 1982;49: 1586–1593.

116. Gill JB, Ruddy TD, Newell JB, et al: Prognostic importance of thallium uptake by the lungs during exercise in coronary artery disease. *N Engl J Med* 1987;317:1485–1489.

117. Weiss AT, Berman DS, Lew AS, et al: Transient ischemic dilation of the left ventricle on stress thallium-201 scintigraphy: A marker of severe and extensive coronary artery disease. *J Am Coll Cardiol* 1987;9:752–759.

118. Taylor GJ, Humphries JO, Mellits ED, et al: Predictors of clinical course, coronary anatomy, and left ventricular function after recovery from acute myocardial infarction. *Circulation* 1980:62:960–970.

119. Roubin GS, Harris PJ, Bernstein L, Kelly DT: Coronary anatomy and prognosis after myocardial infarction in patients 60 years of age and younger. *Circulation* 1983;67:743–749.

120. Varma SK, Gibson RS: Prognostic significance of multivessel disease after non-Q wave infarction *Circulation* 1987;76(Suppl IV):IV-170.

121. Rees JR, Redding VJ: Anastomotic blood flow in experimental myocardial infarction: A new method using ^{133}Xenon clearance for repeated measurements during recovery. *Circ Res* 1971;28: 671–679.

122. Schaper W, Wusten B, Flameng W, et al: Local dilatory reserve in chronic experimental coronary occlusion without infarction: Quantitation of collateral development. *Basic Res Cardiol* 1975;70: 159–173.

123. The Risk Group: Risk of myocardial infarction and death during treatment with low dose aspirin and intravenous heparin in men with unstable coronary artery disease. *Lancet* 1990;336:827–830.

124. Wallentin S: Aspirin (75 mg/day) after an episode of unstable coronary artery disease: Long term effects on the risk for myocardial infarction occurrence of severe angina and the need for revascularization. *J Am Coll Cardiol* 1991;18:1587–1593.

125. Theroux P, Ouimet H, McCans J, et al: Aspirin, heparin, or both to treat unstable angina. *N Engl J Med* 1988;319:1105–1111.

126. Lewis HD, Hjemdahl-Monsen CE, Cairns J, et al: Role of antithrombotic therapy in unstable angina, myocardial infarction and sudden death. *N Engl J Med* 1983;309:396–403.

127. Cairns JA, Gent M, Singer J, et al: Aspirin, sulfinpyrazone, or both in unstable angina: Results of a Canadian multicenter trial. *N Engl J Med* 1985; 313:1369–1375.

128. Balsano F, Rizzon P, Violi F, et al: Antiplatelet treatment with ticlopidine in unstable angina. A controlled multicenter clinic trial. *Circulation* 1990; 82:17–26.

129. Klint CR, Knatterud GI, Stamler J, et al: Persantine–aspirin reinfarction study: II, Secondary coronary prevention with persantine and aspirin. *J Am Coll Cardiol* 1986;7:251–259.

130. Ambrose JA, Hjemdahl-Monsen CE, Borrico S, et al: Angiographic demonstration of a common link between unstable angina pectoris and non-Q wave acute myocardial infarction. *Am J Cardiol* 1988;61:244–247.

131. Fuster V, Badiman L, Badiman JJ, et al: The pathogenesis of coronary artery disease and the acute coronary syndromes. *N Engl J Med* 1992; 326:242–250, 310–318.

132. SCATI Group: Randomised controlled trial of subcutaneous calcium-heparin in acute myocardial infarction. *Lancet* 1989;2:182–186.

133. Mahan EF, Chandler JW, Rogers WJ, et al: Heparin and infarct coronary artery patency after streptokinase in acute myocardial infarction. *Am J Cardiol* 1990;65:967–972.

134. Bleich SD, Nichols TC, Schumacher RR, et al: Effect of heparin on coronary arterial patency after thrombolysis with tissue plasminogen activator in acute myocardial infarction. *Am J Cardiol* 1990;66:1412–1417.

135. Hsia J, Hamilton WP, Kleiman N, et al: A comparison between heparin and low-dose aspirin as adjunctive therapy with tissue plasminogen activator for acute myocardial infarction. *N Engl J Med* 1990;323:1433–1437.

136. Cohen M, Adams PC, Parry G, et al: Combination antithrombotic therapy in unstable rest angina and non-Q wave infarction in nonprior aspirin users: Primary endpoint analysis from the ATACS trial. *Circulation* 1994;89:81–88.

137. Cohen M, Parry G, Adams PC, et al: Prospective evaluation of a prostacyclin-sparing aspirin formulation and heparin/warfarin in aspirin users with unstable angina or non-Q wave myocardial infarction at rest. The Antithrombotic Therapy in Acute Coronary Syndromes Research Group. *Eur Heart J* 1994;15:1196–1203.

138. Gruppo Italiano per lo Studio della Streptochinasi nell' Infarto Miocardico (GISSI): Effectiveness of intravenous thrombolytic treatment in acute myocardial infarction. *Lancet* 1986;1:397–402.

139. ISIS-2 Collaborative Group: Randomized trial of intravenous streptokinase, oral aspirin, both or neither among 17,187 cases of suspected acute myocardial infarction. *Lancet* 1988;2:349–352.

140. The TIMI 3A Investigators: Early effects of tissue-type plasminogen activator added to conventional therapy on the culprit coronary lesion in patients presenting with ischemic cardiac pain at rest: Results of the thrombolysis in myocardial ischemia (TIMI 3A) trial. *Circulation* 1993;87:38–52.

141. The TIMI-3B Investigators: Effects of tissue plasminogen activator and a comparison of early invasive and conservative strategies in unstable angina and non-Q wave myocardial infarction: Results of the TIMI-3B trial. *Circulation* 1994;89: 1545–1556.

142. Waters D, Lam JYT: Is thrombolytic therapy striking out in unstable angina? *Circulation* 1992; 86:1642–1644.

143. Karlsson JE, Berglund U, Bjorkholm A, et al: Thrombolysis with recombinant human tissue-type plasminogen activator during instability in coronary artery disease: Effect on myocardial ischemia and need for coronary revascularization. *Am Heart J* 1992;124:1419–1426.

144. Bar FW, Verheugt FW, Col J, et al: Thrombolysis in patients with unstable angina improves the angiographic but not the clinical outcome: Results of UNASEM, a multicenter, randomized, placebo-controlled, clinical trial with anistreplase. *Circulation* 1992;86:131–137.

145. Grip L, Bone D, Holmgren A, et al: Late thrombolysis followed by antithrombotic treatment in acute myocardial infarction: Effect of therapy evaluated with thallium 201 SPECT. *Eur Heart J* 1993;14:1050–1055.

146. Ambrose JA, Almeida OD, Sharma SK, et al: Adjunctive thrombolytic therapy during angioplasty for ischemic rest angina: Results of the TAUSA trial. *Circulation* 1994;90:69–77.

147. Mizuno K, Satumora K, Miyamoto A, et al: Angioscopic evaluation of coronary artery thrombi in acute coronary syndromes. *N Engl J Med* 1992; 326:287–291.

148. Jang IK, Gold HK, Ziskind AA, et al: Differential sensitivity of erythrocyte-rich and platelet-rich arterial thrombi to lysis with recombinant tissue-type plasminogen activator: A possible explanation for resistance to coronary thrombolysis. *Circulation* 1989;79:920–928.

149. Parise P, Agnelli G: Thrombus resistance to lysis and reocclusion: The role of platelets. *Blood Coagul Fibrinolysis* 1991;2:749–758.

150. Yusuf S, Wittes J, Friedman L, et al: Overview of results of randomized clinical trials in heart disease: Unstable angina, heart failure, primary prevention with aspirin, and risk factor modification. *JAMA* 1988;260:2259–2263.

151. Jugdutt BI, Warnica JW: Intravenous nitroglycerin therapy to limit myocardial infarct size, expansion, and complications. Effect of timing, dosage and infarct location. *Circulation* 1988;78: 906–919.

152. Gunnar RM, Bourdillon PD, Dixon DW, et al. Guidelines for the early management of patients with acute myocardial infarction. *J Am Coll Cardiol* 1990;16:249–292.

153. Yusef S, Peto R, Lewis J, et al: Beta blockade during and after myocardial infarction: An overview of the randomized trials. *Prog Cardiovasc Dis* 1985; 27:335.

154. Norwegian Multicenter Study Group: Timolol-induced reduction in mortality and reinfarction in patients surviving acute myocardial infarction. *N Engl J Med* 1981;304:801.

155. β-Blocker Heart Attack Trial Research Group: A randomized trial of propranolol in patients with acute myocardial infarction: I, Mortality results. *JAMA* 1982;147:1707.

156. Yusef S, Witles J, Probstfield J: Evaluating effects of treatment in subgroups of patients within a clinical trial: The case on non-Q wave myocardial infarction and beta blockers. *Am J Cardiol* 1990;66:220–222.

157. Gheorghiade M, Schultz L, Tilley B, et al: Effects of propranolol in non-Q wave acute myocardial infarction in the beta blocker heart attack trial. *Am J Cardiol* 1990;66:129–133.

158. The MIAMI Trial Research Group: Mortality results. *Am J Cardiol* 1985;56(Suppl G):12.

159. Overskeid K, Abrahamsen AM, Frisvold OI, et al: Letter to the editor. *N Engl J Med* 1981;305:407.

160. Gibson RS, Young PM, Boden WE, et al: Prognostic significance and beneficial effect of diltiazem on the incidence of early recurrent ischemia after non-Q wave myocardial infarction: Results from the multicenter diltiazem reinfarction study. *Am J Cardiol* 1987;60:203–209.

161. The Multicenter Diltiazem Postinfarction Trial Research Group: The effect of diltiazem on mortality and reinfarction after myocardial infarction. *N Engl J Med* 1988;319:385–392.

162. Boden WE: Management of non-Q wave myocardial infarction: Role of diltiazem versus β-blocker therapy. *J Cardiovasc Pharm* 1990;16(Suppl 6):55–60.

163. Gibson RS: Current status of calcium channel-blocking drugs after Q wave and non-Q wave myocardial infarction. *Circulation* 1989;80(Suppl IV):IV-107–IV-119.

164. Madsen JK, Hansen JF: Mortality of patients excluded from the Danish Verapamil Infarction Trial II. The DAVIT-II Study Group. *Eur Heart J* 1993;14:377–379.

165. Gøtzsche CO, Søgaard P, Ravkilde J, et al: Effects of captopril on left ventricular systolic and diastolic function after acute myocardial infarction. *Am J Cardiol* 1992;70:156–160.

166. James IM, Dickenson EJ, Gurgoyne W, et al: Treatment of hypertension with captopril: Preservation of regional blood flow and reduced platelet aggregation. *J Hum Hypertens* 1988;2:21–25.

167. Kiowski W, Zuber M, Elasser S, et al: Coronary vasodilation and improved myocardial lactate metabolism after angiotensin converting enzyme inhibition with enalopril in patients with congestive heart failure. *Am Heart J* 1991;122:1382–1388.

168. Ontkean MT, Gay R, Greenberg B: Effects of chronic captopril therapy on endothelium-derived relaxing factor activity in heart failure. *J Am Coll Cardiol* 1992;19(Suppl A):768–774.

169. DeFeyter PJ, Serruys PW, Soward A, et al: Coronary angioplasty for early postinfarction unstable angina. *Circulation* 1986;74:1365–1370.

170. Safian RD, Snyder LD, Snyder BA, et al: Usefulness of percutaneous transluminal coronary angioplasty for unstable angina pectoris after non-Q wave acute myocardial infarction. *Am J Cardiol* 1987;59:263–266.

171. Gottlieb SO, Walford GD, Ouyang P, et al: Initial and late results of coronary angioplasty for early postinfarction unstable angina. *Cathet Cardiovasc Diagn* 1987;13:93–99.

172. Holt GW, Gersh BJ, Holmes DR, et al: Results of percutaneous transluminal coronary angioplasty for angina pectoris early after acute myocardial infarction. *Am J Cardiol* 1988;61:1238–1242.

173. Suryapranata H, Beatt K, DeFeyter DE, et al: Percutaneous transluminal coronary angioplasty for angina pectoris after non-Q wave acute myocardial infarction. *Am J Cardiol* 1988;61:240–243.

174. Bellamy GR, McEniery PT, Zaidi AR, Hollman J: Percutaneous transluminal angioplasty after non-Q wave infarction. *Cleve Clin J Med* 1989;56: 141–145.

175. Alfonso R, Macaya C, Iniquez A, et al: Percutaneous transluminal coronary angioplasty after non-Q wave myocardial infarction. *Am J Cardiol* 1990;65:835–839.

176. Suryapranta H, Serruys PW, Beatt K, et al: Recovery of regional myocardial dysfunction after successful coronary angioplasty early after a non-Q wave infarction. *Am Heart J* 1990;120:261–269.

177. Goldberg RJ, Gore JM, Gurwitz JH, et al: The impact of age on the incidence and prognosis of initial acute myocardial infarction: The Worcester heart attack study. *Am Heart J* 1989;117:543–549.

178. Benhorin J, Andrews M, Carleen E, et al: Occurrence, characteristics and prognostic significance of early postacute myocardial infarction angina pectoris. *Am J Cardiol* 1988;62:679–685.

179. Schuster EH, Bulkley BH: Ischemia at a distance after acute myocardial infarction: A cause of early postinfarction angina. *Circulation* 1980;62:509–515.

180. Madigan N, Rutherford BD, Barnhorst DA, Danielson GK: Early saphenous vein grafting after subendocardial infarction: Immediate surgical results and late prognosis. *Circulation* 1977;56 (Suppl II):II-1–II-3.

181. Jones EL, Waites TF, Craver JM, et al: Coronary bypass for relief of persistent pain following acute myocardial infarction. *Ann Thorac Surg* 1981;32: 33–43.

182. Roberts AJ, Sanders JH, Moran JH, et al: The efficacy of medical stabilization prior to myocardial revascularization in early refractory postinfarction angina. *Ann Surg* 1983;197:91–98.

183. Nunley DL, Grunkemeier GL, Teply JF, et al: Coronary bypass operation following acute complicated myocardial infarction. *J Thorac Cardiovasc Surg* 1983;85:485–491.

184. Williams DB, Ivey TD, Bailey WW, et al: Postinfarction angina: Results of early revascularization. *J Am Coll Cardiol* 1983;2:859–864.
185. Breyer RH, Engelman RM, Rousou JA, Lemeshow S: Postinfarction angina: An expanding subset of patients undergoing coronary artery bypass. *J Thorac Cardiovasc Surg* 1985;90:532–540.
186. Singh AK, Rivera R, Cooper GN, Karlson KE: Early myocardial revascularization for postinfarction angina: Results and long-term follow-up. *J Am Coll Cardiol* 6:1121–1125.
187. Kouchoukos NT, Murphy S, Philpott T, et al: Coronary artery bypass grafting for postinfarction angina pectoris. *Circulation* 1989;79(Suppl I): I-68–I-72.
188. Gardner TJ, Stuart RS, Green PS, et al: The risk of coronary bypass surgery for patients with postinfarction angina. *Circulation* 1989;79(Suppl I): I-79–I-80.
189. Kennedy JW, Ivey TD, Misbach G, et al: Coronary artery bypass graft surgery early after acute myocardial infarction. *Circulation* 1989;79(Suppl I): I-73–I-78.
190. Sintek CF, Pfeffer TA, Khonsari S: Surgical revascularization after acute myocardial infarction. *J Thorac Cardiovasc Surg* 1994;107:1317–1322.
191. Mark DB, Nelson CL, Califf RM, et al: Continuing evolution of therapy for coronary artery disease: Initial results from the era of coronary angioplasty. *Circulation* 1994;89:2105–2025.
192. Mock MB, Reeder GS, Schaff HV, et al: Percutaneous transluminal coronary angioplasty versus coronary artery bypass: Isn't it time for a randomized trial? *N Engl J Med* 1985;312:916–919.
193. Editorial: BARI, CABRI, EAST, GABI and RITA: Coronary angioplasty on trial. *Lancet* 1990;335:1315–1316.
194. Hlatky MA, Cotugno HE, Mark DB, et al: Trends in physician management of uncomplicated acute myocardial infarction. *Am J Cardiol* 1988;61: 515–558.
195. Gibson RS, Beller GA: Value of predischarge myocardial perfusion scintigraphy, in Topol EJ, et al (eds.): *Artherosclerosis and Coronary Artery Disease.* New York, Raven Press, chapter 69.
196. Mueller H, Cohen L, Williams D, et al: Subgroup analysis of the TIMI-2 study. *J Am Coll Cardiol* 1991;17:167A.
197. Ellis SG, Mooney MR, George BS, et al: Randomized trial of late elective angioplasty versus conservative management for patients with residual stenoses after thrombolytic treatment of myocardial infarction. *Circulation* 1992;86:1400–1406.
198. The TIMI Study Group: Comparison of invasive and conservative strategies after treatment with intravenous tissue plasminogen activator in acute myocardial infarction: Results of the thrombolysis in myocardial infarction (TIMI) phase II trial. *N Engl J Med* 1989;320:618–627.
199. Barbash GI, Roth A, Hod H, et al: Randomized controlled trial of late in-hospital angiography and angioplasty versus conservative management after treatment with recombinant tissue-type plasminogen activator in acute myocardial infarction. *Am J Cardiol* 1990;66:538–545.
200. Feit F, Mueller HS, Braunwald E, et al: Thrombolysis in myocardial infarction (TIMI) phase II trial: Outcome comparison of a "conservative strategy" in community versus tertiary hospitals. *J Am Coll Cardiol* 1990;16:1529–1534.
201. Rogers WJ, Babb JD, Baim DS, et al: Selective versus routine predischarge coronary arteriography after therapy with recombinant tissue-type plasminogen activator, heparin and aspirin for acute myocardial infarction. *J Am Coll Cardiol* 1991;17:1007–1016.
202. SWIFT (Should We Intervene Following Thrombolysis?) Trial Study Group: SWIFT trial of delayed elective intervention v conservative treatment after thrombolysis with anistreplase in acute myocardial infarction. *Br Med J* 1991;302:555–560.
203. Williams DO, Braunwald E, Knatterud G, et al: One-year results of the thrombolysis in myocardial infarction investigation (TIMI) phase II trial. *Circulation* 1992;85:533–542.
204. Arnold AR, Simoons ML, Detry JM, et al: Prediction of mortality following hospital discharge after thrombolysis for acute myocardial infarction: Is there a need for coronary angiography? *Eur Heart J* 1993;14:306–315.

19

Thrombolytic Therapy: A Critical Review of Clinical Trials

Kevin R. Kruse, MD, Robert M. Califf, MD, and E. Magnus Ohman, MD

The last two decades have witnessed a dramatic change in the management of acute myocardial infarction. From a conservative approach of bed rest and few therapeutic interventions, there has evolved a multifaceted strategy comprising pharmacological agents, emergency cardiac catheterization, and early cardiac rehabilitation. This evolution has been facilitated by many large, properly conducted clinical trials. The appropriate use of statistical methods has further enhanced our knowledge and allowed previous studies to be pooled and summarized to add strength to new observations (1).

Since the concept was formulated that thrombotic occlusion of a coronary artery was the culprit in an acute myocardial infarction (2–4) and that agents that induce a fibrinolytic state could dissolve this clot (5), a substantial experience has been gained about the impact of different thrombolytic agents on patency of the infarct-related artery, left ventricular function, and mortality. With more than 150,000 patients entered into various clinical trials, thrombolytic therapy for acute myocardial infarction is probably the most thoroughly studied pharmacological intervention in medical history. The purpose of this chapter is to review the major clinical trials of thrombolytic therapy in acute myocardial infarction.

HISTORICAL PERSPECTIVE

The major thrombolytic agents that have been subjected to large randomized clinical trials include streptokinase (SK), urokinase (UK), tissue-type plasminogen activator (t-PA), single-chain urokinase-type plasminogen activator (scuPA), anisoylated plasminogen–streptokinase activator complex (APSAC), and recombinant plasminogen activator (r-PA) (see Ch. 1). Detailed descriptions and overviews of drug development for thrombotic disease have been published by Mueller and Scheidt (6) and by Sherry and Marder (7). Although the first description of proteolytic activity was attributed to human urine in the 1800s, it was not until the 1940s and 1950s that the agent responsible for this activity (urokinase) was purified (8–10). Urokinase was first studied for the treatment of pulmonary embolism and thrombosed venous catheters. In the 1930s, the next thrombolytic agent (streptokinase) was discovered as a product of β-hemolytic streptococci (11). The concept that acute coronary thrombus was responsible for myocardial infarction led to an increased interest in the use of fibrinolytic agents (2). In 1958, Fletcher, Sherry, and colleagues wrote the first report on the use of intravenous streptokinase in acute myocardial infarction (12).

During the 1960s and 1970s, many small trials examined the use of intravenous thrombolytic therapy. Unfortunately, the small number of patients and wide inclusion criteria resulted in most studies showing little clinical benefit and frequent hemorrhagic complications. A meta-analysis of 33 trials of streptokinase and urokinase was reported in 1985 by Yusuf and colleagues (13) and provided the first evidence from patient outcomes that thrombolytic therapy could reduce mortality in patients presenting with an acute myocardial infarction.

The report of the successful intracoronary infusion of streptokinase by Rentrop and colleagues (14) in a patient who developed an acute occlusion during a diagnostic cardiac catheterization was followed by a number of studies on the intracoronary use of thrombolytic therapy. Although most studies of small numbers of patients failed to document a reduction in mortality, one exception was the Western Washington Study, which showed a significant mortality reduction in patients with anterior wall myocardial infarctions (15). These and other studies led to the 1982 FDA approval of both streptokinase and urokinase for the intracoronary treatment of acute myocardial infarction. A number of limitations of the intracoronary application of thrombolytic therapy became evident. The logistics of performing acute cardiac catheterization for all patients with an acute myocardial infarction were apparent. The delay in achieving recanalization of the infarct-related artery was also recognized. This delay may have explained the lack of improvement in global left ventricular function in the Western Washington Study of intracoronary streptokinase (16), as it became evident that minimizing the delay from onset of symptoms to therapy was an important factor for myocardial salvage (17).

These factors led to the development of other, more fibrin-specific thrombolytic agents in an effort to improve clot lysis while avoiding hemorrhagic complications. The design of anisoylated plasminogen–streptokinase activator complex (APSAC) was reported in 1981 (18), and the cloning of tissue-type plasminogen activator (t-PA) from *E. coli* expressing human DNA-derived melanoma cells was accomplished in 1983 (19). Multiple large clinical trials in the 1980s compared the efficacy of thrombolytic agents versus standard therapy. The results of these trials and others led to FDA approval of intravenous streptokinase and t-PA in 1987 and APSAC in 1989 for the treatment of acute myocardial infarction. Thrombolytic therapy is now considered standard care in the treatment of patients who present with acute myocardial infarction.

Additional efforts have focused on determining the role and timing of adjunctive mechanical interventions (20,21). By the early 1980s, cardiac catheterization could be performed acutely, and in selected patients angioplasty was attempted in combination with thrombolytic therapy (22). A number of studies followed, indicating the relative success with the combination of angioplasty and streptokinase (23), urokinase (24), or tissue-type plasminogen activator (25). These studies allowed a better understanding of the pathophysiology of myocardial infarction and reperfusion. The relative role of angioplasty after thrombolytic therapy in acute myocardial infarction was subsequently addressed in four studies, all of which observed no benefit on either mortality or resting left ventricular function (26–29). The role of acute angioplasty during thrombolytic therapy appears to be confined to patients in whom restoration of coronary artery patency fails (30–32). Ellis et al randomized a small number of patients who failed to achieve early arterial patency in the setting of acute anterior myocardial infarction and showed a trend toward enhanced clinical outcome with a strategy of acute cardiac catheterization and "rescue" angioplasty compared with a conservative approach (33). On the other hand, a strategy of primary angioplasty in acute myocardial infarction has been associated with a high success rate with good long-term outcome (34,35) (see Ch. 22). Thus the role of acute cardiac catheterization and mechanical revascularization in acute myocardial infarction is a complex issue that requires further evaluation.

A second generation of randomized clinical trials was undertaken in the late 1980s and early 1990s to determine which thrombolytic agent (streptokinase, APSAC, or t-PA) resulted in improved survival in patients presenting with an acute myocardial infarction. Although these mega-trials provided important information that has helped define the current role of thrombolytic therapy, there is still considerable controversy over which thrombolytic agent provides the optimal risk-to-benefit-to-cost profile. Current clinical and research efforts are directed toward improving clinical outcomes through earlier treatment strategies, improved thrombolytic agents, and optimal adjunctive therapies.

THROMBOLYTIC AGENTS

The coagulation system functions under a complex and incompletely understood interaction between clot formation and dissolution (36,37). Fibrin, a major component of the thrombus, is the target for thrombolytic agents. The essential step of fibrinolysis is initiated when plasminogen activators convert the proenzyme plasminogen to the proteolytic enzyme plasmin. All thrombolytic agents function as plasminogen activators and are classified as fibrin-specific or non-fibrin-specific based on their binding characteristics to plasminogen-bound fibrin. Once formed, plasmin facilitates clot lysis by cleaving fibrin to produce fibrin degradation products. In low concentrations, plasmin is rapidly inactivated by α_2-antiplasmin; plasminogen activators are inactivated by plasminogen-activator inhibitors (PAI). During therapeutic thrombolysis, however, the conversion of plasminogen to plasmin overwhelms the endogenous inhibitors (α_2-antiplasmin and PAI), resulting in a systemic thrombolytic state. Thrombolytic agents differ in their pharmacological characteristics and in the degree to which they activate plasma plasminogen to form plasmin (38–46). The main characteristics of the plasminogen activators that have been studied in clinical trials are shown in Table 19–1.

Non-Fibrin-Specific Agents

Streptokinase is a protein product of β-hemolytic streptococcus. It is not an enzyme but binds noncovalently with plasminogen to form an activator complex. The complex allows for conversion of other plasminogen molecules to plasmin. Streptokinase has a pharmacological half-life of 23 minutes. Anisoylated plasminogen–streptokinase activator complex (APSAC) is a preformed complex of plasminogen and streptokinase. Spontaneous deacylation occurs in plasma and is required for the complex to become active. The half-life is determined by the rate of deacylation and is 95 minutes in the commercial product. Both streptokinase and APSAC have relative antigenicity and therefore can induce neutralizing antibodies.

Urokinase (UK) is an endogenous compound that is produced by the renal and vascular endothelial cells and is secreted in the urine. Urokinase is a low molecular weight, two-chain enzyme that has a half-life of 14 minutes. scuPA is a single-chain urokinase plasminogen activator, also known as prourokinase.

Fibrin-Specific Agents

Tissue-type plasminogen activator (t-PA) is a naturally occurring enzyme synthesized by endothelial cells. The commercial compound is produced by recombinant DNA technology. Human melanoma

Table 19–1. Characteristics of Plasminogen Activators

	Plasminogen Binding	Half-Life (min)	Fibrinogen Depletion	Fibrin Specificity	Antigenicity
Streptokinase	Indirect	23	4+	–	Yes
t-PA, alteplase	Direct	5	1–2+	++	No
Urokinase	Direct	14	3+	–	No
APSAC, anistreplase	Indirect	95	3+	+	Yes
scuPA, prourokinase	Indirect	9, 114*	1–2+	++	No
r-PA, reteplase	Direct	15	2–3+	++	No
Staphylokinase	Indirect	6, 37*	1+	++	Yes

t-PA = tissue-type plasminogen activator, APSAC = anisoylated plasminogen–streptokinase activator complex, scuPA = single-chain urokinase plasminogen activator, r-PA = recombinant plasminogen activator.

*Biphasic plasma clearance.

cell DNA for tissue-type plasminogen activator is genetically inserted into an established mammalian cell culture. Since t-PA has a binding site for fibrin, it attaches to thrombus preferentially and facilitates the conversion of clot-bound plasminogen to plasmin. At therapeutic dose levels, however, t-PA loses some degree of its fibrin specificity and activates circulating plasminogen. t-PA is cleared primarily by the liver and has a half-life of 5 minutes. A newer, nonglycosylated plasminogen activator (r-PA) is also produced by recombinant DNA techniques, but it lacks the N-terminal sequence for the finger, epidermal growth factor, and kringle-I domains of t PA. This results in greater thrombolytic potency and a longer half-life (approximately 15 minutes), allowing for bolus therapy.

Newer thrombolytic agents under development include staphylokinase (47), mutants or deletion molecules of t-PA that have altered half-lives and higher affinity for fibrin (48–50), nitrosylated t-PA (51), and conjugated plasminogen activators and monoclonal antibodies (42,43,50). The attachment of a fibrin antibody to a thrombolytic agent could markedly enhance the fibrin specificity (52,53). In addition, monoclonal antibodies to the glycoprotein IIb/IIIa receptor could be coupled directly to thrombolytic agents for improved lysis of platelet-rich clot (54). Although these third-generation conjugated thrombolytic agents have yet to be studied in randomized clinical trials, they provide hope for improved thrombolysis with a reduction in systemic complications.

CLINICAL ENDPOINTS

Multiple well-designed randomized clinical trials have now established thrombolytic therapy as a standard treatment for patients who present with an acute myocardial infarction. However, the progression from experimental animal studies to clinical trials required the establishment of acceptable efficacy and safety endpoints (55). Although the most important endpoint for any study of acute myocardial infarction must be mortality (56), the number of patients required to study this endpoint for different thrombolytic agents is in the tens of thousands. Although large clinical trials must be performed, mega-trials such as GISSI-2 (57), ISIS-3 (58), and GUSTO-I (59) cannot be conducted for every new promising thrombolytic agent. Hence there is a need to develop surrogate endpoints that either alone or in combination can serve to differentiate or add supportive data to the knowledge of the effectiveness of therapeutic agents.

Since the use of thrombolytic therapy in acute myocardial infarction leads to higher patency of the infarct-related artery, limitation of infarct size, and improved survival, many studies have used patency and left ventricular function as "surrogate" endpoints. Unfortunately, nonfatal endpoints can be fraught with errors relating to subjectivity and incompleteness of measurement. Clinical endpoints frequently used in thrombolytic trials include angiographic patency and reocclusion rates, left ventricular function, composite clinical, hematological, or physiological measurements, hemorrhagic events, and cost-effectiveness (Table 19–2). The major problem with these endpoints is that they are not of equal importance and a therapy could have a positive effect with regard to one endpoint and a negative effect with regard to another.

MORTALITY

Thrombolytic trials conducted between 1959 and 1979 were small and did not convincingly demonstrate a reduction in mortality. Yusuf reported a meta-analysis of 24 of these trials and demonstrated a 22% reduction in mortality for patients treated with thrombolysis ($p < 0.001$) (13). To confirm these findings, larger collaborative multicenter randomized trials were organized.

Streptokinase

The efficacy of streptokinase was evaluated in four large multicenter trials, summarized in Table 19–3 and Fig. 19–1. The Gruppo Italiano per lo Studio della Streptochinasi nell'Infarto Miocardico (GISSI-1) trial was an open-label study randomizing 11,806 patients to receive 1.5 million units of streptokinase over 1 hour or standard medical therapy (60). Patients had electrocardiographically documented ST segment elevation or depression and symptoms for less than 12 hours. There was no

Table 19–2. Clinical Endpoints

Mortality	Hemorrhagic Complications
Angiographic	Hemorrhagic stroke
Patency/TIMI flow grade	Major bleeding
Reocclusion	Hematological Measurements
Physiological Measurements	Thrombin Activity
Myocardial enzymes	Fibrinopeptide A (FPA)
Electrocardiographic	Thrombin–antithrombin complex (TAT)
Technetium sestamibi/Thallium	Fragment 1.2 (F1.2)
Contrast echocardiography	Fibrinolysis
Ventricular function	Fibrinogen
Left ventriculography	D-dimer
Echocardiogram	Plasminogen-activator inhibitor
MUGA	Platelet Activity
Composite Clinical	Platelet aggregation
Reinfarction, recurrent ischemia	Bleeding time
Congestive heart failure, stroke	Platelet factor 4 (PF4)
Cost-effectiveness	Platelet flow cytometry

MUGA = multigated equilibrium radionuclide angiography.

difference in baseline characteristics. Adjunctive drug therapy was administered at the physician's discretion and included aspirin (14%), heparin (62%), beta blockers (8%), nitrates (37%), and calcium channel blockers (48%). An overall 18% reduction in in-hospital (14- to 21-day) mortality was seen for active treatment versus standard therapy (10.7% vs. 13.0%, $p = 0.0002$). The relative reduction in mortality was time dependent, decreasing from 47% in patients treated within 1 hour, to 23% for those treated within 3 hours, to 17% for those treated within 6 hours of symptom onset. There was no significant reduction in mortality in the 1,946 patients randomized after 6 hours of symptoms. The reduction in mortality that was observed early (in-hospital) was maintained over 12 months: 17.2% in the streptokinase group versus 19.0% in controls, $p = 0.008$ (61).

The Intravenous Streptokinase in Acute Myocardial Infarction (ISAM) study was a double-blind trial that randomized 1,741 patients with ST elevation to treatment with streptokinase or placebo (62). There was an nonsignificant 11% reduction in 21-day mortality with streptokinase therapy (6.3% vs. 7.1%, p = NS). Only 48% of the patients eligible for inclusion were eventually randomized, and 1.3% of screened patients died before randomization. The nonsignificant difference was possibly related to the

Table 19–3. Mortality Trials of Streptokinase

	GISSI-1 (60)	ISAM (62)	ISIS-2 (63)	EMERAS (64)
Number of patients	11,806	1,741	17,187	3,568
Number of sites	176	38	417	236
Dose/Duration	1.5 MU/1 h	1.5 MU/1 h	1.5 MU/1 h	1.5 MU/1 h
Enrollment period	2/84–6/85	3/82–3/85	3/85–12/87	1/88–1/91
Placebo-blinding	No	Yes	Yes	Yes
Age criteria	All	<75 y	All	All
Symptoms	<12 h	<6 h	<24 h	6–24 h
ECG criteria	ST ↑ or ↓	ST ↑	None	None
Aspirin	±	Yes	Randomized	Yes
Heparin	±	IV	±	±
Mortality follow-up	In-hospital	21 d	35 d	35 d

ECG = electrocardiographic, MU = million units, IV = intravenous.

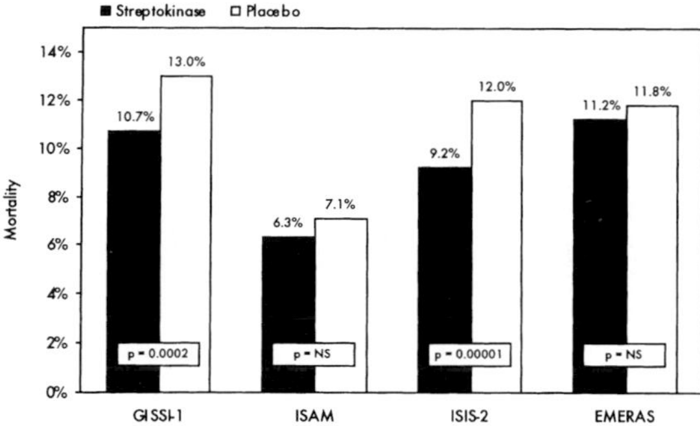

Figure 19–1. Short-term mortality after acute myocardial infarction in mortality trials of streptokinase. The lengths of follow-up were: in-hospital for GISSI-1 (60), 21 days for ISAM (62), 35 days for ISIS-2 (63), and 35 days for EMERAS (64). NS = not statistically significant.

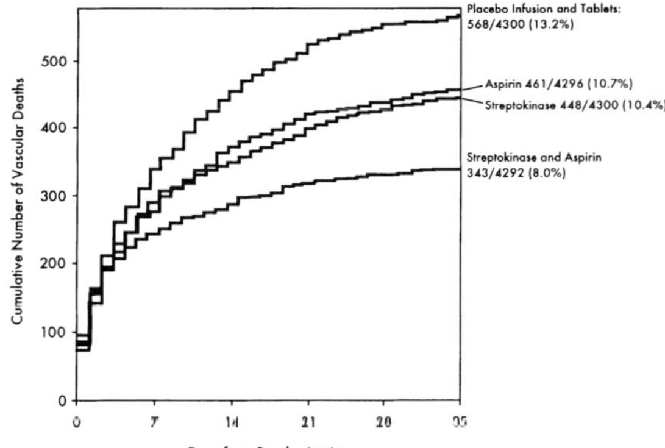

Figure 19–2. Short-term mortality with streptokinase, aspirin, both, or neither in ISIS-2. *Reprinted from ISIS-2 Collaborative Study Group (63), with permission of The Lancet, Ltd.*

smaller sample size and the large number of excluded patients, which resulted in a lower event rate.

The second International Study of Infarct Survival (ISIS-2) was the largest double blind, placebo controlled study of intravenous streptokinase in suspected myocardial infarction (63). In this study 17,187 patients in 417 hospitals, with symptoms of less than 24 hours duration, were randomized in a 2 × 2 factorial design to aspirin alone (162.5 mg per day for 1 month), streptokinase alone (1.5 MU over 1 hour), both, or neither. There were no entry criteria other than the physician's clinical suspicion of an acute myocardial infarction. Patients randomized to streptokinase had a 25% reduction in 35-day vascular mortality compared with those who received placebo (9.2% vs. 12.0%, < 0.001). The study also showed that aspirin alone could reduce vascular mortality by 23% ($p < 0.001$). Importantly, the effect of aspirin in combination with streptokinase was even more pronounced, with a 42% reduction (8.0% vs. 13.2%, $p < 0.001$) in vascular mortality at 35 days compared with neither agent (Fig. 19–2). The additional benefits from aspirin administration included reduced rates of reinfarction, cardiac arrest, cardiac rupture, stroke, and all-cause mortality. Similar to the GISSI-1 study, the reduction in mortality from thrombolytic therapy was more pronounced in patients treated earlier; however, patients treated late (5 to 24 hours) also had a significant reduction in mortality. Three other findings from this large study are noteworthy: (i) the reduction in mortality was seen in all patient subsets (that is, inferior and anterior infarctions, old and young patients, men and women, diabetics and nondiabetics), (ii) patients with clinically suspected infarction and ST segment elevation or left bundle branch block on the electrocardiogram received the greatest reduction in mortality, and (iii) long-term follow-up (out to 2 years) showed a sustained survival benefit in favor of streptokinase and aspirin (82.6% vs. 78.4% for placebo) (Fig. 19–3). This large study supported the use of thrombolytic therapy in combination with aspirin for all subsets of patients with acute myocardial infarction.

The Estudio Multicentrico Estreptoquinasa Republicas de America del Sur (EMERAS) Collaborative Group randomized 4,534 patients in a double-blind fashion to streptokinase or placebo up to 24 hours after symptom onset (64). Once the results of ISIS-2 were known, only patients presenting within 6 to 24 hours of symptom onset were randomized ($n = 3{,}568$). The 35-day mortality was not significantly different between streptokinase and placebo (11.2% vs. 11.8%).

Tissue-Type Plasminogen Activator

The effect of t-PA in reducing mortality in patients with suspected acute myocardial infarction

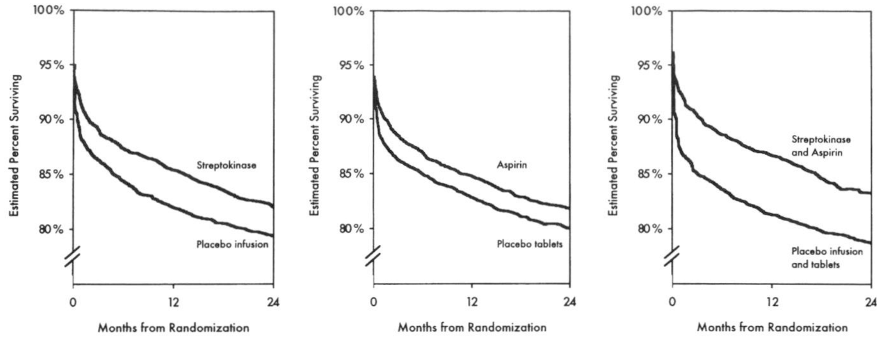

Figure 19–3. Long-term mortality after acute myocardial infarction in ISIS-2. *Reprinted from the ISIS-2 Collaborative Study Group (63), with permission of The Lancet, Ltd.*

was examined in the Anglo-Scandinavian Study of Early Thrombolysis (ASSET), in which 5,011 patients were randomized to receive t-PA (100 mg over 3 hours) plus intravenous heparin, or placebo (65,66) (Table 19–4 and Fig. 19–4). The entry criteria did not require electrocardiographic evidence of myocardial infarction. Despite a definite diagnosis of myocardial infarction in only 58% of patients at discharge, there was a significant 26% reduction in mortality at 30 days in patients randomized to t-PA (7.2% vs. 9.8%, $p = 0.001$). Of note is that patients received no aspirin or other antiplatelet agents in this study. In a subsequent study of t-PA in acute myocardial infarction by the European Cooperative Study Group (ECSG-5), in which all patients received aspirin (250 mg) in addition to intravenous heparin, the reduction in mortality was 51% at 14 days in patients randomized to 100 mg t-PA (95% confidence interval, −76% to 1%) (67). Although this study provided promising results, it was not powered to detect a statistically significant reduction in mortality.

The Late Assessment of Thrombolytic Efficacy (LATE) study evaluated the effect of thrombolysis (t-PA 100 mg over 3 hours) in patients presenting between 6 and 24 hours from symptom onset (68). A total of 5,711 patients were randomized in this double-blind, placebo-controlled trial. By intention-to-treat analysis, there was no significant reduction in mortality at 35 days of follow-up (8.9% vs. 10.3%). However, in the patients treated within 12 hours of symptom onset (a subgroup prospec-

Table 19–4. Mortality Trials of t-PA, APSAC, and Urokinase

	t-PA		APSAC	Urokinase
	ASSET (65)	LATE (68)	AIMS (69)	USIM (71)
Number of patients	5,011	5,711	1,258	2,201
Number of sites	52	230	39	89
Dose/Duration	100 mg/3 h	100 mg/3 h	30 U/5 min	2-1 MU boluses
Enrollment period	11/86–2/88	4/89–2/92	9/85–10/87	4/86–9/88
Placebo-blinding	Yes	Yes	Yes	No
Age criteria	≤75 y	All	≤75 y	All
Symptoms	<5 h	6–24 h	<6 h	<4 h
ECG criteria	None	ST ↑ or ↓	ST ↑	ST ↑
Aspirin	±	Yes	±	±
Heparin	IV	±	IV	IV
Mortality follow-up	30 d	35 d	30 d	In-hospital

APSAC = anisoylated plasminogen–streptokinase activator complex, ECG = electrocardiographic, MU = million units, IV = intravenous.

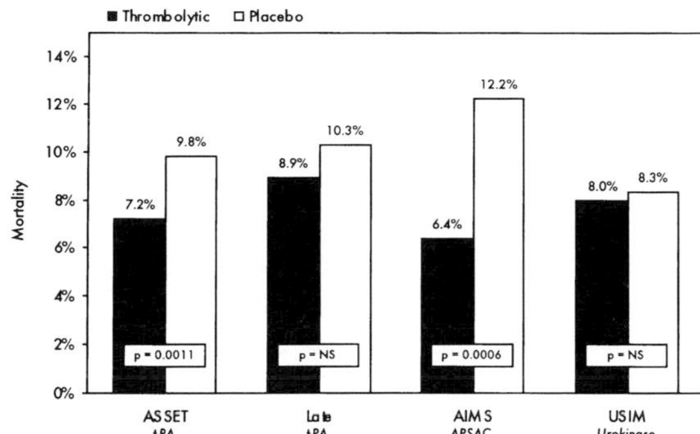

Figure 19–4. Short-term mortality after acute myocardial infarction in mortality trials of tissue-type plasminogen activator (t-PA), anisoylated plasminogen–streptokinase activator complex (APSAC), and urokinase. Follow-up was 30 days in ASSET (65,66), 35 days in LATE (68), 30 days in AIMS (69,70), and in-hospital in USIM (71). NS = not statistically significant.

tively defined for analysis), there was a 25.6% reduction in mortality (8.9% vs. 12.0%, $p = 0.02$).

Anisoylated Plasminogen–Streptokinase Activator Complex

The only large mortality study of APSAC in patients with acute myocardial infarction, the Anistreplase Intervention Mortality Study (AIMS), was terminated prematurely, after the second interim analysis (880 of 2,000 patients planned) showed a significant reduction in mortality in patients randomized to APSAC (69,70). The study required electrocardiographic evidence of myocardial infarction; all patients received intravenous heparin followed by oral anticoagulation and were discharged on timolol unless contraindicated. A report of 1,258 patients available at the termination of the study showed that patients randomized to APSAC (30 U over 5 minutes) had a 51% reduction in mortality (6.4% vs. 12.2%, $p = 0.0006$) after 30 days of follow-up. Similar to the ISIS-2 study, the greatest reduction in mortality was seen in older patients and in those individuals treated within 6 hours of symptom onset. The 1-year follow-up data from AIMS also showed that the reduction in mortality was maintained.

Urokinase

The Urochinasi per la Sistemia nell'Infarto Miocardico (USIM) Collaborative Trial is the largest randomized study of urokinase plus intravenous heparin versus intravenous heparin alone (71). This study was neither placebo-controlled nor powered to detect a difference in mortality. Complete follow-up of 2,201 patients showed no significant difference in in-hospital mortality (8.0% vs. 8.3%).

Pooled Analysis

In 1994 the Fibrinolytic Therapy Trialists' (FTT) Collaborative Group reported an overview of all randomized trials of more than 1,000 patients comparing thrombolytic therapy with conventional therapy (72). A pooled analysis of 58,600 patients showed an 18% reduction in 35-day mortality (9.6% vs. 11.5%, $p = 0.00001$). On the day of randomization, however, thrombolytic therapy was associated with significantly higher mortality (2.4% vs. 1.9%, $p = 0.001$); the beneficial effect of fibrinolytic therapy did not emerge until days 2 through 35 after randomization. Although this analysis reinforced the benefit of thrombolytic therapy, it provided important information regarding the selection of patients and helped to determine the indications and contraindications for thrombolytic therapy in clinical practice (see the section Patient Selection).

Comparative Trials

Given the documented reduction in mortality in these trials, it would have been unethical to enroll further patients in placebo-controlled thrombolytic trials. Thus it became increasingly important to evaluate the efficacy of new thrombolytic agents via comparative studies with other endpoints such as patency, left ventricular function, reocclusion, and clinical events during hospitalization.

To address the question of whether one thrombolytic agent was more effective in reducing mortality in acute myocardial infarction, many comparative thrombolytic trials have been conducted (73–83). However, to show a reduction in 30-day mortality (from an estimated 8% to 10% "control" rate) requires very large numbers of patients. For example, a randomized clinical trial of more than 6,600 patients (3,300 in each group) would be required to show (with 80% power) that a treatment reduces mortality by 20% compared with the "control" treatment (assuming that the "control" population has a 10% mortality rate). Three such megatrials have been conducted: GISSI-2, ISIS-3, and GUSTO-I.

The GISSI-2/International Study was a multicenter, randomized, open-label trial designed to compare streptokinase (1.5 MU over 60 minutes) with standard t-PA (100 mg over 3 hours) (57,84,85) (Fig. 19–5). Entry criteria included symptoms for less than 6 hours, electrocardiographic evidence of acute myocardial infarction, and no contraindication to thrombolytic therapy. There was no upper age limit for inclusion in the study. Patients were also randomized to receive subcutaneous heparin (given in a dose of 12,500 U twice daily) versus placebo, starting 12 hours after the beginning of thrombolytic infusion. The effectiveness of the anticoagulation was not monitored. In addition, all patients received 325 mg aspirin per day. Early beta-blockade (atenolol) was instituted in 23% of patients. There was no significant difference in in-hospital mortality between patients randomized to streptokinase (8.5%) and those given t-PA (8.9%). Similarly, there was no significant difference in major in-hospital events, except for a higher incidence of strokes in the patients who received t-PA (1.3% vs. 0.9%, RR 1.41, 95% CI 1.09–1.83) and more major bleeding (>2 units of blood transfused) in patients who received streptokinase (0.6% t-PA vs. 0.9% streptokinase, RR 0.67, 95% CI 0.49–0.91). The overall results from this large study are difficult to interpret because of the late administration of subcutaneous heparin in only half the patients.

The second large randomized study (ISIS-3) was a multicenter, double-blind trial that enrolled patients thought by their physicians to have "clear" indications for thrombolysis into one of three treatment arms: streptokinase 1.5 MU infused over 60 minutes, t-PA (duteplase) 0.60 MU/kg infused over 4 hours, or APSAC 30-U bolus infused over 5 minutes (58) (Fig. 19–6). Eligible patients included those with a clinically suspected acute myocardial infarction with symptoms for up to 24 hours. There were no electrocardiographic or age criteria

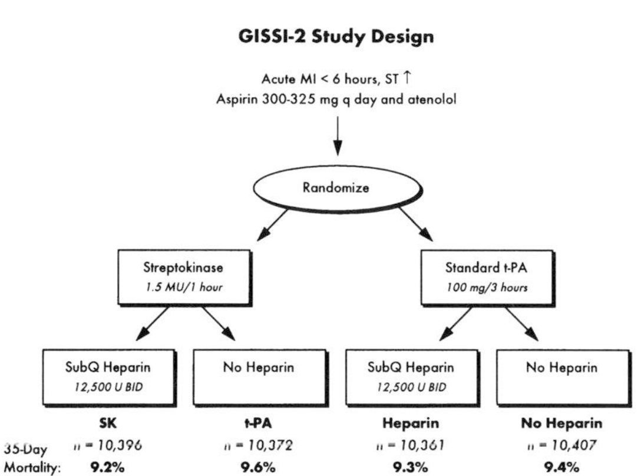

Figure 19–5. Study design of the GISSI-2/International Study. The study was a 2 × 2 factorial design with patients randomized to receive streptokinase (SK) 1.5 million units over 1 hour, or tissue-type plasminogen activator (t-PA) 100 mg over 3 hours, followed by subcutaneous (SubQ) heparin 12,500 units twice daily (BID) beginning 12 hours after the start of the thrombolytic infusion versus placebo. In addition, 36% of patients received early intravenous atenolol followed by daily oral beta-blockade.

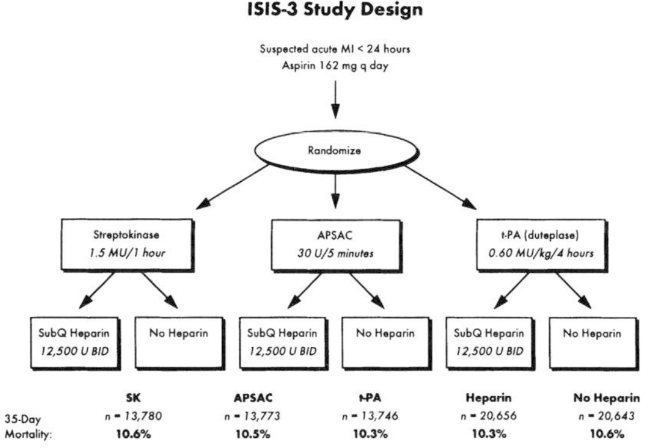

Figure 19–6. Study design of the ISIS-3 trial. The study was a 3 × 2 factorial design, in which patients were randomized to receive one of three thrombolytic agents—streptokinase (SK), anisoylated plasminogen–streptokinase activator complex (APSAC), or tissue-type plasminogen activator (t-PA)—with further randomization to subcutaneous (SubQ) heparin twice daily (BID) versus placebo. In a separate arm, physicians randomized patients to thrombolytic therapy (any of the three agents) or conventional therapy if they were uncertain of the benefit of thrombolytic therapy for a particular patient.

for patient enrollment. Physicians were asked whether a patient had "clear" or "uncertain" indications for thrombolysis. Patients with an "uncertain" indication (no ST segment elevation, presentation >6 hours after pain onset, relative contraindication) were randomized to thrombolytic therapy (streptokinase, t-PA, or APSAC) or standard therapy.

Patients were further randomized in a factorial design to subcutaneous heparin (12,500 U twice daily) to be started 4 hours after the start of thrombolytic therapy (see Ch. 20). All patients were to receive aspirin at a dose of 162 mg/day. The report of 41,299 patients randomized to thrombolytic therapy was published in 1992. There was no difference in 35-day mortality among the three thrombolytic agents (streptokinase 10.6%, APSAC 10.5%, and t-PA 10.3%). The subset analysis of 25,836 patients who presented within 6 hours of symptom onset with ST elevation also showed no difference in mortality (streptokinase 10.0%, t-PA 9.6%, and APSAC 9.9%). Further, a composite analysis of the GISSI-2 and ISIS-3 trials did not demonstrate a significant reduction in mortality between treatment groups (58) (Fig. 19–7).

Since the results of these large randomized trials showed no significant difference in mortality among thrombolytic agents, many physicians were uncertain about which agent to use (86). The areas of concern over interpreting the results focused on the open-label design and the wide entry criteria (no qualifying electrocardiographic criteria and symptom duration up to 24 hours) of GISSI-2 and the use of an alternative t-PA therapy (duteplase) for ISIS-3. More recent studies had shown that a front-loaded t-PA dosing regimen resulted in improved 90-minute patency rate, a lower rate of reocclusion, and possibly a lower mortality (79,87, 88). In the front-loaded regimen, t-PA was administered as a 15-mg bolus, followed by 0.75 mg/kg over 30 minutes, then 0.50 mg/kg over the last 60 minutes (total 100 mg over 90 minutes). The Rapid Administration of Alteplase in Myocardial Infarction (RAAMI) trial showed improved patency rates at 60 minutes (76% vs. 62%) and 90 minutes (82% vs. 75%) in patients who received accelerated-dose t-PA (88). The t-PA versus Anistreplase (APSAC) Patency Study (TAPS) (79) showed similar results with an improved early patency rate (90-minute patency, 84% vs. 70%) and a lower in-hospital mortality rate (2.4% vs. 8.1%) for accelerated t-PA.

In addition, both ISIS-3 and GISSI-2 had randomized patients to receive subcutaneous heparin either 4 hours (ISIS-3) or 12 hours (GISSI-2) after the start of lytic infusion. The collective results of several angiographic patency trials of intravenous heparin (89–93) had suggested that the combination of t-PA and intravenous heparin resulted in an improved angiographic patency rate. The use of subcutaneous heparin may have hampered the ability to achieve and maintain patency, resulting in a loss of any potential survival advantage for t-PA.

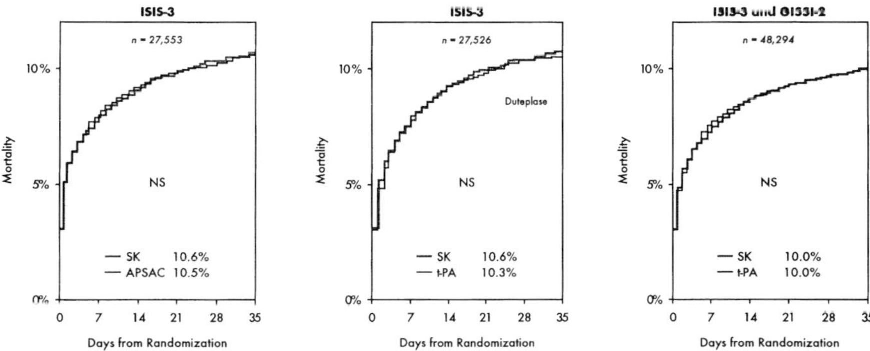

Figure 19–7. Cumulative short-term mortality after acute myocardial infarction: comparative trials of streptokinase (SK), anisoylated plasminogen–streptokinase activator complex (APSAC), and tissue-plasminogen activator (t-PA). NS = not significant. *From ISIS-3 Collaborative Group (58), with permission of The Lancet, Ltd.*

These concerns prompted the organization of the Global Utilization of Streptokinase and t-PA for Occluded Coronary Arteries (GUSTO-I) trial to test the hypothesis that early and sustained infarct-vessel recanalization is associated with better survival (59). The study was designed as a multicenter (1,081 hospitals), open-label trial with randomization to one of four thrombolytic regimens: streptokinase and subcutaneous heparin, streptokinase and intravenous heparin, accelerated t-PA and intravenous heparin, or t-PA, streptokinase, and intravenous heparin (94) (Fig. 19–8). Entry criteria included electrocardiographic signs (≥0.1 mV of ST segment elevation in two or more limb leads or ≥0.2 mV in two or more contiguous precordial leads) and presentation within 6 hours of symptom onset. There was no upper age limit. Aspirin (≥160 mg) was given acutely followed by a daily dose of 160 to 325 mg. Patients without contraindication received intravenous atenolol (10 mg) followed by oral therapy (50–100 mg daily). Intravenous beta blocker therapy was administered to 46% of patients; oral therapy was given to 71%. The 30-day mortality for each treatment arm is displayed in Fig. 19–9 (94). Accelerated administration of t-PA with intravenous heparin was associated with a 14% relative reduction in the risk of death (1% absolute reduction) over the two streptokinase-only strategies (6.3% vs. 7.3%, $p = 0.001$). This represents 10 lives saved per 1,000 patients treated. When compared separately with each streptokinase group, t-PA therapy showed a persistent reduction in mortality. The use of combination therapy (t-PA–streptokinase) showed no significant difference compared with the other treatment strategies.

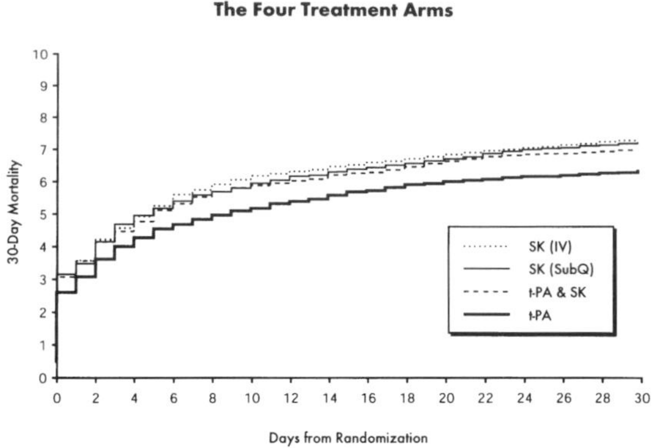

Figure 19–9. Short-term mortality in the GUSTO-I trial. Patients who received accelerated tissue-type plasminogen activator (t-PA) had significantly lower 30-day mortality than those who received streptokinase (SK) with either intravenous (IV) or subcutaneous (SubQ) heparin or the combination of t-PA and streptokinase with intravenous heparin. *From Califf and Topol (94), with permission.*

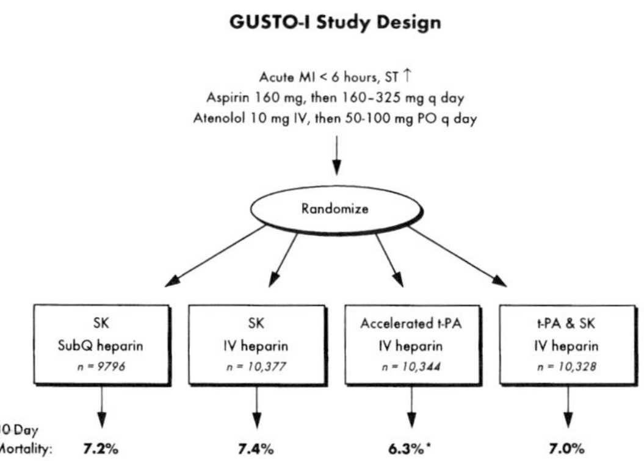

Figure 19–8. Study design of the GUSTO-I trial. The original design included the two experimental arms and one reference arm, in which patients received streptokinase (SK) with intravenous (IV) heparin. When the results of the ISIS-3 trial were reported, the second reference arm, streptokinase with subcutaneous (SubQ) heparin, was added. MI = myocardial infarction, t-PA = tissue-type plasminogen activator. *From Califf and Topol (94), with permission.*

Although t-PA was associated with an excess of hemorrhagic strokes (0.70% vs. 0.51%, $p = 0.03$) (59,95), the accelerated t-PA group maintained an advantage over the streptokinase-only groups for a combined endpoint of death or disabling stroke (6.9% vs. 7.8%, $p = 0.006$) (Fig. 19–10). This represents the prevention of death and disabling stroke in 9 patients per 1,000 treated. The results of GUSTO-I have raised much controversy, particularly with regard to the cost-effectiveness of widespread accelerated t-PA use, which is more expensive and complex to administer. However, these results support the notion that accelerated t-PA improves survival and provides an overall net clinical benefit. As will be discussed in later sections, the enhanced survival with accelerated t-PA was

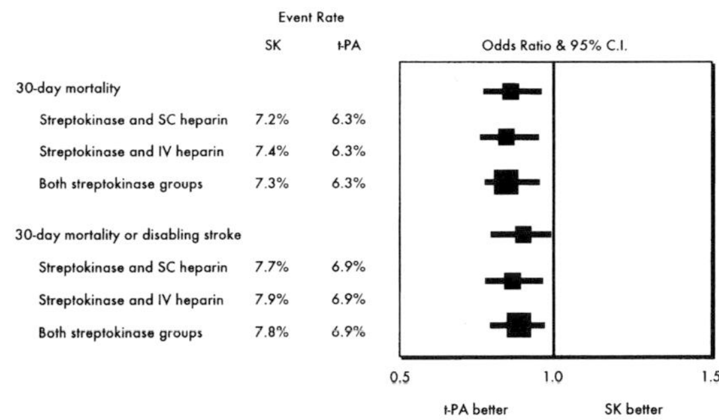

Figure 19–10. Odds ratios and 95% confidence intervals (CI) for reductions in 30-day mortality and 30-day mortality or disabling stroke among patients in the GUSTO-I trial who received accelerated t-PA versus streptokinase with subcutaneous (SC) or intravenous (IV) heparin. Adapted from The GUSTO Investigators, **N Engl J Med,** 1993;329:677.

evident by 24 hours and correlated with the ability to achieve early, complete reperfusion as defined by the presence of Thrombolysis in Myocardial Infarction (TIMI) grade 3 flow (see Table 19–5). Of note, accelerated t-PA therapy was associated

Table 19–5. Classification of TIMI (Thrombolysis in Myocardial Infarction) Flow in the Infarct-Related Coronary Artery

Flow Grade	Description
TIMI Grade 0	No perfusion; there is no anterograde flow beyond the point of occlusion.
TIMI Grade 1	Penetration without perfusion; contrast passes beyond obstruction but fails to opacify the entire coronary bed during the cineangiogram.
TIMI Grade 2	Partial perfusion; contrast passes across and opacifies the coronary bed distal to obstruction, but the rates of entry and clearance of dye are perceptibly slower than those of the opposite, unobstructed arterial bed.
TIMI Grade 3	Complete perfusion; antegrade flow and clearance of dye occur as promptly as in the uninvolved bed in the same vessel or in the opposite artery.

Data from Chesebro et al (80).

with fewer arrhythmias and less left ventricular dysfunction (congestive heart failure, cardiogenic shock, and sustained hypotension), but similar rates of reinfarction, recurrent ischemia, and angiographic reocclusion, compared with streptokinase.

Another agent subjected to comparative trials was r-PA. The RAPID trial was a randomized, open-label evaluation of r-PA versus t-PA with angiographic patency as the primary endpoint (96). A total of 660 patients presenting within 6 hours of acute myocardial infarction were randomized to one of four treatment arms: standard-dose t-PA (100 mg over 3 hours), r-PA as a single 15-MU bolus, r-PA as a 10-MU bolus followed by 5 MU 30 minutes later, and r-PA as a 10-MU bolus followed by 10 MU 30 minutes later. The group that received the two 10-MU boluses had a higher rate of TIMI grade 3 flow at 60 minutes (51% vs. 33%, $p < 0.01$) and 90 minutes (63% vs. 49%, $p < 0.05$) than the standard t-PA group. Although the trial was not powered to detect a difference in mortality, the 30 day mortality observed with 10 MU boluses of r-PA was 1.9%, while patients randomized to standard-dose t-PA had a 3.9% mortality. The RAPID-2 trial randomized 324 patients within 12 hours of an acute myocardial infarction to r-PA or accelerated t-PA as used in the GUSTO-I trial (97). More patients receiving r-PA (two 10-MU boluses) achieved TIMI grade 3 flow at 60 minutes (51% vs. 37%, $p < 0.01$) and at 90 minutes (60% vs. 45%, $p < 0.05$). The administration of r-PA resulted in a 35-day mortality rate of 4.1% compared with 8.4% for accelerated t-PA ($p = 0.11$). The International Joint Efficacy Comparison of Thrombolytics (INJECT) study was a double-blind trial that randomized 6,010 patients to either r-PA (two 10-MU boluses) or streptokinase (1.5 MU over 1 hour), both with intravenous heparin (98). There was a nonsignificant 0.5% absolute reduction in 30-day mortality for r-PA compared with streptokinase (8.9% vs. 9.4%, $p = 0.48$). To establish the efficacy of r-PA, the GUSTO-III trial has a proposed enrollment of approximately 15,000 in a 2:1 randomization to r-PA (two 10-MU boluses, 30 minutes apart) or accelerated t-PA therapy, with 30-day mortality as the primary endpoint.

PATENCY

The status of the infarct-related artery during and after acute myocardial infarction is recognized as an important prognostic factor. Angiographic flow criteria of the Thrombolytic in Myocardial Infarction (TIMI) Study Group are summarized in Table 19–5 (80). Recanalization is defined as progression from documented TIMI grade 0 or 1 flow to TIMI grade 2 or 3 flow after thrombolytic therapy. The use of immediate cardiac catheterization to document coronary flow status prior to thrombolytic therapy causes inherent delays. Therefore, instead of recanalization rates, patency rates at 60 to 90 minutes after thrombolytic therapy are usually evaluated. Infarct artery patency has been defined as the presence of TIMI grade 2 or 3 flow at the time of angiography, which can include lesions that were never occluded, underwent spontaneous reperfusion, or became recanalized due to therapy. It is therefore desirable to assess patency within the first few hours, because spontaneous lysis in the infarct-related artery can occur over time (2).

A pooled analysis of 14,124 angiographic observations from 58 studies of streptokinase, standard t-PA, accelerated t-PA, or APSAC provides important information about their relative effects on patency (Fig. 19–11) (99). At 90 minutes, accelerated t-PA had the highest patency rate (84%), followed by APSAC (70%), standard-dose t-PA (70%), streptokinase (51%), and no thrombolytic therapy (21%). By 24 hours, a "catch-up" phenomenon had occurred; all thrombolytic strategies had similar patency rates, ranging from 80% to 86%. This may be due to different reocclusion rates, delayed recanalization, spontaneous reperfusion, or bias due to exclusion of patients who did not survive until follow-up angiography. The results of the GUSTO-I angiographic substudy confirmed these findings (100) (Fig. 19–12). The 90-minute angiogram again documented that accelerated t-PA was associated with the highest patency rate (81%), followed by t-PA with streptokinase (73%), streptokinase with intravenous heparin (60%), and streptokinase with subcutaneous heparin (54%). A catch-up phenomenon was also observed by 24 hours with patency rates of 77% to 94%. The ability simply to achieve

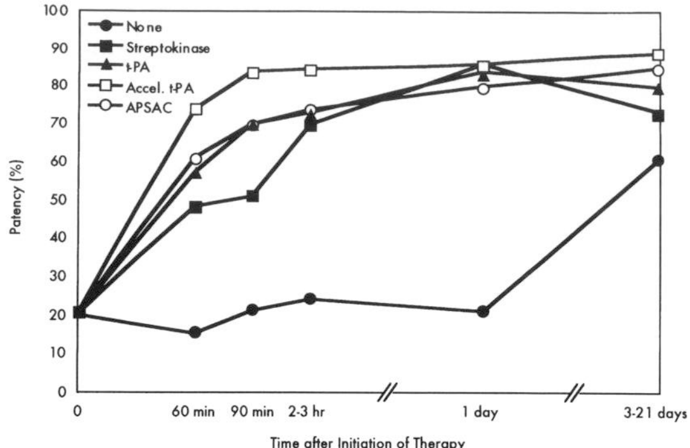

Figure 19–11. Pooled analysis of 14,124 angiographic observations from 58 studies of streptokinase, standard t-PA, accelerated t-PA (Accel t-PA), or anisoylated plasminogen–streptokinase activator complex (APSAC). Accelerated t-PA was associated with the highest rate of 90-minute patency (TIMI grade 2 or 3 flow). *From Granger et al (99), with permission.*

TIMI grade 2 or 3 flow may overestimate the efficacy of thrombolytic reperfusion, however.

Complete Reperfusion

The concept of "optimal" reperfusion has emerged, challenging the concept of angiographic patency as acceptable reperfusion (101,102) (see Ch. 21). In this construct, the ultimate goal is to obtain rapid and sustained reperfusion at the tissue level.

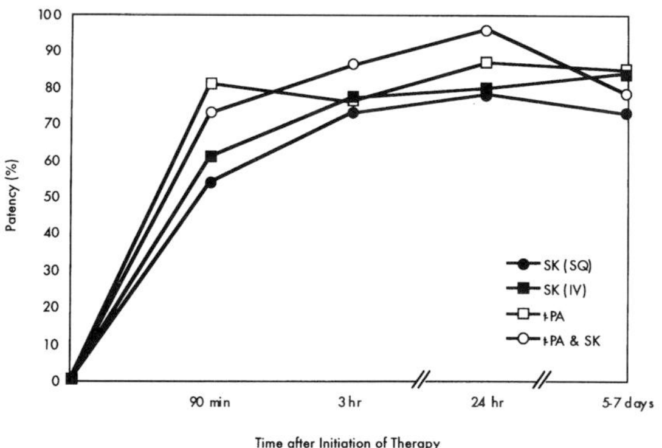

Figure 19–12. Patency in the GUSTO-I angiographic substudy. Accelerated t-PA (t-PA) was again associated with the highest rate of TIMI grade 2 or 3 flow at 90 minutes, although a "catch-up" phenomenon was noted at later times. IV = intravenous, SQ = subcutaneous, SK = streptokinase. *Data from Simes et al (100).*

The potential benefits of restored tissue-level myocardial perfusion include the limitation of infarct expansion, salvage of hibernating myocardium, improvement in ventricular healing and remodeling, limitation of ventricular dilation, maintenance of electrical stability, and ultimately, improved survival.

Recent reports have confirmed that TIMI grade 2 flow does not represent effective myocardial recanalization. A retrospective analysis of four German multicenter studies evaluated the impact of infarct-related artery reperfusion on mortality (103). In this report, 907 patients had an angiogram of the infarct-related artery 90 minutes after the initiation of thrombolytic therapy. In-hospital mortality of patients with partial reperfusion (TIMI grade 2 flow) was not significantly different from that of patients with an occluded (TIMI grade 0 or 1 flow) infarct-related artery (6.6% vs. 7.1%). In contrast, patients with complete reperfusion (TIMI grade 3 flow) had a 2.7% in-hospital mortality, a 60% reduction ($p = 0.01$).

The TEAM-2 and TEAM-3 (Thrombolysis trial of Eminase in Acute Myocardial infarction) studies (78,104) also challenged the concept that TIMI grade 2 anterograde flow should be regarded as patent. In these studies, the ventriculographic, enzymatic, and electrocardiographic outcomes with TIMI grade 2 flow did not differ from those with TIMI grade 0 or 1 flow. TIMI grade 3 flow, however, was associated with improved ejection fraction, more rapid and smaller enzyme peaks, and a lower QRS score.

In an angiographic substudy of the GUSTO-I trial (100), 1,210 patients were randomized to a 90-minute angiogram after initiation of treatment. Figure 19–13 summarizes the angiographic data and subsequent associated 30-day mortality. The patients with TIMI grade 2 flow had a 30-day mortality of 7.9%, which did not represent a statistically significant survival advantage over TIMI grade 1 (9.2%) or TIMI grade 0 flow (8.4%). However, TIMI grade 3 flow resulted in a reduction in 30-day mortality to 4.0% ($p < 0.01$).

The ability of a thrombolytic agent to achieve and maintain TIMI grade 3 flow is therefore critical and should result in improved survival. In GUSTO-I, accelerated t-PA was associated with

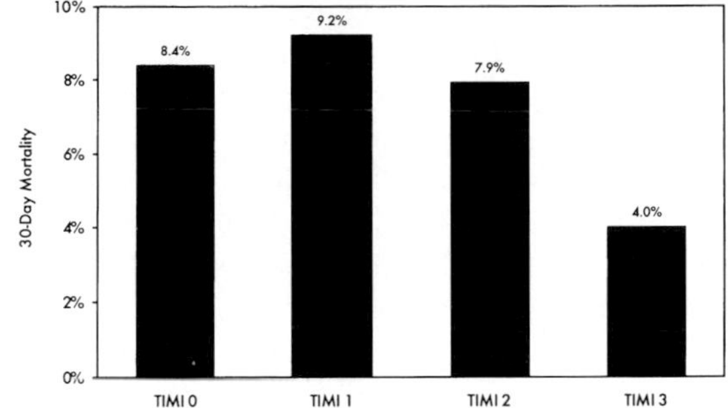

Figure 19–13. Mortality at 30 days versus Thrombolysis in Myocardial Infarction (TIMI) flow grade at 90 minutes in the GUSTO-I angiographic substudy. TIMI grade 3 flow at 90 minutes was associated with significantly lower mortality ($p < 0.01$). *Data from Simes et al (100).*

the highest incidence of TIMI grade 3 flow (54%) at 90-minute angiography. In comparison, only 29% of patients who received streptokinase with subcutaneous heparin had TIMI grade 3 flow (Fig. 19–14). Logistic regression analysis showed that TIMI grade 3 flow was associated with a significant reduction in 30-day mortality with an odds ratio of 0.44 in relation to TIMI grade 0 or 1 flow ($p = 0.007$). After adjusting for important prognostic risk factors (sex, age, previous myocardial infarction, myocardial infarction location, height, systolic blood pressure, and heart rate), TIMI grade 3 flow

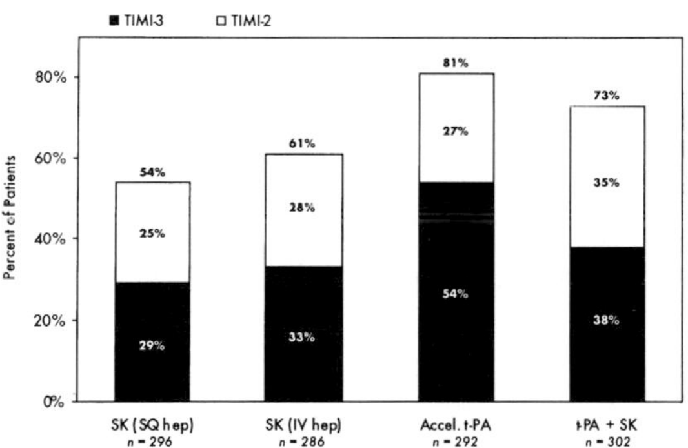

Figure 19–14. TIMI flow grades for patients who received accelerated t-PA (Accel. t-PA), streptokinase (SK) with subcutaneous heparin (SQ hep) or intravenous heparin (IV hep), or combination t-PA and streptokinase with intravenous heparin (t-PA + SK) in the GUSTO-I angiographic substudy. A significantly larger proportion of patients who received accelerated t-PA achieved TIMI grade 3 flow at 90 minutes ($p < 0.001$). *Data from Simes et al (100).*

remained a significant predictor of 30-day mortality ($p = 0.015$). Based on this finding, a model was developed to predict 30-day mortality based on the 90-minute angiographic coronary TIMI flow grade achieved by each of the thrombolytic strategies (100) (Fig. 19–15). There was a high degree of correlation ($r = 0.97$) between the observed and the predicted mortality.

This observation across multiple trials reinforces the concept that the early restoration of TIMI grade 3 flow results in improved survival. Accordingly, there is room for much improvement, since accelerated t-PA therapy is associated with 46% incomplete reperfusion (TIMI grade 0, 1, or 2 flow). In addition, there are likely patients within the TIMI grade 3 subgroup who do not achieve adequate tissue-level perfusion. Therefore, further improvements in thrombolytic and adjunctive therapy are required, not only to achieve a higher rate of TIMI grade 3 flow but also to ensure adequate reperfusion at the myocardial tissue level.

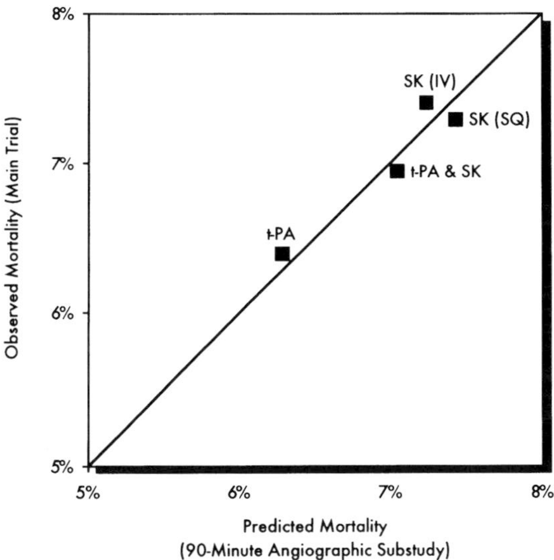

Figure 19–15. Plot of predicted versus observed 30-day mortality based on 90-minute TIMI flow grade in the GUSTO-I angiographic substudy, where points lying on the diagonal represent a perfect match. The proportion of squared error explained (R^2) was 0.92. Predicted results were based on the 1,210 patients in the angiographic substudy; observed results are for the 39,811 patients in the main trial. t-PA = accelerated t-PA, SK = streptokinase, IV = intravenous heparin, SQ = subcutaneous heparin, t-PA & SK = combination t-PA and streptokinase with intravenous heparin. *Reprinted from Simes et al (100), with permission.*

It should be kept in mind, however, that the clinical determinants of mortality are complex and multifactorial (105,106). A predictive model was developed using baseline clinical characteristics from the GUSTO-I trial. Multivariable analysis identified many characteristics (age, systolic blood pressure, Killip class, heart rate, infarct location, previous myocardial infarction, height, time to treatment, history of diabetes, weight, smoking status, choice of thrombolytic therapy, previous bypass surgery, hypertension, and prior cerebrovascular disease) that were significantly associated with mortality. From these routinely collected clinical factors, a statistical model was developed that provides accurate predicted mortality rates (105).

Sustained Reperfusion

Early reperfusion is essential, but the coronary blood flow must also be maintained. Reocclusion after thrombolytic therapy has been angiographically defined as a change from TIMI grade 2 or 3 flow at baseline to TIMI grade 0 or 1 flow at follow-up. Comparison of reocclusion rates among trials is difficult since the follow-up duration has varied greatly. In addition, the angiogram provides only a "snapshot" at a particular time and does not take into account cyclical flow variations or intermittent coronary occlusions.

Many clinical trials have documented the importance of sustained coronary perfusion. In four sequential Thrombolysis and Angioplasty in Myocardial Infarction (TAMI) trials, reocclusion within 7 days occurred in 12.4% of 810 patients and resulted in substantial morbidity and greater in-hospital mortality (11.0% vs. 4.5%, $p = 0.01$) compared with patients who had sustained coronary reperfusion (107). Another work has studied a noninvasive means of assessing the status of the infarct-related artery, by analyzing ST segment shifts on continuous computer-assisted electrocardiography (108,109). Reperfusion was marked by ST segment recovery after thrombolytic therapy, and dynamic episodes of ST segment reelevation can noninvasively document inadequate tissue-level perfusion. Previous studies have documented reduced infarct size and improved mortality when ST segment recovery is complete and sustained (110–112).

Reocclusion rates with various thrombolytic agents have been compared in several clinical trials (see Ch. 20). A pooled analysis of 8,288 angiographic observations reported a reocclusion rate of 3.0% for APSAC, 11.8% for standard t-PA, 4.2% for streptokinase, and 6.0% for accelerated t-PA (113). Unfortunately, direct comparisons are difficult due to the use of different treatment protocols, definitions, and follow-up intervals. The GUSTO-I trial (114) provided the largest angiographic follow-up comparing thrombolytic strategies and defined reocclusion as the change from TIMI grade 2 or 3 flow at 90 minutes to TIMI grade 0 or 1 flow at the follow-up (5- to 7-day) angiogram. In the 586 patients with paired angiograms suitable for analysis, there was no significant difference among thrombolytic agents: 5.5% for streptokinase with intravenous heparin, 6.4% for streptokinase with subcutaneous heparin, 5.9% for accelerated t-PA, and 4.9% for t-PA–streptokinase. The RAPID-1 and -2 trials have provided preliminary data concerning the reocclusion rate for r-PA. In RAPID-1, there was a slight trend in favor of r-PA (2.9% vs. 7.8%, $p = 0.12$) over standard t-PA therapy (96). This was not seen, however, when r-PA was compared with the accelerated t-PA strategy studied in the RAPID-2 trial (9.0% vs. 7.0%, $p = 0.61$) (97). The overall reocclusion rate for r-PA was 6.0%, which is similar to the rate observed in the GUSTO-I angiographic substudy.

Predictors of Reocclusion

Previous studies have implicated lesion morphology (115–117), stenosis severity (117–122), TIMI grade 2 flow (115,123), presence of collaterals, type of thrombolytic (83,113,124,125), and adjunctive therapy (63,90–92) as predictors of reocclusion (see Ch. 20). In the GUSTO-I angiographic substudy, the overall reocclusion rate from the 90-minute angiogram to the 5- to 7-day angiogram was 5.6% in the 586 patients who had angiograms suitable for analysis. There were no early angiographic criteria (TIMI flow grade, thrombus, lesion morphology, or percent diameter stenosis) identified that predicted subsequent reocclusion (114, 126). In the TIMI-4 trial, reocclusion occurred in 5% of 278 patients from 90-minute angiography to follow-up at 18 to 36 hours. Angiographic predictors of reocclusion included TIMI grade 2 flow, ulcerated lesions, and presence of collateral vessels (118). In the Antithrombotics in the Prevention of Reocclusion in Coronary Thrombolysis (APRICOT) trial (119), patients presenting with acute myocardial infarction were randomized to therapy with streptokinase or APSAC; patency was determined within 48 hours after initiating thrombolysis. A second angiographic study was performed after 3 months to determine late reocclusion rates. Of the 284 patients who had a patent infarct-related artery within 48 hours, 248 underwent a repeat angiogram at 3 months. Multivariate analysis showed that culprit lesion stenosis severity was an independent risk factor for reocclusion (OR 2.31, 95% CI 1.28 to 4.18, $p = 0.006$). Reocclusion was noted in 42% of lesions with >90% stenosis compared with a 23% reocclusion rate in lesions with ≤90% stenosis. The ability to predict reocclusion has implications in the direct management (use of adjunctive medical therapies, length of hospital stay) of postinfarction patients treated with thrombolytic therapy.

Angiographic endpoints, including early (60- to 90-minute) TIMI flow grade and reocclusion rates, have been shown to correlate with clinical outcome and mortality in large randomized thrombolytic trials (100,107). These endpoints should therefore be considered as essential supportive data to determine the potential effectiveness of a thrombolytic agent.

THROMBOLYTIC THERAPY AND INFARCT SIZE

In the prethrombolytic era, measurement of the release of cardiac enzymes such as creatine kinase MB (MBCK) was used as a noninvasive measure of myocardial damage. Controversy arose when similar measurements were applied to patients who had received thrombolytic therapy (127) (see Ch. 8). However, Hermens and colleagues have shown that the amount of MBCK released from necrotic myocardium can be completely recovered in serum by measuring the cumulative cardiac enzyme release in a biexponential analysis (128). Three studies have examined cumulative release of enzyme in patients randomized to thrombolytic therapy or placebo, with remarkably similar results. In the ISAM study, 1,741 patients were randomized to streptokinase or placebo (62). The integrated area of MBCK release was significantly lower (approximately 9%, $p = 0.02$) in the patients who received streptokinase. The effect was particularly noticeable in patients treated within 3 hours (16%, $p = 0.001$). In the European Cooperative Study of t-PA and placebo, the cumulative release of α-hydroxybutyrate was examined in 702 patients (67). Patients who received t-PA had a 20% reduction in infarct size compared with patients randomized to placebo ($p = 0.018$). Though neither of these studies used any independent measure of infarct size, the data concur that thrombolytic therapy reduces infarct size if given within 6 hours of symptom onset, and the effect is particularly prominent if therapy is given earlier. Finally, the GUSTO-I enzyme substudy enrolled 553 patients from 15 hospitals (129). Infarct size was defined as the cumulative release of α-hydroxybutyrate dehydrogenase (HBDH) activity per liter of plasma over the first 72 hours after onset of symptoms. Patients treated with accelerated t-PA or combination t-PA–streptokinase therapy had a 12% smaller infarct size compared with the streptokinase-only groups (3.88 g-Eq/L vs. 4.39 g-Eq/L, $p = 0.043$). An important observation was that the infarct size as measured by HBDH release correlated with angiographic 90-minute patency rates and the left ventricular function data. Median infarct size at 72 hours was 3.72 g-Eq/L with TIMI grade 3 flow, 4.35 g-Eq/L with TIMI grade 2 flow, and 5.07 g-Eq/L in patients with TIMI grade 0 or 1 flow ($p = 0.024$ for grade 3 vs. grade 0 or 1 flow). There was an inverse relationship between enzyme infarct size and measures of left ventricular function 5 to 7 days after myocardial infarction. This study confirms that achieving early coronary patency (regardless of the method) will salvage myocardium, preserve left ventricular function, and improve survival.

Infarct size has also been evaluated by using the 12-lead electrocardiogram. A QRS score has been validated against anatomic infarct size in the prethrombolytic era. Its validity has not been confirmed in patients with successful reperfusion; nevertheless, this QRS score has been used in two studies (130,131). In both there was substantial overlap in the QRS scores of patients with and without successful reperfusion, though there was a trend toward less myocardial damage as assessed by the electrocardiogram in both studies. In another study, very early administration (within 1.5 hours) of thrombolytic therapy was associated with smaller infarct size, as assessed both by a QRS score and by enzymatic release, compared with later administration (132). The enhanced myocardial salvage, measured by the QRS score, has also been linked to the degree of reperfusion in the infarct-related artery (133).

LEFT VENTRICULAR FUNCTION

Since the function of the left ventricle, as measured by ejection fraction, has been documented as the single most important prognostic indicator of survival after acute myocardial infarction (134), some investigators have argued that left ventricular function should be the primary endpoint for the investigation of any thrombolytic agent (135). This approach has some advantages; the use of a continuous variable such as ejection fraction allows small studies to detect treatment differences, and ejection fraction can be determined both noninvasively and during cardiac catheterization with a high level of accuracy and reproducibility.

However, the use of left ventricular ejection fraction as a primary endpoint in reperfusion trials also poses many problems (136–138). Studies have documented a complex relationship between ejection fraction and infarct size (139). Further, if a thrombolytic agent is effective in reducing mortality, more patients with very poor left ventricular function are likely to survive. A paradox is therefore created in that a greater reduction in mortality will allow an increasing proportion of patients with lower ejection fractions to be included for analysis (136). Some have suggested that an arbitrary ejection fraction value be assigned for patients who did not survive. Contrarily, examination of ejection fraction after thrombolytic therapy may overestimate the effectiveness of a treatment strategy, as it is least likely to be performed in patients with the worst prognoses (32). This issue becomes particularly relevant when ejection fraction is measured by left ventriculography during cardiac catheterization, where the proportion of technically inadequate studies can approach 20%. For example, in the TIMI-1 study only 145 of 290 patients had adequate ventriculograms. Patients without ventriculograms had a significantly higher mortality (11% vs. 2%), more congestive heart failure (23% vs. 12%), and a higher incidence of cardiogenic shock (9% vs. 2%) (140). Furthermore, the different methods for measuring left ventricular function are not directly interchangeable; radionuclide ventriculography generally reports lower ejection fractions after myocardial infarction (137).

The ejection fraction represents global left ventricular function, including both infarct zone and noninfarct zone data (141). In the early phase of infarction, there is compensatory hyperkinesis of the noninfarct zone, which regresses over the first 3 days (142,143). During the same period, recovery of function in the infarct zone takes place (144). Nonetheless, noninfarct-zone function remained the most powerful predictor of in-hospital mortality in the TAMI studies (145). Thus there appears to be a complex relationship between mortality and regional myocardial function. A therapy that results in a large increase in myocardial salvage may improve global ejection fraction by only a smaller relative percentage (146) (Fig. 19–16). Norris and White (135) have argued that the end-systolic volume is a better predictor of survival than ejection fraction. Left ventricular dilation, as measured by end-systolic volumes occurring after infarction, may be a more sensitive index because it accounts for this complex relationship between hyperkinesis and dilation.

Most clinical trials of thrombolytic therapy have included some measure of global left ventricular function. Some selected studies are listed in Table 19–6 (27,62,67,77,147–154). A pooled analysis of all randomized trials does show that patients randomized to thrombolytic agents generally have an improvement in ejection fraction at various time points compared with controls (99) (Fig. 19–17). However, it appears that there is not a consistent re-

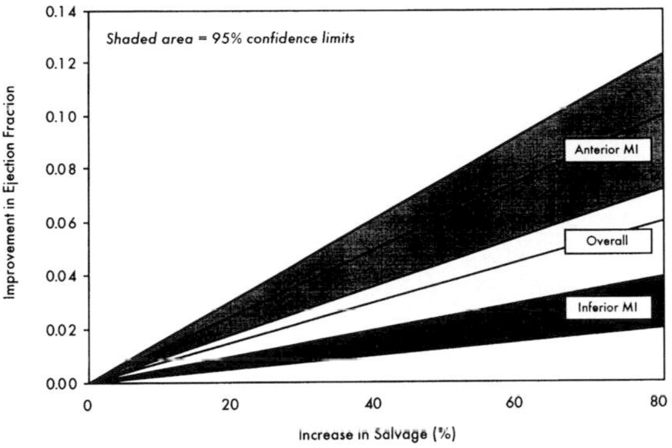

Figure 19–16. Expected improvement in ejection fraction for anterior and inferior myocardial infarction (MI) as a function of the percent increase in myocardial salvage over that with existing therapy. *From Gibbons et al (146), with permission.*

lationship between changes in mortality and changes in ejection fraction in individual studies (138) (Fig. 19–18). This speaks clearly to the inadequacy of left ventricular function as a surrogate endpoint in reperfusion studies.

The ability of left ventricular function to improve over time due to the salvage of "stunned" myocardium and the loss of noninfarct-zone compensatory hyperkinesis has been examined in several trials (27,80,152,155–157). The largest report of serial paired ventriculographic data summarized the results of the TAMI trials (155). Although there was no significant difference in global ejection fraction from the acute study to the 7-day study (51.2 ± 11% vs. 51.9 ± 11%, $p = 0.19$), regional wall motion in the infarct zone did improve over time. Multivariable analysis identified reduced acute ejection fraction, reduced acute noninfarct-zone regional function, presence of TIMI grade 3 flow, and resolution of chest pain prior to cardiac catheterization as independent predictors for improvement in the left ventricular ejection fraction at follow-up. There was no correlation with time from onset of symptoms to initiation of thrombolytic therapy.

Studies have compared the effects of different thrombolytic agents on the preservation of left ventricular function (77,83,140,158). In the TIMI-1 study, in which patients were randomized to receive intravenous streptokinase or t-PA, left ventricular function was assessed by contrast ventriculography (140). Complete data were available for only 50%

Table 19–6. Thrombolytic Therapy and Left Ventricular Function: Randomized Studies

Trial	*N*	Day Assessed	Method	Technically Adequate (%)	Ejection Fraction (%) Active	Ejection Fraction (%) Placebo	Mortality (%) Active	Mortality (%) Placebo
Streptokinase								
ISAM (62)	1,741	21–28	CV	49	57	54	6.3	7.1
					$p < 0.005$			
Western Washington (147,148)	368	10 ± 7	CV	46	54	51	6.3	9.6
					$p = 0.056$			
		56 ± 42	RN	56	51	47		
					$p = 0.08$			
White et al (77a)	219	21	CV	89	59	53	2.5	12.9*
					$p = 0.005$			
ECSG (149)	533	10–20	RN	32	48	44	5.9	11.7
					$p = 0.003$			
Tissue Plasminogen Activator								
Guerci et al (27)	138	10	RN	85	53	46	5.6	7.6
					$p < 0.02$			
National Heart Foundation (150)	144	7	CV	72	58	52	9.6	4.2
					$p = 0.04$			
TICO (151)	145	21	CV	87	61	54	5.4	5.6
					$p = 0.006$			
		21	CV	88	52	48		
					$p = 0.08$			
ECSG (67)	721	10–22	CV	80	51	49	2.8	5.7*
					$p < 0.05$			
TPAT (152)	115	9	RN	90	54	48	5.1	8.9
					$p < 0.02$			
Anisoylated Plasminogen–Streptokinase Activator Complex								
APSIM (153)	231	4	CV	90	53	47	6.3	5.0
					$p = 0.002$			
		19 ± 2	RN	77	43	39		
					$p = 0.04$			
Meinertz et al (154)	313	14–21	CV	82	53	54	5.6	13.0*
					p = NS			

RN = radionuclide angiography, CV = contrast left ventriculography, NS = not statistically significant.
*Significant reduction in mortality.

of the patients randomized. There were no significant differences in either baseline ejection fraction (streptokinase 48 ± 12% vs. t-PA 49 ± 10%) or discharge ejection fraction (streptokinase 49 ± 12% vs. t-PA 50 ± 9%). Both agents were similarly effective in preservation of infarct-zone function. The relative improvement in infarct-zone function was significantly better in patients who had collateral circulation to this region.

White and colleagues randomized 270 patients to either streptokinase or t-PA within 6 hours of onset of symptoms of acute myocardial infarction (77). Contrast left ventriculography was performed in 89% at 3 weeks. The ejection fraction was identical in both groups at 58 ± 12%. The end-systolic volume was 61 ± 29 ml in the streptokinase group and 66 ± 31 ml in the t-PA group. The mortality among patients assigned to streptokinase was 7.4% compared with 3.7% for t-PA treated patients. Other events were similarly distributed. The GAUS and TAMI-5 studies compared left ventricular function after treatment with t-PA or urokinase. Both studies showed no significant difference in ejection fraction between treatment groups.

The angiographic substudy of the GUSTO-I trial examined global ejection fraction and other indices of ventricular function and salvage (114). In this angiographic substudy, 2,431 patients were

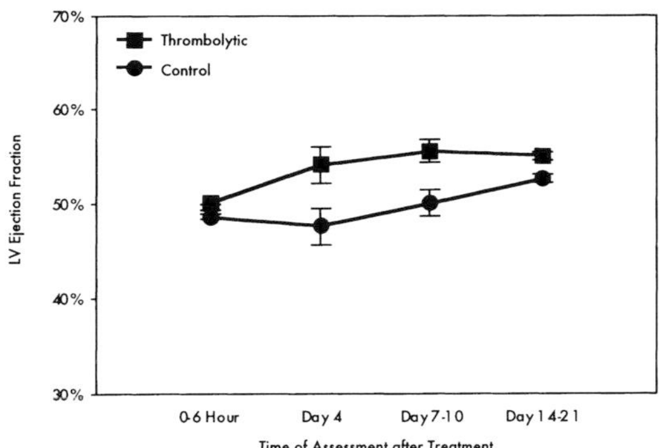

Figure 19–17. Pooled analysis of left ventricular (LV) ejection fraction from randomized trials of thrombolytic therapy versus control. Thrombolytic therapy results in a significantly higher ejection fraction at each time point (all $p \leq 0.001$). *Reprinted from Granger et al (99), with permission.*

randomly assigned to one of the four thrombolytic treatment arms (streptokinase with subcutaneous heparin or streptokinase, accelerated t-PA, or t-PA–streptokinase with intravenous heparin). After the initiation of thrombolysis, patients were subsequently randomized to cardiac catheterization at

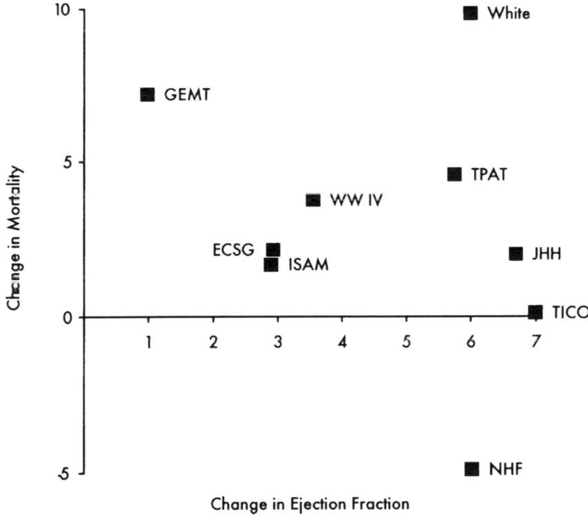

Figure 19–18. Relationship between improvement in ejection fraction and reduction in mortality in 10 placebo-controlled thrombolytic trials. An inconsistent association is noted; however, most of these trials were not powered to detect a difference in mortality. *Reprinted from Califf et al (138), with permission.* For each trial, see reference as follows: GEMT (154), ECSG (67), ISAM (62), WWIV (16), White (77), TPAT (152), JHH (27), TICO (151), and NHF (150).

one of four times (90 minutes, 180 minutes, 24 hours, or 5 to 7 days). The group assigned to the 90-minute angiogram had a follow-up angiogram performed at 5 to 7 days to allow for paired analysis. A total of 967 patients underwent 90-minute angiography, and 733 angiograms were obtained at 5 to 7 days. There was no statistically significant difference in global ejection fraction between the groups at any time frame.

Four other measure of left ventricular function were analyzed, including end-systolic volume index (ml/m^2), regional wall motion (mean excursion of the most abnormal 50% of chords in the infarct region, expressed as the number of standard deviations per chord), number of abnormal chords (number of consecutive chords in the infarct zone >2 standard deviations below the norm), and the percentage of patients with no abnormal chords in the infarct zone. At 90 minutes, the group given t-PA had less depression of regional wall motion in the ischemic zone, fewer abnormal chords, and a larger proportion of patients with preserved wall motion than those given streptokinase. When the 5- to 7-day follow-up angiograms were compared, the regional wall motion and number of abnormal chords remained better in the t-PA group.

Although ejection fraction was not useful for differentiation among treatment groups, it was still a powerful predictor of clinical outcome. Among patients with an ejection fraction above 45%, the 30-day mortality was 3.9%. Conversely, an ejection fraction of less than 45% at 90 minutes was associated with a mortality of 14.7%. Another interesting association was seen between early patency rates and ventricular function. At 90 minutes, TIMI grade 3 flow was associated with a higher global ejection fraction (62 ± 14%) than grade 2 (56 ± 15%), grade 1 (55 ± 15%), or grade 0 flow (55 ± 15%). This improvement was seen in all other measures of left ventricular function and was maintained at the 5- to 7-day angiogram.

HEMORRHAGIC COMPLICATIONS

The use of any plasminogen activator in humans during acute myocardial infarction results in a higher incidence of bleeding complications. A number of factors need to be considered in an analysis of these complications. A major bleeding complication may be defined either on clinical grounds (e.g., life-threatening gastrointestinal bleeding) or as a measure (e.g., absolute decrease in hematocrit of >15%) (159). The latter definition depends on the threshold of the individual physician for administering transfusions after thrombolytic therapy, while the former does not allow for hematological consequences and cannot be quantified. To compare bleeding complications in different studies, the same definitions should be applied to all patients; unfortunately, this is seldom the case. The Landefeld index was developed to overcome these limitations and is defined as the number of packed red blood cell units transfused + (change in hematocrit/3) (160) (see Ch. 20).

A number of baseline characteristics affect hemorrhagic propensity after thrombolytic administration. In general, patients who are female, older, or lighter than average, or who have a history of hypertension are more likely to suffer from greater blood loss (161). Patients who undergo more invasive procedures (acute cardiac catheterization, intraaortic balloon pump insertion, acute coronary artery bypass grafting) also have a higher likelihood of hemorrhagic complications (161). Though the incidence of bleeding complications can be somewhat reduced by adjusting the dose of the thrombolytic agent to the weight of the patient (162), the previously mentioned categories of patients remain more likely to suffer major hemorrhagic complications. In the GUSTO-I trial (59), the incidence of severe or life-threatening bleeding was not statistically different among treatment groups and ranged from 0.3% to 0.6%. The requirement for packed red cell transfusion was lowest in the t-PA group (10%), followed by the streptokinase with subcutaneous heparin (11%), the t-PA–streptokinase (12%), and the streptokinase with intravenous heparin (12%) groups. The bleeding event rates observed in the GUSTO-I trial are similar to data from previous large randomized clinical trials; there does not appear to be a significant difference among thrombolytic agents. Future research should focus on reduction of the bleeding complications associated with thrombolysis, particularly reducing the need for blood transfusions.

The most devastating hemorrhagic complication of thrombolytic therapy is intracranial bleeding. This complication has an associated mortality rate of approximately 40% to 50% and results in significant disability in up to half of the survivors (95,163,164). A pooled analysis of 58,600 patients reported by the FTT Collaborative Group summarized the incidence of stroke after thrombolytic therapy (72). Fibrinolytic therapy was associated with an excess of any stroke within 35 days (1.2% vs. 0.8%, $p < 0.001$) compared with control. The rate of hemorrhagic stroke was also significantly higher with thrombolysis (0.4% vs. 0.1%, $p < 0.001$). Hemorrhagic strokes occurred with an increased incidence early (<24 hours) after initiation of thrombolytic therapy. The overall and hemorrhagic stroke rates in the large randomized clinical trials of various thrombolytic agents are summarized in Table 19–7.

Because of the catastrophic consequences of stroke, prevention is essential. Several risk factors for stroke have been reported (163,165–169), although most studies have had limited power to detect a true difference. These risk factors include advanced age, elevated systolic blood pressure, lower body weight, female sex, history of hypertension, history of cerebrovascular accident or dementia, facial or head trauma within 2 weeks, atrial fibrillation, type and dose of thrombolytic agent, prior anticoagulation, and adjunctive therapy. In the GUSTO-I trial, there were 592 adverse cerebrovascular events (1.4%) in the 41,021 patients randomized (95), of which 268 were primary intracranial hemorrhages. Multivariable logistic regression analysis identified several characteristics that predicted an increased risk for intracranial hemorrhage. The factors include (in decreasing order of association) age, weight, prior cerebrovascular disease, diastolic blood pressure, combination t-PA–streptokinase therapy, hypertension, accelerated t-PA therapy, and systolic blood pressure. Identification of higher-risk patient groups may allow consideration of alternative reperfusion strategies such as direct angioplasty.

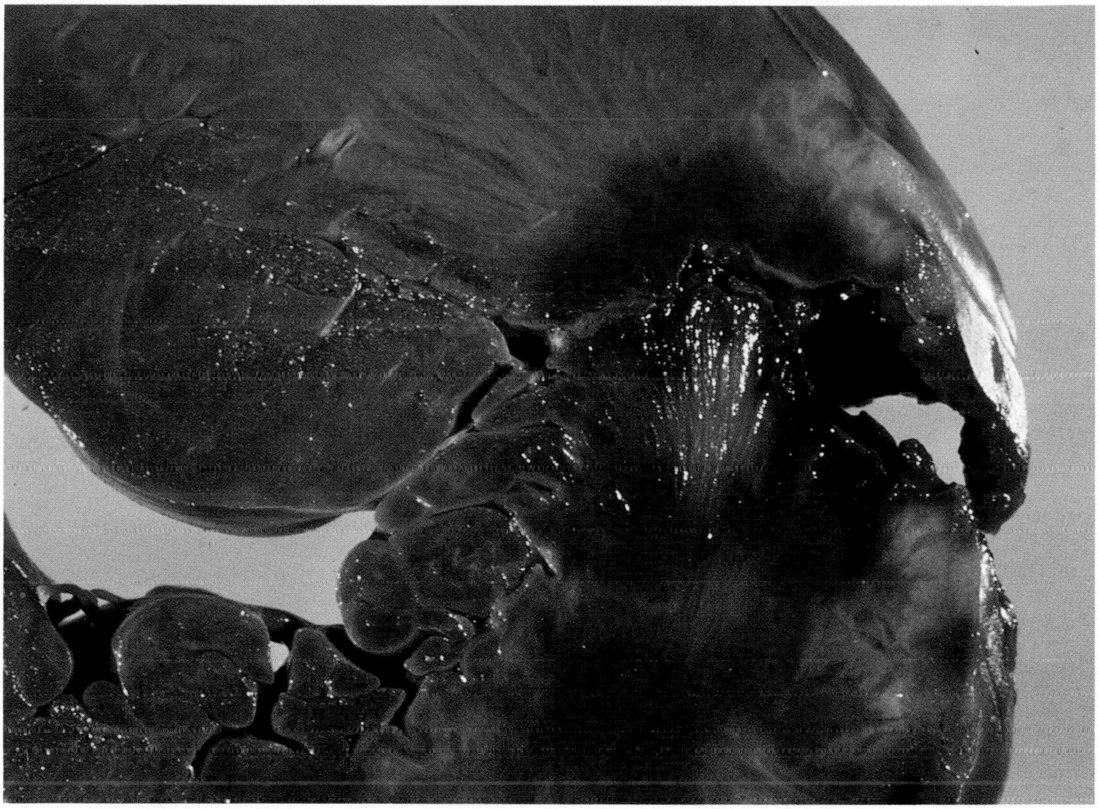

PLATE 1 Autopsy specimen showing a complete rupture of the lateral wall of the left ventricle. The rupture takes a serpiginous path through an area of hemorrhagic infarction.

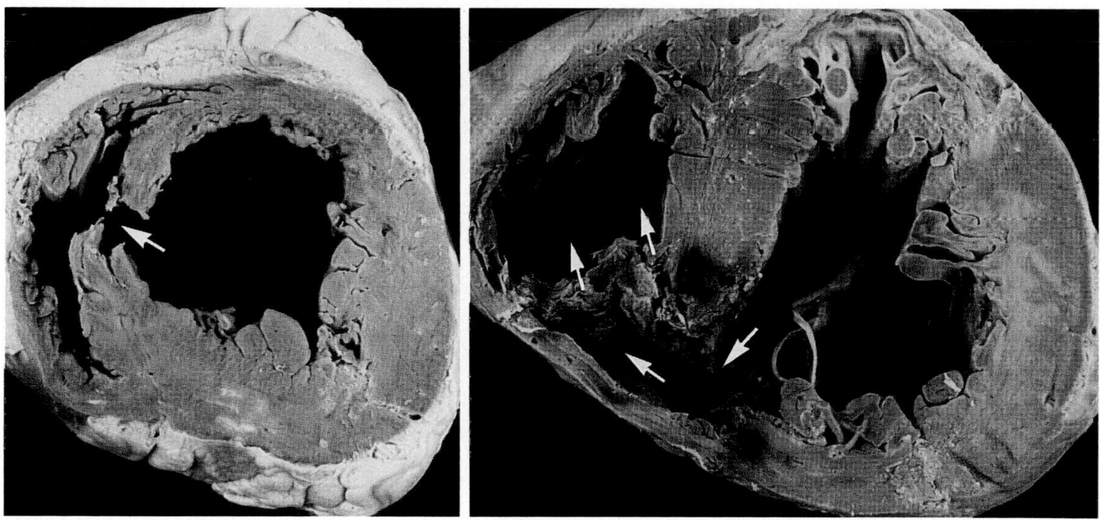

PLATE 2 Autopsy specimens of postinfarction ventricular septal rupture. Apical rupture is simple, with straight rupture tract (arrow, **left**). Inferobasal rupture is complex, with serpiginous rupture tract (arrows, **right**).

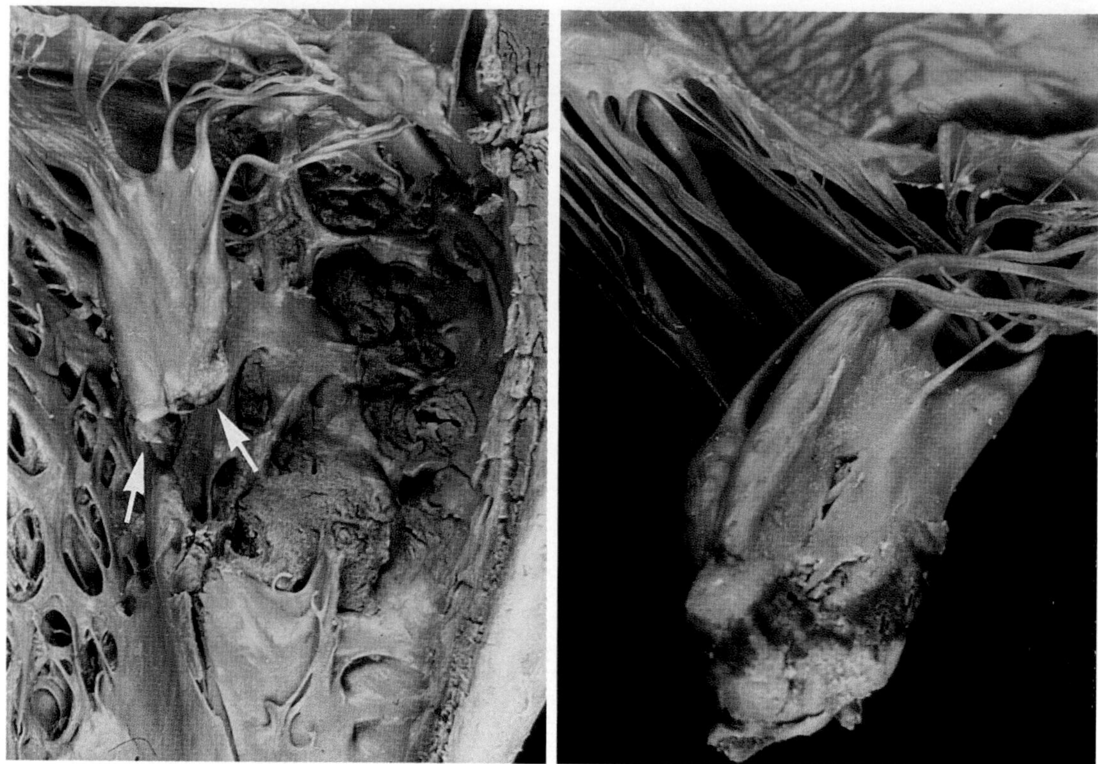

PLATE 3 Autopsy specimen showing postinfarction rupture of the posteromedial mitral papillary muscle. The entire papillary muscle head is ruptured (arrows, **left**). Chordae tendineae tend to become twisted (**right**).

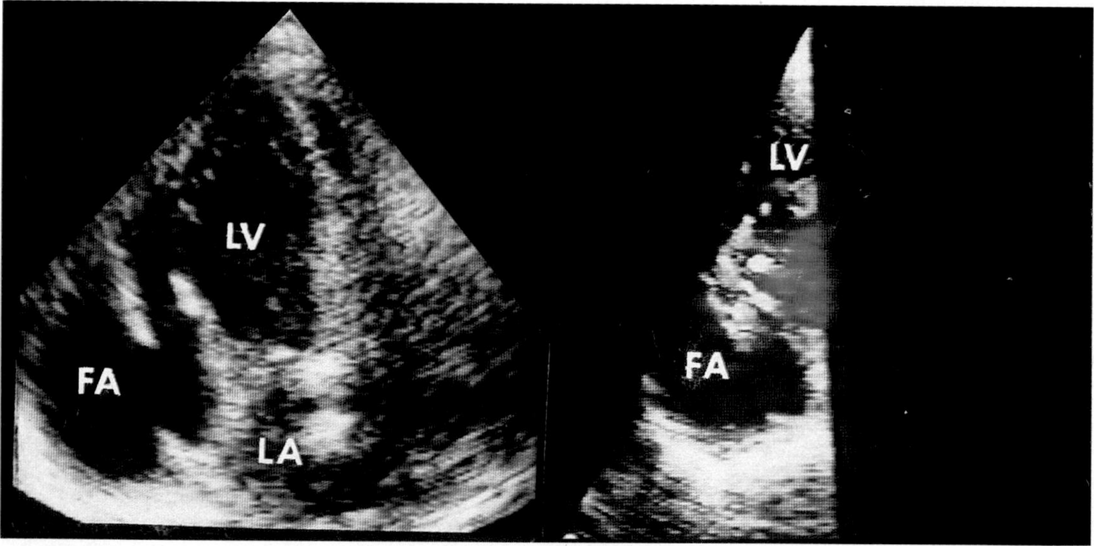

PLATE 4 Precordial echocardiogram from a patient with a false aneurysm. *Top*, Black-and-white still-frame image from a modified apical four-chamber view. There is a large communication between the left ventricle (LV) and the false aneurysm (FA). LA = left atrium. *Bottom,* Color-flow image of the site of communication in early systole (*left*) in which a mosaic color is shown to extend from the left ventricle into the false aneurysm. During late systole (*right*), a blue color extends well into the false aneurysm, indicating direct communication between the left ventricle and the false aneurysm.

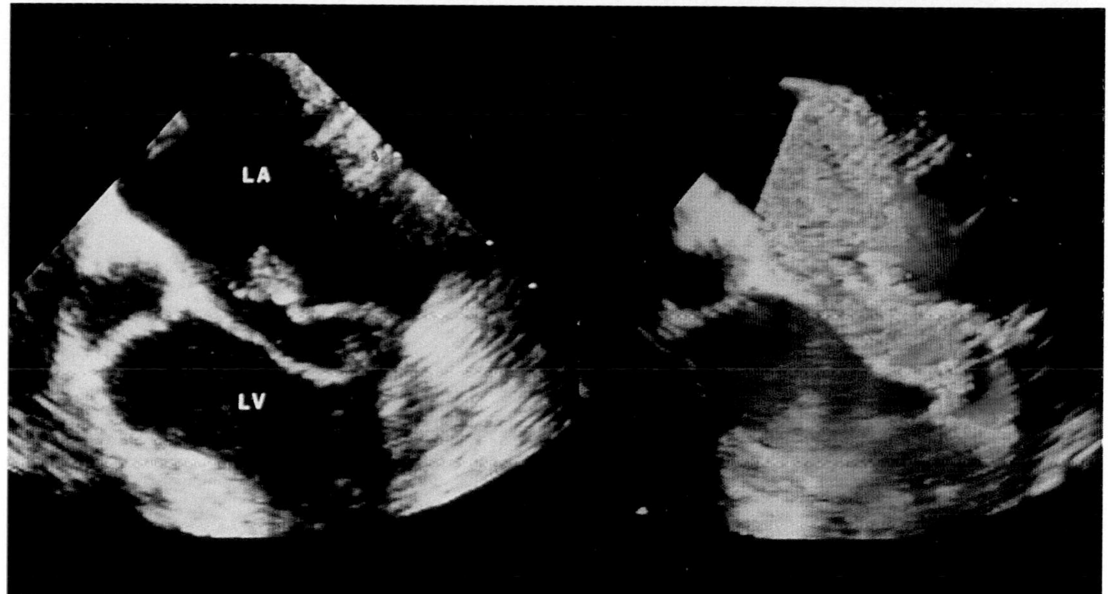

PLATE 5 Transesophageal echocardiogram of a patient with complete rupture of a papillary muscle. *Left,* Black-and-white still-frame image in which the head of the papillary muscle can be visualized attached to the posterior leaflet. There is complete loss of coaptation of the anterior and posterior mitral valve leaflets. *Right,* Color-flow imaging during systole in which there is a wide jet of mitral regurgitation, indicating a significant degree of mitral regurgitation from the papillary muscle rupture. LV = left ventricle, LA = left atrium.

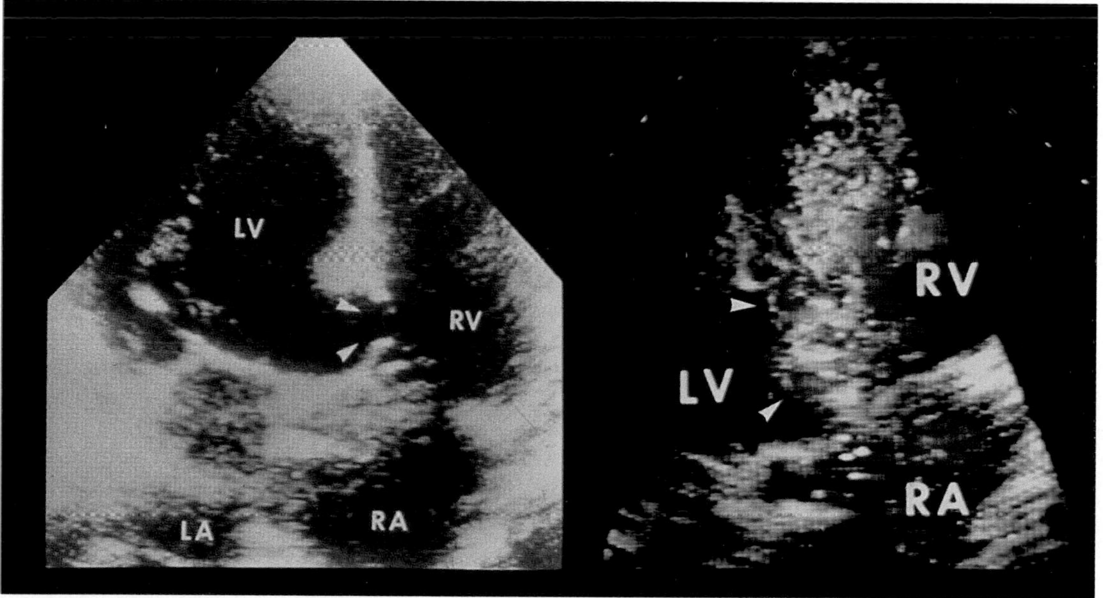

PLATE 6 Precordial two-dimensional echocardiographic image from a patient with a ventricular septal defect of the inferior septum at the basal level. *Left,* Still-frame black-and-white image from the four-chamber apical view. The white arrows indicate communication between the left ventricle (LV) and the right ventricle (RV). *Right,* Color-flow still-frame image that shows a large mosaic pattern emanating from the area of the septal rupture (arrows) into the right ventricle, indicating a right-to-left shunt. LA = left atrium, RA = right atrium.

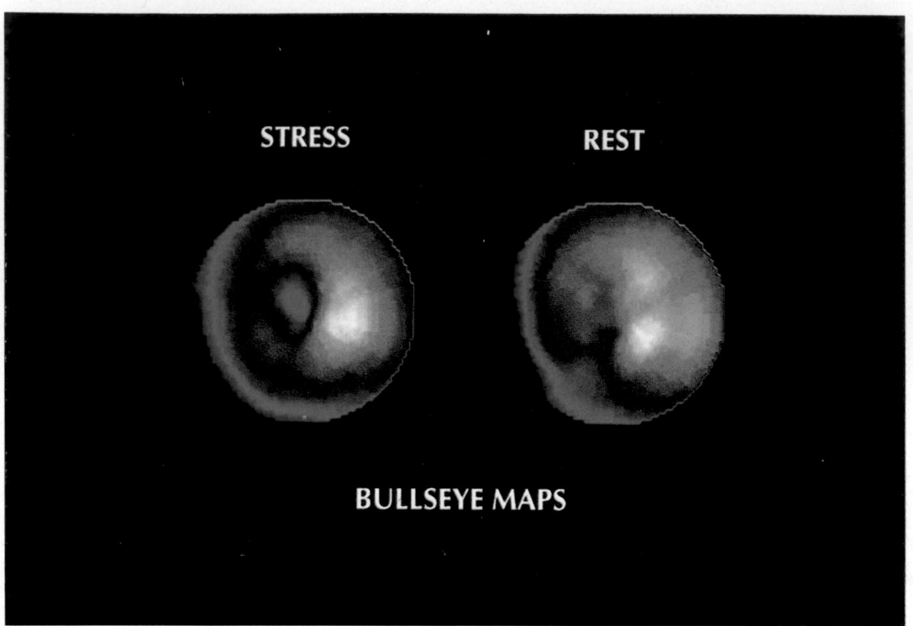

PLATE 7 Technetium-99*m* sestamibi bull's-eye polar map displays at stress (left) and at rest (right) in a patient with a significant left anterior descending coronary artery stenosis. Note the defect in the apex and anteroseptal region at stress, which demonstrates partial reversibility on the resting bull's-eye plot.

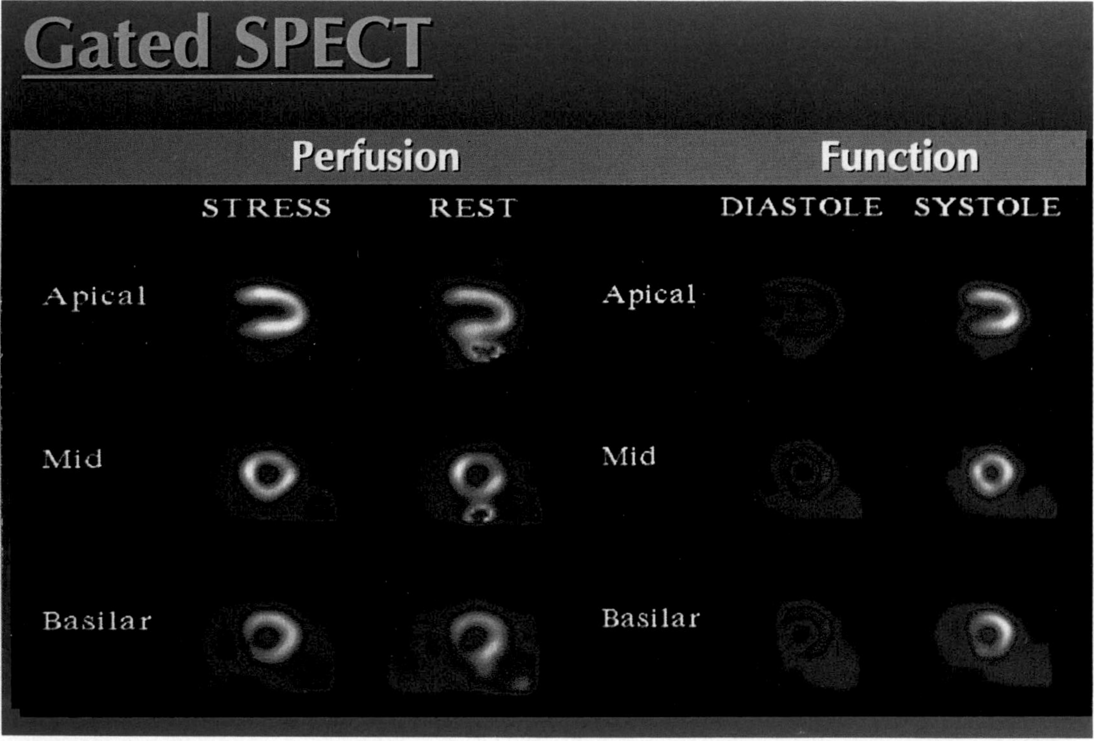

PLATE 8 An example of a patient with a normal gated ^{99m}Tc sestamibi SPECT imaging study. The stress and rest perfusion images are shown on the left, with the vertical long-axis (top row), mid short-axis (middle row), and basilar short-axis (bottom row) tomograms displayed. Note only some basilar septal thinning, which shows no evidence for reversibility. The gated end-diastolic and end-systolic images from the stress study, shown on the right, demonstrate uniform systolic thickening in all myocardial segments reflected by the increased brightness on the end-systolic tomograms (right column).

Table 19–7. Stroke Rates

Agent	Trial	*N*	Overall Stroke Rate (%)	Hemorrhagic Stroke Rate (%)
t-PA	ASSET (65)	2,512	1.1	0.3
	LATE (68)	2,825	2.3	0.8
	ISIS-3 (58)	13,569	1.4	0.7
	GISSI-2 (57)	10,372	1.3	0.4
	GUSTO-I (95)	10,376	1.6	0.7
	RAPID-1, -2 (96,97)	309	3.2	2.3
	Total	**39,855**	**1.47**	**0.61**
Streptokinase	ISIS-2 (63)	8,592	0.7	0.1
	EMERAS (64)	2,234	1.5	0.8
	GISSI-2 (57)	10,396	1.9	0.3
	ISIS-3 (58)	13,607	1.0	0.2
	GUSTO-I* (59)	20,213	1.3	0.5
	INJECT (98)	2,971	1.0	0.4
	Total	**57,823**	**1.09**	**0.35**
APSAC	AIMS (69)	624	1.3	0.3
	ISIS-3 (58)	13,599	1.3	0.6
	Total	**14,223**	**1.27**	**0.54**
r-PA	RAPID-1, -2 (96,97)	323	0.9	0.6
	INJECT (98)	2,965	1.2	0.8
	Total	**3,288**	**1.19**	**0.76**

*Pooled streptokinase arms.

THE OPEN ARTERY CONCEPT

Although the importance of early, sustained coronary reperfusion has been discussed, the concept of the open artery theory and the mechanisms for improved survival should be reviewed (170–174). Multiple studies have shown improvement in long-term survival in patients discharged with a patent infarct-related artery; however, the mechanisms behind this benefit have not been clearly defined. These mechanisms have previously been classified as time dependent or non time dependent. The reduction in mortality with very early reperfusion is attributed to myocardial salvage with preservation of left ventricular function. Previous animal reperfusion studies have confirmed this time dependent salvage of jeopardized myocardium (139,175). By 2 hours, less than 50% of ischemic myocardium remains viable; this decreases to less than 20% after 6 hours of coronary occlusion. Therefore, the contribution of myocardial salvage as a mechanism for reduction in mortality decreases quickly over time.

Other factors that were previously considered non–time dependent, including improved healing and remodeling, less cavity dilation, reduced wall stress, lower rates of ventricular aneurysm formation and cardiac rupture, maintenance of a conduit for collateral blood supply, and increased myocardial electrical stability, are listed in Table 19–8. These factors should probably be considered only "less" time dependent, because they exert a greater contribution to the survival benefit of later reperfusion. The concept of the open artery hypothesis is

Table 19–8. Potential Mechanisms for Mortality Reduction with Thrombolytic Therapy

Time Dependent
Myocardial salvage
Preservation of left ventricular function
Less Time Dependent
Improved healing and remodeling
Less cavity dilation and reduced wall stress
Lower rates of ventricular aneurysm formation and cardiac rupture
Maintenance of a conduit for collateral blood supply
Increased myocardial electrical stability

Table 19–9. Importance of Patency in Long-Term Mortality After Myocardial Infarction

Study (Year)	n	Intervention	Follow-up (months)	Mortality (%)	
				Open Artery	Closed Artery
Kennedy (1985)	134	Lytic	12	5	15
Dalen (1988)	289	Lytic	12	8	15
Mathey (1988)	227	Lytic	48	16	37
Simoons (1989)	234	Lytic + PTCA	36	9	33
Kander (1989)	293	Lytic + PTCA	21	6	6
Taylor (1992)	180	Lytic	74	6	19
Brodie (1992)	348	PTCA	40	5	7
Moliterno (1992)	200	PTCA,CABG	42	2	16
Total (95% CI)	1,917			7 (6–9)	18 (15–21)

Lytic = intravenous thrombolytic therapy, PTCA = percutaneous transluminal coronary angioplasty, CABG = coronary artery bypass surgery, CI = confidence interval. *Data from Ohman and Christenson (176).*

intriguing, but complex and poorly understood. Future research will undoubtedly provide a greater understanding of the mechanisms of survival benefit from early versus late coronary reperfusion. The long-term importance of patency of the infarct-related artery at the time of discharge is underscored by observational studies (Table 19–9) with a lower long-term mortality with sustained reperfustion (176).

PATIENT SELECTION

Appropriate patient selection is important, so that the maximum number of patients can benefit from reperfusion therapy without suffering serious or life-threatening complications (177,178). Inclusion and exclusion criteria for thrombolysis have undergone considerable evolution over the last 10 years; the composite results of thousands of patients randomized in various protocols have provided important efficacy and safety data for many patient subgroups. The FTT Collaborative Group results can aid in the selection of patients who would benefit from thrombolysis (72). These pooled data reinforce the need for electrocardiographic changes suggestive of acute myocardial infarction, the importance of early treatment (with significant benefit extending to 12 hours after symptom onset), and the benefit to multiple patient populations (elderly patients, women, and diabetics) (Fig. 19–19). The American College of Cardiology and the American Heart Association have published guidelines for the use of thrombolytic therapy (179). The current criteria for and contraindications to thrombolytic therapy are summarized in Table 19–10.

Although the majority of patients who suffer a myocardial infarction are ineligible for thrombolytic therapy, the percentage of eligible patients who are treated is disappointingly low and varies between 20% and 60% (180). The proportion of treated patients is difficult to determine and varies depending on how the infarct population is defined. Previous reports have used retrospective analyses based on a discharge diagnosis of myocardial infarction. In the GUSTO-I trial, data from 106 North American hospitals were collected on patients with MBCK-documented myocardial infarction. Of the 637 patients with such a diagnosis, only 31% were treated with thrombolytic therapy. However, many of these patients were ineligible according to the criteria listed in Table 19–10. Among the fully eligible patients (those with electrocardiographic criteria, presentation within 12 hours of symptom onset, and no contraindications), the majority (85%) received thrombolytic therapy (181). With increased awareness and improved treatment strategies, the proportion of patients treated should continue to increase.

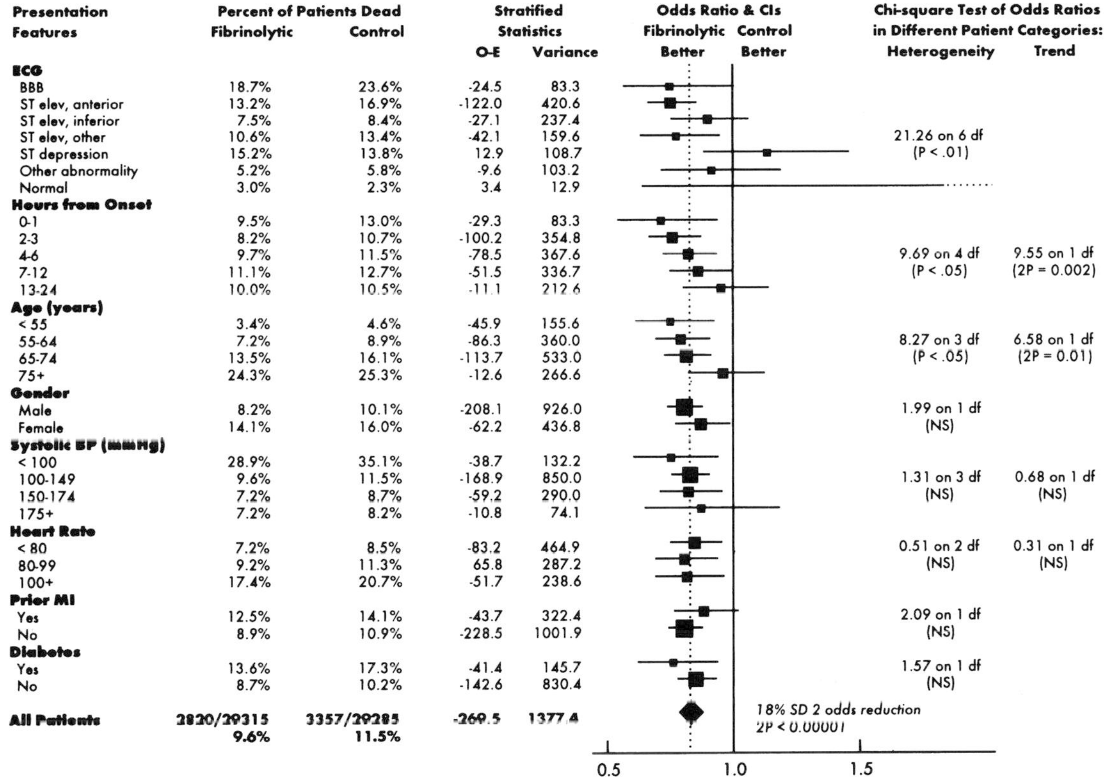

Presentation Features	Percent of Patients Dead: Fibrinolytic	Percent of Patients Dead: Control	Stratified Statistics: O-E	Stratified Statistics: Variance	Chi-square Test of Odds Ratios in Different Patient Categories: Heterogeneity	Trend
ECG						
BBB	18.7%	23.6%	-24.5	83.3		
ST elev, anterior	13.2%	16.9%	-122.0	420.6		
ST elev, inferior	7.5%	8.4%	-27.1	237.4		
ST elev, other	10.6%	13.4%	-42.1	159.6	21.26 on 6 df	
ST depression	15.2%	13.8%	12.9	108.7	(P < .01)	
Other abnormality	5.2%	5.8%	-9.6	103.2		
Normal	3.0%	2.3%	3.4	12.9		
Hours from Onset						
0-1	9.5%	13.0%	-29.3	83.3		
2-3	8.2%	10.7%	-100.2	354.8		
4-6	9.7%	11.5%	-78.5	367.6	9.69 on 4 df	9.55 on 1 df
7-12	11.1%	12.7%	-51.5	336.7	(P < .05)	(2P = 0.002)
13-24	10.0%	10.5%	-11.1	212.6		
Age (years)						
< 55	3.4%	4.6%	-45.9	155.6		
55-64	7.2%	8.9%	-86.3	360.0	8.27 on 3 df	6.58 on 1 df
65-74	13.5%	16.1%	-113.7	533.0	(P < .05)	(2P = 0.01)
75+	24.3%	25.3%	-12.6	266.6		
Gender						
Male	8.2%	10.1%	-208.1	926.0	1.99 on 1 df	
Female	14.1%	16.0%	-62.2	436.8	(NS)	
Systolic BP (mmHg)						
< 100	28.9%	35.1%	-38.7	132.2		
100-149	9.6%	11.5%	-168.9	850.0	1.31 on 3 df	0.68 on 1 df
150-174	7.2%	8.7%	-59.2	290.0	(NS)	(NS)
175+	7.2%	8.2%	-10.8	74.1		
Heart Rate						
< 80	7.2%	8.5%	-83.2	464.9	0.51 on 2 df	0.31 on 1 df
80-99	9.2%	11.3%	65.8	287.2	(NS)	(NS)
100+	17.4%	20.7%	-51.7	238.6		
Prior MI						
Yes	12.5%	14.1%	-43.7	322.4	2.09 on 1 df	
No	8.9%	10.9%	-228.5	1001.9	(NS)	
Diabetes						
Yes	13.6%	17.3%	-41.4	145.7	1.57 on 1 df	
No	8.7%	10.2%	-142.6	830.4	(NS)	
All Patients	2820/29315 9.6%	3357/29285 11.5%	-269.5	1377.4		

Figure 19–19. Indications for fibrinolytic therapy in suspected acute myocardial infarction. Most patient subgroups appear to benefit from early thrombolysis. BBB = bundle branch block, CIs = confidence intervals, df = degrees of freedom, NS = not significant, O–E = observed minus expected, SD = standard deviation. *From the Fibrinolytic Therapy Trialists' (FTT) Collaborative Group (72), reprinted with permission of The Lancet, Ltd.*

The pooled results of trials have reinforced that the benefit of thrombolytic therapy in the treatment of acute myocardial infarction is time dependent (72) (Fig. 19–20). The ability to obtain early, sustained coronary perfusion results in improved myocardial salvage and enhanced clinical outcome. Although much emphasis has focused on developing thrombolytic and adjunctive treatment strategies to improve reperfusion time, there is also a need for decreasing any delays that may occur from symptom onset to reperfusion.

The individual components of delay are shown in Fig. 19–21 and can be divided into patient, transport, and in-hospital delays, and drug perfusion time (182–184). Various educational campaigns directed toward high-risk groups have emphasized the need to seek early medical attention for symptoms suggestive of acute myocardial infarction (185–190). This deserves particular attention since patient delays are quite variable and can be extreme.

The second area of delay involves transportation time. To significantly shorten treatment time, several investigations have targeted this time period for possible therapeutic interventions (191,192). The prehospital administration of thrombolytic therapy was studied in the Grampian Region Early Anistreplase Trial (GREAT) (192,193), the Myocardial Infarction Triage and Intervention (MITI) Project (194), and the European Myocardial Infarction Project (EMIP) (195). A meta-analysis of all randomized prehospital thrombolytic trials shows a significant 16% reduction in mortality ($p = 0.01$): mortality in the hospital-

Table 19–10. Patient Selection for Thrombolytic Therapy

Criteria
Chest pain >20 minutes consistent with acute myocardial infarction
Electrocardiographic
ST segment elevation of at least 0.1 mm in at least two contiguous leads
Left bundle branch block with clinical characteristics of acute myocardial infarction
Patient presentation within 12 hours of symptom onset
Expanded population subsets
Elderly (no upper age limit)
Controlled hypertension
Nontraumatic cardiopulmonary resuscitation (<10 minutes)
Contraindications (Absolute)
Active internal bleeding
Aortic dissection
Acute pericarditis
History of serious bleeding tendency
Major surgery head trauma, or stroke within 6 months
Traumatic cardiopulmonary resuscitation
Prior intracranial bleeding, cerebral neoplasm, or other major intracranial pathology
Contraindications (Relative)
Recent surgery or gastrointestinal bleeding (<2 months)
Severe, persistent hypertension (diastolic blood pressure >100 mm Hg)
Pregnancy, or within 1 month postpartum
Recent major trauma (<2 weeks), including cardiopulmonary resuscitation with rib fractures
Vascular puncture in a noncompressible site

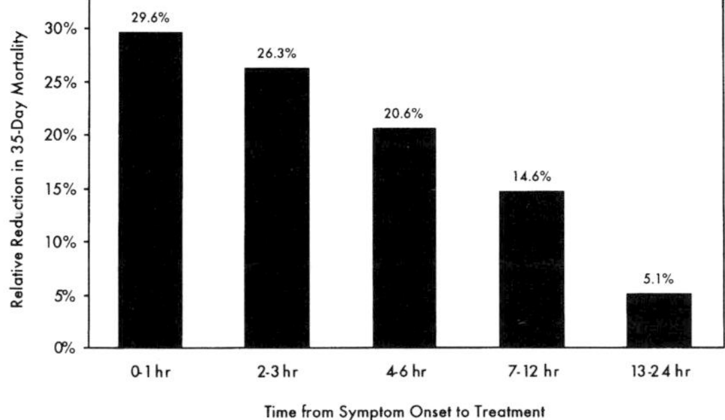

Figure 19–20. Decrease in mortality reduction with increasing time to thrombolytic treatment. *Data from the Fibrinolytic Therapy Trialists' (FTT) Collaborative Group (72).*

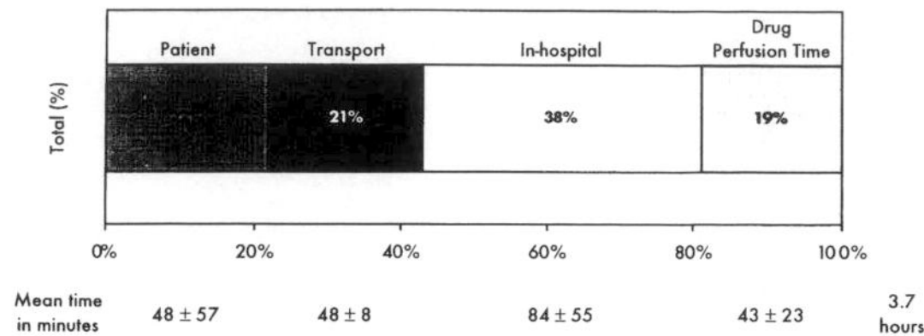

Figure 19–21. Components of delay until reperfusion is achieved. *Reprinted from Gersh and Anderson (182), with permission.*

thrombolysis group was 10.8% (357 of 3,316) compared with 9.0% (295 of 3,291) in the prehospital-thrombolysis group (196). Although these results are promising, there are many limitations of prehospital administration of thrombolytic therapy, including the need for skilled personnel, maintenance of a stock of drugs, overall cost, and the potential for misdiagnosis and litigation.

Strategies to limit in-hospital delays are also critical. Various protocols, procedures, and training programs have attempted to improve "door-to-needle" time. A GUSTO-I substudy examined the reasons for delay and subsequently randomized hospitals to a team approach to treatment or to control. The mean time to initiation of thrombolytic therapy was improved from 70 minutes to 63 minutes ($p = 0.015$) (197). Undoubtedly, future research efforts will focus on improving the time to therapy and developing more effective thrombolytic and adjunctive medical strategies to restore coronary flow. Caution must be maintained with the use of more potent regimens, however, due to the risk of unintended complications, particularly hemorrhagic stroke.

REPEAT THROMBOLYSIS

The use of thrombolytic therapy in acute myocardial infarction restores coronary perfusion, decreases infarct size, and improves mortality. However, once coronary flow is restored, the underlying unstable atherosclerotic plaque can cause reocclusion. Reocclusion can be clinically silent, result in ischemia, or lead to reinfarction. Pooled analysis of large randomized clinical trials has documented a slightly higher reinfarction rate among patients treated with thrombolytic therapy; the pooled reinfarction rates were 3.2% for t-PA (57–59,65,68), 3.4% for streptokinase (57–60,62–64,84), and 3.7% for APSAC (58,70) compared with a 2.7% incidence for patients in the control arms. In the GUSTO-I trial (198), reinfarction within 30 days of the index infarction occurred in 4% of patients (1,628 of 41,021). There was no significant difference in reinfarction rates among the four treatment strategies, and the average time from index infarction to reinfarction was 4 days. Patients who suffered reinfarction had a significantly higher 30-day mortality, ranging from 17% to 20%, compared with the overall observed mortality rates of 6.3% to 7.4%. Other studies confirm this observation and also have found reinfarction to be a predictor of increased long-term mortality (199,200).

From these observations, it is clear that specific strategies to prevent and treat this complication must be developed. Strategies to prevent reinfarction include recognition of high-risk groups, continuous electrocardiographic monitoring, and adjunctive pharmacological approaches. Reinfarction after thrombolytic therapy should be treated with the same urgency as the initial myocardial infarction. Studies of repeat thrombolytic therapy have shown improvement in clinical outcomes after reinfarction without an increased incidence of hemorrhagic stroke (201 204). In the GUSTO-I trial, patients with reinfarction who underwent repeat thrombolysis had a 30-day mortality of 11% compared with 24% in patients who did not receive repeat infusions (205).

Special consideration must be given to the repeat use of thrombolytic agents known to induce an immune response: streptokinase, APSAC, and staphylokinase. Antibody titers 34 weeks after administration of streptokinase are sufficiently high to completely inhibit a repeated standard dose of streptokinase (175). This observation has led to the recommendation that streptokinase administration not be repeated within 1 year; instead, administration of a nonantigenic agent (t-PA, r-PA, urokinase, or scuPA) is recommended (41).

ADJUNCTIVE THERAPIES

The ISIS-II study showed clearly that antiplatelet therapy with aspirin significantly improved the outcome of patients when it was combined with intravenous streptokinase (see Ch. 12). This opened an avenue for exploring potent antiplatelet/antithrombin therapies in acute myocardial infarction. A higher patency rate has been suggested for intravenous heparin in patients receiving t-PA therapy, and a 9% reduction (odds ratio 0.91, 95% confidence interval 0.59–1.39) in-hospital mortality was shown in a recent pooled analysis of six randomized controlled trials (206). However, this same analysis showed a significantly higher rate of hemorrhagic complications when t-PA and intravenous heparin were combined (206). Since no studies have examined the use of front-loaded t-PA alone, intravenous heparin should also be administered if t-PA is given in this way, but future randomized trials should examine the risk-to-benefit ratio of intravenous heparin administration with more potent thrombolytic strategies.

The value of intravenous heparin in conjunction with nonspecific fibrinolytic agents such as streptokinase and APSAC has also been explored in randomized trials. In the GUSTO-I trial, there was no difference in 30-day mortality in the patients assigned to subcutaneous versus intravenous heparin (7.2% versus 7.4%) (59). Furthermore, there was no significant difference in rate of stroke or intracranial hemorrhage between these two groups of patients. The rates of recurrent ischemia and reinfarction were also similar. The value of intravenous heparin in conjunction with APSAC was explored in the Duke University Clinical Cardiology Studies (DUCCS)-I trial. In this study, there was no evidence of a benefit in patients who received intravenous APSAC with intravenous heparin over those who received APSAC with placebo. There was, moreover, a significant increase in hemorrhagic events in the patients who received intravenous heparin (207). Thus, from this evidence, along with the lack of benefit shown with the addition of subcutaneous heparin to streptokinase or APSAC therapy in both the GISSI-2 and ISIS-3 studies, we can conclude that antithrombin therapy with intravenous heparin adds little when streptokinase or APSAC is being used (see Ch. 20).

There has been renewed interest in the use of more potent antithrombin therapies in conjunction with streptokinase. Early dose-ranging trials of antithrombin agents such as hirulog (208) and efegatran (Weaver WD, personal communication) have been performed. All of the trials to date have suggested slightly higher rates of TIMI grade 3 flow or patency at 90-minute angiography. However, these strategies have not been evaluated in large clinical trials, and the safety of this approach has yet to be explored (see Ch. 20).

A variety of antithrombin therapies have also been evaluated with front-loaded t-PA treatment. A careful dose-ranging trial by the TIMI investigators showed that hirudin was associated with not only slightly improved patency rates at 90 minutes (in comparison with heparin) but also lower rates of mortality, recurrent ischemia, and reinfarction (209). A subsequent large randomized trial of intravenous hirudin in acute ischemic syndromes noted an excess rate of intracranial hemorrhage in patients assigned hirudin plus t-PA or streptokinase (210). Subsequent reduction of the dose and exclusion of patients who had histories of stroke led to an enhanced safety profile.

In the GUSTO-IIb trial, 12,142 patients with acute coronary syndromes were randomly assigned to 72 hours of therapy with either heparin or hirudin (211). Although patients randomized to hirudin had a significant reduction in death and myocardial infarction at 24 hours, this therapeutic benefit was not sustained. At 30 days, the primary endpoint of death or nonfatal myocardial infarction occurred in 9.8% of the heparin group versus 8.9% of the hirudin group ($p = 0.058$). Of the 4,131 patients who presented with ST-segment elevation, 74% received thrombolytic therapy with either t-PA (70%) or streptokinase (30%). The 30-day mortality or reinfarction rate was 11.3% for the heparin group versus 9.9% for the hirudin group ($p = 0.13$). The role of antithrombin therapy in conjunction with thrombolytic therapy awaits further cost-benefit and other data analyses.

Given the considerable benefit of adding aspirin to streptokinase, modification of platelet activation during acute myocardial infarction has been investigated. An early dose-ranging experience with prostacyclins failed—the risk of hemorrhage increased, and no clinical benefit was shown (212). Subsequently, a chimeric antibody to the platelet glycoprotein IIb/IIIa receptor (which is the final pathway of platelet activation, leading to aggregation) has been evaluated. In an initial early dose-ranging trial (213), this antibody (c7E3 Fab) was given after a standard 3-hour dose of t-PA. Although this trial was too small to provide firm estimates on either clinical outcomes or hemorrhagic events, it did suggest that when the therapy was administered shortly after the cessation of t-PA, a better clinical outcomes profile was observed. More recently, Integrilin™, a glycoprotein IIb/IIIa receptor blocker, has been evaluated in a dose-ranging trial in combination with front-loaded t-PA. In this early experience, it was noted that substantial platelet activation occurs in patients receiving t-PA in acute myocardial infarction (214). Continued evaluation has suggested superior patency and TIMI grade 3 flow rates in patients receiving Integrilin™ with front-loaded t-PA, aspirin, and heparin versus those receiving placebo with the same therapies (215). Furthermore, this has been accompanied by a significant reduction in ischemia as detected by 24-hour ST segment monitoring (216). There are limited data on the use of streptokinase in conjunction with potent antiplatelet therapies, although this is under investigation in the Phase III PARADIGM trial. Thus antiplatelet therapies appear to be associated with higher patency rates and possible reductions in ischemia, although the safety profiles of these agents will need to be explored in larger clinical investigations.

Adjunctive therapies such as potent antithrombin/antiplatelet agents appear to have much to offer in the future, given that only half of patients receiving thrombolytic therapy achieve successful reperfusion at the tissue level (101). The challenges for clinical investigation in this field are finding the appropriate dose with various thrombolytic therapies as well as establishing an adequate safety profile in larger patient populations. Despite these caveats, the adjunctive therapies have much to offer to improve outcomes in patients with acute myocardial infarction who receive thrombolytic therapy.

CONCLUSIONS

The results of multiple clinical trials have documented the ability of fibrinolytic agents to reduce mortality in patients with acute myocardial infarction. This clinical benefit is achieved by early establishment of rapid, complete coronary reperfusion. Data suggest that restoring tissue-level reperfusion results in myocardial salvage, improved left ventricular function, and increased electrical stability. Future research will focus on earlier treatment, developing noninvasive methods to detect reperfusion, achieving more rapid, complete, and sustained coronary perfusion (with more potent thrombolytic, antiplatelet, or antithrombin agents), preventing reperfusion injury, reducing complications, and developing cost-effective treatment strategies.

REFERENCES

1. Yusuf S, Wittes J, Friedman L: Overview of results of randomized clinical trials in heart disease: I. Treatments following myocardial infarction. *JAMA* 1988;260:2088–2093.
2. DeWood MA, Spores J, Notske R, et al: Prevalence of total coronary occlusion during the early hours of transmural myocardial infarction. *N Engl J Med* 1980;303:897–902.
3. Libby P: Molecular bases of the acute coronary syndromes. *Circulation* 1995;91:2844–2850.
4. Kawai C: Pathogenesis of acute myocardial infarction, novel regulatory systems of bioactive substances in the vessel wall. *Circulation* 1994;90:1033–1043.
5. Chazov EL, Matteeva LS, Mazaev AV, et al: Intracoronary administration of fibrinolysis in acute myocardial infarction. *Ter Arkh* 1976;48:8–19.
6. Mueller RL, Scheidt S: History of drugs for thrombotic disease: discovery, development, and directions for the future. *Circulation* 1994;89:432–449.
7. Sherry S, Marder VJ: Thrombosis, fibrinolysis, and thrombolytic therapy: A perspective. *Prog Cardiovasc Dis* 1991;34:89–100.
8. MacFarlane RG, Pilling J: Fibrinolytic activity in normal urine. *Nature* 1947;159:779.
9. Williams JRB: The fibrinolytic activity of the urine. *Br J Exp Pathol* 1951;32:530–537.
10. Sobel GW, Mohler SR, Jones NW, Dowdy ABC, Guest MM: Urokinase: An activator of plasma profibrinolysin extracted from urine. *Am J Physiol* 1952;171:768–769.
11. Tillett WS, Garner RL: The fibrinolytic activity of streptococci. *J Exp Med* 1933;58:485–502.
12. Fletcher AP, Alkjaersig N, Smyrniotis FE, Sherry S: Treatment of patients suffering from early, myocardial infarction with massive and prolonged streptokinase therapy. *Trans Assoc Am Physicians* 1958;71:287–296.
13. Yusuf S, Collins R, Peto R, et al: Intravenous and intracoronary fibrinolytic therapy in acute myocardial infarction: Overview of results on mortality, reinfarction and side effects from 33 randomised controlled trials. *Eur Heart J* 1985;6:556–585.
14. Rentrop KP, Blanke H, Karsch KR, et al: Acute myocardial infarction: Intracoronary application of nitroglycerin and streptokinase. *Clin Cardiol* 1979;2:354–363.
15. Kennedy JW, Ritchie JL, Davis KB, Fritz JK: Western Washington randomized trial of intracoronary streptokinase in acute myocardial infarction. *N Engl J Med* 1983;309:1477–1482.
16. Ritchie JL, Davis KB, Williams DL, Caldwell J, Kennedy JW: Global and regional left ventricular function and tomographic radionuclide perfusion: The Western Washington Intracoronary Streptokinase in Myocardial Infarction Trial. *Circulation* 1984;70:867–875.
17. Mathey DG, Sheehan FH, Schofer J, Dodge HT: Time from onset of symptoms to thrombolytic therapy: A major determinant of myocardial salvage in patients with acute transmural infarction. *J Am Coll Cardiol* 1985;6:518–525.
18. Smith RAG, Dupe RJ, English PD, et al: Fibrinolysis with acyl-enzymes: A new approach to thrombolytic therapy. *Nature* 1981;290:505–508.
19. Pennica D, Holmes WE, Kohr WJ, et al: Cloning and expression of human tissue-type plasminogen activator cDNA in *E. coli*. *Nature* 1983;301:214–221.
20. Williams DO, Sharaf BL, McKendall GR: An overview of trials investigating the role of adjunctive mechanical revascularization with thrombolysis. *Cor Art Dis* 1992;3:109–116.
21. Labinaz M, Ellis SG, Phillips HR III, Ohman EM: The role of angioplasty after successful thrombolysis for acute myocardial infarction. *Cor Art Dis* 1994;5:399–406.

22. Meyer J, Merx W, Schmitz H, et al: Percutaneous transluminal coronary angioplasty immediately after intracoronary streptolysis of transmural myocardial infarction. *Circulation* 1982;66:905–913.
23. Stack RS, O'Connor CM, Mark DB, et al: Coronary perfusion during acute myocardial infarction with a combined therapy of coronary angioplasty and high-dose intravenous streptokinase. *Circulation* 1988;77:151–161.
24. Yasuno M, Saito Y, Ishida M, et al: Effects of percutaneous transluminal coronary angioplasty: Intracoronary thrombolysis with urokinase in acute myocardial infarction. *Am J Cardiol* 1984;53:1217–1220.
25. Topol EJ, O'Neill WW, Langburd AB, et al: A randomized, placebo-controlled trial of intravenous recombinant tissue-type plasminogen activator and emergency coronary angioplasty in patients with acute myocardial infarction. *Circulation* 1987;75:420–428.
26. Topol EJ, Califf RM, George BS, et al: A randomized trial of immediate versus delayed elective angioplasty after intravenous tissue plasminogen activator in acute myocardial infarction. *N Engl J Med* 1987;317:581–588.
27. Guerci AD, Gerstenblith G, Brinker JA, et al: A randomized trial of intravenous tissue plasminogen activator for acute myocardial infarction with subsequent randomization to elective coronary angioplasty. *N Engl J Med* 1987;317:1613–1618.
28. Simoons ML, Arnold AE, Betriu A, et al: Thrombolysis with tissue plasminogen activator in acute myocardial infarction: No additional benefit from immediate percutaneous coronary angioplasty. *Lancet* 1988;1:197–203.
29. TIMI Study Group: Comparison of invasive and conservative strategies after treatment with intravenous tissue plasminogen activator in acute myocardial infarction. Results of the Thrombolysis in Myocardial Infarction (TIMI) phase II trial. *N Engl J Med* 1989;320:618–627.
30. Fung AY, Lai P, Topol EJ, et al: Value of percutaneous transluminal coronary angioplasty after unsuccessful intravenous streptokinase therapy in acute myocardial infarction. *Am J Cardiol* 1986;58:686–691.
31. Califf RM, Topol EJ, George BS, et al: Characteristics and outcome of patients in whom reperfusion with intravenous tissue-type plasminogen activator fails: Results of the Thrombolysis and Angioplasty in Myocardial Infarction (TAMI) I trial. *Circulation* 1988;77:1090–1099.
32. O'Connor CM, Mark DB, Hinohara T, et al: Rescue coronary angioplasty after failure of intravenous streptokinase in acute myocardial infarction: In-hospital and long-term outcomes. *J Invas Cardiol* 1989;1:85–89.
33. Ellis SG, da Silva ER, Heyndrickx G, et al: Randomized comparison of rescue angioplasty with conservative management of patients with early failure of thrombolysis for acute anterior myocardial infarction. *Circulation* 1994;90:2280–2284.
34. Topol EJ: Coronary angioplasty for acute myocardial infarction. *Ann Intern Med* 1988;109:970–980.
35. Rothbaum DA, Linnemeier TJ, Landin RJ, et al: Emergency percutaneous transluminal coronary angioplasty in acute myocardial infarction: A 3 year experience. *J Am Coll Cardiol* 1987;10:264–272.
36. Haire WD: Pharmacology of fibrinolysis. *Chest* 1992;4:91S–97S.
37. Robbins KC: Fibrinolytic therapy: Biochemical mechanisms. *Thromb Haemost* 1991;17:1–6.
38. Henkin J, Marcotte P, Yang H: The plasminogen–plasmin system. *Prog Cardiovasc Dis* 1991;34:135–164.
39. Marder VJ, Sherry S: Thrombolytic therapy: Current status (first of two parts). *N Engl J Med* 1988;318:1512–1520.
40. Jalihal S, Morris GK: Antistreptokinase titres after intravenous streptokinase. *Lancet* 1990;1:184–185.
41. Cross D, White H: Antistreptokinase titres after intravenous streptokinase. *Lancet* 1990;1:534.
42. Berger H, Pizzo SV: Preparation of polyethylene glycol tissue plasminogen activator adducts that retain functional activity: Characteristics and behavior in three animal species. *Blood* 1988;71:1641–1647.
43. Bang NU: Tissue-type plasminogen activator mutants—theoretical and clinical considerations. *Circulation* 1989;79:1391–1392.
44. Runge MS, Quertermous T, Haber E: Plasminogen activators, the old and the new. *Circulation* 1989;79:217–224.
45. Koster RW, Cohen AF, Hopkins GR, Beier H, Gunzler WA, van der Wouw PA: Pharmacokinetics and pharmacodynamics of saruplase, an unglycosylated single-chain urokinase-type plasminogen activator, in patients with acute myocardial infarction. *Thromb Haemost* 1994;72:740–744.

46. Collen D, Van de Werf F: Coronary thrombolysis with recombinant staphylokinase in patients with evolving myocardial infarction. *Circulation* 1993;87: 1850–1853.

47. Collen D, DeCock F, Stassen J: Comparative immunogencity and thrombolytic properties toward arterial and venous thrombi of streptokinase and recombinant staphylokinase in baboons. *Circulation* 1993;87:996–1006.

48. Collen D, Lignen HR, Gold HK: Towards better thrombolytic therapy. *Prog Cardiovasc Dis* 1991;34: 101–112.

49. Stassen JM, Nystrom A, Hoylaerts M, Collen D: Antithrombotic effects of thrombolytic agents in a platelet-rich femoral vein thrombosis model in the hamster. *Circulation* 1995;91:1330–1335.

50. Lijnen HR, Collen D. New strategies in the development of thrombolytic agents. *Thromb Res* 1991; 58:69–72.

51. Stamler JS, Simon DI, Jaraki O, et al: S-nitrosylation of tissue type-plasminogen activator confers vasodilatory and antiplatelet properties on the enzyme. *Proc Natl Acad Sci USA* 1992;89:8087–8091.

52. Holvoet P, Dewerchin M, Stassen JM, et al: Thrombolytic profiles of clot-targeted plasminogen activators, parameters determining potency and initial and maximal rates. *Circulation* 1993;87: 1007–1016.

53. Collen D, Dewerchin M, Stassen JM, Kieckens L, Lijnen HR: Thrombolytic and pharmacokinetic properties of conjugates of urokinase-type plasminogen activator with a monoclonal antibody specific for cross-linked fibrin. *Fibrinolysis* 1989;3: 197–202.

54. Bode C, Meinhardt G, Runge MS, et al: Platelet-targeted fibrinolysis enhances clot lysis and inhibits platelet aggregation. *Circulation* 1991;84:805–813.

55. Conti CR: Brief overview of the end points of thrombolytic therapy. *Am J Cardiol* 1991;67:8E–10E.

56. Califf RM: Why are large-scale trials needed? *Cor Art Dis* 1992;3:92–95.

57. The International Study Group: In-hospital mortality and clinical course of 20,891 patients with suspected acute myocardial infarction randomised between alteplase and streptokinase with or without heparin. *Lancet* 1990;336:71–75.

58. ISIS-3 Collaborative Group: ISIS-3: A randomised comparison of streptokinase vs tissue plasminogen activator vs anistreplase and of aspirin plus heparin vs aspirin alone among 41,299 cases of suspected acute myocardial infarction. ISIS-3 (Third International Study of Infarct Survival) Collaborative Group. *Lancet* 1992;339:753–770.

59. The GUSTO Investigators: An international randomized trial comparing four thrombolytic strategies for acute myocardial infarction. *N Engl J Med* 1993;329:673–682.

60. Gruppo Italiano per lo Studio della Streptochinasi nell'Infarto Miocardico (GISSI): Effectiveness of intravenous thrombolytic treatment in acute myocardial infarction. *Lancet* 1986;1:397–402.

61. Gruppo Italiano per lo Studio della Streptochinasi nell'Infarto Miocardico (GISSI): Long-term effects of intravenous thrombolysis in acute myocardial infarction: Final report of the GISSI study. *Lancet* 1987;2:871–874.

62. The ISAM Study Group: A prospective trial of intravenous streptokinase in acute myocardial infarction (ISAM). Mortality, morbidity, and infarct size at 21 days. *N Engl J Med* 1986;314:1465–1471.

63. ISIS-2 (Second International Study of Infarct Survival) Collaborative Group: Randomised trial of intravenous streptokinase, oral aspirin, both, or neither among 17,187 cases of suspected acute myocardial infarction: ISIS-2. *Lancet* 1988;2:349–360.

64. EMERAS (Estudio Multicentrico Estreptoquinasa Republicas de America del Sur) Collaborative Group: Randomised trial of late thrombolysis in patients with suspected acute myocardial infarction. *Lancet* 1993;342:767–772.

65. Wilcox RG, von der Lippe G, Olsson CG, Jensen G, Skene AM, Hampton JR: Trial of tissue plasminogen activator for mortality reduction in acute myocardial infarction. Anglo-Scandinavian Study of Early Thrombolysis (ASSET). *Lancet* 1988;2: 525–530.

66. Wilcox RG, von der Lippe G, Olsson CG, Jensen G, Skene AM, Hampton JR: Effects of alteplase in acute myocardial infarction: 6-month results from the ASSET study. Anglo-Scandinavian Study of Early Thrombolysis. *Lancet* 1990;335:1175–1178.

67. Van de Werf F, Arnold AE, for the European Cooperative Study Group: Intravenous tissue plasminogen activator and size of infarct, left ventricular function, and survival in acute myocardial infarction. *Br Med J* 1988;297:1374–1379.

68. LATE Study Group: Late assessment of thrombolytic efficacy (LATE) study with alteplase 6–24 hours after onset of acute myocardial infarction. *Lancet* 1993;342:759–766.

69. AIMS Trial Study Group: Effect of intravenous APSAC on mortality after acute myocardial infarction: Preliminary report of a placebo-controlled clinical trial. *Lancet* 1988;1:545–549.
70. AIMS Trial Study Group: Long-term effects of intravenous anistreplase in acute myocardial infarction: Final report of the AIMS study. AIMS Trial Study Group. *Lancet* 1990;335:427–431.
71. Rossi P, Bolognese L, on behalf of Urochinasi per la Sistemica nell'Infarto Miocardico (USIM) Collaborative Group: Comparison of intravenous urokinase plus heparin versus heparin alone in acute myocardial infarction. *Am J Cardiol* 1991;68: 585–592.
72. Fibrinolytic Therapy Trialists' (FTT) Collaborative Group: Indications for fibrinolytic therapy in suspected acute myocardial infarction: Collaborative overview of early mortality and major morbidity results from all randomised trials of more than 1000 patients. *Lancet* 1994;343:311–322.
73. Pacouret G, Charbonnier B, Curien ND, et al: Invasive reperfusion study. II. Multicentre European randomized trial of anistreplase vs streptokinase in acute myocardial infarction. *Eur Heart J* 1991;12: 179–185.
74. Verstraete M, Bernard R, Bory M, et al: Randomised trial of intravenous recombinant tissue-type plasminogen activator versus intravenous streptokinase in acute myocardial infarction. Report from the European Cooperative Study Group for Recombinant Tissue-type Plasminogen Activator. *Lancet* 1985;1:842–847.
75. Anderson JL, Becker LC, Sorensen SG, et al: Anistreplase versus alteplase in acute myocardial infarction: Comparative effects on left ventricular function, morbidity and 1-day coronary artery patency. The TEAM-3 Investigators. *J Am Coll Cardiol* 1992;20:753–766.
76. PRIMI Trial Study Group: Randomised double-blind trial of recombinant pro-urokinase against streptokinase in acute myocardial infarction. PRIMI Trial Study Group. *Lancet* 1989;1: 863–868.
77. White HD, Rivers JT, Maslowski AH, et al: Effect of intravenous streptokinase as compared with that of tissue plasminogen activator on left ventricular function after first myocardial infarction. *N Engl J Med* 1989;320:817–821.
77a. White HD, Norris RM, Brown MA, et al: Effect of intravenous streptokinase on left ventricular function and early survival after acute myocardial infarction. *N Engl J Med* 1987;317:850–855.
78. Anderson JL, Sorensen SG, Moreno FL, et al: Multicenter patency trial of intravenous anistreplase compared with streptokinase in acute myocardial infarction. The TEAM-2 Study Investigators. *Circulation* 1991;83:126–140.
79. Neuhaus KL, von Essen R, Tebbe U, et al: Improved thrombolysis in acute myocardial infarction with front-loaded administration of alteplase: Results of the rt-PA–APSAC patency study (TAPS). *J Am Coll Cardiol* 1992;19:885–891.
80. Chesebro JH, Knatterud G, Roberts R, et al: Thrombolysis in Myocardial Infarction (TIMI) Trial, Phase I: A comparison between intravenous tissue plasminogen activator and intravenous streptokinase. *Circulation* 1987;76:142–154.
81. Bassand JP, Cassagnes J, Machecourt J, et al: Comparative effects of APSAC and rt-PA on infarct size and left ventricular function in acute myocardial infarction. A multicenter randomized study. *Circulation* 1991;84:1107–1117.
82. Magnani B: Plasminogen Activator Italian Multicenter Study (PAIMS): Comparison of intravenous recombinant single-chain human tissue-type plasminogen activator (rt-PA) with intravenous streptokinase in acute myocardial infarction. *J Am Coll Cardiol* 1989;13:19–26.
83. Neuhaus KL, Tebbe U, Gottwik M, et al: Intravenous recombinant tissue plasminogen activator (rt-PA) and urokinase in acute myocardial infarction: Results of the German activator urokinase study (GAUS). *J Am Coll Cardiol* 1988;12:581–587.
84. Gruppo Italiano per lo Studio della Sopravvivenza nell'Infarto Miocardico: GISSI-2: A factorial randomised trial of alteplase versus streptokinase and heparin versus no heparin among 12 490 patients with acute myocardial infarction. *Lancet* 1990;336: 65–71.
85. GISSI-2: Six-month survival in 20,891 patients with acute myocardial infarction randomised between alteplase and streptokinase with or without heparin. GISSI-2 and International Study Group. Gruppo Italiano per lo Studio della Sopravvivenza nell'Infarto Miocardico. *Eur Heart J* 1992;13:1692–1697.
86. Topol EJ: Which thrombolytic agent should one choose? *Prog Cardiovasc Dis* 1991;34:165–178.
87. Neuhaus KL, Feuerer W, Jeep-Tebbe S, Niederer W, Vogt A, Tebbe U: Improved thrombolysis with a modified dose regimen of recombinant tissue-type

plasminogen activator. *J Am Coll Cardiol* 1989;14: 1566–1569.

88. Carney RJ, Murphy GA, Brandt TR, et al: Randomized angiographic trial of recombinant tissue-type plasminogen activator (alteplase) in myocardial infarction. RAAMI Study Investigators. *J Am Coll Cardiol* 1992;20:17–23.

89. Topol EJ, George BS, Kereiakes DJ, et al: A randomized controlled trial of intravenous tissue plasminogen activator and early intravenous heparin in acute myocardial infarction. *Circulation* 1989;79: 281–286.

90. Hsia J, Hamilton WP, Kleiman N, Roberts R, Chaitman BR, Ross AM: A comparison between heparin and low-dose aspirin as adjunctive therapy with tissue plasminogen activator for acute myocardial infarction. Heparin–Aspirin Reperfusion Trial (HART) Investigators. *N Engl J Med* 1990;323: 1433–1437.

91. Bleich SD, Nichols TC, Schumacher RR, Cooke DH, Tate DA, Teichman SL: Effect of heparin on coronary arterial patency after thrombolysis with tissue plasminogen activator in acute myocardial infarction. *Am J Cardiol* 1990;66:1412–1417.

92. de Bono DP, Simoons ML, Tijssen J, et al: Effect of early intravenous heparin on coronary patency, infarct size, and bleeding complications after alteplase thrombolysis: Results of a randomised double blind European Cooperative Study Group trial. *Br Heart J* 1992;67:122–128.

93. Thompson PL, Aylward PE, Federman J, et al: A randomized comparison of intravenous heparin with oral aspirin and dipyridamole 24 hours after recombinant tissue-type plasminogen activator for acute myocardial infarction. National Heart Foundation of Australia Coronary Thrombolysis Group. *Circulation* 1991;83:1534–1542.

94. Califf RM, Topol EJ: The paradigm of acute reperfusion and the GUSTO-I trial, in Califf RM, Mark DB, Wagner GS (eds): *Acute Coronary Care*. St. Louis, Mosby-Year Book, Inc., 1995, pp 69–83.

95. Gore JM, Granger CB, Sloan MA, et al: Stroke after thrombolysis: Mortality and functional outcomes in the GUSTO-I trial. *Circulation* 1995;92: 2811–2818.

96. Smalling RW, Bode C, Kalbfleisch J, et al: More rapid, complete, and stable coronary thrombolysis with bolus administration of reteplase compared with alteplase infusion in acute myocardial infarction. *Circulation* 1995;91:2725–2732.

97. Weaver WD, Bode C, Burnett C, et al: Reteplase vs alteplase patency investigation during myocardial infarction trial (RAPID 2) (abstract). *J Am Coll Cardiol* 1995;25:87A.

98. International Joint Efficacy Comparison of Thrombolytics: Randomised, double-blind comparison of reteplase double-bolus administration with streptokinase in acute myocardial infarction (INJECT): Trial to investigate equivalence. *Lancet* 1995;346:329–336.

99. Granger CB, Califf RM, Topol EJ: Thrombolytic therapy for acute myocardial infarction. A review. *Drugs* 1992;44:293–325.

100. Simes RJ, Topol EJ, Holmes DR Jr, et al: Link between the angiographic substudy and mortality outcomes in a large randomized trial of myocardial reperfusion: Importance of early and complete infarct artery reperfusion. *Circulation* 1995; 91:1923–1928.

101. Lincoff AM, Topol EJ: Illusion of reperfusion: Does anyone achieve optimal reperfusion during acute myocardial infarction? *Circulation* 1993;88: 1361–1374.

102. Kennedy JW: Optimal management of acute myocardial infarction requires early and complete reperfusion. *Circulation* 1995;91:1905–1907.

103. Vogt A, von Essen R, Tebbe U, Feuerer W, Appel KF, Neuhaus KL: Impact of early perfusion status of the infarct-related artery on short-term mortality after thrombolysis for acute myocardial infarction: retrospective analysis of four German multicenter studies. *J Am Coll Cardiol* 1993;21: 1391–1395.

104. Anderson JL, Karagounis LA, Becker LC, Sorensen SG, Menlove RL, for the TEAM-3 Investigators: TIMI perfusion grade 3 but not grade 2 results in improved outcome after thrombolysis for myocardial infarction: Ventriculographic, enzymatic, and electrocardiographic evidence from the TEAM-3 study. *Circulation* 1994;87:1829–1839.

105. Lee KL, Woodlief LH, Topol EJ, et al: Predictors of 30-day mortality in the era of reperfusion for acute myocardial infarction: Results from an international trial of 41,021 patients. *Circulation* 1995;91:1659–1668.

106. Volpi A, DeVita C, Franzosi MG, et al: Determinants of 6-month mortality in survivors of myocardial infarction after thrombolysis. Results of the GISSI-2 data base. *Circulation* 1993;88:416–429.

107. Ohman EM, Califf RM, Topol EJ, et al: Consequences of reocclusion after successful reperfusion therapy in acute myocardial infarction. TAMI study group. *Circulation* 1990;82:781–791.

108. Krucoff MW, Croll MA, Pope JE, et al: Continuous 12-lead ST segment recovery analysis in the TAMI 7 Study: Performance of a noninvasive method for real time detection of failed myocardial reperfusion. *Circulation* 1993;88:437–446.

109. Krucoff MW, Croll MA, Pope JE, et al: Continuously updated 12-lead ST-segment recovery analysis for myocardial infarct artery patency assessment and its correlation with multiple simultaneous early angiographic observations. *Am J Cardiol* 1993;71:145–151.

110. Barbash GI, Roth A, Hod H, et al: Rapid resolution of ST elevation and prediction of clinical outcome in patients undergoing thrombolysis with alteplase (recombinant tissue-type plasminogen activator): Results of the Israeli Study of Early Intervention in Myocardial Infarction. *Br Heart J* 1990;64:241–247.

111. Mauri F, Gasparini M, Barbonaglia L, et al: Prognostic significance of the extent of myocardial injury in acute myocardial infarction treated by streptokinase (the GISSI trial). *Am J Cardiol* 1989; 63:1291–1295.

112. Krucoff MW, Trollinger KM, Veldkamp RF, et al, for the TAMI 9 Study Group: Detection of recurrent ischemia with continuous electrocardiographic monitoring: Early risk stratification following thrombolytic therapy. *Circulation* 1992; 86(Suppl):I-4.

113. Barbagelata NA, Granger CB, Oqueli E., et al: TIMI grade 3 flow and reocclusion after intravenous thrombolytic therapy: a pooled analysis. *Am Heart J* 1997 (in press).

114. The GUSTO Angiographic Investigators: The effects of tissue plasminogen activator, streptokinase, or both on coronary-artery patency, ventricular function, and survival after acute myocardial infarction. *N Engl J Med* 1993;329:1615–1622.

115. Wall TC, Mark DB, Califf RM, et al: Prediction of early recurrent myocardial ischemia and coronary reocclusion after successful thrombolysis: A qualitative and quantitative angiographic study. *Am J Cardiol* 1989;63:423–428.

116. Davies SW, Marchant B, Lyons JP, et al: Irregular coronary lesion morphology after thrombolysis predicts early clinical instability. *J Am Coll Cardiol* 1991;18:669–674.

117. Gash AK, Spann JF, Sherry S, et al: Factors influencing reocclusion after coronary thrombolysis for acute myocardial infarction. *Am J Cardiol* 1986; 57:175–177.

118. Gibson CM, Cannon CP, Piana RN, et al: Angiographic predictors of reocclusion after thrombolysis: Results from the Thrombolysis in Myocardial Infarction (TIMI) 4 Trial. *J Am Coll Cardiol* 1995; 25:582–589.

119. Veen G, Meyer A, Verheugt FWA, et al: Culprit lesion morphology and stenosis severity in the prediction of reocclusion after coronary thrombolysis: Angiographic results of the APRICOT study. *J Am Coll Cardiol* 1993;22:1755–1762.

120. Serruys PW, Wijns W, van den Brand M, et al: Is transluminal coronary angioplasty mandatory after successful thrombolysis? *Br Heart J* 1983;50: 257–265.

121. Badger RS, Brown BG, Kennedy JW, et al: Usefulness of recanalization to luminal diameter of 0.6 millimeter or more with intracoronary streptokinase during acute myocardial infarction in predicting "normal" perfusion status, continued arterial patency and survival at one year. *Am J Cardiol* 1987;59:519–522.

122. Harrison DG, Ferguson DW, Collins SM, et al: Rethrombosis after reperfusion with streptokinase: Importance of geometry of residual lesions. *Circulation* 1984;69:991–999.

123. Grines CL, Topol EJ, Bates ER, Juni JE, Walton JA Jr, O'Neill WW: Infarct vessel status after intravenous tissue plasminogen activator and acute coronary angioplasty: Prediction of clinical outcome. *Am Heart J* 1988;115:1–7.

124. Barbagelata A, Granger CB, Topol EJ, et al: Frequency, significance, and cost of recurrent ischemia after thrombolytic therapy for acute myocardial infarction. *Am J Cardiol* 1995;76: 1007–1013.

125. Anderson JL: Reperfusion, patency and reocclusion with anistreplase (APSAC) in acute myocardial infarction. *Am J Cardiol* 1989;64:12A–17A.

126. Reiner JS, Lundergan CF, van den Brand M, et al: Early angiography cannot predict postthrombolytic coronary reocclusion: Observations from the GUSTO angiographic study. *J Am Coll Cardiol* 1994;24:1439–1444.

127. Roberts R: Enzymatic estimation of infarct size—thrombolysis induced its demise: Will it now rekindle its renaissance. *Circulation* 1990;81:707–710.

128. Hermens WT, van der Veen FH, Willems GM, et al: Complete recovery in plasma of enzymes lost from the heart after permanent coronary artery occlusion in the dog. *Circulation* 1990;81:649–659.

129. Baardman T, Hermens WT, Lenderink T, et al: Differential effects of tissue plasminogen activator and streptokinase on infarct size and on rate of enzyme release—influence of early infarct related artery patency—the GUSTO enzyme substudy. *Eur Heart J* 1996;17:237–246.

130. Timmis AD, Griffin B, Crick JCP, et al: The effects of early coronary patency on the evolution of myocardial infarction: A prospective arteriographic study. *Br Heart J* 1987;58:345–351.

131. Hogg KL, Lees KR, Hornung RS, et al: Electrocardiographic evidence of myocardial salvage after thrombolysis in acute myocardial infarction. *Br Heart J* 1989;61:489–495.

132. Koren G, Weiss AT, Hasin Y, et al: Prevention of myocardial damage in acute myocardial ischemia by early treatment with intravenous streptokinase. *N Engl J Med* 1985;313:1384–1389.

133. Clemmensen P, Ohman EM, Sevilla DC, et al: Importance of early and complete reperfusion to achieve myocardial salvage after thrombolysis in acute myocardial infarction. *Am J Cardiol* 1992;70:1391–1396.

134. Multicenter Post-Infarction Research Group: Risk stratification and survival after myocardial infarction. *N Engl J Med* 1983;309:321–336.

135. Norris RM, White HD: Therapeutic trials in coronary thrombosis should measure left ventricular function as primary endpoint of treatment. *Lancet* 1988;1:104–106.

136. Van de Werf F: Discrepancies between the effects of coronary reperfusion on survival and left ventricular function. *Lancet* 1989;1:1367–1369.

137. Sheehan FH: Measurement of left ventricular function as an endpoint in trials of thrombolytic therapy. *Cor Art Dis* 1990;1:13–22.

138. Califf RM, Harrelson-Woodlief L, Topol EJ: Left ventricular ejection fraction may not be useful as an end point of thrombolytic therapy comparative trials. *Circulation* 1990;82:1847–1853.

139. Reimer KA, Lowe JE, Rasmussen MM, Jennings RB: The wave-front phenomenon of ischemic cell death: Myocardial infarct size versus duration of coronary occlusion in dogs. *Circulation* 1977;56:786–794.

140. Sheehan FH, Braunwald E, Canner P, et al: The effect of intravenous thrombolytic therapy on left ventricular function: A report on tissue-type plasminogen activator and streptokinase from the Thrombolysis in Myocardial Infarction (TIMI Phase I) trial. *Circulation* 1987;75:817–829.

141. Sheehan FH, Bolson EL, Dodge HT, Mathey DG, Schofer J, Woo HW: Advantages and applications of the centerline method for characterizing regional ventricular function. *Circulation* 1986;74:293–305.

142. Stack RS, Phillips HR, Grierson DS, et al: Functional improvement of jeopardized myocardium following intracoronary streptokinase infusion in acute myocardial infarction. *J Clin Invest* 1983;72:84–95.

143. Schmidt WG, Sheehan FH, von Essen R, Uebis R, Effert S: Evolution of left ventricular function after intracoronary thrombolysis for acute myocardial infarction. *Am J Cardiol* 1989;63:497–502.

144. Sheehan FH, Doerr R, Schmidt WG, et al: Early recovery of left ventricular function after thrombolytic therapy for acute myocardial infarction: An important determinant of survival. *J Am Coll Cardiol* 1988;12:289–300.

145. Grines CL, Topol EJ, Califf RM, et al: Prognostic implications and predictors of enhanced regional wall motion of the noninfarct zone after thrombolysis and angioplasty therapy of acute myocardial infarction. The TAMI Study Groups. *Circulation* 1989;80:245–253.

146. Gibbons RJ, Christian TF, Hopfenspirger M, Hodge DO, Bailey KR: Myocardium at risk and infarct size after thrombolytic therapy for acute myocardial infarction: Implications for the design of randomized trials of acute intervention. *J Am Coll Cardiol* 1994;24:616–623.

147. Kennedy JW, Martin GV, Davis KB, et al: The Western Washington Intravenous Streptokinase in Acute Myocardial Infarction Randomized Trial. *Circulation* 1988;77:345–352.

148. Ritchie JL, Cerqueira M, Maynard C, Davis K, Kennedy JW: Ventricular function and infarct size: The Western Washington Intravenous Streptokinase in Myocardial Infarction Trial. *J Am Coll Cardiol* 1988;11:689–697.

149. Simoons ML, Serruys PW, van den Brand M, et al: Early thrombolysis in acute myocardial infarction: Limitation of infarct size and improved survival. *J Am Coll Cardiol* 1986;7:717–728.

150. National Heart Foundation of Australia Coronary Thrombolysis Group: Coronary thrombolysis and myocardial salvage by tissue plasminogen activator given up to 4 hours after onset of myocardial infarction. *Lancet* 1988;1:203–208.

151. O'Rourke M, Baron D, Keogh A, et al: Limitation of myocardial infarction by early infusion of recombinant tissue-type plasminogen activator. *Circulation* 1988;77:1311–1315.

152. Armstrong PW, Baigrie RS, Daly PA, et al: Tissue plasminogen activator: Toronto (TPAT) placebo-controlled randomized trial in acute myocardial infarction. *J Am Coll Cardiol* 1989;13:1469–1476.

153. Bassand JP, Machecourt J, Cassagnes J, et al: Multicenter trial of intravenous anisoylated plasminogen streptokinase activator complex (APSAC) in acute myocardial infarction: Effects on infarct size and left ventricular function. *J Am Coll Cardiol* 1989;13:988–997.

154. Meinertz T, Kasper W, Schumacher M, Just H: The German multicenter trial of anisoylated plasminogen streptokinase activator complex versus heparin for acute myocardial infarction. *Am J Cardiol* 1988;62:347–351.

155. Harrison JK, Califf RM, Woodlief LH, et al: Systolic left ventricular function after reperfusion therapy for acute myocardial infarction: An analysis of determinants of improvement. *Circulation* 1993;87:1531–1541.

156. Belenkie I, Knudtson ML, Roth DL, et al: Relation between flow grade after thrombolytic therapy and the effect of angioplasty on left ventricular function: A prospective randomized trial. *Am Heart J* 1991;121:407–416.

157. Sheehan FH, Thery C, Durand P, Bertrand ME, Bolson EL: Early beneficial effect of streptokinase on left ventricular function in acute myocardial infarction. *Am J Cardiol* 1991;67:555–558.

158. Califf RM, Topol EJ, Stack RS, et al: Evaluation of combination thrombolytic therapy and timing of cardiac catheterization in acute myocardial infarction. Results of thrombolysis and angioplasty in myocardial infarction—phase 5 randomized trial. TAMI Study Group. *Circulation* 1991;83:1543–1556.

159. Mueller HS, Rao AK, Forman SA: Thrombolysis in myocardial infarction (TIMI): Comparative studies of coronary reperfusion and systemic fibrinogenolysis with two forms of recombinant tissue-type plasminogen activator. *J Am Coll Cardiol* 1987;10:479–490.

160. Landefeld CS, Cook EF, Flatley M, Weisberg M, Goldman L: Identification and preliminary validation of predictors of major bleeding in hospitalized patients starting anticoagulation therapy. *Am J Med* 1987;82:703–713.

161. Berkowitz SD, Granger CB, Pieper KS, et al., for the Global Utilization of Streptokinase and Tissue Plasminogen Activator for Occluded Coronary Arteries (GUSTO) I Investigators: Incidence and predictors of bleeding following contemporary thrombolytic therapy for myocardial infarction. *Circulation* 1997; (in press).

162. Topol EJ, George BS, Kereiakes DJ, et al: Comparison of two dose regimens of intravenous tissue plasminogen activator for acute myocardial infarction. *Am J Cardiol* 1988;61:723–728.

163. de Jaegere PP, Arnold AA, Balk AH, Simoons ML: Intracranial hemorrhage in association with thrombolytic therapy: Incidence and clinical predictive factors. *J Am Coll Cardiol* 1992;19:289–294.

164. Kase CS, Pessin MS, Zivin JA, et al: Intracranial hemorrhage after coronary thrombolysis with tissue plasminogen activator. *Am J Med* 1992;92:384–390.

165. O'Connor CM, Califf RM, Massey EW, et al: Stroke and acute myocardial infarction in the thrombolytic era: Clinical correlates and long-term prognosis. *J Am Coll Cardiol* 1990;16:533–540.

166. Gore JM, Sloan M, Price TR, et al: Intracerebral hemorrhage, cerebral infarction, and subdural hematoma after acute myocardial infarction and thrombolytic therapy in the Thrombolysis in Myocardial Infarction study: Thrombolysis in Myocardial Infarction, Phase II, pilot and clinical trial. *Circulation* 1991;83:448–459.

167. Maggioni AP, Franzosi MG, Santoro E, et al: The risk of stroke in patients with acute myocardial infarction after thrombolytic and antithrombotic treatment. *N Engl J Med* 1992;327:1–6.

168. Simoons ML, Maggioni AP, Knatterud G, et al: Individual risk assessment for intracranial haemorrhage during thrombolytic therapy. *Lancet* 1993;342:1523–1528.

169. Granger C, White H, Simoons M, et al: Risk factors for stroke following thrombolytic therapy: Case-control study from the GUSTO trial (abstract). *J Am Coll Cardiol* 1995;25:232A.

170. Califf RM, Topol EJ, Gersh BJ: From myocardial salvage to patient salvage in acute myocardial in-

farction: The role of reperfusion therapy. *J Am Coll Cardiol* 1989;14:1382–1388.

171. Tiefenbrunn AJ, Sobel BE: Timing of coronary recanalization, paradigms, paradoxes, and pertinence. *Circulation* 1992;85:2311–2315.

172. Hohnloser SH, Franck P, Klingenheben T, Zabel M, Just H: Open infarct artery, late potentials, and other prognostic factors in patients after acute myocardial infarction in the thrombolytic era: A prospective trial. *Circulation* 1994;90:1747–1756.

173. Kim CB, Braunwald E: Potential benefits of late reperfusion of infarcted myocardium. The open artery hypothesis. *Circulation* 1993;88:2426–2436.

174. Fortin DF, Califf RM: Long-term survival from acute myocardial infarction. Salutary effect of an open coronary vessel. *Am J Med* 1990;88:9N–15N.

175. Bergmann SR, Lerch RA, Fox KAA, et al: Temporal dependence of beneficial effects of coronary thrombolysis characterized by positron tomography. *Am J Med* 1982;73:573–581.

176. Ohman EM, Christenson RH: Noninvasive assessment of myocardial reperfusion and reocclusion, in Topol EJ, Serruys PW (eds): *Current Review of Interventional Cardiology*. Philadelphia, Current Medicine, 1994m pp 6:1–6.15.

177. Simoons ML, Arnold AER: Tailored thrombolytic therapy. A perspective. *Circulation* 1993;88: 2556–2564.

178. Anderson HV, Willerson JT: Thrombolysis in acute myocardial infarction. *N Engl J Med* 1993; 329:703–709.

179. Gunnar RM, Chairman: ACC/AHA guidelines for the early management of patients with acute myocardial infarction: A report of the American College of Cardiology/American Heart Association task force on assessment of diagnostic and therapeutic cardiovascular procedures (subcommittee to develop guidelines for the early management of patients with acute myocardial infarction). *Circulation* 1990;82:664–707.

180. Maynard C, Weaver WD, Litwin PE, et al: Hospital mortality in acute myocardial infarction in the era of reperfusion therapy (the Myocardial Infarction Triage and Intervention project). *Am J Cardiol* 1993;72:877–882.

181. Granger C, Moffie I, for the GUSTO Investigators: Under use of thrombolytic therapy in North America has been exaggerated: Results of the GUSTO MI registry (abstract). *Circulation* 1994; 90(Suppl I):I-324.

182. Gersh BJ, Anderson JL: Thrombolysis and myocardial salvage: Results of clinical trials and the animal paradigm—paradoxic or predictable. *Circulation* 1993;88:296–306.

183. Kereiakes DJ, Weaver WD, Anderson JL, et al: Time delays in the diagnosis and treatment of acute myocardial infarction: A tale of eight cities. *Am Heart J* 1990;120:773–779.

184. Newby LK, Rutsch WR, Califf RM, et al., for the GUSTO-I Investigators: Time from symptom onset to treatment and outcomes after thrombolytic therapy *J Am Coll Cardiol* 1996;27:1646–1655.

185. Ho MT: Delays in the treatment of acute myocardial infarction: An overview. *Heart Lung* 1991;20: 566–570.

186. Dracup K, Moser DK: Treatment-seeking behavior among those with signs and symptoms of acute myocardial infarction. *Heart Lung* 1991;20: 570–575.

187. Herlitz J, Hartford M, Blohm B, et al: Effect of a media campaign on delay times and ambulance use in suspected acute myocardial infarction. *Am J Cardiol* 1989;64:90–93.

188. Mitic WR, Perkins RRT: The effect of a media campaign on heart attack delay and decision times. *Can J Public Health* 1984;75:414–418.

189. Ho MT, Eisenberg MS, Litwin PE: Delay between onset of chest pain and seeking medical care: The effect of public education. *Ann Emerg Med* 1989;18:727–731.

190. Alonzo AA: The impact of the family and lay others on care-seeking during life-threatening episodes of suspected coronary artery disease. *Soc Sci Med* 1986;22:1297–1311.

191. Weaver WD, Eisenberg MS, Martin JS, et al: Myocardial Infarction Triage and Intervention project—phase I: Patient characteristics and feasibility of prehospital initiation of thrombolytic therapy. *J Am Coll Cardiol* 1990;15:925–930.

192. The GREAT Group: Feasibility, safety, and efficacy of domiciliary thrombolysis by general practitioners: Grampian Region Early Anistreplase Trial. *Br Med J* 1992;305:548–553.

193. Rawles J: Halving of mortality at 1 year by domiciliary thrombolysis in the Grampian Region Early Anistreplase Trial (GREAT). *J Am Coll Cardiol* 1994;23:1–5.

194. Weaver DW, Cerqueira M, Hallstrom AP, et al: Prehospital-initiated vs hospital-initiated thrombolytic

therapy: The Myocardial Infarction and Triage Intervention trial. *JAMA* 1993;1211–1216.

195. European Myocardial Infarction Project Group: Prehospital thrombolytic therapy in patients with suspected acute myocardial infarction. *N Engl J Med* 1993;329:383–389.

196. Fath-Ordoubadi F, Al-Mohammad A, Huehns TY, Beatt KJ: Meta-analysis of randomized trials of prehospital versus hospital thrombolysis (abstract). *Circulation* 1994;90(Suppl I):I-324.

197. Kline EM, Smith DD, Martin JS, et al: In-hospital treatment delays in patients treated with thrombolytic therapy: A report of the GUSTO time to treatment substudy (abstract). *Circulation* 1992;86(Suppl I):I-702.

198. Ohman EM, Armstrong PW, Guerci AD, Vahanian A, for the GUSTO Trial Investigators: Reinfarction after thrombolytic therapy: Experience from the GUSTO trial (abstract). *Circulation* 1993; 88(Suppl I):I-490.

199. Kornowski R, Goldbourt U, Zion M, et al: Predictors and long-term prognostic significance of recurrent infarction in the year after a first myocardial infarction. *Am J Cardiol* 1993;72:883–888.

200. Mueller HS, Forman SA, Menegus MA, Cohen LS, Knatterud GL, Braunwald E: Prognostic significance of nonfatal reinfarction during 3-year follow-up: Results of the Thrombolysis in Myocardial Infarction (TIMI) phase II clinical trial. *J Am Coll Cardiol* 1995;26:900–907.

201. White HD, Cross DB, Williams BF, Norris RM: Safety and efficacy of repeat thrombolytic treatment after acute myocardial infarction. *Br Heart J* 1990;64:177–181.

202. Simoons ML, Arnout J, van den Brand M, Nyssen K, Verstraete M: Retreatment with alteplase for early signs of reocclusion after thrombolysis. The European Cooperative Study Group. *Am J Cardiol* 1993;71:524–528.

203. Barbash GI, Hod H, Roth A, et al: Repeat infusions of recombinant tissue-type plasminogen activator in patients with acute myocardial infarction and early recurrent myocardial ischemia. *J Am Coll Cardiol* 1990;16:779–783.

204. Purvis JA, McNeil AJ, Roberts MJD, et al: First-year follow-up after repeat thrombolytic therapy with recombinant-tissue plasminogen activator for myocardial reinfarction. *Cor Art Dis* 1992;3: 713–720.

205. Barbash GI, Ohman EM, White HD, Granger C, Califf RM, for the GUSTO Investigators: Rescue thrombolysis for suspected reinfarction following thrombolytic therapy: Experience from the GUSTO trial (abstract). *J Am Coll Cardiol* 1994;23: 29A.

206. Mahaffey KW, Granger CB, Collins R, et al: Overview of randomized trials of intravenous heparin in patients with acute myocardial infarction treated with thrombolytic therapy. *Am J Cardiol* 1996;77:551–556.

207. O'Connor CM, Meese R, Carney R, et al: A randomized trial of intravenous heparin in conjunction with anistreplase (anisoylated plasminogen streptokinase activator complex) in acute myocardial infarction: The Duke University Clinical Cardiology Study (DUCCS) 1. *J Am Coll Cardiol* 1994; 23:11–18.

208. Theroux P, Perez-Villa F, Waters D, Lesperance J, Shabani F, Bonan R: Randomized double-blind comparison of two doses of hirulog with heparin as adjunctive therapy to streptokinase to promote early patency of the infarct-related artery in acute myocardial infarction. *Circulation* 1995;91: 2132–2139.

209. Cannon CP, McCabe CH, Henry TD, et al: A pilot trial of recombinant desulfatohirudin compared with heparin in conjunction with tissue-type plasminogen activator and aspirin for acute myocardial infarction: Results of the Thrombolysis in Myocardial Infarction (TIMI) 5 trial. *J Am Coll Cardiol* 1994;23:993–1003.

210. The Global Use of Strategies to Open Occluded Coronary Arteries (GUSTO) IIa Investigators: Randomized trial of intravenous heparin versus recombinant hirudin for acute coronary syndromes. *Circulation* 1994;90:1631–1637.

211. GUSTO-IIb (Global Utilization of Strategies to Open Occluded Coronary Arteries in Acute Coronary Syndromes) results. Presented at the 45th Annual Scientific Sessions of the American College of Cardiology, Orlando, Florida, March 26, 1996.

212. Topol EJ, Ellis SG, Califf RM, et al: Combined tissue-type plasminogen activator and prostacyclin therapy for acute myocardial infarction. *J Am Coll Cardiol* 1989;14:877–884.

213. Kleiman NS, Ohman EM, Califf RM, et al: Profound inhibition of platelet aggregation with monoclonal antibody 7E3 Fab following thrombolytic

therapy: Results of the TAMI 8 pilot study. *J Am Coll Cardiol* 1993;22:381–389.

214. Ohman EM, Kleiman NS, Talley JD, et al: Simultaneous platelet glycoprotein IIb/IIIa integrin blockade with accelerated tissue plasminogen activator in acute myocardial infarction (abstract). *Circulation* 1994;90(Suppl I):I-564.

215. Ohman EM, Kleiman NS, Gacioch G, et al., for the IMPACT-AMI Investigators: Combined accelerated tissue-plasminogen activator and platelet glycoprotein IIb/IIIa integrin receptor blockade with Integrilin™ in acute myocardial infarction: Results of a randomized, placebo-controlled, dose-ranging trial. *Circulation* 1996, (in press).

216. Krucoff MW, Ohman EM, Trollinger KM, et al: Beneficial impact of a platelet inhibitor, integrelin, on parameters of continuous 12-lead ST-segment recovery during myocardial infarction. (Abstract). *Circulation* 1996;92(Suppl I):I-416.

20

Antithrombotic Therapy in Acute Myocardial Infarction: Enhancement of Thrombolysis, Reduction of Reocclusion, and Prevention of Thromboembolism

Richard Gallo, MD, Mark W. I. Webster, MB, ChB, Valentin Fuster, MD, PhD, and James Chesebro, MD

Atherosclerotic plaque disruption with subsequent thrombosis is the predominant cause of acute myocardial infarction (1–3). Early administration of thrombolytic agents recanalizes the occluded coronary artery and provides the basis for the salvage of ischemic myocardium, reduction of infarct size, preservation of myocardial function, and reduction of early and late mortality in acute myocardial infarction. We discuss the rationale and plan for antithrombotic and antiplatelet therapy in acute myocardial infarction, review the clinical studies of treatment with or without thrombolysis, and review the role of antithrombotic therapy in the prevention of arterial thromboembolism.

Acute myocardial infarction usually results from the occlusion of a major epicardial coronary artery (4,5) (see Ch. 2). Thrombolytic and antithrombotic agents limit the extent of myocardial infarction by dissolving thrombus, maintaining a patent artery, and thus limiting the duration of coronary occlusion. A thrombus overlying a disrupted plaque exposes highly thrombogenic lipid gruel and tissue factor from within the arterial plaque and arterial collagen (types I and III) (6,7). These structures activate platelets and both the extrinsic and intrinsic pathways of coagulation (Figs. 20–1, 20–2, and 20–3). The coagulation cascade generates thrombin, which activates platelets, converts fibrinogen to fibrin, and activates factor XIII to crosslink fibrin and stabilize the thrombus. Thrombin also activates factor V to Va, thereby exerting positive feedback on the coagulation cascade. Factor Va forms part of the prothrombinase complex (and is assembled with factor Xa, prothrombin, and calcium on phospholipid such as the platelet membrane), which amplifies thrombin generation by 300,000 times that of factor Xa alone (8) (Fig. 20–3). Thrombin and collagen are the most potent agonists of platelet activation in vitro; studies using a specific thrombin inhibitor such as hirudin confirm the central role of thrombin in platelet-thrombus deposition in vivo after deep arterial injury (9,10).

Assessment of reperfusion is difficult because it requires angiography both before and after the thrombolytic agent is administered. Most studies

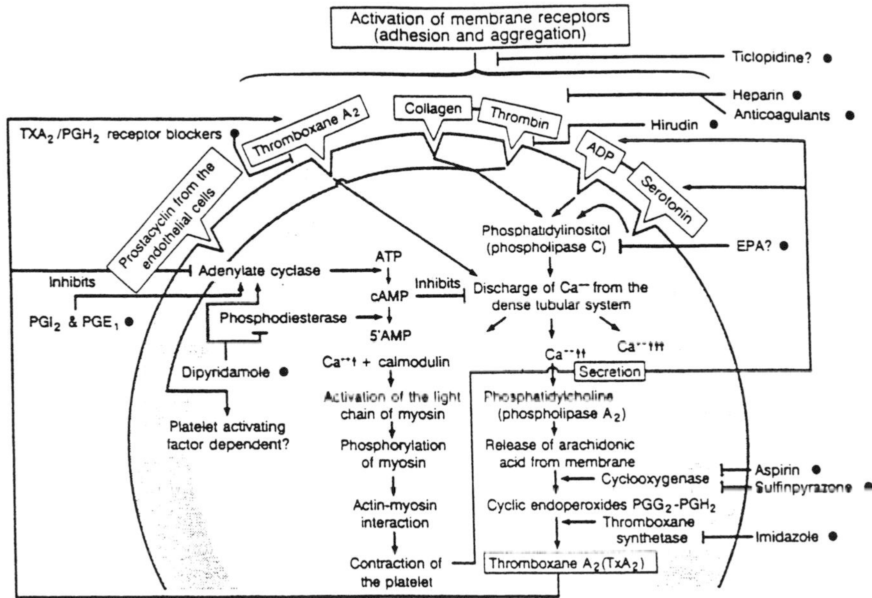

Figure 20–1. Mechanisms of platelet activation and presumed sites of action of various platelet inhibitor agents. Platelet agonists lead to the mobilization of calcium (Ca^{2+}), which mediates platelet activation through metabolic pathways dependent on thrombin and collagen (primary or strong agonists) and adenosine diphosphate (ADP), serotonin, and thromboxane A_2 (TXA_2) (secondary or weak agonists). Cyclic adenosine monophosphate (AMP) inhibits calcium mobilization from the dense tubular system. Thrombin and collagen may independently activate platelets by means of platelet activating factor. ATP = adenosine triphosphate, EPA = eicosapentaenoic acid, PG = prostaglandin. *Modified from Stein et al: Platelet inhibitor agents in cardiovascular disease: An update. J Am Coll Cardiol 1989;14:816, with permission.*

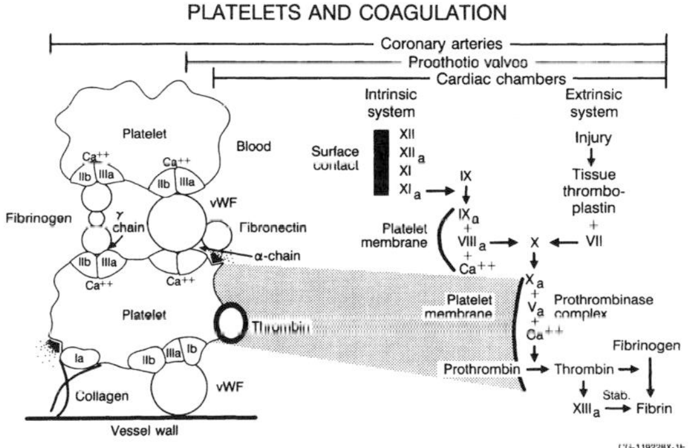

Figure 20–2. Biochemical interactions between platelet membrane receptors, vessel wall, and adhesive macromolecules during platelet adhesion and aggregation (left). Also depicted are the intrinsic and extrinsic systems of the coagulation cascade and their interaction with the platelet membrane (right), such as via both platelet and coagulation processes. Ca^{2+} = calcium, vWF = von Willebrand factor, Ia = glycoprotein Ia, Ib = glycoprotein Ib, IIb/IIIa = glycoprotein IIb/IIIa, XL = crosslinked. *Modified from Stein et al: Antithrombotic therapy in cardiac disease: An emerging approach based on pathogenesis and risk. Circulation 1989;80:1502, with permission.*

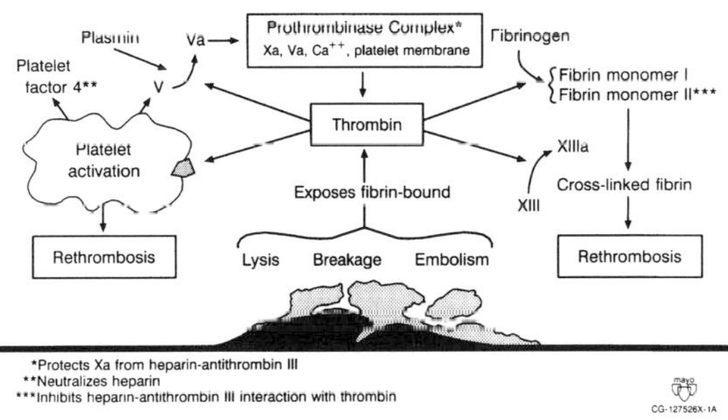

Figure 20–3. Disturbance of thrombus by lysis (endogenous or exogenous), mechanical breakage, or spontaneous embolism exposes thrombin bound to fibrin. Thrombin activates platelets, activates factor V to Va (which leads to generation of more thrombin via the prothrombinase complex), converts fibrinogen to fibrin I and II, and activates factor XIII to XIIIa (which crosslinks fibrin). These processes combine to produce rethrombosis. Heparin may only partially prevent rethrombosis, because factor Xa within the prothrombinase complex is protected from heparin–antithrombin III, platelet factor 4 neutralizes heparin, and fibrin monomer II inhibits heparin–antithrombin III.

report vessel patency rather than reperfusion, but this endpoint is influenced by the incidence of subtotal occlusion, endogenous lysis, and time from symptom onset to lytic therapy. DeWood and colleagues demonstrated coronary occlusion in 87% of patients studied within 4 hours of the onset of symptoms [average 80% occluded within 7 hours (11)], but only 65% of those studied from 12 to 24 hours (12). Angiography is required to determine reperfusion or patency and subsequent reocclusion because noninvasive endpoints are not sufficiently sensitive to determine these endpoints. Reinfarction is less frequent than reocclusion but is of greater clinical importance, since it relates to both the myocardium in jeopardy and that salvaged by thrombolysis. Reocclusion after thrombolysis is, in part, related to the thrombolytic agent or agents used (including the dosage and rapidity of administration), the adequacy of lysis, and especially the adequacy of concurrent antithrombotic therapy.

THROMBOLYTIC AGENT AND ADMINISTRATION REGIMEN

Currently, the most feasible and accessible treatment of patients with acute myocardial infarction is thrombolytic therapy with strategies that produce an early and sustained coronary artery recanalization with net clinical benefits outweighing adverse effects (see Ch. 19). Multiple clinical trials have shown that the open artery has a major impact on long-term survival (12–16). Therefore, the best lytic strategy will be that which most quickly reperfuses the infarct-related artery to normal flow (within 90 minutes or less), minimizing mortality and myocardial necrosis.

Patency

Randomized trials of thrombolytic therapy were reviewed in Ch. 19. Early trials comparing arterial reperfusion and patency rates showed that recombinant tissue-type plasminogen activator (t-PA) was more effective at reperfusion within 90 minutes than streptokinase (11,17). When data from the Thrombolysis in Myocardial infarction (TIMI-1) (11) and European Cooperative Study Group (ECSG) (17) trials are combined, 90-minute patency rates for lytic treatment within 3 hours of onset of symptoms were 81% with t-PA and 55% with streptokinase. Beyond 3 hours, patency was 67% with t-PA and 42% with streptokinase (18).

In the absence of adequate anticoagulation, the higher initial patency of t-PA appears offset by more frequent reocclusions (19–21). Usual heparin doses do not appear to improve reperfusion or initial patency, although they do sustain patency. Similar trials with streptokinase are not available, but with the use of streptokinase and urokinase it has been shown that the aPTT is inversely related to the frequency of recurrent ischemic events (22). In patients receiving streptokinase, inadequate heparin for 3 weeks resulted in a lower patency and more stenosis than adequate heparin, despite all patients receiving aspirin (23).

In the GUSTO angiographic substudy (13), a higher incidence of normal flow was present with accelerated rt-PA (54% with TIMI grade 3 flow) compared with streptokinase/IV heparin (32%) or streptokinase/SC heparin (29%). The 90-minute patency (TIMI flow grade 2 or 3) was significantly higher in the accelerated rt-PA group (80.8%) versus 73.1% in the streptokinase + rt-PA group with IV heparin, 61% in the streptokinase/IV heparin group, and 56% in the streptokinase/SC heparin group. At 3 hours, 24 hours, and 5–7 days, there were no significant differences in patency rates among groups. The angiographic incidence of reocclusion on *heparin plus aspirin* was the lowest reported and similar in all four groups (4.9–6.4% from 90 minutes to 5–7 days) and thus documents the importance and safety of combined heparin plus aspirin.

Mortality

In a comparison of nonaccelerated rt-PA and streptokinase without the immediate use of intravenous heparin, ISIS-3 and GISSI-2 failed to show any difference in either mortality or ejection fraction (24,25) (see Ch. 19). However, in GUSTO, the use of front-loaded rt-PA with intravenous heparin and aspirin reduced 30-day mortality from myocardial infarction by 1.0%, from 7.3% to 6.3%, compared with other streptokinase strategies, representing a 14% proportionate reduction (26). There was a higher incidence of total stroke in the front-loaded rt-PA group (1.55% versus 1.22%), but the net clinical benefit favored the front-loaded rt-PA group over the combined streptokinase groups (6.9% versus 7.8%). GISSI-1 and ISIS-3 demonstrated that thrombolysis with streptokinase compared with placebo saved 26 lives per 1,000 myocardial infarctions treated (27,28). GUSTO showed that an accelerated rt-PA strategy with heparin plus aspirin saved an additional 10 lives per 1,000 patients treated (26).

There is now considerable evidence supporting rapid reperfusion in the treatment of acute MI. With successful reperfusion in the Western Washington Intracoronary Streptokinase trial 1-year mortality was 2.5%, compared with 14.5% when reperfusion did not occur (29). In the TIMI-1 trial, patients who achieved reperfusion at 90 minutes following the start of thrombolytic therapy had a 1-year mortality of 8.1%, compared with 14.8% for patients who remained occluded (30). Since this initial trial, coronary flow after thrombolysis has been graded according to the TIMI system: TIMI grade 3 being normal, brisk flow; TIMI grade 2 being full patency but delayed flow compared with other normal arteries; TIMI grade 1 being penetration of thrombus but incomplete patency; TIMI grade 0 being no flow or penetration of thrombus (28). Combining the results from four angiographic trials comparing TIMI flow to 30–42 day mortality (13,31–34), patients with TIMI grade 3 have the lowest mortality at 3.3%, compared with 6.6% for TIMI grade 2, and 9.5% for TIMI grade 0 or 1 (35,36a).

With this in mind, it must be clarified that 90-minute patency is not necessarily tantamount to reperfusion (36b). Yet several investigators have noted that although either TIMI grade 2 or 3 flow is equated with patency, achievement of TIMI grade 3 flow better correlates with an improved clinical outcome (36c–36e). In these studies TIMI grade 2 flow was shown to be no better, and, perhaps, even worse than TIMI grade 0 or 1 flow. For example, the TEAM-2 investigators demonstrated that those patients with TIMI grade 3 flow after thrombolysis achieved a better outcome as measured by indices of myocardial infarction (36c). Similarly, the GUSTO angiographic study demonstrated that TIMI grade 3 flow at 90 minutes is a significant predictor of 30-day mortality ($p < .01$). In this trial TIMI grade 3 flow was associated with a mortality rate of 4.4% (13).

Earlier treatment is also associated with improved survival. In the GISSI-1 trial (27), there was a 50% improvement in mortality in patients treated within the first hour of their myocardial infarction. The MITI trial (37) upheld these results, demonstrating a mortality of 1.2% for patients treated within the first 70 minutes compared with 8.7% for those treated between 70 minutes and 3 hours; similar results were seen in the European Myocardial Infarction Project (EMIP) (38) and the Grampian Region Early Anistreplase Trial (GREAT) (39a), which were both designed to evaluate early prehospital thrombolytic therapy. In the recent meta-analysis from the Fibrinolytic Therapy Trialists (FTT) Collaborative Group it was calculated that there are 1.6/1000 lives saved for each hour earlier treatment is initiated (39b). In the GUSTO trial, 30-day mortality was 4.3% in patients who received front-loaded rt-PA less than 2 hours after chest pain (versus 5.4% for streptokinase), compared with 5.5% in patients treated between 2 and 4 hours (versus 6.7% for streptokinase), and 8.8% in patients receiving rt-PA between 4 and 6 hours (9.3% for streptokinase) (13).

Limitations of Thrombolytic Therapy

The success of thrombolysis has not been complete. Despite intensive efforts to improve the time to treatment, and use of aggressive thrombolytic strategies, resistance to recanalization is still observed in 19% of patients, TIMI grade 3 flow occurs in only 54% at best with accelerated rt-PA (13), acute coronary reocclusion occurs in at least 5–7%, and substantial bleeding in 0.8–1.5% including rates of intracerebral bleeding in the order of 0.5–0.9% (26,40a,b). Therefore, the efficacy of thrombolytic therapy can be considerably improved. The use of potent and specific anticoagulant and antiplatelet agents as adjuvant therapy to thrombolysis is one attempt at improving the efficacy of thrombolysis.

RATIONALE FOR ANTITHROMBOTIC AND ANTIPLATELET THERAPY DURING AND AFTER THROMBOLYSIS

Importance of Thorough Lysis

The key goal of thrombolytic therapy is to activate the plasminogen system to form plasmin, the enzyme which lysis the fibrin clot. However, as a thrombus undergoes fibrinolysis several local and systemic factors are activated that can lead to reocclusion. It is this balance between thrombolysis and thrombosis where antithrombotic therapy comes into play. The lesion dimensions following thrombolysis are in large part determined by the extent of lysis and influence of shear forces at the site of the lesion. Shear force is a measure of the difference in flow between the center and the periphery of the vessel and has a major influence on subsequent platelet deposition, thrombus growth, and reocclusion. Shear force is related directly to the flow velocity and inversely to the third power of the lumen diameter. At high shear rates, cell membrane ADP is increased and red cells push platelets to the periphery. Platelet deposition occurs mainly at the site of maximal stenosis on exposed arterial media or atherosclerotic plaque (Fig. 20–4) (41–43). Fibrin deposition also increases with shear force, but relative to platelets increases downstream of the stenosis where flow separation and eddy currents also lead to red cell deposition within the tail of thrombus (43).

Angiographic studies document that residual stenosis is a major determinant of subsequent reocclusion in patients receiving only heparin with thrombolytic therapy. In the TIMI-1 study, a minimal lumen diameter of <0.6 mm was associated with reocclusion in 28% of vessels, compared with only 3% if the diameter was >0.6 mm (11). All patients received adjuvant heparin but not aspirin.

Healthy vascular endothelium produces vasocoactive substances that influence the vascular tone and hence coronary dimensions at the site of the lesion and elsewhere. Endothelium-derived relaxing

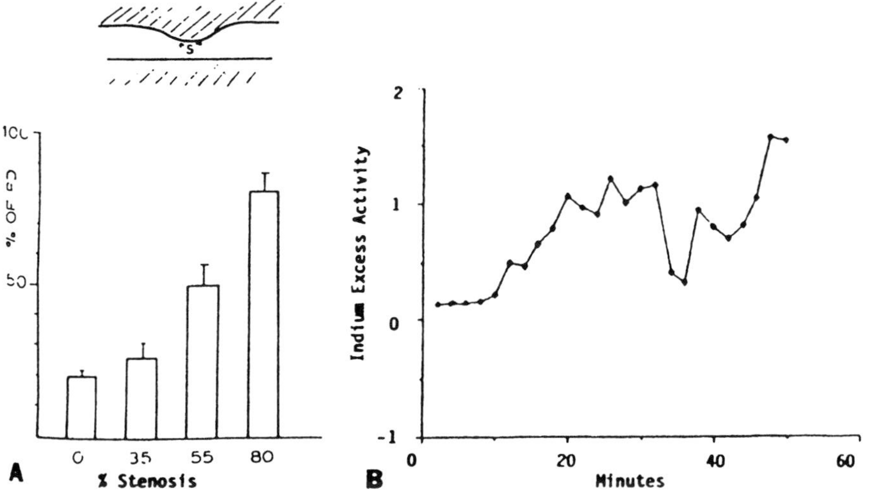

Figure 20–4. Ex vivo perfusion demonstrates the importance of stenosis severity on platelet deposition. Blood from a catheterized carotid artery of a pig is perfused through a chamber containing arterial media (similar to deep injury) with various degrees of eccentric stenosis. Platelet deposition (PD) on the peak of the stenosis (S) is depicted as a percentage of total PD on the exposed tissue (left). A continuous scintigraphic image of PD is recorded in an area of 80% stenosis (right). There is initial thrombus growth (1), embolism (2), and subsequent accelerated regrowth (3). *Modified from Fuster et al: Insights into the pathogenesis of acute ischemic syndromes. Circulation 1988:77:1217, with permission.*

factor (EDRF) is released in response to increased coronary flow, acetylcholine, and thrombin (44). Other agonists include adenosine diphosphate and serotonin, which may be released from platelet-dense granules. These agonists will vasodilate in the presence of normal endothelium, but they vasoconstrict in the presence of dysfunctional or denuded endothelium (45). The vascular endothelium also releases prostacyclin, which, like EDRG, has both vasodilator and powerful antiplatelet effects, and endothelin (46), which is longer-acting and produces vasoconstriction (3). Thrombin also releases endothelin from the arterial wall (3).

Platelets and thus arterial thrombi contain significant quantities of vasoconstrictor substances, especially thromboxane A_2 and serotonin (3). Experimentally, the severity of vasoconstriction correlated with the degree of platelet deposition after deep arterial injury produced by balloon dilation (47). Antiplatelet therapy with aspirin, a drug that inhibits thromboxane synthesis but has no direct vasodilator effects, reduces this vasoconstriction. Deep arterial injury is produced in humans at the time of plaque disruption or coronary angioplasty; this injury has been associated with severe vasoconstriction at the site of injury and in the vessel downstream (48,49).

It is important to maximize thrombolysis to reduce the amount of residual thrombus and thereby reduce the shear force at the site of the lesion. This in turn reduces platelet deposition, the amount of vasoconstrictor substances, and the consequent adverse rheology. Vasodilation with nitrates will also reduce this adverse shear force.

Activation of Thrombosis During Thrombolysis

There is now extensive evidence that thrombosis occurs simultaneously with endogenous and exogenous thrombolysis (50). Active thrombin bound to fibrin and in situ fibrin degradation have been demonstrated within pathologic thrombi by immunohistochemical stains (51). Residual mural thrombus following thrombolysis has a highly active surface, probably because of fibrin-bound thrombin; this surface is more thrombogenic than deeply injured arterial wall (52,53). In addition, plasmin generated during thrombolysis acts on factor V to produce proteolytic fragments with procoagulant activity (54), and it activates factor V to Va, which contributes to accelerated thrombin generation via the prothrombinase complex as discussed earlier (Fig. 20–3).

With thrombolysis, numerous studies have shown that platelets are activated either directly by the thrombolytic agent, or, indirectly through thrombin and, perhaps plasmin (55a-d–57). Platelet-rich thrombi have been shown in-vitro to be much less sensitive to thrombolysis. Jang et al (56) showed in a rabbit model using the femoral artery, that it is easier to thrombolyse fibrin and red blood cell-rich thrombi with rt-PA than platelet-rich thrombi. In fact the concentration of rt-PA required to lyse the platelet-rich thrombi was ten times greater than that needed for the fibrin-rich thrombi. Platelet activation during thrombolysis with streptokinase or rt-PA leads to the generation of thromboxane A_2; metabolites of thromboxane A_2 have been detected in plasma and urine in experimental and clinical studies (55,56). Streptokinase may also induce antibodies that aggregate platelets, adding to the thrombus burden (57).

Markers of activated coagulation indicating thrombin activity can be detected in the plasma and include fibrinopeptide A (FPA), which is released with the conversion of fibrinogen to fibrin (Figs. 20–5 and 20–6) or with generation by plasma levels of thrombin–antithrombin III (TAT), or prothrombin fragment 1.2 (F1.2), (Fig. 20–5). Elevated levels occur during both streptokinase and rt-PA infusions, and they decrease following the infusion (58–61), or with the co-administration of heparin (61–63). TAT is increased 15 minutes after infusion of rt-PA or a combination of urokinase and pro-urokinase (64). Patients with persistently elevated levels at 120 minutes were more likely to have angiographic reocclusion 24 to 36 hours later.

Thrombosis and thrombolysis are opposing, dynamic, and simultaneous processes; inhibiting one enhances the other (50). Thus adjunctive therapy with anticoagulant, antiplatelet, and especially both agents contributes to the lasting efficacy of thrombolysis with reduction of residual thrombus.

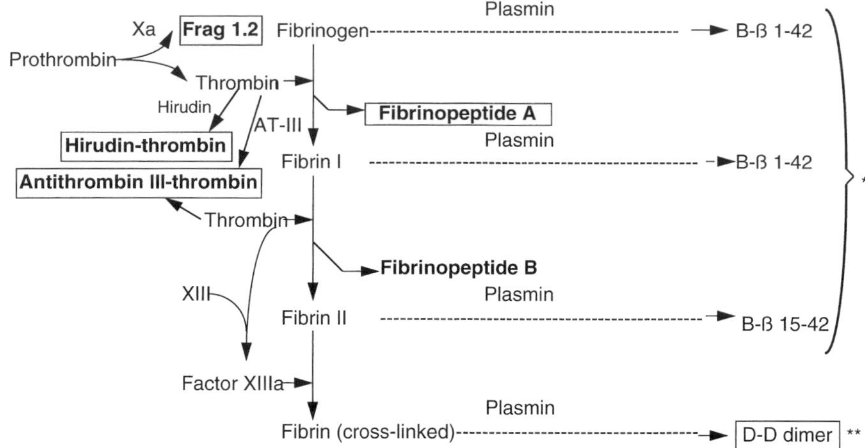

Figure 20–5. This diagram depicts formation of biochemical markers during conversion of prothrombin to thrombin, and fibrinogen to fibrin, and during thrombolysis. These markers can be measured in plasma and indicate the extent of the ongoing chemical conversions.

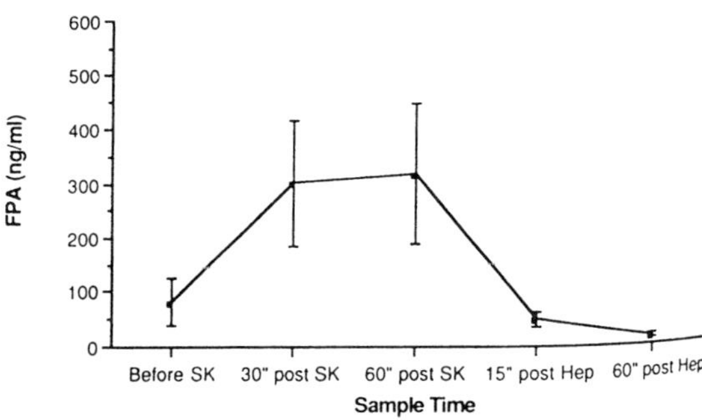

Figure 20–6. Response of fibrinopeptide A to streptokinase (SK) and heparin (Hep) in 19 patients with acute myocardial infarction. The fibrinopeptide A level is markedly elevated immediately after streptokinase, but it declines promptly after heparin. *Adapted from Eisenberg et al (58), with permission.*

ADJUVANT ANTITHROMBOTIC THERAPY DURING THROMBOLYSIS

A-Antithrombins

The propensity of a freshly fibrinolysed thrombus to undergo rethrombosis has led to the development of conjunctive antithrombotic agents. Such therapy can be targeted at the thrombin molecule (such as heparin, low-molecular weight heparin, hirudin and its derivatives, argatroban, etc.) and its precursors (i.e. tissue factor pathway inhibitor, tick associated peptide, etc.), or the platelet (aspirin, dipyridamole, ticlopidine, GP IIb/IIIa antagonists, prostacyclin, inhibitors of thromboxane or serotonin synthesis or receptor antagonists, etc.) (64b, c).

I. Heparin

Thrombin, produced by activation of the coagulation cascade, is the strongest agonist for platelet activation and deposition (8,9). Specific thrombin inhibition can prevent the formation of platelet-rich thrombi after deep arterial injury (9,10), suggesting that thrombin plays a key role in arterial thrombosis. The need for thrombin inhibitors such as heparin is justified by the need to reduce reocclusion and limit the increase in thrombin activity accompanying thrombolysis (58,60–62).

The anticoagulant response to heparin varies greatly among patients with thrombotic diseases for several reasons (65). First, the concentration of heparin-binding proteins varies greatly among different patients. These binding proteins and receptor sites on endothelium must be saturated before therapeutic plasma levels can be achieved. Thus the initial dose of heparin is critical for either intravenous or subcutaneous administration. Second, natural inhibitors of heparin that may be released from thrombus (both platelet factor 4 secreted from activated platelets, and fibrin monomer II formed during the conversion of fibrinogen to fibrin inhibit heparin) are more likely to be influential when large amounts of thrombus are present. Third, heparin is a cofactor that acts indirectly by enhancing binding of antithrombin III and heparin cofactor II to thrombin and other coagulation factors. Binding of thrombin to fibrin within a thrombus or to arterial wall matrix masks receptors on thrombin to antithrombin III or heparin cofactor II. Fourth, at usual therapeutic levels (aPTT 60–85 seconds) heparin is more potent for inhibiting fibrin formation than it is against platelet activation and deposition. Fifth, the clinical efficacy of heparin is optimized if the anticoagulant effect is consistently maintained above a defined level of activated partial thromboplastin time (aPTT) usually ranging between 60 and 85 seconds. However, there may be wide variation in the responsiveness of reagents used in the aPTT test between different laboratories (65,66).

Experimentally, heparin produces a dose-dependent reduction in the deposition of platelets and fibrinogen and the incidence of macroscopic mural thrombosis at dosages of 30 to 250 U/kg, administered as a bolus followed by the same dosage per hour, if started prior to deep arterial injury (9). The higher dosages cannot, however, be safely used in humans, and low dosages are only moderately effective (Fig. 20–7). Heparin effectively potentates lysis when used in combination with a thrombolytic agent. In a canine model of arterial thrombosis using an intravascular copper coil to induce thrombosis, pretreatment with heparin (200 or 300 U/kg)

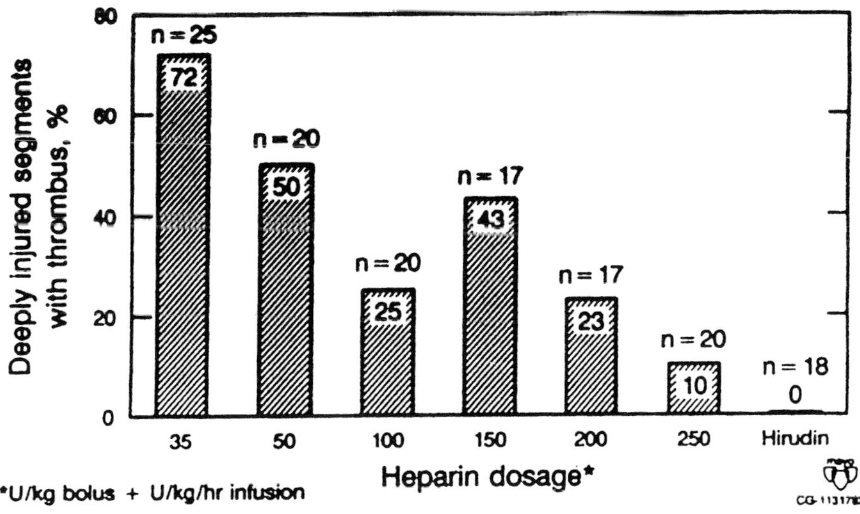

Figure 20–7. Percentage of arterial segments with macroscopic mural thrombus in a porcine carotid model of deep arterial injury produced by balloon dilation. Heparin produced a dose-dependent reduction in mural thrombus formation, from 72% in the lowest to 10% in the highest heparin dosage group. In comparison, hirudin 1 mg/kg bolus followed by 1 mg/kg per hour (which prolonged the aPTT to approximately three times control value) completely abolished mural thrombus formation. *Adapted from Heras et al (9), with permission.*

reduced the time to reperfusion (67,68). In one of the studies thrombus reaccumulated during the t-PA infusion if heparin was discontinued.

An overview of trials from the prethrombolytic era suggests that heparin may be beneficial in acute myocardial infarction. Overall, heparin therapy was associated with a 17% reduction in the risk of death, compared with non-heparin-treated controls, and a 22% reduction in reinfarction (69). Combined results of several major trials using anticoagulant therapy in the *chronic* phase of myocardial infarction in the prethrombolytic era (70–74) showed a significant 21% reduction in mortality, which was attributed mainly to a reduction in venous and arterial thromboembolism. Two newer prospective trials with warfarin are discussed below.

Prior to the GUSTO trial there were five randomized studies evaluating the timing of heparin administration (delayed or at the same time as thrombolysis) with an endpoint of vessel patency: TAMI-3 (75), Bleich (19), HART (20), ECSG-6 (21), Australian (76a) (Table 20–1). In the TAMI-3 study, all patients received intravenous rt-PA (1.5 mg/kg over 4 hours); half of the 134 patients were also randomly allocated to a single bolus of heparin 10,000 U. Infarct-related vessel patency was assessed at 90 minutes and was 79% in both treatment groups (75). Limitations of the study include its relatively small size, the dosage regimen of a single bolus without a subsequent infusion, and a 20-minute delay in initiating heparin therapy in patients receiving rt-PA plus heparin compared with rt-PA alone. There was no increased incidence of bleeding complications in patients receiving heparin in addition to rt-PA.

In a study by Bleich and colleagues (19), 83 patients with acute myocardial infarction were given t-PA 100 mg over 3 hours. Forty-one patients were randomly assigned to t-PA alone and 42 to t-PA with heparin (5000-U bolus followed by 1000 U per hour, titrated to prolong the activated partial thromboplastin time [aPTT] to 1.5 to 2 times control). Angiography at a mean of 57 hours after therapy demonstrated improved patency of the infarct-related artery (IRA) in those who received heparin plus t-PA (71% patent), compared with those who received t-PA alone (44% patent, $p < 0.02$). One patient who received heparin had a major bleeding episode. The Heparin Aspirin Reperfusion Trial (HART) (20) was a randomized trial to compare IRA patency between patients receiving intravenous heparin versus low-dose aspirin given with rt-PA (100 mg) in acute myocardial infarction. An-

Table 20–1. Heparin as Adjunctive Therapy with rt-PA After Acute Myocardial Infarction

Study	No. of Patients	Protocol	Results
Bleich et al	84	rt-PA + IV heparin vs. rt-PA	Improved infarct-related artery patency (71 vs. 43%)
TAMI-3 (73)	134	rt-PA + IV heparin vs. rt-PA (heparin was received by all patients for 24 hrs)	No difference in 90-min patency
Australian National Heart Foundation (76)	202	All patients received rt-PA & IV heparin for 24 hrs. Then, IV heparin vs. aspirin + dipyridamole	No difference in 7-day infarct-related patency
HART (20)	205	rt-PA + IV heparin (7 days) vs. rt-PA + aspirin 80 mg/day (7 days)	Improved infarct-related patency at 18 hrs (82 vs. 52%), but no difference in reocclusion at 7 days
ECSG-6 (21)	652	rt-PA + heparin vs. rt-PA	Improved infarct-related patency at 80 hrs (83 vs. 75%)
GISSI-2 (25)	10,372	rt-PA + SC heparin vs. rt-PA (heparin started 12 hrs after thrombolysis)	No difference in 30-day mortality (9.2 vs. 8.7%)
ISIS-3 (24)	13,746	rt-PA + SC heparin vs. rt-PA (heparin started 4 hrs after thrombolysis)	No difference in 30-day mortality (10.5 vs. 11.0%)

giography was performed at a mean of 18 hours after starting t-PA. In patients receiving heparin but not aspirin, those with an activated partial thromboplastin time (aPTT) less than 45 seconds had an infarct-related patency rate of 45%; in those with an aPTT greater than 45 seconds the patency rate was 88%; finally, in those with aPTT values greater than 60 seconds, the patency rate was 95% (p = 0.025). This study and others document the importance of a therapeutic aPTT in maintaining adequate perfusion of the IRA. The ECSG-6 (21) study demonstrated that in those patients with an aPTT >2 times control at 3–36 hours, patency at a mean of 81 hours was 90% as compared to 80% and 72% for those patients whose aPTT was 1.3–2.0 or <1.3 times control, respectively. It is noteworthy that in this study only 32% of patients achieved a therapeutic aPTT. Lastly, Kaplan et al showed that the aPTT level in patients treated with conjunctive heparin therapy was inversely correlated with recurrent ischemic events (76b).

Further angiographic support for use of intravenous heparin after thrombolysis with rt-PA comes from the Sixth Trial of the European Cooperative Study Group (ECSG-6) (21). This study randomly assigned 652 patients with an acute myocardial infarction treated with rt-PA and aspirin to either concomitant intravenous heparin or placebo. Patients treated with heparin had a higher patency rate after 2 to 5 days (83% versus 75%, p = 0.02), but a similar mortality rate. In those with aPTT > 2× control, patency was 90%, and with aPTT < 1.2× control, patency was 72%.

The Australian National Heart Foundation trial also compared heparin with aspirin after thrombolysis (76a). A total of 241 patients were treated with rt-PA and a 24-hour intravenous infusion of heparin, then randomly assigned to either continued intravenous heparin or aspirin (300 mg) plus dipyridamole (300 mg) daily for 7 days. This study showed no difference in mortality or bleeding after 1 month or coronary artery patency after 7–10 days in the heparin versus the aspirin/dipyridamole groups (81.1% versus 80.2%). These studies taken together show that the main benefit of heparin in conventional doses, especially when the aPTT is >60 seconds or 2× control, appears to be reduction of early reocclusion rather than enhancement of the acute lytic effect of rt-PA.

No clinical mortality trials of adequate size have assessed heparin as the sole adjunctive therapy to thrombolysis. After aspirin was effective in the ISIS-2 trial (28), no heparin trial could be designed without comparison of heparin and aspirin. The SCATI (Studio sulla Calciparina nell'angina e nella trombosi ventricolare nell'infarto) trial (77) is the only study providing data showing benefit in short-term survival rate when subcutaneous heparin (12,500 U SC every 12 hours during hospitalization) was added to streptokinase in the absence of aspirin (Table 20–2). No patients received aspirin in this trial. The mortality in 433 patients receiving

Table 20–2. Heparin as Adjunctive Therapy to Streptokinase in Acute Myocardial Infarction

Study	No. of Patients	Protocol	Results
SCATI (77)	433	SK + SC heparin, until discharge (no aspirin)	Reduction of in-hospital mortality (4.6% vs. 8.6%)
GISSI-2 (25) including International Study	10,396	SK + SC heparin vs. SK alone (heparin started 12 hrs after thrombolysis)	Slight reduction in 30-day mortality (7.9% vs. 9.2%, NS)
ISIS-3 (24)	13,780	SK + SC heparin vs. SK alone (heparin started 4 hrs after thrombolysis)	No difference in 30-day mortality (10.3% vs. 10.6%)
GUSTO (26)	20,251	SK + SC heparin vs. SK + IV heparin (heparin started 4 hrs after thrombolysis)	No difference in 30-day mortality (7.2% vs. 7.4%)

SK: Streptokinase
SC: Subcutaneous
IV: Intravenous

thrombolysis with streptokinase (1,500,000 U over 1 hour) during the in-hospital period was 8.8% in the control group and 4.5% in the heparin treated group (p = 0.05). However, almost all bleeding complications were seen in the heparin treated group (4.4%). Patients given heparin without thrombolysis showed a trend toward reduced in-hospital mortality that was not statistically significant (7.7% with heparin administration and 11.7% in the control group, p = 0.10). Of those patients given streptokinase, there was a trend toward reduced recurrent myocardial ischemia with heparin administration, but little difference in the rate of nonfatal reinfarction (Fig. 20–8).

Despite being designed to primarily assess the effect of streptokinase, aspirin, or both on the mortality following an acute myocardial infarction, the large ISIS-2 study (28) also reported on the effect of heparin administration on clinical endpoints. Heparin administration was planned at entry, but it was not randomized, and there were no details on the dosages or frequency of administration. Despite these limitations, heparin therapy was associated with a beneficial effect on vascular mortality. During the first 35 days following the infarction, mortality was 8.3% in patients treated with intravenous heparin compared with 9.0% for subcutaneous heparin and 10.1% for those not receiving heparin. Additionally, the benefit was largely in those patients who received streptokinase and aspirin (Table 20–3). Heparin administration was, however, associated with an increased incidence of bleeding (1.1%, 0.5%, 0.3% for intravenous, subcutaneous, and no heparin, respectively).

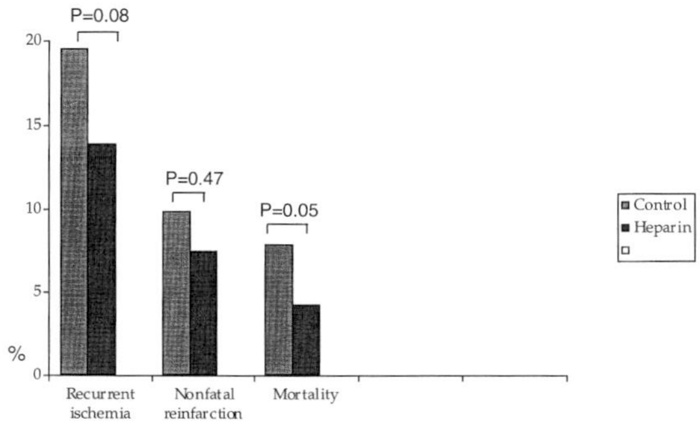

Figure 20–8. Major in-hospital endpoints in patients receiving streptokinase in the SCATI study (77).

The pilot randomized study for ISIS-2 (78) was small (619 patients) and studied the effect of heparin when started 12 hours after thrombolytic therapy. Streptokinase (1,500,000 U over 1 hour) was followed by either heparin 1,000 U/hour starting 12 hours later or matching placebo. Despite the numbers being too small for definite conclusions, heparin therapy with or without streptokinase was associated with a trend toward reduced reinfarction (2.2% compared with 4.5% in those not receiving heparin). There was no difference in mortality or bleeding complications between the treatment groups.

The combined results of the large ISIS-3 (24) and GISSI-2 (25) trials also indicated a small reduction in mortality in patients assigned to subcutaneous heparin, but this effect was apparent only during the in-hospital treatment period while patients were on treatment (0.5% mortality benefit during first 7 days). Off treatment, there was no difference in mortality during follow-up, and reinfarction rates were not reduced. The delay (4 hours in ISIS-3 and 12 hours in GISSI-2), low unmonitored dose, and subcutaneous mode of administration of heparin in these two trials likely led to subtherapeutic aPTT's during the first 24–48 hours, when the risk of reocclusion is highest, and may have vitiated any potential benefit of early reperfusion from rt-PA.

Both the principle and angiographic substudy of the GUSTO trial (13,26) have provided information about the benefits and risks of heparin plus aspirin administration after thrombolysis but, as planned, did not provide a control group without heparin. This study randomly assigned 41,021 patients into four treatment groups: (i) accelerated rt-PA plus intravenous heparin, (ii) streptokinase plus subcutaneous heparin, (iii) streptokinase plus intravenous heparin, or (iv) both thrombolytic agents (nonaccelerated rt-PA and lower-dose streptokinase) with intravenous heparin; all patients received 160 mg aspirin daily. Essentially, the results showed no clinical benefit from immediate intravenous heparin versus subcutaneous heparin for streptokinase when added to aspirin (8.2% versus 7.9%) in terms of mortality and nonfatal stroke. Furthermore, there was no significant difference in patency rates between the use of intravenous hep-

Table 20–3. Effect of Heparin Therapy "Planned at Entry" on 35-Day Vascular Mortality in Each of the Treatment Groups in the ISIS-2 Study

	Mortality, % (*n* = total patients)			
Heparin	Streptokinase and Aspirin	Streptokinase	Aspirin	Double Placebo
IV	6.4 (1,024)	8.3 (2,054)	8.7 (2,048)	13.1 (1,023)
SC	7.6 (1,805)	9.0 (3,601)	9.4 (3,605)	13.5 (1,800)
none	9.6 (1,463)	10.1 (2,937)	9.8 (2,934)	12.9 (1,477)

arin or subcutaneous heparin with streptokinase. There was no beneficial effect on mortality with the combined use of thrombolytics over standard-dose streptokinase and subcutaneous heparin (mortality and nonfatal stroke rates, 7.9% versus 7.9%). Accelerated-dose rt-PA plus intravenous heparin resulted in an absolute reduction of 1.0%, from 7.3% to 6.3%, mortality over the other streptokinase strategies. Half of the benefit was present at 24 hours after starting therapy and persisted at 1 month. This accounted for a 19% reduction in early mortality with accelerated rt-PA (15). The mechanism by which accelerated rt-PA plus intravenous heparin produced a better outcome appears related to a rapid, complete, and maintained restoration of coronary blood flow (TIMI grade 3 flow) in the infarct-related artery (see earlier discussion). These important results strongly support the hypothesis that earlier and sustained reperfusion leads to improved survival. The combined use of heparin plus aspirin resulted in the lowest angiographic reocclusion rates so far reported, 4.9–6.4% at 5–7 days for all thrombolytic groups (13).

Thrombolytic agents such as streptokinase, urokinase, or APSAC are nonspecific fibrinolytics, and they convert plasminogen to plasmin, deplete fibrinogen, plasminogen, and factor V and VIII (40b,79). It is unclear how this systemic lytic state relates to possible reduction of reocclusion in view of continued reocclusion after both streptokinase and rt-PA when heparin alone is used post lysis (11), and the very low rates of reocclusion when both heparin and aspirin are used after any thrombolysis (13,80).

Several important issues concerning the use of heparin as adjuvant therapy in thrombolysis remain unresolved (40). First, it is not clear whether the differences in efficacy observed between the accelerated rt-PA regimen used in the GUSTO trial and the conventional protocol used in the GISSI-2 and ISIS-3 trials are due to the more aggressive heparin plus aspirin regimen or to a more aggressive thrombolysis strategy. Second, the GUSTO trial assessed the benefits of intravenous heparin versus subcutaneous heparin with streptokinase plus aspirin (it found no difference in mortality rates), but it did not do the same for rt-PA or other thrombolytics. However, large-scale randomized trials of mortality comparing intravenous heparin versus no heparin after thrombolysis with rt-PA do not make sense because of the high reocclusion rate without heparin. Third, the issue of duration of heparin treatment after thrombolytic therapy is unresolved. Although the Australian National Heart Trial (76) and the rt-PA Heparin Duration Trial (81) showed that heparin beyond 24 hours was no more effective than an adequate antiplatelet regimen in maintaining infarct-related vessel patency, the occlusion rates of 13–20% in both groups were high, and residual thrombus in 17–21% by angiography (which underestimates thrombus) suggests that long-term anticoagulation plus aspirin is likely necessary.

II. Oral Anticoagulants

Pooled data from randomized trials performed in the prethrombolytic era indicate that oral anticoagulants in the acute phase of myocardial infarction reduce mortality by more than 20% (74). Heparin followed by oral warfarin therapy for 1 month after myocardial infarction may produce further lysis of the residual coronary thrombus (92). This will reduce the shear force at the site of the lesion, lessening the likelihood of reocclusion, and may reduce progression of the original coronary lesion. The recent APRICOT (Antithrombotics in the

Prevention of Reocclusion in Coronary Thrombolysis) trial (83) was designed to determine angiographic characteristics predictive of reocclusion after successful thrombolysis with streptokinase or anoisoylated plasminogen–streptokinase activator complex (APSAC), and the antithrombotic effects of three regimens (aspirin 325 mg vs. coumadin, international normalized ratio [INR] 2.8–4.0, vs. placebo) on angiographic and clinical outcomes in 248 patients. After 3 months aspirin appeared slightly better than coumadin in reducing angiographic reocclusion, reinfarction, and mortality. However, the low dose of heparin (20,000 U/24 hours) preceding and while starting coumadin therapy (when 5 of the 7 reinfarctions on coumadin occurred) and the subtherapeutic INRs (<2.8) in 22% of patients leaving the hospital on coumadin necessitate repeating the study.

The ATACS (Antithrombotic Therapy in Acute Coronary Syndromes Research Group) trial (84) compared combined therapy with aspirin (162.5 mg/day) and anticoagulation (intravenous heparin, then warfarin, INR 2–3) versus aspirin alone in patients with unstable angina and non-Q wave myocardial infarctions. This study showed a significant reduction in recurrent ischemic events in the combination group versus aspirin alone (10.5% vs. 27%, $p = 0.004$). Bleeding complications were slightly higher in the combination therapy group.

The WARIS (Warfarin Re-Infarction Study) trial (85), was a placebo-controlled study of 1,214 patients followed for 37 months after myocardial infarction, and it showed that warfarin compared with placebo in the secondary prevention of myocardial infarction significantly reduced (placebo vs. warfarin) mortality from 20% in the placebo to 15% in the warfarin group, reinfarction from 20% to 14%, and cerebrovascular accidents from 7% to 3%. The reduction in reinfarction from 5.1% in the placebo to 2.3% in the warfarin group over 37 months was confirmed in a lower risk of postinfarction patients by the ASPECT study (86). The encouraging results of the ATACS, WARIS, and ASPECT trials now necessitate a direct comparison between warfarin, aspirin, and combination therapy in myocardial infarction. The Coumadin Aspirin Reinfarction Study (CARS) is an ongoing trial comparing combined low-dose aspirin and warfarin therapy versus aspirin therapy alone in secondary prevention of myocardial infarction, death, and stroke after myocardial infarction.

Aspirin

Thrombolysis produces marked platelet activation (55,56). Possible mechanisms include exposure of thrombin bound to fibrin on the surface of the thrombus (Fig. 20–3), formation of plasmin, and direct or indirect actions on the platelet or through stimulation of other procoagulant systems on the surface of the thrombus (63). The dose required to effectively block platelet aggregation is a subject of debate. Some studies such as the Dutch-TIA trial concluded that a dose as low as 30 mg/day is all that is needed and may, in fact, be better than a larger dose due to inhibition of platelet synthesis of thromboxane, without blocking endothelial cell synthesis of prostacyclin (87b). Nevertheless, it is currently recommended to give 162.5–325 mg of aspirin immediately, in conjunction with thrombolysis, and daily thereafter (87c).

The large and definitive ISIS-2 study (28) in patients with prolonged chest pain with or without electrocardiographic changes clearly confirmed the clinical efficacy of aspirin combined with streptokinase. More than 17,000 patients with suspected acute myocardial infarction presenting within 24 hours of the onset of symptoms were enrolled. A 2×2 factorial design was used to evaluate streptokinase (1,500,000 U over 1 hour), aspirin 160 mg/day, and a combination of the two agents. The major endpoint was 5-week vascular mortality, which was reduced 25% by streptokinase alone, 23% by aspirin alone, and 42% by both agents compared with placebo ($p < 0.0001$) (Fig. 20–9). The benefit on mortality evident at 35 days persisted throughout a median follow-up of 15 months. The beneficial effect of aspirin was probably related to a reduction of early reinfarction rate and spontaneous or streptokinase-induced reperfusion. The in-hospital reinfarction rate was 3.7% in patients receiving streptokinase alone compared with 2.9% in those given placebo. However, the group allocated to streptokinase plus aspirin had a reinfarction rate of only 1.8%, suggesting that aspirin is beneficial in the prevention of reocclusion

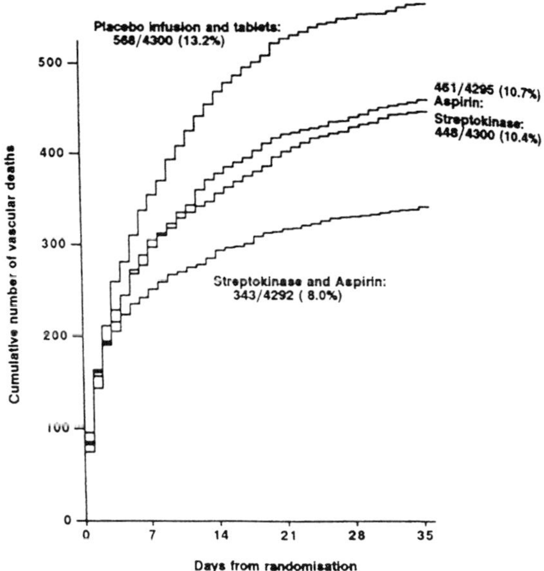

Figure 20–9. Effect of aspirin, streptokinase, both, or neither on 35-day vascular mortality in the ISIS-2 study (28).

after thrombolysis. Major bleeding complications (requiring blood transfusions) occurred in 0.6% of those receiving streptokinase plus aspirin, compared with 0.5% receiving streptokinase alone, and 0.3% in the placebo group. Streptokinase plus aspirin was associated with a reduced incidence of stroke (including fatal and disabling strokes) during the in-hospital period. The stroke incidence was 0.6% with streptokinase plus aspirin, 0.7% with streptokinase alone, and 1.0% with placebo. Hemorrhagic strokes were slightly more frequent during the first 24 hours in the combined streptokinase plus aspirin group; this was more than offset by a reduced incidence of nonhemorrhagic stroke during the remainder of hospitalization. A meta-analysis by Roux et al of 32 trials including 4930 patients treated with either rt-PA or streptokinase demonstrated that aspirin reduces angiographic reocclusion from 25% to 11%, and recurrent ischemia from 41% to 25% (80). A longer follow-up of patients in the ISIS-2 trial showed that the early mortality benefit achieved with aspirin persists at least four years later (87d).

Not all patients included in the ISIS-2 study had a confirmed myocardial infarction. The entry criteria were liberal enough so that a number of patients with noncardiac chest pain and unstable angina, a condition known to benefit from aspirin therapy (88–91), were undoubtedly included. This limitation was unlikely to alter the overall conclusions because of the large size of the study. Aspirin is of definite benefit in combination with streptokinase and now has an established place in the acute management of myocardial infarction.

Nitrates

Vasoconstriction at the site of a coronary lesion increases the local shear force and consequently platelet deposition, a major contributing factor to rethrombosis (see Ch. 12). Nitrates produce a nonendothelium-dependent vasodilation that reduces the shear force and may additionally enhance delivery of the thrombolytic agent to the site of thrombosis. There is also experimental evidence that intravenous nitroglycerin has a significant in vivo antiplatelet effect (92). In a porcine model of deep arterial injury by balloon dilation, an infusion of nitroglycerin titrated to reduce the mean arterial pressure by 10% also significantly reduced platelet deposition.

Nitroglycerin inhibits platelet aggregation in humans (93) and may also enhance coronary artery patency in humans. An angiographic study demonstrated an 88% patency rate of the infarct-related artery following intracoronary streptokinase and intracoronary nitroglycerin, compared with 73% following intracoronary streptokinase alone (94). If data from the first three European Cooperative combined studies evaluating rt-PA are pooled, a trend toward increased vessel patency was noted in those patients who received nitrates during the 6 hours prior to thrombolysis (95).

In the recently reported GISSI-3 (96) trial, the systematic administration of nitrates (intravenous for the first 24 hours, followed by 10 mg of transdermal glyceryl trinitrate daily for 6 weeks), although shown not to cause any unfavorable clinical events, did not show any independent effect on improving survival or ventricular function after acute myocardial infarction. The ISIS-4 trial (97) similarly failed to document benefit of nitrates 5 weeks after acute myocardial infarction, but it showed somewhat fewer deaths on days 0–1. However, because of delayed administration up to several hours and because many patients in the control group received nitrates for symptomatic ischemia, the interpretation of results from these two trials is complicated.

Newer Antithrombotic Therapy

Antithrombins

Thrombin is the most potent activator of platelets (9,10,98); it also converts fibrinogen to fibrin and activates factors V, VIII, and XIII, the last of which crosslinks fibrin for stabilization of the thrombus. Active thrombin binds to subendothelial extracellular matrix. After binding, it is protected from inactivation by the relatively large size of the antithrombin III–heparin complex (99).

Hirudin, a specific thrombin inhibitor, isolated from the saliva of the European leech, documents the important role of thrombin in the thrombotic response to deep arterial injury. Hirudin has the greatest binding affinity of any antithrombin (Kd 2×10^{-13} for recombinant hirudin). It inhibits platelet aggregation to thrombin but not thromboxane, ADP, or collagen. Thrombin inhibition with hirudin reduces fibrin deposition at lower doses (aPTT, $1.7 \times$ control), and at higher doses (aPTT, $>2\times$ control) hirudin can totally eliminate mural thrombosis and reduces platelet deposition to a single layer or less (99). Hirudin binds to thrombin with 1:1 stoichiometry, so that the plasma concentration of hirudin required to prevent thrombus formation totally is proportional to the amount of thrombin generated (100–102a).

The powerful and specific antithrombin action of hirudin compared with heparin markedly reduced platelet, fibrin(ogen), and thrombus deposition in deeply injured porcine carotid arteries (9,99). Heparin and hirudin prolonged the aPTT to twice the control value. Thrombosis in the heparin treated animals was present in 57% of segments, whereas no thrombus was found in the hirudin treated group (Fig. 20–7). Quantitative platelet deposition was markedly decreased and limited to a single layer by hirudin compared with extensive, multilayered platelet deposition in pigs treated with heparin (9).

Although both heparin and hirudin are antithrombin drugs, their efficacy in arterial thrombosis is very different. Heparin is a cofactor of antithrombin III; heparin–antithrombin III only partially inhibits new thrombin formation and new fibrin polymerization in arteries. Heparin, unlike hirudin, is inhibited by fibrin II monomer and platelet factor 4, released from activated platelets, and is 50 times less effective at partially inhibiting fibrin-bound compared with free thrombin. On the other hand, hirudin totally inhibits fibrin-bound and free thrombin at the same dosage (98–104).

Hirudin binding induces conformational changes to thrombin and blocks its coagulant activity. Thrombin activates platelets by binding to the thrombin receptor on the platelet membrane and producing a proteolytic degradation of GP V (102a,103,105). Hirudin's high affinity for thrombin and the platelet thrombin receptor can induce thrombin displacement from platelets (106). This may explain the efficient endogenous lysis of thrombus with hirudin (107). The hirudin molecule is about one-tenth the size of the heparin–antithrombin III (AT III) complex, and it easily binds thrombin-bound fibrin compared with the masking of receptors to AT III on fibrin-bound thrombin (103,104). There is no naturally occurring inhibitor of hirudin. Renal elimination is the route of clearance (100,102). The prevention of thrombosis and the "dethrombosis" of platelet by hirudin documents the pivotal role of thrombin in the activation of platelets and maintenance of arterial thrombi (9,99,107,108). Unlike heparin, hirudin totally blocks growth of mural thrombus at high and low shear rates (9,99). By totally blocking growth of thrombus, hirudin also enhances lysis by endogenous tissue-type plasminogen activator (rt-PA) or urokinase. This strategy of prolonged antithrombotic therapy to reduce intravascular thrombus and improve lumen diameter may be useful after thrombolysis for myocardial infarction or as primary antithrombotic therapy for patients with unstable angina or non-Q wave myocardial infarction (102b).

The TIMI-5 trial (32) randomized 246 patients to standard dose heparin versus one of four dose of hirudin (bolus 0.15–0.6 mg/kg, followed by a continuous infusion of 0.05–0.2 mg/kg hour) in combination with front loaded rt-PA. The primary end point, TIMI grade 3 flow at 90 minutes and 18–36 hours, was 61.8% in the hirudin group and 49.4% in the heparin group ($p = 0.07$). This trend became highly significant at 18–36 hours where patency was 98% in the hirudin group and 89% in the heparin group ($p = 0.01$). Furthermore, reocclusion occurred in only 1.6% of patients vs. 6.7% for heparin. The incidence of in-hospital death or reinfarction was only 6.8% for hirudin, as compared to 16.7% for heparin ($p = 0.02$). The composite endpoint of death myocardial infarction, severe CHF or cardiogenic shock was similarly reduced with hirudin (19.0% vs. 9.3%, $p = 0.03$). Lastly, the incidence of major spontaneous hemorrhage was infrequent, and more common in the heparin group (4.7% vs. 1.2%).

The HIT-I trial (109a) randomized 143 patients to hirudin (bolus 0.1–0.15 mg/kg, infusion 0.07–0.15 mg/kg/hour) in combination with front loaded rt-PA. TIMI grade 3 flow at 60 minutes was present in 50%, 57% and 61% of patients respectively. This percentage increased to 72%, 76% and 92% at 36–48 hours. Reocclusion occurred in 6.7%, 5.6%, and 1.2% of patients, with reinfarction in 0.0%, 4.8% and 1.2% of patients. The incidence of bleeding was 0.05, 2.4%, and 2.4% in the respective group.

The TIMI-6 study, (109b) a non-angiographic trial, reported findings from the combination of hirudin (with similar dosing to TIMI-5) or heparin and streptokinase in 193 patients. The composite endpoint of death, CHF, or cardiogenic shock was 17.6% in the heparin group compared to 21.6%, 9.7%, and 11.6% with the respective hirudin doses suggesting that a dose of 0.1 mg/kg/hr was the optimal dose.

Two angiographic pilot studies from the Montreal Heart Institute evaluated hirulog in combination with streptokinase (110a,b). Lidon et al randomized 45 patients to hirudin 0.5 mg/kg/hour for 12 hours followed by 0.1 mg/kg/hour for 5 days or standard dose heparin (aPTT 2-2.5 times control). Patency of the IRA at 90 minutes was significantly better in the hirudin treated patients (77% vs. 47%, $p < 0.05$) (102). Furthermore, TIMI grade 3 flow was 67% in the IRA compared to 40% for heparin ($p = 0.08$). Theroux et al evaluated hirulog at dose of either 0.5 or 1.0 mg/kg/hr, and found that both patency and TIMI grade 3 flow were improved, though there was no dose response effect (110b).

In spite of these promising initial results, three recent trials of hirudin in acute coronary syndromes suggest that patients with acute coronary problems may have higher blood levels (111–113) than stable patients (100) which may cause bleeding especially if the aPTT is > 100 during thrombolytic therapy. The TIMI-9A (112), and GUSTO-IIa (112) trials all showed that hirudin in combination with front loaded rt-PA resulted in a significant increase in hemorrhagic stroke and bleeding complications as did heparin if used in larger doses. Despite these important safety concerns, which are addressed by decreasing the dose to maintain the aPTT at 60–85 sec, specific thrombin inhibition has attractive advantages over heparin. The GUSTO IIb and TIMI-9B studies are currently ongoing with a lower dose of hirudin (0.1 mg/kg bolus and 0.1 mg/kg/hr infusion) which is not causing excess bleeding.

Antiplatelet Therapy

Despite it wide use, safety and low cost, aspirin has limited effect on in vivo inhibition of platelet aggregation. Aspirin irreversibly inhibits cyclooxygenase and production of platelet thromboxane (114a). However, two remaining pathways of platelet activation, one dependent on ATP and collagen, and the other on thrombin, remain unaffected. Several platelet inhibitors have been identified, but only antagonists to the receptor involved in the final common pathway of platelet aggregation (glycoprotein IIb/IIIa receptor) have reached the clinical trial stage (114b).

Unlike aspirin, antagonists of the GP IIb/IIIa platelet membrane receptor, completely abolish platelet aggregation at a dosage where there is more than 80% binding (114b). This has led to the development of several different types of drugs including peptides (e.g. Integrelin, and MK383), non-peptides (e.g. lamifiban, xemlofiban, tirolifiban), and antibodies (e.g. c7E3) (114d, e).

The monoclonal antibody 7E3 is the only anti–glycoprotein IIb/IIa that is commercially available for complex angioplasty after myocardial infarction (115,116). This monoclonal antibody has been shown to accelerate initial thrombolysis and prevent thrombosis in the canine model (117,118). In the eight Thrombolysis and Angioplasty in Myocardial Infarction trial (TAMI-8) (119), 60 patients received rt-PA for acute myocardial infarction followed by 7E3 at escalating doses and variable times (3, 6, and 15 hours after thrombolysis). All patients received aspirin and intravenous heparin. Angiography was performed 24 hours after therapy. There was evidence of improved infarct-related vessel patency in the group receiving 7E3 (92% vs. 56%, $p = 0.03$). This favorable result came at a cost of increased hemorrhagic complications (27% of patients). However, it was important to note that none of these bleeding complications included hemorrhagic strokes. Significant thrombocytopenia occurred in two of the first four patients.

A subgroup analysis of patients with myocardial infarction who received c7E3 during high-risk angioplasty in the recent EPIC trial, demonstrated a significant reduction in recurrent ischemic events with no recurrent infarction or revascularization at 6 months of follow-up (116). There are currently two randomized trials under way evaluating conjunctive therapy with GP IIb/IIIa antagonists in conjunction with rt-PA (Integrelin in one trial, and lamifiban in the other) (79a). Preliminary data from the Integrelin study demonstrated nearly complete restoration of TIMI grade 3 flow in the 110 patients evaluated, with fewer reinfarctions, and a low incidence of bleeding (119b).

The recent EPILOG trial (Evaluation of PTCA to improve Long-term Outcome by c7E3 GP IIb/IIIa Receptor Blockade) and CAPTURE trial (Chimeric 7E3 Antiplatelet Therapy in Unstable Angina Refractory to Standard Treatment) were prematurely terminated because of positive findings at interim analysis. Efficacy of 7E3 was found to exceed a predetermined stopping level for both studies (119c).

One question which remains to be resolved is whether heparin is necessary at all with these agents. Currently we are evaluating this question using the ex-vivo perfusion chamber in patients undergoing high-risk angioplasty with c7E3. The recently started PARAGON study will evaluate this question in patients with unstable angina.

ARTERIAL THROMBOEMBOLISM

Most systemic emboli occurring soon after a myocardial infarction originate from a left ventricular (LV) mural thrombus (120–132). More than 90% of thrombi develop in patients suffering an anterior Q wave myocardial infarction, particularly if the cardiac apex is involved and has an akinetic or dyskinetic wall motion. Other contributing factors to the formation of thrombi include local inflammation, stasis of blood in a dyskinetic region of the left ventricle, and a generalized hypercoagulable state present soon after an acute infarct (59,132–137). The majority of thrombi develop in the first 48-hours (two-thirds), and 83% (in the largest series) (121–127,131,138) initially develop in the first week following the infarct. Ventricular thrombi are intermediate in composition between arterial and venous thrombi; they contain abundant platelets and significant fibrin from the blood stasis in the region of abnormal wall motion.

Autopsy studies, despite an inherent selection bias, first suggested that anticoagulation may be beneficial. Left ventricular thrombi were found in more than 50% of patients not treated with anticoagulants, compared with 20% to 25% of those anticoagulated (72,139).

More recently, two-dimensional echocardiography (with a sensitivity and specificity of 85% to 90% for detecting left ventricular thrombi) (121–127,131, 138,140) has become the method of choice for following changes in thrombus morphology, including the effect of anticoagulation. Six prospective, randomized, controlled studies evaluated anticoagulation, starting within 12 to 36 hours of the onset of symptoms, in patients with anterior Q wave infarcts (Table 20–4) (77,123,130,142–144). The two largest studies (77,130) employed a fixed regimen of heparin, 12,500 U twice daily; the other smaller studies used heparin (adjusted for the aPTT) (123) or heparin followed by warfarin (142–144). Combining data from all six studies, anticoagulation halves the in-hospital incidence of left ventricular thrombus

Table 20–4. Randomized Studies on the Effect of Early Anticoagulation on Left Ventricular Thrombi in Acute Anterior Myocardial Infarction

				Left Ventricular Thrombi		Emboli	
Author	Study Entry	Echo-cardiography	Treatment	Treated	Control	Treated	Control
Nordrehaug (144)	<12 hrs	at discharge	heparin/warfarin*	0/26	7/27	0/26	1/27
Arvan (143)	<12 hrs	10 days	heparin/warfarin*	4/13	6/17	1/13	1/17
Davis (142)	<12 hrs	14 days	heparin/warfarin*+	14/25	15/27	0/25	1/27
Gueret (123)	<12 hrs	at discharge	heparin*	8/21	13/25	1/21	1/25
Turpie (130)	<36 hrs	4–7 days	heparin++δ	10/95	28/88	1/95	4/88
SCATI (77)	<24 hrs	at discharge	heparin++	19/107	34/93	0/107	2/93
				55/287 (19%)	103/277 (37%)	3/287 (1%)	10/277 (4%)
				$p < 0.001$		$p = 0.04$	

*Adjusted for aPTT, prothrombin time.

+Control group received heparin 5,000 U three times daily, 18/27 also received warfarin.

++12,500 U twice daily.

δControl group received heparin 5,000 U twice daily.

formation, from 37% in the control group to 19% in patients who were anticoagulated. The delay in initiating anticoagulation with heparin, lack of a bolus, or both probably accounts for the relatively high incidence of ventricular thrombi in those anticoagulated.

The Canadian study (130), which used a fixed heparin dosage, found that treatment efficacy correlated with the plasma heparin level and the prolongation of the aPTT, suggesting that a dosage adjusted for the aPTT may have been even more effective. The control group received low-dose heparin, which was not effective at preventing thrombus formation. They also noted that beta blocker therapy was associated with a significant increase in the incidence of thrombi (28% compared with 15% in those not taking beta blockers, $p = 0.01$). This has been observed by others (145) and probably relates to the negative inotropic effect of these drugs.

The other large study, from the SCATI group in Italy (77), is relevant to the current clinical practice because more than half of the patients (enrolled within 6 hours of the onset of symptoms) were also given streptokinase. Thrombolytic agents may prevent mural thrombus if myocardium is salvaged and wall motion is preserved, by lysing any newly formed thrombus. However, thrombolysis enhances thrombin generation (58,59), may increase thrombosis, and has had little impact on the incidence of left ventricular thrombosis (146). Since systemic thrombolysis has become standard treatment for myocardial infarction, there have been seven studies evaluating the role of thrombolytics in the prevention of left ventricular thrombosis (126,146–151). Six of the seven studies reported a trend in favor of thrombolysis, with only one achieving statistical significance. In a recent meta-analysis evaluating the impact of thrombolytics on ventricular thrombosis after an acute myocardial infarction, data from six of these studies did show a favorable trend in the thrombolytic treated group, but it did not attain statistical significance (152).

Alternatively, thrombolytic agents have been used in an attempt to dissolve ventricular thrombi (153–155). This approach may actually enhance thrombosis by exposing fibrin-bound thrombin, enhancing further thrombin generation, or it may cause systemic embolization of a penduncalated or freely mobile thrombus.

Left ventricular mural thrombus formation has been used as a surrogate endpoint for arterial embolism because the embolic event rate is low (approximately 10–15% of the incidence of LV thrombus) and no recent study has had sufficient power to detect a reduction in emboli with anticoagulation. However, the large, randomized studies from the Medical Research Council (71) and Veterans' Administration (72) provide strong evidence that anticoagulation is beneficial. Systemic emboli (cerebral plus peripheral) were reduced from 3.4% to 1.3% with anticoagulation in the former, and from 5.4% to 0.8% in the latter.

The more recent studies have focused on those with anterior Q wave infarcts, the group of patients at particular risk for left ventricular thrombus formation and embolism. If the in-hospital embolic event rates from the six recent, randomized studies are combined, the incidence of clinically recognized systemic embolism is approximately 4% in the control group and 1% in those anticoagulated (Table 20–4). The peak incidence of embolism is during the first 7–10 days postinfarct; most of the remaining emboli will occur during the next 3 months. Beyond 3 months, emboli are generally associated with persistent, severe, global left ventricular dysfunction but not with isolated localized dyskinesis (156). Anticoagulation is most effective if commenced immediately, because two-thirds of thrombi form within 48 hours and emboli may occur before thrombus is visible by echocardiography. In addition, anticoagulation appears to be more effective at preventing thrombus formation than in lysing preexisting thrombi.

Anticoagulation was still found to be of benefit in two randomized studies of patients with established thrombi (157,158). Thrombus characteristics associated with an increased likelihood of embolism include large size, protrusion into the luminal cavity, and especially, free intracavity motion (126). Echocardiographic thrombus features frequently change spontaneously over time (123). Many thrombi disappear during anticoagulation, but a few recur soon after the anticoagulants are stopped (159). It is not known whether late thrombus recurrence has an associated increased embolic risk. Patients with a left ventricular aneurysm but no diffuse contraction abnormality have an incidence of emboli beyond 3 months after infarction of less than 1%/year and thus do not appear to require anticoagulation (156). Because starting oral anticoagulation without therapeutic heparin coverage increases the incidence of LV thrombus, therapeutic heparin (aPTT 55–85 seconds) should always be given until the INR has attained a therapeutic level of 2.0–3.0 for 2 days (160).

Antiplatelet agents are of little benefit in preventing left ventricular thrombi. Two studies, one using aspirin 100 mg/day and the other aspirin plus dipyridamole (161,162) started within 12–24 hours of a myocardial infarct, found no reduction in the incidence of thrombus formation.

VENOUS THROMBOEMBOLISM

Much of our current knowledge of the natural history of deep vein thrombosis comes from studies performed in the 1960s and early 1970s, when the management of acute myocardial infarction included prolonged bedrest. Deep leg vein thrombosis begins soon after the infarct (50% develop within 72 hours and 75% within 5–7 days), but it usually takes another 2 or 3 days to propagate proximally into the popliteal, femoral, or iliac vessels (163–168). This occurs in approximately one-quarter of calf vein thrombi; conversely, the greatly majority (90–95%) of proximal thrombi arise from the calf veins (167,168). Prevention of iliofemoral thrombosis is of major importance because, if untreated, 40–50% will embolize to the lungs. Overall, 10% of deep calf vein thrombi will lead to clinical pulmonary embolism, of which one-third will prove fatal.

The risk of venous thromboembolism appears similar to that following major surgery, another condition associated with a temporary hypercoagulable state (169). Factors associated with an increased risk of deep vein thrombosis include heart failure (particularly cardiogenic shock), prolonged immobilization, age over 70 years, previous deep vein thrombosis, obesity, and varicose veins (163, 164,170,171).

Early mobilization should reduce the incidence of calf vein thrombosis and, more importantly, proximal extension and embolism. This was confirmed in one study using ^{125}I-labeled fibrinogen to detect venous thrombosis. Leg vein thrombi occurred in 9% of patients mobilized within 1 to 3 days of their infarct, compared with 63% of those randomly allocated to bedrest for 5 days (170). This study also documented the importance of heart failure as a major additional risk factor; 22% of those mobilized early and 80% of those mobilized late who had heart failure also had deep vein thrombosis.

The large Medical Research Council (71) and Veterans' Administration (72) studies of anticoagulation following acute myocardial infarction reported an incidence of clinically detected pulmonary embolism of approximately 5% in untreated patients, which was reduced to 2% with anticoagulation (of moderate intensity only). Anticoagulation also reduces deaths from pulmonary embolism and the incidence of pulmonary embolism or infarction detected at autopsy. However, these studies were performed in the era of prolonged immobilization and have limited relevance to current practice.

An alternative treatment that has been evaluated extensively in surgical patients is subcutaneous heparin 5,000 U, two or three times daily. The main effect of low-dose heparin is to increase the rate of antithrombin III–mediated inactivation of activated factor Xa, thereby reducing subsequent amplification of the intrinsic coagulation cascade (172–177). This regimen is not effective in the presence of brisk thrombin generation, and so it must be given early as prophylaxis to prevent thrombus formation. It produces little, if any, prolongation of the aPTT, so that it does not require monitoring, and the risk of bleeding, even in patients undergoing surgery, is not increased (172). Low-dose heparin, started within 12 to 18 hours of a myocardial infarction and continued for 10 days, reduces the incidence of venous thrombosis from 23% in control patients to 4% in those treated (176–181). This benefit was also evident in subgroups at particular risk for thrombosis, such as patients with heart failure. Similar findings emerge from studies of patients following major surgery, in whom a reduction in the incidence of pulmonary embolism has also been demonstrated (172–175,178).

Apart from preventing pulmonary embolism, it is possible that effective prophylaxis of venous thrombosis may also reduce the incidence of systemic emboli. Approximately 30% of the population have a patent foramen ovale (182), and it now appears that paradoxical embolism is an underrecognized cause of stroke, at least in younger patients, and may occur in the absence of pulmonary hypertension (183,184).

SUMMARY AND RECOMMENDATIONS

Thrombosis and thrombolysis are dynamic, opposing, and simultaneously occurring processes. There is immediate activation of the coagulation cascade and platelet activation with coronary thrombosis, with further activation after exogenous thrombolysis. Oral aspirin and parenteral heparin have individually been shown to improve mortality when combined with thrombolytic therapy in acute myocardial infarction, probably by reducing simultaneous thrombosis and subsequent reocclusion.

Streptokinase, urokinase, and anisolylated plasminogen–streptokinase activator complex (APSAC) are nonspecific fibrinolytic agents producing a secondary anticoagulant effect due to an extensive depletion of fibrinogen and coagulation factors. Unless the patient has acute transmural anterior infarction with a risk of left ventricular thrombus, the immediate requirement for additional anticoagulation with heparin may not be necessary. For patients receiving rt-PA as thrombolytic therapy, full intravenous heparin is necessary for the maintenance of arterial patency. Because rt-PA is more fibrin specific, inducing less depletion of fibrinogen and coagulation factors, and because of its relatively short half-life, the need for immediate additional anticoagulation with heparin assumes a major role in preventing reocclusion. The very low rates of reocclusion in the GUSTO trial when heparin plus aspirin was used in all patients (4.9–6.3% over 5–7 days) and the important need to maintain arterial patency suggest that this combined therapy should be used during the first 5–7 days of hospitalization.

Aspirin (160–325 mg) and thrombolytic therapy should be administered immediately. All patients with an acute myocardial infarction with ST elevation in two or more leads who are seen within 6 or even 12 hours of onset of symptoms and who have no specific contraindications should receive immediate thrombolytic therapy. The choice of thrombolytic therapy is much less important for ultimate survival than the delay in the initiation of treatment and onset of symptoms. To accelerate lysis and prevent reocclusion, antithrombotic agents must be administered simultaneously or very early after thrombolytic therapy. Adjunctive intravenous heparin should be used immediately when rt-PA is used. The initial dose of heparin is critical for all routes of administration. To achieve immediate therapeutic levels of intravenous or subcutaneous heparin, an average bolus of 5,000 U is necessary, followed by an infusion of 1,000 U/hour starting immediately with or before rt-PA treatment. Heparin infusion should subsequently be adjusted to maintain the aPTT at 60–85 seconds for 24 to 72 hours, followed by subcutaneous heparin (approximately 15,000 to 17,000 U every 12 hours) to prolong the aPTT to 60–85 seconds for the remainder of hospitalization. For subcutaneous administration, adequate anticoagulant response is not achieved in the first 24 hours unless a starting dose of at least 17,500 U every 12 hours is used or a 5,000 U IV bolus is given with 12,500 U subcutaneously. When switching from intravenous heparin to subcutaneous dosing, the intravenous infusion should overlap for 2 hours after the subcutaneous dose.

Patients with a severe residual stenosis or angiographically identified thrombus following thrombolysis are at particular risk for reocclusion and should be empirically anticoagulated with warfarin for 2 to 3 months to minimize residual stenosis and occlusion. While on warfarin (international normalized ratio [INR] 2.0 to 3.0 as in the ATACS study) the aspirin dosage should be reduced to 80 mg/day. Patients who develop recurrent angina or ischemia, heart failure, or a positive exercise test are possible candidates for coronary angiography and possible revascularization.

Early institution of systemic anticoagulation with full-dose intravenous or subcutaneous heparin is highly recommended for patients with large anterior myocardial infarctions or any extensive infarction involving the apex. It is not necessary to wait for echocardiographic documentation prior to the initiation of anticoagulation, since this may delay therapy when it is most beneficial. Anticoagulation should consist of heparin, titrated to prolong the aPTT to 60–85 seconds throughout hospitalization regardless of whether left ventricular thrombus is evident by echocardiography. Although the in-hospital period carries the greatest risk for embolism, these patients should probably be anticoagulated with warfarin to prolong the prothrombin time to an INR of 2.0 to 3.0. Oral anticoagulation should be continued for 3 months postinfarction, particularly if a predischarge echocardiogram demonstrates the presence of a thrombus, apical dyskinesis or akinesis.

Patients at continued high risk beyond the first 3 months after myocardial infarction include those patients with left ventricular failure (ejection fraction <30%), a prior history of systemic embolization, or the presence of atrial fibrillation. Indefinite treatment with warfarin is recommended in these patients.

All patients with an acute myocardial infarction are at increased risk for venous thromboembolism. Early mobilization after myocardial infarction is essential for preventing deep vein thrombosis. Low-dose subcutaneous heparin (5,000 U every 12 hours) is indicated, especially for patients at higher risk of thromboembolism such as those with ventricular dysfunction, with shock, requiring prolonged immobilization (>3 days), who are older or obese, or with a history of deep vein thrombosis or pulmonary embolism.

More potent inhibitors of platelets and the coagulation cascade, such as monoclonal antibodies to glycoprotein IIb/IIIa and the specific thrombin inhibitor hirudin, show considerable promise for the future. Until the efficacy and safety of these newer therapies are evaluated, heparin and aspirin have an established and important role in the acute management of myocardial infarction.

REFERENCES

1. Falk E: Plaque rupture with severe preexisting stenosis precipitating coronary thrombosis: Characteristics of coronary atherosclerosis plaques underlying fatal occlusive thrombi. *Br Heart J* 1983;50: 127–134.

2. Fuster V, Stein B, Ambrose JA, Badimon L, Badimon JJ, Chesebro JH: Atherosclerosis plaque rupture and thrombosis: Evolving concepts. *Circulation* 1990;(Suppl II):II-47–II-59.
3. Fuster V, Badimon L, Badimon JJ, Chesebro JH: The pathogenesis of coronary artery disease and the acute coronary syndromes, Parts 1 & 2. *N Engl J Med* 1992;326:242–250,310–318.
4. Davies MJ, Thomas AC: Plaque fissuring—the cause of acute myocardial infarction, sudden ischemic death and crescendo angina. *Br Heart J* 1985;53:363–373.
5. Davies MJ, Bland JM, Hangartner JRW, et al: Factors influencing the presence or absence of acute coronary thrombi in sudden ischaemic death. *Eur Heart J* 1989;10:203–208.
6. Drake TA, Morrissey JH, Edgington TS: Selective cellular expression of tissue factor in human tissues: Implications for disorders of hemostasis and thrombosis. *Am J Pathol* 1989;134:1087–1097.

7a. Drake TA, Morrissey JH, Edgington TS: Immunohistochemical detection of tissue factor in human atherosclerotic plaques. *Circulation* 1989;80:II-182.

7b. Falk E, Shah PK, Fuster V: Coronary plaque disruption. *Circulation* 1995;92:657–71.

7c. Toschi V, Gallo R, Lettino M, Fernandez-Ortiz A, Fallon J, Nemerson Y, Chesebro JH, Fuster V, Badimon JJ: Tissue factor predicts the thrombogenicity of human atherosclerotic plaque components. *Circulation* 1995;92:I–112.

8a. Mann KG, Tracy PB, Nesheim ME: Assembly and function of prothrombinase complex on synthetic and natural membranes, in Oates JA, Harwiger J, Ross R (eds): *Interaction of Platelets with the Vessel Wall.* Washington, DC, American Physiologic Society, 1985, pp 47–57.

8b. Kamat SG, Kleiman NS: Platelets and platelet inhibitors in acute myocardial infarction. *Cardiology Clinics,* 1995;13:435–447.

9. Heras M, Chesebro JH, Penny WJ, et al: Effects of thrombin inhibition on the development of acute platelet-thrombus deposition during angioplasty in pigs: Heparin versus recombinant hirudin, a specific thrombin inhibitor. *Circulation* 1989;79: 657–665.
10. Jang IK, Gold HK, Ziskind AA, et al: Prevention of platelet-rich arterial thrombosis by selective thrombin inhibition. *Circulation* 1990;81:219–225.
11. Chesebro JH, Knatterud G, Roberts R, et al: Thrombolysis in Myocardial Infarction (TIMI) trial, phase I: A comparison between intravenous tissue plasminogen activator versus intravenous streptokinase. *Circulation* 1987;76:142–154.

12a. DeWood MA, Spores J, Notske R, et al: Prevalence of total coronary occlusion during the early hours of transmural myocardial infarction. *N Engl J Med* 1980;303:897–902.

12b. Reiner JS, Lundergran CL, van den Brand M, et al, for the GUSTO angiographic investigators (1994): Early angiography cannot predict post thrombolytic coronary reocclusion: Observations from the GUSTO angiographic study. *J Am Coll Cardiol* 24:1439–1444.

12c. Gibson CM, Cannon CP, Piana RN, et al (1995): Angiographic predictors of reocclusion after thrombolysis: Results from the Thrombolysis in Myocardial Infarction (TIMI) 4 Trial. *J Am Coll Cardiol* 25:582–589.

13. The GUSTO Angiographic Investigators: The effects of tissue plasminogen activators, streptokinase, or both on coronary-artery patency, ventricular function, and survival after acute myocardial infarction. *N Engl J Med* 1993;329:1615–1622.
14. Braunwald E: The open-artery theory is alive and well. *N Engl J Med* 1993;329:1650–1652.
15. Topol EJ: Validation of the early open infarct vessel hypothesis. *Am J Cardiol* 1993;72:40G–45G.
16. Kennedy JW: Optimal management of acute myocardial infarction requires early and complete reperfusion. *Circulation* 1995;91:1905–1907.
17. Verstraete M, Bernard R, Bonz M, et al: Randomized trial of intravenous recombinant tissue-type plasminogen activator versus intravenous streptokinase in acute myocardial infarction. *Lancet* 1985;1: 842–847.
18. Chesebro JH, Braunwald E, Knatterud G: Thrombolytic therapy. *N Engl J Med* 1988;139:1542–1543.
19. Bleich SD, Nichols TC, Schumacher RR, Cooke DH, Tate DA, Teichman SL: Effects of heparin on coronary arterial patency after thrombolysis with tissue plasminogen activator in acute myocardial infarction. *Am J Cardiol* 1990;66:1412–1417.
20. Hsia J, Hamilton WP, Kleinman N, et al: A comparison between heparin and low-dose aspirin as adjunctive therapy with tissue plasminogen activator for acute myocardial infarction. *N Engl J Med* 1990;323:1433–1437.
21. de Bono DP, Simoons ML, Tijssen J, et al: Effect of early intravenous heparin on coronary patency, infarct size and bleeding complications after alteplase

thrombolysis: Results of a randomized double-blind European Cooperative Study Group trial. *Br Heart J* 1992;67:122–128.

22. Kaplan K, Davison R, Parker M, et al: Role of heparin after intravenous thrombolytic therapy for acute myocardial infarction. *Am J Cardiol* 1987;59: 241–244.
23. Cuccia C, Volterrami M, Volpini M, et al: Relationship between anticoagulation level, ischemic events and angiographic characteristics of the infarct-related artery following streptokinase in patients with acute myocardial infarction. *J Am Coll Cardiol* 1992;19:92A.
24. ISIS-3 (Third International Study of Infarct Survival) Collaborative Group: ISIS-3: A randomized comparison of streptokinase vs tissue plasminogen activator vs anistreplase and of aspirin plus heparin vs aspirin alone among 41,299 cases of suspected acute myocardial infarction. *Lancet* 1992;339: 753–770.
25. Gruppo Italiano per lo Studio della Sopravivenza Nell'Infarto Miocardico: GISSI-2: A factorial randomized trial of alteplase versus streptokinase and heparin versus no heparin among 12,490 patients with acute myocardial infarction. *Lancet* 1990;336: 65–71.
26. The GUSTO (Global Utilization of Streptokinase in Occluded Arteries) Investigators: An international randomized trial comparing four thrombolytic strategies for acute myocardial infarction. *N Engl J Med* 1993;329:673–682.
27. Gruppo Italiano per lo Studio della Sopravivenza nell'Infarto Miocardico (GISSI): Effectiveness of intravenous thrombolytic treatment in acute myocardial infarction. *Lancet* 1986;1:397–402.
28. ISIS-2 (Second International Study of Infarct Survival) Collaborative Group: Randomized trial of intravenous streptokinase, oral aspirin, both, or neither among 17,187 cases of suspected acute myocardial infarction: ISIS-2. *Lancet* 1988;2:349–360.
29. Kennedy JW, Ritchie JL, Davis KB, Stadius ML, Maynard C, Fritz JK: The Western Washington Randomized Trial of Intracoronary Streptokinase in acute myocardial infarction: A 12 month follow-up report. *N Engl J Med* 1985;312:1073–1078.
30. TIMI Study Group: The thrombolysis in Myocardial Infarction (TIMI) Trial; Phase I findings. *N Engl J Med* 1985;312:932–936.
31. Cannon CP, McCabe CH, Diver DJ, et al, and the TIMI 4 Investigators: Comparison of front-loaded recombinant tissue-type plasminogen activator, anistreplase and combination thrombolytic therapy for acute myocardial infarction: Results of the Thrombolysis in Myocardial Infarction (TIMI 4) trial. *J Am Coll Cardiol* 1994;24:1602–1610.
32. Canon CP, McCabe CH, Henry TD, et al, for the TIMI 5 Investigators: A pilot trial of recombinant desulfatohirudin compared with heparin in conjunction with tissue-type plasminogen activator and aspirin for acute myocardial infarction: Results of the Thrombolysis in Myocardial Infarction (TIMI) 5 trial. *J Am Coll Cardiol* 1994;23:993–1003.
33. Lincoff AM, Ellis SG, Galeana A, et al, for the TAMI Study Group: Is a coronary artery with TIMI grade 2 flow "pattern"? Outcome in Thrombolysis and Angioplasty in Myocardial Infarction (TAMI) Trial. *Circulation* 1992;86(Suppl I):I-268.
34. Vogt A, von Eisen R, Tebbe U, et al: Impact of early perfusion status of the infarct-related artery on short term mortality after thrombolysis for acute myocardial infarction: Retrospective analysis of four German multicenter studies. *J Am Coll Cardiol* 1993;21:1391–1395.
35. Cannon CP, Braunwald E: GUSTO, TIMI and the case for reperfusion. *Acta Cardiol* 1994;49:1–8.

36a. Cannon CP, Antman EM, Walls R, Braunwald E: Time as an adjunctive agent to thrombolytic therapy. *J Thromb Thrombolysis* 1994;1:27–34.

36b. Lincoff AM, Topol EJ: Illusion of reperfusion: Does anyone achieve optimal reperfusion during acute myocardial infarction? *Circulation* 1993;87: 1792–1805.

36c. Kargounis L, Sorensen SG, Menlove RL, et al: Does thrombolysis in myocardial infarction perfusion grade 2 represent a mostly patent artery or a mostly occluded artery? Enzymatic and electrocardiographic evidence from the TEAM-2 study. *J Am Coll Cardiol* 1992;19:1–10.

36d. Simes RJ, Topol EJ, Holmes DR, et al, for the GUSTO investigators: Link between the angiographic substudy and mortality outcomes in a large randomized trial of myocardial reperfusion: Importance of early and complete infarct artery reperfusion. *Circulation* 1995;91:1923–1928.

36e. Ohman EM, Califf RM, Topol EJ, et al: Consequences of reocclusion after successful reperfusion therapy in acute myocardial infarction. *Circulation* 1990;82:781–791.

37. Weaver WD, Cerqueira M, Hallstrom AP, et al, for the MITI Project Group: Prehospital-initiated vs

hospital-initiated thrombolytic therapy: The Myocardial Infarction Triage and Intervention Trial. *JAMA* 1993;270:1211–1216.

38. The EMIP Group: Pre-hospital thrombolytic therapy in patients with suspected acute myocardial infarction. *N Engl J Med* 1993;329:383–389.

39a. GREAT Group: Feasibility, safety, and efficacy of domiciliary thrombolysis by general practitioners: Grampian Region Early Antistreplase Trial. *Br Med J* 1992;305:548–553.

39b. Fibrinolytic Therapy Trialists' (FTT Collaborative Group): Indications for fibrinolytic therapy in suspected acute myocardial infarction: Collaborative overview of early mortality and major morbidity results from all randomized trials of more than 1000 patients. *Lancet* 1994;343:311–322.

40a. Fernandez-Ortiz A, Jang IK, Fuster V: Antiplatelet and antithrombin therapy. *Cor Art Dis* 1994;5: 297–305.

40b. Collen D: Fibrin-Selective Thrombolytic Therapy for Acute Myocardial Infarction. *Circulation* 1996; 93:857–865.

41. Badimon L, Badimon JJ: Mechanism of arterial thrombosis in nonparallel streamlines: Platelet thrombi grow at the apex of stenotic severely injured vessel wall. Experimental study in the pig model. *J Clin Invest* 1989;84:1134–1144.

42. Badimon L, Badimon JB, Galvez, Chesebro JH, Fuster V: Influence of arterial damage and wall shear rate on platelet deposition: Ex vivo study in a swine model. *Arteriosclerosis* 6:3312–3319.

43. Mailhac A, Badimon JB, Fallon JT, et al: Effect of an eccentric severe stenosis on fibrin(ogen) deposition on severely damaged vessel wall in arterial thrombosis: Relative contribution of fibrin(ogen) and platelets. *Circulation* 1994;90:988–996.

44. Luscher TF: Endothelium-derived relaxing and contracting factors: Potential role in coronary artery disease. *Eur Heart J* 1989;10:847–857.

45. Vanhoutte PM, Shimokawa H: Endothelium-derived relaxing factor and coronary vasospasm. *Circulation* 1989;80:1–9.

46. Yanagisawa M, Kurihara H, Kimura S, et al: A novel potent vasoconstrictor peptide produced by vascular endothelial cells. *Nature* 1988;332: 411–415.

47. Lam JYT, Chesebro JH, Steele PM, et al: Is vasospasm related to platelet deposition? Relationship in a porcine preparation of arterial injury in vivo. *Circulation* 1987;75:243–248.

48. Fischell TA, Nellessen U, Johnson DE, et al: Endothelium-dependent arterial vasoconstriction after balloon angioplasty. *Circulation* 1989;79: 899–910.

49. Wilson RF, Laxson DD, Lesser JR, White CW: Intense microvascular constriction after angioplasty of acute thrombotic coronary arterial lesions. *Lancet* 1989;1:807–811.

50. Chesebro JH, Fuster V: Dynamic thrombosis and thrombolysis: Role of antithrombins. *Circulation* 1991;83:1815–1817.

51. Francis CW, Markham RE, Marder VJ: Demonstration of in situ fibrin degradation in pathologic thrombi. *Blood* 1984;63:1216–1224.

52. Meyer B, Badimon JJ, Mailhac A, Fernandez-Ortiz et al: Inhibition of growth of thrombus on fresh mural thrombus: Targeting optimal therapy. *Circulation* 1994;90:2432–2438.

53. Badimon L, Lassila R, Badimon J, et al: Residual thrombus is more thrombogenic than severely damaged vessel wall. *Circulation* 1988;78:II-118.

54. Lee CD, Mann KG: Activation and inactivation of human factor V by plasmin. *Blood* 1989;73: 185–190.

55a. Fitzgerald DJ, Catella F, Roy L, Fitzgerald GA: Marked platelet activation in vivo after intravenous streptokinase in patients with acute myocardial infarction. *Circulation* 1989;80:1718–1725.

55b. Kerins DM, Roy L, Fitzgerald GA, Fitzgerald DJ: Platelet and vascular function during coronary thrombolysis with tissue-type plasminogen activator. *Circulation* 1989;80:1718–1725.

55c. Lucore CL, Sobel BE: Interactions of tissue-type plasminogen activator with plasma inhibitors and their pharmacologic implications. *Circulation* 1988; 77:660–669.

55d. Golino P, Ashton JH, Glas-Greenwalt P, et al (1988): Mediation of reocclusion by thromboxane A2 and serotonin after thrombolysis after thrombolysis with tissue-type plasminogen activator in a canine preparation of coronary thrombosis. *Circulation* 77:678–684.

56. Kerins DM, Roy L, Fitzgerald GA, Fitzgerald DJ: Platelet and vascular function during coronary thrombolysis with tissue-type plasminogen activator. *Circulation* 1989;80:1718–1725.

57. Vaughan DE, Van Houtte E, Declerck PJ, et al: Prevalence and mechanism of streptokinase-induced platelet aggregation. *Circulation* 1989;80: II-218.

58. Eisenberg PR, Sherman LA, Jaffe AS: Paradoxic elevation of Fibrinopeptide A after streptokinase: Evidence for continued thrombosis despite intense fibrinolysis. *J Am Coll Cardiol* 1987;10: 527–529.

59. Merlini PA, Bauer KA, Manucci PM, et al: Persistent activation of coagulation mechanism in unstable angina and myocardial infarction. *Circulation* 1994;90:61–68.

60. Owen J, Friedman KD, Grossman BA, et al: Thrombolytic therapy with tissue plasminogen activator or streptokinase induces transient thrombin activity. *Blood* 1988;72:616–620.

61. Merlini PA, Bauer KA, Oltrona L, et al: Thrombin generation and activity during thrombolysis and concomitant heparin therapy in patients with acute myocardial infarction. *J Am Coll Cardiol* 1995;25: 203–209.

62. Rapold HJ: Promotion of thrombin activity by thrombolytic therapy without simultaneous anticoagulation. *Lancet* 1990;335:481–482.

63. Aronson DL, Chang P, Kessler CM: Platelet-dependent thrombin generation after in vitro fibrinolytic treatment. *Circulation* 1992;85:1706–1712.

64a. Gulba DC, Barthels M, Reil GH, Lichtlen PR: Thrombin antithrombin-III complex level as early predictor of reocclusion after successful thrombolysis. *Lancet* 1988;2:97.

64b. Weitz JI, Califf RM, Ginsberg JS, et al: New antithrombotics. *Chest* 1995;108:471–485.

64c. Cannon CP: Thrombin inhibitors in acute myocardial infarction. *Cardiology Clinics* 1995;13:421–433.

65. Hirsh J: Heparin. *N Engl J Med* 1991;324: 1565–1574.

66. Hirsh J, Fuster V: Guide to anticoagulant therapy: Part 1: Heparin; Part 2: Oral anticoagulants. *Circulation* 1994;89:1449–1480.

67. Cercek B, Lew AS, Hod H, et al: Enhancement of thrombolysis with tissue-type plasminogen activator by pretreatment with heparin. *Circulation* 1986; 74:583–587.

68. Tomaru T, Uchida Y, Nakamura F, et al: Enhancement of arterial thrombolysis with native tissue-type plasminogen activator by pretreatment with heparin or baroxobin: An angiographic study. *Am Heart J* 1989;117:275–281.

69. MacMahon S, Collins R, Knight C, et al: Reduction in major morbidity and mortality by heparin in acute myocardial infarction. *Circulation* 1988;78: II-98.

70. Wright IS, Marple CD, Beck DF: Report of the committee for the evaluation of anticoagulants in the therapy of coronary thrombosis with acute myocardial infarction. *Am Heart J* 1948;36:801–815.

71. Assessment of short-term anticoagulation administration after cardiac infarction. Report of the working party on anticoagulant therapy in coronary thrombosis to the Medical Research Council. *Br Med J* 1969;1:335–342.

72. Veterans Administration Cooperative Clinical Trial: Anticoagulants in acute myocardial infarction. *JAMA* 1973;225:724–729.

73. Drapkin A, Merskey C: Anticoagulant therapy after acute myocardial infarction: Relation of therapeutic benefit to patient's age sex and severity of infarction. *JAMA* 1972;222:541–548.

74. Chalmers TC, Matta RJ, Smith H, et al: Evidence favoring the use of anticoagulants in the hospital phase of acute myocardial infarction. *N Engl J Med* 1977;297:1091–1096.

75. Topol EJ, George BS, Kereiakes DJ, et al: A randomized controlled trial of intravenous tissue plasminogen activator and early intravenous heparin in acute myocardial infarction. *Circulation* 1989;79: 281–286.

76a. Thompson PL, Aylward PE, Federman J, et al, for the National Heart Foundation of Australia Coronary Thrombolysis Group: A randomized comparison of intravenous heparin with oral aspirin and dipyridamole 24 hours after recombinant tissue-type plasminogen activator for acute myocardial infarction. *Circulation* 1991;83:1534–1542.

76b. Kaplan K, Davison R, Parker M, et al: Role of heparin after intravenous thrombolytic therapy for acute myocardial infarction. *Am J Cardiol* 1987;59: 241–244.

77. The SCATI (Studio sulla caliparina nee'angina e nella trombosi ventricolare nell'infarto) Group: Randomized controlled trial of subcutaneous calcium-heparin in acute myocardial infarction. *Lancet* 1989; 2:182–186.

78. ISIS Pilot Study Investigators: Randomized factorial trial of high-dose intravenous streptokinase, of oral aspirin and of intravenous heparin in acute myocardial infarction. *Eur Heart J* 1987;8:634–642.

79. Collen D, Lijnen HR: Basic and clinical aspects of fibrinolysis and thrombolysis. *Blood* 1991;78: 3114–3124.

80. Roux S, Christeller S, Ladin E: Effects of aspirin on coronary reocclusion and recurrent ischemia after

thrombolysis: A meta analysis. *J Am Coll Cardiol* 1992;19:671–677.

81. Flynn M, Weth D, Gudipati R, et al, for the rt-PA Heparin Duration Trial Investigators: Influence of heparin duration on coronary angiographic characteristics in patients receiving accelerated weight-adjusted rt-PA dosing for acute myocardial infarction. *Circulation* 1993;88:I-201.

82. Nakagawa S, Hanada Y, Koiwaya Y, Tanaka K: Angiographic features in the infarct-related artery after intracoronary urokinase followed by prolonged anticoagulation. Role of ruptured atheromatous plaque and adherent thrombus in acute myocardial infarction in vivo. *Circulation* 1988;78:1335–1344.

83. Meijer A, Verheugt FW, Weter CJ, et al: Aspirin versus coumadin in the prevention of reocclusion and recurrent ischemia after successful thrombolysis: A prospective placebo-controlled angiographic study. Results of the APRICOT study. *Circulation* 1993;87:1524–1530.

84. Cohen M, Adams PC, Parry G, et al, and the Antithrombotic Therapy in Acute Coronary Syndromes Research Group: Combination antithrombotic therapy in unstable rest angina and non-Q wave infarction in non prior aspirin users. Primary end points analysis from the ATACS trial. *Circulation* 1994;1:81–88.

85. Smith P, Arnesen H, Holme I, for the WARIS trial: The effect of warfarin on mortality and reinfarction after myocardial infarction. *N Engl J Med* 1990; 323:147–152.

86. ASPECT Research Group: Effect of long-term oral anticoagulant treatment on mortality and cardiovascular morbidity after myocardial infarction. Anticoagulants in the Secondary Prevention of Events in Coronary Thrombosis (ASPECT) Research Group. *Lancet* 1994;343:499–503.

87a. Baigent C, Collins R, for the ISIS Collaborative Group: ISIS 2: 4 year mortality follow-up of 17187 patients after fibrinolytic and antiplatelet therapy in suspected acute myocardial infarction. *Circulation* 1993;88:I-291.

87b. The Dutch TIA Trial Study Group: A comparison of two doses of aspirin (30 mg vs. 283 mg a day) in patients after a transient ischemic attack or minor ischemic stroke. *N Eng J Med* 1991;325:1261–1266.

87c. Cairns JA, Fuster V, Gore J, et al: Coronary thrombolysis. *Chest* 1995;108:401S–423S.

87d. Baigent C, Collins R, for the ISIS Collaborative Group: ISIS 2: 4 year mortality follow-up of 17,187 patients after fibrinolytic and antiplatelet therapy in suspected acute myocardial infarction. *Circulation* 1993;88:I–291.

88. Lewis HD, Davis JW, Archibald DG, et al: Protective effect of aspirin against acute myocardial infarction and death in men with unstable angina: Results of a Veterans Administration Cooperative Study. *N Engl J Med* 1983;309:396–403.

89. Cairns JA, Gent M, Singer J, et al: Aspirin, sulfinpyrazone, or both in unstable angina. *N Engl J Med* 1985;313:1369–1375.

90. Theroux P, Ouimet H, McCans J, et al: Aspirin, heparin, or both to treat acute unstable angina. *N Engl J Med* 1988;319:1105–1111.

91. The RISC Group: Risk of myocardial infarction and death during treatment with low-dose aspirin and intravenous heparin in men with unstable coronary artery disease. *Lancet* 1990;336:827–830.

92. Lam JYT, Chesebro JH, Fuster V: Platelets vasoconstriction and nitroglycerin during arterial wall injury. A new antithrombotic role for an old drug. *Circulation* 1988;78:712–716.

93. Lascoste LL, Theroux P, Lidon RM, Colucci R, Lam JY: Antithrombotic properties of transdermal nitroglycerin in stable angina pectoris. *Am J Cardiol* 1994;73:1058–1062.

94. Rentrop KP, Feit F, Blanke H, et al: Effects of intracoronary streptokinase and intracoronary nitroglycerin infusion on coronary angiographic patterns and mortality in patients with acute myocardial infarction. *N Engl J Med* 1984;311:1457–1463.

95. Brower RW, Arnold AER, Lubsen J, Verstraete M: Coronary patency after intravenous infusion of recombinant tissue type plasminogen activator in acute myocardial infarction. *J Am Coll Cardiol* 1988; 11:681–688.

96. GISSI 3: Effects of lisinopril and transdermal glyceryl trinitrate singly and together on 6-week mortality and ventricular function after acute myocardial infarction. Gruppo Italiano per lo Studio della Sopravivenza nell' Infarcto Miocardico. *Lancet* 1994; 343:1115–1122.

97. ISIS-4 Investigators: A randomised factorial trial assessing early oral captopril, oral mononitrate, and intravenous magnesium sulphate in 58,050 patients with suspected acute myocardial infarction. ISIS-4 (Fourth International Study of Infarct Survival) Collaborative Group. *Lancet* 1995;345:669–685.

98. Bar-Shavit R, Eldor A, Voldavsky I: Binding of thrombin to subendothelial extracellular matrix:

Protection and expression of functional properties. *J Clin Invest* 1989;84:1096–1104.

99. Heras M, Chesebro JH, Webster MWI, et al: Hirudin, heparin and placebo during deep arterial injury in the pig. The in vivo role of thrombin in platelet-mediated thrombosis. *Circulation* 1990; 82:1476–1484.

100. Zoldhelyi P, Webster MWI, Fuster V, et al: Recombinant hirudin in patients with chronic stable coronary artery disease. Safety half-life, and effect on coagulation parameters. *Circulation* 1993;88: 2015–2022.

101. Chesebro JH, Webster MWI, Zoldhelyi P, Roche PC, Badimon L, Badimon JJ: Antithrombotic therapy in the progression of coronary artery disease. *Circulation* 1992;86(Suppl III):III-100–III-110.

102a. Markwardt F, Kaiser B, Novak G: Studies on antithrombotic effects of recombinant hirudin. *Thromb Res* 1989;54:377–388.

102b. Mruk JS, Zoldhelyi P, Webster MWI, Heras M, Grill DE, Holmes DR, Fuster V, Chesebro JH: Does antithrombotic therapy influence residual thrombus after thrombolysis of platelet-rich thrombus? Effects of recombinant Hirudin, heparin, or aspirin. *Circulation* 1996;93:792–799.

103. Weitz JI, Hudoba M, Massel D, Maraganore J, Hirsh J: Clot-bound thrombin is protected from inhibition by heparin–antithrombin III but is susceptible to inactivation by antithrombin III–independent inhibitors. *J Clin Invest* 1990;86: 385–391.

104. Massel DR, Hudoba M, Weitz JI: Clot-bound thrombin is protected from heparin inhibition. A potential mechanism for rethrombosis after lytic therapy. *Circulation* 1989;89:II-420.

105. Seiss W: Molecular mechanisms of platelet activation. *Physiol Rev* 1989;69:58–178.

106. Tam SW, Fenton JW, Detweiler TC: Dissociation of thrombin from platelets by hirudin. *J Biol Chem* 1979;254:8723–8725.

107. Chesebro JH, Rao AK, Schwartz D, et al: Endogenous thrombolysis and recanalization of occluded aortocoronary vein grafts with recombinant hirudin in patients with unstable angina. *Circulation* 1994;90:I-568.

108. Wysokinski WE, McBane RD, Hassinger ML, Stewart ML, Chesebro JH, Owen WG: "Dethrombosis": Effect of thrombin inhibition on thrombus propagation and maintenance (abstract). *Thromb Haemost* 1993;69:692.

109a. Neuhaus KL, Niederer W, Wagner J, et al, for the ALKK-Study Group: HIT (Hirudin for the improvement of thrombolysis): Results of a dose escalation study. *Circulation* 1993;88:I-292.

109b. Lee LV, for the TIMI 6 Investigators: Initial experience with hirudin and streptokinase in acute myocardial infarction: Results of the Thrombolysis in Myocardial Infarction (TIMI) 6 Trial. *Am J Cardiol* 1995;75:7–13.

110a. Lidon-Corbi RM, Theroux P, Lesperance J, et al: A pilot, early angiographic patency study using a direct thrombin inhibitor as adjunctive therapy to streptokinase in acute myocardial infarction. *Circulation* 1994;89:1557–1566.

110b. Theroux P, Perez-Villa F, Waters D, et al: Randomized double-blind comparison of two doses of hirulog with heparin as adjunctive therapy to streptokinase to promote early patency of the infarct-related artery in acute myocardial infarction. *Circulation* 1995;91:2132–2139.

111. Antman EM: Hirudin in acute myocardial infarction. Safety report from the Thrombolysis and Thrombin Inhibition in Myocardial Infarction (TIMI) 9A trial. *Circulation* 1994;90:1624–1630.

112. The Global Use of Strategies to Open Occluded Coronary Arteries (GUSTO)-IIa Investigators: Randomized trial of intravenous heparin versus recombinant hirudin for acute coronary syndromes. *Circulation* 1994;90:1631–1637.

113. Neuhaus KL, van Essen R, Tebbe U, et al, for the ALKK investigators: Safety observations from the pilot phase of the randomized r-hirudin for Improvement of Thrombolysis (HIT-III) Study. *Circulation* 1994;90:1638–1642.

114a. Patrono C: Aspirin as an antiplatelet drug. *N Engl J Med* 1994;330:18.1287–1294.

114b. Coller BS: Blockade of platelet GPIIb/IIIa receptors as an antithrombotic strategy. *Circulation* 1995;92:2374–2380.

115. Coller BS: A new murine monoclonal antibody reports an activation-dependent change in the conformation and/or microenvironment of platelet glycoprotein IIb/IIIa complex. *J Clin Invest* 1985;76:101–108.

116. EPIC Study Investigators: Use of a monoclonal antibody directed against the platelet glycoprotein IIb/IIIa receptor in high-risk coronary angioplasty. *N Engl J Med* 1994;330:956–961.

117. Coller BS, Folts JD, Scrudder LE, Smith SR: Antithrombotic effect of a monoclonal antibody to the

platelet glycoprotein IIb/IIIa receptor in an experimental animal model. *Blood* 1986;68:783–786.

118. Harker LA: New antithrombotic strategies for resistant thrombotic processes. *J Clin Pharmacol* 1994;34:3–16.

119. Kleinman NS, Ohman M, Califf R, et al: Profound inhibition of platelet aggregation with monoclonal antibody 7E3 Fab after thrombolytic therapy. Results of the Thrombolysis and Angioplasty in Myocardial Infarction (TAMI) 8 pilot study. *J Am Coll Cardiol* 1993;22:381–389.

120. Weinrich DJ, Burke JF, Pauletto FJ: Left ventricular mural thrombosis complicating acute myocardial infarction. *Ann Intern Med* 1984;100:789–794.

121. Asinger RW, Mikell FL, Elsperger J, Hodges M: Incidence of left-ventricular thrombosis after acute myocardial infarction: Serial evaluation by two-dimensional echocardiography. *N Engl J Med* 1981;305:297–302.

122. Spirito P, Bellotti P, Chiarella F, et al: Prognostic significance and natural history of left ventricular thrombi in patients with acute myocardial infarction: A two-dimensional echocardiographic study. *Circulation* 1985;72:774–780.

123. Gueret P, Dubourg O, Ferrier A, et al: Effects of full dose heparin on the development of left ventricular thrombosis in acute myocardial infarction. *J Am Coll Cardiol* 1986;8:419–426.

124. Keating EC, Gross SA, Schlamowitz RA, et al: Mural thrombi in myocardial infarctions. Prospective evaluations by two dimensional echocardiography. *Am J Med* 1984;74:989–995.

125. Johannessen KA, Nordrehaug JE, von der Lippe G: Left ventricular thrombosis and cerebrovascular accident in acute myocardial infarction. *Br Heart J* 1984;51:553–556.

126. Keren A, Goldberg S, Gottlieb S, et al: Natural history of left ventricular thrombi: Their appearance and resolution in the posthospitalization period of acute myocardial infarction. *J Am Coll Cardiol* 1990;15:790–800.

127. Domenicucci S, Bellotti P, Chiarella F, et al: Spontaneous morphologic changes in left ventricular thrombi: A prospective two dimensional echocardiographic study. *Circulation* 1985;72:774–780.

128. Domenenicucci S, Chiarella F, Bellotti P, et al: Early appearance of left ventricular thrombi after acute myocardial infarction: A marker of higher in hospital mortality in patients not treated with antithrombotic drugs. *Eur Heart J* 1990;11:51–58.

129. Kothari AJ, Packowski K, Baker KM, et al: Ventricular thrombi in acute myocardial infarction: Incidence, complications and effect of anticoagulation (abstract). *J Am Coll Cardiol* 1984;3:601.

130. Turpie AG, Robinson JG, Doyle DJ, et al: Comparison of high-dose with low-dose subcutaneous heparin to prevent left ventricular mural thrombosis in patients with acute myocardial infarction. *N Engl J Med* 1989;320:352–357.

131. Visser CA, Kan G, Lie KI, et al: Left ventricular thrombus following acute myocardial: A prospective serial echocardiographic study of 96 patients. *Eur Med J* 1983;4:333–337.

132. Meltzer RS, Visser CA, Fuster V: Intracardiac thrombi and systemic embolization. *Ann Intern Med* 1986;104:689–698.

133. Mikell FL, Asinger RW, Elsperger KJ, et al: Regional stasis of blood in the dysfunctional left ventricle: Echocardiographic detection and differentiation from early thrombosis. *Circulation* 1982;66: 755–763.

134. Maze SS, Kotler MN, Parry WR: Flow characteristics in the dilated left ventricle with thrombi. *J Am Coll Cardiol* 1989;13:873–881.

135. Delemarre J, Visser CA, Bot H, et al: Prediction of apical thrombus formation in acute myocardial infarction based on left ventricular spatial flow pattern. *J Am Coll Cardiol* 1990;15:355–360.

136. Johnson RC, Crissman RS, Didio LJ: Endocardial alterations in myocardial infarction. *Lab Invest* 1979;40:183–193.

137. Hochman JS, Platia EB, Bulkey BH: Endocardial abnormalities in left ventricular aneurysms: A clinicopathologic study. *Ann Intern Med* 1984; 100:29–35.

138. Judgutt BI, Sivaram CA, Wortman C, et al: Prospective two-dimensional echocardiographic evaluation of left-ventricular thrombus and embolism after acute myocardial infarction. *J Am Coll Cardiol* 1989;13:554–564.

139. Hilden T, Raaschou F, Iversen K, Schwartz M: Anticoagulants in acute myocardial infarction. *Lancet* 1961;2:327–331.

140. Ezekowitz MD, Wilson DA, Smith EO, et al: Comparison of indium-111 platelet scintigraphy and two-dimensional echocardiography in the diagnosis of left ventricular thrombi. *N Engl J Med* 1982;306:1509–1513.

141. Asinger RW, Mikell FL, Sharma B, et al: Observations on detecting left-ventricular thrombus

with two-dimensional echocardiography: Emphasis on avoidance of false positive diagnosis. *Am J Cardiol* 1981;47:145–156.

142. Davis MJE, Ireland MA: Effect of early anticoagulation on the frequency of left ventricular thrombi after anterior wall acute myocardial infarction. *Am J Cardiol* 1986;57:1244–1247.
143. Avran S, Boscha K: Prophylactic anticoagulation for left ventricular thrombi after anterior wall acute myocardial infarction. *Am J Cardiol* 1986;57: 1244–1247.
144. Nordrehaug JE, Johannessen KA, von der Lippe G: Usefulness of high dose anticoagulants in preventing left ventricular thrombus in acute myocardial infarction. *Am J Cardiol* 1985;55:1491–1493.
145. Johannessen KA, Nordrehaug JE, von der Lippe G: Increased occurrence of left ventricular thrombi during early treatment with timolol in patients with acute myocardial infarction. *Circulation* 1987;75:151–155.
146. Vecchio C, Chiarella F, Lupi G, et al: Left ventricular thrombus in anterior acute myocardial infarction after thrombolysis. A GISSI-2 connected study. *Circulation* 1991;84:512–519.
147. Eigler N, Maurer G, Shah PK: Effect of early systemic thrombolytic therapy on left ventricular mural thrombus formation in acute anterior myocardial infarction. *Am J Cardiol* 1984;54:261–263.
148. Held AC, Gore JM, Paraskos J, et al: Impact of thrombolytic therapy on left-ventricular mural thrombi in acute myocardial infarction. *Am J Cardiol* 1988;62:310–311.
149. Natarajan D, Hotchandani RK, Nigam PD: Reduced incidence of left ventricular thrombi with intravenous streptokinase in acute myocardial infarction: Prospective evaluation by cross-sectional echocardiography. *Int J Cardiol* 1988;20:201–207.
150. Lupi G, Domenicucci S, Chiarella F, et al: Influence of thrombolytic treatment followed by full dose anticoagulation on the frequency of left ventricular thrombi in acute myocardial infarction. *Am J Cardiol* 1989;64:588–590.
151. Bhatnager SK, Al-Yusuf AR: Effects of intravenous recombinant tissue type plasminogen activator therapy on the incidence and associations of left ventricular thrombus in patients with a first acute Q wave anterior myocardial infarction. *Am Heart J* 1991;122:1251–1256.
152. Vaitkus PT, Baranathan ES: Embolic potential, prevention and management of mural thrombus complicating myocardial infarction: A meta-analysis. *J Am Coll Cardiol* 1993;22:1004–1009.
153. Kremer P, Fiebig R, Tilsner V, et al: Lysis of mobile left ventricular thrombi with urokinase. *Circulation* 1985;72:112–118.
154. Shenoy MM, Friedman SA, Dhar S, et al: Streptokinase lysis of intraventricular thrombus and pulmonary emboli with resolution of acquired intracardiac shunt. *Ann Intern Med* 1985;103:65–66.
155. Keren A, Medina A, Gottlieb S, et al: Lysis of mobile left ventricular thrombi during acute myocardial infarction with urokinase. *Am J Cardiol* 1987;60:1180–1181.
156. Lapeyre AC, Steel PM, Kazmier FJ, et al: Systemic embolism in chronic left ventricular aneurysm: Incidence and role of anticoagulation. *J Am Coll Cardiol* 1985;6:534–538.
157. Tramarin R, Pozzoli M, Febo O, et al: Two-dimensional echocardiographic assessment of anticoagulant therapy in left ventricular thrombosis early after acute myocardial infarction. *Eur Heart J* 1986;7:482–492.
158. Kouvaras G, Chronopoulos G, Soufras G, et al: The effects of long term antithrombotic treatment on left ventricular thrombi in patients after an acute myocardial infarction. *Am Heart J* 1990;119:73–78.
159. Johannessen KA, Nordrehaug JE, von der Lippe G: Left ventricular thrombi after short term high dose anticoagulants in acute myocardial infarction. *Eur Heart J* 1987;8:975–980.
160. Kontny F, Dale J, Abildgaard U, Hegrenaes L, Lem P, Morstol T: Adverse effect of warfarin in acute myocardial infarction: Increased left ventricular thrombus without heparin. *Eur Heart J* 1993;14:1040–1043.
161. Funke Kupper AJ, Verheugt FWA, et al: Effect of low dose acetylsalicylic acid on the frequency and hematologic activity of left ventricular thrombus in anterior wall acute myocardial infarction. *Am J Cardiol* 1989;63:917–920.
162. Johannessen K-A, Stratton JR, Taulow E, et al: Usefulness of aspirin plus dipyridamole in reducing left ventricular thrombus formation in anterior wall acute myocardial infarction. *Am J Cardiol* 1989;63:101–102.
163. Weinmann EE, Salzman EW: Deep vein thrombosis. *N Engl J Med* 1994;331:1630–1641.
164. Hirsh J, Hull RD: Diagnosis of venous thrombosis, in *Venous Thromboembolism: Natural History, Diag-*

nosis, and Management. Boca Raton, FL, CRC Press, 1987, pp 23–28.

165. Nicolaides AN, Kakkar VV, Renney JTG, et al: Myocardial infarction and deep-vein thrombosis. *Br J Surg* 1968;55:742–747.

166. Maurer BJ, Wray R, Shillingford JP: Frequency of venous thrombosis after myocardial infarction. *Lancet* 1971;2:1385–1387.

167. Kakkar VV, Howe CT, Flanc C, et al: Natural history of postoperative deep-vein thrombosis. *Lancet* 1969;2:230–232.

168. Flanc C, Kakkar VV, Clarke MB: The detection of venous thrombosis of the legs using ^{125}I-labeled fibrinogen. *Br J Surg* 1968;55:742–747.

169. Ygge J: Changes in blood coagulation and fibrinolysis during the postoperative period. *Am J Surg* 1970;119:225–232.

170. Miller R, Lies JE, Caretta RF, et al: Prevention of lower extremity venous thrombosis by early mobilization: Confirmation in patients with acute myocardial infarction by 125I-fibrinogen uptake and venography. *Ann Inter Med* 1976;84:700–703.

171. Simmons AV, Sheppard MA, Cox AF: Deep venous thrombosis after myocardial infarction: Predisposing factors. *Br Heart J* 1973;35:623–625.

172. Hirsh J: Antithrombotic therapy in deep-vein thrombosis and pulmonary embolism. *Am Heart J* 1992;123:1115–1122.

173. Clagett GP, Anderson FA, Levine MN, et al: Prevention of venous thromboembolism. *Chest* 1992; 102(Suppl 4):391S–407S.

174. Kakkar VV, Corrigan TP, Fossard DP: Prevention of fatal postoperative pulmonary embolism by low doses of heparin: An international multicenter trial. *Lancet* 1975;2:45–51.

175. Clagett GP, Reisch JS: Prevention of venous thromboembolism in general surgical patients: Results of a meta-analysis. *Ann Surg* 1988;208: 227–240.

176. Handley AJ: Low dose heparin after myocardial infarction. *Lancet* 1972;2:623–624.

177. Gallus AS, Hirsh J, Tuttle RJ, et al: Small subcutaneous doses of heparin in the prevention of deep-vein thrombosis. *N Engl J Med* 1973;288: 545–551.

178. Warlow C, Beattie AG, Terry G, et al: A double blind trial of low doses of subcutaneous heparin in the prevention of deep-vein thrombosis. *Lancet* 1973;1:934–936.

179. Emerson PA, Marks P: Preventing thromboembolism after myocardial infarction: effect of low dose heparin or smoking. *Br Med J* 1977;1: 18–20.

180. Handley AJ, Emerson PA, Flemming PR: Heparin in the prevention of deep-vein thrombosis after myocardial infarction. *Br Med J* 1972;2:436–438.

181. Wray R, Maurer B, Shillingford J: Prophylactic anticoagulant therapy in the prevention of calf-vein thrombosis after myocardial infarction. *N Engl J Med* 1973;288:815–817.

182. Hagen PT, Scholz DG, Edwards WD: Incidence and size of patient foramen ovale during the first 10 decades of life: An autopsy study of 965 normal hearts. *Mayo Clin Proc* 1984;59:17–20.

183. Lechat P, Mas JL, Lascault G, et al: Prevalence of patent foramen ovale in patients with stroke. *N Engl J Med* 1988;318:1148–1152.

184. Webster MWI, Chancellor AM, Smith HJ, et al: Patent foramen ovale in young stroke patients. *Lancet* 1988;2:11–12.

21

Pathogenesis and Modification of Myocardial Stunning and Reperfusion Injury

Mervyn B. Forman, MB, BCh, PhD, FRCP (Ed), and John J. Murray, MD, PhD

The rationale for reperfusion therapy in humans was provided by the observation that occlusion of a major epicardial artery in the experimental model resulted in various gradations of ischemia in the occluded bed, with the most severe reduction occurring in the subendocardium. This produces a "wavefront" progression of irreversible myocardial injury extending from the subendocardium to subepicardium with increasing durations of ischemia (1,2). The rapidity of this progression depends on the severity of ischemia, the area of the occluded bed, and myocardial oxygen consumption during ischemia (2,3). A major determinant of the severity of ischemia is the extent of collateral blood supply, which is species dependent. In animals with an inherent good collateral circulation such as the dog, myocardial salvage can be achieved if reperfusion is established within 3 to 6 hours of ischemia (1,2). Conversely, in animals with poor collateral circulation, such as rabbits and pigs, total necrosis of the risk region is present within 1 hour of ischemia (4,5).

Acute myocardial infarction is a serious, life-threatening event with morbidity and mortality related to the degree of left ventricular dysfunction. Therapy directed to reduction of infarct size and preservation of ventricular function therefore has important clinical implications. The use of numerous thrombolytic agents and percutaneous transluminal coronary angioplasty (PTCA) has established reperfusion therapy as routine treatment of acute myocardial infarction. Multiple randomized trials have demonstrated that early and sustained reperfusion results in marked reduction in the incidence of sudden death and decreases long-term cardiac mortality (6–12). In contrast in trials utilizing endpoints related to infarct size and ventricular function, the benefit of thrombolytic therapy compared with conventional therapy has been less consistent (8,13–17). Numerous explanations have been proposed to explain the apparent discrepancy between improvement in late ventricular function and reduction in mortality (18,19).

Early reperfusion (<1.5 or <3.5 hours) failed to prevent Q waves on electrocardiography or persistent defects on thallium tomographic images, respectively (15,16). Marked variability has also been observed in myocardial salvage, particularly with anterior myocardial infarctions, utilizing technetium-99*m* sestamibi as the perfusion agent (20, 21). One possible explanation is that reperfusion itself may also produce deleterious effects on the ischemic myocardium limiting its potential to reduce infarct size, so-called reperfusion injury (22,23). This would not preclude other potential benefits of restoration of blood flow, which could decrease cardiac morbidity and mortality by increasing scar thickness and accelerating postinfarct ventricular remodeling, thereby reducing infarct expansion and aneurysm formation and decreasing the incidence of ventricular arrhythmias (24–26).

Similarly, improvements in global left ventricular function have been modest, with the greatest increase occurring in patients undergoing successful reperfusion within 3 hours (18). While the failure to show dramatic improvement in ventricular function following thrombolytic therapy may be related to a small amount of salvage, it may also be secondary to a delay in recovery secondary to postischemic left ventricular dysfunction, so-called myocardial stunning (20,27). This chapter reviews numerous biochemical and structural abnormalities associated with regional ischemia and reperfusion. Postulated mechanisms that may be involved in the potentiation of myocardial stunning and reperfusion injury are described. Finally, the role of numerous therapeutic interventions that may enhance myocardial salvage and hasten the recovery of ventricular function of viable myocytes after successful reperfusion are discussed.

DEFINITIONS

Early reperfusion remains the most effective way of reducing infarct size and improving ventricular function in experimental models and humans. In the late 1970s, however, it was suggested that reperfusion itself may also produce deleterious effects on the previously ischemic myocardium (28). Studies in the experimental preparation have demonstrated that reperfusion can produce lethal ventricular arrhythmias (reperfusion arrhythmias) and prolonged left ventricular dysfunction of reversibly injured myocytes (myocardial stunning), and result in the conversion and/or acceleration of lethal injury of potentially viable myocardial and endothelial cells (reperfusion injury) (22,23,27,29–31).

Reperfusion Arrhythmias

Reperfusion arrhythmias refer to the induction of various arrhythmias at the onset of reperfusion. These include premature ventricular beats, accelerated idioventricular rhythms, ventricular tachycardia, and ventricular fibrillation (29,32). They may occur after resolution of coronary spasm, after spontaneous or drug-induced thrombolysis, and after reflow following ischemic arrest from cardiac surgery (33). Although ventricular fibrillation is frequently observed after 30 minutes of regional ischemia in the canine model, it is less common in patients after successful thrombolytic therapy (32,34). This is probably related to the controlled reperfusion that occurs in humans as a result of residual thrombus and/or stenosis, in comparison with the experimental model in which reperfusion is rapid and complete. Numerous mechanisms have been proposed including activation of alpha and beta receptors, disturbances of ionic hemostasis, particularly of calcium and potassium, and the generation of highly reactive oxygen species (35–37). These mechanisms are not mutually exclusive since peroxidation of cellular membranes by free radicals could alter calcium homeostasis and critical ion channels (38,39). These mechanisms and potential therapeutic implications are discussed in detail in Chapter 14.

Myocardial Stunning

Since its original description by Heyndrickx in 1975, numerous experimental and clinical observations have shown that myocardial functional recovery after coronary occlusion and reperfusion may require hours to several weeks (27,30,40). Such postischemic dysfunction has been termed myocardial stunning and occurs in the absence of histologically detectable necrosis (27,30,41) (see Ch. 3). It should be regarded as an entity separate from contractile abnormalities occurring during temporary periods of ischemia and from those associated with irreversible injury. Experimental observations demonstrate that the degree of ischemia is an important determinant in both severity and time to recovery of ventricular function (42). Myocardial stunning is a potentially reversible phenomenon provided an adequate time is allowed for the contractile function to recover. Stunning has been recorded after brief episodes of ischemia (5 to 15 minutes), emphasizing that it occurs in reversibly injured cells (27,30,41). Longer periods of ischemia

(40 to 120 minutes), however, may also cause stunning as a result of nonlethal injury to the epicardial border zone surrounding infarcted myocardium (43,44). Myocardial stunning has been observed in many clinical situations including exercise-induced angina, following prolonged episodes of coronary spasm, after reperfusion of acute myocardial infarction, and after global ischemia for cardiac surgery (30).

Reperfusion Injury

Since the description of reperfusion injury in 1977 by Hearse, numerous experimental studies have attempted to determine the importance and pathophysiology of this entity (28) (see Ch. 3). Although reperfusion injury is potentially the most serious deleterious consequence of reperfusion, it remains the most controversial (45). Reperfusion injury is defined as reperfusion-induced conversion of reversibly injured myocardial and endothelial cells to irreversibly injured cells (23). This implies that cells that were potentially viable just before reperfusion undergo lethal injury during the perireperfusion period. This phenomenon should be distinguished from the entity of acceleration of necrosis of cells that were already irreversibly injured at the time of reperfusion. Conclusive proof that reperfusion injury is an important contributor to ultimate infarct size in vivo would require the demonstration that a significant population of cells that are viable just before reperfusion undergo irreversible injury in the early reperfusion period. Preliminary histologic evidence for this phenomenon has recently been provided in the rabbit model. Death of myocytes by apoptosis, a process producing internuclear DNA fragmentation, was only observed in animals undergoing reperfusion after regional ischemia and not in animals with persistent ischemia (46). Rapid advances in the area of positron emission tomography may allow detection of this phenomenon in the intact animal in the future; however, three further observations in the experimental preparation lend strong support to the occurrence of this entity. First, the administration of various therapeutic agents at the time of or soon after reperfusion has been shown to significantly enhance myocardial salvage (47–50). Second, reperfusion results in new and accelerated ultrastructural changes in the endothelium of capillaries within the ischemic region, compared with equivalent durations of permanent ischemia (51,52). Third, agents that attenuate structural and functional changes in the microvasculature after reperfusion also result in a significant reduction in infarct size in the experimental model (53,54). Although stunning and reperfusion injury may occur in both regional and global ischemic preparations, their occurrence in regional ischemic models is emphasized in this chapter.

METABOLIC, BIOCHEMICAL, AND STRUCTURAL CHANGES ASSOCIATED WITH ISCHEMIA AND REPERFUSION

Metabolic Consequences of Ischemia

The limited energy reserves in the myocardium coupled with the high energy requirements mandate a constant supply of oxygen and substrates to myocardial cells to maintain normal metabolic and contractile function (55,56) (see Ch. 3). The normal myocardium preferentially utilizes free fatty acids that are metabolized via β oxidation to yield 72 moles of adenosine triphosphate (ATP) per mole of fatty acid (56). High-energy phosphate (HEP) stores in the myocardium are limited and exist predominately in the form of ATP and creatine phosphate (CP) (55). Myocardial ischemia is associated with the cessation of oxidative phosphorylation such that alternative metabolic pathways are activated in an attempt to maintain cellular levels of HEP. The low levels of citrate, ATP, and CP present in ischemic tissue in conjunction with increased concentrations of inorganic phosphates results in activation of various metabolic steps involved in anaerobic glycolysis, resulting in enhancement of this pathway as an alternative source of HEP (57). This mechanism is relatively inefficient, producing less than 10% of the ATP required for normal myocardial function and therefore is unable to sustain myocardial viability for prolonged periods (55). Furthermore, continued ischemia results in progressive acidosis due to the accumulation of protons, for example $NADPH_2$ and lactic acid, with eventual inhibition of glycolysis as an alternative energy source (57). Small quantities of ATP are also produced during myocardial ischemia via dephosphorylation of CP. The limited stores of CP in conjunction with inefficiency of anaerobic glycolysis results in a rapid depletion of HEP during ischemia, such that 80% of creatine phosphate is lost within minutes of regional ischemia and greater than half of ATP by 15 minutes (58).

Although the energy requirements of myocardial cells are decreased during ischemia, ATP continues to be utilized to maintain essential metabolic functions of the cells, such as removal of sodium and replenishment of calcium in the sarcoplasmic reticulum (59). The inability of the mitochondria to phosphorylate ATP results in the accumulation of adenosine diphosphate (ADP) and adenosine monophosphate (AMP) (58). AMP is metabolized via 5-nucleotidase, predominantly found in the membranous fraction of the cell, to adenosine, which is then deaminated to inosine in the interstitium (60). Once AMP is degraded to adenosine, nucleoside transport systems facilitate the loss of nucleoside molecules, such as adenosine and inosine, from ischemic myocardial cells (61). Inosine is catabolized to hypoxanthine and xanthine by enzymes localized predominantly in endothelial cells. It has been proposed that the xanthine oxidase pathway may produce large amounts of oxygen-derived free radicals at reperfusion (62).

Restoration of HEP following reperfusion of viable cells can occur via nucleotide salvage pathways that are metabolically rapid or through a slow de novo synthetic pathway (Fig. 21–1) (63). Phosphoribosyl pyrophosphate (PRPP) is an essential component of the de novo pathway and is also a substrate in two of the three salvage pathways. A limited supply of PRPP following ischemia associated with rapid washout of adenine nucleotides during reperfusion results in slow replenishment of high-energy phosphates (64). Experimental studies have shown that following a 15-minute coronary occlusion, ATP levels may remain significantly depressed even after 5 days of reperfusion (64).

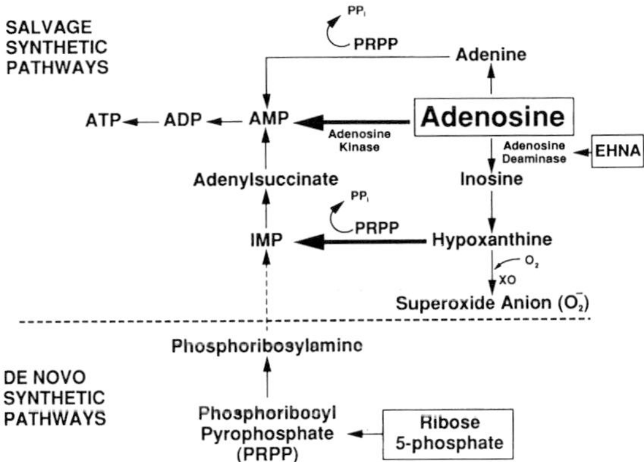

Figure 21–1. Flow diagram illustrating salvage and de novo synthetic pathways in the production of ATP. The salvage pathways that are kinetically most active are thought to be adenosine and hypoxanthine. Adenosine would result in more rapid restoration of high-energy stores, since it can immediately be converted to adenosine monophosphate (AMP) by adenosine kinase. In contrast, the administration of inosine would require more biochemical pathways and would depend on phosphoribosyl pyrophosphate (PRPP) as a substrate, which may be depleted following ischemia and reperfusion. A limited supply of PRPP would also result in the conversion of hypoxanthine to oxygen-derived free radicals through the xanthine oxidase pathway. Repletion of ATP through de novo synthesis is slow, also requiring a number of intermediary metabolites and the presence of PRPP. EHNA = erythro-9-[2-hydroxy-3-nonyl] adenine; IMP = inosine monophosphate; XO = xanthine oxidase.

Abnormalities of Fluid and Electrolyte Homeostasis

Reperfusion could potentially exacerbate myocardial injury by causing explosive cell swelling, interstitial edema, and myocardial hemorrhage (65–68). Myocardial ischemia results in the rapid depletion of high-energy phosphate stores with rapid development of intracellular acidosis (69,70). This leads to inactivation of the sodium–potassium–adenosine triphosphatase pump, with loss of transmembrane ionic homeostasis and slow net gain in tissue water with ischemic times longer than 40 minutes (71). Animals subjected to 15 minutes of ischemia develop only mild tissue edema and increased tissue water 20 minutes after reperfusion (72). After more prolonged ischemic times, reperfusion is associated with explosive cellular swelling secondary to a marked increase in intracellular water, sodium, and calcium (65,66,73). The ultrastructural changes observed in irreversibly injured myocytes are chromatin clumping and margination, with ultimate development of shrunken nuclei, disruption of sarcolemmal membranes, and formation of blebs (72). The myofibrils undergo fragmentation, and sarcoplasmic reticulum and transverse tubules are dilated and disrupted. The mitochondria contain amorphous and granular flocculent densities, a hallmark of irreversible injury (74). These observations suggest that the severe abnormalities in fluid and electrolyte homeostasis probably occur in a cell that has already undergone lethal injury at the time of reperfusion. Another hallmark of reperfused myocardium is the presence of contraction band necrosis at the border zones within 2 minutes of reperfusion, which increases with longer durations of reperfusion. Contraction band necrosis may be induced by hypokalemia or hypomagnesemia, hypoxia, and reoxygenation and in the calcium paradox phenomenon (75).

Myocardial Hemorrhage

Macroscopic hemorrhage is invariably present in the subendocardium in the experimental model with ischemic times greater than 40 minutes (76). As microvascular damage lags behind myocyte injury, red cell extravasation does not occur with short ischemic periods (<60 minutes) in the dog (52). Myocardial hemorrhage has been observed at autopsy in patients who underwent successful reperfusion therapy with thrombolytic agents or with surgical revascularization (77). The possibility that hemorrhage itself at reperfusion could lead to extension of myocardial necrosis was suggested (78). Subsequent studies have revealed that hemorrhage occurs exclusively in areas of irreversible injury and is surrounded by a rim of nonhemorrhagic necrotic myocardium (79–81). These experimental observations have also been confirmed in humans (82). Hemorrhage, therefore, is most likely not an important determinant of reperfusion injury and also does not delay healing of infarcted tissue.

Calcium/Oxygen Paradox

The calcium paradox was described by Zimmerman et al in 1967 (83). These investigators noted that exposure of the isolated heart to brief periods of a calcium-free perfusate was followed by extensive tissue injury as manifested by enzyme leakage and contraction band formation when the hearts were reexposed to a calcium-replete solution. Similar observations were made by Hearse and colleagues with the introduction of oxygen to isolated hearts that had been exposed to a period of hypoxia (oxygen paradox) (84). A unifying hypothesis is that both perturbations resulted in an inability of the sarcolemma to regulate calcium homeostasis on reexposure to oxygen and calcium. Calcium overload has been postulated to activate phospholipases and proteases, accelerate adenosine triphosphate depletion through calcium-activated adenosine triphosphatases, and accelerate free radical formation through xanthine oxidase, thereby facilitating further cellular injury (62,85). Although cellular calcium homeostasis is disturbed during brief episodes of ischemia with free cytosolic calcium rising several-fold within 10–15 minutes, the myocardial cells' ability to regulate calcium recovers soon after reperfusion (86). Massive calcium overload occurs with reperfusion after prolonged ischemia in irreversibly injured cells, probably as a result of severe functional and structural changes in the plasmalemma and not from specific abnormalities of specific calcium channels (72). Ultrastructural changes include contraction band necrosis of myofibrils and the appearance of amorphous dense bodies in the mitochondria that are thought to represent denatured proteins and/or proteins and lipids. Granular densities that appear on reperfusion are believed to be composed of calcium and phosphorus (65).

The precise role of calcium in the pathogenesis of myocardial reperfusion injury remains unproven. Exposure of the heart to a calcium-free environment would only occur in the setting of cardioplegia with calcium-free solutions. Administration of calcium channel blockers prior to reperfusion has failed to consistently enhance myocardial salvage, suggesting that calcium entry through voltage-regulated calcium channels does not significantly contribute to reperfusion injury. Extensive calcium overload therefore probably occurs only in cells that have already undergone lethal injury. Possible sources include uncontrolled release by intracellular organelles and/or entry through a sarcolemmal membrane that has lost its ability to regulate ion exchange. In contrast, calcium appears to play a role in the contractile dysfunction (myocardial stunning) after brief episodes of ischemia that have not resulted in irreversible injury to myocardial cells (30). Although the exact mechanisms remain unknown, activation of protein kinases generated by increased intracellular calcium levels during ischemia in conjunction with the production of cytotoxic free radicals on reperfusion may induce abnormalities in intracellular calcium processing and contractile proteins (30).

Free Radicals

Free radicals are molecules with an unpaired electron and are therefore highly reactive and cytotoxic (87) (see Ch. 3). They may be involved in a larger number of pathologic processes, including radiation and hyperoxic lung injury, drug toxicity, and myocardial ischemic–reperfusion injury (88–91). In the heart, free radicals have been postulated to play a role in the pathogenesis of reperfusion arrhythmias, myocardial stunning, and reperfusion injury (22,30,33).

Molecular oxygen (O_2) is a stable compound because it contains paired electrons, rendering it far less reactive. Although most of molecular oxygen is tetravalently reduced to water, a small amount is univalently reduced to highly reactive free radicals. Potential sources in normal biological systems include the mitochondrial electron transport system, the endoplasmic reticulum in microsomes, peroxisomes, and the formation of prostanoid substances (87). Oxygen-derived free radicals include singlet oxygen, superoxide ion (O_2^-), the hydroxyl radical ($\cdot OH$), and their intermediary hydrogen peroxide (H_2O_2) (62,87). The superoxide ion appears to be an important initiator of subsequent free radical production, as it can react with iron in either the Haber–Weiss or Fenton reaction to form hydroxyl radicals, and it may generate additional iron-containing free radicals by releasing iron from ferritin stores (92). Free radicals can react with other cellular elements to cause protein degradation and lipid peroxidation (93,94). Lipid peroxidation increases cellular damage by causing formation of lipid hydroperoxides and aldehydes that interact with protein sulfhydryl groups, perpetuating cellular damage (87).

Cells contain numerous mechanisms for preventing damage by free radicals (95). The primary mechanism of clearance of superoxide ion from biological systems is superoxide dismutase (95). This enzyme's critical role can be appreciated when one considers that the cascade-like production of reactive species results from superoxide ion generation. Dismutation of superoxide ion by superoxide dismutase produces hydrogen peroxide, which requires further enzyme reduction. Cytoplasmic enzymes, glutathione peroxidase, and catalase provide the final detoxification steps in the reduction of hydrogen peroxide to water (95). Glutathione peroxidase appears to be a more effective enzyme than catalase in protecting myocardial cells from hydrogen peroxide–mediated damage (96). Glutathione peroxidase can also metabolize lipid hydroperoxides to less reactive hydroxy fatty acids. There is no known endogenous cellular defense mechanism for clearing hydroxyl radicals.

Although the quantities of free radical scavenging enzymes in specific cell types in the myocardium are unknown, recent studies have demonstrated a loss of these protective intracellular antioxidant systems with acute myocardial ischemia (97). In addition, cellular hypoxia has been associated with several biochemical and physiologic changes that may provoke free radical production when oxygen and blood elements are reintroduced into the ischemic bed at reperfusion. Recent studies using electron paramagnetic resonance spectroscopy have shown increased myocardial levels of oxygen free radicals in both regional and global ischemic models (98,99). Although the exact cellular source of free radicals remains to be determined, possibilities include nicotinamide adenine dinucleotide phosphate (NADPH) oxidase, cyclooxygenase and lipoxygenase pathways from activated neutrophils, autocatalytic lipid peroxidation, and intracellular sources (xanthine oxidase, aldehyde oxidase, flavoproteins, and the mitochondrial electron transport chain) (62,94,100). Iron appears to be an important factor in enhancing free radical cytotoxicity: it causes formation of hydroxyl radical, is essential for starting and propagating lipid peroxidation, and has been shown to enhance reperfusion injury and reperfusion-induced arrhythmias in isolated ischemic heart preparations (92,101). The superoxide anion may also to act as a neutrophil chemoattractant, possibly via interaction with a lipid noncovalently bound to albumen (101).

Neutrophils

Neutrophils play an important role in the acute inflammatory response to tissue injury and have recently been implicated in causing reperfusion injury in the myocardium and other organs (100,102, 103). Neutrophil activation occurs early during myocardial ischemia, as demonstrated by the presence of numerous neutrophil chemotactic factors in the cardiac lymph from the reperfused bed (104,105). Tissue injury appears to be a prerequisite for neutrophil infiltration, since only ischemic periods of longer than 40 minutes result in a 3–4 fold increase in neutrophil counts in the reperfused myocardium (106). The time course and distribution of neutrophil infiltration after 60 minutes of regional ischemia in the dog has been described utilizing radiolabelled cells. The greatest extent of infiltration occurs during the first hour of reperfusion with preferential localization to the subendocardium (107). These findings have recently been extended utilizing fluorescent videomicroscopy to visualize neutrophil adhesion to epicardial microvessels in vivo (107a). Sixty minutes of regional ischemia followed by a reperfusion significantly increased neutrophil adhesion to coronary microvessels compared to ischemia alone. Neutrophil accumulation increased within 10 minutes of reperfusion and maximized approximately 1 hour into reperfusion (107a). The time course of neutrophil adhesion and infiltration appears to correlate with levels of chemotactic factors present in cardiac lymph (104,105). In contrast, neutrophil infiltration is observed only after 4–6 hours in the permanent occlusion model, predominately at the border of the ischemic zone (108). The essential initiating step in this accumulation includes interaction of the neutrophil with vascular endothelial cells (adhesion) (103). This is followed by activation, diapedesis, and extravascular migration into surrounding myocytes.

The exact mechanism(s) responsible for neutrophil activation and accumulation in reperfused tissue is unknown but is probably secondary to changes in both neutrophils and endothelial cells. These changes are initiated by the presence of numerous inflammatory mediators present in the reperfused myocardium. Activation of the complement cascade occurs during the early phase of ischemia even in the absence of reperfusion (109, 110). The complement fraction C1q localizes to the ischemic myocardium in vivo, and C5a is found in cardiac lymph (105,110). Activated neutrophils contain an enzyme that cleaves C5 into an active chemoattricant fragment (111). Exposure of neutrophils to various chemoattractants derived from a variety of sources causes the cell to become more spherical and induces increased expression of the CD11b/CD18 receptor, which promotes adhesion, aggregation, and chemotaxis (112,113). The importance of the CD18 receptor in early localization of neutrophils in reperfused tissue is illustrated by the observation that monoclonal antibodies to the receptor significantly attenuate their infiltration during the first hour of reperfusion (107).

Ongoing neutrophil activation is mediated by a number of other chemotactic cytokines produced both by neutrophils [interleukin 1, tumor necrosis factor (TNF)] and other cell types such as interleukin 8 from endothelial cells (114,115). These compounds produce an increase in cytosolic calcium in the neutrophil, leading to activation of phospholipases and generation of arachidonate products from cyclooxygenase and lipoxygenase enzymes and the phospholipid, platelet activating factor (PAF) (116). Both leukotriene B_4 and PAF are potent chemoattractants and also enhance vascular smooth tone, potentiate platelet aggregation, promote endothelial permeability, and modulate proteolytic enzyme release (114). Activated neutrophils can also release phospholipid A_2 into the environment, thereby enhancing the production of eicosanoids and PAF by other cells (117–119). The importance of leukotrienes in the inflammatory response is suggested by the observation that lipoxygenase inhibitors attenuate neutrophil infiltration into reperfused myocardium and reduce infarct size (120).

Although the processes are complex, calcium appears to play a role as a second messenger in the secretion of cytotoxic substances from activated neutrophils (121). These substances include numerous potent proteolytic enzymes and reactive oxygen species. Exposure of neutrophils to chemoattractant factors such as leukotriene B_4 and C5a results in release of enzymes from azurophilic and specific granules via reverse endocytosis (121). Neutrophil activation causes a greatly enhanced oxygen uptake by the cells (respiratory burst), resulting in the production of large quantities of reactive oxygen species because of the univalent reduction of oxygen by NADPH oxidase (122). These species include superoxide anion, hydrogen peroxide, hydroxyl radical, hydrochlorous acid, and chloramines (123). Normal endothelial and myocardial cells are protected from oxidant injury by numerous endogenous enzymes that are depleted by ischemia (97, 123). Both lysosomal enzymes, such as elastase, and reactive oxygen species have been shown to damage endothelial cell basement membranes in vitro (124,125). Neutrophil-derived oxidants may also inactivate antiproteases such as α_1-antitrypsin present in the plasma (126). Neutrophil degranulation and free radical release may therefore permit an unchecked activity of proteolytic enzymes on endothelial and myocyte membranes.

VASCULAR CHANGES

Physiology of Normal Myocardial Endothelium

Endothelial cells account for an exceptionally high surface area in the heart (1,000 cm^2/g) and form a continuous lining of the vasculature (127,128). They are attached to blood vessels by subendothelium, which consists of an organized matrix of molecules including collagen, elastin, fibronectin, and von Willibrand's factor secreted by endothelial cells themselves (129). Endothelial cells also secrete β_2 integrins (VLA-2, VLA-3), which bind collagen to sites on the endothelial cell (129). The endothelial cell provides a selective barrier separating intravascular and extravascular spaces and is therefore in a position to regulate the transfer of nutrients to myocytes, the diapedesis of leukocytes, and the interaction between circulating vasoactive substances and vascular smooth muscle.

Recent evidence has shown that the endothelial cell is metabolically very active and plays an important role in regulating microcirculatory flow. These involve substances that both inhibit and activate the coagulation pathway. Endothelial cells produce numerous antiplatelet factors (prostacyclin, adenosine, endothelium-derived relaxing factor), proaggregatory factors (thromboxane A_2), anticoagulation factors [tissue-type plasminogen activator (t-PA), thrombomodulin, protein S, antithrombin III, heparin sulfate] and procoagulation factors (plasminogen activator inhibitor, factor V, factor VIII, and tissue factor) (129–134). The fragile balance between these factors could be altered by reperfusion-induced damage to the endothelium, resulting in inappropriate intravascular thrombus formation.

Recent advances in endothelial physiology have revealed that numerous vasoactive compounds are produced by endothelial cells that regulate vascular responses. These include nitric oxide (NO) and NO-containing compounds, endothelins, prostacyclin, adenosine, smooth muscle cell hyperpolarizing factors, and angiotensins (130,131,133,135). Endothelial cells have surface receptors for many vasoactive compounds including acetylcholine, histamine, serotonin, catecholamines, bradykinin, and adenine nucleotides, reflecting the integral involvement of the endothelium in regulating vascular smooth muscle tone (128,133,136). The functionally intact endothelium releases endothelium-derived relaxing factor (EDRF) when exposed to these chemical agonists (129,133). EDRF appears to be indistinguishable from nitric oxide, has a short half-life (6 to 50 seconds), and produces smooth muscle relaxation by increasing cyclic guanosine 3′,5′-monophosphate (GMP) (129,133). NO is synthesized from the conversion of L-arginine to cit rulline by a constitutive and inducible form of NO synthase (129). Although it has been suggested that EDRF represents a number of nitroso compounds, NO appears to be the active form of EDRF

(129,137). NO is a free radical and is rapidly inactivated by superoxide anions. It is readily diffusible ad- and abluminally, where it has numerous physiologic effects. These include relaxation of vascular smooth muscle in large and small arteries, veins, and microvessels, inhibition of platelet aggregation, and reduction in neutrophil activation and adherence to endothelial cell surfaces (129,130,133, 133a,133b). It may also scavenge reactive oxygen species and attenuate thrombin-induced PAF synthesis in endothelial cells (133,138). Infusion of L-arginine has been shown to reduce neutrophil infiltration, preserve endothelial function and enhance myocardial salvage in experimental models of regional ischemia and reperfusion (133a,133c).

The vasoregulatory role of endothelial cells has recently been heightened by the isolation and purification of a 21-amino-acid peptide termed endothelin (ET), which appears to be the most potent vasoconstrictor discovered, with a potency 10 times that of angiotensin II (129,135,139). Three families of endothelin have been identified (ET-1, ET-2, ET-3), which are formed from an intermediate biological precursor, pre-endothelin, which then undergoes cleavage by a converting enzyme (129,140). Endothelial cells appear to be the most abundant source of ET-1; the production is stimulated by both mechanical factors such as shear stress or by a number of substances including thrombin, tumor growth factor beta (TGF_{β}), angiotensin II, and interleukin 1 (135,140). Two distinct ET receptor subtypes have been identified: ET_A, which is selective for ET-1 and found in vascular smooth muscle; and ET_B, which is localized on endothelial cells and is a nonselective receptor (140). Activation of the ET_A receptor results in an intense sustained vasoconstriction by increasing cellular calcium from both intra- and intercellular sources (129). ET_B activation mediates vasodilation by increasing EDRF and/or PGI_2 production and by activation of the calcium-activated K^+ channel (129). It is now recognized that a marked vascular variation in receptor distribution occurs in different species, and that ET_B activation can elicit both a dilator and constrictor response (140). Elevated plasma levels of ET have been found in experimental models of reperfusion and in patients undergoing thrombolysis (141–143). Recently a several-fold increase in messenger RNA for ET-1 was found in rabbit myocardium undergoing 30 minutes of ischemia followed by 180 minutes of reperfusion (144). Similarly, a twofold increase in de novo synthesis of ET-1 has been demonstrated in pigs reperfused after 90 minutes of regional ischemia, but not in animals with permanent ischemia (143). In situ hybridization revealed that cardiomyocytes, and not endothelial cells, are the source of ET-1 production (143). However, the precise role of this peptide in reperfusion injury remains unknown, since disparate results on infarct size reduction have been found in various animal models utilizing ET antibodies and both selective and nonselective receptor antagonists (143–149,149a).

Other vasoactive compounds produced by endothelial cells include prostacyclin and angiotensin, endothelium-derived hyperpolarizing factors (EDHFs), and endothelium-derived constricting factor (EDCF) (129,130,133). The chemical nature of the latter two compounds are yet to be determined, but they appear to modulate more immediate vascular responses (129). Prostacyclin is synthesized from arachidonic acid and produces smooth muscle relaxation, disaggregates platelets, and acts as a profibrinolytic agent (129,132,150). Angiotensin I is synthesized by endothelial cells and is then converted to angiotensin II by angiotensin converting enzyme (ACE) in the cell. ACE also inactivates bradykinin, a peptide that stimulates the release of NO and prostacyclin (129).

The endothelium also plays a pivotal role in the myocardial metabolism of adenine nucleotides (151). Vascular endothelial cells, via their capacity to release and take up adenosine, are responsible for the maintenance of constant plasma levels of this nucleoside in the coronary circulation (136,151). Adenosine is a potent coronary arteriolar vasodilator and may be an important regulator of coronary blood flow (137). Adenosine disaggregates platelets and inhibits their release of thromboxane (134). Adenosine is also an important modulator of neutrophil function since it markedly reduces superoxide anion generation and inhibits adherence of activated neutrophils to cultured endothelial cells (152–154).

The endothelium also modulates local inflammatory and immune responses. Neutrophil adherence, activation, and migration involve an interplay between expression of adhesion molecules by endothelial cells, neutrophil activation, and local cytokine activity. Exposure of endothelial cells to thrombin, interleukin, and TNF induces the expression of molecules on the endothelial cell surface (selectin-E) and intracellularly (ICAM-1) that increase neutrophil adhesiveness to endothelial cells (129,155). The presence of cytokines (IL-1, TNF, and TGF) also stimulates endogenous endothelial production of interleukins 1 and 8 and PAF (129,156). Endothelial-derived PAF upregulates the CD11b/CD18 complex, thereby increasing neutrophil adherence to the vessel wall, and also their responsiveness to chemotactic factors (129). Interleukin 8 regulates transendothelial migration of neutrophils through the endothelial barrier (129). Endothelial cells are also known to produce several factors that inhibit neutrophil attachment, including adenosine, prostacyclin, and cyclic adenosine monophosphate (130,131,150). The balance between induction and suppression of neutrophil adherence is related to the physiologic or pathologic environment, and further work is required to unravel the regulator signals of these cellular interactions.

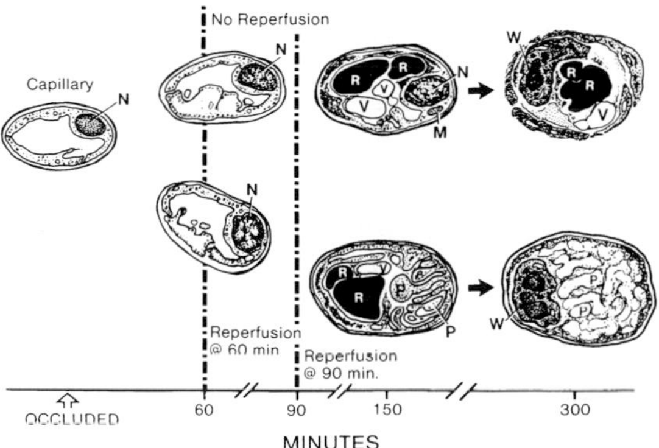

Figure 21–2. Sequential changes in microvasculature after varying periods of ischemia. *Bottom:* After 60 minutes of ischemia, endothelial cells are swollen, and there is a decrease in pinocytotic vesicles; nuclei (N) show condensation and margination of nuclear chromatin. Vertical dash lines represent the critical period of ischemia when the no reflow phenomenon is observed on reperfusion. Endothelial changes increase with longer duration of ischemia (90 minutes) followed by reperfusion. There is severe capillary damage with large intraluminal protrusions (P), absent or decreased pinocytotic vesicles, membrane-bound vesicles (V), and capillary obstruction with red (R) and white (W) cell plugging. Vessels ultimately rupture with fibrin and platelet deposition and red and white cell extravasation. *Top:* With permanent coronary occlusion, intravascular protrusions are less pronounced; however, membrane-bound vesicles and red and white cell plugging with fibrin deposition are prominent but are seen only after longer durations of ischemia. Usually at this phase endothelial cells start to disintegrate.

Pathological Changes in Endothelium with Ischemia and Reperfusion

Histological Changes

A marked disparity is noted in the progression of ultrastructural changes between myocytes and endothelial cells with comparable periods of permanent ischemia (51,52,157) (see Ch. 2). Whereas myocytes in the subendocardium manifest changes of irreversible injury after 40 minutes of ischemia, only mild swelling of endothelial cells in small vessels is observed, suggesting that the latter cell is more resistant to ischemia (52). After 60 minutes of ischemia, 20% of endothelial cells manifest focal swelling with loss of pinocytotic vesicles, which increases to 40% after 90 to 180 minutes of ischemia (Fig. 21–2). After more prolonged periods of ischemia (180 to 360 minutes) progressive changes are noted, which include margination of nuclear chromatin and mild swelling of cytoplasm with occasional vesicle formation. Longer durations of permanent ischemia are associated with capillary obstruction secondary to red and white cell accumulation and occasional endothelial protrusions (157) (Figs. 21–2 and 21–3). In contrast, reperfusion is associated with marked acceleration of vascular injury (22,23,51). Reperfusion after 45 to 90 minutes of ischemia results in explosive endothelial swelling of the microvasculature. Histologic changes range from mild capillary endothelial cell swelling, loss of pinocytotic vesicles, blebs, and cytoplasmic protrusions to breaks in endothelial cells, disruption of the basement membrane, and red cell and neutrophil plugging, which result in capillary obstruction (51) (see Figs. 21–2 and 21–3). Reperfusion is also associated with a rapid increase in neutrophil infiltration with ischemic times greater than 40

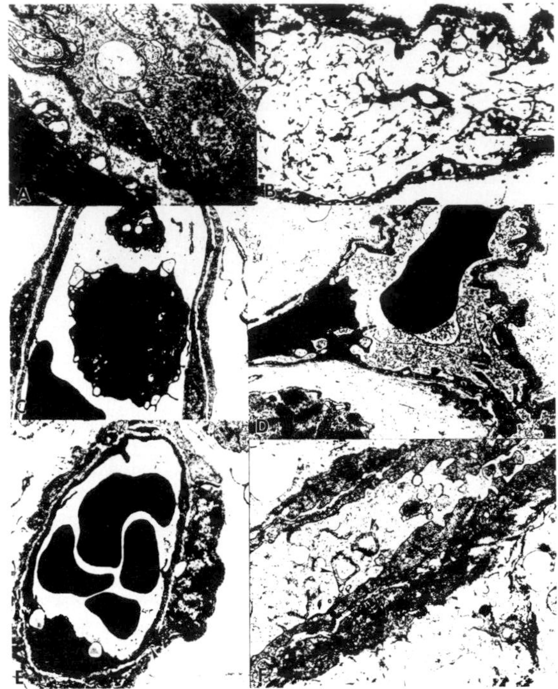

Figure 21–3. Electron micrographs of (**A**) border zones from a permanent 3-day coronary occlusion model; (**B,C**) blood reperfusion infarct after 90 minutes of occlusion; (**D,E**) intracoronary infusion of perfluorochemical after 90 minutes of reperfusion; and (**F**) intracoronary infusion of adenosine after 90 minutes of coronary occlusion. **A.** Endothelial cell swelling (arrows) with intraluminal membrane-bound bodies (arrowheads) in the border zone of a permanent coronary occlusion infarct at 3 days. **B.** Marked endothelial swelling with cellular protrusions (arrowheads) that are totally obstructing the capillary lumen. **C.** Polymorphonuclear leukocytes and endothelial cell within capillary lumen, which is a prominent feature of reperfused infarcts. **D,E.** Animal treated with perfluorochemical showing only mild endothelial swelling and membrane-bound structures (**D,** arrowhead) with prominent pinocytotic vesicles (**E,** arrowhead). **F.** Capillary from an animal treated with adenosine. Note mild endothelial swelling and the increase in endothelial cell folds (arrowhead) (**A,** ×8,600; **B,** ×20,000; **C,** ×7,700; **D,** ×7,700; **E,** ×12,000; **F,** ×20,330).

minutes in the canine model (106,107). Intravascular neutrophils may "plug" up to 27% of the capillaries, and this is associated with a decrease in regional blood flow (158). Endothelial cell damage associated with capillary obstruction by blood elements contributes to the continual decrease in blood flow to areas of ischemic myocardium even after the onset of reperfusion—the no reflow phenomenon (159). The release of vasoactive substances by neutrophils, platelets, and endothelial cells may further perpetuate the no reflow phenomenon.

Functional Changes

Experimental studies utilizing different animal species have shown that the endothelium both from large and small coronary vessels is markedly dysfunctional following regional ischemia and reperfusion. Abnormalities in endothelial-dependent relaxation are observed within 2.5 minutes of reperfusion and are maximal at 180 minutes (160). Several studies support a key role of the neutrophil in the pathogenesis of endothelial dysfunction since the administration of different antineutrophil agents (Fluosol, adenosine, prostacyclin, antibodies to Mac-1) preserve endothelial vasodilatory responses after reperfusion (53,54,160). Although the exact mechanism whereby neutrophils mediate functional abnormalities remains unknown, generation of superoxide anion during the early stage of reperfusion may act as a precipitating mechanism, since administration of superoxide dismutase (SOD) preserved endothelial vasodilatory reserve (161).

Regional ischemia and reperfusion have also recently been shown to significantly increase the release of the potent vasoconstrictor peptide endothelin-1 from the previously ischemic bed (141,142). Increased messenger RNA for endothelin-1 is present in the myocardium shortly after reperfusion (143,144). Intravenous infusion of adenosine at reperfusion, in a dose previously found to be cardioprotective, suppresses this release during the early reperfusion period (144). The precise role of this peptide in the pathogenesis of myocardium reperfusion injury remains to be determined.

In summary, three observations strongly support the hypothesis that endothelial cell dysfunction plays a pivotal role in extending myocardial necrosis following reperfusion. First, ischemia without reperfusion does not result in impairment of endothelial-dependent relaxation (160,162). Second, the administration of various pharmacologic agents that preserve endothelial function have also been shown to significantly enhance salvage following reperfusion (53,54,161). Third, ischemic preconditioning, a potent anti-ischemic mechanism, also prevents endothelial dysfunction following reperfusion (162).

Neutrophil–Endothelial Interactions

The recent identification of numerous adhesive molecules that regulate various interactions between endothelial cells and neutrophils has considerably increased our understanding of these key cellular elements in the acute inflammatory process (see Table 21–1). These molecules, which are expressed over a variable time period, result in an orchestrated sequence of events involving neutrophils and endothelial cells at the site of inflammation. The initial phase of neutrophil contact is slowing or rolling of the cells in venules, followed by activation and firm adherence to the endothelial cells, and finally transmigration through endothelial cell junctions into the myocardium. Three families of adhesion molecules have been identified, and each plays an important role in modulating the various stages of the acute inflammatory response. They include (i) the selectin family, (ii) the immunoglobulin family, and (iii) the integrins. A detailed description of these molecules can be found in numerous recent review articles (155,163–165). In the following few paragraphs, a brief overview of these molecules is given, emphasizing their potential role in the reperfused ischemic myocardium.

Selectins

The selectins are a recently identified family of glycoproteins that are expressed on the surface of blood cells and endothelial cells and mediate the initial phase of neutrophil adhesion, namely rolling. They include L-selectin expressed on neutrophils, E-selectin on endothelial cells, and P-selectins on platelets and endothelial cells. All three selectins recognize a common carbohydrate ligand, the oligosaccharide known as sialyl Lewis^x, although this may not be the only ligand for the selectins. P-selectin is stored in α granules of platelets and in Weibel–Palade bodies of endothelial cells and is rapidly redistributed to the surface of the endothelial cells that have been exposed to thrombin, leukotriene C_4, or free radicals. A recent in vivo study in the feline model of regional ischemia demonstrated that endothelial P-selectin was maximally expressed 20 minutes after reperfusion predominately in postcapillary venules and persisted for up to 170 minutes after reperfusion (165a). L-selectin is constitutively expressed by neutrophils and is rapidly downregulated from the cell surface on exposure of the neutrophil to numerous neutrophil activating agents. This event follows the kinetics of upregulation of Mac-1 from intracellular stores, illustrating a close link between these two adhesion molecules. E-selectin (ELAM) is expressed only after de novo synthesis 3–6 hours after activation of endothelial cells by various cytokines (TNFα, interleukin 1β). An in vivo study showed that expression of E-selectin was only minimally increased after 4½ hours of reperfusion suggesting it does not play an important role in the early inflammatory response following myocardial ischemia/reperfusion (165a). P- and L-selectins are responsible for initial neutrophil rolling on endothelial cells, which slows down the neutrophil in the microvasculature, especially venules, allowing other adhesion molecules to become operative. Monoclonal antibodies to both P- and L-selectins have been shown to attenuate neutrophil infiltration and reduce infarct size in the experimental model of ischemia/reperfusion (166,167).

β_2 or Leukocyte Integrins

The CD18 integrin family includes three structurally related α, β heterodiamers, CD11/CD18 (LFA), CD11b/CD18 (Mac-1), and CD11c/CD18 (p150.95). They were among the first adhesion molecules identified and play an important role in solidifying the adhesion processes by increasing adhesion of neutrophils to each other (aggregation) and to endothelial cells. They also assist in neutrophil migration, antigen presentation, and neutrophil effector functions. They are capable of interacting with a large number of ligands, including the immunoglobulin superfamily (ICAM), complement, and fibrinogen. Integrins are rapidly upregulated from intracellular granules in neutrophils when they are exposed to compounds produced from stimulated endothelial cells, namely platelet activating factor (PAF) and interleukin 8. Both inflammatory mediators are synthesized by endothelial cells within minutes after being exposed to thrombin, LTC_4, TNFα, and other agonists, where they upregulate CD11b by binding to specific surface receptors. The important role of the integrins in the pathogenesis of myocardial reperfusion injury is illustrated by infarct salvage in the canine model

Table 21–1. Principle Receptors Involved in Modifying Neutrophil–Endothelial Interactions Following Myocardial Ischemia and Reperfusion

Receptor	Primary Distribution	Ligand	Time to Peak Expression	Modifiers	Function
Selections					
L-Selectin (CD62L)	Neutrophil	CD34, GlyCAM-1 MAdCAM-1	constitutive	Rapidly shed on PMN activation	PMN rolling with adherence
P-Selectin (CD62P)	Endothelial Cell Platelet	siayl-Lewis^x and others	10–20 min	Complement, LTC_4, histamine, thrombin, IL-1, and TNFα increase expression	PMN rolling with adherence
E-Selectin (CD62E)	Endothelial Cell	siayl-Lewis^x and others	3–6 hours	IL-1, TNFα, and LPS increase expression	PMN rolling with adherence
Immunoglobulin					
ICAM-1 (CD54)	Endothelial Cell	Mac-1, LFA-1	12–24 hours	IL-1, TNFα, LPS increase expression	PMN adherence with transmigration
ICAM-2 (CD102)	Endothelial Cell	LFA-1	constitutive	———	PMN adherence with transmigration
PECAM-1 (CD31)	Endothelial Cell Neutrophil Platelets	PECAM	constitutive	———	PMN extravasation Endothelial integrity
β_2 Integrins					
LFA (CD11a/CD18)	Lymphocyte Neutrophil	ICAM-1 ICAM-2	constitutive	IL-8, C5a, PAF, LTB_4, and TNFα rapidly increase affinity	PMN adherence with transmigration
Mac-1 (CD11b/CD18)	Neutrophil	ICAM-1 iC3b, fibronectin	minutes	IL-8, C5a, PAF, LTB_4, and TNFα increase expression	PMN adherence with transmigration PMN aggregation
P150,95 (CD11c/CD18)	Neutrophil	iC3b, fibronectin	minutes	IL-8, C5a, PAF, LTB_4, and TNFα increase expression	PMN adherence with transmigration

C5a = enzymatically generated fragment of fifth component of complement with anaphylactoid activity; iC3b = inactive fragment of third component of complement; GlyCAM = glycosylation-dependent cell adhesion molecule; IL-1 = interleukin 1; IL-8 = interleukin 8; ICAM = intracellular adhesion molecule; LFA = lymphocyte function antigen; LPS = lipopolysaccharide; LTB_4 = leukotriene B_4; LTC_4 = leukotriene C_4; Mac-1 = macrophage-1 glycoprotein; MAdCAM = mucosal addressin cell adhesion molecule; PMN = polymorphonuclear neutrophil; PAF = platelet activating factor; PECAM = platelet endothelial cell adhesion molecule; TNF = tumor necrosis factor utilizing monoclonal antibodies to CD11/CD18 glycoprotein complex (168,169).

IMMUNOGLOBULIN FAMILY

These are a group of immunoglobulins, expressed by endothelial cells, that play a role in neutrophil adhesion and diapedesis. They include ICAM-1, ICAM-2, and PECAM-1. ICAM-1 is present in low levels at basal conditions and can be greatly upregulated in response to interleukin 1 and TNF within 1–2 hours and persists for days. Reperfusion appears to be an important prerequisite for increased expression of ICAM-1 in vivo. In the canine model of regional ischemia, increased message for ICAM-1 and interleukin 6 were observed in the same viable myocardial cells in the border zones of the infarct only in animals undergoing reperfusion (170). While the message for interleukin peaked within 3 hours of reperfusion, ICAM-1 increased progressively over the 24-hour reperfusion period (171). ICAM-2 is constitutively expressed and does not appear to be modified by cytokines. ICAM-1 and ICAM 2 are responsible for adhesion and migration of neutrophils by interacting with β_2 integrins. Migration of neutrophils through endothelial cell junctions is also mediated by another adhesion molecule of the immunoglobulin family, known as platelet–endothelial adhesion molecule-1 (PECAM-1). Monoclonal antibodies to ICAM-1 reduce neutrophil infiltration and infarct size in the experimental model of regional ischemia (172).

SUMMARY

Multiple adhesion molecules sequentially mediate the recruitment of neutrophils to sites of tissue injury through their attachment to endothelial cells. This is a three-step process: (i) initial rolling of neutrophils on endothelial cells to overcome intracellular shear stress forces mediated by selectin molecules, (ii) further adhesion and attachment mediated by the integrin–immunoglobulin pathway, and (iii) transmigration of neutrophils through endothelial cell junctions to sites of tissue injury. Exaggerated and prolonged activation of this natural defense mechanism may occur following reperfusion of ischemic but viable myocardium, resulting in lethal injury to endothelial and myocardial cells. This hypothesis is supported by the observation that monoclonal antibodies to these molecules enhance salvage in animal models of myocardial ischemia and reperfusion.

Complement

The complement system, which forms an important part of the humoral defense mechanism and is a primary mediator of the inflammatory response, consists of a number of proteins that circulate in an inactive form in the plasma (115). Myocardial ischemia and reperfusion have been shown to activate both the classical and alternative pathways through interaction of complement components with disrupted myocytes and through the release by activated neutrophils of proteases and oxygen free radicals, respectively (114,115). A number of regulatory proteins have been identified that modulate various active components of the complement system. A detailed review of complement activation and its regulation have been published recently (173). A brief overview of the role of complement in myocardial ischemia and reperfusion is presented in the next few paragraphs.

A huge body of experimental and clinical evidence has demonstrated that complement activation occurs following myocardial ischemia and reperfusion. Components of complement have been documented in the myocardium in experimentally induced myocardial ischemia and appear to correlate with neutrophil accumulation (110). The ability of cardiac lymph obtained from the ischemic bed in the dog to activate complement is abolished by the addition of anti-C5a serum (105). Elevated levels of complement components in the plasma and myocardium have been found in patients following myocardial infarction (173). Administration of agents that reduce levels of complement, such as cobra venom factor, administration of a soluble complex of the complement receptor type 1 (CRT), which accelerates the decay of numerous complement complexes, or infusion of a C1 esterase inhibitor (C1 INH) which blocks the classic complement pathway in its first step, have been shown to enhance myocardial salvage following reperfusion (174,175,175a). The findings suggest that inappropriate activation of complement significantly contributes to myocardial necrosis following reperfusion.

Complement could accelerate tissue injury following ischemia by two main pathways: amplification of the inflammatory process through neutrophil activation, and by acting as a direct cytotoxin through generation of a complex of complement fragments (C5b-9) known as the membrane attack complex (MAC) (115,173). The generation of various cleavage products of complement, particularly C5a, initiates the early inflammatory response by increasing vascular permeability, producing smooth muscle contraction, and acting as a potent chemoattractant for neutrophils (115,173). C5a also promotes neutrophil adherence, oxygen free radical generation, and proteolytic enzyme release. Complement plays an important role in neutrophil adherence to vascular endothelial cells. C5a and other cytokines result in an increased expression of CD11b/CD18 glycoprotein receptor (Mac-1) on neutrophils. Deposition of the degranulation product of C3b, iC3b, in endothelial cells results in the formation of an important receptor for Mac-1 (115). Thus complement plays a key role in the initial interaction of neutrophils to endothelial cells through rapid induction of the Mac-1 glycoprotein on neutrophils and its corresponding receptor on the endothelial cell, resulting in subsequent neutrophil activation and vascular injury. Complement may also produce direct injury to cells through the generation of MAC (115,173). MAC inserts into the membrane bilayer, allowing the bidirectional flow of macromolecules with resultant cell death (115,173). In addition to its cytotoxic effect, MAC can also amplify the inflammatory response by increasing expression of P-selectin on neutrophils (164,173). Complement activation appears to play an essential role in the initiation and maintenance of the inflammatory response through recruitment, adherence, and activation of neutrophils to endothelial cells after an ischemic insult. This, in conjunction with its direct cytotoxic effects, supports its role as a mediator of myocardial injury.

Although the complement system is believed to be the most important source of inflammatory mediators after ischemia, a number of other chemotactic cytokines also play a role in the inflammatory response. These include interleukin 1 from neutrophils, interleukin 8 synthesized from endothelial cells after exposure to TNF or IL-1, PAF from platelets and endothelial cells, and leukotriene B_4 from neutrophils. In addition to neutrophil recruitment, these compounds can also modify other pathways in the inflammatory response, such as upregulation of neutrophil integrins and induction of neutrophil migration by IL-8 (114).

MECHANISMS OF STUNNING AND REPERFUSION INJURY

Stunning

Numerous theories have been proposed to explain the phenomenon of myocardial stunning.

Insufficient Energy Production and/or Utilization

Numerous experimental studies utilizing both in vivo and in vitro models of regional and global ischemia have demonstrated a rapid depletion of HEPs, particularly creatine phosphate and ATP (58,64,176). Although creatine phosphate rapidly normalizes following relief of ischemia and may exceed preischemic levels ("overshoot"), replenishment of ATP stores may take days depending on the duration and severity of the preceding ischemic episode (30,64,177). Myocardial stunning is also associated with decreased myofibrillar creatinine kinase activity and decreased free ADP required to produce ATP at the contraction site (30). Recovery of adenine nucleotides occurs in two phases in ischemic cells and is determined by the availability of essential substrates required for the salvage and de novo synthetic pathways (63,178). Enhancement of total myocardial ATP stores has been shown to correlate with improvement of contractile function of the stunned myocardium in some studies (178). However, replenishment of total myocardial ATP stores does not appear to be mandatory to improve myocardial stunning, since a marked and sustained increase in contractility can be achieved with inotropic agents (30,178,179).

Abnormalities of Coronary Vasodilatory Reserve

Ten to fifteen minutes of regional ischemia results in increased microvascular permeability and impaired endothelial-dependent relaxation in isolated coronary rings from dogs undergoing regional ischemia (180,181). Bolli et al reported an increase in coronary vascular resistance and impaired vasodilatory response in the microvasculature following 15 minutes of ischemia in the intact dog (181). Augmentation of coronary blood flow with papaverine and dipyridamole has been shown to significantly improve postischemic ventricular dysfunction (182). The mechanism remains unknown but may be due to alleviation of heterogeneous microvascular flow secondary to vasospasm or mechanical plugging, increased myofiber stretch, washout of toxic metabolites formed during ischemia such as hydrogen ions and lactate, or enhancement of the metabolic substrate of viable cells by enhanced oxygen delivery.

Abnormalities of Intracellular Calcium Homeostasis

Calcium overload has been proposed as a possible cause of myocardial stunning (see Ch. 3). Cytosolic free calcium increases after 9–10 minutes of ischemia and precedes the loss of plasma membrane structural integrity (183,184). The mechanism remains unclear but may be secondary to decreased calcium uptake by the sarcoplasmic reticulum or secondary to increase in intracellular Na^+ mediated through Na^+–Ca^{2+} exchange (30,185). Since Na^+–Ca^{2+} exchange is inhibited by acidosis, normalization of pH in reperfusion may enhance calcium entry via this exchange mechanism. The exact mechanisms whereby calcium induces contractile dysfunction remain unknown, but enhanced calcium entry at reperfusion could activate phospholipases or increase the generation of reactive oxygen species via the xanthine oxidase pathway (62).

Sarcoplasmic reticulum obtained from stunned myocardium demonstrates abnormalities in calcium transport and a decrease in activation of calcium and magnesium -ATPase (186). In a Langgendorf preparation of global ischemia, a shift in maximal calcium-activated pressure has been observed that may reflect either decreased myofilament calcium sensitization or a decrease in calcium transients (187). Therefore, sarcoplasmic reticulum dysfunction secondary to calcium overload during early reperfusion could perpetuate ventricular dysfunction by diminishing contractile protein activation through attenuated calcium release during systole. The importance of calcium in the pathogenesis of myocardial stunning is further supported by the observation that selective administration of calcium antagonists into the reperfused bed improves ventricular function in doses that do not alter systemic hemodynamics or regional myocardial blood flow (188).

Role of Oxygen-Derived Free Radicals

Numerous studies support the hypothesis that oxygen-derived free radicals play an important role in the pathogenesis of myocardial stunning (30,189) (see Ch. 3). First, the addition of free radicals to in vivo and in vitro preparations reduces contractile function (190,191). Second, increased quantities of free radicals have been demonstrated in global and regional ischemic models utilizing electron paramagnetic resonance spectroscopy and spin trapping agents (189,192). Finally, improvement in contractile function in the experimental preparation has invariably been shown by the addition of free radical scavenging enzymes or by agents that inhibit the function of free radicals (30). The exact source of free radicals remains to be determined, but they could be produced from autoxidation of catecholamines, by autocatalytic lipid peroxidation, and via intramyocardial sources, such as xanthine oxidase and the mitochondrial electron transport chain (62,94,100). The xanthine oxidase pathway appears not to play an important role in humans since xanthine oxidase is either absent or present in minute quantities in the human myocardium (193). Although the role of neutrophils, another potential source of free radicals, remains controversial, induction of neutropenia or administration of "anti-neutrophil" agents have invariably failed to prevent contractile dysfunction (194). Furthermore, the brief period of ischemia required to produce stunning does not activate neutrophils or increase their infiltration into the ischemic myocardium.

A series of experiments have been published by Bolli and colleagues exploring the role of oxygen radicals in a canine model of stunned myocardium (30,194a). These studies indicate that (i) although all three oxygen species (superoxide anion, hydrogen peroxide, hydroxyl radical) contribute to myocardial stunning the hydroxyl radical appears to play an important role after repetitive ischemia, (ii) free radical contractile dysfunction occurs within the initial 60 seconds following reperfusion, (iii) recurrent brief episodes of ischemia result in cumulative depression of contractility caused by recurrent bursts of free radical generation associated with each episode of reperfusion, and (iv) the beneficial effects of SOD and catalase persist for 24 hours in the conscious model.

Summary

The exact pathogenesis of myocardial stunning remains to be elucidated. Recent evidence suggests that both calcium- and oxygen-derived free radicals play an important role in the etiology of myocardial stunning. Both calcium overload through activation of degradative enzymes and production of cytosolic free radicals at reperfusion could exacerbate injury to subcellular structures such as the sarcolemma and contractile proteins. This may result in altered calcium homeostasis and sensitivity, producing abnormal excitation–contraction coupling with subsequent contractile dysfunction.

Reperfusion Injury

Current experimental evidence suggests that microvascular damage plays a pivotal role in reducing the potential benefit of successful reperfusion (23,49,51–54,195). This results in a progressive decrease in blood flow to areas of potentially viable myocytes, suggesting a dynamic process of microcirculatory failure (23,159,160). Although the exact mechanisms remain speculative, functional and histologic studies support a role for the neutrophil in mediating endothelial cell injury (106,114,196).

Reperfusion is associated with an exaggerated degree of endothelial disruption not present in preparations of permanent occlusion with comparable durations of ischemia (51,52,79,157). Mechanical obstruction by endothelial cell protrusions, circulating blood elements, and/or functional endothelial derangements may be involved (49,53,54, 157,158,160). Endothelium-dependent relaxation involving both epicardial vessels and the coronary microvasculature is significantly impaired after reperfusion (53,54,160,161,197). A recent study has also demonstrated that endothelium-independent vascular responses may be abnormal, possibly as a result of mechanical obstruction of the microvasculature by neutrophil or concomitant injury of smooth muscle cells in muscular arterioles (54).

Neutrophils appear to be important mediators of vascular injury. Neutrophils studied ex vivo demonstrate enhanced chemotaxis and lysozyme degranulation after reperfusion (196,198). Reperfusion after greater than 40 minutes of ischemia results in a rapid influx of these activated neutrophils into the ischemic bed (106,107,158). These cells could cause tissue injury by release of reactive oxygen species such as superoxide anion and hydrochlorous acid from myeloperoxidase, and via numerous potent proteolytic enzymes (121,122). The induction of neutropenia in reperfusion models attenuates neutrophil infiltration into the ischemic myocardium and reduces infarct size (199). Further evidence for the role of neutrophils in microvascular injury is suggested by the observation that agents that suppress neutrophil function result in preservation of both the functional and the structural integrity of the endothelium (53,54,160).

A hypothetical scheme that illustrates potential mechanisms whereby the neutrophil may mediate vascular injury is shown in Fig. 21–4. Under basal conditions, inhibition of neutrophil–endothelial cell interactions is mediated by negative glycocalyx on endothelial cells in conjunction with the production of numerous anti-inflammatory mediators. During ischemia, changes occur in both endothelial cells and neutrophils that enhance their interaction in the perireperfusion period. Ischemia results in the depletion of endogenous inflammatory and vasodilatory substances associated with the deposition of complement, and possible increased expression of adhesion molecules on endothelial cells and neutrophils, which amplifies their interaction. The introduction of oxygen and cellular elements into an immunologically primed vascular bed at reperfusion results in enhanced neutrophil–endothelial cell interactions associated with further activation of the neutrophil to secrete chemotactic factors, vasoconstrictor, and cytoxic compounds (reactive oxygen species, proteolytic enzymes). This causes progressive endothelial injury and further mechanical

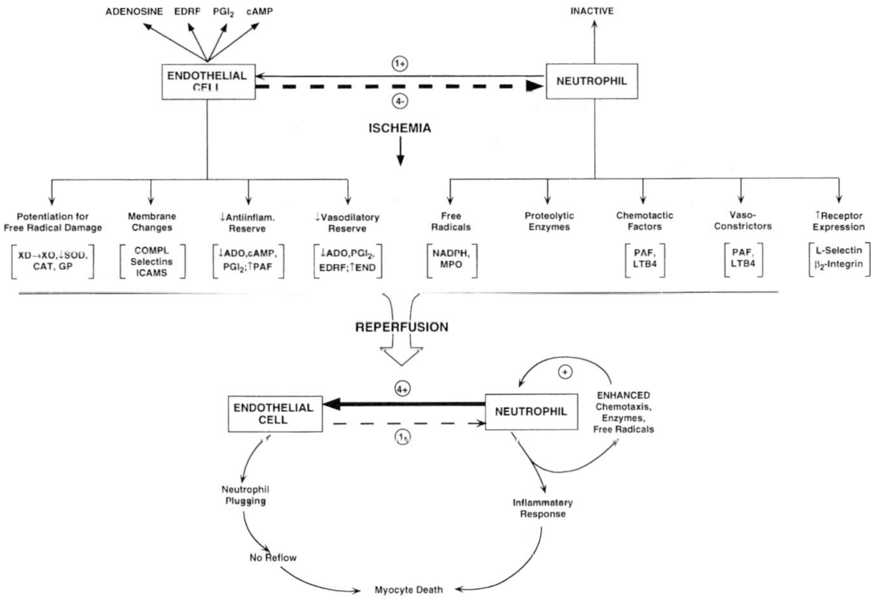

Figure 21–4. Schematic diagram illustrating potential role of endothelial cells and neutrophils in pathogenesis of myocardial reperfusion injury. For explanation, see text. ADO = adenosine; cAMP = cyclic adenosine monophosphate; COMPL = complement; CAT = catalase; EDRF = endothelium-derived relaxation factor; END = endothelin; GP = glutathione peroxidase; ICAMS = intracellular adhesion molecules; LTB_4 = leukotriene B_4; MPO = myeloperoxidase; NADPH = nicotinamide adenine dinucleotide phosphate; PAF = platelet activating factor; PGI_2 = prostacyclin; XD = xanthine dehydrogenase; XO = xanthine oxidase.

plugging of capillaries with neutrophils and other blood elements, thereby decreasing blood flow to potentially viable myocytes (no reflow phenomenon) and resulting in irreversible necrosis of these cells (reperfusion injury).

THERAPEUTIC INTERVENTIONS IN EXPERIMENTAL PREPARATIONS

Myocardial Stunning

Free Radical Agents

A large number of anti–free radical agents have been assessed predominately in the canine model of regional ischemia (189,200–213). These include free radical scavenging enzymes superoxide dismutase (SOD) and catalase, drugs that inhibit the enzyme xanthine oxidase (allopurinol and its active metabolite oxypurinol), iron chelators (desferoxamine), and oxygen free radical–scavenging agents (dimethylthiourea, mercaptopropionyl glycine [MPG], and N-acetylcysteine). The majority of these studies have shown beneficial effects confirming that free radicals play an important role in myocardial stunning in the experimental model. Although the exact mechanisms whereby free radicals mediate stunning remain to be determined, these cytotoxic compounds appear to induce contractile abnormalities during the first 60 seconds following reperfusion. This is supported by observations of Bolli et al, where desferoxamine and MPG only attenuated stunning if given prior to reperfusion but not after 60 seconds of reperfusion (189).

Calcium Channel Blockers

Since an excessive uptake of calcium during the reperfusion period has been postulated to contribute to contractile dysfunction of the stunned myocardium, numerous studies have attempted to investigate the effects of various calcium channel blockers on this phenomenon (214,215). Because in some studies the calcium channel blocker was given during the ischemic period, the protective effect noted could have been related to a reduction in ischemic severity caused by enhanced collateral blood flow or to the blocker's effects on systemic hemodynamics, which could alter ventricular loading conditions. Additional studies in which calcium channel blockers were administered, both locally and after 30 minutes of reperfusion, suggest that altered calcium homeostasis may be involved in the pathophysiology of myocardial stunning (188).

Adenosine

Adenosine is an endogenous nucleoside produced from the breakdown of adenine triphosphate (ATP), which possesses a number of complex cellular and metabolic effects that could ameliorate postischemic contractile dysfunction. These mechanisms have been recently reviewed and are illustrated in Fig. 21–5 (178). Intracoronary adenosine administered continuously during and after reperfusion significantly attenuates myocardial stunning for up to 4 hours in the canine model undergoing a single episode of regional ischemia (215a). Most of current information known about the effect of adenosine or "adenosine-like" agents in contractile function pertains to the state of ATP stores and regional blood flow. Although the beneficial effects of adenosine may also be mediated by improvement in the metabolic substrate of the ischemic cell, restoration of calcium homeostasis, and a reduc-

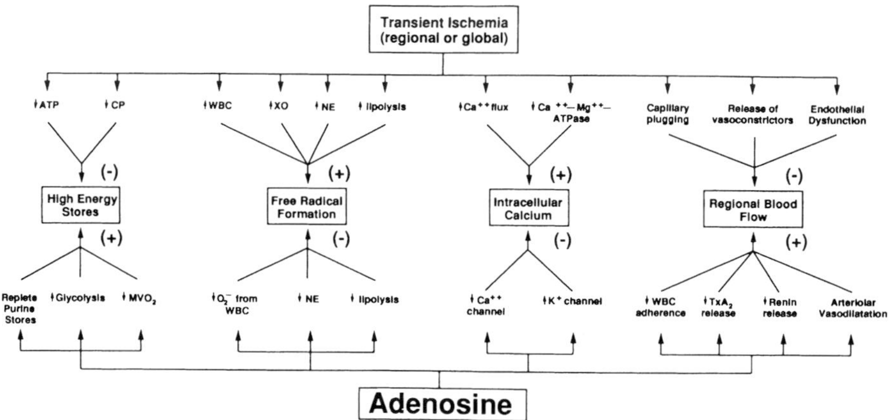

Figure 21–5. Schematic diagram of potential mechanisms of action of adenosine in reducing myocardial stunning. Transient regional or global ischemia followed by reperfusion results in depletion of myocardial high-energy stores and increased production of oxygen-derived free radicals via neutrophils, the xanthine oxidase pathway, autoxidation of catecholamines, and products of lipid peroxidation. Free radical–mediated injury may also contribute to abnormalities in calcium homeostasis. A reduction in subendocardial blood flow associated with reduced vasodilatory reserve is also observed in the stunned myocardium. Endogenous release of adenosine during ischemia may preserve cell viability by enhancing anaerobic glycolysis and decreasing myocardial oxygen consumption. Reperfusion results in a rapid washout of various adenine nucleosides, including adenosine. Administration of adenosine could accelerate the recovery of contractile function through a number of mechanisms. Adenosine may enhance intracellular ATP levels via the salvage pathway while conserving utilization through its negative inotropic effect. Adenosine could also reduce free radical–mediated injury by inhibiting superoxide anion release from neutrophils and decreasing catecholamine release and lipid peroxidation. Adenosine also blocks calcium-dependent channels and therefore may restore intracellular calcium homeostasis. Finally, adenosine may enhance oxygen delivery and washout of "toxic" metabolites through arteriolar vasodilation and antiplatelet and antineutrophil effects. ATP = adenosine triphosphate; ATPase = adenosine triphosphatase; Ca^{++} = calcium ions; CP = creatine phosphate; Mg^{++} = magnesium ions; MVO_2 = myocardial oxygen consumption; NE = norepinephrine; O_2^- = superoxide anion; T_XA_2 = thromboxane A_2; WBC = white blood cell; XO = xanthine oxidase. *Reprinted with permission from Forman and Velasco (178).*

tion in oxygen free radicals, further studies are needed to clarify these mechanisms.

The administration of adenine, inosine, and drugs that increase endogenous adenosine levels by inhibiting its degradation such as erythro-9-[2-hydroxy-3-nonyl] adenine (EHNA) have been shown to accelerate ATP repletion after both regional and global ischemia (216–219). Infusions of ribose that increase the level of 5-phosphoribosyl-1-pyrophosphate, a major limiting factor for the biosynthesis of adenine nucleotides, or 5-amino-4-imidazolcarboxamide ribose (AICAR), which bypasses the initial metabolic processes in the salvage pathways, have also been shown to increase myocardial ATP levels (177,220). Mauser et al compared the infusions of adenosine, AICAR, and ribose in the intact dog undergoing 45 minutes of regional ischemia and 3 hours of reperfusion (221). The most striking increase in adenine nucleotide synthesis was observed with adenosine (90-fold increase), which resulted in significantly higher myocardial ATP levels 3 hours after reperfusion. A significant increase in ATP in the reperfused myocardium has also been shown in both the intact and isolated globally ischemic heart with adenosine deaminase inhibitor EHNA and EHNA combined with the adenine nucleotide transport blocker p-nitrobenzyl thioinosine (NBMPR) (218,222,223).

Some studies have also shown a correlation between repletion of ATP levels and improvement of contractile function of the stunned myocardium. Administration of adenosine in the cardioplegia solution in isolated rabbit hearts undergoing 120 minutes of global ischemia significantly repleted ATP, and this was associated with an improvement in both systolic and diastolic functional parameters of ventricular function (219). Foker et al reported that the combination of adenine and EHNA restored ATP levels to 88% of the preischemic levels in dogs undergoing 20 minutes of ischemia followed by 30 minutes of cardiopulmonary bypass, and this was associated with an improved cardiac output while the animals were in bypass (222). Replenishment of total myocardial ATP stores appears not to be mandatory to improve stunning, since contractility can be restored with the administration of inotropic agents (224,225). One possible explanation is that adenosine may modify the functions of various cells and metabolic processes thought to play a role in the pathogenesis of myocardial stunning (Fig. 21–5) (178). Bolli et al reported an increase in coronary vascular resistance and impaired vasodilatory response in the microcirculation following 15 minutes of ischemia in the intact dog (181). Selective enhancement of coronary blood flow with numerous vasodilators significantly improves ventricular function after repetitive short periods of regional ischemia (182). Therefore, the potent coronary arteriolar vasodilatory effects of adenosine may account for its beneficial effects on myocardial stunning. This is supported by the study of Ledingham et al showing that the addition of adenosine in the reperfusate of isolated rat hearts undergoing 3 hours of hypothermic ischemic arrest increased ventricular function and coronary blood flow without a concomitant increase in myocardial ATP stores (226).

Reperfusion Injury

Methodologic Concerns

Several considerations need to be addressed when interpreting the results of experimental studies and extrapolating the data to humans. The anatomic and physiologic differences between acute occlusion of normal canine coronary arteries and that of chronically diseased human coronary vessels allow for only crude comparisons. The speed of reperfusion is usually immediate and complete in the experimental model, whereas it is slower and incomplete in humans. Further studies are needed to investigate if slow reperfusion influences either the severity or the time course of reperfusion injury.

The marked variability in experimental preparations from different laboratories may also influence the final results of a therapeutic intervention. The failure in some studies to measure collateral blood flow, an important determinant of cell necrosis in the canine model, could lead to spurious results if the treated group by chance had higher ischemic flows. Open chest anesthetized preparations would be expected to undergo accelerated cell necrosis as a result of the higher myocardial oxygen consumption and potential activation of neutrophils and the sympathetic nervous system, compared with conscious closed chest preparations. Other methodologic variables include duration of ischemia and reperfusion, method of determination of irreversible injury, and presence of a residual stenosis in the culprit vessel. Finally, differences in the dose, timing, and duration of the various pharmacologic agents may affect the efficacy of the drug. Administration of agents before or throughout the ischemic period would not allow differentiation of whether the drug was beneficial during the ischemic or reperfusion period. The wide disparity in experimental studies therefore makes interpretation of pharmacologic strategies extremely difficult.

Adenosine

Pharmacology of Adenosine

Adenosine is an endogenous nucleoside produced from the degradation of adenosine triphosphate (ATP) (136). A continual release of adenosine occurs from the heart, which is related to myocardial metabolism. This release is facilitated during myocardial ischemia, resulting in the accumulation of adenosine diphosphate (ADP) and adenosine monophosphate (AMP) due to inability of mitochondria to rephosphorylate ATP (58). Adenosine formation occurs following ischemia by either dephosphorylation of 5′-AMP by 5′-nucleotidase present in the cell membrane or cytoplasm and by hydrolysis of S-adenosylhomocysteine (SAH) by SAH hydrolase (227). These enzymes are regulated by metabolic factors such as ATP, ADP, and inorganic phosphate and by neurohumoral factors such as noradrenalin (227). Inactivation of adenosine deaminase and adenosine kinase may also contribute to adenosine production. Adenosine nucleoside transport systems facilitate the loss of both nucleotides from ischemic myocyte, and adenosine is then deaminated to inosine in the interstitium (228). Further depletion of adenine nucleotides, including adenosine, occurs with reperfusion due to rapid washout of these compounds. Inosine is catabolized to hypoxanthine and xanthine by xanthine oxidase localized predominately in endothelial cells. Restoration of ATP following reperfusion of viable cells can occur via nucleoside salvage pathways that are metabolically rapid or through a slow de novo synthesis pathway (178). Administration of endogenous adenosine would result in rapid restoration of ATP, since it can be immediately converted to AMP via adenosine kinase (Fig. 21–1) (178).

The effects of adenosine are mediated by purinergic type 1 (P_1) receptors located on the cell surface (229). To date, three distinct P_1 receptors—A_1, A_2, and A_3 adenosine receptors—have been well characterized by pharmacological and molecular biological criteria (229,230). All three receptors belong to the superfamily of receptors containing seven transmembrane spanning domains, and all three are coupled to regulatory G proteins (231). Subtypes of the A_1 (A_{1a} and A_{1b}) and A_2 (A_{2a} and A_{2b}) have been proposed and may have significance regarding the development of more specific agonists for therapeutic use (229,230). The A_1 and A_3 receptors are negatively linked to adenylyl cyclase via G_i, whereas A_{2a} and A_{2b} receptors are positively coupled to adenylyl cyclase via G_s. In addition, A_1 receptors are coupled to potassium channels (activate), calcium channels (inhibit), and phospholipase C (stimulate) (231). Cardiomyocytes contain A_1 and A_2 receptors (the subtype of the A_2 receptor in cardiomyocytes remains unclear), and coronary arteries contain A_1, A_{2a}, and A_{2b} receptors and are found predominately in the myocardium and coronary vasculature. Although the messenger RNA for A_3 receptors is present in the heart, the exact cell types expressing this message have not been resolved, and the physiological significance of A_3 receptors is unknown (232). Pharmacological evidence suggests the existence of additional adenosine receptor subtypes in cardiovascular tissues, e.g., an A_4 receptor in coronary arteries and an atypical A_2 receptor on platelets; however, these receptor subtypes have not been cloned, and their existence is controversial (229,230).

Rationale for Use of Adenosine as a Cardioprotective Agent Following Ischemia/Reperfusion

Although the exact cause of myocardial reperfusion injury remains to be elucidated, numerous mechanisms have been proposed. These include neutrophil-mediated myocardial and endothelial cell injury, generation of cytotoxic oxygen-derived free radicals, a progressive decrease in microvascular flow to the reperfused bed (no reflow phenomenon), alterations in calcium homeostasis, and ongoing depletion of high-energy phosphate stores (22,23,31,38). The diverse physiological properties of adenosine, coupled with increased concentrations in the ischemic myocardium, suggest that it may play on important role in regulating and protecting the myocardium in the setting of ischemia and reperfusion. The potential pathways implicated in the pathogenesis of myocardial reperfusion injury and the effect of adenosine on these mechanisms are illustrated in Fig. 21–6.

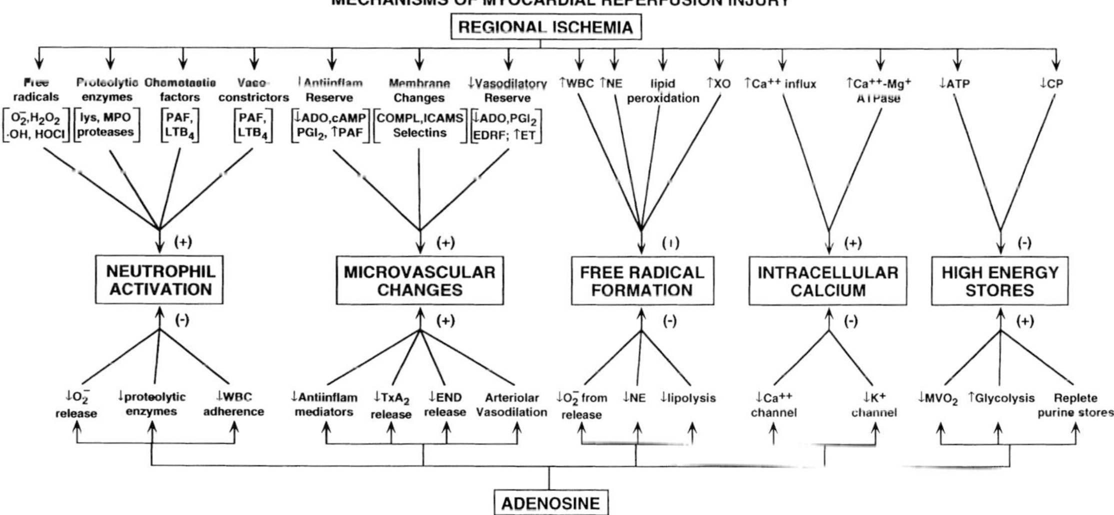

Figure 21–6. Schematic diagram of potential mechanisms of action of adenosine on myocardial reperfusion injury. Regional ischemia followed by reperfusion results in activation of neutrophils to release free radicals and various proteolytic enzymes and vasoconstrictors. Ischemia is also associated with changes in endothelial cells such as deposition of complement, expression of leukocyte adhesion molecules, and depletion of endogenous anti-inflammatory and vasodilator reserves. An increased propensity for the production of oxygen-derived free radicals may occur following ischemia/reperfusion through neutrophils, auto-oxidation of catecholamines, the xanthine oxidase pathway, and products of lipid peroxidation. The introduction of oxygen and neutrophils with reperfusion into an immunologically compromised bed may therefore result in further endothelial and myocardial injury. Reperfusion results in further depletion of high-energy stores through the rapid washout of various adenine nucleotides including adenosine. Administration of exogenous adenosine could ameliorate myocardial reperfusion injury through a number of mechanisms. Adenosine could reduce neutrophil-mediated cellular injury during reperfusion by inhibiting neutrophil adhesion to endothelial cells and by decreasing the production of free radicals and proteolytic enzymes. The potent arteriolar vasodilator properties of adenosine could reverse the effects of various vasoconstrictor substances present in the reperfused bed. Furthermore, restoration of the anti-inflammatory and vasodilator functions of endothelial cells through ATP repletion and oxygen delivery would maintain regional blood flow following reperfusion. Adenosine could also reduce free radical–mediated injury by inhibiting superoxide anion release from neutrophils, decrease catecholamine release, and reduce lipid peroxidation. Adenosine also blocks calcium-dependent channels and may therefore restore intracellular calcium homeostasis. Finally, adenosine could enhance intracellular ATP levels via the salvage pathway while conserving utilization through its negative inotropic effect. ADO = adenosine; ATP = adenosine triphosphate; ATPase = adenosine triphosphatase; Ca^{++} = calcium ions; CP = creatine phosphate; COMPL = complement; EDRF = endothelium-derived relaxing factor; ET = endothelin; ICAMS = intracellular cardiac adhesion molecules; LTB_4 = leukotriene; lys = lysozyme; Mg^+ = magnesium ions; MPO = myeloperoxidase; MVO_2 = myocardial oxygen consumption; NE = noradrenaline; O_2^- = superoxide anion; PAF = platelet activating factor; PGI_2 = prostacyclin; TxA_2 = thromboxane A_2; WBC = white blood cell; XO = xanthine oxidase.

Preservation of Microvascular Blood Flow

Although the mechanisms responsible for microvascular injury with subsequent decrease in myocardial blood flow are complex and diverse, adenosine would appear to be a crucial counterregulatory compound in the maintenance of microcirculatory flow due to its numerous pharmacological actions. First, adenosine could decrease mechanical obstruction of capillary channels caused by neutrophil and endothelial cell debris by reducing neutrophil adherence and neutrophil-mediated cellular damage via activation of A_2 receptors (152,153). Second, the potent arteriolar vasodilator properties of adenosine would oppose the effects of vasoconstrictor substances present in the vascular bed after reperfusion, such as endothelin, leukotrienes, and platelet activating factor (136). Third, adenosine could reduce the release of vasoconstrictor substances produced by activated platelets and neutrophils via stimulation of A_2 receptors (134,233). Furthermore, A_1 receptor–mediated inhibition of noradrenaline release from sympathetic nerve endings and reduced renin release would also decrease the vasoconstrictor burden on the reperfused bed (234). Finally, adenosine may hasten repletion of endogenous vasodilator and anti-inflammatory compounds produced by endothelial cells by restoring the metabolic machinery of these cells through replenishment of ATP stores or by enhancing oxygen delivery through arteriolar vasodilatation (136,219,221).

Neutrophil Effects

Recent studies have shown that adenosine is an important modulator of neutrophil function. Both adenosine and adenosine analogues markedly inhibit superoxide anion production by neutrophils through A_2 receptor activation (154). Adenosine also reduces neutrophil adherence and cytotoxicity to cultured endothelial cells via stimulation of the A_2 receptor (152,153). Although adenosine facilitates neutrophil chemotaxis in vitro via the A_1 receptor, in vivo studies have shown decreased numbers of neutrophils in the reperfused bed in animals receiving exogenous adenosine (49,54,235). These observations suggest that with pharmacological doses of adenosine, A_2 receptor stimulation mediates the antineutrophil action of adenosine. The protective effects of adenosine on myocardial reperfusion injury may therefore be mediated in part by its effects on neutrophils.

Effects on Oxygen-Derived Free Radicals

Although free radicals do not appear to play major role in the pathogenesis of reperfusion injury, adenosine possesses a number of physiological effects that may reduce free radical formation following ischemia. Adenosine has been shown to reduce superoxide anion production by neutrophils in vitro via an interaction with the A_2 receptor (154,234). Inhibition of norepinephrine release from sympathetic nerve endings (A_1 receptor–mediated) and reduced formation of thromboxane from platelets (A_2 receptor–mediated) may also reduce free radical generation via autoxidation of catecholamines or from arachidonate, thereby limiting the degree of lethal myocardial injury (134,234). Adenosine also decreases lipolysis (A_1 receptor–mediated), which could stabilize cellular membranes and prevent further lipid peroxidation (236). Adenosine may also decrease the production of superoxide anion after reperfusion through the enzyme xanthine oxidase by further reducing ATP degradation. Therefore, the multiple effects of adenosine on free radical generation in reperfused tissue suggest that it would be useful in limiting free radical–induced reperfusion injury after regional ischemia.

Effects on Calcium Homeostasis

It is well known that activation of A_1 receptors opens potassium channels (K_{ATP}) in the myocardium (237). Since opening of K_{ATP} channels would hyperpolarize myocardial cells and consequently reduce calcium via voltage-regulated calcium channels, it is possible that adenosine could ameliorate reperfusion injury via this mechanism. In support of this view, recent experiments indicate that (i) protection from reperfusion injury by ischemic preconditioning is mediated by activation of A_1 receptors by endogenous adenosine (238); (ii) the protective effects of ischemic preconditioning are blocked by glibenclamide, an antagonist of K_{ATP} channels (239); and (iii) RP 52891, a K_{ATP} channel opener, reduces reperfusion injury (239). In addition to opening K_{ATP} channels, activation of A_1 receptors would inhibit catecholamine-induced activation of adenylate cyclase, which in turn would decrease intracellular levels of cAMP, reduce activation of protein kinase A, decrease phosphorylation of the calcium slow channel, and attenuate the flux of calcium through this channel.

Effects on Metabolic Substrate

Adenosine initiates numerous metabolic events that could be beneficial in the setting of ischemia and reperfusion. Adenosine would appear to be the most efficient way of restoring ATP levels in viable but energy deficient cells following myocardial ischemia. Adenosine would bypass many of the preliminary reactions in the salvage pathways, thereby accelerating its conversion to AMP through the enzyme adenosine kinase (Fig. 21–1) (240). Adenosine also has higher affinity for the nucleoside transporter compared with other adenine nucleotides, further enhancing its potential to replenish high-energy phosphates (241). This has been confirmed in preparations of both regional and global ischemia in which adenosine with or without an adenosine deaminase inhibitor resulted in a rapid increase in ATP levels following reperfusion (178).

Adenosine may also maintain cell viability by increasing cellular uptake of glucose independently of its vasodilator action by enhancing anaerobic glycolysis (242,243). The antilipolytic effect of adenosine would stabilize cellular membranes, thereby decreasing intracellular lactate production and acidosis (236). Myocardial ischemia is also associated with increased levels of endogenous catecholamines, thereby increasing myocardial oxygen consumption through stimulation of β-adenoreceptors (244). Adenosine may reduce oxygen consumption, thereby conserving high-energy phosphates through its negative inotropic and chronotropic effects and by inhibiting noradrenaline release from sympathetic nerve endings through activation of A_1 receptors (234,245).

Mimicking an Endogenous Protective Mechanism—Adenosine Is the Mediator of Preconditioning

Further support for the role of adenosine as an important endogenous cardioprotective agent has been provided by experimental evidence that it mediates the phenomenon of preconditioning. Preconditioning refers to the observation that a brief period of ischemia renders the myocardium resistant to infarction following a subsequent more prolonged episode of ischemia (246). Infusion of adenosine or A_1 receptor agonists have been shown to mimic the protective effects of preconditioning in a number of animal models, including rabbits, dogs, pigs, and rats (247–249). A preliminary study suggests that A_3 receptors may also play a role (250). The exact mechanism whereby A_1 receptor activation mediates preconditioning remains unknown. Occupancy of the A_1 receptor is known to activate protein kinase C, which modulates the function of many proteins within cells by phosphorylation. Activators or inhibitors of protein kinase C mimic or abolish the anti-ischemic effects of preconditioning, respectively (251). A_1 receptors also open K_{ATP} channels, which could protect the ischemic cell by reducing the action potential duration and thereby slowing ATP utilization (237,252). Opening of K_{ATP} channels may also reduce calcium influx through voltage-activated calcium channels, which would also conserve energy stores and also might reduce calcium-induced injury. The important role of K_{ATP} channels is supported by recent experimental evidence that the administration of glibenclamide, a blocker of K_{ATP} channels, abolishes the cardioprotective effects of preconditioning and that pinacidil, a potassium channel opener, reproduces the infarct size reduction of preconditioning (239). While the exact mechanisms of preconditioning remain to be determined, these studies strongly support a critical role of adenosine, particularly through the A_1 receptor, as an important endogenous cardioprotective compound in the setting of myocardial ischemia and reperfusion.

Effects of Adenosine on Reperfusion Injury in Experimental Models of Regional Ischemia

Canine Model

Since the pharmacological actions of adenosine counteract many of the proposed mechanisms of reperfusion injury, we initially evaluated the nucleoside in a closed chest canine preparation of reperfusion subjected to 90 minutes of proximal left anterior descending coronary artery occlusion and 24 hours of reperfusion (49,195). Selective intracoronary administration of adenosine at 3.75 mg/min for 60 minutes *after* reperfusion produced a 75% reduction in infarct size expressed as a percent of the risk region when compared with blood reperfused controls (Fig. 21–7A). This was associated with improvement in regional ventricular function in the ischemic zone. Regression analysis of infarct size and collateral blood flow measured with radioactive microspheres showed a definite inverse relationship in control animals, whereas in adenosine treated animals infarct size was small irrespective of flow (Fig. 21–7B). The difference between the regression lines was greatest at low collateral flow, suggesting a greater benefit of treatment following severe ischemia. These findings have been confirmed by Hofmeister et al in the open chest canine model of left circumflex occlusion (253).

Additional studies were performed using intracoronary adenosine as a probe to determine the time course of reperfusion injury in the canine model. Animals underwent 40 minutes (group I), 120 minutes (group II), and 180 minutes (group III) of coronary occlusion and 24–72 hours of reperfusion (254,255). The risk region was defined in vivo with Monastral blue, and the area of necrosis histochemically with triphenyltetrazolium chloride and histologically with Mallory's trichrome stain. Animals randomly received either adenosine (3.75 mg/min) in the left main coronary artery for the first 60 minutes of reperfusion or blood reperfusion alone (control). Infarct size was significantly reduced in the adenosine treated animals subjected to 40 minutes and 120 minutes of regional ischemia, but not in animals undergoing 180 minutes of ischemia (Fig. 21–8). Adenosine improved regional myocardial blood flow 3 hours after reperfusion and reduced neutrophil plugging and vascular damage in group I and group II animals only. These observations confirm and extend our previous findings, where intracoronary adenosine reduced infarct size after 90 minutes of ischemia (49). This study shows that reperfusion-induced injury has a limited time course, and that adenosine is only effective when given following 40, 90, and 120 minutes of ischemia but not after 180 minutes.

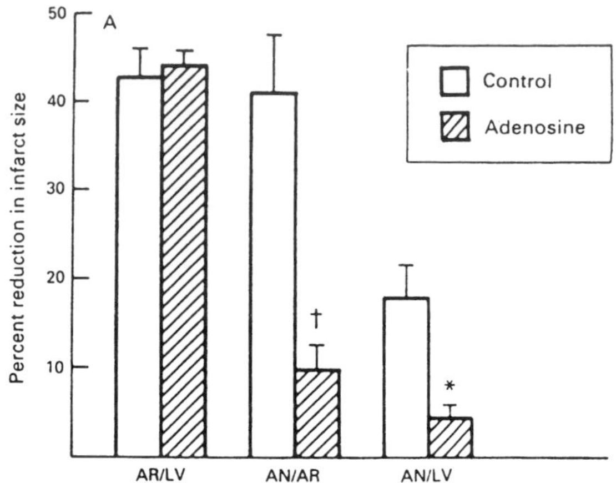

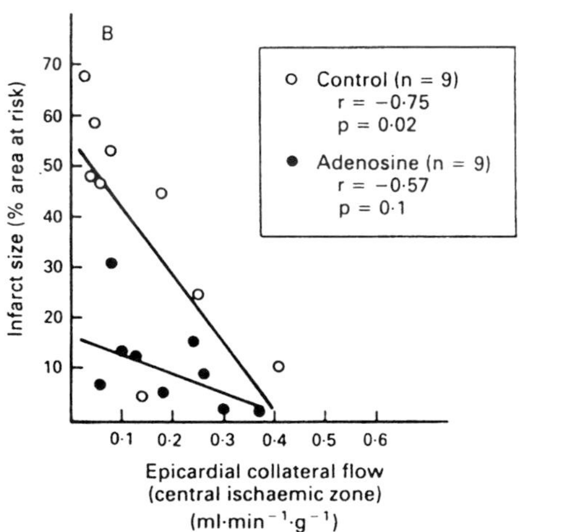

Figure 21–7. Intracoronary adenosine at 3.75 mg/min infused for 1 hour after reperfusion in animals undergoing 90 minutes of left anterior descending coronary artery occlusion resulted in a significant decrease in infarct size (AN) expressed both as a percentage of area at risk (AR) or total left ventricle (LV). $*p = 0.002$, $\dagger p < 0.001$. **B.** Relation between infarct size expressed as a percentage of area of risk and collateral blood flow in control and adenosine treated animals. In control animals an inverse relationship was noted, whereas in adenosine treated animals infarct size was small irrespective of flow.

Since pharmacological interventions may delay the process of myocardial necrosis for 24–72 hours, it is essential that the effects of a drug be determined over a prolonged reperfusion period. Furthermore, the clinical applicability of intracoronary administration of drugs would be limited. In animals subjected to 90 minutes of proximal left anterior descending coronary artery occlusion, in-

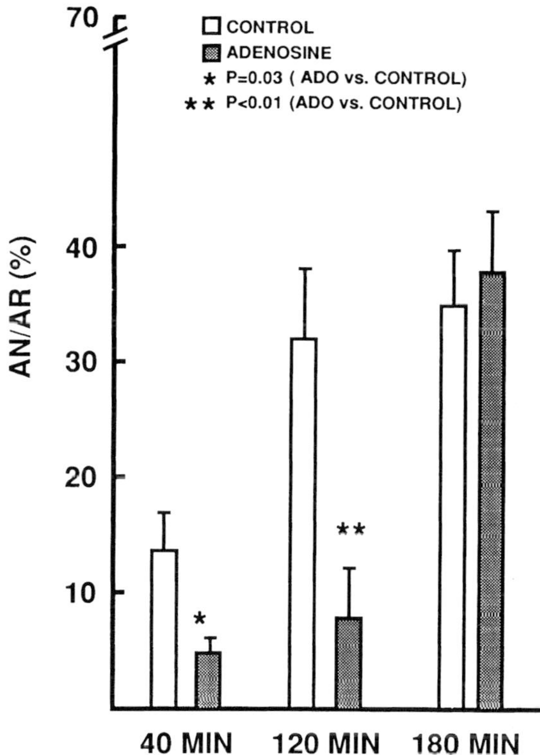

Figure 21–8. Selective infusion of adenosine significantly reduced infarct size (AN) expressed as a percentage of the area at risk (AR) in group I (40 minutes) and group II (120 minutes) of regional ischemia. Adenosine failed to enhance myocardial salvage after 180 minutes ischemia (group III).

travenous adenosine (0.15 mg/kg/min) infused for 150 minutes after reperfusion significantly reduced infarct size as a percentage of the anatomical area at risk 72 hours after reperfusion [35.3(SEM 4.3)% in controls vs. 17.1(4.3)% in treated animals, $p < 0.01$] (50). This was associated with improved regional ventricular function using a computerized radial shortening method at 72 hours [5.5(2.0)% in controls vs. 17.3(3.5)% in treated animals, $p < 0.01$]. No significant effects on heart rate or blood pressure were noted during adenosine infusion. Therefore, intravenous adenosine results in a sustained reduction in reperfusion injury in the canine model.

RABBIT MODEL

Our previous studies had shown that large doses of intracoronary and intravenous adenosine significantly attenuate myocardial reperfusion injury in a highly collateralized model. To evaluate the effect of adenosine in a model with inherently poor collaterals, various doses of intravenous adenosine given during the first 60 minutes of reperfusion were evaluated in the rabbit model subjected to 30 minutes of occlusion of the left circumflex artery and 48 hours of reperfusion (256). The low (0.1 mg/min), intermediate (0.3 mg/min), and high (0.55 mg/min) doses significantly reduced histologically determined infarct size as a percentage of the perfusion bed [control: 52.0(4.6)%; low: 35.3(4.1)%; intermediate: 31.7(4.6)%; high: 31.3(4.6)%]. Both the intermediate and high doses of adenosine, but not the low dose, significantly decreased mean blood pressure.

The failure to observe a dose–response effect on infarct size reduction suggests that the drug may be acting on circulating formed elements, which would be exposed to high levels of the nucleoside as they pass by the tip of the infusion catheter. These findings suggest that myocardial reperfusion injury plays an important role in limiting myocardial salvage in a model with poorly established collateral blood flow. A study by Goto et al using a similar model failed to show a reduction in infarct size with intravenous adenosine in doses of 0.3 and 0.7 mg/min (257). The reasons for this discrepancy may be related to the severe systemic hypotension produced by the larger dose, resulting in possible extension of ischemic injury due to failure to augment postischemic regional blood flow. The failure to show a cardioprotective effect with the lower (nonhypotensive) dose may be due to the use of low doses of lidocaine. In contrast, Thorton et al found protection in the rabbit model with the A_1 agonists phenyl isopropyl adenosine and cyclopentyladenosine when delivered prior to ischemia (249).

Potential Mechanisms of Action of Adenosine

EFFECTS ON VASCULAR INJURY AND NO REFLOW PHENOMENON

Numerous studies have shown that reperfusion accelerates structural and functional changes in the vasculature of the previously ischemic bed, resulting in a progressive decrease in blood flow (no reflow phenomenon) (31,51,53,54). Selective administration of adenosine in a dose previously shown to reduce infarct size significantly preserved endothelium-dependent and -independent vasodilator reserve in the dog subjected to 2 hours of coronary occlusion. A progressive decrease in blood flow to the inner two-thirds of the reperfused bed was observed at 3 and 24 hours after reperfusion in control animals. In contrast, blood flow was maintained in adenosine treated animals and was similar to baseline values up to 24 hours after reperfusion (Fig. 21–9) (54,195). Ultrastructural analysis showed extensive microvascular injury in capillaries of the subendocardium associated with luminal plugging by endothelial cell projections, neutrophils, platelets, and red cells in control animals. These changes were attenuated after adenosine treatment, with relative preservation of endothelial cells and only occasional obstruction of capillaries by cellular elements (Fig. 21–3F). These and other studies from our laboratory suggest that prevention of microvascular injury by adenosine may preserve reversibly injured myocytes following restoration of blood flow to the previously ischemic myocardium (49, 54,195).

The mechanisms responsible for the progressive decrease in regional blood flow are complex and not fully defined. Both mechanical factors—such as leukostasis, platelet aggregation, and/or vascular disruption—and humoral mediators may be involved (141,158,195) The antineutrophil and antiplatelet effects of adenosine may account for its protective effect on the vasculature (134,152–154). Intravascular and interstitial neutrophil infiltration is significantly reduced in animals treated with exogenous adenosine (49,54).

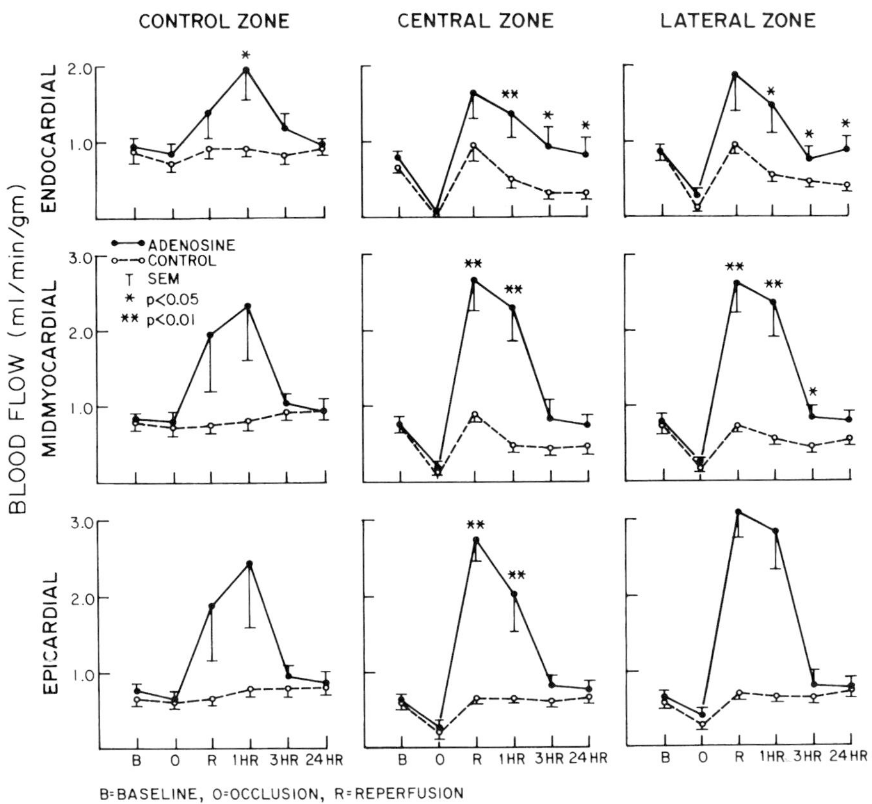

Figure 21–9. Serial changes in regional myocardial blood flow in control and adenosine treated animals after 120 minutes of ischemia. The progressive decrease in flow noted in the endocardial regions in the central and lateral ischemic zones in the control group was compatible with the no reflow phenomenon. Flow in the adenosine group was significantly higher at 3 and 24 hours and was similar to the baseline flow. Bars = SEM; B = baseline; O = occlusion; R = reperfusion.

Adenosine may also prevent microvascular spasm by reversing the effects of numerous vasoconstrictor mediators released from damaged endothelial cells, activated platelets, and neutrophils in the reperfused bed. The isolation of a potent vasoconstrictor peptide from endothelial cells suggests that endothelin may play a role in microvascular hypoperfusion following relief of myocardial ischemia. While regional myocardial ischemia in vivo results in a progressive and parallel increase in coronary sinus and aortic levels of endothelin, a further significant release in coronary sinus levels was demonstrable during the early reperfusion period (141). Preliminary studies have shown that intravenous adenosine in previously determined cardioprotective doses suppresses cardiac release of endothelin (142). The mechanism responsible for this suppression and the ultimate role of endothelin on myocardial reperfusion injury await further clarification.

The Protective Effects of Adenosine are Receptor-mediated

The protective effects of adenosine on myocardial reperfusion injury could be mediated through activation of extracellular receptors or through a nonreceptor mechanism such as replenishment of the ATP pool. To address this, we compared the efficacy of various doses of adenosine with a selective A_1 receptor agonist (cyclopentyladenosine) and a selective A_2 receptor agonist (CGS 21680C) in the rabbit model (Fig. 21–10) (258). A significant reduction in infarct size was noted with all three doses of adenosine, intermediate and low doses of cyclopentyladenosine, and the high and intermediate doses of CGS 21680C. Furthermore, all three

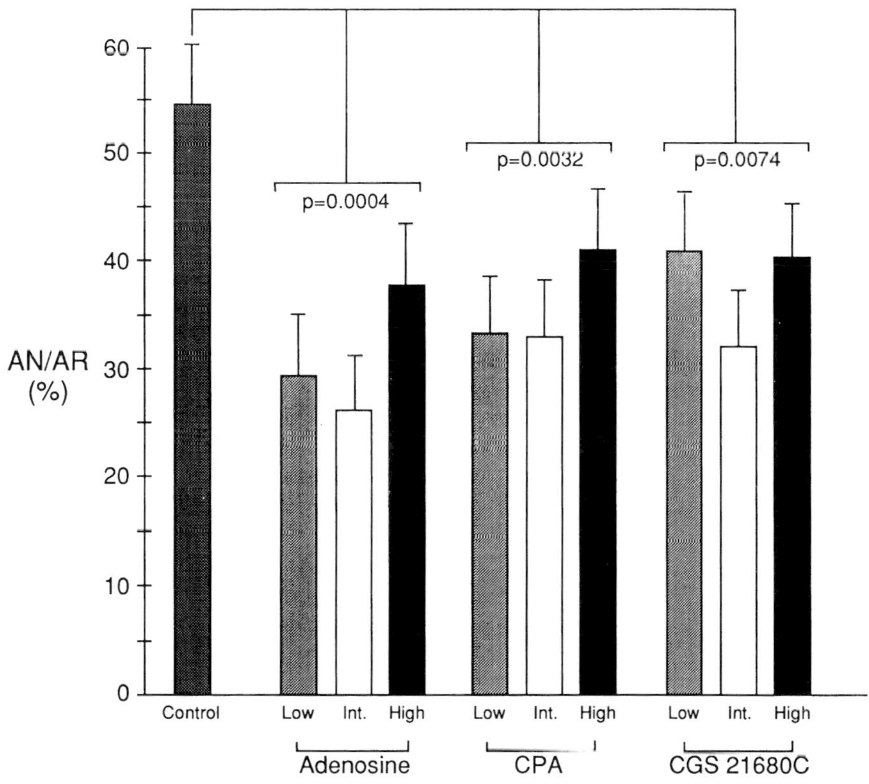

Figure 21–10. Effect of serial doses of adenosine, selective A_1 agonist cyclopentyladenosine (CPA) and selective A_2 agonist (CGS 21680C) on infarct size expressed as a percentage of risk region (AN/AR) in rabbits undergoing 30 minutes of circumflex coronary artery occlusion and 48 hours of reperfusion. Note that all three adenosine receptor agonists afforded similar degrees of protection. *Reprinted by permission from Norton et al (258).*

adenosine receptor agonists afford degrees of protection that were not statistically different. This study shows that intravenous infusions of very low doses of adenosine enhance myocardial salvage, and that this protection is receptor-mediated. The contribution of each receptor type to myocardial protection was not determined in this study, since it is conceivable that local concentrations of each agent may have been high at the infusion site, thereby negating the selectivity of each agonist on formed elements such as neutrophils and platelets. This hypothesis may also explain the equal efficacy of remarkably small does of adenosine in reducing reperfusion injury.

Perfluorochemicals

Perfluorochemicals are substances with a small particle size, low viscosity, and high oxygen-carrying capacity (259). The role of one perfluorochemical preparation, Fluosol, an emulsion of two perfluorocarbons, a detergent Pluronic F-68 (poloxamer 188), and phospholipids, on myocardial reperfusion injury has been investigated in a closed chest canine model of regional ischemia. Intracoronary administration of Fluosol, 5 to 10 minutes *after* the onset of reperfusion, resulted in a pronounced (≈60%) reduction in infarct size both at 24 hours and 2 weeks after reperfusion, and this was associated with a significant enhancement in both global and regional ventricular function (Figs. 21–11 and 21–12) (47,260). Enhanced salvage has also been reported by Schaer et al with administration of the drug without blood during the first 15 minutes of reperfusion (261). Similar beneficial effects have been observed with intravenous administration of Fluosol during the last 30 minutes of a 90-minute occlusion period in the dog (196,198). Intravenously administered Fluosol has similarly been shown to attenuate myocardial reperfusion injury in the rabbit model (262).

Further studies have been performed in an attempt to clarify the mechanisms whereby Fluosol reduces myocardial reperfusion injury. Preservation of endothelial structure and endothelial-dependent relaxation of large and small vessels was found 1

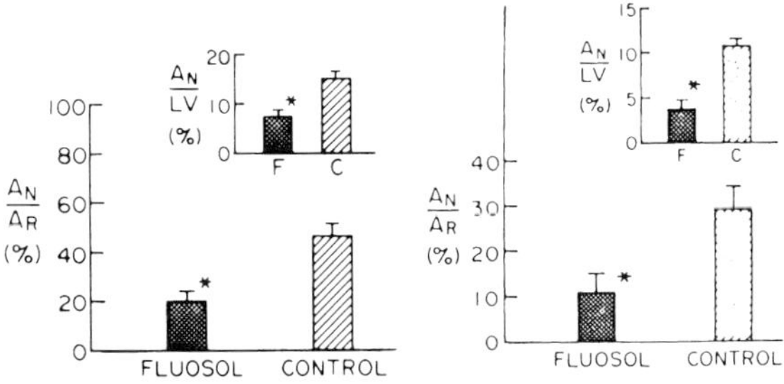

Figure 21–11. Infarct size (A_N) expressed as a percentage of area at risk (A_R) or as a percentage of the total left ventricle (LV) in control and perfluorochemical treated animals determined 24 hours (**left**) and 2 weeks (**right**) after reperfusion. A significant reduction in infarct size is present in the treated group.

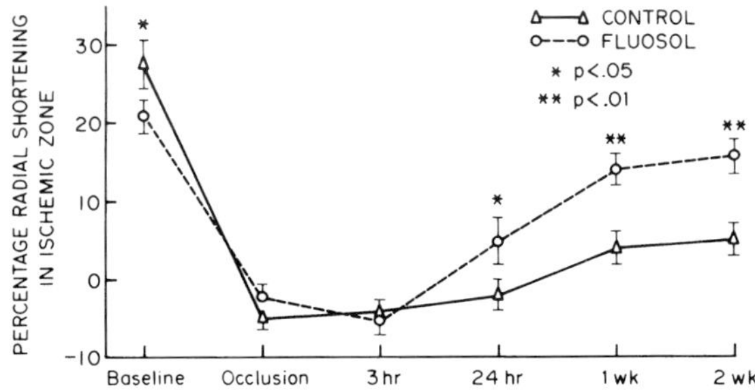

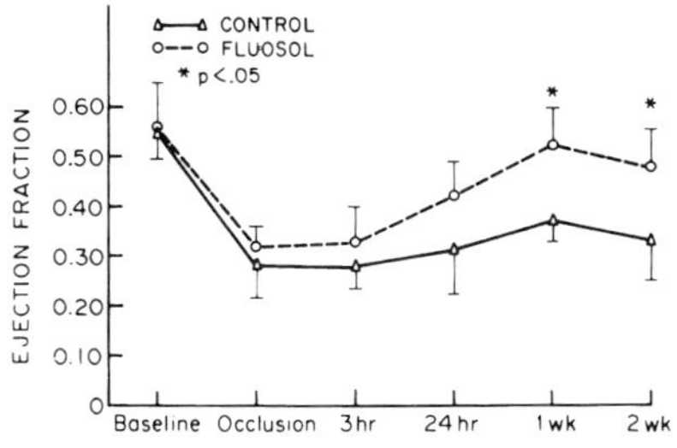

Figure 21–12. Serial percentage radial shortening in the ischemic zone during the experimental protocol in animals subjected to 90 minutes of regional ischemia and 2 weeks reperfusion. Animals were randomized to an infusion of intracoronary perfluorochemical or saline after reperfusion (**top**). Significant improvement in shortening was already apparent at 24 hours after reperfusion in perfluorochemical treated animals, and they continued to show even greater improvement of regional ventricular function over the 2-week period compared with control animals. Significantly greater improvement in ejection fraction was noted in the perfluorochemical treated animals 1 and 2 weeks after reperfusion (**bottom**). *Reprinted from Forman et al (260), with permission.*

hour after reperfusion in the Fluosol animals (Fig. 21–13) (53). Fluosol markedly attenuates neutrophil infiltration into reperfused tissue and reduces neutrophil plugging of capillaries (Figure 21–3D, E) (196,198). Studies of neutrophil function ex vivo revealed a reduction in chemotaxis and lysosome degranulation for up to 24 hours in cells from animals treated with Fluosol (196,198). Inhibition of neutrophil adherence and cytotoxicity to endothelial cell cultures subjected to anoxia is observed when stimulated neutrophils are pretreated with Fluosol (263). These studies suggest that Fluosol, predominately through its effects on the neutrophil, inhibits neutrophil-mediated microvascular damage, thereby enhancing myocardial salvage after ischemia and reperfusion. This is supported by in vivo experiments that Fluosol reduces infarct size without concomitant administration of oxygen (264).

Recent studies have elucidated the mechanism of Fluosol's effects on neutrophils. Neutrophils preincubated with Fluosol, even in concentrations lower than obtained in vivo, manifested enhanced superoxide anion production and lysozyme degranulation within 5 minutes of exposure to the drug, and this effect was entirely attributable to the detergent component, poloxamer 188 (265). This is supported by a recent study showing that prolonged infusion of poloxamer 188 results in a sustained reduction in infarct size in the dog (266). The stimulation of neutrophils by Fluosol was found to result directly from phagocytosis and indirectly from activation of the alternative pathway of complement (267). The mechanism whereby Fluosol reduces reperfusion injury appears to be due to stimulation and subsequent "deactivation" of neutrophils peripherally, which reduces their cytotoxic potential in the reperfused myocardium.

These observations provide definite proof that neutrophil-mediated vascular damage is an important mechanism in the pathogenesis of reperfusion injury. Administration of a potent "antineutrophil" agent after reperfusion significantly attenuated vascular injury, and this is associated with enhanced myocardial salvage. These findings suggest that perfluorochemicals may provide a novel form of therapy to enhance myocardial salvage after successful reperfusion.

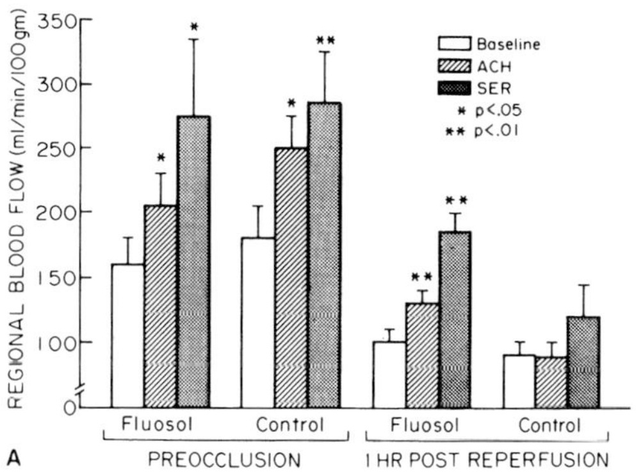

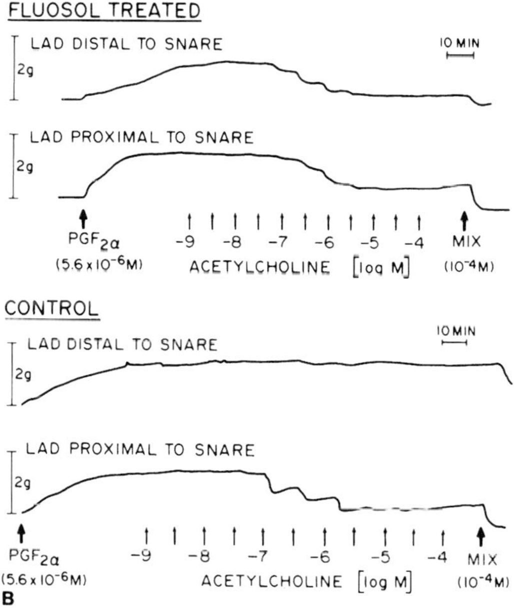

Figure 21–13 **A.** Regional myocardial blood responses in vivo measured with xenon-133 in perfluorochemical and control animals subjected to 90 minutes of regional ischemia and 1 hour of reperfusion. Acetylcholine (ACH) and serotonin (SER) were infused into the left anterior descending coronary artery (LAD) before occlusion and at 1 hour after reperfusion. Note that before occlusion both endothelium-dependent agonists produced a significant increase in flow in both groups. After reperfusion, however, only perfluorochemical treated animals had a significant increase from baseline flow. **B.** Comparative vascular responses of arterial rings to acetylcholine in animals treated with intracoronary perfluorochemical and saline (control). Note loss of relaxation response of the control animal in ischemic (distal to snare) artery, whereas in the perfluorochemical treated animal the ischemic vessel relaxes as well as the proximal (nonischemic) vessel. *Reprinted from Forman et al (53), with permission.*

Free Radical Agents

Numerous studies have attempted to evaluate the role of oxygen-derived free radicals in reducing reperfusion injury in experimental models of reperfusion. Agents evaluated include the free radical scavenging enzymes superoxide dismutase and catalase, xanthine oxidase inhibitors (allopurinol and oxypurinol), agents that scavenge the hydroxyl radical (N-2-mercaptopropionyl glycine and N-acetylcysteine), and the iron chelator desferrioxamine (48,268–285). The literature reflects a wide discrepancy on the effects of these agents on myocardial protection following reperfusion. The majority of the studies in which the drug was given just prior to or after reperfusion, where important determinants of infarct size were measured, and when the animals were reperfused for at least 24 hours, have failed to show a beneficial effect on infarct size reduction in the canine model. Further studies are required using a standardized model and protocol in various laboratories to conclusively address the question whether free radicals are important mediators of this phenomenon. At the present, experimental studies do not clearly support an important role of free radicals in the pathogenesis of myocardial reperfusion injury.

Calcium Channel Blockers

The efficacy of a wide variety of calcium channel blockers has been explored in experimental models of reperfusion (286). These studies have demonstrated inconsistent effects on infarct size reduction. In the majority of studies, these agents were given either before or during the ischemic period. Some degree of myocardial preservation has been observed in animals with high collateral blood flow and small areas of ischemia, suggesting that the agents may delay cell necrosis in areas of moderate ischemia (286). Verapamil failed to prevent the reduction in endothelium-dependent vasodilatory reserve or to decrease neutrophil infiltration in the intact animal (287). Furthermore, calcium channel blockers only partially decrease excessive calcium influx in supraphysiologic doses (288). Calcium channel blockers are therefore unlikely to have a major beneficial effect on myocardial reperfusion injury. They may prove beneficial when used as adjunctive therapy to delay the deleterious effects of ischemia prior to the restoration of blood flow with thrombolytic agents or balloon angioplasty.

Antineutrophil Agents

Reperfusion injury may be mediated by the rapid and indiscriminate influx of activated neutrophils into the reperfused bed, resulting in further vascular and myocardial cell injury. This hypothesis is supported by earlier studies that demonstrated myocardial salvage in animals rendered neutropenic with neutrophil antiserum, antimetabolites (hydroxyurea), or leukocyte-depleting filters (102, 199,289). These interventions produce numerous other physiologic effects such as depletion of other cell types, complement activation, and release of adenosine, which could influence reperfusion injury (114). Further studies utilizing nonsteroidal anti-inflammatory drugs (ibuprofen), inhibitors of the lipoxygenase and cyclooxygenase pathways (such as nafazatron, BW 755C), prostacyclin analogues (iloprost and taprosline), prostaglandin E, PAF antagonists, and complement-modifying drugs (cobra venom factor, which depletes various complement fractions, complement receptor type I, which accelerates the decay of various complement complexes, and a C1 esterase inhibitor which blocks the classical pathway), have resulted in infarct size reduction in reperfusion models (102, 174,175,175a). Following the recent identification of a number of adhesion molecules that regulate the interaction between neutrophils and endothelial cells, a number of studies have been performed utilizing various monoclonal antibodies to these receptors. Administration of antibodies against both the α and β subunit of the glycoprotein molecule on neutrophils have invariably resulted in infarct size reduction in various animal models including dogs, cats, and primates (168,169). This has been associated with reduced neutrophil infiltration and preservation of endothelial-dependent relaxation in some studies (168). However, in one study administration of an antibody to the common β-subunit of the glycoprotein receptor failed to reduce infarct size 3 hours after reperfusion in dogs (290). Antibodies to P- and L-selectin glycoproteins on neutrophils and to the immunoglobulin receptor expressed on endothelial cells (ICAM-1) have also shown cardioprotective effects (166,167,172). Administration of a soluble oligosaccharide, a counter receptor for selectins, also reduced infarct size in the feline model of regional ischemia (291). Infusion of a stable synthetic sphingosine derivative, N,N,N-trimethylsphingosine (TMS) which attenuates P-selectin expression on endothelial cells and reduces neutrophil adherence to the endothelium significantly attenuated myocardial necrosis following reperfusion in the cat (291a). Since the majority of these studies were performed with short reperfusion times, it is unclear whether these interventions would result a sustained reduction in infarct size. Nevertheless, they provide further evidence that neutrophil-mediated vascular and myocardial damage play an important role in limiting myocardial salvage following experimental ischemia and reperfusion.

Nitric Oxide Donors

Experimental studies have demonstrated that endothelial dysfunction manifested as reduced nitric oxide (NO) release occurs soon after reperfusion and is associated with rapid accumulation of neutrophils into the reperfused bed (161,133a). NO possesses numerous anti-inflammatory properties which could ameliorate myocardial reperfusion injury. These include inhibition of neutrophil adhesion and activation, inhibition of platelet aggregation and adhesion and stabilization of microvascular permeability (133a,133b). NO would also maintain microcirculatory flow following reperfusion by dilating vascular smooth muscle and suppressing the release of the potent vasoconstrictor endothelin-1 (133a,133b). Recently a number of NO donor pharmacologic agents have been developed which are able to release NO into the reperfused myocardium without requiring extensive cellular metabolism. Preliminary experimental studies utilizing a number of different NO donors have shown cardioprotective effects in the canine and feline models of regional ischemia after short durations of reperfusion (133a,133c). Further long term studies are required to evaluate the ultimate role of these agents in enhancing myocardial salvage following reperfusion of the ischemic myocardium.

CLINICAL STUDIES

Myocardial Stunning

Myocardial stunning has been demonstrated in various settings associated with ischemia and reperfusion in humans and may be associated with increased morbidity and mortality. Although stunning can be reversed with inotropic agents, these invariably increased myocardial oxygen demand, which may be detrimental in patients with severe coronary artery disease. Prevention of myocardial stunning would be preferable in this setting and in patients with severe left ventricular dysfunction. No definitive studies have been performed in humans to assess the efficacy of the numerous pharmacologic agents (antioxidants, calcium antagonists, "adenosine-like" agents) that have shown promise in the experimental model. Preliminary studies in patients undergoing global ischemia during coronary bypass surgery have shown improved ventricular function when adenosine or SOD has been added to the cardioplegic solution. Further evaluation of agents to prevent postischemic ventricular dysfunction appears warranted.

Reperfusion Injury

The best endpoint needed to optimize detection of an improvement in myocardial salvage in humans beyond reperfusion alone remains to be determined. Technetium-99*m* sestamibi is a new radiopharmaceutical that distributes according to myocardial blood flow and has minimal redistribution. It has been shown to closely correlate with pathologically determined risk regions and infarct size in the experimental model (292). Gibbons and coworkers have shown in a number of studies that (i) sestamibi detected myocardial salvage following successful reperfusion, (ii) myocardium at risk and myocardial salvage are significantly greater in anterior than inferior infarctions, and (iii) salvage in inferior infarction is associated with a small improvement in global ejection fraction (20).

Only a few clinical studies have been performed to investigate the existence and contribution of reperfusion injury to myocardial salvage in patients treated with thrombolytic agents or emergency balloon angioplasty. The majority of the studies have utilized global ejection fraction or regional wall motion abnormalities as an endpoint to evaluate the efficacy of adjunctive therapy beyond reperfusion alone. Differences in ejection fraction would be difficult to detect, particularly in studies that have included a significant percentage of inferior infarctions (20). Since myocardial stunning may persist for weeks to months following successful reperfusion, the utilization of regional wall motion as an index of salvage may prove insensitive, particularly when employed in the early reperfusion period (293). Therefore, interpretation of the majority of a few currently available clinical studies is problematic.

Studies using intravenous captopril and the prostacyclin analogue Iloprost in conjunction with tissue-type plasminogen activator (t-PA) failed to demonstrate improved regional and global ejection fraction 7–10 days after thrombolytic therapy (294,295). A randomized placebo-controlled trial utilizing superoxide dismutase intravenously in patients with anterior infarction reperfused with angioplasty within 4 hours also did not improve regional and global ejection fraction measured at 4 to 6 weeks after angioplasty (296). Oral administration of captopril at the time of streptokinase infusion in approximately 300 patients experiencing a first anterior myocardial infarction was associated with a significant reduction in enzymatically determined infarct size and reduced clinical heart failure (297).

Three studies have recently explored the role of the perfluorochemical Fluosol and its detergent component poloxamer 188 as an adjunctive therapy to reperfusion strategies. In a small but well-controlled study, a 30-minute intracoronary infusion of Fluosol *after* successful angioplasty in patients with a first large anterior myocardial infarction significantly improved regional and global ventricular function and reduced infarct size utilizing thallium tomographic imaging 10–12 days after angioplasty (Fig. 21–14) (298). In a larger open-labeled trial utilizing t-PA, intravenous Fluosol in an identical dose failed to produce beneficial effects utilizing similar endpoints (299). The reasons for these discordant results are speculative. Possible explanations include failure to confirm exact time of reperfusion angiographically, inclusion of a large population of inferior infarctions, and failure to determine infarct size, a primary endpoint, in a large number of patients with anterior infarctions. In a randomized double-blind trial of 113 patients treated with intravenous t-PA or streptokinase, Schaer et al have shown that a 48-hour infusion of the detergent component of Fluosol, poloxamer-188, significantly im-

A.

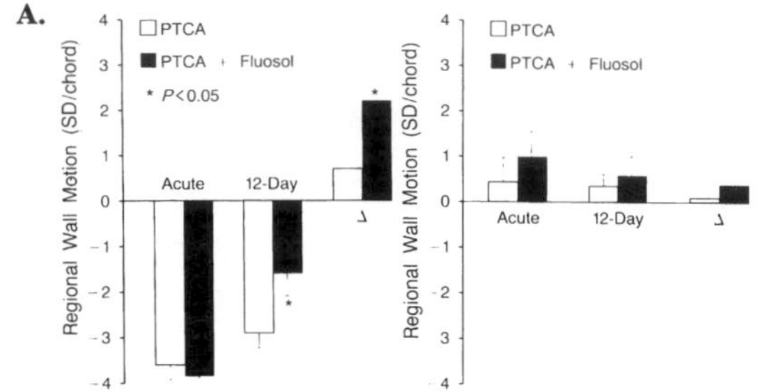

B.

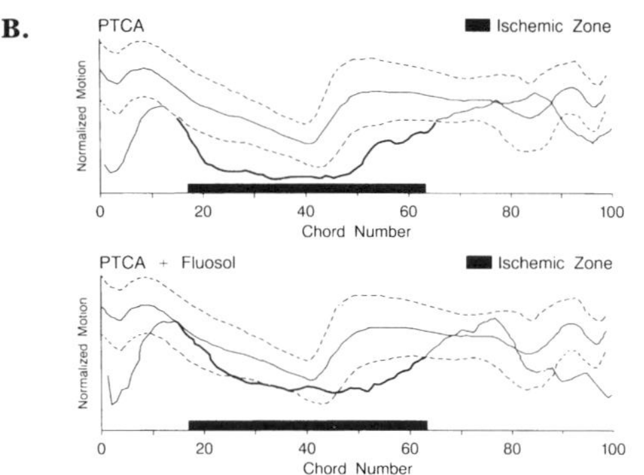

Figure 21–14 **A.** Regional wall motion in the central ischemic (left panel) and nonischemic regions (right panel) expressed as standard deviation (SD) per chord is illustrated. Note that before reperfusion, regional wall motion was similar in both groups in the central ischemic zone (derived from 50% of the chords lying in the infarct-related artery territory whose motion was most depressed compared with the normal patient group). Twelve days after angioplasty (PTCA), a significant improvement was observed in Fluosol treated patients, such that wall motion was within the normal population range. Relative hyperkinesia was noted in the nonischemic region in both groups acutely and at 12 days. **B.** This graph illustrates normalized wall motion (solid light line) and 2 SD from the mean (interrupted lines) for a normal group utilizing the centerline method. Mean wall motion in the ischemic zone for the angioplasty (PTCA) group (upper panel) and angioplasty plus Fluosol group (lower panel) is shown by the dark line at 12 days after reperfusion. The ischemic zone was defined by the chords that fell below the normal range before angioplasty. In the angioplasty group (upper panel), wall motion remains <2 SD from the mean, whereas >50% of the chords in the Fluosol group (lower panel) fall within 2 SD of the mean. *Reprinted from Forman et al (298), with permission.*

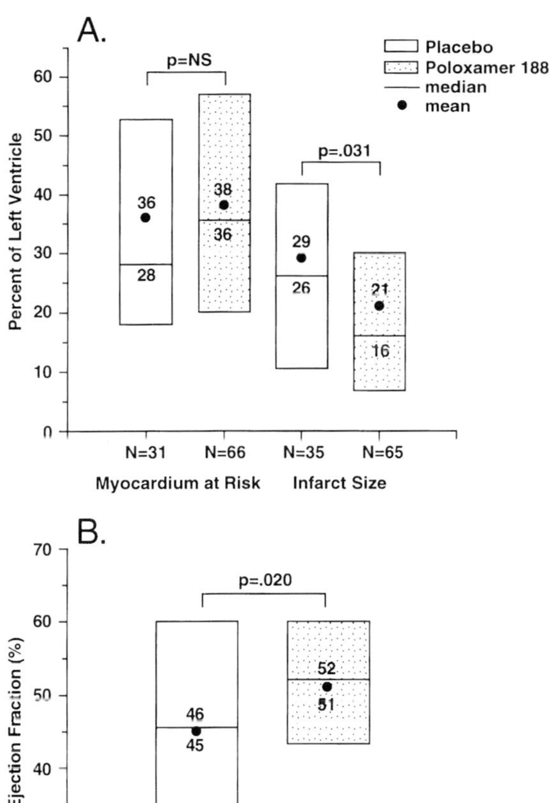

Figure 21–15 **A.** Bar graph demonstrating the myocardium at risk and myocardial infarct size (expressed as a percentage of the left ventricle) in poloxamer 188 and placebo treated patients reperfused with intravenous streptokinase or t-PA. Measurements were obtained by SPECT sestamibi scanning before reperfusion (myocardium at risk) and 5 to 7 days postinfarction (infarct size). The lower and upper borders of the box are the interquartile ranges (25th and 75th percentiles). NS indicates not statistically significant. **B.** Bar graph demonstrating the global left ventricular ejection fraction in poloxamer 188 and placebo treated patients. Measurements were obtained by radionuclide angiography performed 5 to 7 days postinfarction. The lower and upper borders of the box represent the interquartile ranges. *Reprinted by permission from Shaer et al (300).*

proved myocardial salvage utilizing acute and delayed sestamibi tomographic imaging, and this was associated with improvement in global ejection fraction (Fig. 21–15) (300). A large-scale trial is currently being performed in an attempt to confirm these initial observations. Studies are also in progress to evaluate the potential role of intravenous adenosine in conjunction with both t-PA and emergent angioplasty in reducing reperfusion injury.

CONCLUSIONS

Timely reperfusion remains the optimal approach in the treatment of evolving myocardial infarction. This can best be achieved with the early administration of various potent thrombolytic agents. Prolonged ischemia may be inevitable in approximately one-third of patients in whom thrombolysis is unsuccessful and who require either mechanical or surgical revascularization. The administration of agents that delay irreversible cell necrosis (calcium channel blockers, beta blockers) in this subset may result in enhanced myocardial salvage provided reperfusion can be achieved. The introduction of oxygen and cellular elements after reperfusion triggers deleterious events that result in prolonged ventricular dysfunction of viable myocytes (stunning) or reduce the amount of potentially salvageable myocardium (reperfusion injury). Experimental studies suggest that oxygen-derived free radicals play an important role in myocardial stunning, possibly by altering intracellular calcium shifts and or myofilament sensitivity. Although the stunned myocardium responds to inotropic agents, amelioration of stunning may be clinically indicated in patients with severe left ventricular dysfunction or in those with severe multivessel disease, in whom agents that increase myocardial oxygen consumption would be contraindicated. Animal studies suggest that anti–free radical agents and calcium channel antagonists may be useful therapeutic agents in humans.

Experimental studies have demonstrated that microvascular damage plays an important role in the pathogenesis of reperfusion injury. Reperfusion enhances the infiltration of activated neutrophils into the ischemic bed, and neutrophil plugging of capillary lumens in association with explosive endothelial swelling of capillaries results in a progressive decrease in blood flow. Current experimental studies do not conclusively support a role for oxygen-derived free radicals in reperfusion injury. Therapeutic agents that modify the interaction between neutrophils and the endothelium have shown promising results in experimental preparations of reperfusion. Perfluorochemical, adenosine, and various antineutrophil agents result in reduced infarct size in the experimental model. Clinical trials with these agents appear warranted to determine the role of reperfusion injury in limiting myocardial salvage in patients undergoing reperfusion within the first few hours of a thrombotic event.

ACKNOWLEDGMENTS

This work was supported in part by grants from the National Heart, Lung and Blood Institute (2 R01 HL 40892-05A1) and General Medical Institute (2 P50 GM 15431) of the National Institutes of Health. The expert review of this chapter by Dr. Edwin K. Jackson is greatly appreciated.

REFERENCES

1. Reimer KA, Lowe JE, Rasmussen MM, Jennings RB: The wavefront phenomenon of ischemic cell death: 1. Myocardial infarct size vs. duration of coronary occlusion in dogs. *Circulation* 1977;56: 786–794.
2. Reimer KA, Jennings RB: The "wavefront phenomenon" of myocardial ischemic cell death: II, Transmural progression of necrosis within the framework of ischemic bed size (myocardium at risk) and collateral flow. *Lab Invest* 1979;40:633–644.
3. Lowe JE, Reimer KA, Jennings RB: Experimental infarct size as a function of the amount of myocardium at risk. *Am J Pathol* 1978;90:363–380.
4. Schaper W, Binz K, Sass S, Winkler B: Influence of collateral blood flow and of variations in MVO_2 on tissue-ATP content in ischemic and infarcted myocardium. *J Mol Cell Cardiol* 1987;19:19–37.
5. Connelly CM, Vogel WM, Hernandez YM, Apstein CS: Movement of the necrotic wavefront after coronary occlusion in the rabbit. *Am J Physiol* 1982; 243:H682–H690.
6. Gruppo Italiano per lo Studio della Streptochinasi nell' Infarto Miocardico (GISSI): Effectiveness of intravenous thrombolytic treatment in acute myocardial infarction. *Lancet* 1986;1:397–401.
7. ISIS-2 (Second International Study of Infarct Survival) Collaborative Group: Randomized trial of intravenous streptokinase, oral aspirin, both or neither among 17,187 cases of suspected acute myocardial infarction: ISIS-2. *Lancet* 1988;2:350–360.
8. Wilcox RG, Von der Lippe G, Olsson CG, et al: Trial of tissue plasminogen activator for mortality reduction in acute myocardial infarction: Anglo-Scandinavian Study of Early Thrombolysis (ASSET). *Lancet* 1988;2:525–530.
9. AIMS Trial Study Group: Effect of intravenous APSAC on mortality after acute myocardial infarction: Preliminary report of a placebo-controlled clinical trial. *Lancet* 1988;1:545–549.
10. The International Study Group: In hospital mortality and clinical course of 20,891 patient with suspected acute myocardial infarction randomized between anteplase and streptokinase without heparin. *Lancet* 1990;336:71–75.
11. Third International Study of Infarct Survival (ISIS-3): A randomized comparison of streptokinase versus tissue plasminogen activation versus antetreplase and of aspirin plus heparin versus aspirin among 41,299 cases of suspected acute myocardial infarction. *Lancet* 1992;339:753–770.
12. The GUSTO Investigators: An international randomized trial comparing four thrombolysis strategies for acute myocardial infarction. *N Engl J Med* 1993;29:673–682.
13. The ISAM Study Group: A prospective trial of intravenous streptokinase in acute myocardial infarction (ISAM): Mortality, morbidity, and infarct size at 21 days. *N Engl J Med* 1986;314:1465–1471.
14. Serruys PW, Simoons ML, Suryapranata H, et al: Prevention of global and regional left ventricular function after early thrombolysis in acute myocardial infarction. *J Am Coll Cardiol* 1986;7:729–742.
15. Koren G, Weiss AT, Hasin Y, et al: Prevention of myocardial damage in acute myocardial ischemia by early treatment with intravenous streptokinase. *N Engl J Med* 1985;313:1384–1389.
16. Ritchie JL, Cerqueira M, Maynard C, et al: Ventricular function and infarct size: The Western Washington intravenous streptokinase in myocardial infarction trial. *J Am Coll Cardiol* 1988;11:689–697.
17. Simoons ML, Seryys PW, van der Brand M, et al: Early thrombolysis in acute myocardial infarction limitations of infarct size and improved survival. *J Am Coll Cardiol* 1986;7:717–728.
18. Van de Werf F: Discrepancies between the effects of coronary reperfusion on survival and left ventricular function. *Lancet* 1989;1:1367–1368.
19. Califf RM, Topol EJ, Gersh BJ: From myocardial salvage to patient salvage in acute myocardial infarction: The role of reperfusion therapy. *J Am Coll Cardiol* 1989;14:1382–1388.

20. Gibbons, RJ, Christian TF, Hopfenspirger M, Hodge DO, Bailey KR: Myocardium at risk and infarct size after thrombolytic therapy for acute myocardial infarction. Implications for the design of randomized trials of acute intervention. *J Am Coll Cardiol* 1994;24:616–623.
21. Christian TF, Gibbon RJ, Gersh BJ: The effect of infarct location on myocardial salvage assessed by Tc-99m isonitrile. *J Am Coll Cardiol* 1991;17: 1303–1308.
22. Braunwald E, Kloner RA: Myocardial reperfusion: A double edged sword. *J Clin Invest* 1985;76: 1713–1719.
23. Forman MB, Virmani R, Puett DW: Mechanisms and therapy of myocardial reperfusion injury. *Circulation* 1990;81(Suppl IV):IV-69–IV-78.
24. Hochman JS, Choo H: Limitation of myocardial infarction expansion by reperfusion independent of myocardial salvage. *Circulation* 1987;75:299–306.
25. Arnold JMO, Antman EM, Przyklenk K: Differential effects of reperfusion in incidence of ventricular arrthymias and recovery of ventricular function at 4 days following coronary occlusion. *Am Heart J* 1987;113:1055 1065.
26. Hale SL, Kloner RA: Left ventricular topographic alterations in the completely healed rat infarct by early and late reperfusion. *Am Heart J* 1988;116: 1508–1513.
27. Braunwald E, Kloner RA: The stunned myocardium: Prolonged, postischemic ventricular dysfunction. *Circulation* 1982;66:1146–1149.
28. Hearse DJ: Reperfusion of the ischemic myocardium. *J Mol Cell Cardiol* 1977;9:605–616.
29. Arnold JMO, Antman EM, Przyklenk K, et al: Differential effects of reperfusion on incidence of ventricular arrhythmias and recovery of ventricular function at 4 days following coronary occlusion. *Am Heart J* 1987;133:1055–1065.
30. Bolli R: Mechanism of myocardial "stunning." *Circulation* 1990;82:723–738.
31. Forman MB, Puett DW, Virmani R: Endothelial and myocardial injury during ischemia and reperfusion: Pathogenesis and therapeutic implications. *J Am Coll Cardiol* 1989;13:450–459.
32. Balke CW, Kaplinsky E, Michelson EL, et al: Reperfusion ventricular tachyarrhythmias: Correlation with antecedent coronary artery occlusion tachyarrhythmias and duration of myocardial ischemia. *Am Heart J* 1981;101:449–455.
33. Hearse DJ, Tosaki A: Free radicals and reperfusion induced arrhythmias: Protection by spin trap agent PBN in the rat heart. *Circ Res* 1987;60: 375–383.
34. Califf RM, O'Neil W, Stack RS, et al: Failure of simple clinical measurements to predict perfusion status after intravenous thrombolysis. *Ann Intern Med* 1988;108:658–662.
35. Sheridan DJ, Penkoske PA, Sobel BE, et al: Alpha adrenergic contributions to dysrhythmia during myocardial ischemia and reperfusion in cats. *J Clin Invest* 1980;65:161–171.
36. Harris AS: Potassium and experimental coronary occlusion. *Am Heart J* 1966;71:797–802.
37. Bernier M, Hearse DJ, Manning AS: Reperfusion-induced arrhythmias and oxygen-derived free radicals: Studies with "anti-free radical" interventions and a free radical–generating system in the isolated perfused rat heart. *Circ Res* 1986;58:331–340.
38. Opie LH: Reperfusion injury and its pharmacologic modification. *Circulation* 1989;80:1049–1062.
39. Hearse DJ, Bolli R: Reperfusion-induced injury. Manifestations, mechanisms and clinical relevance. *Cardiovasc Res* 1992;26:101–108.
40. Heyndrickx GR, Millard RW, McRitchie RJ, et al: Regional myocardial functional and electrophysiological alterations after brief coronary artery occlusion in conscious dogs. *J Clin Invest* 1975;56: 978–985.
41. Heyndrickx GR, Baig H, Nellens P, et al: Depression of regional blood flow and wall thickening after brief coronary occlusions. *Am J Physiol* 1978;234:H653–H659.
42. Bolli R, Patel BS, Hartley CJ, et al: Nonuniform transmural recovery of contractile function in stunned myocardium. *Am J Physiol* 1989;257: H375–H385.
43. Lavallee M, Cox D, Patrick TA, Vatner SF: Salvage of myocardial function by coronary artery reperfusion 1, 2 and 3 hours after occlusion in conscious dogs. *Circ Res* 1983;53:235–247.
44. Bush LR, Buja LM, Samowitz W, et al: Recovery of left ventricular segmental function after long-term reperfusion following temporary coronary occlusion in conscious dogs. *Circ Res* 1983;53:248–263.
45. Zughaib ME, Tang X-L, Sun J-Z, Bolli R: Myocardial reperfusion injury. Fact or myth? A 1993 appraisal of a seemingly endless controversy. *Ann NY Acad Sci* 1994;723:218–228.
46. Gottlieb RA, Burleson KO, Kloner RA, Babior BM, Engler RL: Reperfusion injury includes apoptosis in rabbit cardiomyocytes. *J Clin Invest* 1994; 94:1621–1628.

47. Forman MB, Bingham S, Kopelman HA, et al: Reduction of infarct size with intracoronary perfluorochemical in a canine preparation of reperfusion. *Circulation* 1985;71:1060–1068.

48. Ambrosio G, Becker LC, Hutchins GM, et al: Reduction in experimental infarct size by recombinant human superoxide dismutase: Insights into the pathophysiology of reperfusion injury. *Circulation* 1986;74:1424–1433.

49. Olafsson B, Forman MB, Puett DW, et al: Reduction of reperfusion injury in the canine preparation by intracoronary adenosine: Importance of the endothelium and the no-reflow phenomenon. *Circulation* 1987;76:1135–1145.

50. Pitarys CJ II, Virmani R, Vildibill HD, Jackson EK, Forman MB: Reduction of myocardial reperfusion injury by intravenous adenosine administered during the early reperfusion period. *Circulation* 1991;83:237–247.

51. Kloner RA, Ganote CE, Jennings RB: The "no-reflow" phenomenon after temporary occlusion in the dog. *J Clin Invest* 1974;54:1496–1508.

52. Armiger LC, Gavin JB: Changes in the microvascular of ischemic and infarcted myocardium. *Lab Invest* 1975;33:51–56.

53. Forman MB, Puett DW, Bingham SE, et al: Preservation of endothelial cell structure and function by intracoronary perfluorochemical in a canine preparation of reperfusion. *Circulation* 1987;76: 469–479.

54. Babbitt DG, Virmani R, Forman MB: Intracoronary adenosine administered after reperfusion limits vascular injury after prolonged ischemia in the canine model. *Circulation* 1989;80: 1388–1399.

55. Reimer KA, Jennings RB: Myocardial ischemia, hypoxia and infarction, in Fozzard HA (ed): *The Heart and Cardiovascular System.* New York, Raven Press, 1986, pp 1133–1201.

56. Neely JR, Morgan HE: Relationship between carbohydrate and lipid metabolism and energy balance of the heart. *Ann Rev Physiol* 1974;36:413–459.

57. Opie LH: Myocardial ischemia—metabolic pathways and implications of increased glycolysis. *Cardiovasc Drugs Ther* 1990;4:777–790.

58. Jennings RB, Reimer KA, Hill ML, Mayer SE: Total ischemia in dog hearts, in vitro: 1. Comparison of high energy phosphate production, utilization, and depletion, and of adenine nucleotide catabolism in total ischemia in vitro vs. severe ischemia in vivo. *Circ Res* 1981;49:892–900.

59. Reimer KA, Jennings, RB, Hill ML: Total ischemia in dog hearts, in vitro. 2. High energy phosphate depletion and associated defects in energy metabolism, cell volume regulation and sarcolemmal integrity. *Circ Res* 1981;49:901–911.

60. Schrader J: Metabolism of adenosine and sites of production in the heart, in Berne RM, Rall TW, Rubio R (eds): *Regulatory Function of Adenosine.* The Hague, Martinus/Nijhoff Publishers, 1983, pp 133–156.

61. Clanachan AS, Heaton TP, Parkinson FE: Drug interactions with nucleoside transport systems, in Gerlach E, Becker BF (eds): *Topics and Perspectives in Adenosine Research.* Berlin, Springer-Verlag, 1987, pp 118–130.

62. McCord JM: Oxygen-derived free radicals in postischemic tissue. *N Engl J Med* 1985;312: 159–163.

63. Pasque MK, Spray TL, Pellom GL, et al: Ribose-enhanced myocardial recovery following ischemia in the isolated working rate heart. *J Thorac Cardiovasc Surg* 1982;83:390–398.

64. DeBoer LWV, Ingwall JS, Kloner RA, Braunwald E: Prolonged derangements of canine myocardial purine metabolism after a brief coronary occlusion not associated with anatomic evidence of necrosis. *Proc Natl Acad Sci USA* 1980;77:5471–5475.

65. Jennings RB, Reimer KA: Factors involved in salvaging ischemic myocardium: Effect of reperfusion of arterial blood. *Circulation* 1983;68(Suppl I): I-25–I36.

66. Jennings RB, Reimer KA: Lethal myocardial ischemic injury. *Am J Pathol* 1981;103:241–255.

67. Powers ER, DiBona DR, Powell WJ Jr: Myocardial cell volume and coronary resistance during diminished coronary perfusion. *Am J Physiol* 1984;247: H467–H477.

68. Higginson LAJ, Beanlands DS, Navi RC, et al: The time course and characterization of myocardial hemorrhage after coronary reperfusion in the anesthetized dog. *Circulation* 1983;67:1024–1031.

69. Nees S, Gerbes AL, Willerhausen-Zonnchen B, Cerlach E: Purine metabolism in cultured coronary endothelial cells, in *Purine Metabolism in Man, III. Adv Exp Med Biol* 1980;122B:25–30.

70. Jennings RB, Reimer KA, Hill ML, Mayer SE: Total ischemia in dog hearts in vitro: Comparison of high energy phosphate production, utilization and depletion and of adenosine nucleotide catabolism in total ischemia in vitro vs severe ischemia in vivo. *Circ Res* 1981;49:892–900.

71. Whalen DA Jr, Hamilton DG, Ganote CE, et al: Effect of a transient period of ischemia on myocardial cells: 1. Effects on cell volume regulation. *Am J Pathol* 1974;74:381–397.

72. Jennings RB, Schaper J, Hill ML, et al: Effects of reperfusion late in the phase of reversible ischemic injury: Changes in cell volume, electrolytes, metabolites and ultrastructure. *Circ Res* 1985;56: 262–278.

73. Shen AC, Jennings RB: Myocardial calcium and magnesium in acute ischemic injury. *Am J Pathol* 1972;67:417–434.

74. Jennings RB, Ganote CE: Structural changes in the myocardium during acute ischemia. *Circ Res* 1974;35(Suppl 3):156–172.

75. Ganote CE: Contraction band necrosis and irreversible myocardial injury. *J Mol Cell Cardiol* 1983; 15:67–73.

76. Higginson LAJ, White F, Heggtveit HA, et al: Determinants of myocardial hemorrhage after coronary reperfusion in the anesthetized dog. *Circulation* 1982;65:62–69.

77. Becker LC, Ambrosio E: Myocardial consequences of reperfusion. *Prog Cardiovasc Dis* 1987;30:23–44.

78. Bresnahan GF, Roberts R, Shell WE, et al: Deleterious effects due to hemorrhage after myocardial reperfusion. *Am J Cardiol* 1974;33:82–86.

79. Kloner RA, Rude RE, Carlson N, et al: Ultrastructural evidence of microvascular damage and myocardial cell injury after coronary artery occlusion: Which comes first? *Circulation* 1980;62:945–952.

80. Kloner RA, Ellis SG, Lange R, et al: Studies of experimental coronary artery reperfusion: Effects on infarct size, myocardial function, biochemistry, ultrastructure and microvascular damage. *Circulation* 1983;68(Suppl I):I-8–I-15.

81. Fishbein MC, Y-Rit J, Lando U, et al: The relationship of vascular injury and myocardial hemorrhage to necrosis after reperfusion. *Circulation* 1980;62: 1274–1279.

82. Kao K-J, Hackel DB, Kong Y: Hemorrhagic myocardial infarction after streptokinase treatment for acute coronary thrombosis. *Arch Pathol Lab Med* 1984;108:121–124.

83. Zimmerman ANE, Daems W, Hulsmann WC, et al: Morphological changes of heart muscle caused by successive perfusion with calcium-free and calcium-containing solutions (calcium paradox). *Cardiovasc Res* 1967;1:201–209.

84. Hearse DJ, Humphrey SM, Bullock CR: The oxygen paradox and the calcium paradox: Two facets of the same problem? *J Mol Cell Cardiol* 1978;10: 641–668.

85. Nayler WG, Panagiotopoulos S, Elz JS, Sturrock WJ: Fundamental mechanisms of action of calcium antagonists in myocardial ischemia. *Am J Cardiol* 1987;59:75B–83B.

86. Marban E: Pathogenetic role of calcium in stunning. *Cardiovasc Drugs Ther* 1991;5:891–894.

87. Del Maestro RF: An approach to free radicals in medicine and biology. *Acta Physiol Scand* 1980; 492(Suppl):153–168.

88. Southorn PAQ, Powis G: Free radicals in medicine: II, Involvement in human disease. *Mayo Clin Proc* 1988;63:390–408.

89. Davies KJ, Doroshow JH: Redox cycling of anthracyclines by cardiac mitochondria: 1, Anthracycline radical formation by NADH dehydrogenase. *J Biol Chem* 1986;261:3060–3067.

90. Cohen MV: Free radicals in ischemic and reperfusion myocardial injury: Is this the time for clinical trials? *Ann Intern Med* 1989;111:918–931.

91. Kloner RA, Przyklenk K, Whittaker P: Deleterious effects of oxygen radicals in ischemia reperfusion: Resolved and unresolved issues. *Circulation* 1989;80: 1115–1127.

92. Thomas CE, Morehouse LA, Aust SD: Ferritin and superoxide-dependent lipid peroxidation. *J Biol Chem* 1985;260:3275–3280.

93. Benedetti A, Comporti N, Esterbauer H: Identification of 4-hydroxynonenal as a cytotoxic product originating from the peroxidation of liver microsomal lipids. *Biochim Biophys Acta* 1980;620:281–296.

94. Tribble DL, Aw TY, Jones DP: The pathophysiological significance of lipid peroxidation in oxidative cell injury. *Hepatology* 1987;7:377–386.

95. Fridovich I: Superoxide radical: An endogenous toxicant. *Annu Rev Pharmacol Toxicol* 1983;23:239–257.

96. Fantone JC, Ward PA: Role of oxygen-derived free radicals and metabolites in leukocyte-dependent inflammatory reactions. *Am J Pathol* 1982;107: 397–418.

97. Ferrari R, Ceconi C, Curello S, et al: Oxygen-mediated myocardial damage during ischaemia and reperfusion: Role of the cellular defenses against oxygen toxicity. *J Mol Cell Cardiol* 1985;17: 937–965.

98. Zweier JL, Flaherty JT, Weisfeldt ML: Direct measurement of free radical generation following reperfusion of ischemic myocardium. *Proc Natl Acad Sci USA* 1987;84:1404–1407.

99. Bolli R, Patel BS, Jeroudi MO, et al: Demonstration of free radical generation in "stunned" myocardium of intact dogs with the use of the spin trap-α-phenyl—N-tert-butyl nitrone. *J Clin Invest* 1988;82:476–485.

100. Engler R: Granulocytes and oxidative injury in myocardial ischemia and reperfusion. *Fed Proc* 1987;46:2395–2396.

101. McCord JM: Oxygen-derived radicals: A link between reperfusion injury and inflammation. *Fed Proc* 1987;46:2402.

102. Mullane KM, Read N, Salmon JA, Moncada S: Role of leukocytes in acute myocardial infarction in anesthetized dogs: Relationship to myocardial salvage by anti-inflammatory drugs. *J Pharmacol Exp Ther* 1984;228:510–522.

103. Harlan JM: Leukocyte–endothelial interactions. *Blood* 1985;65:513–525.

104. Dreyer WJ, Smith CW, Michael LH, et al: Canine neutrophil activations by cardiac lymph obtained during reperfusion of ischemic myocardium. *Circ Res* 1989;65:1751–1762.

105. Dreyer WJ, Michael LH, Nguyen T, et al: Kinetics of C5a release in cardiac lymph of dogs experiencing coronary artery ischemia-reperfusion injury. *Circ Res* 1992;71:1518–1524.

106. Go LO, Murry CE, Richard VJ, et al: Myocardial neutrophil accumulation during reperfusion after reversible or irreversible ischemic injury. *Am J Physiol* 1988;255 (*Heart Circ Physiol* 24): H1188–H1198.

107. Dreyer WJ, Michael LH, Wist S, et al: Neutrophil accumulation in ischemic canine myocardium. Insights into time course, distribution and mechanisms of localization during early reperfusion. *Circulation* 1991;84:400–411.

107a. Sheridan FM, Cole PG, Ramage D: Leukocyte adhesion to the coronary microvasculature during ischemia and reperfusion in an in vivo canine model: *Circulation* 1996;93:1784–1787.

108. Sommers HM, Jennings RB: Experimental acute myocardial infarction—histologic and histochemical studies of early myocardial infarcts induced by temporary or permanent occlusion of a coronary artery. *Lab Invest* 1964;13:1491–1503.

109. Pickard RN, O'Rourke RA, Cronford, et al: Complement localization and mediation of ischemic injury in baboon myocardium. *J Clin Invest* 1980;66:1050–1060.

110. Rossen RD, Swain JL, Michael LH, et al: Selective accumulation of the first component of complement and leukocytes in ischemic canine heart muscle: A possible initiator of an extra myocardial metabolism of ischemic injury. *Circ Res* 1985;57:119–130.

111. Ward PA, Hill JH: C5 chemotactic fragments produced by an enzyme in lysosomal granules of neutrophils. *J Immunol* 1970;104:535–543.

112. Hoffstein ST, Friedman RS, Weissmann G: Degranulation, membrane addition and shape change during chemotactic factor-induced aggregation of human neutrophils. *J Cell Biol* 1982;95: 234–241.

113. Harlan JM, Killen PD, Senecal FM, et al: The role of neutrophil membrane glycoprotein GP-150 in neutrophil adherence to endothelium *in vitro*. *Blood* 1985;66:176–178.

114. Hansen PR: Role of neutrophils in myocardial ischemia and reperfusion. *Circulation* 1995;91: 1872–1885.

115. Homeister JW, Lucchesi BR: Complement activation and inhibition in myocardial ischemia and reperfusion injury. *Ann Rev Pharmacol Toxicol* 1994; 34:17–30.

116. Korchak HM, Vienne K, Rutherford LEW, Weissmann G: Neutrophil stimulation: Receptor, membrane, and metabolic events. *Fed Proc* 1984; 43:2749–2754.

117. Lanni C, Becker EL: Release of phospholipase A_2 activity from rabbit peritoneal neutrophils by F-Met-Leu-Phe. *Am J Pathol* 1983;113:90–94.

118. Marclouf JA, Murphy RC: Transcellular metabolism of neutrophil-derived leukotriene A_4 by human platelets. *J Biol Chem* 1988;263:174–181.

119. Fermark SJ, Cannon PJ: Endothelial cell leukotriene C_4 synthesis results from intercellular transfer of leukotriene A_4 synthesized by polymorphonuclear leukocytes. *J Biol Chem* 1986;261: 16466–16472.

120. Mullane KM, Salmon JA, Kraemer R: Leukocyte-derived metabolites of arachidonic acid in ischemia-induced myocardial injury. *Fed Proc* 1987; 46:2422–2433.

121. Goldstein IM: Neutrophil degranulation, in Synderman R (ed): *Contemporary Topics in Immunobiology: Regulation of Leukocyte Function,* vol. 14. New York, Plenum Press, 1984, pp 189–219.

122. Babior BM: The respiratory burst of phagocytes. *J Clin Invest* 1984;73:599–601.

123. Guarnieri C, Flamigni F, Caldarera CM: Role of oxygen in the cellular damage induced by reoxygenation of hypoxic heart. *J Mol Cell Cardiol* 1980;12:797–808.

124. Smedly LA, Tonnesen MG, Sandhaus RA, et al: Neutrophil-mediated injury to endothelial cells: Enhancement by endotoxin and essential role of neutrophil elastase. *J Clin Invest* 1986;77: 1233–1243.

125. Sacks T, Moldow CF, Craddock PR, et al: Oxygen radicals mediate endothelial damage by complement-stimulated granulocytes. *J Clin Invest* 1978; 61:1161–1167.

126. Carp H, Janoff A: In vitro suppression serum elastase-inhibitory capacity by reactive oxygen species generated by phagocytosing polymorphonuclear leukocytes. *J Clin Invest* 1979;63: 793–797.

127. Simionescu M, Simionescu N: Isolation and characterization of endothelial cells from the heart microvasculature. *Microvasc Res* 1978;16:426–452.

128. Gerlach E, Nees S, Becker BF: The vascular endothelium: A survey of some newly evolving biochemical and physiological features. *Basic Res Cardiol* 1984;80:459–474.

129. Davies MG, Hagen P-O: The vascular endothelium. A new horizon. *Ann Surgery* 1993;218: 593–609.

130. Kaiser L, Sparks HV Jr: Endothelial cells: Not just a cellophane wrapper. *Arch Intern Med* 1987;147: 569–573.

131. Nees S, Gerlach E: Adenine nucleotide and adenosine metabolism in cultured coronary endothelial cells: Formation and release of adenine compounds and possible functional implications, in Berne RM, Rall TW, Rubio R (eds): *Regulatory Function of Adenosine*. The Hague, Boston, London, Martinus Nijhoff Publishers, 1983, pp 347–360.

132. Aiken JW, Gorman RR, Shebuski RJ: Prevention of blockage of partially obstructed coronary arteries with prostacyclin correlates with inhibition of platelet aggregation. *Prostaglandins* 1979;17: 483–494.

133. Brenner BM, Troy JL, Ballermann BJ: Endothelium-dependent vascular responses: Mediators and mechanisms. *J Clin Invest* 1989;84:1373–1378.

133a. Lefer DJ: Myocardial protective actions of nitric oxide donors after myocardial ischemia and reperfusion. *New Horizons* 1995;3:105–112.

133b. Loscalzo J, Welch G: Nitric oxide and its role in the cardiovascular system. *Progress in Cardiovascular diseases.* 1995;38:87–104.

133c. Lefer AM: Attenuation of myocardial ischemia-reperfusion injury with nitric oxide replacement therapy. *Am Thorac Surg* 1995;60:847–851.

134. Tanabe M, Terashita Z, Nishikawa K, Hirata M: Inhibition of coronary circulatory failure and thromboxane A_2 release during coronary occlusion and reperfusion. *J Cardiovasc Pharmacol* 1984; 6:442–448.

135. Rubanyi GM, Botelho LHP: Endothelins. *FASEB J* 1991;5:2713–2720.

136. Berne RM: The role of adenosine in the regulation of coronary blood flow. *Circ Res* 1980;47: 807–813.

137. Palmer RMJ, Ferrige AL, Moncada S: Nitric oxide release accounts for the biological activity of endothelium-derived relaxing factor. *Nature* 1987; 327:524–528.

138. Feigl EO: EDRF—a protective factor? *Nature* 1988;331:490–491.

139. Yanagisawa M, Kurihara H, Kimura S, et al: A novel potent vasoconstrictor peptide produced by vascular endothelial cells. *Nature* 1988;322: 411–415.

140. Yanagisawa M: The endothelin system. A new target for therapeutic intervention. *Circulation* 1994;89:1320–1322.

141. Velasco CE, Turner M, Kondo T, et al: Enhanced local endothelin release following myocardial ischemia and reperfusion contributes to "no-reflow." *Am Heart J* 1994;128:441–451.

142. Velasco CE, Jackson EK, Morrow JA, et al: Intravenous adenosine suppresses cardiac release of endothelin after myocardial ischemia and reperfusion. *Cardiovasc Res* 1993;27:121–128.

143. Tønnessen T, Saleh D, Naess PA, Janagisawa M, Christensen G: Increased in vivo expression and production of endothelin-1 by porcine cardiomyocytes subjected to ischemia. *Circ Res* 1995;76: 767–772.

144. Vitola JV, Forman MB, Holsinger JP, et al: Role of endothelin in the rabbit model of myocardial infarction: effect of receptor antagonists. *J Cardiovasc Pharm* 1996 (in press).

145. Watanabe T, Suzuki N, Shinamoto N, Fujino M, Imada A: Contribution of endogenous endothelin to the extension of myocardial infarct size in rats. *Circ Res* 1991;69:370–377.

146. Watanabe T, Awane Y, Ikeda S, et al: Pharmacology of a non-selective ET_A and ET_B receptor antagonist, TAK-044, and the inhibition of myocardial infarct size in rats. *Br J Pharmacol* 1995; 114:949–954.

147. Grover GJ, Dzworczyk S, Parham CS: The endothelin-1 receptor antagonist BQ-123 reduces

infarct size in a canine model of coronary occlusion and reperfusion. *Cardiovasc Res* 1993;27:1613–1618.

148. Velasco CE, Yanagisawa M, Williamson JL, Triana JF: Cardioprotective action of endothelin-1 during ischemia. *Circulation* 1993;88:I-544.

149. Velasco CE, Yanagisawa M: Endothelins protect the ischemic myocardium. *J Am Coll Cardiol* 1994; 23(Suppl):30A.

149a. Wang Q-D, Li X-S, Lundberg JM, Pernow J: Protective effects of non-peptide endothelin receptor antagonist bosentan on myocardial ischemia and reperfusion injury in the pig. *Cardiovascular Research* 1995;29:805–812.

150. Boxer L, Allen J, Schmidt M, et al: Inhibition of polymorphonuclear leukocyte adherence by prostacyclin. *J Lab Clin Med* 1980;95:672–678.

151. Sparks HV Jr, Bardenheuer H: Regulation of adenosine formation by the heart. *Circ Res* 1986;58:193–201.

152. Cronstein BN, Levin RI, Belanoff J, et al: Adenosine: An endogenous inhibitor of neutrophil-mediated injury to endothelial cells. *J Clin Invest* 1986;78:760–770.

153. Norton ED, Forman MB, Jackson EK, Hoover RL: Adenosine: A physiologic modulator of neutrophil–endothelial interactions (abstract). *Circulation* 1989;80:11–15.

154. Cronstein BN, Kramer SB, Weissmann G, Hirschhorn R: Adenosine: A physiologic modulator of superoxide anion generation by human neutrophils. *J Exp Med* 1983,158:1160–1177.

155. Carlos TM, Harlan JM: Leukocyte endothelial adhesion molecules. *Blood* 1994;34:2068–2101.

156. Camussi G, Aglietta M, Malavasi F, et al: The release of platelet-activating factor from human endothelial cells in culture. *J Immunol* 1983;131: 2397–2403.

157. Gavin JB, Thomson RW, Humphrey SM, Herdson PB: Changes in vascular morphology associated with the no-reflow phenomenon in ischemic myocardium. *Virchow Arch* 1983;399:325–332.

158. Engler RL, Dahigren MD, Morris D, et al: Role of leukocytes in the response to acute myocardial ischemia and reflow in dogs. *Am J Physiol* 1986;251: H314–H323.

159. Ambrosio G, Weisman HF, Mannisi JA, et al: Progressive impairment of regional myocardial perfusion after initial restorative of postischemic blood flow. *Circulation* 1989;80:1846–1865.

160. Lefer AM, Tsao PS, Lefer DJ, Ma X-L: Role of endothelial dysfunction in the pathogenesis of reperfusion injury after myocardial ischemia. *FASEB J* 1991;5:2029–2034.

161. Tsao PS, Aoki H, Lefer DJ, Johnson G III, Lefer AM: Time course of endothelial dysfunction and myocardial injury during myocardial ischemia and reperfusion in the rat. *Circulation* 1990;82: 1402–1412.

162. Richard V, Kaeffer N, Tron C, Thuillez C: Ischemic preconditioning protects against coronary endothelial dysfunction induced by ischemia and reperfusion. *Circulation* 1994;89:1254–1261.

163. Lefer AM, Weyrich AS, Buerke M: Role of selectins, a new family of adhesion molecules, in ischemia-reperfusion injury. *Cardiovasc Res* 1991;28: 289–294.

164. Bevilacqua MP, Nelson RM, Munnori G, Cecconi O: Endothelial–leukocyte adhesion molecules in human disease. *Ann Rev Med* 1994;45:361–378.

165. Kishmoto T, Rothlein R: Integrins, ICAMS, and selections: Role and regulation of adhesion molecules in neutrophil recruitment to inflammatory sites. *Adv Pharmacol* 1994;25:117–168.

165a. Weyrich AS, Buerke M, Albertine KH, Lefer AM: Time course of coronary vascular endothelial adhesion molecule expression during reperfusion of the ischemic feline myocardium. *J Leukoc Biol* 1995;57:45–55.

166. Weyrich AS, Ma X-I, Lefer DJ, Albertine KH, Lefer AM: In vivo neutralization of P-selectins protects feline heart and endothelium in myocardial ischemia and reperfusion injury. *J Clin Invest* 1993;91:2620–2629.

167. Ma X-L, Weyrich AS, Lefer DJ, et al: Monoclonal antibody to L-selectin attenuates neutrophil accumulation and protects ischemia reperfused cat myocardium. *Circulation* 1993;88:649–658.

168. Ma-X-L, Tsao PS, Lefer AM: Antibody to CD-18 exerts endothelial and cardiac protective effects in myocardial ischemia and reperfusion. *J Clin Invest* 1991;88:1237–1243.

169. Simpson PJ, Todd RF, Mickelson JK, et al: Sustained limitation of myocardial reperfusion injury by a monoclonal antibody that alters leukocyte function. *Circulation* 1990;81:226–237.

170. Youker KA, Hawkins HK, Kukiela GL, et al: Molecular evidence for induction of intracellular adhesion molecule-1 in the viable border zone associated with ischemia–reperfusion injury of the dog heart. *Circulation* 1994;89:2736–2746.

171. Kukielka GL, Youker KA, Hawkins HK, et al: Regulations of ICAM-1 and IL-6 in myocardial

ischemia: Effect of reperfusion. *Ann NY Acad Sci* 1994;723:258–270.

172. Ma X-L, Lefer DJ, Lefer AM, Rothlein R: Coronary endothelial and cardiac protective effects of a monoclonal antibody to intracellular adhesion molecule-1 in myocardial ischemia and reperfusion. *Circulation* 1992;86:937–946.

173. Kilgore KS, Friedrichs GS, Homeister JW, Lucchesi BR: The complement system in myocardial ischemia/reperfusion injury. *Cardiovasc Res* 1994;28: 437–444.

174. Maroko PR, Carpenter CB, Chiariello M, et al: Reduction by cobra venom factor of myocardial necrosis after coronary infusion. *J Clin Invest* 1978; 61:661–670.

175. Weisman HF, Bartow T and MK Leppo, et al: Soluble human complement receptor type I: In vivo inhibitor of complement suppressing postischemic myocardial inflammation and necrosis. *Science* 1990;249:146–151.

175a. Buerke M, Murohora T, Lefer AM: Cardioprotective effects of a C1 esterase inhibitor in myocardial ischemia and reperfusion. *Circulation* 1995;91: 393–402.

176. Reimer KA, Hill ML, Jennings RB: Prolonged depletion of ATP and of the adenine nucleotides following reversible myocardial ischemic injury in dogs. *J Mol Cell Cardiol* 1981; 13:229–239.

177. Swain JH, Hines JJ, Sabina RL, Holmes FW: Accelerated repletion of ATP and GTP pools in postischemic myocardium using a precursor of purine de novo synthesis. *Circ Res* 1982;5: 102–105.

178. Forman MB, Velasco CE: Role of adenosine in the treatment of myocardial stunning. *Cardiovasc Drug Ther* 1991;5:901–908.

179. Bolli R, Zhu W-X, Myers ML, et al: Beta-adrenergic stimulation reverses postischemic myocardial dysfunction without producing subsequent functional deterioration. *Am J Cardiol* 1985;56: 964–968.

180. Dauber IM, VanBenthuysen KM, McMurtry IF, et al: Functional coronary microvascular injury evident as increased permeability due to brief ischemia and reperfusion. *Circ Res* 1990;66: 986–998.

181. Bolli R, Triana JF, Jeroudi MO: Prolonged impairment of coronary vasodilation after reversible ischemia: Evidence for microvascular "stunning." *Circ Res* 1990;67:332–343.

182. Stahl LD, Aversano TR, Becker LC: Selective enhancement of function of stunned myocardium by increased flow. *Circulation* 1986;74:843–851.

183. Steenbergen C, Murphy E, Levy L, London RE: Elevation in cytosolic free calcium concentration early in myocardial ischemia in perfused rat heart. *Circ Res* 1987;60:700–707.

184. Marban E, Kitakze M, Kusuoka H, Porterfield JK, Yuo DT, Chacko VP: Intracellular free calcium concentration measured with ^{19}F NMR spectroscopy in intact ferret hearts. *Proc Natl Acad Sci USA* 1987;86.6005–6009.

185. Nayler WG: Basic mechanisms involved in the protection of the ischemic myocardium. *Drugs* 1991;42:21–27.

186. Krause SM, Jacobus WE, Becker LC: Alternations in cardiac sarcoplasmic reticulum calcium transport in the postischemic "stunned" myocardium. *Circ Res* 1989;65:526–530.

187. Kusuoka H, Porterfield JK, Weisman HF, Weisfeldt ML, Marban E: Pathophysiology and pathogenesis of stunned myocardium: Depress Ca_2^+ activation of contraction as a consequence of reperfusion-induced cellular calcium overload in ferret hearts. J Clin Invest 1987;79:950–961.

188. Przyklenk K, Ghafari GB, Eitzman DT, Kloner RA: Nifedipine administered after reperfusion ablates systolic contractile dysfunction of postischemic "stunned" myocardium. *J Am Coll Cardiol* 1989;13:1176–1183.

189. Bolli R, Jeroudi MO, Patel BS, et al: Marked reduction of free radical generation and contractile dysfunction by antioxidant therapy begun at the time of reperfusion: Evidence that myocardial "stunning" is a manifestation of reperfusion injury. *Circ Res* 1989;65:607–622.

190. Burton KP: Superoxide dismutase enhances recovery following myocardial ischemia. *Am J Physiol* 1985;248:H637–H643.

191. Przyklenk K, Whittaker P, Kloner RA: Direct evidence that oxygen free radicals cause contractile dysfunction in vivo (abstract). *Circulation* 1988; 78(Suppl II):II-264.

192. Zweier JL, Flaherty JT, Weisfeldt ML: Direct measurement of free radical generation following reperfusion of ischemic myocardium. *Proc Natl Acad Sci USA* 1987;84:1404–1407.

193. Eddy LJ, Stewart JR, Jones HP, et al: Free radical producing enzyme xanthine oxidase is undetectable in human hearts. *Am J Physiol* 1987;253: 11709–11711.

194. Bolli R: Role of neutrophils in myocardial stunning after brief ischemia: The end of a six year old controversy (1987–1993). *Cardiovasc Res* 1993; 27:728–730.

194a. Bolli R, Zughaib M, Li X-Y, et al: Recurrent ischemia in the canine heart causes recurrent bursts of free radical production that have a cumulative effect on contractile function. A pathophysiological basis for chronic myocardial "stunning." *J Clin Invest* 1995;96:1066–1084.

195. Forman MB, Velasco CE, Jackson EK: Adenosine attenuates reperfusion injury following regional myocardial ischemia. *Cardiovasc Res* 1993;27:9–17.

196. Forman MB, Pitarys CJ, Vildibill HD, et al: Pharmacologic perturbation of neutrophils by Fluosol-DA results in a sustained reduction in infarct size in the canine model of reperfusion. *J Am Coll Cardiol* 1992;19:205–216.

197. Ku DD: Coronary vascular reactivity after acute myocardial ischemia. *Science* 1982;218:576–578.

198. Bajaj AK, Cobb MA, Virmani R, et al: Limitation of myocardial reperfusion injury by intravenous perfluorochemicals: Role of neutrophil activation. *Circulation* 1989;79:645–656.

199. Romson JL, Hook BG, Kunkel SL, et al: Reduction of the extent of ischemic myocardial injury by neutrophil depletion in the dog. *Circulation* 1983;67:1016–1023.

200. Myers ML, Bolli R, Lekich RF, et al: Enhancement of recovery of myocardial function by oxygen–free radical scavengers after reversible regional ischemia. *Circulation* 1985;72:915–921.

201. Asinger RW, Petersen DA, Elsperger KJ, et al: Longterm recovery of LV wall thickening after one hour of ischemia is not affected when superoxide dismutase and catalase are administered during the first 45 minutes of reperfusion (abstract). *J Am Coll Cardiol* 1988;11:163A.

202. Bolli R, Zhu W-X, Hartley CJ, et al: Attenuation of dysfunction in the postischemic "stunned" myocardium by dimethylthiourca. *Circulation* 1987; 76:458–468.

203. Bolli R, Patel BS, Zhu W-X, et al: The iron chelator desferrioxamine attenuates postischemic ventricular dysfunction. *Am J Physiol* 1987;253: H1372–H1380.

204. Charlat ML, O'Neill PG, Egan JM, et al: Evidence for a pathogenic role of xanthine oxidase in the "stunned" myocardium. *Am J Physiol* 1987; 252:H566–H577.

205. Farber NE, Vercellotti GM, Jacob HS, et al: Evidence for a role of iron-catalyzed oxidants in functional and metabolic stunning in the canine heart. *Circ Res* 1988;63:351–360.

206. Forman MB, Puett DW, Cates CU, et al: Glutathione redox pathway and reperfusion injury: Effect of N-acetylcysteine on infarct size and ventricular function. *Circulation* 1988;78:202–213.

207. Gross GJ, Farber NE, Hardman HF, et al: Beneficial actions of superoxide dismutase and catalase in stunned myocardium of dogs. *Am J Physiol* 1986;250:H372–H377.

208. Myers ML, Bolli R, Lekich RF, et al: N-2-mercaptopropionyl glycine improves recovery of myocardial function after reversible regional ischemia. *J Am Coll Cardiol* 1986;8:1161–1168.

209. Stewart JR, Crute SL, Loughlin V, et al: Prevention of free radical–induced myocardial reperfusion injury with allopurinol. *J Thorac Cardiovasc Surg* 1985;90:68–72.

210. Nejima J, Knight DR, Fallon JT, et al: Superoxide dismutase reduces reperfusion arrhythmias but fails to salvage regional function or myocardium at risk in conscious dogs. *Circulation* 1989;79:143.

211. Przyklenk K, Kloner RA: "Reperfusion injury" by oxygen-derived free radicals: Effect of superoxide dismutase plus catalase, given at the time of reperfusion, on myocardial infarct size, contractile function, coronary microvasculature, and regional myocardial blood flow. *Circ Res* 1989;64:86–96.

212. Przyklenk K, Kloner RA: Superoxide dismutase plus catalase improve contractile function in the canine model of the "stunned myocardium." *Circ Res* 1986;58:148–156.

213. Vanhaecke J, Van de Werf F, Jank I-K, et al: Despite superoxide dismutase treatment, postischemic contractile dysfunction persists after 4 hrs of reperfusion (abstract). *J Am Coll Cardiol* 1988;11:164A.

214. Przyklenk K, Kloner RA: Effect of verapamil on post-ischemic "stunned" myocardium: Importance of the timing of treatment. *J Am Coll Cardiol* 1988;11:616–623.

215. Taylor AL, Colino P, Buja LM, Eckels RM: Is postischemic systolic dysfunction primarily caused by reperfusion? *Circulation* 1987;76(Suppl IV):IV-228.

215a. Sekili (548).

216. DeWitt DF, Jochim KE, Behrendt DM: Nucleotide degradation and functional impairment

during cardioplegia: Amelioration by inosine. *Circulation* 1983;67:171–178.

217. Henrichs KJ, Matsuoka H, Schaper W: Enhanced post-ischemic ATP repletion by pharmacological inhibition of nucleoside washout and catabolism. *J Cardiovasc Pharm* 1988;11:694–700.

218. Reibel DK, Rovetto MJ: Myocardial adenosine salvage rates and restoration of ATP content following ischemia. *Am J Physiol* 1979;237: H247–H252.

219. Bolling SF, Bies LD, Bove HL, Gallagher KP: Augmenting intracellular adenosine improves myocardial recovery. *J Thorac Cardiovasc Surg* 1990;99: 469–474.

220. Zimmer HG: Normalization of depressed heart function in rats by ribose. *Science* 1983;23:81–82.

221. Mauser M, Hoffmeister JM, Nienaber C, Schaper W: Influence of ribose, adenosine, and "AICAR" on the rate of myocardial adenosine triphosphate synthesis during reperfusion after coronary artery after occlusion in the dog. *Circ Res* 1985;56: 220–280.

222. Foker JE, Einzig S, Wang T: Adenosine metabolism and myocardial preservation: Consequences of adenosine catabolism on myocardial high-energy compounds and tissue blood flow. *J Thorac Cardiovasc Surg* 1980;50:506–516.

223. Abd-Elfattah AS, Jessen ME, Lekven J, Doherty NE III, Brunsting LA, Wechsler AS: Myocardial reperfusion injury: Role of myocardial hypoxanthine and xanthine in free radical–mediated reperfusion injury. *Circulation* 1988;78:(Suppl III): III-224–III-235.

224. Arnold JMO, Braunwald E, Sandor T, Kloner RA: Inotropic stimulations of reperfusion myocardium: Effects on infarct size and myocardial function. *J Am Coll Cardiol* 1985;6:1026–1034.

225. Becker LC, Levine JH, DiPaula AF, Guarnieri T, Aversano T: Reversal of dysfunction in postischemic stunned myocardium by epinephrine and postextrasystolic potentiation. *J Am Coll Cardiol* 1986;7:580–589.

226. Ledingham S, Katayama O, Lachno D, Patel N, Yacoub M: Beneficial effect of adenosine during reperfusion following prolonged cardioplegic arrest. *Cardiovas Res* 1990;24:247–253.

227. Kitakaze M, Huri M, Kamada T: Role of adenosine and its interaction with 2 adrenoceptor activity in ischemic and reperfusion injury of the myocardium. *Cardiovasc Res* 1993;27:18–27.

228. Schrader J: Metabolism of adenosine and sites of production in the heart, in Berne RM, Rall TW, Rubio R (eds): *Regulating Function of Adenosine.* The Hague, Martins/Nijhoff Publishers, 1983, pp 133–156.

229. Dnziel HH, Westfall DP: Receptors for adenosine nucleotides and nucleotides: Subclassification, distribution and molecular characterization. *Pharmacol Rev* 1994;46:450–466.

230. Tucker AL, Linden J: Cloned receptors and cardiovascular responses to adenosine. *Cardiovasc Res* 1993;27:62–67.

231. Ramkumar V, Pierson G, Stiles GL: Adenosine receptors: Clinical implications and biochemical mechanisms. *Prog Drug Res* 1988;32:196–245.

232. Sajjadi FG, Firestein CS: cDNA cloning and sequence analysis of the human A3 adenosine receptor. *Biochem Biophys Acta* 1993;1179:105–107.

233. Schrier DJ, Imre KM: The effects of adenosine agonists of human neutrophil function. *J Immunol* 1986;137:3284–3289.

234. Richardt G, Waas W, Kranzhomig R, Mayer E, Schomig A: Adenosine inhibits exocytotic release of endogenous noradrenalin in rat heart: A protective mechanism in early myocardial ischemia. *Circ Res* 1987;61:117–123.

235. Cronstein BN, Daguma L, Nichols D, Hutchinson AJ, Williams M: The adenosine/neutrophil paradox resolved: Human neutrophils possess both A_1 and A_2 receptors that promote chemotaxis and inhibit O_2 generation, respectively. *J Clin Invest* 1990;85:1150–1157.

236. Fredholm BB: Methods used to study the involvement of adenosine in the regulation of lipolysis, in Paton DM (ed): *Methods in Pharmacology.* New York, Plenum Press, 1985, pp 337–357.

237. Schubert P: Synaptic and non-synaptic modulation by adenosine: A differential action of K- and Ca-fluxes, in Stafanovich V, Rudolphi K, Schubert P (eds): *Adenosine: Receptor and Modulation of Cell Function.* Oxford, IRL Press, 1985, pp 117–129.

238. Liu GS, Thorton J, Van Winkle DM, Stanley AWH, Olsson RA, Downey JM: Protection against infarction afforded by preconditioning is mediated by A_1 adenosine receptors in the rabbit heart. *Circulation* 1991;84:350–356.

239. Gross GJ, Auchampach JA: Blockade of ATP-sensitive potassium channels prevents myocardial preconditioning in dogs. *Circ Res* 1992;70: 223–233.

240. Pasque MK, Spray TL, Pellom GL, et al: Ribose-enhanced myocardial recovery following ischemia in the isolated working rat heart. *J Thorac Cardiovasc Surg* 1982;83:390–398.

241. Clanachan AS, Heaton TP, Parkinson FE: Drug interactions with nucleoside transport systems, in Gerlach E, Becker BF (eds): *Topics and Perspectives in Adenosine Research.* Berlin, Springer-Verlag, 1984, pp 118–130.

242. Wyatt DA, Edmunds MC, Rubio R, Berne RM, Lasley RD, Mentzer RM: Adenosine stimulates glycolytic flux in isolated perfused rate hearts by A_1-adenosine receptors. *Am J Physiol* 1989;257: H1952–H1957.

243. Mainwaring R, Lasley R, Rubio R, Wyatt DA, Mentzer RM: Adenosine stimulates glucose uptake in the isolated rat heart. *Surgery* 1988;103: 445–449.

244. Carlsson L, Abrahamsson T, Almgren O: Local release of noradrenaline during acute ischemia. An experimental study in the isolated perfused rat heart. *J Cardiovasc Pharmacol* 1985;7:791–798.

245. Pelleg A, Belardinelli L: Cardiac electrophysiology and pharmacology of adenosine: Basic and clinical aspects. *Cardiovasc Res* 1993;27:54–61.

246. Murry CE, Jennings RB, Reimer KA: Preconditioning with ischemia: A delay of lethal cell injury in ischemic myocardium. *Circulation* 1986;74: 1124–1136.

247. Van Winkle DM, Chien GL, Wolff RA, Soifer BE, Davis RF: Intracoronary infusion of R-phenylisopropyl adenosine prior to ischemia/ reperfusion reduces myocardial infarct size in swine (abstract). *Circulation* 1992;86(Suppl I):I-213.

248. Auchampach JA, Gross GJ: Adenosine A_1 receptors, K_{ATP} channels and ischemic preconditioning in dogs. *Am J Physiol* 1993;284:H1327–H1336.

249. Thorton JD, Liu GS, Olsson RA, Downey JM: Intravenous pretreatment with A_1-selective adenosine analogues protects the heart agonist infarction. *Circulation* 1992;85:659–665.

250. Liu GS, Richards SC, Olson RA, Mullune K, Walsh RS, Downey JM: Evidence that the adenosine A_3 receptor may mediate the protection afforded by preconditioning in the isolated rabbit heart. *Cardiovasc Res* 1994;28:1057–1061.

251. Downey JM, Cohen, MV, Ytrehus K, Liu Y: Cellular mechanisms in ischemic preconditioning. The role of adenosine and protein kinase C. *Ann NY Acad Sci* 1994;723:82–98.

252. Downey JM: An explanation for the reported observation that ATP dependant potassium channel openers mimic preconditioning. *Cardiovasc Res* 1993;27:1565.

253. Homeister JW, Hoff PT, Fletcher DD, Fantone JC, Lucchesi BR: Combined adenosine and lidocaine administration limits myocardial reperfusion injury. *Circulation* 1990;82:595–608.

254. Velasco CE, Turner M, Cobb MA, Virmani R, Forman MB: Myocardial reperfusion injury in the canine model after 40 minutes of ischemia: Effect of intracoronary adenosine. *Am Heart J* 1991;122: 1561–1570.

255. Babbitt DG, Virmani R, Vildibill HD, Norton ED, Forman MB: Intracoronary adenosine administration during reperfusion following 3 hours of ischemia: Effects on infarct size, ventricular function, and regional myocardial blood flow. *Am Heart J* 1990;120:808–818.

256. Norton ED, Jackson EK, Virmani R, Forman MB: Effect of intravenous adenosine on myocardial reperfusion injury in a model with low myocardial blood flow. *Am Heart J* 1991;122: 1283–1291.

257. Goto M, Miura T, Iliodoromitis EK, et al: Adenosine infusion during early reperfusion failed to limit myocardial infarct size in a collateral deficient species. *Cardiovasc Res* 1991;25:943–949.

258. Norton ED, Jackson EK, Turner MB, Virmani R, Forman MB: The effects of intravenous infusions of selective A_1-receptor and A_2-receptor agonists on myocardial reperfusion injury. *Am Heart J* 1992;123:332–338.

259. Forman MB, Ingram DA, Murray JJ: Role of perfluorocarbon emulsions in the treatment of myocardial reperfusion injury. *Am Heart J* 1992;124: 1347–1357.

260. Forman MB, Puett DW, Wilson BH, et al: Beneficial long-term effect of intracoronary perfluorochemical on infarct size and ventricular function in a canine reperfusion model. *J Am Coll Cardiol* 1987;9:1082–1090.

261. Schaer GL, Karas SP, Santoian EC, et al: Reduction in reperfusion injury by blood-free reperfusion after experimental myocardial infarction. *J Am Coll Cardiol* 1990;15:1385–1393.

262. Virmani R, Kolodgie FD, Osmilowski A, Forman MB: Effect of perfluorochemical Fluosol®-DA on myocardial infarct healing in the rabbit. *Am J Cardiovasc Pathol* 1990;3:69–80.

263. Babbitt DG, Forman MB, Jones RL, et al: Prevention of neutrophil-mediated injury to endothelial cells by perfluorochemical. *Am J Pathol* 1990;136: 1445–1459.

264. Vitola JV, Ingram DA, Holsinger JP, et al: Fluosol reduces myocardial reperfusion injury by prolonged suppression of neutrophils by its detergent component (RheothRx) and not by enhancing O_2 delivery. *J Am Coll Cardiol* 1994;25:103A.

265. Ingram DA, Forman MB, Murray JJ: Phagocytic activation of human neutrophils by the detergent component of Fluosol®. *Am J Pathol* 1992;140: 1081–1087.

266. Schaer GL, Hursey TL, Abrahams SL, et al: Reduction in reperfusion induced necrosis in dogs by RheothRx injection (poloxamer 188 N.F.) a hemorheological agent that alters neutrophil function. *Circulation* 1994;90:2964–2975.

267. Ingram DA, Forman MB, Murray JJ: Activation of Complement by Fluosol® attributable to the pluronic micelle structure. *J Cardiovasc Pharmacol* 1993;22:456–461.

268. Gallagher KP, Buda AJ, Pace D, et al: Failure of superoxide dismutase and catalase to alter size of infarction in conscious dogs after 3 hours of occlusion followed by reperfusion. *Circulation* 1986; 73:1065–1076.

269. Jolly SR, Kane WJ, Bailie MB, et al: Canine myocardial reperfusion injury: Its reduction by the combined administration of superoxide dismutase and catalase. *Circ Res* 1984;54:277–285.

270. Patel B, Jeroudi MO, O'Neill PG, et al: Human superoxide dismutase fails to limit infarct size after 2h ischemia and reperfusion (abstract). *Circulation* 1988;78(Suppl II):11–373.

271. Richard VJ, Murry CE, Jenninqs RB, Reimer KA: Therapy to reduce free radicals during early reperfusion does not limit the size of myocardial infarcts caused by 90 minutes of ischemia in dogs. *Circulation* 1988;78:473–480.

272. Uraizee A, Reimer KA, Murry CE, et al: Failure of superoxide dismutase to limit size of myocardial infarction after 40 minutes of ischemia and 4 days of reperfusion in dogs. *Circulation* 1987;75:1237–1248.

273. Werns SW, Shea MJ, Driscoll EM, et al: The independent effects of oxygen radical scavengers on canine infarct size: Reduction by superoxide dismutase but not catalase. *Circ Res* 1985;56:895–898.

274. Tamura Y, Chi L, Driscoll EM, et al: Superoxide dismutase conjugated to polyethylene glycol provides sustained protection against myocardial ischemia reperfusion injury in canine heart. *Circ Res* 1988;63:946–959.

275. Tanaka M, FitzHarris GP, Stoler RC, et al: PEG-SOD plus catalase does not limit infarct size after 90 minutes of ischemia and four days of reperfusion in dogs. *Circulation* 1989;89:II–296.

276. Chambers DE, Parks DA, Patterson G, et al: Xanthine oxidase as a source of free radical damage in myocardial ischemia. *J Mol Cell Cardiol* 1985;17: 145–152.

277. Werns SW, Shea MJ, Mitsos SE, et al: Reduction of the size of infarction by allopurinol in the ischemic-reperfused canine heart. *Circulation* 1986; 73:518–524.

278. Reimer KA, Jennings RB: The failure of the xanthine oxidase inhibitor allopurinol to limit infarct size after ischemia and reperfusion in dogs. *Circulation* 1985;71:1069–1075.

279. Puett DW, Forman MB, Cates CU, et al: Oxypurinol limits myocardial stunning but does not reduce infarct size after reperfusion. *Circulation* 1987;76:678–686.

280. Kinsman JM, Murry CE, Richard VJ, et al: The xanthine oxidase inhibitor oxypurinol does not limit infarct size in a canine model of 40 minutes of ischemia with reperfusion. *J Am Coll Cardiol* 1988;12:209–217.

281. Miura T, Downey JM, Hotta D, Imura O: Effect of superoxide dismutase plus catalase on myocardial infarct size in rabbits. *Can J Cardiol* 1988;4:407–411.

282. Mitsos SE, Askew TE, Fantone JC, et al: Protective effects of N-2-mercaptopropionyl glycine against myocardial reperfusion injury after neutrophil depletion in the dog: Evidence for the role of intracellular-derived free radicals. *Circulation* 1986;73:1077–1086.

283. Reddy BR, Wynne J, Kloner RA, Przyklenk K: Desferrioxamine fails to provide sustained protection against ischemia reperfusion injury. *Circulation* 1989;89:II–239.

284. Horowitz LD, Fennessey PV, Shikes RH, Kong Y: Marked reduction in myocardial infarct size due to prolonged infusion of an antioxidant during reperfusion. *Circulation* 1994;89:1792–1801.

285. Näslund U, Häggmark S, Johansson G, Marklund SL, Reiz S: Limitation of myocardial infarct size by superoxide dismutase as an adjunct to reperfusion after different durations of occlusion in the pig. *Circulation* 1990;66:1294–1301.

286. Kloner RA, Braunwald E: Effects of calcium antagonists on the infarcting myocardium. *Am J Cardiol* 1987;59:84B–94B.

287. Metha JL, Nichols WW, Donnelly WH, et al: Impaired canine coronary vasodilator response to acetylcholine and bradykinin after occlusion-reperfusion. *Circ Res* 1989;64:43–54.

288. Nayler WG, Panagiotopoulos S, Elz JS, Daly MJ: Calcium-medicated damage during post-ischemic reperfusion. *J Mol Cell Cardiol* 1988;20(Suppl 11): 41–54.

289. Mullane KM, Salmon JA, Kraemer R: Leukocyte-derived metabolites of arachidonic acid in ischemia-induced myocardial injury. *Fed Proc* 1986; 45:2422–2433.

290. Tanaka M, Books SE, Richard VJ, et al: Effect of anti-CD18 antibody on myocardial neutrophil accumulation and infarct size after ischemia and reperfusion in dogs. *Circulation* 1993; 87:526–535.

291. Buerke M, Weyrich AS, Zheng Z, Gaeta FC, Forrest MJ, Lefer AM: Sialyl Lewis^{x}-containing oligosaccharide attenuates myocardial reperfusion injury in cats. *J Clin Invest* 1994;93:1140–1148.

291a. Murohara T, Buerke M, Margiotta J, et al: Myocardial and endothelial protection by TMS in ischemia-reperfusion injury. *Am J Physiol* (*Heart Circ Physiol* 38) 1995;269:H504–H514.

291b. Sekili S, Jeroudi MO, Tang X-L, Zughaib M, San J-Z, Bolli R: Effect of adenosine on myocardial "stunning" in the dog. *Circ Res* 1995;76:82–94.

292. Decoster RM, Wijns W, Cauwe F, Robert A, Bechers C, Melin JA: Area at risk determination by technetium-99m-hexakis-2-methoxyisobutyl isonitrile in experimental reperfusion myocardial infarction. *Circulation* 1990;82:2152–2162.

293. Galli M, Marcassa C, Bolli R, et al: Spontaneous delayed recovery of perfusion and contraction after the first 5 weeks after anterior infarction. Evidence for the presence of hibernating myocardium in the infarcted area. *Circulation* 1994;90: 1386–1397.

294. Nabel EG, Topol EJ, Galeana A, et al: A randomized, double-blind, controlled, pilot trial of combined early intravenous captopril and tPA therapy in acute myocardial infarction (abstract). *Circulation* 1989;80:II-112.

295. Topol EJ, Ellis SG, Califf RM, et al: Combined tissue-type plasminogen activator and prostacyclin therapy for acute myocardial infarction. *J Am Coll Cardiol* 1989;14:877–884.

296. Flaherty JT, Pitt B, Gruber JW, et al: Recombinant human superoxide dismutase (h-SOD) fails to improve recovery of ventricular function in patients undergoing coronary angioplasty for acute myocardial infarction. *Circulation* 1994;89:1987–1991.

297. Kingma JH, van Gilst WH, Peels CH, Dambrink J-HE, Verheugt FWA, Wielenga RP: Acute intervention with captopril during thrombolysis in patients with first anterior myocardial infarction. Results from the captopril and thrombolysis study (CATS) *Eur Heart J* 1994;15:898–907.

298. Forman MB, Perry JM, Wilson BH, et al: Demonstration of myocardial reperfusion injury in humans: Results of a pilot study utilizing acute angioplasty with perfluorochemical in anterior myocardial infarction. *J Am Coll Cardiol* 1991;18: 911–918.

299. Wall TC, Califf RM, Blankenship J, et al: Intravenous Fluosol in the treatment of acute myocardial infarction. Results of the thrombolysis and angioplasty in myocardial infarction 9 trial. *Circulation* 1994;90:114–120.

300. Shaer GL, Spaccavento LJ, Browne KF et al: Beneficial effects of RheothRx® injection in patients receiving thrombolytic therapy for acute myocardial infarction. Results of a randomized double-blind placebo-controlled trial *Circulation* 1996;94: 298–307.

22

The Role of Percutaneous Transluminal Coronary Angioplasty in Acute Myocardial Infarction

David R. Holmes, Jr, MD, and Bernard J. Gersh, MB, ChB, DPhil, FRCP

The role of percutaneous transluminal coronary angioplasty (PTCA) in the management of patients with acute myocardial infarction continues to evolve and grow as scientific data on performance and outcome expands (Fig. 22–1) (1–28). Acute PTCA as sole therapy is clearly feasible, achieves a high initial patency rate, and is particularly promising when the infarction is associated with hemodynamic instability (Fig. 22–2) (29–32). PTCA can also be used *after* lytic therapy to treat persistent occlusions or a severe residual stenosis. The latter use may contribute to reocclusion, which occurs in approximately 15% of patients. Nonetheless, there are potentially deleterious consequences of PTCA in the setting of acute infarction that are related to the complex vascular "milieu" comprising plaque fissuring, platelet aggregation, and intravascular thrombus (33–36) (see Chs. 4 and 20). Prior thrombolytic therapy produces another complicating factor for PTCA because of the potential for extension of procedure-related intramural dissections or hematomas (Fig. 22–3).

The issues surrounding PTCA during acute myocardial infarction are extremely complex, in regard to both its specific role and its timing (11,19,21,23,37–40). The ultimate contribution of the technique remains to be established. Ongoing trials in different patient subsets will continue to provide important information; the availability and access to facilities, reimbursement strategies, and costs will be additional determinants (41–43). Results of trials of PTCA in combination with new adjunctive drugs such as adenosine to enhance myocardial salvage will also provide important new information.

The goal of reperfusion for acute myocardial infarction is to maximize reperfusion rates, enhance myocardial salvage, reduce recurrent ischemia, and minimize complications associated with many of the currently available therapeutic strategies. For each of these goals, PTCA has the potential to play an important role.

PRIMARY DILATION

Primary dilation without the concomitant use of thrombolytic therapy has been widely used for the treatment of acute myocardial infarction. Early information on outcome came from individual clinical series without the benefit of controlled trials (Table 22–1) (10–16,25,44). O'Neill et al (10) reported on the first trial of primary dilation for the treatment of acute myocardial infarction. In this

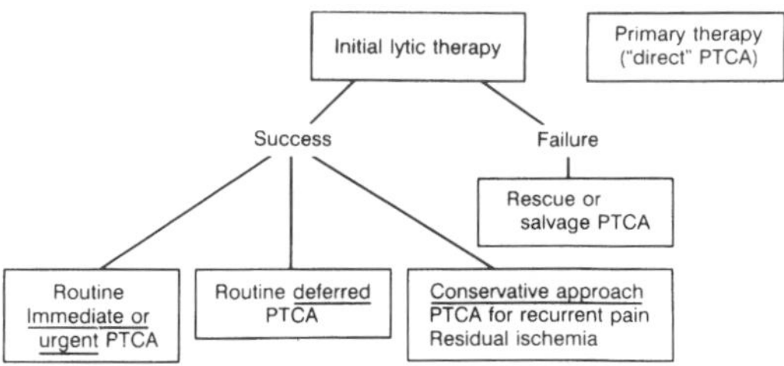

Figure 22–1. Potential applications for PTCA during acute myocardial infarction.

initial series comparing primary PTCA with intracoronary streptokinase, PTCA was successful in 83% of the 29 patients in whom it was attempted. The late reocclusion rate was 8.3%, and in-hospital mortality was 6.8%. The 83% reperfusion rate was similar to that achieved in the 29 patients who received intracoronary streptokinase. The data, however, suggested that PTCA was superior to intracoronary streptokinase for improving left ventricular function and decreasing recurrent ischemia.

Despite the lack of randomized controlled trials, throughout the mid and late 1980s accumulated data have shown primary dilation to be an effective treatment for acute myocardial infarction, and in many institutions, primary dilation became the treatment of choice. This was based on the reported series involving a total of more than 1,000 patients that documented angiographic reperfusion rates of 83% to 95%; the reperfusion rates documented with intravenous thrombolysis were substantially lower—approximately 50% with streptokinase and anisoylated streptokinase–plasminogen activator complex (APSAC) and 70% to 75% with t-PA (8,45–55). In addition, TIMI grade 3 rates of perfusion were substantially better with PTCA than with thrombolysis. Several studies have documented that the greatest incremental benefit effect of reperfusion is seen with TIMI grade 3 flow, not TIMI grade 2 flow.

Direct (primary) PTCA not only yields excellent reperfusion rates but also has been documented to result in improved left ventricular function, assessed with both global and regional techniques (10,14, 25). Rothbaum et al (14) documented that the average improvement in left ventricular ejection fraction was 13 ± 12% in patients with successful angioplasty for lesions of the left anterior descending coronary artery and 10 ± 12% for lesions of the right or circumflex coronary arteries. The extent of the improvement in global ejection fraction is as good as and may be even somewhat greater than that generally documented with intravenous lytic therapy. Other authors have also documented improvement in global ejection fraction with primary PTCA (10,25). O'Neill et al (10) documented a greater improvement in ejection fraction with PTCA

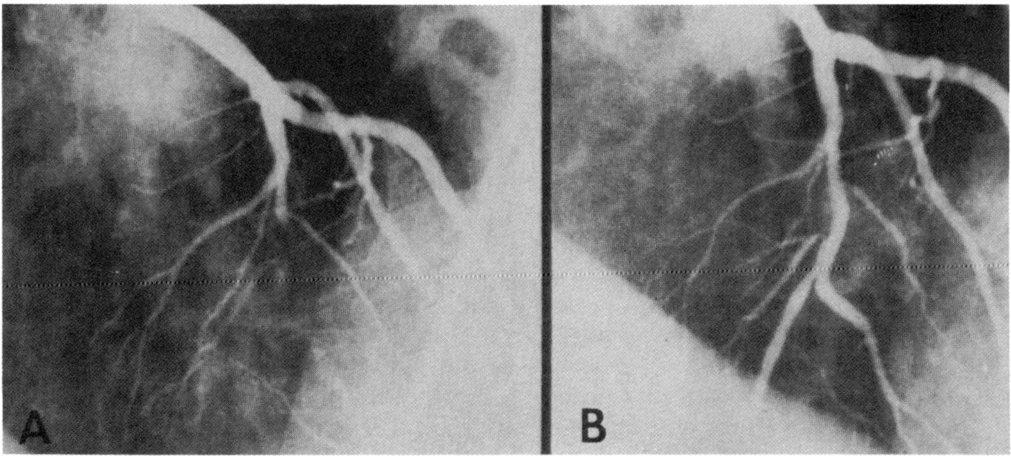

Figure 22–2. Dilation used as primary therapy during acute infarction. **A.** Left anterior descending coronary artery is occluded at baseline with evolving large anterior infarction. **B.** Primary dilation results in excellent improvement and successfully restores flow.

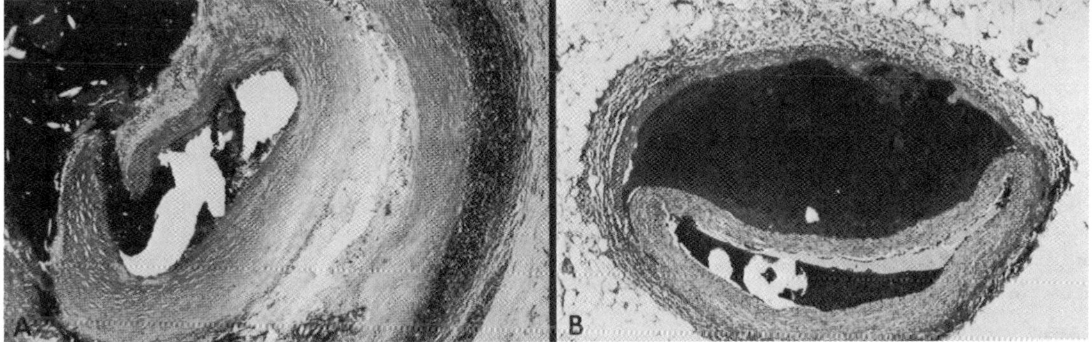

Figure 22–3. Postmortem photomicrographs of left anterior descending coronary artery from a patient who underwent combined lytic therapy and dilation for acute myocardial infarction. **A.** Dissection through the wall with development of large hematoma (10 o'clock position). **B.** Hematoma is propagated distally, resulting in vessel closure. (Hematoxylin-eosin; ×10.) *Courtesy of Dr. William D. Edwards.*

than with intracoronary lytic therapy. Whether this apparently greater improvement in left ventricular function is related to the speed of reperfusion with PTCA, completeness of reperfusion with a less severe residual stenosis than with lytic therapy, or patient selection criteria cannot be determined without a controlled randomized trial. Nonetheless, the concept that PTCA might provide better improvement in left ventricular function than lytic therapy remains intriguing and should be pursued.

There are other theoretical advantages to direct primary PTCA. The pathologic and morphologic features of the infarcted area may be altered differently by PTCA and by lytic therapy (see Ch. 2). Waller et al (33) documented a decreased incidence of hemorrhagic infarction with primary dilation compared with lytic therapy or with PTCA and lytic therapy, but this is controversial (Fig. 22–4). In contrast, data from Olson et al (34), at the Mayo Clinic, did not, however, document a significant increase in the incidence of hemorrhagic infarction in patients receiving thrombolytic therapy compared with those who had PTCA alone (see Ch. 2). The significance of hemorrhagic as opposed to "anemic" infarction is unclear because, in a 1989 review, Davies (35) concluded that the evidence to implicate an increased risk of myocardial rupture due to hemorrhagic infarction after thrombolytic therapy was inconclusive. There is also the theoretical potential that hemorrhagic dissection in the infarct-related artery could be reduced when PTCA is used alone compared with PTCA combined with lytic therapy, but data to substantiate this concept are as yet unavailable.

Table 22–1. Reported Success Rates of Primary PTCA for Acute Myocardial Infarction

Author	Year	No. of patients	Success rate, %
Kimura et al (13)	1984	58	88
O'Neill et al (10)	1986	29	83
Rothbaum et al (14)	1987	151	87
Miller et al (16)	1987	81	92
Marco et al (15)	1987	43	95
Zolnick et al (17)	1988	61	85
O'Keefe et al (25)	1989	500	94

An equally important theoretical advantage with primary dilation is the potential for reducing some of the bleeding complications of lytic therapy, particularly at vascular access sites. In all series of patients receiving lytic therapy and catheterization, the incidence of hemorrhage requiring transfusions or even local surgical repair is substantial. For example, Stack et al (8) studied outcomes in patients undergoing PTCA after high-dose streptokinase. In their study of 216 patients, 55% had a groin hematoma, 41% had a decrease in the hematocrit value to less than 30%, and 40% required a transfusion. Primary dilation, although it requires heparin and is combined with aspirin, offers the attractive possibility of a decreased incidence of bleeding.

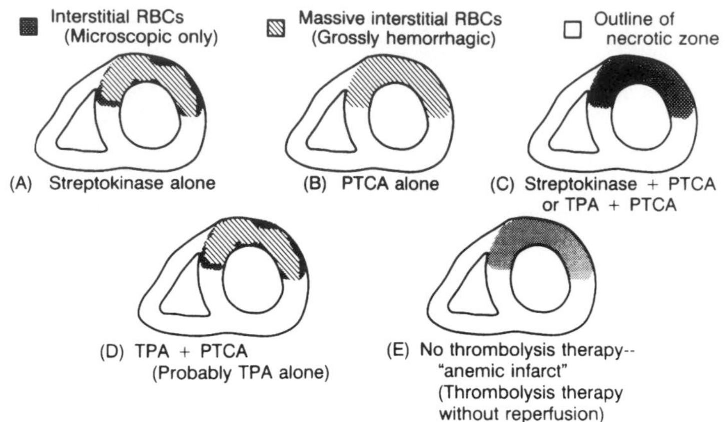

Figure 22–4. Relationship between the type of reperfusion therapy and the myocardial pathology after infarction. *Reprinted from Waller et al (33), with permission of the American College of Cardiology.*

Primary dilation is not without disadvantages. Reocclusion after dilation for acute myocardial infarction has been well documented (3,5,6,10–15, 25,44,45,50,55–58). The presence of a large mass of intracoronary thrombus and the residual thrombogenic substrate with plaque fissuring has been found to be associated with an increased incidence of acute closure syndromes with PTCA (Fig. 22–5) (59). Use of adequate heparin as well as aspirin could decrease this, as may other approaches, such as hirudin, platelet IIb/IIIa glycoprotein-receptor blockers, and antibodies to von Willebrand factor (60–64) (see Ch. 20). If reocclusion with thrombus is documented, intracoronary lytic therapy may then be helpful, but evidence to date is anecdotal.

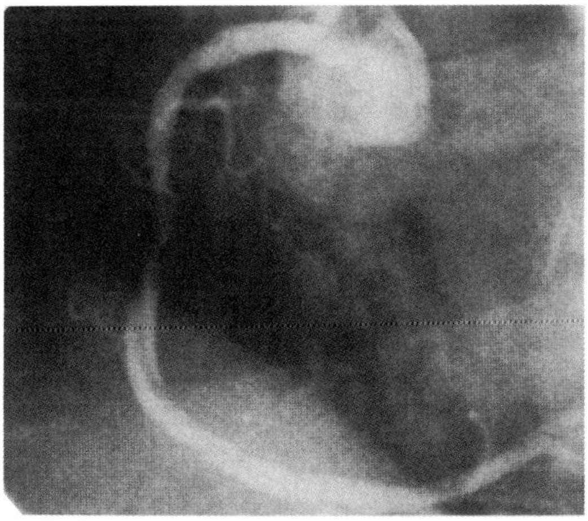

Figure 22–5. Left anterior oblique view of right coronary artery in a patient with acute infarction after lytic therapy and PTCA. Identification of the large intraluminal thrombus is associated with an increased incidence of reocclusion.

Another concern with primary dilation applies to the patient in whom obstruction is predominantly due to thrombus, in whom the underlying residual stenosis may not be sufficiently severe to warrant dilation. It is noteworthy that in the Thrombolysis in Myocardial Infarction (TIMI) and Thrombolysis and Angioplasty in Myocardial Infarction (TAMI) experience, approximately 15% of patients had relatively mild residual stenoses of less than 50% to 60% after thrombolysis (3,18).

Most problematic are concerns related to access to the catheterization laboratory and to trained personnel; these are very relevant and should not be underestimated. The logistics of these problems are daunting and the costs are great, at least when compared with primary lytic therapy. Given the relatively "narrow window" during which reperfusion is likely to salvage significant amounts of myocardium, most patients will be unable to be treated with primary dilation. Nonetheless, in those centers with easy access and trained personnel, primary dilation for acute myocardial infarction is an excellent approach that increases the possibility of achieving reperfusion rates greater than those currently obtainable with conventional regimens of lytic therapy alone; it also increases the potential for enhanced myocardial salvage.

With the large body of observational data available, there was an increasing need for randomized trials comparing direct angioplasty with thrombolysis. Such trials were planned and have been completed. The numbers of patients are still relatively small compared with the very large number of patients in the thrombolysis trials, but some important questions have been answered. None of these trials were designed with death as the primary endpoint. In a recent meta-analysis of seven trials of primary angioplasty versus thrombolytic therapy (including the initial PTCA versus intracoronary streptokinase trials), Michels has documented that at 6 weeks, 21 of 571 patients (3.7%) treated with PTCA had died compared with 37 of 574 patients in the thrombolytic group (6.4%) (odds ratio 0.56; 95% CI, 0.33 to 0.96). The reduction in mortality was particularly evident among the higher-risk patients who were older and had higher rates of anterior infarction. In lower-risk patients, there was substantially less improvement in mortality because the thrombolytic group also had low mortality. For the combined endpoint of death or nonfatal reinfarction at 6 weeks, there was also a similar reduction in events in patients being treated by PTCA (6.1% versus 11.0%, odds ratio 0.53; 95% CI, 0.35 to 0.85).

Patients in these trials randomized to the PTCA arm also had decreased bleeding including stroke, less recurrent ischemia, and shorter hospital stays. Data on left ventricular function was not concordant in all studies. Myocardial salvage was the primary endpoint in the Mayo Clinic trial. This was assessed using technetium-99*m* isonitrile (sestamibi). In this study, there was no difference in myocardial salvage between patients treated with direct angioplasty versus the group treated with thrombolytic therapy.

There is limited data available on the longer-term follow-up of these patients. In the PAMI trial, the predictors of in-hospital and 6-month outcome were assessed by Stone et al. (JACC, 1995;25: 370–377). In their analysis, the most powerful multivariate correlate of freedom from recurrent ischemic events was primary angioplasty (10.3% versus 28.0%, $p = 0.0001$). This independent beneficial effect was maintained at 6 months. In the Mayo Clinic trial, at 1 year late follow-up events of death or nonfatal reinfarction were low in both groups.

The Primary Angioplasty Registry (PAR), while not a randomized trial, prospectively enrolled and followed up 258 patients treated with direct angioplasty for acute myocardial infarction at one of six centers. These investigators found that improved clinical outcomes after direct angioplasty were maintained out to 6 months. (Circulation 1994;25: 156–162).

Recently, the results of the PAM-2 trial have been reported. This multicenter study evaluated outcomes and risk stratification in patients presenting within 12 hours of symptom onset of acute myocardial infarction. High-risk patients defined by age >70 years, ejection fraction <45%, three-vessel disease, suboptimal PTCA, significant ventricular arrhythmias, or vein graft occlusion were randomized to PTCA with or without placement of an intraaortic balloon pump; low-risk patients were randomized to stepdown unit admission and early dismissal versus CCU admission and conventional dismissal at ≥5 days. Preliminary results have documented an extraordinarily good outcome, with in-hospital mortality in the high-risk patients of 3.7% and in the low-risk patients of only 0.4%. These striking results further document the excellent outcome that can be achieved with direct angioplasty.

The GUSTO IIb study has been recently completed and presented in abstract form. An integral part of this study included a substudy comparing direct angioplasty versus thrombolytic therapy. This study has the advantage that it includes multiple centers from several different countries and a large enough number of patients to be powered to detect a mortality difference between primary PTCA and thrombolytic therapy as a primary endpoint. Eleven thousand thirty-eight patients were randomized: 573 to accelerated tPA and 565 to primary angioplasty. Preliminary assessment of the results documented no significance in 30-day death [5.7% with PTCA; 7% with tPA ($p = 0.37$); nonfatal reinfarction (4.5% with PTCA; 6.5% with tPA ($p = 0.13$)] or in nonfatal stroke [0.2% with PTCA and 0.9% with tPA ($p = 0.20$)]. Nonetheless, there was a difference in the combined endpoint of death, reinfarction and nonfatal stroke which occurred in 9.6% of patients treated with primary angioplasty versus 13.7% with tPA ($p = 0.30$). Further data analysis is underway. It is the largest trial and the one which included the largest number of centers and operators, these findings may reflect practice outcomes more accurately than the smaller more selected series. Although these data still demonstrate a trend in favor of primary angioplasty, this is not as marked a difference as has been noted in prior studies.

In addition to "routine" primary dilation, primary dilation is the treatment of choice for reperfusion therapy in three specific areas. First, in patients in whom thrombolytic therapy is contraindicated, dilation is an excellent option. The list of absolute or relative contraindications for thrombolytic therapy is relatively long. In affected patients, the risks of therapy outweigh the potential benefits of thrombolysis. In the GISSI-1 trial, approximately 20% of patients with suspected acute myocardial infarction had a contraindication to lytic therapy (69). In the Anglo-Scandinavian Study of Early Thrombolysis (ASSET) trial, 17.8% had one or more similar contraindications to lytic therapy (70). In these patients, if the clinical goal is to achieve acute reperfusion, PTCA provides the best option given the logistic constraints of acute coronary bypass graft surgery. In an analysis of the outcome of primary coronary angioplasty in patients with a contraindication to thrombolysis, Himbert et al (AJC 1993;71:377–381) studied 45 patients. Overall mortality in this high-risk group was 9%, which is improved relative to historical cohorts of patients with similar contraindications to thrombolytic therapy.

Second, dilation should be considered as primary therapy for acute myocardial infarction in patients with hemodynamic instability or cardiogenic shock (29–32,72,73). Historical cohort reports documented mortality rates ranging from 60% to 90% with conventional therapy, and thrombolysis alone has not been shown to improve survival (74–76). In the GISSI-1 trial, patients with Killip class III or IV at the time of presentation with acute myocardial infarction showed no improvement in survival with streptokinase therapy compared with the control group (69). In contrast, impressive evidence suggests that acute PTCA reduces mortality in comparison with historical controls, particularly if patency can be maintained (29–32). Although the numbers of patients are small, successful PTCA is accompanied by an acute survival of 60% to 70% (Fig. 22–6). This contrasts with the rate in patients with cardiogenic shock and unsuccessful dilation, in whom survival is 18%, and is similar to what would have been expected from historical controls (29). In our own experience, 45 patients with cardiogenic and acute myocardial infarction showed a similar trend. In patients with successful PTCA, 71% of patients survived to hospital dismissal. This result was in marked contrast to that in patients with unsuccessful PTCA, in whom the in-hospital mortality was 71%. It must be remembered that surgical therapy in these patients, particularly those with mechanical complications such as mitral regurgitation or ventricular septal defect, is also associated with improved outcome (77,78).

Cardiogenic shock has been evaluated in the GUSTO trial. In this trial, cardiogenic shock was documented in 2,972 (7.2%) of the total series. This patient group, however, accounted for 58% of all mortality in the entire trial. An aggressive strategy of angiography and reperfusion was associated with improved in-hospital survival. (JACC 1995;26:668–674). In the patients who developed

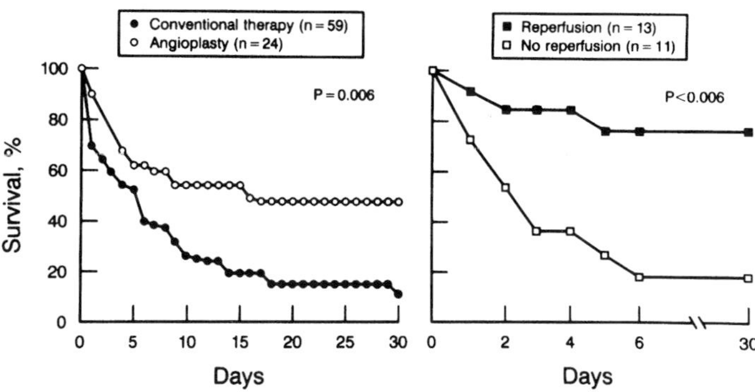

Figure 22–6. Effect of PTCA on survival in patients with cardiogenic shock. When reperfusion is successful (right), survival is significantly improved. *Reprinted from Lee et al (29), with permission of the American Heart Association.*

shock in hospital and were then treated with PTCA, the mortality was 32%, compared with patients treated without aggressive reperfusion, in whom the mortality was 61% ($p < 0.001$).

Third, dilation is a logical form of primary therapy for patients in whom the diagnosis of acute myocardial ischemia or myocardial infarction is suspected but insufficiently documented either clinically or electrocardiographically to warrant the administration of thrombolytic therapy. In this situation, emergency coronary angiography and left ventricular angiography can substantiate the diagnosis by documenting regional wall motion abnormalities and a thrombotically occluded coronary artery in the distribution of the ventriculographic abnormalities. Diagnostic confirmation can be followed by immediate dilation.

PTCA AFTER LYTIC THERAPY

Given the issues of access and patient transfer and the potential need to treat the residual stenosis after lysis of the thrombus, there has been understandable interest in the application of PTCA after lytic therapy (Fig. 22–1) (3–6,8,18,19,21,56,58). This approach has been the subject of multiple trials that are complex in design. In the majority r-tPA has been used, but in addition, APSAC and streptokinase have been studied. In the evaluation of the role of PTCA after lytic therapy, the status of the infarct-related artery is a crucial factor to be considered. If patent, it would appear from several trials that enthusiasm for "routine" PTCA is declining. However, in the event of persistent occlusion after lytic therapy, PTCA is a logical and appealing option.

Identification of Arterial Patency After Lytic Therapy

The ability to differentiate patients with successful reperfusion from those without has major clinical implications and remains a pivotal area of investigation (80,81). Previously, it was believed that therapeutic efficacy could be accurately assessed on the basis of clinical indicators such as relief of pain, resolution of ST segment elevation, and reperfusion arrhythmias. The limitations of these indices were, however, highlighted by a 1988 systematic evaluation of patients enrolled in the TAMI trials (Table 22–2). Complete resolution of ST segment elevation was by far the most specific indicator of reperfusion, indicating restored patency in approximately 95% of cases. However, this factor was very insensitive and was seen in only approximately 5% of patients (80). Thus conventional approaches to recognize reperfusion in large numbers of patients, although specific, are highly insensitive.

Other techniques of noninvasively identifying reperfusion are under investigation. New approaches utilizing electrocardiographic monitoring and beat-to-beat analysis of regional ST segment elevation hold promise (82,83). Biochemical approaches also hold promise for the early detection of reperfusion (84–93) (see Ch. 8). Analyses of creatine kinase isoforms and frequent serial determinations of creatine kinase MB fractions with assays that provide results within minutes may allow such early detection. The early detection of myoglobin in the serum as an index of acute reperfusion is under evaluation (90). Until the efficacy of these methods has been documented, acute angiographic assessment remains the standard for determination of the patency of the infarct-related artery after thrombolytic therapy. Given the logistic constraints and the bleeding complications associated with this approach, the urgent need to establish noninvasive techniques for assessing the patency of the infarct-related artery is self-evident.

Table 22–2. Assessment of Reperfusion After r-tPA in 386 Patients

Factor	% of pt	Patency, % of pt
ST segment		
Unchanged	56	63
Improved	38	84
Resolved	6	96
Chest pain		
Unchanged/worse	20	60
Improved	51	71
Resolved	29	84
Arrhythmia		
None 64	72	
Ventricular arrhythmia	7	75

Data from Califf et al (80).

Role of PTCA After Intravenous Thrombolytic Therapy with Patent Infarct-Related Artery

Three pivotal early studies documented the role of PTCA after intravenous thrombolytic therapy with a patent infarct-related artery: TAMI, TIMI, and the European Cooperative Study Group (ECSG) (Table 22–3) (3–6,9,18,19,58). These randomized trials all addressed the role and timing of an invasive strategy with PTCA after administration of r-tPA. Despite differences in specific aspects of trial design and in the administered doses of r-tPA, the overall conclusions from the trials were surprisingly similar and emphasize the value of carefully designed randomized trials in that at the onset, the intuitive opinion of many was that immediate or "early" PTCA would be the logical next step after apparently successful thrombolytic therapy.

TAMI-I

The TAMI-I trial enrolled 386 patients who underwent angiography 90 minutes after administration of 150 mg of r-tPA; after demonstration of a patent infarct-related artery, the patients were randomly assigned to *immediate* PTCA or to a strategy of deferred PTCA 7 to 10 days later. Patients with persistent occlusion after lytic therapy were treated with PTCA but were excluded from the randomized trial.

The major endpoint of the trial was predismissal left ventricular function, and this did not differ between the two groups; neither experienced a significant change in predismissal ejection fraction in comparison with baseline (Table 22–4). The mortality rate was 4% in patients undergoing *immediate* angioplasty and 1% in the deferred PTCA group, but these rates were not significantly different. Reocclusion rates were similar in both groups: 11% with immediate PTCA and 13% with deferred PTCA. However, the success rates of PTCA were higher and the need for emergency coronary bypass graft surgery was lower in the deferred PTCA group. In addition, the deferred PTCA group had a lower requirement for blood transfusions and a lower incidence of acute closure. A striking finding was that in 14% of patients in the deferred PTCA group, who initially had a high-grade residual stenosis after thrombolytic therapy, the stenosis at the time of follow-up angiography before dismissal was less than 50% and did not require any intervention. Presumably, this reflected further dissolution of thrombus. The conclusion from this trial was that in patients with "initially successful thrombolysis and suitable coronary-artery anatomy, immediate angioplasty offers no clear advantage over delayed elective angioplasty" (3).

Table 22–3. Strategies for Three Studies of Thrombolysis for Acute Myocardial Infarction

Study	No. of patients	Dose of rtPA, mg	Catheterization	PTCA
TIMI-IIA	389	150* 100	Immediate vs.18–48 hr	Immediate vs. 18–48 hr
TAMI	386	150	Immediate	Immediate vs. 7 days later
ECSG	367	100	Immediate vs. before dismissal	Immediate vs. none
TIMI-IIB	3,262	150†	Routine, 18–48 hr later vs. no arteriography unless there was evidence of recurrent spontaneous or exercise-induced ischemia	18–48 hr later if anatomy suitable vs. no PTCA unless evidence of recurrent spontaneous or exercise-induced ischemia

*The first one-third of the patients received 150 mg; this dose was subsequently changed to 100 mg.

†In 520 patients, 150 mg was used; in the remaining 2,742 patients, 100 mg was used.

ECSG, European Cooperative Study Group; TAMI, Thrombolysis and Myocardial Infarction; TIMI (IIA and IIB), Thrombolysis in Myocardial Infarction.

Table 22–4. PTCA Performance and Outcome in Three Studies of Thrombolysis for Acute Myocardial Infarction

	TIMI-IIA		TAMI		ECSG	
	Immediate PTCA	18–48 hr PTCA	Immediate PTCA	Elective PTCA	Immediate PTCA	Noninvasive
No. of patients	195	194	99	98	183	184
PTCA performed, no. of patients	141	107	99	35	168	. . .
PTCA successful, %	84	92	85	94	90	. . .
Complication, %						
Transfusion	20	7.2	22	18	10	4
Reinfarction	6.7	4.1	. . .	. . .	4	7
Reocclusion	. . .	. . .	11 (NS)	13	12.5 (NS)	11
CABG within 24 hr of PTCA	4.3	1.9	7 (0.17)	2	. . .	. . .
Dismissal ejection fraction, %	50.3	49.0	53 (NS)	56	51	51
In-hospital mortality, %	7.2 (NS)	5.7	4 (0.37)	1	7 (0.4)	3

CABG, coronary artery bypass graft surgery; ECSG, European Cooperative Study Group; NS, not significant; TAMI, Thrombolysis and Myocardial Infarction; TIMI, Thrombolysis in Myocardial Infarction. Numbers in parentheses are *p* values.

ECSG Trial

The design of the ECSG trial was somewhat different; it compared the strategy of immediate PTCA after administration of 100 mg of r-tPA with a conservative approach without any intervention in 367 patients (Tables 22–3 and 22–4) (47). Again, the primary endpoint was left ventricular function and estimates of infarct size with enzymatic techniques. As was the case with the TAMI-I trial, there was no difference in ejection fraction between the two groups. The incidence of recurrent ischemia after 24 hours was similar: 13% for the invasive group and 11% for the conservative group. However, the incidence of bleeding and transfusion requirements were higher with the invasive group. In addition, in-hospital mortality was higher in the invasive group than in the noninvasive group—7% and 3%, respectively. Again, the final conclusions of this trial indicated that thrombolytic therapy, combined with immediate PTCA, did not appear to be superior to early noninvasive treatment with r-tPA, heparin, and acetylsalicylic acid in acute myocardial infarction (47).

TIMI Trial

This trial was more complex than the others (4–6,18,50,94). The major aims were to evaluate the role of early PTCA, delayed PTCA, or medical therapy after intravenous thrombolysis with r-tPA. There were two major arms. TIMI-IIA compared emergency PTCA (within 2 hours of r-tPA therapy) with a deferred approach in which catheterization and angioplasty were done 18 to 48 hours later. TIMI-IIB, the second arm, compared routine, deferred PTCA 18 to 48 hours after r-tPA with a conservative strategy in which revascularization was performed only if clinically indicated. Primary endpoints were death, recurrent infarction, and both rest and exercise left ventricular function.

In TIMI-IIA, which compared immediate PTCA with delayed catheterization and angioplasty at 18 to 48 hours, 389 patients were enrolled (Table 22–4) (18). In the *immediate* PTCA group, dilation was performed in only 72%. The most common reason for not attempting PTCA was the angiographer's impression that a lesion was technically unsuitable for dilation (16%). In the *delayed* group, dilation was performed in only 55%. The most frequent reasons for not attempting dilation were the presence of a residual lesion of less than 60% (14% of patients) and the finding of a persistently occluded infarct-related artery (12% of patients). As was the case in the TAMI-I trial, primary success rates were higher in the patients undergoing *delayed* PTCA (92% versus 84%). Patients who had immediate catheterization/PTCA had an increased frequency of bleeding and emergency coronary bypass graft surgery. Despite the early intervention, there was no significant difference in the primary endpoint of ejection fraction between the immediate (50.3%) and the delayed (49%) PTCA group. Given the lack of improvement in left ventricular function and the increased complications, the TIMI investigators concluded that the "immediate performance of coronary arteriography and PTCA compared with delaying these procedures for 18 to 48 hours provides no advantage and may be harmful" (18).

The TIMI-IIB trial compared an invasive strategy with a conservative strategy *after thrombolysis* (6); 3,262 patients were randomized either to an invasive strategy that consisted of routine coronary arteriography 18 to 48 hours after administration of r-tPA followed by routine prophylactic PTCA if the anatomy was suitable or to a conservative strategy in which coronary angiography and PTCA were performed only in the event of recurrent spontaneous or exercise-induced ischemia. The primary endpoints for this part of the trial were survival, death, and recurrent myocardial infarction at 42 days. Although 1,636 patients were assigned to the invasive strategy, PTCA was only attempted in 56.7%, and the success rate was 93% (Fig. 22–7). Conversely, in the conservative group, 13.3% underwent clinically indicated PTCA within 14 days of thrombolytic therapy, and the success rate was 91.7% (Fig. 22–8). When the major endpoints of survival and freedom from recurrent myocardial infarction were analyzed, there was no significant difference between the groups at 42 days (10.9% for the invasive group and 9.7% for the conservative group) or at 1 year (95). In addition, the two groups had no significant differences in either rest or exercise ejection fraction at the time of hospital dismissal or on repeat testing 6 weeks later (Table 22–5). The conclusion of TIMI-IIB was that

> in patients with acute myocardial infarction who were treated with rt-PA and with heparin followed by aspirin, an invasive strategy of coronary arteriography 18 to 48 hours after the onset of symptoms, followed by prophylactic PTCA, offered no advantage in terms of reductions in mortality or reinfarction over a more conservative strategy, according to which these procedures were provided only to patients with recurrent ischemia; the latter strategy was less complex and less costly (6).

It should again be emphasized that during the planning phase of these trials, most investigators thought that early PTCA would be the logical step after the administration of thrombolytic therapy. Subsequently, the conclusions from all three trials

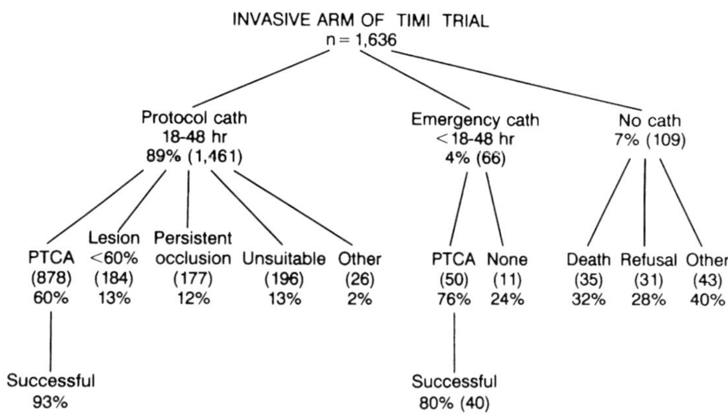

Figure 22–7. Results of catheterization and outcome of PTCA in invasive arm of TIMI trial.

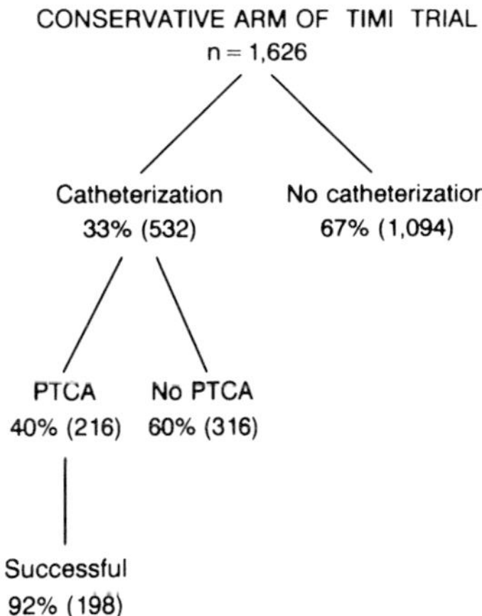

Figure 22–8. Need for catheterization and dilation in conservative arm of TIMI trial.

pointed in a different direction; thus, current investigative efforts are being directed at maximizing thrombolytic reperfusion rates, identifying mechanisms of reocclusion and rethrombosis, and treating persistent occlusion.

It should also be emphasized that there are differences among the three trials. Moreover, the trials were confined, by design, to specific patient subgroups. The results should not be extrapolated to different patient subsets that were not tested. Patients with cardiogenic shock, a subset routinely not included in all of these trials, may benefit substantially from early PTCA. Other patients who were not specifically addressed are those with failed thrombolysis and persistently occluded infarct-related arteries (21,96,97). In addition, none of these trials were designed to evaluate the role of primary dilation or acute coronary bypass graft surgery in acute infarction. In this regard, not all patients who were assigned to the invasive group underwent dilation, and this factor may bias the results. Finally, in all three trials, the thrombolytic drug was r-tPA, which may have affected the early outcome of PTCA.

Subsequent studies have been confirmatory. Michels and Yusuf analyzed the outcome in different groups of patients treated with thrombolytic therapy followed by potential angioplasty. These included (i) immediate PTCA after lytic therapy versus no PTCA; (ii) early PTCA versus no PTCA; (iii) delayed PTCA versus no PTCA; and (iv) immediate PTCA versus delayed PTCA. In each of these groups of studies, there were trends or significant differences with increased risk in the more aggressively treated patients. Routine dilation in addition

Table 22–5. Outcome at 6 Weeks in TIMI-IIB

	Invasive strategy (n = 1,636)	Conservative strategy (n = 1,626)	p value
Primary event, %			
Nonfatal reinfarction	5.9	5.4	0.57
Death	5.2	4.7	0.49
Reinfarction/death	10.9	9.7	0.25
Secondary event, %			
Any adverse event*	13.0	10.6	0.04
Positive ETT at dismissal	12.8	17.7	<0.001
Positive ETT at 6 weeks	16.8	19.4	0.09
Resting ejection fraction at dismissal	50.5	49.9	0.30
Exercise ejection fraction − resting ejection fraction	3.7	3.1	0.06
Resting ejection fraction at 6 weeks	50.0	50.4	0.51
Exercise ejection fraction − resting ejection fraction	3.3	2.3	0.02

ETT, exercise treadmill test.

*Coronary bypass grafting; PTCA, cerebrovascular accident, intracranial hemorrhage.

Data from the TIMI Study Group (6).

to successful thrombolysis, therefore, appears to offer no immediate advantage and may result in increased complications.

The issue of Q wave myocardial infarction has been studied extensively. There is less information on non-Q wave infarction, although that is the subject of current studies. The TIMI-IIIB trial assessed the outcome of t-PA and a comparison of early invasive and conservative strategies in unstable angina and non-Q wave infarction. In this study, 740 patients were randomized to an early invasive approach and 733 to the early conservative approach. There was no difference in the 6-week endpoints of death, nonfatal myocardial infarction, or a positive exercise test; however, patients randomized to an early invasive strategy had a significantly shorter average length of initial hospitalization, required fewer rehospitalization, and had decreased antianginal medication use.

PTCA IN THE SETTING OF FAILED THROMBOLYSIS ("RESCUE" PTCA)

Despite the use of different thrombolytic agents alone or in combination, the "ceiling" for successful reperfusion remains around 70% to 75% (8,45–55). With streptokinase and APSAC, documented reperfusion rates are lower (8,45–55). The failure to achieve acute reperfusion is multifactorial and related to local factors in the arterial wall, failure to achieve sufficiently high concentrations of the lytic agent at the site of thrombus, the presence of inhibitors, and the cell composition of the thrombus (whether platelet rich or red-cell rich) (see Ch. 20). Whatever the cause, the consequences for myocardial salvage are the same; the achievement of a higher rate of reperfusion is a priority for future investigation. Recently, a modified dosing regimen for r-tPA has been described in which the majority of the dose is given early ("front-loaded") with a bolus of 15 mg followed by 50 mg over 30 minutes and then 35 mg over 60 minutes. An initial report documented a 75% patency at 60 minutes and a 90% patency at 90 minutes (99). This would be a major advance if subsequent studies substantiate these findings. Until then, even with the best lytic agent, as many as 25% of patients with acute myocardial infarction characterized by pain and ST segment elevation may receive lytic therapy only to have it fail. In this setting, PTCA may play a very valuable role as a rescue (salvage) procedure, but there is a relative lack of confirmatory data in this important subgroup of patients.

Patients who do not have acute reperfusion appear to constitute a subset with a substantial increase in mortality or morbidity (96,97). In the TAMI-I experience with 386 patients, the mortality rate was 5.2% in those with successful thrombolysis and 10.4% in those with failed thrombolysis. Failed reperfusion with *lytic* therapy also appears to identify a subgroup of patients in whom the results of rescue dilation are also less favorable, with a higher incidence of reocclusion as well as less improvement in left ventricular function.

The success rates of rescue dilation have been generally lower than those with dilation when the infarct-related artery is patent, perhaps a reflection of the extent of residual thrombus (20,21,96,97, 100–105). Furthermore, the failure of lysis may have identified patients in whom the underlying cause of myocardial infarction and coronary occlusion might have been somewhat different, and this could also have influenced the outcome. The early experience with rescue dilation after use of single lytic agents was associated with reperfusion rates of 70% to 75%. The results were the same with streptokinase alone or with r-tPA alone, and they led in part to investigation of combination lytic therapy.

Topol et al (101), in a TAMI study, documented that the combination of r-tPA and urokinase did not affect the initial patency of the infarct-related artery; this finding lent support to the notion that there is a plateau for reperfusion rates. However, the combination did have a substantial impact on the outcome of salvage angioplasty. Patients who received 150 mg of r-tPA and 100,000 units of urokinase had an increased technical success, decreased reocclusion, and improved left ventricular function. The combination of 50 mg of r-tPA and 1.5 mU of streptokinase has been reported (100). In a small number of patients who had rescue dilation after failed angioplasty, sustained patency was achieved in 9 of 10 patients with a decreased incidence of reocclusion. The authors pointed out the cost implications of one-half dose r-tPA and streptokinase compared with full-dose r-tPA and urokinase. If the former combination is equally effective, it will be substantially less costly.

The benefits of rescue (salvage) angioplasty might extend beyond the potential salvage of ischemic myocardium. Given the time delay, which includes time to medical evaluation, administration of the thrombolytic drug, recognition that thrombolysis has failed, and then time to catheterization and completion of dilation, it is unrealistic to expect a dramatic improvement in left ventricular function. Nonetheless, in our experience with rescue angioplasty, even in the absence of any myocardial salvage (as represented by an improvement in left ventricular function), the long-term outcome of the patients was surprisingly good (21). In a group of 34 patients with average predismissal ejection fractions of 36% who had undergone rescue angioplasty, the 4-year survival was 89%. Rescue angioplasty could, therefore, provide a long-term benefit not by salvaging myocardium but by providing a patent artery that could improve ventricular remodeling, altering the electrical substrate for reentrant ventricular arrhythmia, or acting as a source for future collaterals. All are possible mechanisms, but they remain speculative at this time.

The database concerning rescue angioplasty is expanding. Ellis et al evaluated the outcome of 151 patients with anterior infarction treated with thrombolytic therapy that failed, leaving an angiographically documented myocardial infarction. These patients were randomized to either conservative therapy (aspirin, heparin, and vasodilators) or to balloon angioplasty. (Circulation 1994;90: 2280–2284). Angioplasty was technically successful in 92% of randomized patients. The primary endpoint was 1-month ejection fraction. In this study, at 30 days there was no difference in death (5.1% angioplasty, 9.6% conservative, $p = 0.18$), no difference in resting ejection fraction (40 ± 11% and 39 ± 12%, $p = 0.49$), or severe congestive heart failure (1.3% versus 7.0%, $p = 0.11$). Ejection fraction with exercise was moderately improved in the PTCA group (43 ± 15% versus 38 ± 13%, $p = 0.04$).

The CORAMI (Cohort of Reserve Angioplasty in Myocardial Infarction) study group has reported on the outcome of 72 patients who underwent rescue angioplasty. The procedure was successful in 90% of the patients. The in-hospital outcome documented a survival rate of 96%, reocclusion in 7%, and no emergency surgery. Of the 69 survivors, follow-up was available in 65 for a mean duration of 16 ± 12 months. The actuarial survival at 18 months was 92%.

The role of rescue dilation is evolving. As long as there is a substantial rate of failed reperfusion with thrombolytic therapy, rescue dilation will play an important role in the treatment of acute myocardial infarction. This will be enhanced by development of noninvasive markers that can promptly and reliably detect successful or failed thrombolytic reperfusion.

SUMMARY

The role of dilation during myocardial infarction continues to evolve. Although not a panacea, it can play various, very effective roles.

Direct (primary) PTCA is feasible and very effective, with success rates approaching 90%. Reocclusion, particularly of the right coronary artery, is a persistent limitation, as is the case with lytic therapy alone. Several controlled studies are currently under way to compare this approach with lytic therapy alone. At the current time, if facilities and personnel are available, direct primary PTCA is a feasible and valid approach to the treatment of acute myocardial infarction. In addition, in selected patients (for example, those with cardiogenic shock), its role has been well established.

PTCA also has an important role after the administration of lytic therapy. When lytic therapy has failed, rescue (salvage) angioplasty is probably the best and most convenient means to restore flow. With a combination of lytic agents, it is hoped that this approach will become more successful for maintaining the patency of the infarct-related artery with a potential for myocardial salvage and improved long-term outcome. Problems include the current inability to distinguish failed reperfusion reliably and in a timely fashion without the need for urgent angiography in all patients.

When the infarct-related artery is patent after lytic therapy, the role of PTCA is more controversial, and the bulk of accumulated evidence argues against routine use of the procedure. Given that the randomized trials have not shown any advantage to PTCA in this setting, and indeed have even shown increased morbidity and mortality, urgent PTCA is currently contraindicated if the infarct-related artery is patent and the patient is stable. The role of delayed elective PTCA has also been studied. Intuitively, elective dilation of a high-grade residual stenosis in the infarct-related artery seems reasonable, but this approach does not take into account local factors in the milieu of the acute ischemic lesion (such as plaque fissure and thrombus), all of which decrease the likelihood of success with PTCA. In concert, recent data strongly suggest that the intuitive approach may not be optimal and that reperfusion momentum should be avoided. In this setting, PTCA should be performed only if there is recurrent or provocable ischemia. Other long-term studies with attention to risk stratification are needed to identify patients who will benefit from elective delayed PTCA.

REFERENCES

1. Meyer J, Merx W, Schmitz H, et al: Percutaneous transluminal coronary angioplasty immediately after intracoronary streptolysis of transmural myocardial infarction. *Circulation* 1982;66:905–913.
2. Hartzler GO, Rutherford BD, McConahay DR, et al: Percutaneous transluminal coronary angioplasty with and without thrombolytic therapy for treatment of acute myocardial infarction. *Am Heart J* 1983;106: 965–973.
3. Topol EJ, Califf RM, George BS, et al: A randomized trial of immediate versus delayed elective angioplasty after intravenous tissue plasminogen activator in acute myocardial infarction. *N Engl J Med* 1987; 317:581–588.
4. The TIMI Study Group: The Thrombolysis in Myocardial Infarction (TIMI) trial: Phase I findings. *N Engl J Med* 1985;312:932–936.
5. Passamani E, Hodges M, Herman M, et al: The Thrombolysis in Myocardial Infarction (TIMI) phase II pilot study: Tissue plasminogen activator followed by percutaneous transluminal coronary angioplasty. *J Am Coll Cardiol* 1987;10(Suppl B): 51B–64B.
6. The TIMI Study Group: Comparison of invasive and conservative strategies after treatment with intravenous tissue plasminogen activator in acute myocardial infarction: Results of the Thrombolysis in Myocardial Infarction (TIMI) phase II trial. *N Engl J Med* 1989;320:618–627.
7. Guerci AD, Gerstenblith G, Brinker JA, et al: A randomized trial of intravenous tissue plasminogen activator for acute myocardial infarction with subsequent randomization to elective coronary angioplasty. *N Engl J Med* 1987;317:1613–1618.
8. Stack RS, O'Connor CM, Mark DB, et al: Coronary perfusion during acute myocardial infarction with a combined therapy of coronary angioplasty and high-dose intravenous streptokinase. *Circulation* 1988;77:151–161.
9. Topol EJ, Califf RM, Kereiakes DJ, George BS: Thrombolysis and Angioplasty in Myocardial Infarction (TAMI) trial. *J Am Coll Cardiol* 1987; 10(Suppl B):65B–74B.
10. O'Neill W, Timmis GC, Bourdillon PD, et al: A prospective randomized clinical trial of intracoronary streptokinase versus coronary angioplasty for acute myocardial infarction. *N Engl J Med* 1986; 314:812–818.
11. Holmes DR Jr, Smith HC, Vlietstra RE, et al: Percutaneous transluminal coronary angioplasty, alone or in combination with streptokinase therapy, during acute myocardial infarction. *Mayo Clin Proc* 1985;60:449–456.
12. Hartzler GO, Rutherford BD, McConahay DR: Percutaneous transluminal coronary angioplasty: Application for acute myocardial infarction. *Am J Cardiol* 1984;53:117C–121C.
13. Kimura T, Nosaka H, Ueno K, Nobuyoshi M: Role of coronary angioplasty in acute myocardial infarction. *Am Heart J* 1984;107:820–822.
14. Rothbaum DA, Linnemeier TJ, Landin RJ, et al: Emergency percutaneous transluminal coronary angioplasty in acute myocardial infarction: A 3 year experience. *J Am Coll Cardiol* 1987;10:264–272.
15. Marco J, Caster L, Szatmary LJ, Fajadet J: Emergency percutaneous transluminal coronary angioplasty without thrombolysis as initial therapy in acute myocardial infarction. *Int J Cardiol* 1987;15: 55–63.
16. Miller PF, Brodie BR, Weintraub RA, et al: Emergency coronary angioplasty for acute myocardial

infarction: Results from a community hospital. *Arch Intern Med* 1987;147:1565–1570.

17. Zolnick MR, Gersh BJ, Holmes DR Jr: Long-term follow-up after percutaneous transluminal coronary angioplasty during acute myocardial infarction. *Circulation* 1988;78(Suppl II):II-634.
18. The TIMI Research Group: Immediate vs delayed catheterization and angioplasty following thrombolytic therapy for acute myocardial infarction: TIMI II A results. *JAMA* 1988;260:2849–2858.
19. Holmes DR Jr, Topol EJ: Reperfusion momentum: Lessons from the randomized trials of immediate coronary angioplasty for myocardial infarction (editorial). *J Am Coll Cardiol* 1989;14:1572–1578.
20. Fung AY, Lai P, Topol EJ, et al: Value of percutaneous transluminal coronary angioplasty after unsuccessful intravenous streptokinase therapy in acute myocardial infarction. *Am J Cardiol* 1986;58:686–691.
21. Holmes DR Jr, Gersh BJ, Bailey KR, et al: Emergency "rescue" percutaneous transluminal coronary angioplasty after failed thrombolysis with streptokinase: Early and late results. *Circulation* 1990;81 (Suppl IV):IV-51–IV-56.
22. Stack RS, Califf RM, Hinohara T, et al: Survival and cardiac event rates in the first year after emergency coronary angioplasty for acute myocardial infarction. *J Am Coll Cardiol* 1988;11:1141–1419.
23. Topol EJ: The long-term investment of coronary angioplasty for acute myocardial infarction. *J Am Coll Cardiol* 1988;11:1150–1152.
24. Holland KJ, O'Neill WW, Bates ER, Pitt B, Topol EJ: Emergency percutaneous transluminal coronary angioplasty during acute myocardial infarction for patients more than 70 years of age. *Am J Cardiol* 1989;63:399–403.
25. O'Keefe JH Jr, Rutherford BD, McConahay DR, et al: Early and late results of coronary angioplasty without antecedent thrombolytic therapy for acute myocardial infarction. *Am J Cardiol* 1989;64: 1221–1230.
26. Ellis SG, O'Neill WW, Bates ER, Walton JA, Nabel EG, Topol EJ: Coronary angioplasty as primary therapy for acute myocardial infarction 6 to 48 hours after symptom onset: Report of an initial experience. *J Am Coll Cardiol* 1989;13:1122–1126.
27. Ellis SG, O'Neill WW, Bates ER, et al: Implications for patient triage from survival and left ventricular functional recovery analyses in 500 patients treated with coronary angioplasty for acute infarction. *J Am Coll Cardiol* 1989;13:1251–1259.
28. Erbel R, Pop T, Diefenbach C, Meyer J: Long-term results of thrombolytic therapy with and without percutaneous transluminal coronary angioplasty. *J Am Coll Cardiol* 1989;14:276 285.
29. Lee L, Bates ER, Pitt B, Walton JA, Laufer N, O'Neill WW: Percutaneous transluminal coronary angioplasty improves survival in acute myocardial infarction complicated by cardiogenic shock. *Circulation* 1988;78:1345–1351.
30. Shani J, Rivera M, Greengart A, Hollander G, Kaplan P, Lichstein E: Percutaneous transluminal coronary angioplasty in cardiogenic shock (abstract). *J Am Coll Cardiol* 1986;7:149A.
31. Heuser RR, Maddoux GL, Goss JE, Ramo BW, Raff GL, Shadoff N: Coronary angioplasty for acute mitral regurgitation due to myocardial infarction: A nonsurgical treatment preserving mitral valve integrity. *Ann Intern Med* 1987;107: 852–855.
32. Brown TM Jr, Iannone LA, Gordon DF, Wickemeyer WJ, Wheeler WS, Rough RR: Percutaneous myocardial perfusion (PMR) reduces mortality in acute myocardial infarction (MI) complicated by cardiogenic shock (abstract). *Circulation* 1985;72 (Suppl III):III-309.
33. Waller BF, Rothbaum DA, Pinkerton CA, et al: Status of the myocardium and infarct-related coronary artery in 19 necropsy patients with acute recanalization using pharmacologic (streptokinase, r-tissue plasminogen activator), mechanical (percutaneous transluminal coronary angioplasty) or combined types of reperfusion therapy. *J Am Coll Cardiol* 1987;9:785–801.
34. Olson LJ, McGovern TW, Edwards WD, Saber RS, Frye RL, Holmes DR Jr: Early histopathology of reperfusion therapy for myocardial ischemia: Study of 29 autopsied cases. *J Am Coll Cardiol* 1989;13(Suppl):193A.
35. Davies MJ: Successful and unsuccessful coronary thrombolysis. *Br Heart J* 1989;61:381–384.
36. Kloner RA, Alker KJ: The effect of streptokinase on intramyocardial hemorrhage, infarct size, and the no-reflow phenomenon during coronary reperfusion. *Circulation* 1984;70:513–521.
37. Chaitman BR: More on the saga of routine emergency coronary angioplasty for acute myocardial infarction. *J Am Coll Cardiol* 1989;13:1260–1261.
38. Hutter AM Jr: Coronary angioplasty in acute myocardial infarction: Should it be done? To whom? When? *J Am Coll Cardiol* 1989;13:1127–1129.

39. Ryan TJ: Angioplasty in acute myocardial infarction: Is the balloon leaking? *N Engl J Med* 1987; 317:624–626.
40. Topol EJ: Coronary angioplasty for acute myocardial infarction. *Ann Intern Med* 1988;109: 970–980.
41. Laffel GL, Fineberg HV, Braunwald E: A cost-effectiveness model for coronary thrombolysis/ reperfusion therapy. *J Am Coll Cardiol* 1987;10 (Suppl B):79B–90B.
42. Vermeer F, Simoons ML, de Zwaan C, et al: Cost benefit analysis of early thrombolytic treatment with intracoronary streptokinase: Twelve month follow up report of the randomised multicentre trial conducted by the Interuniversity Cardiology Institute of the Netherlands. *Br Heart J* 1988;59: 527–534.
43. Steinberg EP, Topol EJ, Sakin JW, et al: Cost and procedure implications of thrombolytic therapy for acute myocardial infarction. *J Am Coll Cardiol* 1988; 12(Suppl):58A–68A.
44. O'Neill WW, Topol EJ, Pitt B: Reperfusion therapy of acute myocardial infarction. *Prog Cardiovasc Dis* 1988;30:235–266.
45. Tiefenbrunn AJ, Sobel BE: The impact of coronary thrombolysis on myocardial infarction. *Fibrinolysis* 1989;3:1–15.
46. Tennant SN, Dixon J, Venable TC, et al: Intracoronary thrombolysis in patients with acute myocardial infarction: Comparison of the efficacy of urokinase with streptokinase. *Circulation* 1984;69: 756–760.
47. Mathey DG, Schofer J, Sheehan FH, Becher H, Tilsner V, Dodge HT: Intravenous urokinase in acute myocardial infarction. *Am J Cardiol* 1985;55: 878–882.
48. Timmis AD, Griffin B, Crick JCP, Flax JS, Sowton E: An interim report of a double-blind placebo-controlled recanalisation study of anisoylated plasminogen streptokinase activator complex in acute myocardial infarction. *Drugs* 1987;33(Suppl 3):146–150.
49. PRIMI Trial Study Group: Randomised double-blind trial of recombinant pro-urokinase against streptokinase in acute myocardial infarction. *Lancet* 1989;1:863–867.
50. Chesebro JH, Knatterud G, Roberts R, et al: Thrombolysis in Myocardial Infarction (TIMI) trial, phase I: A comparison between intravenous tissue plasminogen activator and intravenous streptokinase; clinical findings through hospital discharge. *Circulation* 1987;76:142–154.
51. Verstraete M, Bernard R, Bory M, et al: Randomised trial of intravenous recombinant tissue-type plasminogen activator versus intravenous streptokinase in acute myocardial infarction. *Lancet* 1985;1:842–847.
52. Verstraeta M, Bleifeld W, Brower RW: Double-blind randomised trial of intravenous tissue-type plasminogen activator versus placebo in acute myocardial infarction. *Lancet* 1985;2:965–969.
53. Kennedy JW, Ritchie JL, Davis KB, Fritz JK: Western Washington randomized trial of intracoronary streptokinase in acute myocardial infarction. *N Engl J Med* 1983;309:1477–1482.
54. Hogg KJ, Gemmill JD, Burns JM, et al: Angiographic patency study of anistreplase versus streptokinase in acute myocardial infarction. *Lancet* 1990;1:254–258.
55. Anderson JL, Rothbard RL, Hackworthy RA, et al: Multicenter Reperfusion Trial of Intravenous anisoylated plasminogen streptokinase activator complex (APSAC) in acute myocardial infarction: Controlled comparison with intracoronary streptokinase in acute infarction: Controlled comparison with IC streptokinase. *J Am Coll Cardiol* 1988; 11:1153–1163.
56. Topol EJ, George BS, Kereiakes DJ, et al: A randomized controlled trial of intravenous tissue plasminogen activator and early intravenous heparin in acute myocardial infarction. *Circulation* 1989;79: 281–286.
57. Verstraete M, Arnold AER, Brower RW, et al: Acute coronary thrombolysis with recombinant human tissue-type plasminogen activator: Initial patency and influence of maintained infusion on reocclusion rate. *Am J Cardiol* 1987;60:231–237.
58. Simoons ML, Arnold AER, Betriu A, et al: Thrombolysis with tissue plasminogen activator in acute myocardial infarction: No additional benefit from immediate percutaneous coronary angioplasty. *Lancet* 1988;1:197–203.
59. Ellis SG, Topol EJ, Galleson L, et al: Predictors of success for coronary angioplasty performed for acute myocardial infarction. *J Am Coll Cardiol* 1988; 12:1407–1415.
60. Fuster V, Stein B, Badimon L, Chesebro JH: Antithrombotic therapy after myocardial reperfusion in acute myocardial infarction. *J Am Coll Cardiol* 1988;12(Suppl):78A–84A.

61. Stein B, Fuster V, Halperin JL, Chesebro JH: Antithrombotic therapy in cardiac disease: An emerging approach based on pathogenesis and risk. *Circulation* 1989;80:1501–1513.

62. Gold HK, Coller BS, Yasuda T, et al: Rapid and sustained coronary artery recanalization with combined bolus injection of recombinant tissue-type plasminogen activator and monoclonal antiplatelet GPIIb/IIIa antibody in a canine preparation. *Circulation* 1988;77:670–677.

63. Haskel EJ, Adams SP, Feigen LP, et al: Prevention of reoccluding platelet-rich thrombi in canine femoral arteries with a novel peptide antagonist of platelet glycoprotein IIb/IIIa receptors. *Circulation* 1989;80:1775–1782.

64. Heras M, Chesebro JH, Penny WJ, Bailey KR, Badimon L, Fuster V: Effects of thrombin inhibition on the development of acute platelet-thrombus deposition during angioplasty in pigs: Heparin versus recombinant hirudin, a specific thrombin inhibitor. *Circulation* 1989;79:657–665.

65. Topol EJ for the GUSTO IIb Investigators: A comparison of recombinant hirudin versus heparin for the treatment of acute coronary syndromes. *J Am Coll Cardiol* 1996;27 (abstr).

69. Gruppo Italiano per lo Studio della Streptochinase nell'Infarto Miocardico (GISSI): Effectiveness of intravenous thrombolytic treatment in acute myocardial infarction. *Lancet* 1986;1:397–401.

70. Wilcox RG, von der Lippe G, Olsson CG, Jensen G, Skene AM, Hampton JR: Trial of tissue plasminogen activator for mortality reduction in acute myocardial infarction: Anglo-Scandinavian study of early thrombolysis (ASSET). *Lancet* 1988;2:525–530.

72. Hands ME, Rutherford JD, Muller JE, et al: The in-hospital development of cardiogenic shock after myocardial infarction: Incidence, predictors of occurrence, outcome and prognostic factors. The MILIS Study Group. *J Am Coll Cardiol* 1989;14:40–46.

73. Killip T: Cardiogenic shock complicating myocardial infarction. *J Am Coll Cardiol* 1989;14:47–48.

74. Scheidt S, Ascheim R, Killip T III: Shock after acute myocardial infarction: A clinical and hemodynamic profile. *Am J Cardiol* 1970;26:556–564.

75. Hurtado L, Santome J, Fernandez C: Acute myocardial infarction with cardiogenic shock. *Arch Inst Cardiol Mex* 1984;54:121–129.

76. Killip T III, Kimball JT: Treatment of myocardial infarction in a coronary care unit: A two year experience with 250 patients. *Am J Cardiol* 1967;20:457–464.

77. Bolooki H: Emergency cardiac procedures in patients in cardiogenic shock due to complications of coronary artery disease. *Circulation* 1989;79(Suppl I):I-137–I-148.

78. Phillips SJ, Kongtahworn C, Skinner JR, Zeff RH: Emergency coronary artery reperfusion: A choice therapy for evolving myocardial infarction: Results in 339 patients. *J Thorac Cardiovasc Surg* 1983;86:679–688.

80. Califf RM, O'Neil W, Stack RS, et al: Failure of simple clinical measurements to predict perfusion status after intravenous thrombolysis. *Ann Intern Med* 1988;108:658–662.

81. Kircher RJ, Topol EJ, O'Neill WW, Pitt B: Prediction of infarct coronary artery recanalization after intravenous thrombolytic therapy. *Am J Cardiol* 1987;59:513–515.

82. Krucoff MW, Jackson YR, Burdette DL, et al: Digital real-time 12-lead ST segment trends: A bedside noninvasive monitor of infarct vessel patency (abstract). *Circulation* 1989;80(Suppl II):II-354.

83. Hogg KJ, Hornung RS, Howie CA, Hockings N, Dunn FG, Hillis WS: Electrocardiographic prediction of coronary artery patency after thrombolytic treatment in acute myocardial infarction: Use of the ST segment as a non-invasive marker. *Br Heart J* 1988;60:275–280.

84. Roberts R: Reperfusion and the plasma isoforms of creatine kinase isoenzymes: A clinical perspective. *J Am Coll Cardiol* 1987;9:464–466.

85. Puleo PR, Perryman MB, Bresser MA, Rokey R, Pratt CM, Roberts R: Creatine kinase isoform analysis in the detection and assessment of thrombolysis in man. *Circulation* 1987;75:1162–1169.

86. Katus HA, Diederich KW, Schwarz F, Uellner M, Scheffold T, Kübler W: Influence of reperfusion on serum concentrations of cytosolic creatine kinase and structural myosin light chains in acute myocardial infarction. *Am J Cardiol* 1987;60:440–445.

87. Garabedian HD, Gold HK, Yasuda T, et al: Detection of coronary artery reperfusion with creatine kinase-MB determinations during thrombolytic therapy: Correlation with acute angiography. *J Am Coll Cardiol* 1988;11:729–734.

88. van der Laarse A, van der Wall EE, van den Pol RC, et al: Rapid enzyme release from acutely infarcted myocardium after early thrombolytic

therapy: Washout or reperfusion damage? *Am Heart J* 1988;115:711–716.

89. de Zwaan C, Willems GM, Vermeer F, et al: Enzyme tests in the evaluation of thrombolysis in acute myocardial infarction. *Br Heart J* 1988;59: 175–183.

90. Ellis AK, Little T, Masud ARZ, Klocke FJ: Patterns of myoglobin release after reperfusion of injured myocardium. *Circulation* 1987;1:25–33.

91. Abendschein D, Seacord LM, Nohara R, Sobel BE, Jaffe AS: Prompt detection of myocardial injury by assay of creatine kinase isoforms in initial plasma samples. *Clin Cardiol* 1988;11:661–664.

92. Seacord LM, Abendschein DR, Nohara R, Hartzler G, Sobel BE, Jaffe AS: Detection of reperfusion within 1 hour after coronary recanalisation by analysis of isoforms of the MM creatine kinase isoenzyme in plasma. *Fibrinolysis* 1988;2:151–156.

93. Tsukamoto H, Hashimoto H, Matsui Y, et al: Detection of myocardial reperfusion by analysis of serum creatine kinase isoforms. *Clin Cardiol* 1988; 11:287–291.

94. Williams DO, Borer J, Braunwald E, et al: Intravenous recombinant tissue-type plasminogen activator in patients with acute myocardial infarction: A report from the NHLBI Thrombolysis in Myocardial Infarction trial. *Circulation* 1986;73:338–346.

95. Williams DO, Braunwald E, Knatterud G, et al: The Thrombolysis in Myocardial Infarction (TIMI) Trial: Outcome at one year of patients randomized to either invasive or conservative management. *Circulation* 1989;80(Suppl II):II-519.

96. Califf RM, Topol EJ, George BS, et al: Characteristics and outcome of patients in whom reperfusion with intravenous tissue-type plasminogen activator fails: Results of the Thrombolysis and Angioplasty in Myocardial Infarction (TAMI) I trial. *Circulation* 1988;77:1090–1099.

97. O'Connor CM, Mark DB, Hinohara T, et al: Rescue coronary angioplasty after failure of intravenous streptokinase in acute myocardial infarction: In-hospital and long-term outcomes. *J Inv Car* 1989;1:85–95.

99. Neuhaus K-L, Feuerer W, Jeep-Tebbe S, Niederer W, Vogt A, Tebbe U: Improved thrombolysis with a modified dose regimen of recombinant tissue type plasminogen activator. *J Am Coll Cardiol* 1989;14:1566–1569.

100. Grines CL, Nissen SE, Booth DC, et al: Efficacy, safety and cost effectiveness of a new thrombolytic regimen for acute myocardial infarction using half dose tPA with full dose streptokinase. *J Am Coll Cardiol* 1989;14:573–581.

101. Topol EJ, Califf RM, George BS, et al: Coronary arterial thrombolysis with combined infusion of recombinant tissue-type plasminogen activator and urokinase in patients with acute myocardial infarction. *Circulation* 1988;77:1100–1107.

102. Baim DS, Braunwald E, Feit F, et al: The Thrombolysis in Myocardial Infarction (TIMI) Trial Phase II: Additional information and perspectives. *J Am Coll Cardiol* 1990;15:1188–1192.

103. Özbek C, Dyckmans J, Sen S, Schieffer H, and the SIAM Study Group. Comparison of invasive and conservative strategies after treatment with streptokinase in acute myocardial infarction. Results of a randomised trial (SIAM). *J Am Coll Cardiol* 1990;15(Suppl A):63A.

104. Califf RM, Topol EJ, George BS, et al: TAMI 5: A randomized trial of combination thrombolytic therapy and immediate cardiac catheterization (abstract). *Circulation* 1989;80(Suppl II):II-418.

105. Baim DS, Diver DJ, Knatterud GL, and the TIMI II-A Investigators: PTCA "salvage" for thrombolytic failures—implications from TIMI II-A (abstract). *Circulation* 1988;78(Suppl II):II-112.

23

Acute Myocardial Infarction: The Role of Bypass Surgery

Hartzell V. Schaff, MD

INTRODUCTION

Operation for mechanical complications of myocardial infarction (MI) is discussed in Chapter 16, and this chapter reviews isolated, direct coronary artery bypass (CAB) during and early following acute MI. In the United States, approximately 13% of patients treated for acute MI will undergo CAB prior to hospital dismissal, and in the Global Utilization of Streptokinase and Tissue Plasminogen Activator for Occluded Coronary Arteries trial (GUSTO-I), use of CAB early after infarction varied from 9% to 17% in different geographical regions (1). Utilization of CAB early after MI also differs by country (2). In general, invasive procedures are employed more often when patients are initially admitted to facilities where cardiac catheterization is available compared with centers without catheterization laboratories (1).

Geographical differences in utilization of invasive procedures early after MI correlate directly with rates of cardiac catheterization (see Ch. 30). For example, in Texas, 15% of Medicare patients with acute MI underwent CAB within 90 days of infarction compared with 13% in New York; yet for patients with three diseased vessels or stenosis of the left main coronary artery, rates of CAB were similar (3). It is of interest that this same study found a much greater difference in utilization of coronary angioplasty after MI (15% versus 7%) compared with CAB.

Patients with acute MI may be referred for operation in an effort to limit size of the MI, to prevent early reinfarction when critical coronary lesions are discovered on angiography, or to control symptoms of unstable angina. Surgical revascularization may also be recommended for patients who have had successful reperfusion by thrombolysis or balloon recanalization but are left with residual, critical stenoses in the infarct-related artery and/or other major vessels. Cardiac surgeons are called on to treat an increasing number of such patients as a result of the widespread acceptance of acute intervention and early angiography after MI.

A final consideration that may prompt surgical referral is suspicion of hibernating myocardium in patients with left ventricular failure. The concept of reversible ischemic injury is well established, and some patients with left ventricular dysfunction after MI may benefit from surgical revascularization in terms of recovery of ventricular function even when the operation is performed after the critical 24 to 48 hours following acute injury. Indeed, Dreyfus and colleagues reported that survival of patients with ischemic cardiomyopathy having revascularization exceeds 85% at 2 years, and measured ejection fraction improved from 23% to 39% (4). Care should be taken in extrapolation of these very good results, because none of the patients were operated on early after MI, and all had myocardial viability documented by thallium scintigraphy and/or positron emission tomography.

PATHOPHYSIOLOGIC CONSIDERATIONS

The general availability of thrombolytic therapy and balloon angioplasty has relegated CAB to a secondary role for initial therapy for reperfusion of MI. It should be noted, however, that early studies of surgical treatment of acute MI by DeWood and colleagues (5–12) contributed importantly to our understanding of the pathophysiology of acute ischemic syndromes and established the safety of early angiography and CAB in selected patients. Further, there are possible physiologic advantages of controlled surgical reperfusion compared with angioplasty or thrombolytic therapy, and operation may be beneficial in certain subsets of patients who are not candidates for conventional treatment.

Traditional views of reversibility of myocardial damage were based on controlled laboratory experiments of ischemia and reperfusion of isolated myocardial segments in which cell death begins within 20 to 30 minutes of normothermic ischemia. In canine studies of acute coronary occlusion, irreversible myocardial necrosis develops in 60% of the area at risk within 4 hours, and the remaining 40% of area at risk is destroyed 12 to 24 hours after occlusion (see Ch. 2) (13). However, these and other studies (14–20) that attempt to define the course of ischemic myocyte injury in animals suffer from the inability to model the complex interplay of variations in coronary anatomy (and atherosclerotic disease), collateralization, preexisting ischemia, and oxygen demands, which modify infarct size in patients.

Among clinicians there is general acceptance of the potential for reversibility of myocardial dysfunction associated with acute infarction, especially if reperfusion is prompt. Thrombolytic therapy and coronary angioplasty can be instituted more quickly than CAB, but surgical reperfusion offers a unique opportunity to modify conditions of reperfusion and maximize myocardial salvage.

The wide variation in operative methods in coronary artery surgery (21–28) attests to our incomplete understanding of myocardial protection, but several aspects appear critically important for successful reperfusion in acute ischemia. During operation, myocardial ischemia/infarction is limited by instituting full cardiopulmonary bypass with venting of the left ventricle in order to minimize energy expenditure and optimize the myocardial oxygen supply/demand ratio (29,30). Decompression of the left ventricle reduces oxygen consumption of the dyskinetic segment (31), and this is especially important during reperfusion to limit structural damage and ensure immediate functional recovery (Fig. 23–1) (29). As coronary artery bypasses are constructed, the heart should be protected with blood-based cardioplegia, which produces diastolic arrest and can serve as a vehicle for administration of calcium-blocking agents (32), antioxidants such as allopurinol and coenzyme Q10 (33), and metabolic substrates including oxygen, glucose, and glutamate and aspartate (Krebs' cycle intermediates). Further, tissue acidosis can be mitigated by alkaline perfusates, and cell swelling and interstitial edema may be prevented by hyperosmolar perfusion (34). After bypass grafts are opened, the previously ischemic area can be reperfused at optimal pressure

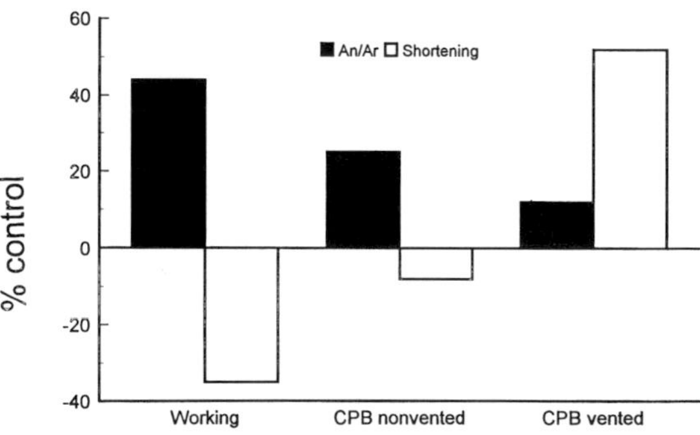

Figure 23–1. After 2 hours of regional ischemia, unmodified reperfusion in a working heart produced a large area of injury (relationship of area of necrosis to area of risk = An/Ar) and marked regional dyskinesia. Reperfusion during cardiopulmonary bypass was most effective with complete venting of the left ventricle. *Modified from Allen et al (29), with permission.*

and flow, with modulation of perfusate composition (35,36).

In addition to providing practical guidelines for clinical practice, laboratory studies of surgical reperfusion challenge fundamental concepts of assessment of ischemic injury (see Ch. 3). For example, postischemic myocardial adenosine triphosphate (ATP) levels do not correlate with functional recovery if reperfusion is controlled and amino acid substrate is added to blood cardioplegia (37). Controlled surgical reperfusion permits functional recovery in myocardium that, by vital staining with triphenyltetrazolium chloride, appears infarcted. Barnard and associates reported that following 2 hours of regional ischemia, the ratio of the area of necrosis to the area of myocardium at risk was similar in hearts with unmodified (medical) reperfusion and in hearts reperfused on cardiopulmonary bypass with blood or cardioplegia (Fig. 23–2) (38). However, systolic function of the reperfused region was dramatically improved with controlled reperfusion during cardiopulmonary bypass. If conditions of reperfusion are controlled, myocardial infarct size correlates directly with duration of ischemia and inversely with return of systolic function in the ischemic zone. As illustrated in Fig. 23–3, controlled reperfusion permits immediate return of regional myocardial function after ischemic intervals as long as 6 hours (39).

Surgical revascularization, when complete, may salvage myocardium by preventing damage to remote areas. When coronary artery disease is limited to the artery supplying the infarcted zone, blood flow to distant regions increases as these segments become hyperdynamic. When remote myocardium is supplied by stenotic arteries, these remote areas may not demonstrate the compensatory increase in contractility, and regional function may diminish (Fig. 23–4) (40). Indeed, ischemia of remote areas may be an important contributing factor to cardiogenic shock following myocardial infarction.

Laboratory experiments have also documented that late return of systolic function is improved by

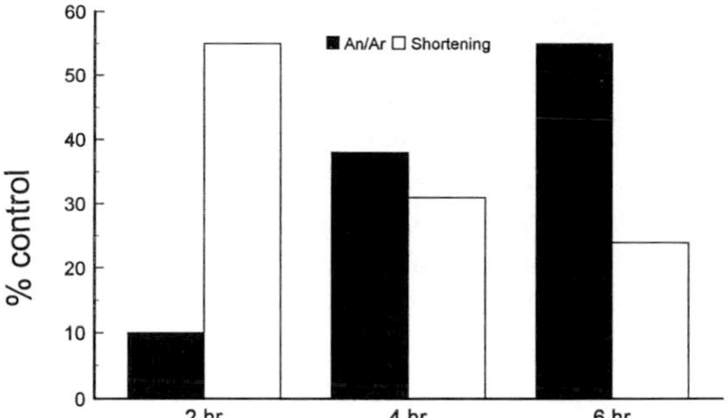

Figure 23–3. Recovery of regional myocardial function immediately after reperfusion. In control (working) hearts reperfused after 2 hours of regional ischemia, there was passive systolic lengthening of the ischemic region. In contrast, hearts regained substantial systolic function after controlled reperfusion on cardiopulmonary bypass even when the ischemic interval extended to 6 hours. *Modified from Allen et al (39), with permission.*

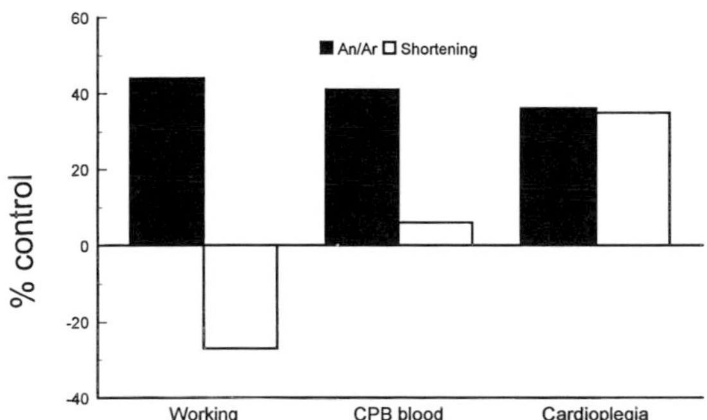

Figure 23–2. Myocardial damage under varied conditions and composition of reperfusion following two hours of regional ischemia. Relationships of area of necrosis to area of risk (An/Ar) were similar in the three groups that differed significantly in percent recovery of systolic shortening. *Modified from Barnard et al (38), with permission.*

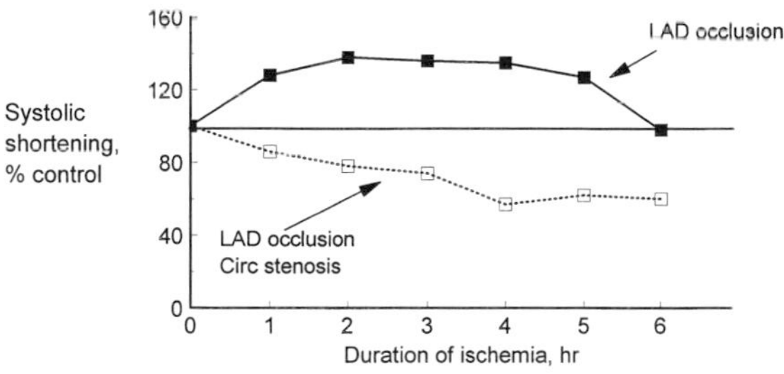

Figure 23–4. With acute occlusion of the left anterior descending coronary artery (LAD), there is enhanced contraction of the zone supplied by the unobstructed circumflex coronary artery (Circ.) If occlusion of the left anterior descending occurs with 50% stenosis of the circumflex coronary artery, regional function in this area is impaired. *Modified from Beyersdorf et al (40), with permission.*

controlled reperfusion. Cheung and colleagues studied reperfusion in a canine model of acute MI, which produced regional dyskinesia during 2-hour occlusion (41). Regional dyskinesia persisted during 2 hours of unmodified reflow, but with substrate-enriched blood cardioplegia and controlled reperfusion, systolic contraction of the "infarcted" area returned. After 7 days, there was similar return of systolic function (approximately 20% of control) in animals with permanent occlusion and those with unmodified reperfusion. Animals with surgical reperfusion, however, regained 50% of preischemic systolic shortening.

CORONARY ARTERY BYPASS AS DEFINITIVE TREATMENT FOR ACUTE MYOCARDIAL INFARCTION

Urgent surgical revascularization for acute MI has not been widely accepted because of logistical and time constraints, uncertainty of the ultimate value of reperfusion in limiting infarct size, and perceived high perioperative risk. The obvious advantages of CAB include immediate restoration of coronary blood flow to jeopardized areas that are not irreversibly injured and potential for revascularization of other diseased arteries. The ultimate goals are to reduce acute in-hospital mortality, which is approximately 10% to 15% in medically treated patients (Table 23–1), and to prevent recurrent angina and infarction.

DeWood and associates (5–12) and Phillips et al (48,49) were early advocates of surgical reperfusion for acute MI. In the experience of DeWood and colleagues with 701 patients undergoing surgical reperfusion for acute MI, early hospital mortality was 4.4% (31/701), and it was higher in the 440 patients with transmural infarction (5.2%) compared with those with non-Q wave infarction (3.1%). This difference in mortality increased during postoperative follow-up extending to 8 years (Fig. 23–5). Additionally, the interval to reperfusion influenced early and late mortality in patients with *transmural* infarctions; survival was significantly better in patients who had restoration of blood flow within 6 hours of chest pain (Fig. 23–6).

The difficulty in making extrapolations from these data has been discussed widely, and Spencer pointed out that myocardial protection was evolving during the study interval, and optimal methods for myocardial salvage were not utilized (50). Also, the series was not consecutive or randomized. In fact, DeWood et al (5) stated, "patients with known extensive preexisting damage (caused by known coronary disease) are usually not recruited aggressively for arteriographic examination and therefore are not offered reperfusion during early myocardial infarction." This selection process necessarily biased results—59% of the transmural infarction patients were in NYHA class I, 25% were in class II,

Table 23–1. Risk of Death Early After Acute MI in Patients Treated in Coronary Care Units

			Mortality	
Study	Time Period	Patients	Current Treatment*	Without Reperfusion**
ASSET (42)	1986–1987	9,955	12.8	14.7
Cairns (43)	1980	810	17.0	17
Cragg (44)	1986–1988	1,374	17.0	19
Ericsson (45)	1984–1985	773	12.9	NR
Goldberg (46)	1975–1988	4,762	18.2	18.9
Total		17,674	13.8 (1,981/14,336)	16.3 (2,077/12,731)

NR, Not reported.

*Current medical treatment includes use of thrombolysis in 10% to 25% of eligible patients.

**Mortality with current therapy, without thrombolysis either because of early study or patients ineligible.

Table modified from Allen et al (47).

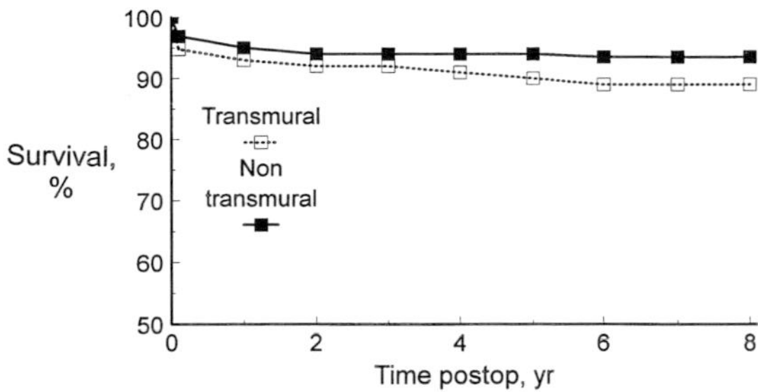

Figure 23–5. Survival following surgical reperfusion for acute myocardial infarction. Patients are stratified according to presence (transmural) or absence (nontransmural) of Q waves on the electrocardiogram. *Modified from DeWood et al (5), with permission.*

and only 10% were in class IV. Only 15% of patients had prior MI, and 29% had single-vessel disease.

To address these possible weaknesses, DeWood and associates performed further analysis of 387 patients having medical or surgical treatment of acute MI who were followed for 10 to 13 years (mean 11.4) (11). Medical and surgical patients had similar distributions for variables such as mean age, sex distribution, previous MI, area of infarction, number of vessels diseased, and clinical classification. The hospital mortality of the medical group was 11.5% (23 of 200) versus 5.8% (11 of 187) for patients having emergency CAB (p = 0.07); early reperfusion (≤6 hours) was associated with an early mortality rate of 2% (2 of 100) versus 11.5% for medically treated patients and 10.3% (9 of 87) for surgically treated patients who had reperfusion more than 6 hours after onset of chest pain.

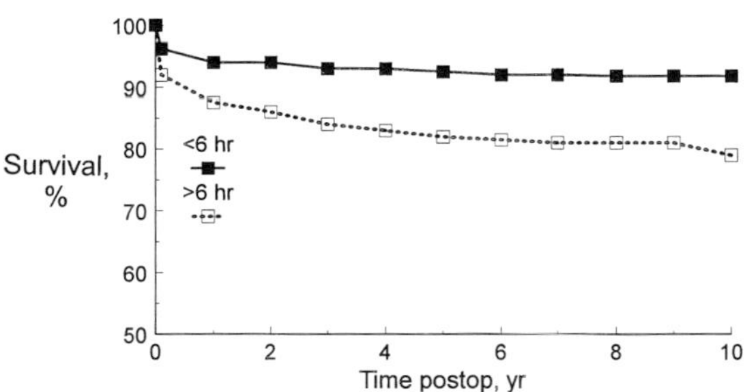

Figure 23–6. Among patients who had surgical reperfusion for transmural myocardial infarction, in-hospital and late survival was significantly better in those who had early reperfusion (≤6 hours) compared with those who had reperfusion later. *Modified from DeWood et al (5), with permission.*

Among survivors of hospitalization, risk of subsequent sudden death in medical patients was 17.5% versus 7.4% in the surgical group (p = 0.01). After adjustment for risk factors by the Cox model, late survival rate of the surgically treated patients was 73% compared with 59% for the medical group (p = 0.0007). There was no difference in late risk of MI in the two groups, but mortality associated with reinfarction was higher in patients who had initial medical therapy—36.6% versus 17.5% (p = 0.04)—and was not influenced by time of reperfusion.

In patients with anterior wall MI, late survival was enhanced by surgical reperfusion before or after the 6-hour mark from onset of chest pain, but regional function was improved only in patients who had reflow established early (12). In contrast, with inferior wall Q wave infarction, overall survival was improved only in patients who had early reperfusion.

The relative importance of time of onset of surgical reperfusion is not completely settled. If all other factors are equal, earlier reperfusion would be expected to result in better outcome and myocardial salvage (see Chs. 2, 9). However, Phillips et al. (48,49) and Kirklin and associates (51) found no relationship between in-hospital mortality and the interval between infarct and operation. Athanasuleas and coworkers analyzed risk factors for early death among 83 patients having CAB during acute evolving MI (52). Time to reperfusion did not influence outcome nor did the infarct-related artery. Overall mortality was 15.6%, and risk was increased in patients with cardiogenic shock, age >65 years, left ventricular ejection fraction ≤0.30, cardiac index ≤2.0 L/min/m^2, and absent collateral coronary blood flow. Other important findings in this study were bypass graft patency rate of 94% and improvement in left ventricular ejection fraction from 39 to 49% ($p < 0.05$). It is likely that refinements in myocardial protection with controlled reperfusion have and will continue to expand the time window for myocardial salvage.

In contrast to the many randomized trials of surgical revascularization for other clinical syndromes of coronary artery disease, there has been only one randomized comparison of medical and surgical treatment of acute MI. Koshal and coworkers studied 68 patients with acute evolving MI who presented within 4 hours of onset of chest pain. Randomly assigned medical and surgical groups were comparable for age, sex, and location of infarct, and CAB was completed at an average interval of 4 ± 1 hours after onset of chest pain (53). There was 1 early and no late deaths among the 34 surgically treated patients (total mortality 2.9%), and 3 early and 4 late deaths among medically treated patients (total mortality 20.6%). Radionuclide global ejection fraction at 48 hours after admission was 45 ± 15% for the medical group versus 50 ± 15% for the surgical group; at 3 months, mean ejection fractions in the two groups were identical (Fig. 23–7). Like DeWood's investigation, this study also suggests some improvement in survival in surgically treated patients, but the authors cautioned that early assessment of left ventricular function in unoperated patients may be misleading because improvement can be expected. An alternative explanation is that ejection fraction of the medically treated group only appears to improve because those who die probably had ventricular dysfunction and were not available for late study.

Few clinical data are available that compare surgical reperfusion versus thrombolysis or percutaneous transluminal coronary angioplasty (PTCA) for acute MI. Patients who have urgent surgical revascularization are highly selected, and many have had unsuccessful thrombolysis and/or angioplasty, which delays operation. Nevertheless, the early outcome of such patients is excellent. Allen and associates (47) summarized results of nine published series of CAB for acute MI (Table 23–2). Although timing of operation and techniques varied, overall mortality was relatively low (5.2%).

When left ventricular failure occurs in MI, risk of hospital death increases dramatically; death occurs in as many as 75% of patients treated with only supportive measures (Table 23–3). Uncontrolled reperfusion by thrombolysis or coronary angioplasty appears to reduce this mortality to 40% to 70%. Although surgical revascularization has been used selectively for patients in cardiogenic shock after MI, early results show survival in approximately 70% of patients, and rigid adherence to principles of controlled reperfusion may yield even better results (see Ch. 13). In Allen's recent report of outcome in 66 patients with preoperative shock having emergency revascularization, early mortality was only 9% (47).

Taken together, these laboratory and clinical studies demonstrate a clear benefit of CAB for acute MI. Myocardium can be salvaged with prompt surgical revascularization, and current methods of controlling reperfusion may further enhance myocardial recovery. However, emergency CAB cannot and should not be applied to all patients, and the greatest clinical challenge in the next decade will be to identify subsets of patients eligible for reperfusion who would be best served by operation.

At present, it seems reasonable to consider emergency CAB for patients with multivessel disease in whom revascularization can be achieved within 6 to 8 hours of chest pain. Others with anterior MI due to occlusion of large anterior descending coronary arteries may also be helped by CAB, especially if reperfusion cannot be accomplished with thrombolysis or percutaneous transluminal coronary angioplasty.

Cardiologists and others who care for patients with acute MI should be aware of the benefits and limitations of reperfusion by CAB. Optimal surgical results and efficient use of facilities require co-

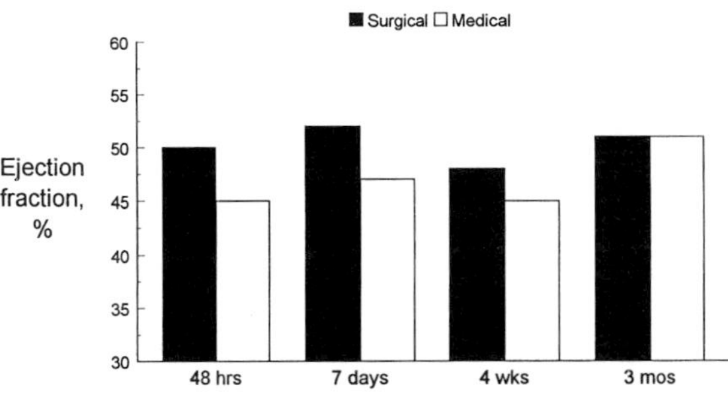

Figure 23–7. Left ventricular ejection fraction obtained by radionuclide angiography at 48 hours, 7 days, 4 weeks, and 3 months following myocardial infarction. The small advantage in ejection fraction in the surgical groups was not maintained 3 months postinfarct because of improvement in ejection fraction in the medically treated patients. *Modified from Koshal et al (53), with permission.*

Table 23–2. Risk of Death Early After Acute Myocardial Infarction in Patients Treated by Coronary Artery Bypass

				Cardiogenic Shock	
Series	No. of Patients	Time (hr)	Mortality (%)	Incidence (%)	Mortality (%)
Ansel (54)	40	0.5–3.0	7.5	NR	NR
DeWood (5)	440	5.3	5.2	9.7	28
Flameng (55)	48	2.8	8.3	46	18.2
Kirklin (51)	35	11.9	2.9	11	0
Koshal (53)	34	4.3	2.9	0	0
Berg (56)	54	<6	3.7	NR	NR
Phillips (57)	261	8	5.7	13	24
Turina (58)	34	Within hours	8.8	NR	NR
Vidne (59)	68	8	1.5	NR	NR
Total	1,014	6	5.2 (53/1,014)	13 (103/818)	23 (24/103)

NR, Not reported.

Table modified from Allen et al (47).

ordination and close communication between cardiologists, angiographers, and surgeons. All too often, CAB is considered only after protracted efforts to establish reperfusion by catheter techniques, and the added ischemic time and trauma to the patient reduce the chance of a satisfactory outcome with operation.

Table 23–3. Incidence and Risk of Death Among Patients with Cardiogenic Shock After Acute Myocardial Infarction

Treatment	No. of Patients	Incidence %* (range)	Mortality (%)
CCU (no reperfusion) (46,60–64)	525	8.8 (7–19)	79
Uncontrolled reperfusion			
Medical			
Thrombolysis (65–67)	514	1.9 (1.6–5)	70
PTCA (68–70)	114	10 (8–13)	43
Surgical			
Failed PTCA (71–78)	150	21 (12–35)	29
Acute MI (5,51,55,57)	103	13 (0–46)	23
Controlled reperfusion (47)	66	42	9

CCU, cardiac care unit; MI, myocardial infarction.

*Average percent.

Table modified from Allen et al (47).

CORONARY ARTERY BYPASS FOR UNSTABLE ANGINA EARLY AFTER MYOCARDIAL INFARCTION

While opinions among cardiac surgeons and cardiologists may differ on the value of CAB for acute reperfusion, clinicians' views on usefulness of surgical revascularization for unstable angina after MI are generally uniform. Reports (79,80) of high operative mortality in unstable patients with acute MI generally reflect early methods of preoperative care, anesthetic management, and myocardial protection, which would be considered inadequate by contemporary standards. Also, we now recognize that there is a continuum of clinical syndromes between unstable angina and completed transmural (Q wave) infarction, and it is likely that some patients in these previous reports had evolving MI rather than reversible ischemia.

Occurrence of angina (or its physiologic equivalent) at rest or with little exercise early after MI identifies patients who have high risk for recurrent infarction or cardiac death. Shuster and Bulkley reported that 6-month mortality was 44% for patients with ischemia in the region of an acute MI and 72% for patients in whom ischemia after acute MI occurred in distant myocardium (81). Other studies suggest that risk of early death is lower in patients with subendocardial MI compared with transmural infarction (9% versus 12%), but risk of reinfarction following subendocardial infarction is 21% within 9 months (82) (see Ch. 18). Marmor and associates found that recurrent infarction developed in 42% of patients with subendocardial infarction, and mortality (16%) was more than twice that observed in patients without recurrent ischemia (83).

Management of patients with unstable postinfarction angina changed radically during the past decade. Roberts and coworkers advocated intensive medical stabilization of patients with postinfarction angina in hopes of lowering operative mortality and perioperative myocardial damage (84). Although angina can be controlled in most instances, such patients will have restricted activities and continued jeopardy from critically narrowed vessels; unless the additional risk of early surgical revascularization is substantial, both physicians and patients prefer definitive revascularization during the same hospitalization. As experience has accumulated, it has become clear that operative risk is acceptably low for most subsets of patients with unstable postinfarction angina.

Table 23–4 summarizes recent published data on operative risk of early CAB for postinfarction angina. Precise estimation of operative risk is difficult because many contemporary surgical reviews of CAB within 30 days of MI have included other clinical subgroups such as those with little or no angina but "compelling anatomy" (proximal high-grade narrowing of one or more of the three major coronary vessels), who may have lower operative mortality, as well as patients with severe left ventricular failure, who have high operative risk. A reasonable estimate of perioperative risk for patients with unstable angina early after MI is 5%.

Patients undergoing surgical revascularization can be stratified further into high- and low-risk groups. As might be expected, the presence of unstable hemodynamic condition and/or angina pectoris that is so severe that intraaortic balloon counterpulsation is required defines patients at highest risk for postoperative death. Naunheim and associates reported an operative risk of 6.1% for patients with unstable postinfarction angina without shock and a risk of 47.8% for revascularization in patients with severe postinfarction ischemia or infarct extension complicated by cardiogenic shock (92). Similarly, Connolly et al found that for patients undergoing CAB within 6 weeks of MI, perioperative mortality was 28% in those with cardiogenic shock compared with 3.7% for those with unstable angina (93).

Even if one accepts the advisability of early operation for unstable postinfarction angina, there remains an important, practical question of whether any delay, e.g., 1 or 2 weeks, will lessen operative mortality and morbidity. Unfortunately, all retrospective studies of timing of operation are flawed by potential bias in patient selection; highly unstable patients and those with large amounts of myocardium in jeopardy are more likely to have urgent

Table 23–4. Outcome of Coronary Artery Bypass for Unstable Angina After Acute Myocardial Infarction

First Author	Year	No. of Pts	Mean Age	Interval MI–CAB	3-VD % Pts	LMCA % Pts	Preop EF	Early Death No.	Risk	70% C.L.
Breyer (85)	1985	75	61	<30d	76%	20%	54%	6	8.0%	4.8%, 11.2%
Jones (86)	1987	107		<30d				9	8.4%	5.6%, 11.2%
Naunheim (87)	1988	185	NA	<30d	NA	NA	NA	12	6.5%	4.6%, 8.4%
Connolly (88)	1988	96	65	<42d	NA	28%	48%	7	7.3%	4.5%, 10.0%
Kouchoukos (89)	1989	240	63	<30d	70%	13%	NA	8	3.3%	2.1%, 4.5%
Gardner (90)	1989	300	62	<30d	NA	NA	47%	15	5.0%	3.7%, 6.3%
Fremes (91)	1991	588	NA	<30d	68%	29%	NA	65	11.1%	8.5%, 13.6%
Total		1,591						122	7.6%	6.4%, 9.0%

NA = data not available; C.L. = 70% confidence limits; 3-VD = three-vessel disease; MI = myocardial infarction; CAB = coronary artery bypass; PO IABP = postoperative intraaortic balloon pump; Periop = perioperative.

revascularization compared with patients with less severe coronary stenoses whose symptoms are reduced by medical treatment. In a study of 145 patients having surgical revascularization within 4 weeks of MI, Katz and colleagues reported an overall operative mortality of 4.4% and a 26% incidence of postoperative cardiac failure (defined as need for intraaortic balloon pumping or catecholamine support exceeding 5 mcg/kg/min or its equivalent) (94). Logistic regression analysis indicated that preoperative left ventricular failure, reduced left ventricular ejection fraction, and preoperative ischemia (need for intravenous nitroglycerin) were independent predictors of postoperative cardiac failure; the time interval between MI and operation was not an important predictor of postoperative cardiac failure.

The combined influence of preoperative left ventricular dysfunction and interval to operation on operative risk was also studied by Hochberg and associates (95). In their series, no early deaths were observed among 50 patients with preoperative ejection fraction greater than 50% who underwent coronary bypass within 4 weeks of MI. When preoperative ejection fraction was less than 50%, however, operative risk was 22% for patients who had revascularization within 7 weeks of infarction, and risk decreased from approximately 50% when operation was undertaken within 2 weeks to 6% when operation was 6 to 7 weeks after MI (Fig. 23–8).

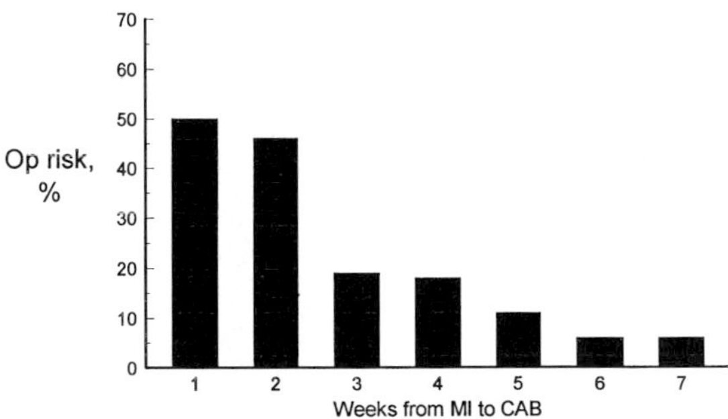

Figure 23–8. Among 124 patients with preoperative ejection fraction less than 0.50, risk of hospital death following coronary artery bypass (CAB) decreased substantially as interval between myocardial infarction (MI) and operation increased. Bars indicate upper 70% confidence interval of proportion. *Data from Hochberg et al (95).*

More recent clinical studies indicate that although there has been a general improvement in early outcome, operative risk for CAB performed within the first few days of acute MI is still higher than that for patients operated on 2 to 4 weeks after infarction (Fig. 23–9) (96). Multivariate analysis suggests that excess mortality of early operation is due to older age of patients and higher prevalence of emergency operation and preoperative renal failure.

Synthesizing these recent studies, we believe that patients with angina following MI should have intensive medical treatment and early angiography. If there is stenosis of the left main coronary artery (≥50%) and/or significant narrowings in two or three major vessels, CAB should be considered. Operation would be performed urgently in all patients who have persistent angina despite optimal medical management, which includes systemic anticoagulation with heparin and intravenous nitroglycerin; the only exceptions to this policy are those patients with advanced age and infirmity and/or serious associated medical illnesses. For patients with multivessel coronary disease whose angina after MI is controlled medically, we generally advise early operation if ventricular function is preserved; revascularization is delayed (2 to 4 weeks) if left ventricular function is significantly impaired (ejection fraction < 40%) in hopes of minimizing operative mortality. This policy seems prudent as long as patients whose operation is postponed can be followed closely.

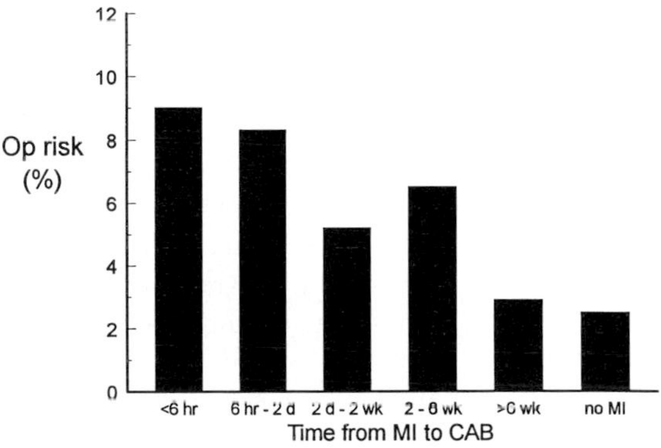

Figure 23–9. Operative risk stratified by interval from acute myocardial infarction to operation. *Data from Creswell et al (96).*

CORONARY ARTERY BYPASS EARLY AFTER THROMBOLYSIS

The emergence of thrombolytic therapy for MI has created a new and expanding subset of patients who are referred for coronary artery revascularization. Efficacy and methods of thrombolysis are discussed in detail in Chapters 19–21 and will not be reviewed here except to restate that successful dissolution of intracoronary thrombus often reveals high-grade fixed obstructions that are prone to reocclusion despite aggressive anticoagulation. Available data (Table 23–3) suggest that approximately 38% of patients treated with thrombolytic agents will undergo CAB during their initial hospitalization (68,97–102). In the Thrombolysis and Myocardial Infarction Trial Phase II (TIMI-II) 11.7% of 3,339 patients underwent coronary bypass surgery within 40 days after entry into the trial, 14% of whom underwent coronary bypass surgery within 24 hours after entry into the trial (107). Indications for operation include residual high-grade stenoses following successful thrombolysis, unsuccessful reperfusion by lytic therapy (or PTCA), and/or discovery of severe, diffuse coronary artery disease (103). In the Thrombolysis and Angioplasty for Myocardial Infarction (TAMI) trial, emergency CAB was performed in 24 of 386 consecutive patients (6%); operation was prompted by left main or equivalent coronary artery disease (7 patients), coronary anatomy unsuitable for angioplasty (4 patients), or unsuccessful angioplasty (13 patients) (101). Other groups have chosen to proceed with CAB in preference to angioplasty as the primary therapy for patients with multivessel coronary disease who have had successful thrombolysis (100).

Perioperative mortality rates were, respectively, 16.7% and 3.9% ($p < .001$) in patients undergoing surgery within 24 hours after entry into the trial or within 24 hours of coronary angioplasty in comparison with patients undergoing operation between 24 hours and 42 days after entry. Perioperative myocardial infarction rates were 5.6% and 6.2% respectively. On multivariate analysis, the only independent predictor of perioperative mortality was bypass surgery within 24 hours after entry or after coronary angioplasty. Among these patients in whom the prevalence of multivessel disease and the use of the internal thoracic artery were lower than in the remaining surgical patients. Among perioperative survivors however, the 1-year mortality rate after discharge was only 2.2% and 1.9% respectively in the two groups (107).

When CAB is undertaken after thrombolysis, risk of postoperative bleeding appears to be related to the interval between lytic therapy and operation. Lee and associates surveyed the literature and determined that there was no increase in postoperative bleeding or mortality in 329 patients who had CAB from 3.3 to 16 days after streptokinase infusion (104). In their institutional experience, however, postoperative blood loss and use of blood and blood products were considerably higher in patients who had revascularization within 12 hours of thrombolysis compared with controls or those who had later operation. In the TIMI-II trial major surgical hemorrhagic events (defined as a blood loss of >5 g/dl) occurred in 74.1% of patients operated on within 24 hours of study entry or coronary angioplasty and in 50.9% of patients undergoing bypass surgery within 24 hours to 42 days of study entry ($p = .002$) (108). The mean number of units transfused were 4.8 ± 4.4 U and 3.5 ± 3.0 U for patients in the two groups respectively (107).

A theoretical advantage of tissue plasminogen activator is clot specificity, which might preserve clotting factors. In the TAMI trial, however, excessive postoperative bleeding was noted in 4 of 24 patients (16.6%, 70% confidence limits 8.8% to 24.6%), and thrombolysis was the probable cause of the bleeding in 2 patients (5.6%, 70% confidence limits 2.5% to 14.1%) (101). The recent availability of the serine proteinase inhibitor, aprotinin, should greatly reduce postoperative bleeding in patients having preoperative thrombolysis. Aprotinin is a powerful antifibrinolytic that reduces postoperative bleeding in patients having primary coronary revascularization as well as in patients having reoperation for CAB (105). Thus aprotinin may be particularly useful to reverse the lytic state in patients having coronary revascularization early after thrombolysis (106).

SUMMARY

Early studies of CAB in acute MI established the effectiveness of early reperfusion in myocardial salvage. Indeed, basic concepts of pathogenesis of infarction and the critical role of intracoronary thrombus in acute coronary syndromes were defined in clinical studies of surgical revascularization. Although thrombolytic agents and PTCA have superseded surgery for most patients with acute infarction, there remains an important role for CAB in patients with unsuccessful reperfusion who have postinfarction angina and in subsets of patients with successful recanalization who have associated critical stenoses in other vessels and/or left main coronary artery narrowing. Surgical revascularization has the unique advantage of control of conditions of reperfusion, and recent laboratory studies indicate that ultimate myocardial salvage is greatly enhanced by optimization of reflow.

REFERENCES

1. Pilote L, Califf RM, Sapp S, et al: Regional variation across the United States in the management of acute myocardial infarction. *N Eng J Med* 1995;333:565–571.
2. Van de Werf F, Topol EJ, Lee KL, et al: Variations in patient management and outcomes for acute myocardial infarction in the United States and other countries: Results from the GUSTO trial. *JAMA* 1995;273:1586–1591.
3. Guadagnoli E, Hauptman PJ Ayanian JZ, et al: Variation in the use of cardiac procedures after acute myocardial infarction. *N Eng J Med* 1995;333:573–578.
4. Dreyfus GD, Duboc D, Blasco A, et al: Myocardial viability assessment in ischemic cardiomyopathy: Benefits of coronary revascularization. *Ann Thorac Surg* 1994;57:1402–1408.
5. DeWood MA, Spores J, Berg R Jr, et al: Acute myocardial infarction: A decade of experience with surgical reperfusion in 701 patients. *Circulation* 1983;68: II-8–II-16.
6. DeWood MA, Spores J, Notske RN, et al: Medical and surgical management of myocardial infarction. *Am J Cardiol* 1979;44:1356–1364.
7. DeWood MA, Heit J, Spores J, et al: Anterior transmural myocardial infarction: Effects of surgical coronary reperfusion on global and regional left ventricular function. *J Am Coll Cardiol* 1983;1:1223–1234.
8. Berg R Jr, Selinger SL, Leonard JJ, et al: Acute evolving myocardial infarction. A surgical emergency. *J Thorac Cardiovasc Surg* 1984;88:902–906.
9. DeWood MA, Berg R Jr: The role of surgical reperfusion in myocardial infarction (review). *Cardiol Clin* 1984;2:113–122.
10. DeWood MA, Selinger SL, Coleman WS, et al: Surgical coronary reperfusion during acute myocardial infarction. *Cardiovasc Clin* 1987;17:91–103.
11. DeWood MA, Notske RN, Berg R Jr, et al: Medical and surgical management of early Q wave myocardial infarction. I. Effects of surgical reperfusion on survival, recurrent myocardial infarction, sudden death and functional class at 10 or more years of follow-up. *J Am Coll Cardiol* 1989;14:65–77.
12. DeWood MA, Leonard J, Grunwald RP, et al: Medical and surgical management of early Q wave myocardial infarction. II. Effects on mortality and global and regional left ventricular function at 10 or more years of follow-up. *J Am Coll Cardiol* 1989; 14:78–90.
13. Reimer KA, Low JE, Rasmussen MM, Jennings RB: The wavefront phenomenon of ischemic cell death. I. Myocardial infarct size vs. duration of coronary occlusion in dogs. *Circulation* 1977;56: 786–794.
14. Kloner RA, Ellis SG, Carlson NV, Braunwald E: Coronary reperfusion for the treatment of acute myocardial infarction: Postischemic ventricular dysfunction. *Cardiology* 1983;70:233–246.
15. Kloner RA, Ellis SG, Lange R, Braunwald E: Studies of experimental coronary artery reperfusion. Effects on infarct size, myocardial function, biochemistry, ultrastructure and microvascular damage. *Circulation* 1983;68(Suppl I):I-8–I-15.
16. Kloner RA, Ganote CE, Jennings RB: The "no-reflow" phenomenon after temporary coronary occlusion in the dog. *J Clin Invest* 1974;54:1496–1508.
17. Kloner RA, Ganote CE, Jennings RB, Reimer KA: Demonstration of the "no-reflow" phenomenon in the dog heart after temporary ischemia. *Recent Adv Stud Cardiac Struct Metab* 1975;10:463–474.
18. Kloner RA, Ganote CE, Whalen DA Jr, Jennings RB: Effect of a transient period of ischemia on

myocardial cells. II. Fine structure during the first few minutes of reflow. *Am J Pathol* 1974;74: 399–422.

19. Jennings RB, Ganote CE, Kloner RA, et al: Explosive swelling of myocardial cells irreversibly injured by transient ischemia. *Recent Adv Stud Cardiac Struct Metab* 1975;6:405–413.
20. Whalen DA Jr, Hamilton DG, Ganote CE, Jennings RB: Effect of a transient period of ischemia on myocardial cells. I. Effects on cell volume regulation. *Am J Pathol* 1974;74:381–397.
21. Wandschneider W, Winter S, Thalmann M, et al: Crystalloid versus blood cardioplegia in coronary by-pass surgery. A prospective, randomized, controlled study in 100 consecutive adults. *J Cardiovasc Surg* 1994;35:85–89.
22. Anderson JR, Hossein-Nia M, Kallis P, et al: Comparison of two strategies for myocardial management during coronary artery operations. *Ann Thorac Surg* 1994;58:768–773.
23. Isomura T, Hisatomi K, Sato T, et al: Interrupted warm blood cardioplegia for coronary artery bypass grafting. *Eur J Card Thorac Surg* 1995;9:133–138.
24. Mezzetti A, Calafiore AM, Lapenna D, et al: Intermittent antegrade warm cardioplegia reduces oxidative stress and improves metabolism of the ischemic-reperfused human myocardium. *J Thorac Cardiovasc Surg* 1995;109:787–795.
25. Savunen T, Kuttila K, Rajalin A, et al: Combined cardioplegia delivery offers no advantage over antegrade cardioplegia administration in coronary surgical patients with a preserved left ventricular function. *Eur J Card Thorac Surg* 1994;8:640–644.
26. Hayashida N, Weisel RD, Shirai T, et al: Tepid antegrade and retrograde cardioplegia. *Ann Thorac Surg* 1995;59:723–729.
27. Calafiore AM, Teodori G, Mezzetti A, et al: Intermittent antegrade warm blood cardioplegia. *Ann Thorac Surg* 1995;59:398–402.
28. Bufkin BL, Mellitt RJ, Gott JP, et al: Aerobic blood cardioplegia for revascularization of acute infarct: Effects of delivery temperature. *Ann Thorac Surg* 1994;58:953–960.
29. Allen BS, Okamoto F, Buckberg GD, et al: Reperfusion conditions: Critical importance of total ventricular decompression during regional reperfusion. *J Thorac Cardiovasc Surg* 1986;92:605–612.
30. Vinten-Johansen J, Buckberg GD, Okamoto F, et al: Superiority of surgical versus medical reperfusion after regional ischemia. *J Thorac Cardiovasc Surg* 1986;92:525–534.
31. Allen BS, Rosenkranz ER, Buckberg GD, et al: High oxygen requirements of dyskinetic cardiac muscle. *J Thorac Cardiovasc Surg* 1986;92:543–552.
32. Allen BS, Okamoto F, Buckberg GD, et al: Reperfusate composition: Benefits of marked hypocalcemia and diltiazem on regional recovery. *J Thorac Cardiovasc Surg* 1986;92:564–572.
33. Okamoto F, Allen BS, Buckberg GD, et al: Reperfusate composition: Supplemental role of intravenous and intracoronary coenzyme Q10 in avoiding reperfusion damage. *J Thorac Cardiovasc Surg* 1986;92:573–582.
34. Okamoto F, Allen BS, Buckberg GD, et al: Reperfusate composition: Interaction of marked hyperglycemia and marked hyperosmolarity in allowing immediate contractile recovery after four hours of regional ischemia. *J Thorac Cardiovasc Surg* 1986;92: 583–593.
35. Allen BS, Buckberg GD, Schwaiger M, et al: Early recovery of regional wall motion in patients following surgical revascularization after eight hours of acute coronary occlusion. *J Thorac Cardiovasc Surg* 1986;92:636–648.
36. Okamoto F, Allen BS, Buckberg GD, et al: Reperfusion conditions: Importance of ensuring gentle versus sudden reperfusion during relief of coronary occlusion. *J Thorac Cardiovasc Surg* 1986;92: 613–620.
37. Rosenkranz ER, Okamoto F, Buckberg GD, et al: Biochemical studies: Failure of tissue adenosine triphosphate levels to predict recovery of contractile function after controlled reperfusion. *J Thorac Cardiovasc Surg* 1986;92:488–501.
38. Barnard RJ, Okamoto F, Buckberg GD, et al: Histochemical studies: Inability of triphenyltetrazolium chloride nonstaining to define tissue necrosis. *J Thorac Cardiovasc Surg* 1986;92:502–512.
39. Allen BS, Okamoto F, Buckberg GD, et al: Immediate functional recovery after six hours of regional ischemia by careful control of conditions of reperfusion and composition of reperfusate. *J Thorac Cardiovasc Surg* 1986;92:621–635.
40. Beyersdorf F, Acar C, Buckberg GD, et al: Studies on prolonged acute regional ischemia. III. Early natural history of simulated single and multivessel disease with emphasis on remote myocardium. *J Thorac Cardiovasc Surg* 1989;98:368–380.

41. Cheung EH, Arcidi JM Jr, Dorsey LM, et al: Reperfusion of infarcting myocardium: Benefit of surgical reperfusion in a chronic model. *Ann Thorac Surg* 1989;48:331–338.

42. Wilcox RG, Olsson CG, Skene AM, et al: Trial of tissue plasminogen activator for mortality reduction in acute myocardial infarction. Anglo-Scandinavian Study of Early Thrombolysis (ASSET). *Lancet* 1988;2:525–530.

43. Cairns JA, Singer J, Gent M, et al: One year mortality outcomes of all coronary and intensive care unit patients with acute myocardial infarction, unstable angina or other chest pain in Hamilton, Ontario, a city of 375,000 people. *Can J Cardiol* 1989;5:239–246.

44. Cragg DR, Friedman HZ, Boneman JD, et al: Outcome of patients with acute myocardial infarction who are ineligible for thrombolytic therapy. *Ann Intern Med* 1991;115:173–177.

45. Ericsson CG, Lindvall B, Olsson G, et al: Trends in coronary care. A retrospective study of patients with myocardial infarction treated in coronary care units. *Acta Med Scand* 1988;224:507–513.

46. Goldberg RJ, Gore JM, Alpert JS, et al: Cardiogenic shock after acute myocardial infarction. Incidence and mortality from a community-wide perspective, 1975 to 1988. *N Engl J Med* 1991;325:1117–1122.

47. Allen BS, Buckberg GD, Fontan FM, et al: Superiority of controlled surgical reperfusion versus percutaneous transluminal coronary angioplasty in acute coronary occlusion. *J Thorac Cardiovasc Surg* 1993;105:864–884.

48. Phillips SJ, Kongtahworn C, Skinner JR, Zeff RH: Emergency coronary artery reperfusion: A choice therapy for evolving myocardial infarction. Results in 339 patients. *J Thorac Cardiovasc Surg* 1983;86: 679–688.

49. Phillips SJ, Zeff RH, Kongtahworn C, et al: Surgery for evolving myocardial infarction. *JAMA* 1982;248:1325–1328.

50. Spencer FC: Emergency coronary bypass for acute infarction: An unproved clinical experiment. *Circulation* 1983;68(Suppl II):II-17–II-19.

51. Kirklin JK, Blackstone EH, Zorn GL Jr, et al: Intermediate-term results of coronary artery bypass grafting for acute myocardial infarction. *Circulation* 1985;72(Suppl II):II-175–II-178.

52. Athanasuleas CL, Geer DA, Arciniegas JG, et al: A reappraisal of surgical intervention for acute myocardial infarction. *J Thorac Cardiovasc Surg* 1987;93: 405–414.

53. Koshal A, Beanlands DS, Davies RA, et al: Urgent surgical reperfusion in acute evolving myocardial infarction. A randomized controlled study. *Circulation* 1988;78(Suppl I):I-171–I-178.

54. Ansel BJ, Walter PJ, Van der Mast M, Vander Sande J: Immediate bypass surgery (0.5–3 h) for evolving myocardial infarction. *Adv Cardiol* 1988;36: 178–188.

55. Flameng W, Sergeant P, Vanhaecke J, Suy R: Emergency aortocoronary bypass surgery: Late effects on infarct size and ventricular function. *Adv Cardiol* 1988;36:195–201.

56. Berg R, Selinger SL, Leonard JJ, et al: Surgical management of acute myocardial infarction, in *Cardiac Surgery*. Philadelphia, FA Davis, 1982, pp 61–74.

57. Phillips SJ, Zeff RH, Skinner JR, et al: Reperfusion protocol and results in 738 patients with evolving myocardial infarction. *Ann Thorac Surg* 1986;41: 119–125.

58. Turina M, von Segesser L: Immediate bypass surgery for evolving myocardial infarction. *Adv Cardiol* 1988;36:213–218.

59. Vidne BA: Emergency coronary artery reperfusion for acute evolving myocardial infarction. *Adv Cardiol* 1988;36:219–225.

60. Hands ME, Rutherford JD, Muller JE, et al: The in-hospital development of cardiogenic shock after myocardial infarction: Incidence, predictors of occurrence, outcome and prognostic factors. The MILIS Study Group. *J Am Coll Cardiol* 1989;14:40–48.

61. Scheidt S, Ascheim R, Killip T III: Shock after acute myocardial infarction. A clinical and hemodynamic profile. *Am J Cardiol* 1970;26:556–564.

62. Chua TS, Koo CC, Tan AT, Ho CK: Mortality trends in the coronary care unit. *Ann Singapore Acad Med* 1990;19:3–8.

63. Killip T III, Kimball JT: Treatment of myocardial infarction in a coronary care unit: A two year experience with 250 patients. *Am J Cardiol* 1967;20: 457–464.

64. Scheidt S, Wilner G, Mueller H, et al: Intra-aortic balloon counterpulsation in cardiogenic shock. Report of a co-operative clinical trial. *N Engl J Med* 1973;288:979–984.

65. GISSI: Effectiveness of intravenous thrombolytic treatment in acute myocardial infarction. *Lancet* 1986;I:397–402.

66. The International Study Group: In-hospital mortality and clinical course of 20891 patients with suspected acute myocardial infarction randomised between alteplase and streptokinase with or without heparin. *Lancet* 1990;336:71–75.
67. Kennedy JW, Gensini GG, Timmis GC, Maynard C: Acute myocardial infarction treated with intracoronary streptokinase: A report of the Society of Cardiac Angiography. *Am J Cardiol* 1985;55: 871–877.
68. Salem BI, Gowda S, Haikal M, et al: Early percutaneous transluminal coronary angioplasty or coronary bypass surgery following thrombolytic treatment of acute myocardial infarction. *Chest* 1987;91: 648–653.
69. Stack RS, Califf RM, Hinohara T, et al: Survival and cardiac event rates in the first year after emergency coronary angioplasty for acute myocardial infarction. *J Am Coll Cardiol* 1988;11:1141–1149.
70. Rothbaum DA, Linnemeier TJ, Landin RJ, et al: Emergency percutaneous transluminal coronary angioplasty in acute myocardial infarction: A 3 year experience. *J Am Coll Cardiol* 1987;10:264–272.
71. Brahos GJ, Baker NH, Ewy G, et al: Aortocoronary bypass following unsuccessful PTCA: Experience in 100 consecutive patients. *Ann Thorac Surg* 1985;40: 7–10.
72. Bredee JJ, Bavinck JH, Berreklouw E, et al: Acute myocardial ischaemia and cardiogenic shock after percutaneous transluminal coronary angioplasty; risk factors for and results of emergency coronary bypass. *Eur Heart J* 1989;10(Suppl H):104–111.
73. Buffet P, Danchin N, Villemot JP, et al: Early and long-term outcome after emergency coronary artery bypass surgery after failed coronary angioplasty. *Circulation* 1991;84(Suppl III):III-254–III-259.
74. Haraphongse M, Na-Ayudhya RK, Burton J, et al: Clinical efficacy of emergency bypass surgery for failed coronary angioplasty. *Can J Cardiol* 1990;6: 186–190.
75. Killen DA, Hamaker WR, Reed WA: Coronary artery bypass following percutaneous transluminal coronary angioplasty. *Ann Thorac Surg* 1985;40: 133–138.
76. Naunheim KS, Fiore AC, Fagan DC, et al: Emergency coronary artery bypass grafting for failed angioplasty: Risk factors and outcome. *Ann Thorac Surg* 1989;47:816–823.
77. Parsonnet V, Fisch D, Gielchinsky I, et al: Emergency operation after failed angioplasty. *J Thorac Cardiovasc Surg* 1988;96:198–203.
78. Reul GJ, Cooley DA, Hallman GL, et al: Coronary artery bypass for unsuccessful percutaneous transluminal coronary angioplasty. *J Thorac Cardiovasc Surg* 1984;88:685–694.
79. Cheanvechai C, Effler DB, Loop FD, et al: Aortocoronary artery graft during early and late phases of acute myocardial infarction. *Ann Thorac Surg* 1973;16:249–260.
80. Dawson JT, Hall RJ, Hallman GL, Cooley DA: Mortality in patients undergoing coronary artery bypass surgery after myocardial infarction. *Am J Cardiol* 1974;33:483–486.
81. Schuster EH, Bulkley BH: Early post-infarction angina. Ischemia at a distance and ischemia in the infarct zone. *N Engl J Med* 1981;305: 1101–1105.
82. Hutter AM Jr, DeSanctis RW, Flynn T, Yeatman LA: Nontransmural myocardial infarction: A comparison of hospital and late clinical course of patients with that of matched patients with transmural anterior and transmural inferior myocardial infarction. *Am J Cardiol* 1981;48: 595–602.
83. Marmor A, Sobel BE, Roberts R: Factors presaging early recurrent myocardial infarction ("extension"). *Am J Cardiol* 1981;48:603–610.
84. Roberts AJ, Sanders JH Jr, Moran JH, et al: The efficacy of medical stabilization prior to myocardial revascularization in early refractory postinfarction angina. *Ann Surg* 1983;197:91–98.
85. Breyer RH, Engelman RM, Rousou JA, Lemeshow S: Postinfarction angina: An expanding subset of patients undergoing coronary artery bypass. *J Thorac Cardiovasc Surg* 1985;90:532–540.
86. Jones RN, Pifarre R, Sullivan HJ, et al: Early myocardial revascularization for postinfarction angina. *Ann Thorac Surg* 1987;44:159–163.
87. Naunheim KS, Kesler KA, Kanter KR, et al: Coronary artery bypass for recent infarction. Predictors of mortality. *Circulation* 1988;78(Suppl I): I-122–I-128.
88. Connolly MW, Gelbfish JS, Rose DM, et al: Early coronary artery bypass grafting for complicated acute myocardial infarction. *J Cardiovasc Surg (Torino)* 1988;29:375–382.

89. Kouchoukos NT, Murphy S, Philpott T, et al: Coronary artery bypass grafting for postinfarction angina pectoris. *Circulation* 1989;79(Suppl I):I-68–I-72.
90. Gardner TJ, Stuart RS, Greene PS, Baumgartner WA: The risk of coronary bypass surgery for patients with postinfarction angina. *Circulation* 1989; 79(Suppl I):I-79–I-80.
91. Fremes SE, Goldman BS, Weisel RD, et al: Recent preoperative myocardial infarction increases the risk of surgery for unstable angina. *J Cardiac Surg* 1991;6:2–12.
92. Naunheim KS, Kesler KA, Kanter KR, et al: Coronary artery bypass for recent infarction. Predictors of mortality. *Circulation* 1988;78(Suppl I): I-122–I-128.
93. Connolly MW, Gelbfish JS, Rose DM, et al: Early coronary artery bypass grafting for complicated acute myocardial infarction. *J Cardiovasc Surg (Torino)* 1988;29:375–382.
94. Katz NM, Kubanick TE, Ahmed SW, et al: Determinants of cardiac failure after coronary bypass surgery within 30 days of acute myocardial infarction. *Ann Thorac Surg* 1986;42:658–663.
95. Hochberg MS, Parsonnet V, Gielchinsky I, et al: Timing of coronary revascularization after acute myocardial infarction. Early and late results in patients revascularized within seven weeks. *J Thorac Cardiovasc Surg* 1984;88:914–921.
96. Creswell LL, Moulton MJ, Cox JL, Rosenbloom M: Revascularization after acute myocardial infarction. *Ann Thorac Surg* 1995;60:19–26.
97. Wilson JM, Held JS, Wright CB, et al: Coronary artery bypass surgery following thrombolytic therapy for acute coronary thrombosis. *Ann Thorac Surg* 1984;37:212–217.
98. Rodewald G, Mathey D, Krebber HJ: Bypass surgery following thrombolytic therapy. *Z Kardiol* 1985;74:143–146.
99. Messmer BJ, von Essen R, Minale C, et al: Intracoronary thrombolysis and early bypass surgery for acute myocardial infarct: Five years' experience. *Thorac Cardiovasc Surg* 1986;34:1–4.
100. Taylor GJ, Moses HW, Katholi RE, et al: Six-year survival after coronary thrombolysis and early revascularization for acute myocardial infarction. *Am J Cardiol* 1992;70:26–30.
101. Kereiakes DJ, Topol EJ, George BS, et al: Favorable early and long-term prognosis following coronary bypass surgery therapy for myocardial infarction: Results of a multicenter trial. TAMI Study Group. *Am Heart J* 1989;118:199–207.
102. Messmer BJ, Uebis R, Rieger C, et al: Late results after intracoronary thrombolysis and early bypass grafting for acute myocardial infarction. *J Thorac Cardiovasc Surg* 1989;97:10–18.
103. Barner HB, Lea JW IV, Naunheim KS, Stoney WS Jr: Emergency coronary bypass not associated with preoperative cardiogenic shock in failed angioplasty, after thrombolysis, and for acute myocardial infarction. *Circulation* 1989;79(Suppl I): I-152–I-159.
104. Lee KF, Mandell J, Rankin JS, et al: Immediate versus delayed coronary grafting after streptokinase treatment. Postoperative blood loss and clinical results. *J Thorac Cardiovasc Surg* 1988;95: 216–222.
105. Lemmer JH Jr, Stanford W, Bonney SL, et al: Aprotinin for coronary bypass operations: Efficacy, safety, and influence on early saphenous graft patency. A multicenter, randomized, double-blind, placebo-controlled study. *J Thorac Cardiovasc Surg* 1994;107:543–553.
106. Efstratiadis T, Munsch C, Crossman D, Taylor K: Aprotinin used in emergency coronary operation after streptokinase treatment. *Ann Thorac Surg* 1991;52:1320–1321.
107. Gersh BJ, Chesebro JH, Braunwald E et al: Coronary Artery Bypass Graft Surgery After Thrombolytic Therapy in the Thrombolysis and Myocardial Infarction Trial, Phase II (TIMI-II), *J Am Coll Cardiol* 1995;25:395–402.

24

The Lungs in Acute Myocardial Infarction

Paul R. Eisenberg, MD, MPH

Pulmonary complications occur frequently in patients with acute myocardial infarction, and they may range from mild dyspnea associated with ischemic symptoms to frank pulmonary edema with acute respiratory failure. Prior pulmonary disease, acute pulmonary complications, and pulmonary vascular disease all may complicate the clinical course of patients with acute myocardial infarction. Often, the management of patients with concomitant pulmonary disease and myocardial infarction must be modified to optimize cardiopulmonary interactions and to avoid deleterious drug side effects on heart and lung function. Effective treatment of patients with myocardial infarction and pulmonary disease requires prompt recognition of acute or chronic pulmonary disease, an understanding of cardiopulmonary interactions, and selection of a management strategy that addresses concerns specific to patients with pulmonary complications.

INITIAL MANAGEMENT OF RESPIRATORY DISTRESS IN ACUTE MYOCARDIAL INFARCTION

Dyspnea is a frequent complaint in patients with acute myocardial infarction, and it may range in severity from mild breathlessness associated with chest discomfort to severe respiratory distress and acute respiratory failure (1). Most often, dyspnea is related to increases in extravascular lung water attributable to increases in pulmonary capillary pressure due to transmitted increases in left atrial pressure (2–7). This results in signs and symptoms of pulmonary edema, the severity of which is related, in part, to the extent to which pulmonary capillary pressure is increased (3). In a minority of patients, the increased pulmonary capillary pressure results in peribronchial edema, which may induce bronchial narrowing with increased airway resistance and wheezing (5,8). Clinical signs of increased extravascular lung water may be obscured in the presence of chronic pulmonary disease. For example, increases in lung water associated with acute myocardial infarction may be difficult to detect in patients with interstitial lung disease (e.g., sarcoidosis, idiopathic pulmonary fibrosis). Similarly, even modest pulmonary edema may result in acute respiratory failure in patients with moderate to severe chronic obstructive airway disease. Even in the absence of obvious pulmonary edema, arterial hypoxemia due to mismatched ventilation and perfusion is common in patients with acute myocardial infarction (3–5,7, 9,10).

Initial Evaluation and Management of Patients with Myocardial Infarction in Respiratory Distress

The initial evaluation and management of patients with acute myocardial infarction and mild to moderate respiratory distress should focus on immediate improvement in oxygenation and subsequent assessment for clinical signs of increased lung water and/or the presence of acute or chronic airflow obstruction. With mild respiratory distress, the chest examination is frequently unremarkable or reveals only basilar late-inspiratory crackles. Occasionally, in patients with prior cardiopulmonary disease or those with reactive airways, mild expiratory wheezing may be heard. Supplemental oxygen provided as 2 to 4 L/min by nasal cannula is often sufficient to relieve hypoxemia in patients with mild respiratory distress. In those with more marked distress, application of a face mask with 60% to 100% oxygen is indicated; often, such patients will need to be intubated (see below). Adequacy of oxygen therapy should be assessed noninvasively with transcutaneous oximetry whenever possible. If the patient is a candidate for treatment with fibrinolytic agents, arterial puncture should be avoided because of the potential for bleeding complications. However, in patients with evidence of acute or chronic airway disease, arterial blood gas analysis may be necessary to assess for hypercapnia and respiratory acidosis.

Moderate to severe respiratory distress in patients with acute myocardial infarction is almost always due to pulmonary edema. Such patients usually present with severe dyspnea, tachypnea, diaphoresis, and when severe, with a cough productive of pink, frothy sputum. End-inspiratory crackles, often extending to the apices of the lungs, are usually present on the chest examination. In some patients wheezing and poor air movement with upper airway rhonchi and gurgles may be predominant features. The cardiac examination usually reveals an S4 gallop. An S3 gallop is infrequent, and when present it may indicate chronic rather than acute left ventricular dysfunction. The jugular venous pressure is often not elevated in patients with acute myocardial infarction, but when elevated, it is indicative of biventricular failure that is often chronic in nature or right ventricular dysfunction. Supplemental 60% to 100% oxygen should generally be administered by face mask to patients who are alert and in only moderate distress. Those who are in severe distress, those in whom respiratory distress or hypoxemia has not improved with initial management (e.g., morphine, nitrates, and so forth), and those whose level of consciousness decreases should be promptly intubated, which will usually require sedation, to relieve the work of breathing and improve oxygenation. Intubation should be by mouth whenever possible, since traumatic nasal intubation may result in significant bleeding complications when aggressive anticoagulant and fibrinolytic regimens are used.

Diagnostic Considerations in Patients with Respiratory Distress and Myocardial Infarction

Severe pulmonary edema in patients with acute myocardial infarction is usually indicative of moderate to severe left ventricular dysfunction and/or significant mitral regurgitation (11–13). Pulmonary edema and hypotension are indicative of cardiogenic shock and are particularly ominous (see Chs. 13 and 16 for additional discussion).

In patients with acute myocardial infarction without evidence of chronic left ventricular dysfunction, pulmonary edema is often indicative of a large infarction with significant acute left ventricular dysfunction and/or acute mitral regurgitation (see Ch. 16). Acute mitral regurgitation may be recognized by the presence of a typical holosystolic murmur, but in many cases the murmur is not present or it is not audible in the initial evaluation. The sudden occurrence of pulmonary edema in patients without chronic left ventricular dysfunction has been referred to as "flash pulmonary edema" (11,14–17). This clinical syndrome is associated with significant proximal left anterior descending, left main, or severe three-vessel coronary disease with an extensive area of myocardium at risk for ischemia or infarction. Often flash pulmonary edema is due to acute ischemic mitral regurgitation.

Pulmonary edema and hypotension in patients with acute infarction are almost invariably indicative of cardiogenic shock (see Ch. 13). Although this clinical syndrome may occur in patients with extensive anterior wall myocardial infarction, frequently it is indicative of acute mitral regurgitation, or less commonly, ventricular septal rupture (see Ch. 16). The physical examination in patients with ventricular septal rupture and acute myocardial infarction usually is remarkable for a holosystolic murmur; often, a thrill can be palpated. The immediate management of patients with cardiogenic shock and pulmonary edema should always include prompt intubation, administration of intravenous vasopressor agents, and in most cases, intra-aortic balloon counterpulsation (see Ch. 16).

The initial evaluation of patients with acute myocardial infarction and respiratory distress should always take into account the possible presence of preexisting pulmonary or cardiac disease. In addition to the history, physical findings such as increased anterior posterior diameter of the chest, decreased breath sounds, prolonged expiratory phase, inspiratory or expiratory wheezing, and the presence of peripheral cyanosis or clubbing are of value in identifying patients with chronic lung disease. In patients with chronic obstructive lung disease, the physical examination is often nonspecific for pulmonary edema because of chronic inspiratory crackles related to airway secretions and wheezing. Wheezing may also be a manifestation of pulmonary edema in patients without a history of chronic lung disease; whether this is due to bronchial edema or increased airway reactivity has not been definitively established. Radiographic findings of pulmonary edema in patients with chronic obstructive lung disease may be atypical because of underlying bullous disease, or chronic interstitial or bronchial radiographic abnormalities (18). Increases in lung water in such patients may be manifest as unilateral pulmonary edema or asymmetric infiltrates; on occasion, significant increases in lung water may not be associated with new pulmonary infiltrates. In patients with chronic interstitial lung disease, increases in intravascular lung water are difficult to distinguish from the underlying pulmonary disease. For reasons stated above, pulmonary artery catheterization is often necessary for the evaluation of the cause of acute respiratory distress in patients with chronic lung disease and acute myocardial infarction.

Initial Management of Myocardial Infarction in Patients with Lung Disease

Initial management of patients with acute myocardial infarction typically includes administration of fibrinolytic agents, intravenous beta blockers, aspirin, and anticoagulants. In patients with chronic lung disease, potential contraindications to thrombolysis include a history of significant hemoptysis or pulmonary alveolar hemorrhage syndrome. Significant chronic hemoptysis is infrequent and is usually associated with severe chronic obstructive lung disease, bronchiectasis, or pulmonary malignancy. Patients with chronic bronchitis or bronchiectasis may have significantly dilated bronchial veins, and they are at risk for significant pulmonary hemorrhage (19–21). The incidence of life-threatening pulmonary hemorrhage in patients with a history of hemoptysis is low, so that although it is reasonable to consider alternative treatments for them (i.e., primary PTCA), thrombolytics may be administered when the potential benefits of reperfusion are greater than the small risk of bronchial bleeding (see Ch. 22). Patients with chronic lung disease and a history of episodes of severe hemoptysis should not be treated with fibrinolytic agents, and often anticoagulants are contraindicated in such patients as well. Pulmonary alveolar hemorrhage syndromes represent an uncertain risk for significant complications with thrombolysis but, fortunately, are infrequently encountered in patients with acute myocardial infarction. The most common clinical syndromes associated with pulmonary hemorrhage are antiglomerular basement membrane syndrome, other pulmonary–renal syndromes, and collagen vascular diseases. The risk of recurrent alveolar hemorrhage is probably low in these patients once they receive treatment for the underlying disease, but alveolar hemorrhage after thrombolysis can occur, and this should be considered before thrombolytic therapy is administered.

The use of intravenous beta blockers in patients with chronic airway disease is somewhat more controversial (see Ch. 12). Patients with a history of asthma, reactive airway disease, or steroid-dependent chronic lung disease should not receive intravenous beta blockers (22–24). However, many patients with chronic obstructive lung disease can be treated with low doses of selective β_1-antagonists, typically intravenous and orally administered metoprolol (25–32). Although the occurrence of acute bronchospasm in selected patients with chronic obstructive lung disease treated with beta blockers is low, the fact that they are not used more routinely in the United States has been attributed, in part, to concern for this complication. In patients with a history of chronic airway disease, frequent examination of the patient after administration of intravenous or oral beta blockers is essential to monitor for the occurrence of bronchospasm.

In patients with asthma, it is important to determine whether there is a history of aspirin sensitivity. Aspirin sensitivity may occur in up to 10% of patients with asthma; such patients often have severe asthma, nasal polyps, and a history of sinusitis and often are steroid dependent (33–35). Administration of aspirin to such patients may precipitate severe acute bronchospasm, or rarely, an anaphylactic reaction. If antiplatelet therapy is necessary, ticlopidine can be considered as an alternative.

Bronchospasm should always be treated in patients with myocardial infarction and respiratory distress, because it increases the work of breathing and when severe promotes acute respiratory failure. β-Agonists delivered by nebulization or metered dose inhalers are the treatment of choice for acute management of bronchospasm in patients with pulmonary edema (36,37). With currently available β_2-specific agonists, tachycardia or arrhythmias are usually not a problem unless high doses are administered (38). In patients with chronic obstructive pulmonary disease, the anticholinergic ipratropium bromide may be more effective for the treatment of bronchospasm than are β-agonists (39–44). Combining ipratropium and β-agonists has been found in some, but not all, studies to be more effective than optimal doses of either agent alone (42, 45–47). Effective use of this anticholinergic may require four to six puffs with a metered dose inhaler. There is no evidence that nebulization of bronchodilators is superior to metered dose inhalers, but for patients with respiratory distress the former may be easier to use. Intravenous aminophylline (theophylline ethylenediamine) may also be of value in treating bronchospasm, particularly if the response to inhaled bronchodilators is suboptimal. Aminophylline also has positive inotropic effects and improves diaphragmatic function (48–53). The usual dose is 5 mg/kg followed by an infusion of 0.3 to 0.5 mg/kg/hr. Blood levels must be monitored closely (at least daily) and should be maintained at 10 to 50 mg/L. Intravenous steroids should not be used to treat bronchospasm in patients with myocardial infarction, because these drugs unfavorably affect myocardial remodeling (54,55).

RESPIRATORY FAILURE IN ACUTE MYOCARDIAL INFARCTION

Mechanisms for Increased Extravascular Lung Water

Multiple potential factors may contribute to increases in extravascular lung water in patients with acute myocardial infarction. The exchange of water between the pulmonary capillaries and interstitium can be described by the Starling equation. A complete discussion of the components of this equation and experimental data supporting their validity is beyond the scope of this chapter, but several excellent in-depth reviews are available (56–58). Briefly, the equation predicts that the flux of fluid from the pulmonary capillaries to the interstitium depends on a balance between hydrostatic and oncotic forces. Hydrostatic forces are typically higher in the capillary than the interstitium, and therefore tend to favor the transudation of water out of the capillaries. Reabsorption of water into the capillaries depends on colloid osmotic forces, which are usually higher in the capillaries. The colloid osmotic pressure is approximately 28 mm Hg, while the intracapillary pressure is normally around

8 mm Hg, so that readsorbtion of water into the intravascular compartment is favored. With increases in pulmonary capillary pressure of more than 20 mm Hg, extravascular lung water accumulates (59–61). Increased hydrostatic pressure appears to mediate pulmonary edema in most patients with myocardial infarction and is attributable to transmitted increases in left atrial pressure (3,13,62).

An important component of the balance between hydrostatic and oncotic pressures is the capillary permeability to proteins. Under normal conditions, intravascular colloid osmotic forces that promote reabsorption of water from the interstitium into the capillaries are maintained by a relatively low permeability of capillaries to intravascular proteins. However, capillary permeability may be altered by intravascular factors and acute lung injury, increasing the interstitial protein content and favoring the accumulation of intravascular lung water (i.e., permeability pulmonary edema) (56,63). Numerous mediators have been described in experimental studies to increase capillary permeability, including but not limited to the following: activated granulocytes, activation of the complement system, reactive oxygen species, endotoxin, platelet activating factor, thromboxane, and potentially, other factors secreted from platelets (56, 63–70). In some studies, acute myocardial infarction has been shown to induce increased pulmonary capillary permeability, but the mechanisms are not clear (66,67,70–72). Coronary reperfusion in one study appeared to exacerbate extravascular lung water accumulation, suggesting that washout of reactive mediators from the infarcted myocardium may induce increases in capillary permeability (73). Administration of fibrinolytic agents to patients with acute myocardial infarction has been shown to induce activation of the complement system (74,75), but other than isolated case reports, there is little evidence that thrombolytic therapy induces pulmonary edema. Although the mechanisms remain undefined, it is important to recognize that a permeability type of pulmonary edema is not uncommon after myocardial infarction (76,77).

The primary mechanism for development of pulmonary edema in association with acute myocardial infarction is an increase in left atrial pressure, which is transmitted to the pulmonary capillaries and results in increased transudation of intravascular water into the pulmonary extravascular compartment (3,13,62). Initially, small increases in the transudation of lung water are thought to be compensated for by increased pulmonary lymphatic flow (56–61). Extravascular water initially accumulates in the peribronchial tissues, but with increasing transudation, lymphatic drainage is insufficient to clear it, and interstitial edema in both the peribronchial and interalveolar tissues develops (stage 1) (60). More marked increases in pulmonary capillary pressure initially result in minimal interstitial fluid accumulation (stage 2), followed by accumulation of intra-alveolar fluid primarily at the corners of the alveolar–capillary membrane, which leads to frank alveolar flooding with severe pulmonary edema (stage 3). Resolution of pulmonary edema depends on lymphatic drainage, which appears to be most efficient in clearing interstitial extravascular lung water (58). Clearance of water from the alveoli also requires an active transport mechanism that may be β-adrenergic dependent (78–82). The rate of resolution of pulmonary edema varies considerably among individuals and may depend on factors such as plasma oncotic pressure, adequacy of lymphatic drainage, central venous pressure, and alterations in pulmonary capillary permeability (56–58,83,84).

Physiologic Responses to Increases in Extravascular Lung Water

Pulmonary physiologic responses to increased extravascular lung water include decreases in total lung capacity (TLC), functional vital capacity (FVC), and expiratory flow rates (FEV_1, FEF_{25-75}, and flow at 50% of vital capacity) (4,5,7,8). In some patients, decreases in expiratory flow rates improve with bronchodilator therapy. Patients with heart failure have been observed to have increased bronchial responsiveness, as defined by a methacholine challenge test, and this has been proposed as a potential mechanism for bronchospasm in response to pulmonary edema (i.e., cardiac asthma) (85,86).

Whether the accumulation of peribronchial and bronchial water is the mechanism for increased bronchial reactivity, or whether such patients have underlying bronchial hyperreactivity, is not known. No evidence of increased bronchial reactivity in patients with heart failure has been gathered (87). Nonetheless, with treatment and resolution of increases in extravascular lung water TLC, FVC, and expiratory flow rates usually return to normal.

The alveolar–arterial oxygen gradient increases in most patients with myocardial infarction, even when there are only minimal increases in extravascular lung water, due to ventilation–perfusion mismatch (3,9,10,88,89). Arterial blood gases in such patients demonstrate a respiratory alkalosis and mild hypoxemia. Alveolar flooding in severe pulmonary edema results in significant right-to-left shunting because of perfusion of alveoli that are not ventilated. When severe intrapulmonary shunting occurs, even administration of 100% inspired oxygen may be insufficient to increase oxygen saturation to greater than 90% in arterial blood. In such patients application of positive end-expiratory pressure will often improve oxygenation by increasing functional residual capacity and improving ventilation of perfused alveoli (90–92). In most patients with acute myocardial infarction, tachypnea increases alveolar ventilation, resulting in hypocapnia. However, in patients with chronic obstructive lung disease or acute bronchospasm, carbon dioxide retention and respiratory acidosis may occur. Acute respiratory muscle fatigue and the administration of morphine and other sedatives to patients with acute myocardial infarction may also precipitate hypercapnia. As noted below, acute respiratory failure in patients with myocardial infarction and pulmonary edema may be associated with an acute respiratory acidosis, often combined with a metabolic acidosis (93,94).

The increased intrapulmonary shunting that occurs in patients with moderate to severe pulmonary edema and the ventilation–perfusion redistribution that occurs because of hypoxic vasoconstriction have important consequences in the pulmonary response to vasoactive medications. For example, hypoxemia may be paradoxically exacerbated by administration of intravenous nitroglycerin, and to a lesser extent nitroprusside, because these agents induce vasodilatation of the pulmonary arteries, antagonizing hypoxic vasoconstriction and resulting in perfusion of poorly ventilated alveoli (95–101). In addition, these and other medications may cause methemoglobinemia, which exacerbates impaired oxygen delivery (102–104).

The presence of significant intrapulmonary shunting in patients with severe pulmonary edema also has important consequences in patients with poor cardiac output and decreased mixed venous oxygen saturation. Such patients, who are typically in cardiogenic shock, may have a sufficiently depressed mixed venous oxygen saturation that admixture of desaturated mixed venous blood with oxygenated blood is insufficient to fully saturate arterial blood, resulting in significant hypoxemia. Improvement in cardiac output with inotropes or afterload reduction may improve arterial oxygen content by increasing the mixed venous oxygen saturation. Similarly, significant anemia may exacerbate hypoxemia in such patients by decreasing oxygen delivery and, thus, the mixed venous oxygen saturation.

Minimal increases in lung water are often not detectable as physiologic abnormalities, alterations in arterial blood gases, or radiographic abnormalities. However, once interstitial edema increases, radiographic abnormalities, including increased interstitial markings, peribronchial tissue prominence, and thickening of interlobular septa (i.e., Kerley B lines), can be appreciated. As pulmonary edema progresses and alveolar flooding occurs, interstitial and alveolar infiltrates are usually present on the chest radiograph (6,13,62,105–115). Although the correlation between measurements of extravascular lung water and the severity of pulmonary edema by chest radiography is poor, in practice radiographic signs of pulmonary edema are sufficiently sensitive and specific to make the diagnosis of increased extravascular lung water in most patients with acute myocardial infarction. Resolution of abnormalities on the chest radiograph with diminution of edema is often delayed compared with the resolution of clinical signs and direct measures of extravascular lung water (i.e., "lag phase") (6,18,112).

Mechanisms for Acute Respiratory Failure Resulting from Pulmonary Edema

Acute respiratory failure in patients with myocardial infarction is usually caused by cardiogenic pulmonary edema (i.e., hydrostatic edema). The accumulation of extravascular lung water in the interstitium and flooding of alveoli result in decreased lung compliance and widening of the alveolar–arterial oxygen gradient. To maintain alveolar ventilation, a greater negative intrathoracic pressure with inspiration and an increase in the respiratory rate must be generated (116). Alveolar flooding results in marked impairment in gas exchange and, as noted above, significant hypoxemia. This is associated with anxiety, severe dyspnea, and tachypnea. The need for greater negative intrathoracic pressures increases the work of breathing, which often rapidly leads to acute respiratory muscle fatigue (117–125). This will occur more rapidly when there are additional factors promoting an increase in the inspiratory work of loading of the diaphragm, such as acute bronchospasm or the presence of chronic obstructive airway disease. Similarly, patients with underlying muscle weakness or decreased respiratory drive will develop respiratory failure more rapidly. The latter may occur immediately with administration of morphine or analgesia for treatment of pulmonary edema. Clinical signs of respiratory muscle fatigue include rapid, shallow breathing, use of accessory respiratory muscles, and paradoxical inspiratory muscle movements in which inspiration is accompanied by chest expansion with abdominal retraction (i.e., abdominal paradox). The development of respiratory muscle fatigue is typically accompanied by hypercapnia, worsening hypoxemia, and either respiratory acidosis alone or a combination of respiratory and lactic acidosis. At this stage, the patient is often confused, and in some cases the level of consciousness rapidly decreases. Prompt intubation is essential to relieve the work of breathing and prevent the progression of hypercapnia and hypoxemia. In patients with acute infarction, hypercapnia and respiratory acidosis may be particularly ominous, and they often precede the development of ventricular arrhythmias and sudden death.

The development of marked negative intrathoracic pressure in patients with pulmonary edema also influences cardiac function, because it increases venous return to the right heart and increases the afterload against which the left ventricle must eject (116,126). As a consequence, with markedly negative pressures, right heart filling and right ventricular end-diastolic volume increases while left ventricular end-diastolic volume decreases. Venous return and right heart filling may be limited by collapse of extrathoracic veins, with large decreases in intrathoracic pressure when central venous pressures are relatively low. The combination of a slight decrease in left ventricular end-diastolic volume and an increase in afterload decreases left ventricular stroke volume. Significant decreases in left ventricular stroke volume with marked negative intrathoracic pressure are usually detectable as inspiratory decreases in the systolic blood pressure of more than 15 mm Hg (i.e., pulsus paradoxus).

Acute respiratory failure may also result from cardiac output that is insufficient to support the work of breathing. In dogs, death due to a marked decrease in cardiac output is preceded by lactic acidosis and respiratory failure (77,127). Similarly, combined lactic and respiratory acidosis have been observed in some patients with myocardial infarction and respiratory failure (93,94). These observations suggest that acute respiratory muscle failure in patients with low cardiac output is due to insufficient oxygen delivery to the respiratory muscles, which may be the mechanism for acute respiratory failure after myocardial infarction in patients with low cardiac output, but without pulmonary edema. Prompt intubation to relieve the work of breathing is often of considerable value in such patients.

Management of Respiratory Failure and Pulmonary Edema

The management of low cardiac output states and cardiogenic pulmonary edema is discussed in Chapter 13 and will not be covered here. Initial pulmonary management of patients with cardiogenic pulmonary edema and respiratory failure usually involves oxygen therapy and mechanical ventilation (88). In patients with mild to moderate pulmonary edema, administration of oxygen by face mask with an inspired oxygen concentration of 40% to 60% is often sufficient to improve hypoxemia and relieve the sensation of dyspnea. Optimization of cardiac function and administration of nitrates, diuretics, and afterload reduction often results in relatively rapid resolution of pulmonary edema. However, in patients with alveolar flooding and severe pulmonary edema, the resolution of pulmonary edema may be relatively slow and often requires several days of support with mechanical ventilation (90–92). Recently, there has been interest in noninvasive methods of mechanical ventilatory support for patients with cardiogenic pulmonary edema in whom rapid resolution is expected with treatment (128). One such approach is to provide continuous positive airway pressure (CPAP) with a tight-fitting face mask (129–131). In one study in which 39 patients were randomly assigned to oxygen or CPAP delivered by face mask, fewer patients receiving CPAP required intubation and mechanical ventilation (132). Another means of providing noninvasive mechanical ventilatory support is the BiPAP ventilator, which provides mechanical ventilatory support with a tight-fitting nasal or combined nasal and mouth mask (128,133). Although these devices may be of value in selected patients, a serious complication of providing positive pressure in this manner is the potential for aspiration with the tight-fitting face mask. Accordingly, in most patients with moderate to severe respiratory distress and significant hypoxemia, prompt intubation is preferable and is generally more effective in reducing the work of breathing and improving oxygenation.

The objectives of mechanical ventilation in patients with acute myocardial infarction and respiratory failure are to decrease the work of breathing and improve arterial oxygenation (90–92). Intubation also establishes a protected airway, which may prevent aspiration in patients with a decreased level of consciousness (134). To decrease the work of breathing, mechanical ventilation must be set to minimize respiratory muscle contractions by the patient (135). This is best and most practically achieved initially by providing intermittent positive-pressure ventilation (IPPV) with the assist-control mode (AC), in which the ventilator assists each respiratory effort by the patient. In many patients with pulmonary edema, this will result in excessive alveolar ventilation, hypocapnea, and a respiratory alkalosis, which is usually best managed by mild sedation of the patient. Tidal volumes should be maintained at approximately 8 to 10 ml/kg; it is not appropriate to decrease them in patients with respiratory alkalosis (135a). However, lower tidal volumes may be used to maintain peak airway pressures less than 45 mm Hg. Usually, a modest respiratory alkalosis is well tolerated and resolves when the pulmonary edema improves. In particularly difficult cases, it may be necessary to use synchronized intermittent mandatory ventilation (SIMV), in which only a preset number of ventilatory efforts are mechanically assisted. The use of this mode will often decrease the minute ventilation (calculated as tidal volume × number of breaths per minute), because the tidal volumes of spontaneous respirations are less than those of assisted breaths. However, with this mode of ventilation the extent of respiratory muscle rest depends on the number of breaths per minute that are assisted. Because this is preset on the ventilator, if the respiratory rate increases, the assisted rate may be insufficient, unless reset, to prevent respiratory muscle fatigue. When properly adjusted, either AC or SIMV at an appropriate rate should significantly decrease the work of breathing.

Intermittent positive pressure on inspiration delivered by a mechanical ventilator improves oxygenation by maintaining larger tidal volumes than those usually present in patients with respiratory failure, therefore optimizing alveolar ventilation (90–92). End-expiratory positive pressure (PEEP) increases functional residual capacity, prevents airway closure, and may improve ventilation of previously poorly ventilated but well-perfused alveoli. As a consequence, modest amounts of PEEP (e.g., 5 cm H_2O) will often decrease intrapulmonary shunting. Initially, patients who are intubated for pulmonary edema should be given 100% inspired oxygen and 3 to 5 cm of H_2O of PEEP. Subsequent adjustments of inspired oxygen concentration should be based on transcutaneous oxygen saturations and arterial blood gas levels. Changes in lung compliance can be measured to determine optimal levels of PEEP, particularly when pressures greater than 10 mm Hg are used.

In patients with pulmonary edema in whom severe hypoxemia does not improve with an inspired oxygen concentration of 60% or more and PEEP of 5 to 10 mm Hg, an alternative mode of ventilation is inverse ratio ventilation (IRV) (92,136). The inspiratory time is greater with IRV than with conventional ventilation and is longer than the expiratory time. This provides a longer interval in which to inflate the lungs, so that the inspiratory flow rate of the gas and peak airway pressures are lower than with conventional ventilation. Because the inspiratory time is longer than the expiratory time, there is the potential for incomplete expiration, resulting in air trapping. Recent studies suggest that the improved oxygenation often achieved with this mode of ventilation in patients with pulmonary edema is attributable in part to incomplete expiration and development of intrinsic or "auto-PEEP." This refers to maintenance of a positive airway pressure during the expiratory phase. In part, because of auto-PEEP and the longer inspiratory time, mean airway pressures are usually only minimally decreased with IRV compared with conventional modes of ventilation. Whether the use of IRV improves oxygenation to a greater extent than does conventional ventilation in patients with pulmonary edema or reduces the incidence of barotrauma is controversial (137–143). A significant disadvantage of IRV is that the patient must be heavily sedated, and on occasion paralyzed, to tolerate this mode of ventilation. Therefore, its use is reserved for patients with pulmonary edema and refractory hypoxemia, when attempts to optimize conventional ventilation have failed.

Clinical Manifestations of Cardiopulmonary Interaction

The cardiovascular consequences of positive-pressure inspiratory ventilation and PEEP depend on the extent to which positive pressure is transmitted to the intrathoracic compartment and left and right ventricular preload (144–149). Increased intrathoracic pressure decreases left ventricular afterload and, therefore, improves left ventricular stroke volume (2,150). This potentially beneficial consequence of positive-pressure ventilation in patients with left ventricular dysfunction may be balanced by the decrease in venous return that occurs with positive intrathoracic pressures. In patients with myocardial infarction and increased central venous and left ventricular end-diastolic pressures, positive-pressure ventilation and PEEP may improve left ventricular stroke volume and cardiac output (151–153). On the other hand, stroke volume may decrease in patients with relatively low left ventricular preload because of the decrease in venous return (139,141,154). The latter mechanism likely accounts for hypotension immediately after initiation of mechanical ventilation in patients who are relatively volume depleted. In most patients with acute myocardial infarction and pulmonary edema, there is left ventricular dysfunction with relatively increased preload that often improves with positive-pressure ventilation. However, hypotension or decreases in cardiac output may occur when very high levels of PEEP are used or if preload is decreased by treatment with vasodilator or diuretics. For this reason, pulmonary artery catheterization is usually necessary in mechanically ventilated patients with significant left ventricular dysfunction after myocardial infarction.

Bedside right heart catheterization measures transmural pressures in the cardiac chambers and pulmonary artery. Negative and positive pressure changes in the thorax associated with mechanical or spontaneous ventilation may influence measured intracardiac transmural pressures. Transmural pressures reflect intravascular and juxtavascular pressures, which for intrathoracic structures are the same as the intrapleural pressure. Since the end of a spontaneous expiration intrapleural pressure approximates 0 mm Hg, the measured pressures accurately reflect the actual intracardiac values. During spontaneous breathing the pressures measured at end-inspiration are higher than those during inspiration. However, in patients on ventilators providing positive-inspiratory pressure, the end-expiratory intracardiac pressures are lower than during inspiration. Similarly, transmission of PEEP to the intrathoracic pressure will increase intracardiac pressures during expiration. The extent to which inspiratory or expiratory airway pressures are transmitted to intrathoracic pressure varies as a function of lung compliance. Inspiratory airway pressures are the mean and peak airway values during delivery of the desired tidal volume and PEEP as set on the ventilator. In the patient with pulmonary edema or adult respiratory distress syndrome, peak airway pressures are typically increased, but because lung compliance is decreased (i.e., "stiff lungs") it is not possible to assess the expected change in intrathoracic pressure during assisted ventilation by measurement of the peak airway pressures, or to assess the impact of PEEP on measured intracardiac pressures during expiration. Accurate assessment of intrathoracic pressure in such patients requires direct measurement, often by intraesophageal manometry.

Under most circumstances, transmitted intrathoracic pressures do not confound interpretation of cardiac hemodynamics. However, at high levels of PEEP, hemodynamic measurements acquired by right heart catheterization may be an inaccurate reflection of actual intracardiac pressures. When levels of PEEP greater than 10 to 15 mm Hg are used, intrapleural pressure may be increased during expiration, resulting in an increase in the transmural pressure and, therefore, an overestimation of actual intracardiac pressures. Because the physiologic effect of PEEP is to decrease venous return and left ventricular afterload, left ventricular end-diastolic volume may actually be decreasing while transmural pulmonary artery occlusive pressure is increasing in response to increased intrapleural pressure. These hemodynamic effects are also exerted by auto-PEEP, which, as noted above, occurs when airway pressures do not return to 0 mm Hg or the level set on the ventilator (154a). This is related to incomplete expiration, often referred to as "air trapping." This may occur inadvertently because of a rapid respiratory rate with insufficient expiratory time or the use of IRV ventilation. The former is the most frequent circumstance in which auto-PEEP may cause a decrease in stroke volume that is not clinically recognized. Sedation of the patient and/or adjustment of the mode of ventilation (e.g., AC to SIMV) or, less frequently, the inspiratory flow rate, usually will decrease the respiratory rate and improve stroke volume.

Although high levels of PEEP or IRV rarely confound interpretation of hemodynamic measurements, this possibility should be considered in certain patients. Removing the patient from mechanical ventilation to obtain hemodynamic measurements is inappropriate, because the physiologic cardiopulmonary interactions change and there is a potential for respiratory decompensation in critically ill patients. A better strategy is to use multiple independent measures to assess trends in hemodynamics in patients in whom cardiopulmonary interactions may be complex. In patients in whom a decrease in preload due to positive-pressure breathing is suspected to contribute to decreases in stroke volume, volume infusion is indicated.

Differential Diagnosis and Management of Persistent Pulmonary Infiltrates

The time course of resolution of pulmonary edema in patients with alveolar flooding and respiratory failure is variable, but there is often a cause for concern when it is delayed more than 48 hours. It may be difficult to distinguish cardiogenic from noncardiogenic pulmonary edema, because the pulmonary artery wedge pressure may be normal by the time invasive hemodynamic measurements are acquired. The resolution of cardiogenic pulmonary edema may be slow, and it is not unusual for some patients to require prolonged mechanical ventilatory support (>48 hours). As noted previously, pulmonary capillary permeability may be increased in some patients with acute myocardial infarction, resulting in a permeability rather than hydrostatic type of pulmonary edema. Patients in whom resolution of pulmonary infiltrates is delayed and who have persistent widening of the alveolar–arterial oxygen gradient after acute myocardial infarction are usually considered to suffer from adult respiratory distress syndrome (ARDS), which is attributed to acute lung injury involving increased alveolocapillary permeability resulting from a large number of recognized predisposing factors, including but not limited to aspiration, gram-negative sepsis, and multiple transfusions (65,155–157). Patients with acute myocardial infarction without one of these more common risk factors for ARDS often present with diffuse bilateral pulmonary infiltrates without a documented increase in the pulmonary artery wedge pressure.

It is critical to exclude *cardiac causes for persistent cardiogenic pulmonary edema* before the diagnosis of ARDS is made. The most common cause of edema is subclinical episodes of cardiac ischemia with transient elevations of left atrial pressure and intermittent mitral regurgitation. Intermittent mitral regurgitation may not be appreciated, even with frequent physical examination or by echocardiography/Doppler studies, in the absence of ischemia. Hence, continuous monitoring for sudden increases in pulmonary artery pressure or the appearance of a V wave on the pulmonary artery wedge pressure tracing is often useful. In general, pulmonary artery catheterization is indicated in patients with persistent pulmonary edema to exclude persistent or intermittent cardiac causes of hydrostatic edema.

The development of pulmonary edema 3 to 5 days after acute myocardial infarction more often heralds a mechanical complication such as *mitral regurgitation* or *subacute ventricular septal rupture* than ARDS (see Ch. 16).

Aspiration pneumonia may complicate the course of intubated patients with myocardial infarction and acute respiratory failure (158–162). Observed aspiration at the time of intubation should be managed conservatively without prophylactic antibiotics and does not require intervention other than tracheal suctioning. If large foreign body or food matter aspiration is suspected, bronchoscopy may be necessary to relieve or prevent airway obstruction. Aspiration of gastric contents may cause a chemical pneumonitis with interstitial pulmonary infiltrates and fever, but this is usually self-limiting and should not be treated with antibiotics. Large-volume gastric aspiration is a risk factor for ARDS, but treatment with steroids has not been shown to be effective in preventing complications and increases the risk for development of bacterial pneumonia. *Bacterial pneumonia* may occur after aspiration and may complicate the course of the patient intubated for pulmonary edema. Signs and symptoms include the persistence or development of new infiltrates 24 to 48 hours after intubation with purulent sputum, a fever, and leukocytosis with left shift. Antibiotic treatment should be aimed at anaerobic organisms in most patients, except those who are edentulous. Treatment for gram-negative organisms should be given in institutionalized patients, those with chronic diseases, and most elderly patients.

Nosocomial pneumonia often complicates the course of the patient with pulmonary edema or ARDS who requires prolonged mechanical ventilatory support (163). Gram-negative organisms, particularly *Pseudomonas* and staphylococcus species, are the usual cause (163b,163c). The possibility of nosocomial pneumonia should be considered in patients who develop new pulmonary infiltrates, new purulent sputum, fever, or leukocytosis while on mechanical ventilation. Antibiotic treatment includes drugs that are effective against gram-negative organisms, usually with two agents that are active against *Pseudomonas* species.

Rarely, *pulmonary embolism* may be associated with diffuse interstitial infiltrates and may be misdiagnosed as pulmonary edema (164–166). Pulmonary emboli may also complicate the course of patients with pulmonary edema and prolonged mechanical ventilation. Although anticoagulation prevents this complication in most patients, it may occur in patients who are inadequately anticoagulated or those who develop heparin antibodies. The diagnosis of pulmonary embolism is often not considered in patients with pulmonary edema, and when not treated embolism may result in death. Aggressive testing with radionuclear ventilation–perfusion imaging and/or pulmonary angiography should be carried out in patients with unexplained pulmonary infiltrates or worsening oxygenation while on mechanical ventilation to rule out pulmonary embolism.

Weaning from Mechanical Ventilation

Most patients who are intubated for pulmonary edema associated with myocardial infarction are weaned rapidly from mechanical ventilation once extravascular lung water has decreased toward normal levels (92). Patients with unstable ischemic symptoms should not be weaned from mechanical ventilation. Clinical indicators of probable success of weaning include all of the following: oxygen saturations of greater than 90% on 50% or less oxygen with PEEP of 5 mm Hg or less, respiratory rate of 12 to 14 breaths per minute or less, tidal volumes during spontaneous ventilation of at least 5 ml per kg body weight, and a minute ventilation of less than 10 L/minute (92a). Some patients who do not meet these criteria may be weaned successfully, and there is considerable controversy as to the best criteria to use. Nonetheless, the majority of patients who meet these conservative criteria will be successfully weaned from mechanical ventilation. Although many techniques have been suggested for determining whether mechanical ventilation can be discontinued, in most patients in whom pulmonary edema has resolved after a myocardial infarction a 30- to 60-minute trial of spontaneous ventilation through the endotracheal tube is sufficient to assess the likelihood of successful extubation. The trial of unassisted breathing can be performed by disconnecting the patient from the ventilator and providing oxygen directly to the endotracheal tube (t-piece) or use of the ventilator oxygen circuit without assisted breaths. The latter approach is used more frequently, but it has the disadvantage of increasing the work of breathing because of resistance in the ventilator circuit and the need to trigger a valve to receive inspiratory flow. Accordingly, it is common to use a low level (5 cm H_2O) of positive airway pressure inspiratory support (PSV) to decrease the work of breathing during the trial. In patients in whom PEEP has been used, this may be provided by maintaining a constant positive pressure in the circuit of 5 cm of H_2O. Increasing the level of inspired oxygen to 10% above that required during mechanical ventilation is also useful in preventing hypoxemia. The patient's respiratory rate, chest examination results, oxygen saturation, cardiac rhythm, and comfort should be closely monitored during the trial. The probability of success in discontinuing mechanical ventilation is greatest when the patient's respiratory rate does not increase significantly and oxygen saturations are stable during the trial. Patients who successfully complete a trial of unassisted ventilation usually can be extubated if the underlying cardiac hemodynamics are optimized and there is no evidence of recurrent ischemia. Before extubation it is useful to reinitiate mechanical ventilation for a short period of time and optimize pulmonary toilet with endotracheal suctioning. Occasionally, extubation may coincide with removal of arterial catheters placed for cardiac catheterization or intra-aortic balloon counterpulsation or with discontinuation of pulmonary artery catheterization. In such patients it is best to extubate before catheter removal. This will ensure vascular access if it is needed and will prevent bleeding complications from arterial catheterization sites when extubation induces coughing.

The most common reason for failure of a spontaneous ventilation trial is that the underlying cardiopulmonary physiology has not been optimized. In such cases treatment should initially be directed at optimization of left ventricular function, treatment of pulmonary edema, and ruling out recurrent or ongoing ischemia. Such patients can be treated with decreasing levels of mechanical ventilatory support by decreasing the number of assisted breaths (SIMV weaning) or decreasing the inspiratory pressure support (PSV weaning). Alternatively, fully assisted ventilatory support may be continued, and one or several daily trials of unassisted breathing can be conducted over increasing time intervals. There is no consensus as to which of these methods results in the least time to extubation, but results of one recent study (168) suggest that a once-daily trial of spontaneous breathing was superior to SIMV or PSV weaning (167–169). It cannot be overemphasized that the most frequent reason for failure of spontaneous breathing trials in patients with acute respiratory failure associated with myocardial infarction is that the underlying disease has not been optimally treated.

Prolonged mechanical ventilation may be necessary in patients with ARDS, slowly resolving acute pulmonary disease, and chronic pulmonary disease. Patients with unstable ischemic heart disease may require frequent reintubation and may not be able to be off of mechanical ventilation for more than 24 hours. In each of these instances tracheostomy may be necessary for long-term management of the airway and to facilitate mechanical ventilation and weaning (170). As a rule, successful weaning from mechanical ventilation usually requires a multidisciplinary approach in which the underlying disease, nutrition, and the general physical condition of the patient are optimally managed (92,171,172).

CHRONIC OBSTRUCTIVE LUNG DISEASE AND MYOCARDIAL INFARCTION

The management of chronic obstructive airways disease (COPD) or asthma is not modified extensively in patients who have suffered a myocardial infarction (173). The majority of COPD and asthma patients are treated as outpatients with inhaled β-agonists and/or ipratropium bromide. In patients with acute infarction or ischemic heart disease, the dose of ipratropium should be optimized before adding or increasing the dose of a β-agonist inhaler. Inhaled ipratropium has been found in most studies to be as or more effective than β-agonists in patients with COPD, with fewer adverse side effects (39–41, 43,174–177). The combination of a β-agonist and ipratropium may be of value in selected patients (45,178,179). Serious cardiac arrhythmias are an uncommon side effect of bronchodilators, but tachycardia may occur with β-agonist inhalers and may provoke cardiac ischemia (38). Tachycardia can be avoided, in part, by the use of low doses of β_2-selective agonists. Oral β-agonists should not be used in patients with recent infarction or unstable ischemia. Intravenous aminophylline or theophylline formulations can be used in patients with COPD or asthma, but plasma theophylline levels should be monitored daily in all patients in the ICU, particularly those who are hemodynamically unstable or have congestive heart failure. Oral steroids, as noted above, may have deleterious effects on myocardial remodeling after infarction and should be avoided (54). Inhaled steroids, which are often used in the treatment of asthma, are not absorbed and can be safely administered to patients with infarction.

A common and difficult problem in managing patients with COPD and ischemic heart disease is determining the cause of acute episodes of dyspnea. Wheezing may be associated with primary airway reactivity or may be secondary to cardiac ischemia and/or elevated left atrial pressure. A chest x-ray is essential in the evaluation of dyspnea and may reveal new infiltrates consistent with pneumonia or pulmonary edema. An ECG should always be obtained in patients with dyspnea after infarction to evaluate for ischemia. Symptomatic management of bronchospasm with inhaled bronchodilators is usually appropriate, even when bronchospasm is secondary to increases in extravascular lung water. However, the possibility that episodes of bronchospasm are attributable to cardiac ischemia should always be vigorously pursued. In some patients, pulmonary artery catheterization is of value in detecting increases in the pulmonary artery pressure or the pulmonary artery occlusive pressure during episodes of ischemia. Pulmonary embolism also needs to be considered in patients with episodes of unexplained dyspnea and bronchospasm.

UNCOMMON PULMONARY COMPLICATIONS OF ACUTE MYOCARDIAL INFARCTION

Hemoptysis and Alveolar Hemorrhage

Hemoptysis in patients who have been treated with fibrinolytic agents or aggressive anticoagulation is often indicative of bronchial malignancy or other disease (21). Moderate to severe hemoptysis can often be managed by withdrawing anticoagulants; rarely, emergency bronchoscopy is indicated (180). Bronchial embolization should be considered in patients with severe hemoptysis that is unresponsive to other measures. Initial evaluation of patients with hemoptysis should include cytologic analysis of sputum specimens and chest computed tomography. Elective bronchoscopy should be deferred after myocardial infarction until the patient has been evaluated for inducible ischemia and treated medically or with a revascularization procedure. In patients in whom coronary bypass surgery is considered, a complete evaluation will often be necessary, including bronchoscopy, which can usually be performed safely with cardiac monitoring.

Alveolar hemorrhage is a very uncommon complication of thrombolytic therapy, but it should be suspected in patients who develop diffuse pulmonary infiltrates of undetermined cause, usually associated with a decrease in hematocrit (19,20). The differential diagnosis in such patients includes cardiogenic or noncardiogenic pulmonary edema, pulmonary embolism, and ARDS. Bloody alveolar fluid on bronchoalveolar lavage is usually diagnostic for alveolar hemorrhage.

REFERENCES

1. Cherniack NS: Dyspnea, in Murray JF, Nadel JA (eds): *Textbook of Respiratory Medicine,* 1st ed. Philadelphia, WB Saunders, 1988, pp 389–396.
2. Pinsky MR, Matuschak GM, Itzkoff JM: Respiratory augmentation of left ventricular function during spontaneous ventilation in severe left ventricular failure by grunting. An auto-EPAP effect. *Chest* 1984;86(2):267–269.
3. Biddle TL, Yu PN, Hodges M, et al: Hypoxemia and lung water in acute myocardial infarction. *Am Heart J* 1976;92(6):692–699.
4. Gray BA, Hyde RW, Hodges M, Yu PN: Alterations in lung volume and function in relation to hemodynamic changes in acute myocardial infarction. *Circulation* 1979;59:551–559.
5. Hales CA, Kazemi H: Clinical significance of pulmonary function tests. Pulmonary function after uncomplicated myocardial infarction. *Chest* 1977; 72(3):350–358.
6. Luepker RV, Caralis DG, Voigt GC, Burns RF, Murphy LW, Warbasse JR: Detection of pulmonary edema in acute myocardial infarction. *Am J Cardiol* 1977;39(2):146–152.
7. McNichol MW, Kirby BJ, Bhoola KD, et al: Pulmonary function in acute myocardial infarction. *Br Med J* 1965;2:1270–1273.
8. Hales CA, Kazemi H: Small airways function in myocardial infarction. *N Engl J Med* 1974;290(14): 761–765.
9. Storstein O, Rasmussen K: The cause of arterial hypoxemia in acute myocardial infarction. *Acta Med Scand* 1968;183(3):193–196.
10. Valentine PA, Fluck DC, Mounsey JP, Reid D, Shillingford JP, Steiner RE: Blood-gas changes after acute myocardial infarction. *Lancet* 1966; 2(468):837–841.
11. Brezins M, Benari B, Papo V, Cohen A, Bursztein S, Markiewicz W: Left ventricular function in patients with acute myocardial infarction, acute pulmonary edema, and mechanical ventilation: Relationship to prognosis. *Crit Care Med* 1993;21(3): 380–385.
12. Gottlieb S, Moss AJ, McDermott M, Eberly S: Interrelation of left ventricular ejection fraction, pulmonary congestion and outcome in acute myocardial infarction. *Am J Cardiol* 1992;69(12):977–984.
13. Kostuk W, Barr JW, Simon AL, Ross J Jr: Correlations between the chest film and hemodynamics in acute myocardial infarction. *Circulation* 1973;48(3): 624–632.
14. Wiener RS, Moses HW, Richeson JF, Gatewood RP Jr: Hospital and long-term survival of patients with acute pulmonary edema associated with coronary artery disease. *Am J Cardiol* 1987;60(1):33–35.
15. Goldberger JJ, Peled HB, Stroh JA, Cohen MN, Frishman WH: Prognostic factors in acute pulmonary edema. *Arch Intern Med* 1986;146(3): 489–493.
16. Stone GW, Griffin B, Shah PK, et al: Prevalence of unsuspected mitral regurgitation and left ventricular diastolic dysfunction in patients with coronary artery disease and acute pulmonary edema associated with normal or depressed left ventricular systolic function. *Am J Cardiol* 1991;67(1):37–41.
17. Graham SP, Vetrovec GW: Comparison of angiographic findings and demographic variables in patients with coronary artery disease presenting with acute pulmonary edema versus those presenting with chest pain. *Am J Cardiol* 1991;68(17): 1614–1618.
18. Eisenberg PR, Hansbrough JR, Anderson D, Schuster DP: A prospective study of lung water measurements during patient management in an intensive care unit. *Am Rev Respir Dis* 1987;136(3): 662–668.
19. Nathan PE, Torres AV, Smith AJ, Gagliardi AJ, Rapeport KB: Spontaneous pulmonary hemorrhage following coronary thrombolysis. *Chest* 1992;101(4):1150–1152.
20. Fishwick D, Taylor R, Brewis RA: Pulmonary haemorrhage associated with thrombolysis (letter). *Respir Med* 1994;88(10):795.
21. Disler LJ, Rosendorff A: Pulmonary hemorrhage following intravenous streptokinase for acute myocardial infarction. *Int J Cardiol* 1990;29(3):387–390.
22. Lammers JW, Muller ME, Folgering HT, van Herwaarden CL: A comparative study on the ventilatory and haemodynamic effects of xamoterol and atenolol in asthmatic patients. *Br J Clin Pharmacol* 1986;22(5):595–602.
23. van Herwaarden CL: Beta-adrenoceptor blockade and pulmonary function in patients suffering from

chronic obstructive lung disease. *J Cardiovasc Pharmacol* 1983;5(Suppl 1):S46–S50.

24. Jenne JW: Beta blockers and COPD. *Chest* 1980; 78(5):675–676.

25. Fogari R, Zoppi A, Tettamanti F, Poletti L, Rizzardi G, Fiocchi G: Comparative effects of celiprolol, propranolol, oxprenolol, and atenolol on respiratory function in hypertensive patients with chronic obstructive lung disease. *Cardiovasc Drugs Ther* 1990;4(4):1145–1149.

26. Tattersfield AE: Beta adrenoceptor antagonists and respiratory disease. *J Cardiovasc Pharmacol* 1986;8 (Suppl 4):S35–S9.

27. Sheppard D, DiStefano S, Byrd RC, et al: Effects of esmolol on airway function in patients with asthma. *J Clin Pharmacol* 1986;26(3):169–174.

28. Clague HW, Ahmad D, Carruthers SG. Influence of cardioselectivity and respiratory disease on pulmonary responsiveness to beta-blockade. *Eur J Clin Pharmacol* 1984;27(5):517–523.

29. Fenster PE, Quan SF, Hanson CD, Coaker LA: Suppression of ventricular ectopy with intravenous metoprolol in patients with chronic obstructive pulmonary disease. *Crit Care Med* 1984;12(1):29–32.

30. Gold MR, Dec GW, Cocca-Spofford D, Thompson BT: Esmolol and ventilatory function in cardiac patients with COPD. *Chest* 1991;100(5):1215–1218.

31. Fenster PE, Hasan FM, Abraham T, Woolfenden J: Effect of metoprolol on cardiac and pulmonary function in chronic obstructive pulmonary disease. *Clin Cardiol* 1983;6(3):125–129.

32. Anderson G, Jariwalla AG, Al-Zaibak M: A comparison of oral metoprolol and propranolol in patients with chronic bronchitis. *J Int Med Res* 1980; 8(2):136–138.

33. Lee TH: Mechanism of aspirin sensitivity. *Am Rev Respir Dis* 1992;145(2 Pt 2):S34–S36.

34. Probst L, Stoney P, Jeney E, Hawke M: Nasal polyps, bronchial asthma and aspirin sensitivity. *J Otolaryngol* 1992;21(1):60–65.

35. Szczeklik A. Aspirin-induced asthma: Pathogenesis and clinical presentation. *Allergy Proc* 1992;13(4): 163–173.

36. Brunnee T, Graf K, Kastens B, Fleck E, Kunkel G: Bronchial hyperreactivity in patients with moderate pulmonary circulation overload. *Chest* 1993; 103(5):1477–1481.

37. Fromm RE Jr, Varon J: Acute exacerbations of obstructive lung disease. What to do when immediate care is crucial. *Postgrad Med* 1994;95(8):101–106.

38. Seider N, Abinader EG, Oliven A: Cardiac arrhythmias after inhaled bronchodilators in patients with COPD and ischemic heart disease. *Chest* 1993; 104(4):1070–1074.

39. Karpel JP: Bronchodilator responses to anticholinergic and beta-adrenergic agents in acute and stable COPD. *Chest* 1991;99(4):871–876.

40. Chapman KR: Anticholinergic bronchodilators for adult obstructive airways disease. *Am J Med* 1991; 91(4A):13S–16S.

41. Easton PA, Jadue C, Dhingra S, Anthonisen NR: A comparison of the bronchodilating effects of a beta-2 adrenergic agent (albuterol) and an anticholinergic agent (ipratropium bromide), given by aerosol alone or in sequence. *N Engl J Med* 1986; 315(12):735–739.

42. LeDoux EJ, Morris JF, Temple WP, Duncan C: Standard and double dose ipratropium bromide and combined ipratropium bromide and inhaled metaproterenol in COPD. *Chest* 1989;95(5): 1013–1016.

43. Braun SR, Levy SF: Comparison of ipratropium bromide and albuterol in chronic obstructive pulmonary disease: A three-center study. *Am J Med* 1991;91(4A):28S–32S.

44. Mann KV, Leon AL, Tietze KJ: Use of ipratropium bromide in obstructive lung disease. *Clin Pharm* 1988;7(9):670–680.

45. Rennard SI: Combination bronchodilator therapy in COPD. *Chest* 1995;107(5 Suppl):171S–175S.

46. Lloberes P, Ramis L, Montserrat JM, et al: Effect of three different bronchodilators during an exacerbation of chronic obstructive pulmonary disease. *Eur Respir J* 1988;1(6):536–539.

47. Patrick DM, Dales RE, Stark RM, Laliberte G, Dickinson G: Severe exacerbations of COPD and asthma. Incremental benefit of adding ipratropium to usual therapy. *Chest* 1990;98(2):295–297.

48. Aubier M: Effect of theophylline on diaphragmatic muscle function. *Chest* 1987;92(1 Suppl):27S–31S.

49. Mahler DA: The role of theophylline in the treatment of dyspnea in COPD. *Chest* 1987;92(1 Suppl): 2S–6S.

50. Matthay RA: Favorable cardiovascular effects of theophylline in COPD. *Chest* 1987;92(1 Suppl): 22S–26S.

51. Matthay RA: Effects of theophylline on cardiovascular performance in chronic obstructive pulmonary disease. *Chest* 1985;88(2 Suppl): 112S–117S.

52. Ramsdell J: Use of theophylline in the treatment of COPD. *Chest* 1995;107(5 Suppl):206S–209S.

53. Vaz Fragoso CA, Miller MA: Review of the clinical efficacy of theophylline in the treatment of chronic obstructive pulmonary disease. *Am Rev Respir Dis* 1993;147(6 Pt 2):S40–S47.

54. Weisman HF, Healy B: Myocardial infarct expansion, infarct extension, and reinfarction: Pathophysiologic concepts. *Prog Cardiovasc Dis* 1987;30(2): 73–110.

55. Silverman HS, Pfeifer MP: Relation between use of anti-inflammatory agents and left ventricular free wall rupture during acute myocardial infarction. *Am J Cardiol* 1987;59(4):363–364.

56. Bernard GR, Brigham KL. Pulmonary edema. Pathophysiologic mechanisms and new approaches to therapy. *Chest* 1986;89(4):594–600.

57. Staub NC: New concepts about the pathophysiology of pulmonary edema. *J Thorac Imaging* 1988; 3(3):8–14.

58. Staub NC: Alveolar flooding and clearance. *Am Rev Respir Dis* 1983;127(5 Pt 2):S44–S51.

59. Hachenberg T, Meyer J, Brussel T, et al: Effective pulmonary capillary pressure in experimental myocardial ischaemia. *Eur Heart J* 1993;14(5):705–711.

60. Staub NC, Nagano H, Pearce ML: Pulmonary edema in dogs, especially the sequence of fluid accumulation in lungs. *J Appl Physiol* 1967;22(2): 227–240.

61. Staub NC: Pulmonary edema. *Physiol Rev* 1974; 54(3):678–811.

62. Biddle TL, Khanna PK, Yu PN, Hodges M, Shah PM: Lung water in patients with acute myocardial infarction. *Circulation* 1974;49(1):115–123.

63. Staub NC: Pulmonary edema due to increased microvascular permeability. *Annu Rev Med* 1981;32: 291–312.

64. Hasegawa N, Husari AW, Hart WT, Kandra TG, Raffin TA: Role of the coagulation system in ARDS. *Chest* 1994;105(1):268–277.

65. Kollef MH, Schuster DP: The acute respiratory distress syndrome. *N Engl J Med* 1995;332(1):27–37.

66. Taniguchi H, Takayama Y, Iwasaka T, et al: Effect of the leukotriene receptor antagonist ONO-1078 on extravascular lung water after coronary ligation in dogs. *Jpn Circ J* 1993;57(2):161–166.

67. Taniguchi H, Iwasaka T, Takayama Y, Sugiura T, Inada M: Role of platelet-activating factor in pulmonary edema after coronary ligation in dogs. *Chest* 1992;102(4):1245–1250.

68. Talbott GA, Sharar SR, Harlan JM, Winn RK: Leukocyte–endothelial interactions and organ injury: The role of adhesion molecules. *New Horiz* 1994;2(4):545–554.

69. Welbourn CR, Young Y: Endotoxin, septic shock and acute lung injury: Neutrophils, macrophages and inflammatory mediators. *Br J Surg* 1992;79(10): 998–1003.

70. Richeson JF, Paulshock C, Yu PN: Non-hydrostatic pulmonary edema after coronary artery ligation in dogs. Protective effect of indomethacin. *Circ Res* 1982;50:301–309.

71. Slutsky RA, Peck WW, Higgins CB: Pulmonary edema formation with myocardial infarction and left atrial hypertension: Intravascular and extravascular pulmonary fluid volumes. *Circulation* 1983; 68(1):164–169.

72. Gee MH, Gwirtz PA, Spath JA: Extravascular lung water content of heart and lungs after acute myocardial ischemia. *J Appl Physiol* 1978;45: 102–108.

73. Slutsky RA, Mattrey RF: Pulmonary edema formation after myocardial infarction and coronary reperfusion: Intravascular and extravascular pulmonary fluid volumes. IV. *Circ Shock* 1984;13(2): 183–191.

74. Agostoni A, Gardinali M, Frangi D, et al: Activation of complement and kinin systems after thrombolytic therapy in patients with acute myocardial infarction. A comparison between streptokinase and recombinant tissue-type plasminogen activator. *Circulation* 1994;90(6):2666–2670.

75. Agostoni A, Gardinali M, Frangi D, et al: Thrombolytic treatment and complement activation. *Ann Ital Med Int* 1994;9(3):178–179.

76. Niederman MS, Fein AM, Sklarck HM, et al: Pulmonary edema with low pulmonary capillary wedge pressure after myocardial infarction: Clinical features and prognostic implications. *J Crit Care* 1989;4:194–201.

77. Aubier M, Viires N, Syllie R, Mozes R, Roussos C: Respiratory muscle contribution to lactica acidosis in low cardiac output. *Am Rev Respir Dis* 1982;126: 648–652.

78. Berthiaume Y, Albertine KH, Grady M, Fick G, Matthay MA: Protein clearance from the air spaces and lungs of unanesthetized sheep over 144 h. *J Appl Physiol* 1989;67(5):1887–1897.

79. Berthiaume Y, Broaddus VC, Gropper MA, Tanita T, Matthay MA: Alveolar liquid and protein clearance

from normal dog lungs. *J Appl Physiol* 1988; 65(2):585–593.

80. Berthiaume Y, Staub NC, Matthay MA: Beta-adrenergic agonists increase lung liquid clearance in anesthetized sheep. *J Clin Invest* 1987;79(2): 335–343.

81. Jayr C, Garat C, Meignan M, Pittet JF, Zelter M, Matthay MA: Alveolar liquid and protein clearance in anesthetized ventilated rats. *J Appl Physiol* 1994;76(6):2636–2642.

82. Sakuma T, Okaniwa G, Nakada T, Nishimura T, Fujimura S, Matthay MA: Alveolar fluid clearance in the resected human lung. *Am J Respir Crit Care Med* 1994;150(2):305–310.

83. Matthay MA: Resolution of pulmonary edema. New insights. *West J Med* 1991;154(3):315–321.

84. Matthay MA: Resolution of pulmonary edema. Mechanisms of liquid, protein, and cellular clearance from the lung. *Clin Chest Med* 1985;6(3): 521–545.

85. Cabanes LR, Weber SN, Matran R, et al: Bronchial hyperresponsiveness to methacholine in patients with impaired left ventricular function. *N Engl J Med* 1989;320(20):1317–1322.

86. Pison C, Malo JL, Rouleau JL, Chalaoui J, Ghezzo H, Malo J: Bronchial hyperresponsiveness to inhaled methacholine in subjects with chronic left heart failure at a time of exacerbation and after increasing diuretic therapy. *Chest* 1989;96(2): 230–235.

87. Seibert AF, Allison RC, Bryars CH, Kirkpatrick MB: Normal airway responsiveness to methacholine in cardiac asthma. *Am Rev Respir Dis* 1989; 140(6):1805–1806.

88. Davidson RM, Ramo BW, Wallace AG, Whalen RE, Starmer CF: Blood-gas and hemodynamic responses to oxygen in acute myocardial infarction. *Circulation* 1973;47(4):704–711.

89. Helmers C, Hofvendahl S, Lundman T, et al: Arterial oxygen and carbon-dioxide tension in patients with acute myocardial infarction. *Cardiology* 1973; 58(6):335–346.

90. Tobin MJ: Mechanical ventilation. *N Engl J Med* 1994;330(15):1056–1061.

91. Hubmayer RD, Abel MD, Rehder K: Physiologic approach to mechanical ventilation. *Crit Care Med* 1990;18:103–113.

92. Schuster DP: A physiologic approach to initiating, maintaining, and withdrawing mechanical ventilatory support during acute respiratory failure. *Am J Med* 1990;88:268–278.

92a. Yang KL, Tobin MJ: A prospective study of indexes predicting the outcome of trials of weaning from mechanical ventilation. *N Engl J Med* 1991; 324:1445–1450.

93. Aberman A, Fulop M: The metabolic and respiratory acidosis of acute pulmonary edema. *Ann Intern Med* 1972;76(2):173–184.

94. Fulop M, Horowitz M, Aberman A, Jaffe ER: Lactic acidosis in pulmonary edema due to left ventricular failure. *Ann Intern Med* 1973;79(2): 180–186.

95. Morley TF, Zappasodi SJ, Belli A, Giudice JC: Pulmonary vasodilator therapy for chronic obstructive pulmonary disease and cor pulmonale. Treatment with nifedipine, nitroglycerin, and oxygen. *Chest* 1987;92(1):71–76.

96. Nomoto Y, Kawamura M: Pulmonary gas exchange effects by nitroglycerin, dopamine and dobutamine during one-lung ventilation in man. *Can J Anaesth* 1989;36(3 Pt 1):273–277.

97. Abrams J: Hemodynamic effects of nitroglycerin and long-acting nitrates. *Am Heart J* 1985;110(1 Pt 2):216–224.

98. Anjou-Lindskog E, Broman L, Broman M, Holmgren A: Effects of nitroglycerin on central haemodynamics and VA/Q distribution during ventilation with FIO_2 = 1.0 in patients after coronary bypass surgery. *Acta Anaesthesiol Scand* 1984;28(1):27–33.

99. Yamakage M, Iwasaki H, Satoh K, Namiki A: Effects of induced hypotension on arterial blood-gases under spontaneous breathing. *Acta Anaesthesiol Scand* 1994;38(4):368–371.

100. Torfgard KE, Ahlner J: Mechanisms of action of nitrates. *Cardiovasc Drugs Ther* 1994;8(5):701–717.

101. Marshall BE, Hanson CW, Frasch F, Marshall C: Role of hypoxic pulmonary vasoconstriction in pulmonary gas exchange and blood flow distribution. 2. Pathophysiology. *Intensive Care Med* 1994; 20(5):379–389.

102. Curry SC, Arnold-Capell P: Toxic effects of drugs used in the ICU. Nitroprusside, nitroglycerin, and angiotensin-converting enzyme inhibitors. *Crit Care Clin* 1991;7(3):555–581.

103. Mansouri A, Lurie AA: Concise review: Methemoglobinemia. *Am J Hematol* 1993;42(1):7–12.

104. Buenger JW, Mauro VF: Organic nitrate-induced methemoglobinemia. *Dicp* 1989;23(4):283–288.

105. Bennett ED, Rees S: The significance of radiological changes in the lungs in acute myocardial infarction. *Br J Radiol* 1974;47(564):879–881.

106. Cutillo AG: The clinical assessment of lung water. *Chest* 1987;92(2):319–325.

107. Halperin BD, Feeley TW, Mihm FG, Chiles C, Guthaner DF, Blank NE: Evaluation of the portable chest roentgenogram for quantitating extravascular lung water in critically ill adults. *Chest* 1985;88(5):649–652.

108. Hublitz UF, Shapiro JH: The radiology of pulmonary edema: Four decades of observation, clinical correlations, and studies of the underlying pathophysiology. *CRC Crit Rev Clin Radiol Nucl Med* 1974;5(3):389–422.

109. Hull R, Bjork L, Cullhed I, Lonnerholm T: Clinical and radiological signs of left ventricular failure in acute myocardial infarction. *Acta Med Scand* 1972;192(3):189–196.

110. Madsen EB, Gilpin E, Slutsky RA, Ahnve S, Henning H, Ross J Jr: Usefulness of the chest x-ray for predicting abnormal left ventricular function after acute myocardial infarction. *Am Heart J* 1984; 108(6):1431–1436.

111. Milne EN: Correlation of physiologic findings with chest roentgenology. *Radiol Clin North Am* 1973;11(1):17–47.

112. Sivak ED, Richmond BJ, O'Donavan PB, Borkowski GP: Value of extravascular lung water measurement vs portable chest x-ray in the management of pulmonary edema. *Crit Care Med* 1983;11(7):498–501.

113. Tattersfield AE, McNicol MW, Shawdon H, Rolfe D: Chest x-ray film in acute myocardial infarction. *Br Med J* 1969;1(666):332–335.

114. Swensen SJ, Peters SG, LeRoy AJ, Gay PC, Sykes MW, Trastek VF: Radiology in the intensive-care unit. *Mayo Clin Proc* 1991;66(4):396–410.

115. Schober OH, Meyer GJ, Bossaller C, Creutzig H, Lichtlen PR, Hundeshagen H: Quantitative determination of regional extravascular lung water and regional blood volume in congestive heart failure. *Eur J Nucl Med* 1985;10(1–2): 17–24.

116. Scharf SM: Cardiovascular effects of airways obstruction. *Lung* 1991;169(1):1–23.

117. Greene KE, Peters JI: Pathophysiology of acute respiratory failure. *Clin Chest Med* 1994;15(1): 1–12.

118. Moxham J: Respiratory muscle fatigue: Mechanisms, evaluation and therapy. *Br J Anaesth* 1990; 65(1):43–53.

119. Ward M, Macklem PT: The act of breathing and how it fails. *Chest* 1990;97(3 Suppl):36S–39S.

120. Aubier M. Respiratory muscle fatigue. *Intensive Care Med* 1989;15(Suppl 1):S17–S20.

121. Aldrich TK: Respiratory muscle fatigue. *Clin Chest Med* 1988;9(2):225–236.

122. Derenne JP, Fleury B, Pariente R: Acute respiratory failure of chronic obstructive pulmonary disease. *Am Rev Respir Dis* 1988;138(4):1006–1033.

123. Tobin MJ: Respiratory muscles in disease. *Clin Chest Med* 1988;9(2):263–286.

124. Roussos C: Function and fatigue of respiratory muscles. *Chest* 1985;88(2 Suppl):124S–132S.

125. Grassino A, Macklem PT: Respiratory muscle fatigue and ventilatory failure. *Annu Rev Med* 1984; 35:625–647.

126. Pinsky MR: Determinants of pulmonary arterial flow variation during respiration. *J Appl Physiol* 1984;56(5):1237–1245.

127. Rutledge FS, Hussain SN, Roussos C, Magder S: Diaphragmatic energetics and blood flow during pulmonary edema and hypotension. *J Appl Physiol* 1988;64(5):1908–1915.

128. Meyer TJ, Hill NS: Noninvasive positive pressure ventilation to treat respiratory failure. *Ann Intern Med* 1994;120(9):760–770.

129. Lin M, Yang YF, Chiang HT, Chang MS, Chiang BN, Cheitlin MD: Reappraisal of continuous positive airway pressure therapy in acute cardiogenic pulmonary edema. Short-term results and long-term follow-up. *Chest* 1995;107(5):1379–1386.

130. Vaisanen IT, Rasanen J: Continuous positive airway pressure and supplemental oxygen in the treatment of cardiogenic pulmonary edema. *Chest* 1987;92(3):481–485.

131. Rasanen J, Heikkila J, Downs J, Nikki P, Vaisanen I, Viitanen A: Continuous positive airway pressure by face mask in acute cardiogenic pulmonary edema. *Am J Cardiol* 1985;55(4):296–300.

132. Bersten AD, Holt AW, Vedig AE, Skowronski GA, Baggoley CJ: Treatment of severe cardiogenic pulmonary edema with continuous positive airway pressure delivered by face mask. *N Engl J Med* 1991;325:1825–1830.

133. Lapinsky SE, Mount DB, Mackey D, Grossman RF: Management of acute respiratory failure due

to pulmonary edema with nasal positive pressure support. *Chest* 1994;105(1):229–231.

134. Kharasch M, Graff J: Emergency management of the airway. *Crit Care Clin* 1995;11(1):53–66.

135. Marini JJ: Strategies to minimize breathing effort during mechanical ventilation. *Crit Care Clin* 1990; 6(3):635–661.

135a. Amato MBP, Barbas CSV, Medeiros DM, et al: Beneficial effects of the "open lung approach" with low distending pressures in acute respiratory distress syndrome. *Am J Respir Crit Care Med* 1995; 152:1835–1846.

136. Fields AI: Newer modes of mechanical ventilation for patients with adult respiratory distress syndrome. *Crit Care Med* 1993;21(9 Suppl): S367–S369.

137. Armstrong BW Jr, MacIntyre NR: Pressure-controlled, inverse ratio ventilation that avoids air trapping in the adult respiratory distress syndrome. *Crit Care Med* 1995;23(2):279–285.

138. Lessard MR, Guerot E, Lorino H, Lemaire F, Brochard L: Effects of pressure-controlled with different I:E ratios versus volume-controlled ventilation on respiratory mechanics, gas exchange, and hemodynamics in patients with adult respiratory distress syndrome. *Anesthesiology* 1994;80(5): 983–991.

139. Mang H, Kacmarek RM, Ritz R, Wilson RS, Kimball WP: Cardiorespiratory effects of volume- and pressure-controlled ventilation at various I/E ratios in an acute lung injury model. *Am J Resp Crit Care Med* 1995;151(3 Pt 1):731–736.

140. Manthous CA, Schmidt GA: Inverse ratio ventilation in ARDS. Improved oxygenation without auto-PEEP. *Chest* 1993;103(3):953–954.

141. Mercat A, Graini L, Teboul JL, Lenique F, Richard C: Cardiorespiratory effects of pressure-controlled ventilation with and without inverse ratio in the adult respiratory distress syndrome. *Chest* 1993;104(3):871–875.

142. Shanholtz C, Brower R: Should inverse ratio ventilation be used in adult respiratory distress syndrome? *Am J Resp Crit Care Med* 1994;149(5): 1354–1358.

143. Valta P, Takala J: Volume-controlled inverse ratio ventilation: Effect on dynamic hyperinflation and auto-PEEP. *Acta Anaesthesiol Scand* 1993;37(4): 323–328.

144. Biondi JW, Schulman DS, Soufer R, et al: The effect of incremental positive end-expiratory pressure on right ventricular hemodynamics and ejection fraction. *Anesth Analg* 1988;67(2):144–151.

145. Pinsky MR: The effects of mechanical ventilation on the cardiovascular system. *Crit Care Clin* 1990; 6(3):663–678.

146. Van Hook CJ, Carilli AD, Haponik EF: Hemodynamic effects of positive end-expiratory pressure. Historical perspective. *Am J Med* 1986;81(2): 307–310.

147. Goertz A, Heinrich H, Winter H, Deller A: Hemodynamic effects of different ventilatory patterns. A prospective clinical trial. *Chest* 1991;99(5): 1166–1171.

148. Pinsky MR: The influence of positive-pressure ventilation on cardiovascular function in the critically ill. *Crit Care Clin* 1985;1(3):699–717.

149. Pinsky MR, Matuschak GM, Klain M: Determinants of cardiac augmentation by elevations in intrathoracic pressure. *J Appl Physiol* 1985;58(4): 1189–1198.

150. Guyatt GH: Positive pressure ventilation as a mechanism of reduction of left ventricular afterload. *Can Med Assoc J* 1982;126(11):1310–1312.

151. Poelaert JI, Visser CA, Everaert JA, Koolen JJ, Colardyn FA: Acute hemodynamic changes of pressure-controlled inverse ratio ventilation in the adult respiratory distress syndrome. A transesophageal echocardiographic and Doppler study. *Chest* 1993;104(1):214–219.

152. Nikki P, Rasanen J, Tahvanainen J, Makelainen A: Ventilatory pattern in respiratory failure arising from acute myocardial infarction. Respiratory and hemodynamic effects of IMV vs IPPV and PEEP vs PEEP. *Crit Care Med* 1982;10:75–81.

153. Rasanen J, Nikki P, Heikkila J: Acute myocardial infarction complicated by respiratory failure. The effect of mechanical ventilation. *Chest* 1984;85:21–28.

154. Chan K, Abraham E: Effects of inverse ratio ventilation on cardiorespiratory parameters in severe respiratory failure. *Chest* 1992;102(5):1556–1561.

154a. Mercat A, Graini L, Teboul JL, Lenique F, et al: Cardiorespiratory effects of pressure-controlled ventilation with and without inverse ratio in the adult respiratory distress syndrome. *Chest* 1993; 104:871–875.

155. Matthay MA: The adult respiratory distress syndrome. Definition and prognosis. *Clin Chest Med* 1990;11(4):575–580.

156. Bernard GR, Artigas A, Brigham KL, et al: Report of the American–European Consensus con-

ference on acute respiratory distress syndrome: Definitions, mechanisms, relevant outcomes, and clinical trial coordination. Consensus Committee. *J Crit Care* 1994;9(1):72–81.

157. Marinelli WA, Ingbar DH: Diagnosis and management of acute lung injury. *Clin Chest Med* 1994;15(3):517–546.

158. Bartlett JG: Anaerobic bacterial infections of the lung and pleural space. *Clin Infect Dis* 1993;16 (Suppl 4):S248–S255.

159. Britto J, Demling RH: Aspiration lung injury. *New Horiz* 1993;1(3):435–439.

160. Tietjen PA, Kaner RJ, Quinn CE: Aspiration emergencies. *Clin Chest Med* 1994;15(1):117–135.

161. DePaso WJ. Aspiration pneumonia. *Clin Chest Med* 1991;12(2):269–284.

162. Finegold SM. Aspiration pneumonia. *Rev Infect Dis* 1991;13(Suppl 9):S737–S742.

163. Craven DE, Steger KA, Barat LM, Duncan RA. Nosocomial pneumonia: Epidemiology and infection control. *Intensive Care Med* 1992;18(Suppl 1): S3–S9.

163b. Kollef MH: Ventilator-associated pneumonia. A multivariate analysis. *JAMA* 1993;270:1965–1970.

163c. Kollef MH, Schuster DP: Ventilator associated pneumonia: Clinical considerations. *AJR* 1994; 163:1031–1035.

164. King MB, Harmon KR: Unusual forms of pulmonary embolism. *Clin Chest Med* 1994;15(3): 561–580.

165. Worsley DF, Alavi A, Aronchick JM, Chen JT, Greenspan RH, Ravin CE: Chest radiographic findings in patients with acute pulmonary embolism: Observations from the PIOPED Study. *Radiology* 1993;189(1):133–136.

166. Yuceoglu YZ, Rubler S, Eshwar KP, Tchertkoff V, Grishman A: Pulmonary edema associated with pulmonary embolism: A clinicopathological study. *Angiology* 1971;22(9):501–510.

167. Brochard L, Rauss A, Benito S, et al: Comparison of three methods of gradual withdrawal from ventilatory support during weaning from mechanical ventilation. *Am J Respir Crit Care Med* 1994; 150(4):896–903.

168. Esteban A, Frutos F, Tobin MJ, et al: A comparison of four methods of weaning patients from mechanical ventilation. Spanish Lung Failure Collaborative Group. *N Engl J Med* 1995;332(6): 345–350.

169. Jounieaux V, Duran A, Levi-Valensi P: Synchronized intermittent mandatory ventilation with and without pressure support ventilation in weaning patients with COPD from mechanical ventilation. *Chest* 1994;105(4):1204–1210.

170. Colice GL: Prolonged intubation versus tracheostomy in the adult. *J Intensive Care Med* 1987;2:85–102.

171. Pingleton SK, Harmon GS: Nutritional management in acute respiratory failure. *JAMA* 1987; 257(22):3094–3099.

172. Benotti PN, Bistrian B: Metabolic and nutritional aspects of weaning from mechanical ventilation. *Crit Care Med* 1989;17(2):181–185.

173. Hagedorn SD: Acute exacerbations of COPD. How to evaluate severity and treat the underlying cause. *Postgrad Med* 1992;91(1):105–107,110–112.

174. Braun SR, McKenzie WN, Copeland C, Knight L, Ellersieck M: A comparison of the effect of ipratropium and albuterol in the treatment of chronic obstructive airway disease. *Arch Intern Med* 1989;149(3):544–547.

175. Karpel JP, Pesin J, Greenberg D, Gentry E: A comparison of the effects of ipratropium bromide and metaproterenol sulfate in acute exacerbations of COPD. *Chest* 1990;98(4):835–839.

176. Tashkin DP, Ashutosh K, Bleecker ER, et al: Comparison of the anticholinergic bronchodilator ipratropium bromide with metaproterenol in chronic obstructive pulmonary disease. A 90-day multi-center study. *Am J Med* 1986;81(5A):81–90.

177. Lakshminarayan S: Ipratropium bromide in chronic bronchitis/emphysema. A review of the literature. *Am J Med* 1986;81(5A):76–80.

178. Anonymous: In chronic obstructive pulmonary disease, a combination of ipratropium and albuterol is more effective than either agent alone. An 85-day multicenter trial. COMBIVENT Inhalation Aerosol Study Group. *Chest* 1994;105(5): 1411–1419.

179. Ikeda A, Nishimura K, Koyama H, Izumi T: Bronchodilating effects of combined therapy with clinical dosages of ipratropium bromide and salbutamol for stable COPD: Comparison with ipratropium bromide alone. *Chest* 1995;107(2): 401–405.

180. Silver MR, Balk RA: Bronchoscopic procedures in the intensive care unit. *Crit Care Clin* 1995; 11(1):97–109.

25

Acute Myocardial Infarction in the Elderly

Dalane W. Kitzman, MD, and Christopher M. O'Connor, MD

BACKGROUND

Aging of the Population and Health Care in the Elderly

The United States, similar to most Western countries, is in the midst of a major change in demographics. Due to a variety of factors, the mean age of the population is increasing significantly. While the change in mean age may appear small, the implications of the change become clearer when the individual age groups are examined. The fastest growth is in the ≥65 years age group. In the United States in 1992, more than 40% of noninterest federal spending goes to this segment of the population, and more than $340 billion was spent on their medical care (1,2).

Furthermore, due to significant declines in mortality in this older group, the greatest growth is seen in the over 85 age group, the so-called "very elderly," "old-old," or "oldest old" (3). By some estimates the population of very elderly will increase 3–4 fold through 2030, while the number of young will increase little. It is the very elderly group that consumes the majority of health care resources, and cardiovascular disease is the most common cause of morbidity and mortality among them. Despite this, very few cardiovascular therapies have been studied systematically in trials in this group (4). Instead, until very recently, older patients were excluded from therapeutic trials for fear they would skew the outcome data. (The question of whether older patients may be different from the middle-aged will be examined in more detail below.) Thus our medical system is least prepared to deal with the group that already accounts for the majority of cardiovascular disease cases and health care expenditures and that is growing the fastest.

Gender interacts demographically with the aging phenomenon. For reasons that remain unclear, women have longer life spans than men (5). By the tenth decade (90–100 years), there are nearly four women living for every man (3). Therefore, the older the age group that is examined, the higher the percentage of women (see Ch. 26).

In treating individual patients, physicians' two main goals are to improve survival (reduce mortality) and reduce symptoms (improve quality of life). In the very elderly, it is appropriate to place greater emphasis on the latter goal and relatively less on the former than when caring for younger patients. The percentage of persons with significant, limiting disabilities increases dramatically with age. The cost of providing care for an independent-living, ambulatory elderly patient is considerably less than for one who is institutionalized. On a personal level, the former enjoys a considerably higher quality of life and is more able to continue to contribute to society. Some therapies aimed at prolonging survival have higher risks of disabling complications in the elderly, but more importantly, they have not been rigorously tested in trials in this population. Therefore, there is good rationale for emphasizing therapy aimed at relieving symptoms, minimizing disability, and maintaining quality of life in the elderly.

Psychosocial issues are encountered more frequently and are more challenging to deal with in the elderly patient. Depression, dementia, noncompliance, isolation, inadequate social support, and dependency are all issues that frequently complicate care of the elderly.

Table 25–1. Normal Age-Related Changes in the Anatomy of the Heart

Myocardium:
Increased heart weight, LV mass, LV wall thickness; mild hypertrophy
Fibrosis, collagen accumulation
Chambers:
LV cavity size decreases, long axis shortens rightward shift and dilation of the aorta,
Dilation of left atrium, senile septum
Valves:
Calcific and fatty degeneration of valve leaflets and annuli
Coronary arteries:
Dilation, tortuousity, and Mockebers's medial calcification (arteriosclerosis)
Conduction system:
Fibrosis and loss of specialized cells and fibers
75% pacemaker cell in SA node lost
Fibrosis of A-V node and left anterior fascicle

AGE-RELATED CHANGES IN THE CARDIOVASCULAR SYSTEM

Knowledge of age-related changes in the cardiovascular system is useful for understanding cardiovascular disease in the elderly and response to therapy.

Anatomy

Most information regarding aging of the normal human heart, particularly from very elderly subjects, has been reported only relatively recently (Table 25–1) (6–16). In patients with no history of hypertension and no evidence of coronary artery disease at autopsy, heart weight, indexed to body size, increases in women but not in men with advancing age (15). The increase in heart weight in women may be due to the small rise in blood pressure or other alterations associated with menopause (5,15).

In the myocardium with aging, there is increased fat deposition (17,18), particularly in the epicardium over the right ventricle and along the atrioventricular groove (19). Epicardial and pericardial fat may partially mimic pericardial effusion on echocardiography (20). With advancing age, there is an increase in interstitial collagen and elastin (18,21,22), seen as diffuse foci of fibrosis. This may cause the increase in myocardial stiffness and decreased diastolic compliance seen with aging, which we will discuss further (23–25). There is a decrease in the number and an increase in the size of cardiac myocytes (26,27). Enlargement, irregularity, and replication of nuclei are commonly present and are indicative of polyploidy (28). Focal basophilic myocardial degeneration, a result of abnormal glycogenolysis, is a near-universal finding in the elderly myocardium (18). Accumulation of lipofuscin, a "wear and tear" pigment, can occupy up to 10% of myocardial volume and give a darkened appearance to the aged myocardium and is often called brown atrophy (29). Senile cardiac amyloid is present, to some degree, in the majority of hearts from persons over age 90 but is uncommon before age 60 (30). The functional significance of these changes is largely uninvestigated (23,26,28,29,31).

By autopsy and echocardiography, left ventricular free wall and ventricular septal thickness increase with age for men and women (15,32) (see Ch. 16). The geometry of the heart appears to change with aging. There is shortening of the long-axis dimension, a mild decrease in the internal systolic and diastolic left ventricular dimensions, dilation and rightward shifting of the aortic root, and dilation of the left atrium (7,33,34).

Several age-related changes occur in the cardiac valves that may be functionally important. The thicknesses of the aortic and mitral leaflets increase (8), particularly along the closure margins (35), and the weight and area of the individual aortic valve cusps increase with age (13). This is associated with collagen deposition and degeneration, lipid accumulation, and focal dystrophic calcification of the leaflets and annuli of the aortic and mitral valves (36). Probably the most common clinical manifestations of these changes are aortic valve sclerosis and mitral annular calicification (7,34). Age-related valvular dilation appears to be associated with degeneration in the valve annuli (35,36). This probably contributes to the age-related multivalvular regurgitation that is seen by Doppler echocardiography in a majority of healthy elderly subjects (37). By age 80, 90% of subjects have multivalvular regurgitation, and the aortic valve is affected earliest and to the greatest extent (37). The degree of valvular regurgitation due to normal aging is trivial or mild. However, age alone is currently the strongest risk factor for isolated severe aortic regurgitation (38), and idiopathic dilation of the aortic annulus is now reported to be the most common cause of aortic regurgitation in patients undergoing aortic valve surgery (39). This is an example of an apparent exaggeration of an expected age-related degenerative change that is associated with a known cardiovascular disorder with important health care implications for our country.

With aging, the coronary arteries become tortuous, independent of heart weight (40), possibly due to hemodynamic drag (41). The effect of age on the size of the coronary arteries is unclear. Autopsy studies suggest an increase in coronary artery diameter with age, while a coronary angiographic study in living subjects indicated a decrease in coronary artery diameter with age, independent of left ventricular mass (42). The number and size of coronary collaterals may increase with age (21), but it is not clear whether this is independent of atherosclerosis. Regardless of age, atherosclerosis is always considered a disease process. However, Mönckeberg's medial calcification (arteriosclerosis) probably represents an age-related degenerative process (43). It is a nearly universal finding in the very old and is independent of gender. In the peripheral vasculature, it may contribute to the age-related elevation in systemic systolic blood pressure and arterial impedance. Because degenerative calcification is so common in the elderly, roentgenographic detection of coronary artery calcification loses predictive value for coronary atherosclerosis in subjects older than 65 years (44).

Aging is accompanied by fibrosis, fatty infiltration, and loss of specialized conducting tissues throughout the conduction system (45–49). From the ages of 20 and 75, the number of pacemaker cells in the sinus node may decrease by 40–90% (47,48). There is also a concomitant loss of fibers in the internodal tracts, and partial loss of the left bundle fascicles originating in the bundle of His. These changes appear to be unrelated to coronary artery disease (47). These age-related changes in normal human hearts may be significant, since they probably underlie the described age-related lengthening of the PR, QRS, and QT intervals and the left-axis deviation seen on the surface electrocardiogram (6,49). In particular, there may be a relationship between these age-related changes and the high prevalence of left anterior fascicular block and Q waves in the anteroseptal leads in the asymptomatic elderly.

Physiology

Most of the information regarding the effect of aging on cardiovascular function has been reported within the previous decade. While there is some controversy in this area, particularly with regard to function during exercise, several general statements can now be made from the preponderance of evidence (Table 25–2).

Effect of Age on Cardiovascular Physiology at Rest

Several important age-related changes have already been discussed briefly, including changes in

Table 25–2. Normal Age-Related Changes in Cardiovascular Physiology

- Cardiac output and stroke volume decline mildly.
- Peak exercise heart rate declines.
- Peak exercise ejection fraction declines.
- Left ventricular stiffness increases; diastolic relaxation decreases.
- Valvular regurgitation develops.
- Prolongation of PR, QRS, QT; left-axis deviation.
- Arteries stiffen; aortic impedance increases.
- Systolic blood pressure increases.

valvular function, conduction, and the potential anatomic substrates for altered diastolic function, one of the most important age-related changes in resting physiology. By comparing young and old beagles using invasive techniques, Templeton et al (50) were the first to demonstrate increased left ventricular stiffness associated with aging. While no comparable studies in human subjects are available, several lines of evidence suggest the same phenomenon occurs in humans. Whether assessed by radionuclide angiography or by Doppler, diastolic left ventricular filling is substantially altered in elderly subjects (51,52).

The age-related changes in the pulsed Doppler diastolic transmitral flow pattern observed have been that of reduced early (E) and increased late atrial (A) flow velocities and are independent of any age-related differences in left ventricular mass, heart rate, blood pressure, and contractility, and independent of loading conditions, suggesting that an altered Doppler diastolic left ventricular filling is a primary, biologic effect of aging (53,54). In patients with normal coronary arteries at catheterization, these alterations were associated with a shift of the left ventricular pressure–volume relation upward and to the left, indicative of reduced left ventricular compliance (55). The significance of age-related alterations in diastolic filling has not been established. However, altered diastolic filling may play a role in the decreased exercise capacity seen in normal older subjects (56) and may lower the threshold for expression of congestive heart failure symptoms in the presence of cardiovascular disease (57–60).

No changes in contractility at rest have been reported in those studies in which it was assessed (61–65). Wall motion abnormalities are invariably associated with cardiac disease and should not be considered normal, even in the very elderly (64,65).

Results from the several investigations (61–63, 66–80) who have studied the effect of age in normal subjects on a number of cardiovascular physiologic measurements at rest are summarized in Table 25–3. While the results are not uniform, the principal observations on average are unchanged or slightly increased heart rate, an increase in systolic blood pressure, no change or a mild decrease in cardiac output and stroke volume, no change in ejection fraction, and increased systemic systolic blood pressure and vascular resistance.

Effect of Age on the Cardiovascular Response During Exercise

One would expect that effects of aging on cardiovascular function would be most apparent during exercise stress. It is known that aging is inescapably accompanied by a significant but highly variable reduction in maximal oxygen consumption (VO_2 max) during exercise, which is independent of both gender and changes in body size. The magnitude of the decline is approximately 3–8% per decade and can be modified but not completely halted or reversed by exercise training (61,62,66,81–87).

A limited number of factors could be responsible for a decline in VO_2 max, including cardiac output (heart rate × stroke volume) and arteriovenous oxygen difference (AVO). Investigators have used a variety of techniques to assess the effect of aging on cardiac output (Table 25–4) (61–63,66,69–72,88). Most investigators who have measured AVO by oximetry, a reliable method, during maximal exercise have documented no difference or an increased AVO in elderly compared with young subjects (Table 25–4). By simple algebra, this suggests that the age-related decline in VO_2 max must be due to reduced cardiac output. This has indeed been the finding reported by virtually all investigators (Table 25–4), including those studying older men and women (61,62,66,88) and beagles (89).

Thus the reduced VO_2 max and exercise capacity seen with aging is due predominately to reduced exercise cardiac output. The mechanism of the age-related decline in exercise cardiac output is primarily an age-related reduction in maximal heart rate (62,90,91). The mechanism of the reduced peak heart rate is unclear, but it may be related in part to an age-related decline in beta-adrenergic sensitivity (92).

Reduced stroke volume reserve probably plays a role in decreased maximal exercise cardiac output and oxygen consumption in elderly subjects as well, since in younger subjects in whom exercise heart rate is limited, either by congenital complete heart block or by beta-adrenergic blockade, stroke volume

Table 25–3. Effect of Age on Cardiovascular Function at Rest

Investigator	*n*	Gender	Age Range	Method		Change per decade					
				BP	CO	HR (b/min)	CO (L/min)	Cl (L/min/m^2)	SV (ml)	SVR (U)	SBP/DBP (mm Hg)
Granath 1964 (69)	42	m	16–83	IA	F	−0.6	−0.39	—	−5.2	+1.23	+5.0/−0.2
Higginbotham (1986) (62)	24	m	20–50	IA	F	+0.1	−0.30	−0.21	−6.1	+1.30	+3.0/−0.7
Kitzman 1989 (61)	86	m + f	20–73	IA	F	0.0	−0.29	−0.15	−4.0	+1.38	+4.2/−0.6
Cournand 1945 (73)	13	m	21–52	—	F	0.0	−0.60	−0.30	−7.2	—	—
Brandfonbrener 1955 (74)	67	m	19–86	—	DD	−2.1	−0.51	−0.23	−5.2	—	—
Julius 1967 (70)	54	m + f	18–69	IA	DD	—	−0.39	—	−6.2	+1.26	+3.4/−0.6
Conway 1971 (71)	27	m + f	20–65	IA	DD	−1.3	−0.30	—	−2.0	+1.57	+9.7/+2.7
Davidson 1990 (67)	47	m + f	24–69	IA	TD	+0.9	−0.32	−0.09	−5.0	+0.59	+2.3/−2.7
Kuikka	69	m	6–78	—	RD	—	—	−0.25	—	—	—
1982 (65)	79	f	—	—		—	—	−0.19	—	—	—
Leithe 1984 (75)	16	m + f	24–70	—	RD	+1.8	—	−0.21	—	+0.53	—
Rodeheffer 1986 (63)	65	m	25–80	—	EGNA	−0.7	+0.14	+0.11	+3.4	—	—
Shannon 1991 (76)	16	m + f	<27–>74	AUT	EGNA	+0.9	+0.15	+0.06	+1.1	+0.40	—
Luisada	84	m	20–89	—	IC	+1.8	−0.21	−0.21	−3.9	—	—
1980	48	f	—	—	IC	+0.4	−0.39	−0.08	−6.2	—	—
Vargas 1982 (77)	17	m + f	<31–>71	OB	IC	+3.6	−0.32	—	−8.8	+1.33	+8.4/+3.0
Smith 1987 (78)	41	m	20–69	AUT	IC	+0.6	−0.13	−0.06	−4.3	+0.780	+1.7/+1.6
Hainsworth 1988 (79)	64	m + f	20–80	AUT	SB	−0.6	−0.33	−0.18	−4.5	+2.33	+5.7/+2.5
Lewis 1938 (80)	100	m	40–89	—	R	+0.1	−0.12	−0.03	−2.1	+1.67	+10.3/+0.7
Ogawa	27	m	23–62	OB	R	+0.6	—	—	—	—	+1.4/−0.3
1992 (66)	28	f	20–72	OB	R	−0.8	—	—	—	—	+3.1/+2.0

AUT = automatic; BP = blood pressure; C = cardiac index; CO = cardiac output; DBP = diastolic blood pressure; DD = dye-dilution; EGNA = equilibrium gated nuclear angiography; f = female; F = direct Fick method; HR = heart rate; IA = intra-arterial; IC = impedance cardiography; m = male; *n* = number of subjects; OB = observer; R = rebreathing technique; RD = radioisotope dilution; SB = single breath technique; SBP = systolic blood pressure; SV = stroke volume; SVR = systemic vascular resistance; TD = thermodilution; — = not available.

Table 25–4. Effect of Age on Cardiovascular Function During Maximal Exercise

Investigator	n	Gender	Age Range	Exercise Test	Method		Change per decade								
					BP	CO	VO_2 (ml/min)	VO_2 (ml/kg/min)	HR (b/min)	CO (L/min)	CI (L/min/m²)	SV (ml)	AVO (ml/L)	SVR (U)	SBP/DBP (mm Hg)
Granath	39	m	16–83	CY, supine	IA	F	−124	—	−5.6	−1.12	—	−3.5	+0.12	—	—
1964 (69)	15	m		CY, sitting	IA	F	−117		−5.0	−1.12		−4.6	+1.79		
Hossack	98(12)*	m	20–73	TR		F	−290	−4.6	−10.7	−1.35	−0.82	−2.2	+1.79	—	+8.0/+1.3
1982 (88)	104(11)	f	20–70	—		F	−191	−4.4	−6.0	−0.53	−0.6	−0.9	—	—	—
Higginbotham															
1986 (62)	24	m	20–50	CY, sitting		F		−3.1	−11.2	−1.32	−0.9	—	+0.07	—	—
Kitzman	82	m + f	20–72	CY, sitting	IA	F	−200		−10.0	−1.50	−0.75	−5.0	+0.02	+1.41	+7.5/+1.2
1989 (61)															
Julius 1967 (70)	54	m + f	18–69	CY, sitting	IA	DD	−235	—	−9.0	−1.26	−0.72	−2.9	−0.55	+1.34	+9.0/+1.2
Conway	27	m + f	20–65	CY, sitting	IA	DD	−125	—	−7.3	−0.97	—	−2.0	−0.23	+1.44	+16.0/+6.0
1971 (71)															
Rodeheffer	61	m + f	25–79	CY, sitting	—	EGNA	—	—	−0.5	−0.5	−0.3	−3.4	—	+0.4	+3.3/+2.0
1984 (63)															
Miyamura	147	m	17–54	CY	—	R	−272	−3.8	−2.4	−1.40	—	−6.5	−4.64	—	—
1973 (72)															
Ogawa	27	m	23–68	TR		R	−240	−3.6	−4.6	−1.0	—	−2.8	−0.36	—	—
1992 (66)	28	f	20–72	TR		R	−200	−3.0	−4.0	−0.7	—	−1.2	−0.31	—	—

Abbreviations: See Table 25–3; AVO = arteriovenous oxygen difference; CY = cycle; TR = treadmill; VO_2 = oxygen uptake; Note ( )* = number of subjects with invasive measurements.

is increased and partially compensates for the reduced heart rate via the Frank–Starling mechanism (increased end-diastolic volume) (93). The effect of aging on end-diastolic volume and the Frank–Starling mechanism during exercise is controversial, since one study (63) showed an increase with aging and another showed no change (62). However, there is agreement that older subjects have lower, rather than higher, stroke volumes at maximal exercise than younger subjects (Table 25–4). An age-related decline in Frank–Starling reserve would be consistent with observations suggesting increased left ventricular diastolic stiffness due to aging.

A lower stroke volume in the elderly could be due to higher end-systolic volume (reduced contractility) and/or lower end-diastolic volume (reduced diastolic filling). Left ventricular end-systolic volume appears to be higher and ejection fraction lower at peak exercise in elderly than in young subjects (61–64). Thus contractile reserve is reduced with aging as well. This may be partially due to increased afterload, since systolic blood pressure, aortic impedance (94), and systemic vascular resistance are higher during exercise in old than young healthy subjects. In evaluating elderly patients for coronary heart disease, particularly with radionuclide angiography, it should be recognized that in healthy elderly the left ventricular ejection fraction does not increase as much from rest to peak exercise as it does in young healthy subjects. In fact, a flat response in elderly men and a mild decline in elderly women should be considered normal (61,64). However, it is important to note that the development of wall motion abnormalities is not normal, even in the presence of a normal ejection fraction response.

Implications of Age-Related Changes in the Cardiovascular System

It is likely that many of the age-related changes discussed above may lower the threshold for clinical disease (95,96) and thus predispose to a variety of cardiovascular disorders in the elderly, including congestive heart failure following myocardial infarction. Longitudinal studies of predefined populations may help to further delineate interactions between normal aging and cardiovascular disease (52,81,97–102).

EPIDEMIOLOGY OF ACUTE MI IN THE ELDERLY

The relationship between age and coronary artery disease has been recognized since the classic autopsy study by White et al in 1950 (103). More than 50% of persons over age 50 were found to have significant stenosis of at least one coronary artery. The severity of stenosis and number of vessels involved increased with each age decile. These trends were confirmed to have continued subsequently in more recent studies (104). While the mechanisms are incompletely understood, it is known that cardiovascular disease incidence in general, including stroke, peripheral arterial disease, and congestive heart failure, increase markedly with age. In the case of ischemic heart disease, the relation with increasing age may be related primarily to the cumulative effects of longer duration of exposure to risk factors. Virtually all known ischemic heart disease risk factors are increased in prevalence and severity among the elderly, including hypertension, dyslipidemia, cigarette use, glucose intolerance, and left ventricular hypertrophy (105).

An important feature of the age relationship in ischemic heart disease is the gender differential (5) (see Ch. 26). While the rate of events is much lower in women than in men (ratio of 1:5) at age 35, the relative increase in event rate with age is greater in women. Thus women "catch up" with men in terms of event rates by age 75–80, when the ratio is 1:1 (106,106a).

A large body of evidence has been collected regarding the clinical outcome of acute myocardial infarction in the elderly from the prethrombolytic era. For example, the Framingham Study found that between the ages of 35 and 95 there was more than an eightfold increase in the rate of ischemic heart disease events (105). In the Worcester Heart Attack Study, the incidence of hospitalization for acute myocardial infarction in patients greater than 75 years of age varied between 0.5% and 1% from 1975 through 1984 (107). This was estimated to be approximately 10 times the incidence seen in patients less than 55 years of age and 2 times the incidence in patients between ages 55 and 65. The data set from the Worcester Heart Attack Study probably underestimated the true incidence by not counting patients who died prior to hospitalization and those with previous myocardial infarction (107). Evidence from several studies suggests that up to 40% of patients greater than age 75 were likely to die prior to arrival at the hospital with their acute myocardial infarction. This contrasts with less than 15% of those less than 45 years of age (108). This is in part due to the atypical presentation and the delays in response to symptoms seen in the elderly population (109). In the Bronx Aging Study, 390 patients between the age of 75 and 85 were followed longitudinally. The annual incidence of acute myocardial infarction was 5.6% over a 7-year period, with 43% of these presenting silently (110). These data were consistent with information from the Framingham Study, in which one-third of the myocardial infarctions in men more than 75 years of age were felt to be silent (101).

The clinical characteristics, demographics, hospital course, and long-term outcome of elderly patients in the prethrombolytic era have been well characterized (105,106). Elderly patients who present with myocardial infarction are more likely to be female, and to have a prior history of hypertension, diabetes, previous myocardial infarction, and angina pectoris as well as congestive heart failure. Their clinical course is notable for a higher rate of non-Q wave myocardial infarction and a higher rate of complications (see Ch. 18). The total creatine phosphokinase (CPK) and myocardial band (MB) levels tend to be lower in the elderly. Therefore, there exists the clinical paradox of more complications in the presence of more non-Q wave myocardial infarction. This may be explained by the difficulty in recognizing Q wave myocardial infarctions in the elderly. The higher rate of previous MI and congestive heart failure, the resultant lower baseline ejection fraction, and the greater prevalence of three-vessel coronary disease all contribute to the higher rates of complications, including reinfarction and death (107,111–113).

The prognosis of acute MI in the elderly is poorer than in younger patients, and it is well known that age is an independent risk factor for cardiovascular death in patients who present with acute myocardial infarction (113,113a,114) (see Ch. 31). In data from the prethrombolytic era, mortality rates ranged from 27% to 50% in the elderly, 2–3 times the rate in younger patients (113,115–119).

Several studies have shown a declining mortality from myocardial infarction for elderly and young, men and women, blacks and whites (109,120,121). In one recent study, older patients had the largest improvements in mortality (120). Improvements in myocardial infarction rate and mortality are related, at least partially, to reductions in risk factors as well as improved medical care in the elderly (68,109).

While overall mortality is lower in the thrombolytic era, the age gradient in mortality still exists (121a,121b) (see Ch. 19). The increased mortality is probably related at least partly to the effect of age on the postinfarction complication rate. Applegate et al and Williams et al found up to 2–3 fold higher rates of congestive heart failure, conduction abnormalities, and atrial fibrillation (116,118). Reduced ejection fraction (122) and inability to perform an exercise stress test (123) appear to be two potent markers of increased mortality in the elderly. Several studies have demonstrated that for any given age myocardial infarction mortality is higher in women than men (106a,120,124). This is of note in the elderly, since as discussed above, women comprise a larger percentage of the older population.

PRESENTATION AND DIAGNOSIS

The ability to diagnose acute myocardial infarction in the elderly depends on the proper interpretation of information obtained from the classic triad of (i) presenting symptoms, (ii) the electrocardiogram (ECG), and (iii) the pattern of cardiac enzyme changes over time. Unfortunately, in each of these categories the features are often atypical in elderly patients.

Symptoms

Several authors have reported that elderly patients with acute myocardial infarction more frequently present with atypical symptoms (125–135) (see Ch. 7). Acute myocardial infarction in the elderly usually presents within the setting of five major symptoms: chest pain, dyspnea, stroke, acute confusion, or syncope. Although the majority of elderly patients (about 60%) present with classic symptoms of myocardial infarction (typical chest pain), a much higher proportion than of younger patients present with no chest pain, and instead with isolated dyspnea (20–30%), syncope (up to 10%), acute confusion (up to 10%), vague constitutional symptoms, or signs and symptoms of stroke (1–2%) or peripheral embolism (125–135). Atypical presentations appear particularly frequent in the very elderly patient.

Even among those elderly patients who present with chest pain, the pattern of chest pain is less likely to be typical or classic in its presentation (125). Often there is no associated diaphoresis, nausea, or vomiting. Additionally, the chest pain may be atypical in character, presenting as a vague discomfort that is poorly localized, often in the throat, between the shoulder blades, or in the upper abdominal region, rather than being crushing or squeezing in sensation. The pain may not radiate at all. Several possible explanations have been offered for the increased incidence of atypical or unusual symptoms in the presentation of acute myocardial infarction. These include the coexistence of diabetes mellitus or other diseases causing peripheral neuropathy, which may mask the perception of cardiac pain in the elderly. In addition, elderly patients may have changes in opiate receptor affinity and an altered pain threshold. Finally, reporting of pain by the elderly may be supressed or masked by the more dramatic symptoms of breathlessness, syncope, stroke, or acute confusion (126–128,131–135).

The frequency of dyspnea in the elderly myocardial infarction patient may be due partly to the normal reduction in left ventricular compliance discussed previously, with subsequently reduced left ventricular cardiac output and increased pulmonary vascular pressure. Because the cardiovascular reserve is decreased, the threshold for symptoms may be reduced. In addition, the elderly more frequently have concurrent illnesses such as chronic lung disease, cerebrovascular disease, previous myocardial infarctions, left ventricular dysfunction, congestive heart failure, and cardiac rhythm and conduction abnormalities, which may exacerbate the symptoms (126–128,132,133).

Neurologic symptoms, which are unusual in young patients as a presenting sign of acute myocardial infarction, are not uncommon in the elderly. This may manifest as syncope, stroke, or acute confusion. The mechanisms for this type of symptom are not well understood. Some have suggested it is due to acute reduction in cardiac output or a result of tachycardias or bradyarrhythmias in the presence of cerebrovascular disease. Other explanations include concurrent hypoxemia, changes in glucose tolerance, or delayed medication clearance (112,126,127,134,136–138). It is known that delirium may accompany any illness in elderly and is often the presenting symptom in the very elderly.

In the setting of an acute stroke, acute myocardial infarction may be concealed by the neurologic deficits. Stroke can occur simultaneously in 1–2% of elderly patients. This particular subgroup of acute myocardial infarction patients has a very high in-hospital mortality, approaching 40–50% (112, 136–138).

Furthermore, a significant proportion of myocardial infarctions in the elderly are clinically unrecognized and are only diagnosed by an incidental electrocardiogram (ECG). By age 85, clinically silent myocardial infarctions comprise 50% of all myocardial infarction events in women (101,106, 139).

Electrocardiogram

Unfortunately, the ECG may more frequently be nondiagnostic or difficult to interpret in the elderly population because of underlying abnormalities such as left bundle branch block, left ventricular strain pattern, and previously recognized or unrecognized myocardial infarction. The increased challenge of interpreting the ECG in such patients may lead to important time delays in initiating treatment. Furthermore, with a higher rate of non-Q wave myocardial infarctions in the elderly, the initial ECG may be more frequently nondiagnostic.

Clinically unrecognized myocardial infarction may have similar prognosis and frequency of subsequent new events as symptomatic myocardial infarction. In addition, patients who have resting ST segment depression post–myocardial infarction have a much higher risk of death over the subsequent 3-year period than those without resting ST segment depression. Because of underlying heart disease and other co-morbidities, however, the elderly are less able to tolerate non-Q wave MIs and may experience many complications usually associated with Q wave myocardial infarction. Thus the ECG must be carefully analyzed to make the appropriate diagnosis (101,126–128,131–133,135, 139–141).

Cardiac Enzymes

Cardiac enzyme profiles may also be atypical in the geriatric population (see Ch. 8). Because the elderly often have decreased total body muscle mass, they may have lower than normal baseline creatine kinase (CK) levels. Thus early measurements of cardiac enzymes in the geriatric population may not be elevated to levels seen in younger patients. In addition, MBCK isoenzymes can be increased despite normal CK levels. Therefore, in the elderly, it is important to compare the current CK measurements with the patient's previous CK measurements, if available. Because the MBCK is the most specific and sensitive measure for the diagnosis of myocardial infarction, it would be unreliable to place considerable weight on the total CK alone. Elderly patients may also have concurrent low-grade chronic myositis, causing further difficulty in the interpretation of the CK profile (127,128,131, 135,140).

THERAPY

Acute Intervention

Once the clinical suspicion of acute myocardial infarction is confirmed in an elderly patient within an appropriate time frame, prompt intervention should be considered. The results of the recent analysis by McClellan et al indicate that the greatest impact on survival following acute myocardial infarction in elderly patients related to aspects of care delivered during the first 24 hours (68). Importantly, some data suggest that there may be small but definite increases in delay times between onset and treatment of myocardial infarction in the elderly compared with younger patients (142,142a). It appears the age-related delays in treatment are due primarily to patient factors, which may be improvable with community-wide health education, rather than to delays once health care providers are notified (142). The pivotal acute interventions in the elderly are thrombolytic therapy and primary coronary angioplasty.

Thrombolytic Therapy

Elderly patients have traditionally been excluded from thrombolytic therapy in practice and in clinical trials because of concern about the risk of drug-related complications, particularly intracranial hemorrhage (4,121a,143–147a) (see Ch. 19). Earlier reports by Lew et al cautioned physicians against the use of intravenous streptokinase in patients over the age of 75, because of a twofold higher incidence of major hemorrhagic complications (148). As experience with the elderly population expanded, it became clear that most major hemorrhages occurred at vascular puncture sites, although intracranial hemorrhage rates were clearly increased in the elderly, and this appeared to occur to a greater extent in patients treated with r-tPA than with streptokinase (136,138,149 153). However, in all the thrombolytic therapy trials, age is not only an independent risk for major hemorrhagic events but also an independent risk factor for mortality (138,150,151,154). Therefore, the increase in hemorrhagic events has to be weighed against the marked advantage of mortality reduction in the elderly treated with thrombolytic therapy. In the Fibrinolytic Therapy Trialists overview, it appeared that the greatest absolute age group benefit of thrombolytic therapy was in the patients over 75 (149). It was clear that while the in-hospital mortality rate was higher in the elderly population, there was a greater reduction in mortality (22.1% mortality in patients treated with placebo versus 17.9% treated with thrombolytic therapy in the elderly group). The overall benefit appeared to be twofold *higher* in the elderly than the young, with about 40 lives saved per 1,000 elderly patients treated with thrombolytic therapy versus 21 lives saved per 1,000 patients treated in the younger group (149). In addition, in the GUSTO-I trial front-loaded r-tPA and heparin had the greatest absolute mortality reduction in the age group over 75 (149,155). Furthermore, this therapy had an approximately 10-fold greater cost-effectiveness ratio versus streptokinase in the over 75 age group compared with the under 40 age group (156). (See Fig. 25–1) Therefore, the data from the large trials suggest that older age, independent of other factors, should probably be seen as an indication, rather than a contraindication, for thrombolytic therapy.

Only one clinical trial focused on the role of thrombolytic therapy in the elderly exclusively (157). Enrollment was limited to those over age 75, and the mean age was 81 years. Although only 69 patients were enrolled, they were randomly assigned to weight-adjusted r-tPA followed by heparin versus heparin and aspirin alone. The patients treated with thrombolytic therapy had a mean follow-up ejection fraction of 52% compared with 42% in the heparin/aspirin control group. There were no other differences in clinical outcomes. Despite the small sample size, this thrombolytic therapy trial of the elderly demonstrated important myocardial salvage in the thrombolytic therapy group (157).

Despite substantial evidence in support of the benefit of thrombolytic therapy in the elderly, it appears to be underutilized in this age group. Montague et al found that 4% of patients over the age of 70 with acute myocardial infarction were treated with thrombolytics compared with 20% of patients younger than 70 ($p < 0.001$) (158). Weaver et al found that 29% of younger patients were treated with thrombolytic drugs compared with only 5% of patients over age 70 (159). Similarly, Rosenthal et al found that after adjusting for other covariates, patients age 75 and over were 12 times less likely to receive thrombolytic therapy than those age 65 and under (160). Although the majority of patients admitted with acute myocardial infarction are now

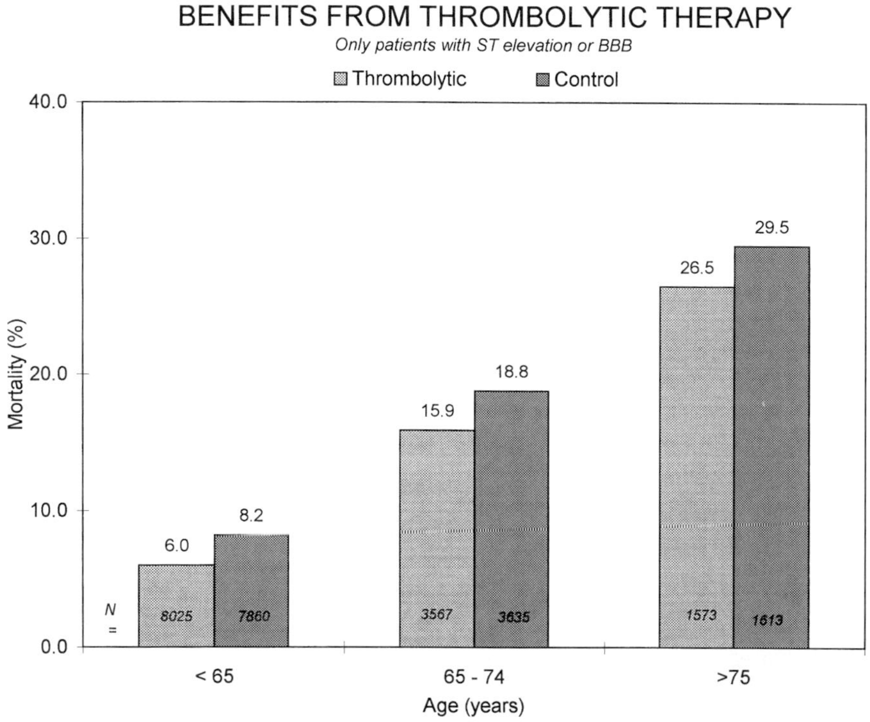

Figure 25–1. The relationship between age and mortality in acute MI patients treated with and without thrombolytic therapy. Data from *Acute Coronary Care, Second Edition,* ed. by Califf RM et al. © 1995 by Mosby-Year Book, Inc. with permission.

over the age of 65, the reasons for underutilization of aggressive therapy in the elderly are unclear. Further efforts to educate health care providers are warranted to increase the use of reperfusion therapy in the elderly (147).

Direct Angioplasty

Given the established risk of major morbidity, particularly hemorrhagic complications with the use of thrombolytic therapy in elderly patients, direct angioplasty has evolved as an alternative therapy or primary therapy for the acute MI patient (see Ch. 22). The first reports were from Holland et al, and revealed high in-hospital mortality and low success rates in patients over 70 years of age (161). Lee reported on 105 elderly patients with a mean age of 75 who received direct percutaneous transluminal coronary angioplasty (PTCA) 5.5 hours after symptom onset (162). Successful initial reperfusion was achieved in 91%. Four patients with failed PTCA underwent emergency bypass surgery, and 10% of the patients had early symptomatic reocclusion of the dilated vessel. There was one death acutely in the catheterization laboratory, and the overall in-hospital mortality rate was 18%; three-vessel coronary disease and cardiogenic shock were the strongest predictors of in-hospital death. Importantly, global ejection fraction improved from 54% to 61% on average. No stroke or intracranial or gastrointestinal hemorrhage occurred in this group of patients. Two patients had significant vascular complications; one required surgical repair and the other required blood transfusion (162). Eckman et al examined 10 case series of direct angioplasty for acute myocardial infarction and reported a mortality rate of 22% (confidence interval, 15–29%) for the 153 patients over the age of 70, which compared favorably with the 17.4% (confidence interval, 17–18%) mortality from previous reports of thrombolytic therapy in this age group (163).

Over the past 5 years there have been four randomized trials of thrombolytic therapy versus angioplasty in acute myocardial infarction. The pooled analysis suggests an advantage in mortality and in-hospital reinfarction and morbidity in patients randomized to PTCA (147,164–167). The most striking results were seen in the Primary Angioplasty in Myocardial Infarction (PAMI) trial, which reported mortality of 6% for PTCA and 15% for thrombolytic therapy in the 150 patients over the age of 65. The stroke rates were 0% and 6%, respectively (164). A definitive assessment of the role of PTCA versus thrombolytic therapy is planned in the GUSTO-IIb substudy in which 1,000 acute MI patients are expected to be randomized in a comparison of angioplasty versus thrombolytic therapy.

In summary, current evidence suggests that in selected patients over the age of 70, primary angioplasty has at least similar mortality rates and lower morbidity rates compared with thrombolytic therapy.

Adjunctive Therapy

Heparin

There appears to be clear evidence that heparin reduces the incidence of recurrent ischemia and reinfarction in the early course of unstable angina, where the probability of death, myocardial infarction, and recurrent unstable angina is greatly reduced by the use of heparin therapy (168) (see Ch. 20). Patients with acute myocardial infarction treated with r-tPA appear to have enhanced infarct artery patency with heparin therapy (169). The role of heparin following streptokinase and anistreplase (APSAC) is less clear, and this strategy probably should not be used routinely (170). Unfortunately, heparin in the elderly is associated with increased risk of hemorrhagic complications (152,153). Because of this risk, heparin use in the elderly is lower than that in younger patients. Of the 3,256 patients with acute myocardial infarction in the Myocardial Infarction Triage Investigation Study Group (MITI), heparin was used in only 35% of those patients over age 75 versus 78% in those under 55 (159).

The first phase of the GUSTO-II study (IIa) was prematurely discontinued because of a higher than expected rate of hemorrhagic stroke, in both the new antithrombin, hirudin, and the heparin groups, particularly in elderly patients (171).

Aspirin

Aspirin therapy has been proven to reduce mortality in acute myocardial infarction. In ISIS-2, patients over 70 years of age achieved particular benefit, with a 21% relative reduction in mortality from 22.3% to 17.6% (172).

Aspirin use in the elderly is associated with a higher incidence of side effects. As the doses increased from 80 mg to 325 mg, the rate of gastrointestinal complications increased twofold, particularly in the elderly patient (173). Unfortunately, utilization of aspirin in acute myocardial infarction is suboptimal, particularly in the elderly with reported rates of 55% in patients over age 75 versus 65% in those under 75 (159,159a).

Coumadin

Coumadin has recently been approved by the FDA as stand-alone anticoagulant therapy following acute myocardial infarction. The Warfarin Reinfarction Study (WARIS) demonstrated the benefit of long-term anticoagulation for cardiac patients, particularly the elderly after acute myocardial infarction (174). Impressively, cerebral vascular events were reduced by 55%, reinfarction by 34%, and overall mortality by 24% as compared with placebo. In addition, the Sixty Plus Reinfarction Study also showed a 27% reduction in mortality in an elderly population with a mean age of 67 years (175). To date, aspirin is still preferred to coumadin because of the lower risk of hemorrhage and the lack of need for monitoring. It is unclear whether warfarin is superior to aspirin following acute myocardial infarction.

Coumadin Plus Aspirin

Currently, four large studies are examining the role of combination therapy (coumadin plus aspirin). Cohen examined the role of the combination of coumadin plus aspirin versus aspirin in unstable angina and demonstrated a reduction in cardiac events with combination therapy in patients with unstable angina (176). The ongoing Coumadin Aspirin Reinfarction Study will enroll 7,000 patients and compare 3 mg of coumadin plus 80 mg of aspirin versus 162 mg of aspirin alone on a combined endpoint of stroke, reinfarction, and death. The data and safety monitoring board has met on several occasions, and there have been no safety concerns raised that were strong enough to recommend premature discontinuation of the trial. In fact, the hemorrhagic complication rates have been low in all patients, with an enrollment age range of up to 90 years (177). These studies will provide further insight into the proper role of coumadin in elderly patients post–myocardial infarction.

Other Platelet Inhibitors

Ticlopidine is a useful alternative antiplatelet therapy for the small percentage of patients who are unable to tolerate aspirin. Ticlopidine appears to interfere with ADP-mediated platelet aggregation and the platelet glycoprotein IIb/IIIa receptor. In an Italian trial of 652 patients with unstable angina, ticlopidine was associated with a 40% reduction in mortality. The combined endpoint of death and nonfatal MI occurred in 7.3% of patients given ticlopidine compared with 13.6% without ticlopidine (178). The drug takes at least 3 days before it becomes effective, however, and it is associated with reversible neutropenia in 2% of patients and severe neutropenia with agranulocytosis in 1% of patients, thus requiring frequent monitoring. The hemorrhagic risk appears less than with aspirin and therefore may be particularly appealing in the elderly (178).

The glycoprotein IIb/IIIa receptor found in the platelet membrane is integral to cellular interactions and cellular adhesions. A chimeric monoclonal antibody to this receptor has been developed for use as an antiplatelet agent. In an unstable angina and angioplasty trial, this therapy was associated with a 28% reduction in the combined rate of death, nonfatal MI, and need for revascularization. This benefit extended out to 6 months (179). Currently, pilot trials are being conducted with oral inhibitors compared with aspirin. These studies include patients over age 70 to determine the safety in the elderly.

Beta Blockers

The role of beta-adrenergic blockade in acute myocardial infarction patients who do not receive thrombolytic therapy has been well established (see Chs. 12,32). Beta blocker therapy reduces infarct size, cardiac rupture, sudden death, reinfarction, ventricular fibrillation, ventricular tachycardia, recurrent ischemia, and overall mortality. Beta-blockade counteracts the increased sympathetic tone resulting in cardiac ischemia, increasing the threshold for ventricular fibrillation and preserving more normal heart rate variability patterns. This may prevent peri–myocardial infarction autonomic instability. Because elderly patients are at greater risk of death, beta blocker therapy has demonstrated a greater effect in this population. For example, in the ISIS-1 trial of 16,027 patients, in which more than 5,000 patients were over age 75, there was a 22% reduction in mortality compared with 4% in those under age 65 (180). The Goteborg Trial of Metoprolol showed a 45% reduction in mortality among patients between 65 and 75 years of age compared with a 21% reduction in those less than 65 years of age (181). Finally, the Metoprolol in Acute Myocardial Infarction (MIAMI) trial exhibited an 18% reduction in mortality with early intravenous metoprolol in elderly patients versus an insignificant trend in younger patients (182). Thus, overall, the early treatment trials show that the younger patients had no significant mortality benefit, but older patients had a 23% reduction in mortality with beta-blockade (180,182).

With respect to treatment later in the course, the BHAT trial examined propranolol versus placebo beginning 5–21 days after infarction (183,184). This trial demonstrated a 34% reduction in mortality in those between the ages of 60 and 69, and only 19% in patients aged 30–59 (183,184). In the Norwegian timolol trial, mortality was diminished by 48% in both the elderly and younger groups (185). At the 6-year follow-up for the timolol study, the beneficial effects of beta blocker therapy persisted in older patients but not in the younger patients (185).

Despite the clear advantage of beta blocker therapy in the elderly population, several studies have suggested that clinicians are still resistant to prescribe these drugs in this patient population (111,186,187,187a). The side effects of beta blockers can be exacerbated in the elderly, particularly congestive heart failure, heart block, hypertension, bronchospasm, impaired glucose metabolism, and depression. However, beta blocker therapy appears to impart benefit even in those with mild congestive heart failure and diabetes mellitus. One study of 4,762 patients hospitalized with acute myocardial infarction in 16 hospitals demonstrated a consistent trend toward reduced use of beta blocker therapy in older patients (186). After adjustment for demographic and clinical variables, it was determined that the independent factors related to the use of beta blocker therapy were the patient's age, prior history of angina, prior history of hypertension, non-Q wave myocardial infarction, no clinical evidence of congestive heart failure or digitalis therapy, in-hospital survival, and the ability to undergo exercise testing. In this study, for example, patients over age 85 were about 25% as likely to have received beta blockers as those under age 55 (186).

These results were similar to those reported by Montague et al, who found a 24% utilization rate of beta blockers in patients age 75 or older versus 39% utilization for patients <75 years of age (158). Smith et al reported similar findings of 27% utilization of beta blocker therapy in patients older than age 75 versus 37% in patients age 65–75 (112). The results of these and other studies suggest that there is considerable room for improvement in the use of beta blocker therapy, particularly in patients who may receive the greatest benefit, i.e., those with large heart attacks with reduced ejection fractions, particularly in the elderly population. Of note, all the beta blocker studies with respect to benefit in the elderly were conducted in the prethrombolytic era. In a recent analysis of the GUSTO database, early intravenous beta blocker therapy was not associated with improvement regardless of age (188). Further research is needed to determine the role of early blockade in elderly patients with acute myocardial infarction who undergo thrombolytic therapy. At this time, there is no evidence that late beta blocker therapy should be excluded from the routine peri–myocardial infarction treatment of the elderly (188).

Calcium Channel Blockers

For some physicians, it has been particularly appealing to use calcium channel blockers when beta blockers are contraindicated secondary to chronic obstructive pulmonary disease (COPD), unstable diabetes mellitus, conduction abnormalities, or clinical congestive heart failure (see Chs. 12,32). However, the results of the Multicenter Diltiazem Post Infarction Trial and other calcium channel blocker trials have demonstrated that these agents can worsen clinical left ventricular systolic function and result in excess mortality (189). In a pooled analysis of 18 calcium channel blocker trials, no benefit of early calcium channel blocker therapy was found in patients with suspected myocardial infarction. In particular, there was no significant decrease in infarction or change in infarct size, reinfarction rates, or overall mortality. The lack of efficacy of these agents appears to be a class effect regardless of age, at least with respect to the first generation calcium channel blockers (190).

In the recently completed Prospective Randomized Amlodipine Survival Evaluation (PRAISE) trial, amlodipine did not increase mortality in patients with significant left ventricular dysfunction with clinical evidence of congestive heart failure. In the group of patients with an ischemic etiology for their congestive heart failure, there was no excess mortality despite the fact that 85% had a documented previous myocardial infarction. The mean ejection fraction was 21%, and half of the patients were older than 65 years. Although no calcium channel blocker can be routinely recommended at this time in the management of early acute myocardial infarction, the late use of newer calcium channel blockers such as amlodipine may merit further investigation (191).

Nitrates

Nitrates and nitroglycerin have been used in the management of acute myocardial infarction patients (see Chs. 12, 32). It is believed that nitroglycerin reduces preload and afterload and may improve collateral blood flow to ischemic myocardial infarction, minimizing infarct size. It may also restore blood flow in the infarct-related artery and release coronary spasm. A pooled analysis of 10 small trials showed a promising 35% reduction in mortality with intravenous nitroglycerin therapy (192).

ISIS-4 and GISSI-3, both recently completed randomized trials of nitroglycerin following acute myocardial infarction, gave further insight in this area (193,194). In ISIS-4, there appeared to be a small and nonsignificant effect on mortality (194). However, in the GISSI-3 study, nitroglycerin afforded a 9% reduction in the combined endpoint of mortality and severe ventricular dysfunction in patients over age 70 (193). Although these studies have been criticized because of the variable use of intravenous nitroglycerin and the high placebo arm "drop-in," long-acting nitrates probably cannot currently be recommended for routine administration post–myocardial infarction.

ACE Inhibitors

Several prospective trials have now shown improved mortality post–myocardial infarction with angiotensin converting enzyme (ACE) inhibitors (see Chs. 12, 29, 32). The studies differ with respect to duration of follow-up. In the SAVE, ARIES, and SMILE trials, in patients with an ejection fraction less than 40% or clinical evidence of heart failure, mortality was significantly reduced in patients receiving ACE inhibitor versus placebo (195–197). In the SAVE trial, mortality was 20% in the treatment group and 25% the placebo group ($p = 0.019$) (195). This reduction in death was greatest in those patients over 64 years of age at 25%, versus an 8% reduction in those less than 55 years. Importantly, the risk of recurrent, fatal, or nonfatal myocardial infarction was also reduced in the captopril treated group. This benefit was also seen in the older patients (195).

In the CONSENSUS-II trial, early intravenous enalapril followed by oral enalapril was associated with a slightly higher mortality in the treatment group (10.2 vs. 9.4%, $p = 0.26$). This result was felt to be due in part to the side effect of early hypotension, particularly in elderly patients (198). However, when oral ACE inhibitor therapy is begun as early as 24 hours, but not within the first 6 hours, it appears to reduce the risk of the development of congestive heart failure and of death (197).

In the three large studies from ISIS-4, GISSI-3, and the Chinese Captopril Study Group, the risk of death following myocardial infarction was significantly reduced at 6 weeks from 7.6% to 7.1%, $p = 0.004$ (193,194,199). These trials document the importance of early ACE inhibition in all myocardial infarction patients. The greatest benefit was in the higher-risk patients, i.e., those with previous myocardial infarction, anterior wall myocardial infarction, and the elderly. Among patients over 70 in the GISSI-3 study, there was a 12% reduction in the combined endpoint of mortality and severe ventricular dysfunction (193).

Complications

Extracranial Hemmorhage

Elderly patients appear to have higher bleeding complication rates than younger patients, particularly after thrombolytic therapy (see Ch. 19). Extracranial hemorrhage occurs most often at the cardiac catheterization site, with hematoma in 25% to 45%, gastrointestinal 4% to 10%, genital urinary 1% to 5%, retroperitoneal <1%, and other causes <1%. Older age is a consistent risk factor for extracranial hemorrhagic complications (150,151,200).

Early studies of the use of intravenous r-tPA followed by heparin reported an increase in the risk of major hemorrhagic events from 8.7% in those younger than 65 to 25% in those older than 70 (150). In the TAMI study group, we found that advanced age was an independent risk factor for development of hemorrhage (151,200). In the GUSTO trial, there was a small but significant age-associated increased risk of noncerebrovascular hemorrhage (155) (Fig. 25–2).

Stroke and Intracranial Hemorrhage

Stroke peri–acute myocardial infarction is associated with extremely high mortality (136,138). Elderly patients given thrombolytic therapy benefit to a greater extent than younger patients, but this occurs at the expense of increased bleeding complications (150). Large randomized trials of acute myocardial infarction and thrombolysis have shown an increased risk of stroke in patients with increasing age (149). The increased risk of stroke in patients over age 70 is felt to be the result of a reduction in the integrity of the cerebrovascular system. In some patients, previous silent cerebral ischemic events may increase the risk for subsequent events after receiving thrombolytic therapy. In addition, cerebral amyloid angiopathy may occur to a much greater extent in the elderly and possibly plays a pathogenic role in some intracranial cerebral hemorrhages associated with thrombolytic therapy (136).

The frequency of cerebral hemorrhage in GISSI-2 and ISIS-3 trials suggested that the increased risk of cerebral hemorrhage in the elderly

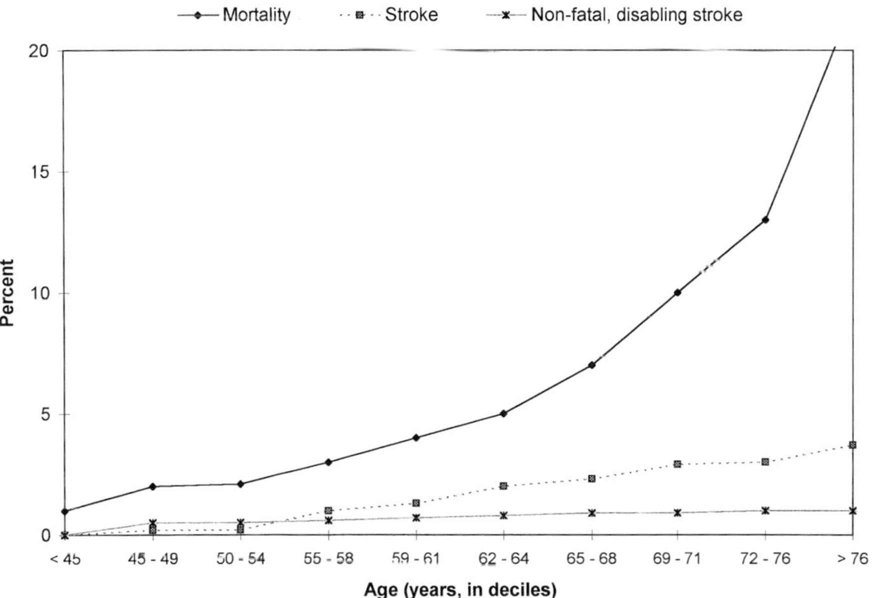

Figure 25–2. The relationship between age, death, total stroke and nonfatal disabling stroke in the GUSTO trial. Data from *Acute Coronary Care, Second Edition*, ed. by Califf RM et al. © 1995 by Mosby-Year Book, Inc. with permission.

was predominately seen in patients treated with r-tPA and less in patients treated with streptokinase (152,153). In a case control study by Simoons et al using the database of six thrombolytic therapy trials, age over 65 was an important independent risk factor for intracranial hemorrhage, with an odds ratio of 2.2. The effect was magnified in elderly patients treated with t-PA (odds ratio 3.2) compared with those treated with streptokinase (odds ratio 1.3) (201). The trend was also seen in the GUSTO-I trial, where the hemorrhagic stroke rate in patients over 75 years was 2.1% with t-PA and 1.2% with streptokinase. However, when the combined endpoint of death and nonfatal disabling stroke was compared between the two treatment arms, r-tPA was still favored because for both thrombolytic agents, the substantial mortality benefit outweighed the strokes that occurred (155).

Delirium

As with any acute illness in the elderly, delirium is a common complication of acute myocardial infarction (118,202–204). It can severely complicate other aspects of management and may be associated with significantly increased mortality (202, 203). Very elderly are particularly prone to develop delirium (202). There is a fivefold increased risk in patients over 80 years of age compared with those under age 80. Some studies suggest that men may be more likely to develop this complication than women. Other risk factors include history of drug use, previous episodes of delirium, and chronic cardiovascular, respiratory, renal, or metabolic illnesses. Patients with preexisting cerebral dysfunction secondary to chronic dementia or prior stroke have less cognitive reserve and are more vulnerable to developing delirium.

In addressing the elderly patient with this complication, a number of organic disturbances must first be excluded; these include infectious etiologies, structural disease of the CNS system, metabolic and endocrine disorders, hypoxemia, and drug therapy. Once these have been excluded, the clinician must consider the possibility of drug withdrawal, as many of the patients have been maintained on chronic benzodiazepenes, alcohol, or barbiturates, which are abruptly withheld during the early post–myocardial infarction period. The combination of acute myocardial infarction and delirium tremens can be particularly lethal; early studies reported greater than 50% mortality in patient who experience delirium tremens (100). Other nonspecific precipitating or contributing factors should also be considered, including sleep deprivation, sensory overload, bereavement, and unfamiliar environment. After searching for and treating organic etiologies and vigorous attempts at ameliorating these nonspecific factors, haloperidol is the drug of choice for the early management of an acute episode of ICU delirium (202–204).

Mechanical Complications

The mechanical complications of papillary muscle rupture and mitral regurgitation, ventricular septal defect, and free wall rupture occur at significantly increased rates in the elderly (116,118) (see Chs. 2–16). These complications usually occur between 1 hour and 7 days postinfarction, with a median of 3 days. Risk factors include female gender and hypertension. Because sudden pulmonary edema or cardiogenic shock resulting from the severe mechanical disadvantage responds poorly to prolonged medical management in these syndromes, they should be managed as surgical emergencies (205). Classic symptoms and physical signs may be obscured by concomitant morbidity or the intensive care environment (noise from ventilators obscuring murmurs); therefore, these diagnoses must be considered whenever a postinfarct patient becomes suddenly or severely unstable hemodynamically (206). Echocardiography should be the initial diagnostic modality and can be performed rapidly at the bedside (207). Transesophageal echocardiography should be considered if optimal images cannot be obtained via the routine, transthoracic route, as it can confirm the diagnosis rapidly and definitively (206,208). Although advanced age increases the risk of perioperative complications, in the absence of significant terminal comorbidities these patients should undergo early cardiac surgery because of the abysmal outcome in the absence of intervention (205,209).

Renal Dysfunction

Approximately 5% of hospitalized patients will develop renal dysfunction during their hospitalization for acute myocardial infarction in the coronary care unit. The elderly are at particularly high risk. Common causes include ischemic acute renal failure, accounting for 50%, contrast nephropathy, and cholesterol emboli (210,211). In addition, nephrotoxins such as ACE inhibitors in those with renal vascular disease, nonsteroidal anti-inflammatory agents, and antibiotics may contribute to renal dysfunction. Increased risk in older patients is due to reduced baseline creatine clearance due to normal aging and a variety of disorders as well as to increased prevalence of generalized vascular disease. Management should include careful volume status management including the use of Swan–Ganz catheterization if necessary. Patients should be weighed daily and a strict log kept of their intake and output to keep them euvolemic. Electrolyte abnormalities should be corrected carefully. When conservative therapy fails, acute renal failure in the coronary care unit requires dialysis.

Cardiopulmonary Resuscitation

Cardiopulmonary resuscitation is needed in 10% of the patients undergoing treatment during hospitalization for acute myocardial infarction. In the Duke CPR series, cardiopulmonary resuscitation was not limited to young patients. Although the return of spontaneous circulation is high in most series at about 50%, the discharge rate is exceedingly low at 5%. In our experience, patients with a cardiovascular etiology have an increased likelihood of survival following resuscitation. Age alone is not an exclusion criterion for the use of CPR, although age plus other co-morbidities (i.e., respiratory failure, renal failure) make the likelihood of recovery from CPR remote (212,212a).

Revascularization

Patient Selection/Cardiac Catheterization

The role of routine cardiac catheterization following acute myocardial infarction remains controversial (see Chs. 30–31). In the TIMI-II trial, equal numbers of patients were identified for bypass surgery using the mandatory cardiac catheterization strategy versus the noninvasive strategy (213). However, this patient population was a relatively low-risk group. In addition, 33% of the patients in the conservative strategy required catheterization during the initial hospitalization, and a total of 60% ultimately required cardiac catheterization in the year following the index infarction (213). The role of noninvasive stress testing after thrombolysis is not clear (see below).

PTCA

As discussed above, primary coronary angioplasty appears promising in the treatment of acute myocardial infarction (see Ch. 22). Its advantages over thrombolytic therapy are multiple, including greater restoration of TIMI grade 3 flow and the lack of hemorrhagic complications. The potential impact of these advantages over thrombolytic therapy are limited because of the need for a 24-hour cardiac catheterization laboratory and because of delays in treatment time in achieving reperfusion. The aggregated results of four randomized prospective trials of PTCA versus thrombolytic therapy demonstrated improved outcome with respect to death, reinfarction, recurrent ischemia, stroke, and hemorrhage. This strategy is particularly appealing to the elderly patients who are at the highest risk for intracranial hemorrhage and other hemorrhagic complications (164). PTCA is an important strategy in patients with cardiogenic shock, a high percentage of whom are elderly (see Ch. 13). In general, average mortality rates in clinical series appear to be reduced to 33% in those achieving a patent infarct-related artery versus 75% in those who continued to have an occluded infarct-related artery. In a series of 97 patients, Carter et al found similar procedural success (80%) and mortality rate in matched patients older versus younger than age 70 (214). The role of primary PTCA should not be confused with the use of PTCA following thrombolytic therapy or rescue PTCA. Although rescue PTCA is useful in some circumstances, such as when myocardial infarction is complicated by shock, it should not be routinely performed.

Elective angioplasty following acute myocardial infarction is indicated for the relief of angina or the reduction of ischemia. The procedural success rate for angioplasty in this setting has improved significantly in the elderly patient population over the past decade, with an angiographic success rate over 95%. Important complications occur at low rates, such as nonfatal myocardial infarction (3%), emergency coronary artery bypass grafting (4%), and procedural mortality (2%). These rates are essentially doubled in patients over age 80 (215). Angioplasty appears to be the preferred approach for recurrent ischemia in patients with one- or two-vessel disease who have preserved left ventricular function. Despite this, Rosenthal et al found that after adjusting for other covariates, patients age 75 and over were eight times less likely to undergo coronary angiography and seven times less likely to undergo coronary angioplasty (160). Although some arguments remain that revascularization in elderly patients post–myocardial infarction does not improve outcome, this is not supported by recent observations (216).

Coronary Artery Bypass Grafting

The role of coronary artery bypass grafting (CABG) in the early stages of acute myocardial infarction is still evolving, and few data are available regarding the elderly (37,217–225) (see Ch. 23). The hospital mortality rate in more than 1,000 patients was approximately 5%, and the surgical reoperation rate was 3% (217,219–225). Age was an independent risk factor of higher mortality. In a small trial with 34 patients randomized to surgical treatment versus medical therapy in acute myocardial infarction, the mortality was 2.9% in the surgically treated patients and 20% in medically treated patients (217). The most common approach is to use coronary artery bypass grafting once the patient has stabilized toward the end of the hospitalization for acute myocardial infarction. Coronary artery bypass grafting is used after thrombolytic therapy in approximately 15% of patients. In the TAMI trial experience of 267 patients who underwent elective bypass surgery, the most common indications for surgery were complex multivessel disease (66%) and recurrent ischemic symptoms with coronary anatomy unsuitable for PTCA (13%). Patients who had bypass surgery deferred 24 hours or more after thrombolytic therapy had fewer red blood cell transfusions and more frequently received internal mammary bypass grafting (226,227). In a multivariable analysis of patients with elective surgery following acute myocardial infarction, Applebaum et al found that only left ventricular ejection fraction less than 30%, preoperative shock, and age greater than 70 were associated with increased in-hospital death (228).

Despite the increased mortality in the elderly, coronary artery bypass grafting remains a suitable alternative and often the preferred strategy for the management of multivessel disease. Although there remains controversy whether CABG should be performed in elderly patients post–myocardial infarction, recent observations suggest that elective revascularization procedures are associated with an acceptable risk in elderly patients without significant co-morbidities and with refractory symptoms (216). The incidences of surgical complications is higher in the elderly, including arrhythmias, renal failure, ventilator dependency, stroke, and infections. In a recent report by Mark et al, patients over age 75 differed considerably in baseline characteristics, which may be responsible, in part, for the differences in outcome (216).

Predischarge Testing

Following uncomplicated acute myocardial infarction, patients usually undergo stress testing in an effort to stratify patients for the risk of subsequent events by assessing provocable ischemia, left ventricular function, and arrhythmias (see Ch. 31). Assessment of submaximal exercise performance may also have the benefit of boosting patient confidence regarding return to physical activity. However, the role of predischarge testing in the elderly is controversial, particularly following thrombolytic therapy. In the prethrombolytic era, ineligibility for a predischarge exercise test carried a poor prognosis (123). Subsequently, in the thrombolytic era, Ciaroni et al examined the prognostic significance during 3.5-year follow-up of exercise treadmill testing performed 14 days after uncomplicated acute MI in 188 patients over age 70 (229). The total mortality was 13.5%, and the predictors of sudden cardiac death included lack of increase in systolic blood pressure, a small increase in double product, low workload, and total exercise duration less than 5 minutes. The degree of ST segment depression was directly and significantly associated with increased risk for cardiac events, including reinfarction, unstable angina, and revascularization. Thus exercise treadmill ECG testing in this population was safe and carried prognostic information.

Data with regard to image-based stress testing are also controversial. In a study by Myers et al of 147 patients over the age of 65 following acute myocardial infarction in which 24 cardiovascular deaths and 3 recurrent myocardial infarctions occurred in 1-year follow-up, knowledge of the exercise test radionuclide angiogram and 24-hour Holter did not improve the prediction of outcome following acute myocardial infarction (230).

More recently, early reports of echocardiography-based techniques have shown promise. Two relatively small studies demonstrated that dobutamine echocardiography can be used to detect viable and ischemic areas of myocardium following thrombolysis for acute myocardial infarction (231, 232). However, these studies included few elderly patients. In a subset analysis of the EPIC study, a multicenter study designed to mimic everyday community hospital experience, dipyridamole echocardiography was performed in 190 elderly patients. Spontaneous clinical events (death, reinfarction, or angina) occurred in 52% of patients with a positive study compared with only 18% of those with a negative study ($p < 0.001$) (233).

In elderly patients with normal rest electrocardiograms, there are currently insufficient data available to confirm whether information gained from radioisotope imaging or echocardiography during exercise testing significantly improve prognostic ability. However, in the patient who is unable to perform an adequate exercise test or who has an abnormal resting electrocardiogram, both conditions being more common in elderly than young patients, an imaging modality is necessary for stress testing. More information is required regarding the utility of stress testing, both exercise and pharmacologic and with and without imaging, after thrombolytic therapy in the elderly.

Cardiac Rehabilitation

Cardiac rehabilitation is a potentially potent intervention for the reduced functional capacity, anxiety, depression, and weaker social support with which elderly survivors of myocardial infarction frequently must cope (see Ch. 33). In general, however, elderly patients are less likely to be referred for cardiac rehabilitation (234,235). Although there are a variety of potential explanations for this, including lack of large-trial data to support this intervention in the elderly age group and the higher frequency of severe communicative (particularly dementia) and mobility disorders, physician bias may also be an important component. In an analysis of 226 coronary artery disease patients, the strength of the physician's recommendation was the most powerful predictor of participation in a cardiac rehabilitation program (234). Another possible explanation for lower participation may be gender. A higher proportion of elderly postinfarct patients are women, and women in general appear less likely to enter a rehabilitation program than men, including in the elderly age group (234,235).

A main component of rehabilitation programs is exercise training. As discussed, even normal aging is accompanied by reduced exercise capacity (62,81, 88). Numerous studies have shown that healthy elderly can significantly increase their exercise capacity through exercise training (82–87,236). Meta-analyses of studies in patients <65 years suggest that rehabilitation is associated with up to 25% reductions in mortality as well as significantly reduced morbidity and increased exercise capacity (238–240). The few comparative data available in patients ≥65 suggest that selected elderly may obtain benefit similar to that of younger patients (241). Exercise training need not necessarily take place within a structured group program; it is also feasible in a home-based format, although fewer outcome data are available for this design.

Another important component of cardiac rehabilitation programs is individual and group counseling, including focused diet and risk factor modification and social adjustment interventions. A British study of 166 consecutive patients 70–97 years old randomly assigned to a special outpatient counseling clinic or usual medical follow-up showed improvements in hospital readmission, depression, anxiety, mobility, and physical function, but no difference in mortality (238). These data suggest that cardiac rehabilitation of one type or another should be a strong consideration in elderly patients with recent myocardial infarction.

Psychosocial Intervention

Psychosocial variables are important risk factors in elderly patients who suffer acute myocardial infarction. Case et al demonstrated that isolation (living alone) after myocardial infarction was much more common in the elderly and an independent risk factor for recurrent events and death (242). In a study by Berkman et al of 194 patients over age 65, lack of emotional support was significantly associated with 6-month mortality with an odds of ratio 2.9 (95% confidence interval, 1.2–6.9) after controlling for severity of infarction and risk factors such as smoking, hypertension, and social demographic factors (243). The two characteristics most closely associated with increased risk of death were age over 75 and lack of emotional support. Thirty-eight percent of patients who reported having no support died in hospital, compared with 12% who had two or more sources of support (243). The Enhancing Recovering Coronary Heart Disease patients (ENRICHD) program is a recently funded National Institutes of Health randomized trial of psychosocial intervention versus usual care to prevent social isolation, depression, and subsequent mortality with nonpharmacologic methods in patients suffering acute myocardial infarction. In this study, there will be particular emphasis on elderly patients who are at the highest risk for these cardiac events because of depression and social isolation (244).

Lipid Lowering Therapy

Recent studies in the general population of patients with hypercholesterolemia have demonstrated that secondary prevention is more cost-effective than primary prevention (see Ch. 36). However, there has been considerable controversy regarding secondary prevention in patients over age 60 (244a). Nearly all studies have excluded elderly patients, even though in the elderly dyslipidemia is an independent risk factor for acute myocardial infarction and is more common than in the young. Therefore, until recently few data were available regarding the role of therapy in this age group. The Stockholm Ischemic Heart Disease Secondary Prevention Study was unique in this regard. In this controlled study, more than 250 of the enrollees (nearly half of the total) were 65 to 70 years old. A 28% reduction in total mortality was seen at the end of 5 years in patients over age 60 treated with combination therapy with clofibrate and niacin (245). Most recently, in the Scandinavian Simvastatin Survival Study ("4S"), simvastatin, an HmG-CoA reductase inhibitor, showed a significant reduction in mortality, nonfatal reinfarction, and the need for revascularization in patients with established coronary heart disease (246). The benefit of therapy was significantly increased in the older compared with the younger age groups. In the patients over age 60 (51% of the total enrollment), the reduction in mortality was 27%. There also appeared to be a significant reduction in nonfatal strokes. Current practice patterns still suggest that cholesterol lowering therapy post–myocardial infarction, particularly in the elderly, is underutilized and in some studies is utilized in less than 10% of patients despite appropriate indications (246).

Heart Failure in the Elderly

A common chronic complication following myocardial infarction is heart failure. Congestive heart failure increases approximately 5–10 fold from middle to old age (247–249), and the prognosis is significantly poorer in elderly than in younger patients, with several-fold higher short- and long-term mortality rates (247,249). Not all of the age-related increase in heart failure is due to ischemic heart disease, since nearly 50% of elderly heart failure patients have normal ejection fractions, suggesting a role of diastolic dysfunction (59,247,249–251). As discussed above, several age-related changes in the cardiovascular system may lower the threshold for expression of heart failure symptoms, lending an explanation for the observation that elderly patients have a higher incidence of peri-infarct and chronic postinfarct congestive heart failure. Relatively little is known regarding whether there are significant age-related differences in pathophysiology or response to therapy of heart failure with respect to age since, similar to trials of other cardiovascular disorders, the elderly have tended to be excluded from prospective trials. There do appear to be modest age-related differences in the hemodynamic and neurohormonal profiles in older patients with heart failure (252). For the present, it is reasonable to treat the elderly postinfarction patient similar to postinfarction patients in general. Results of recent trials (average age of patients 60 years) have shown that therapy with digoxin improves symptoms, exercise tolerance, quality of life, and hemodynamics (253–255); however, information regarding its effect of mortality will await completion of the ongoing DIG trial. Careful attention should be given to dosing of digoxin in the elderly (256). Diuretics also provide symptomatic relief, more rapidly than other medical interventions. As discussed above, angiotensin converting enzyme inhibitors are beneficial in patients with recent anterior myocardial infarction as well as in those with significant left ventricular systolic dysfunction (257,258).

SUMMARY

Several themes have emerged from this discussion. Acute myocardial infarction is more common in the elderly than in the younger population. Elderly patients differ from younger ones because of age-related changes in the cardiovascular system, a higher proportion of women, more severe cardiovascular and other systemic diseases, and a higher rate of atypical presentation. Despite these apparent differences and the high rate of myocardial infarction in the elderly, there is a relative paucity of data from trials that have focused specifically on the elderly. Trial data that are available strongly suggest that even though complication rates from therapy are higher than in the younger population, because the risks from the natural disease course are substantially higher in the elderly, most interventions appear to have enhanced benefit–risk ratios and enhanced absolute benefit in the elderly compared with younger populations. Therefore, if it means avoiding modern therapeutic interventions for acute myocardial infarction, including invasive procedures for selected patients, "gentler" may not always be "kinder" in the elderly patient.

ACKNOWLEDGMENT

The authors gratefully acknowledge the assistance of Vickie Brown and Renee Story in preparing the manuscript.

REFERENCES

1. Samuelson RJ: Sowing more cynicism. *Newsweek* September 1994, p 45.
2. Staff reporter: *Time* October 15, 1993.
3. Manton KG, Soldo BJ: Dynamics of health changes in the oldest old: New perspectives and evidence. *Milbank Memorial Fund Quart* 1985;63:206–285.
4. Gurwitz JH, Col NF, Avorn J: The exclusion of the elderly and women from clinical trials in acute myocardial infarction. *JAMA* 1992;268:1417–1422.
5. Hazzard WR: Biological basis of the sex differential in longevity. *J Am Geriatr Soc* 1986;34:455–471.
6. Kitzman DW, Edwards WD: Age related changes in the anatomy of the normal human heart. *J Gerontol Med Sci* 1990;45:M33–M39.
7. Waller BF, Roberts WC: Cardiovascular disease in the very elderly. Analysis of 40 necropsy patients aged 90 years or over. *Am J Cardiol* 1983;51:403–421.
8. Sahasakul Y, Edwards WD, Naessens JM, Tajik AJ: Age-related changes in aortic and mitral valve thickness: Implications for 2-dimensional echocardiography based on an autopsy study of 200 normal human hearts. *Am J Cardiol* 1988;62:424–430.
9. Howell T: Heart weight among octogenarians. *J Am Geriatr Soc* 1981;29:572–575.
10. Howell TH: Organ weights in nonagenarians. *J Am Geriatr Soc* 1978;26:385–390.
11. Hagen PT, Scholz DG, Edwards WD: Incidence and size of patient foramen ovale during the first 10 decades of life: An autopsy study of 965 normal hearts. *Mayo Clin Proc* 1984;59:17–20.
12. Krovetz LJ: Age-related changes in the size of the aortic valve annulus in man. *Am Heart J* 1974;90:569–574.
13. Silber MA, Roberts WC: Detailed anatomy of the normally functioning aortic valve in hearts of normal and increased weight. *Am J Cardiol* 1985;55:454–461.

14. Lie JT, Hammond PI: Pathology of the senescent heart: Anatomic observations on 237 autopsy specimens of patients 90 to 105 years old. *Mayo Clin Proc* 1988;63:552–564.

15. Kitzman DW, Scholz DG, Hagen PT, Ilstrup DM, Edwards WD: Age-related changes in normal human hearts during the first ten decades. Part II (maturity): A quantitative anatomic study of 765 specimens from subjects 20 to 99 years old. *Mayo Clin Proc* 1988;63:137–146.

16. Schenk KE, Heinze G: Age-dependent changes of heart valves and heart size, in Roy PE, Rona G (eds): *Recent Advances in Studies on Cardiac Structure and Metabolism*. Baltimore, University Park Press, 1975.

17. Reiner L, Mazzoleni A, Rodriguez FL, Freudenthal RP: The weight of the human heart. I. "Normal cases." *Arch Pathol* 1959;68:58–73.

18. McMillan JB, Lev M: The aging heart. I. Endocardium. *J Gerontol* 1959;14:268–283.

19. Waller BF, Block T, Barker BG: The old-age heart: Aging changes of the normal elderly heart and cardiovascular disease in 12 necropsy patients aged 90 to 101 years. *Cardiol Clin* 1984;2:753–779.

20. Savage DD, Garrison RK, Brand F, et al: Prevalence and correlates of posterior extra echocardiographic spaces in a free living population based sample (the Framingham Study). *Am J Cardiol* 1977; 51:1202–1212.

21. Hutchins GM: Structure of the aging heart, in Weisfeldt ML (ed): *The Aging Heart, Its Function and Response to Stress*. New York, Raven Press, 1980.

22. Lenkiewicz JE, Davies MJ, Risen D: Collagen in human myocardium as a function of age. *Cardiovasc Res* 1972;6:549.

23. Lakatta EG, Yin FCP: Myocardial aging: Functional alterations and related cellular mechanisms. *Am J Physiol* 1982;242:H927–H941.

24. Weisfeldt ML: Cardiac failure XVIII: The aging heart. *Hosp Pract* 1985;115–130.

25. Jalil JE, Doering CW, Janicki JS, Shroff SG, Pick R, Weber KT: Influence of increased myocardial collagen on active and passive stiffness in left ventricular hypertrophy (abstract). *J Am Coll Cardiol* 1988; 11:12A.

26. Anversa P, Miler B, Ricci R, Giancarlo G, Olivetti: Myocyte cell loss and myocyte hypertrophy in the aging rat heart. *J Am Coll Cardiol* 1986;8:1441–1448.

27. Pomerance A: Aging and degenerative changes, in Pomerance A, Davies MJ (eds): *The Pathology of the Heart*. Blackwell Scientific Publication, 1975, pp 49–79.

28. Rosenberg B, Pfitzer P: Ploidy in the hearts of elderly patients. *Virchows Arch* 1983;42:19–24.

29. Strehler BL, Mark DD, Mildvan AS, Gee MV: Rate and magnitude of age pigment accumulation in the human myocardium. *J Gerontol* 1959;14: 430–439.

30. Glenner GG: Amyloid deposits and amyloidosis: The B-fibrilloses. *N Engl J Med* 1980;302:1333–1343.

31. Schmucker DL, Sachs HG: Age-dependent alterations in rat ventricular myocardium: A quantitative analysis. *Mech Age Develop* 1985;31:89–101.

32. Gerstenblith G, Frederiksen J, Yin FCP, Fortuin NJ, Lakatta EG, Weisfeldt ML: Echocardiographic assessment of a normal adult aging population. *Circulation* 1977;56:273–278.

33. Gardin JM, Henry WL, Ware JH, Burn C, Borer JS: Echocardiographic measurements in normal subjects: Evaluation of an adult population without clinically apparent heart disease. *J Clin Ultrasound* 1979;7:439–447.

34. Roman MJ, Devereux RB, Kramer-Fox R, O'Loughlin J: Two-dimensional echocardiographic aortic root dimensions in normal children and adults. *Am J Cardiol* 1989;64:507–512.

35. McMillian JB, Lev M: The aging heart. II. The valves. *J Gerontol* 1964;19:1–14.

36. Sell S, Scully RE: Aging changes in the aortic and mitral valves. *Am J Pathol* 1965;46:345–365.

37. Akasaka T, Yoshikawa J, Yoshida K, et al: Age-related valvular regurgitation: A study of pulsed Doppler echocardiography. *Circulation* 1987;76:262.

38. Roman MJ, Devereux RB, Niles NW, et al: Aortic root dilatation as a cause of isolated, severe aortic regurgitation: Prevalence, clinical and echocardiographic patterns and relation to left ventricular hypertrophy and function. *Ann Intern Med* 1987;106: 800–807.

39. Olson LJ, Subramanian R, Edwards WD: Surgical pathology of pure aortic insufficiency: A study of 225 cases. *Mayo Clin Proc* 1984;59:835–841.

40. Hutchins GM, Bulkley BH, Miner MM, Boitnott: Correlation of age and heart weight with tortuosity and caliber of normal human coronary arteries. *Am Heart J* 1977;63:615–622.

41. Robard S: Vascular caliber. *Cardiology* 1975;60:4–49.

42. Leung WH, Stadius ML, Alderman EL: Determinants of normal coronary artery dimensions in humans. *Circulation* 1991;84:2294–2306.

43. Lochman AS, Spray PL, Kerwin BM, Schugoll GI, Roberts WC: Medial calcinosis of Monckeberg: A review of the problem and a description of a patient with involvement of peripheral, visceral, and coronary arteries. *Am J Med* 1976;62:107–112.

44. Uretsky BF, Rifkin RD, Satish SC, Reddy PS: Value of fluoroscopy in the detection of coronary stenosis: Influence of age, sex, and number of vessels calcified on diagnostic efficacy. *Am Heart J* 1988; 115:323–333.

45. Davies MJ, Anderson RH, Becker AE: *The Conduction System of the Heart.* London, Butterworths & Co. Ltd., 1983, pp 16–19,46–70.

46. Eriksson EE, Lev M: Ageing changes in the human AV node, bundle and bundle branches. *J Gerontol* 1952;7:1–7.

47. Davies MJ, Pomerance A: Quantitative study of aging changes in the human sinoatrial node and inernodal tracts. *Br Heart J* 1972;34:150–152.

48. Shiaishi I, Takamatsu T, Minamikawa T, Onouchi Z, Fujita S: Quantitative histological analysis of the human sinoatrial node during growth and aging. *Circulation* 1992;85:2176–2184.

49. Fleg JL, Das DN, Wright J, Lakatta EG: Age-associated changes in the components of atrio-ventricular conduction in apparently healthy volunteers. *J Gerontol Med Sci* 1990;45:M95–M100.

50. Templeton GH, Platt MR, Willcrson JT, Weisfeldt MD: Influence of aging on left ventricular hemodynamics and stiffness in beagles. *Circ Res* 1979;44: 189–194.

51. Miyatake K, Okamoto M, Kinoshita N, et al: Augmentation of atrial contribution to left ventricular inflow with aging as assessed by intracardiac doppler flowmetry. *Am J Cardiol* 1984;54:586–589.

52. Miller TR, Grossman SJ, Schectman KB, Biello DR, Ludbrook PA, Ehsani AA: Left ventricular diastolic filling and its association with age. *Am J Cardiol* 1986;58:531–553.

53. Downes TR, Nomeir AM, Stewart K, Mumma M: Effect of alteration in loading conditions on both normal and abnormal patterns of left ventricular filling in healthy individuals. *Am J Cardiol* 1990;26: 69–82.

54. Kitzman DW, Sheikh KH, Beere PA, Philips JL, Higginbotham MB: Age-related alterations of Doppler left ventricular filling indexes in normal subjects are independent of left ventricular mass, heart rate, contractility, and loading conditions. *J Am Coll Cardiol* 1991;18:1243–1250.

55. Downes TR, Nomeir AM, Smith KM, Stewart KP, Little WC: Mechanism of altered pattern of left ventricular filling with aging in subjects without cardiac disease. *Am J Cardiol* 1989;64:523–527.

56. Levy WC, Cerqueira MD, Abrass IB, Schwartz RS, Stratton JR: Endurance exercise training augments diastolic filling at rest and during exercise in healthy young and older men. *Circulation* 1993;88: 116–126.

57. Sheikh KH, Bashore TM, Kitzman DW, et al: Doppler left ventricular diastolic filling abnormalities in aortic stenosis and their relationship to hemodynamic parameters. *Am J Cardiol* 1989;63: 1360–1368.

58. Kitzman DW, Sullivan MJ: Exercise intolerance in patients with heart failure: Role of diastolic dysfunction. In Lorell BH, Grossman W: Diastolic Relaxation of the Heart. Boston, Kluwer Academic Publishers, 1994;295–302.

59. Gardin JM, Arnold A, Kitzman D, et al: Congestive heart failure with preserved systolic function in a large community-dwelling elderly cohort: The cardiovascular heart study. *J Am Coll Cardiol* 1995.

60. Kitzman DW: Aging and the heart, in Freeman GL (ed): *Developments in Cardiology.* Orlando, FL, WB Saunders, 1994, pp 3–16.

61. Kitzman DW, Sullivan MJ, Cobb FR, Higginbotham MB: Exercise cardiac output declines with advancing age in normal subjects (abstract). *J Am Coll Cardiol* 1989;13(2):241A.

62. Higginbotham MB, Morris KG, Williams RS, et al: Physiologic basis for the age-related decline in aerobic work capacity. *Am J Cardiol* 1986;57:1374–1379.

63. Rodeheffer RJ, Gerstenblith G, Becker LC, Fleg JL, Weisfeldt ML, Lakatta EG: Exercise cardiac output is maintained with advancing age in healthy human subjects: Cardiac dilatation and increased stroke volume compensate for a diminished heart rate. *Circulation* 1984;69:203–213.

64. Port S, Cobb FR, Coleman RE, Jones RH: Effect of age on the response of the left ventricular ejection fraction to exercise. *N Engl J Med* 1980;303: 1133–1137.

65. Kuikka JT, Lansimies: Effect of age on cardiac index, stroke index and left ventricular ejection fraction at rest and during exercise as studied by radiocardiography. *Acta Physiol Scand* 1982;114: 339–343.

66. Ogawa T, Spina RJ, Martin WH, Kohrt WM, Schechtman KB: Effect of aging, sex, and physical

training on cardiovascular responses to exercise. *Circulation* 1992;86:494–503.

67. Davidson WR: Influence of aging on pulmonary hemodynamics in a population free of coronary artery disease. *Am J Cardiol* 1990;65:1454.
68. McClellan M, McNeil BJ, Newhouse JP: Does more intensive treatment of acute myocardial infarction in the elderly reduce mortality. *JAMA* 1994;272:859–866.
69. Granath A, Johsson B, Strandell T: Circulation in healthy old men studied by right heart catheterization at rest and during exercise in supine sitting position. *Acta Med Scand* 1964;176:425.
70. Julius S, Amery A, Whitlock LS, et al: Influence of age on the hemodynamic response to exercise. *Circulation* 1967;36:222.
71. Conway J, Wheeler R, Sannerstedt R: Sympathetic nervous activity during exercise in relation to age. *Cardiovasc Res* 1971;5:577.
72. Miyamura M, Honda Y: Maximum cardiac output related to sex and age. *Jpn J Physiol* 1973;23:645.
73. Cournand RL, Breed ES, Baldwin ED, Richards DW: Measurement of cardiac output in man using the technique of catheterization of the right auricle or ventricle. *J Clin Invest* 1945;24:106–161.
74. Brandfonbrener M, Landowne M, Shock NW: Changes in cardiac output with age. *Circulation* 1955;12:557.
75. Leithe ME, Hermiller JB, Magorien RD, et al: The effect of age on central and regional hemodynamics. *Gerontology* 1984;30:240.
76. Shannon RP, Maher KA, Santinga JT, et al: Comparison of differences in the hemodynamic response to passive postural stress in healthy subjects >70 years and <30 years of age. *Am J Cardiol* 1991;67:1110.
77. Vargas E, Lye M: Physiological responses to postural change in young and old healthy individuals. *Exp Gerontol* 1982;17:45.
78. Smith JJ, Hughes CV, Ptacin MJ, et al: The effect of age on hemodynamic response to graded postural stress in normal men. *J Gerontol* 1987;42:406.
79. Hainsworth R, Al-Shamma YMH: Cardiovascular responses to upright tilting in healthy subjects. *Clin Sci* 1988;74:17.
80. Lewis WH: Changes with age in the cardiac output in adult men. *Am J Physiol* 1938;121:517.
81. Dehn MM, Bruce RA: Longitudinal variations in maximal oxygen intake with age and activity. *J Appl Physiol* 1972;33:805–807.
82. Kitzman DW, Higginbotham MB, Sullivan MS: Aging and the cardiovascular response to exercise. *Cardiol Elderly* 1993;1:543–550.
83. Beere PA, Kitzman DW, Morey M, Higginbotham MB: Peripheral adaptations to exercise training compensate for age related differences in aerobic capacity in healthy men (abstract). *Circulation* 1991; 84(Suppl II):II-186.
84. Morey MC, Cowper PA, Feussner JR, et al: Evaluation of a supervised exercise program in a geriatric population. *J Am Geriatr Soc* 1989;37: 348–354.
85. Martin WH, Ogawa T, Kohrt WM, et al: Effects of aging, gender, and physical training on peripheral vascular function. *Circulation* 1991;84:654–664.
86. Ehsani AA, Ogawa T, Miller TR, Spina RJ: Exercise training improves left ventricular systolic function in older men. *Circulation* 1991;82:96–103.
87. Spina RJ, Ogawa T, Miller TR, Kohrt WM, Ehsani AA: Effect of exercise training on left ventricular performance in older women free of cardiopulmonary disease. *Am J Cardiol* 1993;71:99–194.
88. Hossack KF, Burce RA: Maximal cardiac function in sedentary normal men and women: Comparison of age-related changes. *J Appl Physiol* 1982;53: 799–804.
89. Haidet GC: Dynamic exercise in senescent beagles: Oxygen consumption and hemodynamic responses. *Am J Physiol* 1989;257:H1428–H1437.
90. Kostis JB, Moreyra AE, Amendo MT, DiPietro JD, Cosgrove N, Kuo PT: The effect of age on heart rate in subjects free of heart disease: Studies by ambulatory electrocardiography and maximal exercise stress test. *Circulation* 1982;65:141–145.
91. Lester M, Sheffield LT, Trammell P, Reeves TJ: The effect of age and athletic training on the maximal heart rate during muscular exercise. *Am Heart J* 1968;76:370–376.
92. Stratton JR, Cerqueira MD, Schwaqrtz RS, et al: Differences in cardiovascular responses to isoproterenol in relation to age and exercise training in healthy men. *Circulation* 1992;86:504–512.
93. Sonenblick EH, Braunwald E, Williams JF, Glick G: Effects of exercise on myocardial force–velocity relations in intact unanesthetized man: Relative roles of changes in heart rate, sympathetic activity, and ventricular dimensions. *J Clin Invest* 1967;44: 2051–2062.
94. Yin FCP: Aging and aortic impedence in beagle dogs. *Mech Aging Dev* 1988;42:49–62.

95. Walford GD, Spurgeon HA, Lakatta EG: Diminished cardiac hypertrophy and muscle performance in older compared with younger adult rats with chronic atrioventricular block. *Circ Res* 1988;63:502–511.
96. Isoyama S, Grossman W, Jew JY: Effect of age on myocardial adaptation to volume overload in the rat. *J Clin Invest* 1988;81:1850–1857.
97. Spirito P, Maron BJ: Doppler echocardiography for assessing left ventricular diastolic function. *Ann Intern Med* 1988;109:122–126.
98. Gardin JM, Wong ND, Bommer W, et al: Echocardiographic design of a multicenter investigation of free-living elderly subjects: The Cardiovascular Health Study. *J Am Soc Echocardiogr* 1992;5:63–72.
99. Inouye I, Massie B, Loge D, et al: Abnormal left ventricular filling: An early finding in mild to moderate systemic hypertension. *Am J Cardiol* 1984;53:120–126.
100. Tevel ME, Davidson W, Batterton TD: A critical analysis of mortality associated with delirium tremens. Review of 39 fatalities in a nine year period. *Am J Med Sci* 1961;242:18–29.
101. Kannel WB, Abbott RD: Incidence and prognosis of unrecognized myocardial infarction. An update on the Framingham Study. *N Engl J Med* 1984;311:1144–1152.
102. Nair CK, Thomson W, Ryschon K, Cornelia C, Hee TT, Sketch MH: Long-term follow-up of patients with echocardiographically detected mitral annular calcium and comparison with age- and sex-matched control subjects. *Am J Cardiol* 1989; 63:465–470.
103. White NK, Edwards JE, Dry TJ: The relationship of the degree of coronary atherosclerosis with age, in men. *Circulation* 1950;1:1345–1354.
104. Elveback L, Lie JT: Continued high incidence of coronary artery disease at autopsy in Olmsted County, Minnesota, 1950 to 1979. *Circulation* 1984;70:345–349.
105. Kannel WB, D'Agostino RB: The importance of cardiovascular risk factors in the elderly. *Am J Geriatr Card* 1995;March/April:10–23.
106. Vokonas PS, Kannel WB: Epidemiology of coronary heart disease in the elderly, in Tresch DD, Aronow WS (eds): *Cardiovascular Disease in the Elderly Patient.* New York, Marcel Dekker, Inc., 1994, pp 91–123.
106a. Bueno H, Vidan MT, Almazan A, et al: Influence of sex on the short-term outcome of elderly patients with a first acute myocardial infarction. *Circulation* 1995;92(5):1133–1140.
107. Goldberg RJ, Gore JM, Gurwitz JH, et al: The impact of age on the incidence and prognosis of initial acute myocardial infarction: The Worcester Heart Attack Study. *Am Heart J* 1989;117: 543–549.
108. Wilcox RG, Hampton JR: Importance of age in prehospital and hospital mortality of heart attacks. *Br Heart J* 1980;44:503–507.
109. Pashos CL, Newhouse JP, McNeil BJ: Temporal changes in the care and outcomes of elderly patients with acute myocardial infarction, 1987 through 1990. *JAMA* 1993;270:1832–1836.
110. Nadelmann J, Frishman WH, Ooi WL, et al: Prevalence, incidence, and prognosis of recognized and unrecognized myocardial infarction in persons aged 75 years or older. The Bronx Aging Study. *Am J Cardiol* 1990;66:533–537.
111. Forman DE, Gutierrez BJL, Wei JY: Management of acute myocardial infarction in the very elderly. *Am J Med* 1992;93:315–326.
112. Smith SC, Gilpin E, Ahnve S, et al: Outlook after acute myocardial infarction in the very elderly compared with that in patients aged 65–75 years. *J Am Coll Cardiol* 1990;16:784–792.
113. Tofler GH, Muller JE, Stone PH, et al: Factors leading to shorter survival after acute myocardial infarction in patients ages 65 to 75 years compared with younger patients. *Am J Cardiol* 1988; 62:860–867.
113a. Chung MK, Bosner MS, McKenzie JP, et al: Prognosis of patients > or = 70 years of age with non-Q wave acute myocardial infarction compared with younger patients with similar infarcts and with patients > or = years of age with Q wave acute myocardial infarction. *Am J of Cardiol* 1995; 75(1):18–22.
114. American Heart Association: *1992 Heart and Stroke Facts.* 1991.
115. Peterson ED, Jollis JG, Bebchuk JD, DeLong ER, Muhlbaier LHX, Pryor DB: Changes in mortality after myocardial revascularization in the elderly. *Ann Intern Med* 1994;121:919–927.
116. Applegate WB, Graves S, Collins T, Swwaag RV, Akins D: Acute myocardial infarction in elderly patients. *Southern Med J* 1984;77:1127–1129.
117. Chaturvedi NC, Shivalingappa G, Shanks B, et al: Myocardial infarction in the elderly. *Lancet* 1972;1: 280–281.

118. Williams BO, Begg TB, Semple T, et al: The elderly in a coronary unit. *Br Med J* 1976;2: 451–453.

119. Peterson DR, Thompson DJ, Chinn N: Ischemic heart disease prognosis. A community-wide assessment (1966–1969). *JAMA* 1972;219:1423–1427.

120. Naylor CD, Chen E: Population-wide mortality trends among patients hospitalized for acute myocardial infarction: The Ontario experience, 1981 to 1991. *J Am Coll Cardiol* 1994;24:1431–1438.

121. Udvarhelyi IS, Gatsonis C, Epstein AM, Pashos CL, Newhouse JP, McNeil BJ: Acute myocardial infarction in the medicare population. *JAMA* 1992;268:2530–2536.

121a. Gurwitz JH, Gore JM, Goldberg RJ, et al: Recent age-related trends in the use of thrombolytic therapy in patients who have had acute myocardial infarction. National Registry of Myocardial Infarction. *Annals of Internal Medicine* 1991;124(3):283–91.

121b. Maggioni AP, Maseri A, Fresco C, et al: Age-related increase in mortality among patients with first myocardial infarctions treated with thrombolysis. The Investigators of the Gruppo Italiano per lo Studio della Sopravvivenza nell' Infarcto Miocardico (GISSI-2). *New Eng J of Med* 1993; 329(20):1442–1448.

122. Green SJ, Ong LY, Reiser P, et al: The role of early radionuclide ejection fraction in predicting early mortality after acute myocardial infarction in the elderly. *Mt Sinai J Med* 1985;52:618–622.

123. Deckers JW, Fioretti P, Brower RW, et al: Ineligibility for predischarge exercise testing after myocardial infarction in the elderly: Implications for prognosis. *Eur Heart J* 1984;5:97–100.

124. Fiebach NH, Viscoli CM, Horwitz RI: Differences between women and men in survival after myocardial infarction: Biology or methodology. *JAMA* 1990;263:1092–1096.

125. Solomon CG, Lee TH, Cook EF, et al: Comparison of clinical presentation of acute myocardial infarction in patients older than 65 years of age to younger patients: The multicenter chest pain study experience. *Am J Cardiol* 1989;63:772–776.

126. Black DA: Mental state and presentation of myocardial infarction in the elderly. *Age Aging* 1987; 16:125–127.

127. Bayer AJ, Chadha JS, Farag RR, Pathy MSJ: Changing presentation of myocardial infarction with increasing old age. *J Am Geriatr Soc* 1986;23: 263–266.

128. Bayer AJ: Presentation and management of myocardial infarction in the elderly. *Br J Hosp Med* 1988;40:300.

129. Rodstein M: The characteristics of nonfatal myocardial infarction in the aged. *Arch Intern Med* 1956;98:84.

130. Tinker GM: Clinical presentation of myocardial infarction in the elderly. *Age Aging* 1981;10:237–240.

131. Thompson L, Wood C, Wallagen M: Geriatric acute myocardial infarction: A challenge to recognition, prompt diagnosis, and appropriate care. *Crit Care Nurs Clin N Am* 1992;4:291–299.

132. MacDonald JB: Presentation of acute myocardial infarction in the elderly—a review. *Age Aging* 1984;13:196–200.

133. Liau CS, Hahn LC, Tjung JJ, et al: The clinical characteristics of acute myocardial infarction in aged patients. *J Formosan Med Assn* 1991;90: 122–126.

134. Pathy MS: Clinical presentation of myocardial infarction in the elderly. *Br Heart J* 1967;29:190–199.

135. Aronow WS: Prevalence of presenting symptoms of recognized acute myocardial infarction and of unrecognized healed myocardial infarction in elderly patients. *Am J Cardiol* 1987;60:1182.

136. O'Connor CM, Califf RM, Massey EW, et al: Stroke and acute myocardial infarction in the thrombolytic era: Clinical correlates and long-term prognosis. *J Am Coll Cardiol* 1990;16:533–540.

137. O'Connor CM: Stroke during acute myocardial infarction, in Califf RM, Mark DB, Wagner GS (eds): *Acute Coronary Care,* 1995, pp 635–650.

138. Gore JM, Sloan M, Price TR, et al: Intracerebral hemorrhage, cerebral infarction, and subdural hematoma after acute myocardial infarction and thrombolytic therapy in the Thrombolysis in Myocardial Infarction Study. *Circulation* 1991;83: 448–459.

139. Aronow WS, Starling L, Etienne F, et al: Unrecognized Q wave myocardial infarction in patients older than 64 years in a long-term health-care facility. *Am J Cardiol* 1985;56:483.

140. Gama R, Swain DG, Nightingale PG, Buckley BM: The effective use of cardiac enzymes and electrocardiograms in the diagnosis of acute myocardial infarction in the elderly. *Postgrad Med J* 1990;66:375–377.

141. Aronow WS: Usefulness of resting electrocardiogram in the elderly. *Comprehen Ther* 1992;18:11–16.

142. DeBacker G: Delay times between onset and treatment of acute myocardial infarction in the elderly. *Cardiol Elderly* 1994;2:268–273.

142a. Stone PH, Thompson B, Anderson V, et al: Influence of race, sex, and age on management of unstable angina and non-Q wave myocardial infarction. *JAMA* 1996;275:1104–1112.

143. Chouhan L, Hajar HA, Pomposiello JC: Comparison of thrombolytic therapy for acute myocardial infarction in patients aged <35 and >55 years. *Am J Cardiol* 1993;71:157–159.

144. Himbert D, Steg PG, Juliard JM, Neukirch F, Aumont MC, Gourgon R: Eligibility for reperfusion therapy and outcome in elderly patients with acute myocardial infarction. *Eur Heart J* 1994;15: 483–488.

145. Farnsworth TA: Varying thrombolytic administration rates in elderly patients with acute myocardial infarction. *Br J Clin Pract* 1993;47:305–307.

146. Hendra TJ, Marshall AJ: Increased prescription of thrombolytic treatment to elderly patients with suspected acute myocardial infarction associated with audit. *Br Med J* 1992;304:423–425.

147. Grines CL, Demaria AN: Optimal utilization of thrombolytic therapy for acute myocardial infarction: Concepts and controversies. *J Am Coll Cardiol* 1990;16:223–231.

147a. Malone ML, Sial SH, Battiola RJ, et al: Age-related differences in the utilization of therapies post acute myocardial infarction. *J Am Geriatr Soc* 1995;43:627–633.

148. Lew AS, Hod H, Cercek B, Shah PK, Ganz W: Mortality and morbidity rates of patients older and younger than 75 years with acute myocardial infarction treated with streptokinase. *Am J Cardiol* 1987;59:1–5.

149. Fibrinolytic Therapy Trialists' (FTT) Collaborative Group: Indications for fibrinolytic therapy in suspected acute myocardial infarction: Collaborative overview of early mortality and major morbidity results from all randomized trials of more than 1000 patients. *Lancet* 1994;343: 311–322.

150. Chaitman BR, Thompson B, Wittry MD, et al: The use of tissue-type plasminogen activator for acute myocardial infarction in the elderly: Results from thrombolysis in myocardial infarction phase I, open label studies and the thrombolysis in myocardial infarction phase II pilot study. *J Am Coll Cardiol* 1989;14:1159–1165.

151. Califf RM, Topol EJ, George BS: Hemorrhagic complications associated with the use of intravenous tissue plasminogen activator in treatment of acute myocardial infarction. *Am J Med* 1988; 85:353–359.

152. Gruppo Italiano per lo Studio Della Sopravivenza Nell'Infarto Miocardico: GISSI-2: A factorial randomised trial of alteplase versus streptokinase and heparin versus no heparin among 12,490 patients with acute myocardial infarction. *Lancet* 1990;336:65–71.

153. ISIS-3 (Third International Study of Infarct Survival) Collaborative Group: A randomised comparison of streptokinase versus tissue plasminogen activator versus anistreplase and of aspirin plus heparin versus aspirin alone among 41,299 cases of suspected acute myocardial infarction. *Lancet* 1992;239:753–770.

154. Ohman EM, O'Connor CM, Califf RM: Role of thrombolytic therapy in the treatment of acute myocardial infarction. *Cardiol Elderly* 1993;1: 54–61.

155. The GUSTO Investigators: An international randomized trial comparing four thrombolytic strategies for acute myocardial infarction. *N Engl J Med* 1993;329:673–682.

156. Mark DB, Hlatky MA, Califf RM, et al: Cost effectiveness of thrombolytic therapy with tissue plasminogen activator as compared with streptokinase for acute myocardial infarction. *N Engl J Med* 1995;332:1418–1424.

157. Feit F, Breed J, Anderson JL, et al: A randomized, placebo-controlled trial of tissue plasminogen activator in elderly patients with acute myocardial infarction. *Circulation* 1990;82:666.

158. Montague TJ, Ikuta RM, Wong RY, Bay KS, Teo KK, Davies NJ: Comparison of risk and patterns of practice in patients older and younger than 70 years with acute myocardial infarction in a two year period (1987–1989). *Am J Cardiol* 1991;68: 843–847.

159. Weaver WD, Litwin PE, Martin JS, et al: Effect of age on use of thrombolytic therapy and mortality in acute myocardial infarction: The MITI project group. *J Am Coll Cardiol* 1991;18:657–662.

159a. Krumholz HM, Radford MJ, Ellerbeck EF, et al: Aspirin for secondary prevention after acute myocardial infarction in the elderly: prescribed use and outcomes. *Annals of Internal Medicine* 1996; 124(3):292–298.

160. Rosenthal GD, Fortinsky RH: Differences in the treatment of patients with acute myocardial infarction according to patient age. *J Am Geriatr Soc* 1994;42:826–832.

161. Holland KJ, O'Neill WW, Bates ER, Pitt B, Topol EJ: Emergency percutaneous transluminal coronary angioplasty during acute myocardial infarction for patients more than 70 years of age. *Am J Cardiol* 1989;63:399–403.

162. Lee TC, Laramee LA, Rutherford BD, et al: Emergency percutaneous transluminal coronary angioplasty for acute myocardial infarction in patients 70 years of age or older. *Am J Cardiol* 1990; 66:663–667.

163. Eckman MH, Wong JB, Salem DN, Pauker SG: Direct angioplasty for acute myocardial infarction: A review of clinical subsets. *Ann Intern Med* 1992;117:667.

164. Grines CL, Browne KF, Marco J, et al: A comparison of immediate angioplasty with thrombolytic therapy for acute myocardial infarction. *N Engl J Med* 1993;328:673–679.

165. Zijlstra F, de Boer MJ, Hoorntje JC, et al: A comparison of immediate coronary angioplasty with intravenous streptokinase in acute myocardial infarction. *N Engl J Med* 1993;328:680–684.

166. Gibbons RJ, Holmes DR, Reeder GS, et al: Immediate angioplasty compared with the administration of a thrombolytic agent followed by conservative treatment for myocardial infarction—the Mayo Coronary Care Unit and Catheterization Laboratory Groups. *N Engl J Med* 1993;328: 685–691.

167. Ribeiro EE, Silva LA, Carneiro R, et al: Randomized trial of direct coronary angioplasty versus intravenous streptokinase in acute myocardial infarction. *J Am Coll Cardiol* 1993;22:376–380.

168. Theroux P, Ouimet H, McCans J, et al: Aspirin, heparin, or both to treat unstable angina. *N Engl J Med* 1988;319:1105–1111.

169. Hsia J, Hamilton WO, Kleiman N, Roberts R, Chaitman BR, Ross AMF: A comparison between heparin and low-dose aspirin as adjunctive therapy with tissue plasminogen activator for acute myocardial infarction. *N Engl J Med* 1990; 323:1433–1437.

170. O'Connor CM, Meese R, Carney R, et al: A randomized trial of heparin in conjunction with anistreplase (APSAC) in acute myocardial infarction: The DUCCS 1 Study. *J Am Coll Cardiol* 1993; 23:11–18.

171. The Global Use of Strategies to Open Occluded Coronary Arteries (GUSTO IIA) Investigators: Randomized trial of intravenous heparin versus recombinant hirudin for acute coronary syndromes. *Circulation* 1994;90:1631–1637.

172. ISIS-2 Investigators: Randomized trial of intravenous streptokinase, oral aspirin, both, or neither among 17,187 cases of suspected acute myocardial infarction: ISIS-2. *Lancet* 1988;2:349–360.

173. Antiplatelet Trialist Collaboration: Secondary prevention of vascular disease by prolonged antiplatelet treatment. *Clin Res* 1988;296:320–331.

174. Smith P, Arnesen H, Holme I: The effect of warfarin on mortality and reinfarction after myocardial infarction. *N Engl J Med* 1990;323:147–152.

175. Sixty Plus Reinfarction Study Group, de Vries WA, Loeliger EA, et al: A double-blind trial to assess long-term oral anticoagulation therapy in elderly patients after myocardial infarction. *Lancet* 1980;2:989–994.

176. Cohen M, Adams PC, Parry G, et al: Combination antithrombotic therapy in unstable rest angina and non-Q wave infarction in nonprior aspirin users. *Circulation* 1994;89:81–88.

177. Lee K: Personal communication. 1995.

178. Balsano F, Rizzon P, Violi F, et al: Antiplatelet treatment with ticlopidine in unstable angina: A controlled multicenter clinical trial. *Circulation* 1990;82:17–26.

179. EPIC Investigators: Use of a monoclonal antibody directed against the platelet glycoprotein IIb-IIIa receptor in high risk coronary angioplasty. *N Eng J Med* 1994;330:956–961.

180. ISIS-I (First International Study of Infarct Survival) Collaborative Group: Trial of intravenous atenolol among 16,027 cases of suspected acute myocardial infarction: ISIS-I. *Lancet* 1986;57–66.

181. Herlitz J, Elmfeldt D, Holmberg S, et al: Goteborg Metoprolol Trial: Mortality and causes of death. *Am J Cardiol* 1984;53:9D–14D.

182. MIAMI Trial Research Group: Metoprolol in acute myocardial infarction (MIAMI). *Eur Heart J* 1985;20:19.

183. Beta-Blocker Heart Attack Trial Research Group: A randomized trial of propranolol in patients with myocardial infarction. *JAMA* 1982;247: 1701–1114.

184. Hawkins CM, Richardson DW, Vokonas PS, and the BHAT Research Group: Effect of propranolol in reducing mortality in older myocardial infarction patients. *Circulation* 1983;67:194–197.

185. Norwegian Multicenter Study Group: Timolol-induced reduction in mortality and reinfarction in patients surviving acute myocardial infarction. *N Engl J Med* 1981;304:801–807.

186. Gurwitz JH, Goldberg RJ, Chen Z, Gore JM, Alpert JS: Beta-blocker therapy in acute myocardial infarction: Evidence for underutilization in the elderly. *Am J Med* 1992;93:605–610.

187. Forman DE, Wei JY: Beta-blockers in older patients with myocardial infarction (letter). *JAMA* 1991;226:2222.

187a. Park KC, Forman DE, and Wei JY: Utility of beta-blockade treatment for older postinfarction patients. *J Am Geriatr Soc* 1995;43:747–750.

188. Brener SJ, Cox JL, Pfisterer ME, et al: The potential for unexpected hazard of intravenous beta-blockade for acute myocardial infarction: Results from the GUSTO trial (abtract). *J Am Coll Cardiol* 1995;5A.

189. The Multicenter Diltiazem Postinfarction Trial Research Group: The effect of diltiazem on mortality and reinfarction after myocardial infarction. *N Engl J Med* 1988;319:385–392.

190. Held PH, Yusuf S, Furberg CD: Calcium channel blockers in acute myocardial infarction and unstable angina: An overview. *Br Med J* 1989;299: 92–97.

191. Packer M: Slide presentation at the 44th Annual Scientific Session of the American College of Cardiology, New Orleans, Louisiana, March 19–22, 1995 (abstract).

192. Yusuf S, Collins R, MacMahon S, Peto R: Effect of intravenous nitrates on mortality in acute myocardial infarction: An overview of the randomized trials. *Lancet* 1988;1:1088–1092.

193. Gruppo Italiano per lo Studio della Sopravvivenza nell' Infarto Miocardico: GISSI-3: Effects of lisinopril and transdermal glyceryl trinitrate singly and together on 6-week mortality and ventricular function after acute myocardial infarction. *Lancet* 1994;343:1115–1122.

194. ISIS-4 (Fourth International Study of Infarct Survival) Collaborative Group: ISIS-4: A randomized factorial trial assessing early oral captopril, oral mononitrate, and intravenous magnesium sulphate in 58,050 patients with suspected acute myocardial infarction. *Lancet* 1995;345:669–685.

195. Pfeffer MA, Braunwald E, Moye LA, et al: Effect of captopril on mortality and morbidity in patients with left ventricular dysfunction after myocardial infarction. *N Engl J Med* 1992;327:678–684.

196. The Acute Infarction Ramipril Efficacy (AIRE) Study Investigators: Effect of ramipril on mortality and morbidity of survivors of acute myocardial infarction with clinical evidence of heart failure. *Lancet* 1993;342:821–828.

197. Ambroisioni E, Borghi C, Magnani B, for the Survival of Myocardial Infarction Long-Term Evaluation (SMILE) Study Investigators: The effect of angiotensin-converting-enzyme inhibitor zofenopril on mortality and morbidity after anterior myocardial infarction. *N Engl J Med* 1995;332: 80–85.

198. Swedberg K, Held P, Kjekshus J, Rasmussen K, Ryden L, Wedel HO: Results of the Cooperative New Scandinavian Enalapril Survival Study II (CONSENSUS II). *N Engl J Med* 1992;327: 678–684.

199. Chinese Cardiac Study Collaborative Group: Oral captopril versus placebo among 13,634 patients with suspected acute myocardial infarction: Interim report from the Chinese Cardiac Study (CSS-1). *Lancet* 1995;345:686–687.

200. Sane DC, Califf RM, Topol EJ, et al: Bleeding during thrombolytic therapy for acute myocardial infarction: Mechanisms and management. *Ann Intern Med* 1989;111:1010–1022.

201. Simoons ML, Miggioni AP, Knatterud G, et al: Individual risk assessment for intracranial hemorrhage during thrombolytic therapy. *Lancet* 1993; 342:1523–1528.

202. Lipowski ZJ: Delirium in the elderly patient. *N Engl J Med* 1989;320:578–582.

203. Levekoff SE, Evans DA, Liptzin B, et al: Delirium: The occurrence and persistence of symptoms among elderly hospitalized patients. *Arch Intern Med* 1992;152:334–340.

204. Schor JD, Levkoff SE, Lipsitz LA: Risk factors for delirium in hospitalized elderly. *JAMA* 1992;267: 827–831.

205. Nishimura RA, Schaff HV, Shub C, Gersh BJX, Edwards WD, Tajik AJ: Papillary muscle rupture complicating acute myocardial infarction: Analysis of 17 patients. *Am J Cardiol* 1983;51:373–377.

206. Chandler AH, Nomeir AM, Kitzman DW: Papillary muscle rupture following myocardial infarction: Pivotal role of transesophageal echocardiography in patients with atypical presentations. *Echocardiography* 1995;12:93–98.

207. Buda AG: The role of echocardiography in the evaluation of mechanical complications of acute myocardial infarction. *Circulation* 1991;84:109–121.

208. Oh JK, Seward JB, Khandieria BK, et al: Transesophageal echocardiography in critically ill patients. *Am J Cardiol* 1990;66:1492–1495.

209. Tcheng JE, Jackman JD, Nelson CL, et al: Oucome of patients sustaining acute ischemic mitral regurgitation during myocardial infarction. *Ann Intern Med* 1992;117:18.

210. Davidson CJ, Hlatky M, Morris KG, et al: Cardiovascular and renal toxicity of a nonionic radiographic contrast agent after cardiac catheterization. *Ann Intern Med* 1989;110:119–124.

211. Schwab SJ, Hlatky MA, Pieper KS, et al: Contrast nephrotoxicity: A randomized controlled trial of a nonionic and an ionic radiographic contrast agent. *N Engl J Med* 1995;320:149–153.

212. Thel MC, McNulty S, O'Connor CM: Characteristic mechanisms and outcome of cardiopulmonary arrest in congestive heart failure patients. *J Am Coll Cardiol* 1995;211A.

212a. Brymer C, Gangbar E, O'Rourke K, et al: Age as a determinant of cardiopulmonary resuscitation outcome in the coronary care unit. *J Am Geriatr Soc* 1995;43:634–637.

213. TIMI Study Group: Comparison of invasive and conservative strategies after treatment with intravenous tissue plasminogen activator in acute myocardial infarction. Results of the thrombolysis in myocardial infarction (TIMI) phase II trial. *N Engl J Med* 1989;320:618–627.

214. Carter LF, Stephan WJ, Cavero PGX, et al: Advanced age is not a contraindication for primary infarct angioplasty in patients with cardiogenic shock (abstract). *J Am Coll Cardiol* 1995; 205A–206A.

215. Jackman JD, Navetta FI, Smith JE, et al: Percutaneous transluminal coronary angioplasty in octagenarian as an effective therapy for angina pectoris. *Am J Cardiol* 1991;68:116.

216. Mark DB, Nelson CL, Califf RM, et al: Continuing evolution of therapy for coronary artery disease: Initial results from the era of coronary angioplasty. *Circulation* 1994;89:2015–2025.

217. Koshal A, Beanlands DS, Davies RA, et al: Urgent surgical reperfusion in acute evolving myocardial infarction: A randomized controlled study. *Circulation* 1988;78:I-17–I-18.

218. Pfeffer JM, Pfeffer MA, Fishbein MC, Frohlich ED: Cardiac function and morphology with aging in the spontaneously hypertensive rat. *Am J Physiol* 1979;237:H461–H468.

219. DeWood MA, Leonard J, Grunwald RP, et al: Medical and surgical management of early Q wave myocardial infarction: II. Effects of mortality and global and regional left ventricular function at 10 or more years of follow-up. *J Am Coll Cardiol* 1989; 14:78–90.

220. Phillips S, Zeft R, Skinner J: Reperfusion protocol and results in 738 patients with evolving myocardial infarction. *Ann Thorac Surg* 1986;41:119–125.

221. Phillips S: Surgery in evolving acute myocardial infarction, in Roberts A, Conti CR (eds): *Current Surgery of the Heart.* Philadelphia, JB Lippincott, 1987, pp 247–256.

222. VanHecke J, Flameng W, Sergent P: Emergency bypass surgery: Late effects on size of infarction and ventricular function. *Circulation* 1985;72 (Suppl II):II-179–II-184.

223. Berg R, Selinger S, Leonard J: Immediate coronary bypass surgery for acute myocardial infarction. *J Cardiovasc Surg* 1981;81:483–487.

224. Katz N, Wallace R: Emergency coronary bypass surgery: Indications and results, in Rackley CE (ed): *Advances in Critical Care Cardiology.* Philadelphia, FA Davis, 1986, pp 67–72.

225. Athanasuleas CL, Geer DA, Araciniega JG, et al: A reappraisal of surgical intervention for acute myocardial infarction. *J Thorac Cardiovasc Surg* 1987;93:405–414.

226. Kereiakes DJ, Topol EJ, Califf RM, et al: Favorable early and long-term prognosis following coronary bypass surgery therapy for long-term prognosis following coronary bypass surgery therapy for myocardial infarction: Results of a multicenter trial. *Am Heart J* 1989;118:199–206.

227. Kereiakes DJ, Califf RM, George BS, et al: Comparison of immediate and long-term outcome of patients having emergent or deferred coronary bypass surgery following intravenous thrombolytic therapy for acute myocardial infarction (abstract). *J Am Coll Cardiol* 1991;17:246A.

228. Applebaum R, House R, Rademaker A, et al: Coronary artery bypass grafting within thirty days

of acute myocardial infarction. *J Thorac Cardiovasc Surg* 1991;102:745–752.

229. Ciaroni S, Delonca J, Righetti A: Early exercise testing after acute myocardial infarction in the elderly: Clinical evaluation and prognostic significance. *Am Heart J* 1993;126:304–311.

230. Myers MG, Baigrie RS, Charlat ML, Morgan CD: Are routine non-invasive tests useful in prediction of outcomes after myocardial infarction in elderly people. *Lancet* 1993;342:1069–1072.

231. Previtali M, Poli A, Lanzarini L, Fetiveau R, Mussini A, Ferrario M: Dobutamine stress echocardiography for assessment of myocardial viability and aschemia in acute myocardial infarction treated with thrombolysis. *Am J Cardiol* 1993;72:124G–130G.

232. Smart SC, Sawada S, Ryan T, et al: Low-dose dobutamine echocardiography detects reversible dysfunction after thrombolytic therapy of acute myocardial infarction. *Circulation* 1993;88:405–415.

233. Camerieri A, Picono E, Landi P, et al: Prognostic value of dipyridamole echocardiography early after myocardial infarction in elderly patients. *J Am Coll Cardiol* 1993;22:1809–1815.

234. Ades PA, Waldmann ML, McCann WJ, Weaver SO: Predictors of cardiac rehabilitation participation in older coronary patients. *Arch Intern Med* 1992;152:1033–1035.

235. Ades AA, Waldmann ML, Polk DM, Coflesky JT: Referral patterns and exercise response in the rehabilitation of female coronary patients ages >62 years. *Am J Cardiol* 1992;69:1422–1425.

236. Seals DR, Hagberg JM, Hurley BF, Ehsani AA, Holloszy JO: Endurance exercise training in older men and women. *J Appl Physiol* 1984;57:1024–1029.

238. Nielsen H: Cardiac rehabilitation after acute myocardial infarction in the elderly. *Cardiol Elderly* 1994;2:290–300.

239. O'Connor GT, Buring JE, Yusuf S, et al: An overview of randomized trials of rehabilitation with exercise after myocardial infarction. *Circulation* 1989;80:234–244.

240. Oldridge NB, Guyatt GH, Fischer ME, Rimm AA: Cardiac rehabilitation after myocardial infarction. *JAMA* 1988;260:945–950.

241. Ades PA, Hanson JS, Gunther PGS, Tonino RP: Exercise conditioning in the elderly coronary patient. *J Am Geriatr Soc* 1987;35:121–124.

242. Case RB, Moss AJ, Case N, McDermott M, Eberly S: Living alone after myocardial infarction. *JAMA* 1992;267:515–519.

243. Berkman LF, Leo-Summers L, Horwitz RI: Emotional support and survival after myocardial infarction. *Ann Intern Med* 1992;117:1003–1009.

244. Williams R: Personal communication. 1995.

244a. Paul SD, O'Gara PT, Mahjoub ZA, et al: Geriatric patients with acute myocardial infarction: Cardiac risk factor profiles, presentation, thrombolysis, coronary interventions, and prognosis. *Am Heart J* 1996;131:710–715.

245. Carlson LA, Rosemhamer G: Reduction of mortality in the Stockholm Ischaemic Heart Disease Secondary Prevention Study by combined treatment with clofibrate and nicotinic acid. *Acta Med Scand* 1988;223:405–418.

246. Scandinavian Simvastatin Survival Study Group: Randomized trial of cholesterol lowering in 4444 patients with coronary heart disease: The Scandinavian Simvastatin Survival Study (4S). *Lancet* 1994;344:1383–1389.

247. Schocken DD, Arrieta MI, Leaverton PE, Ross EA: Prevalence and mortality rate of congestive heart failure in the United States. *J Am Coll Cardiol* 1992;20:301–306.

248. Kannel WB: Epidemiological aspects of heart failure. *Cardiol Clin* 1989;7(1):1–9.

249. McKee PA, Castelli WP, McNamara PM, Kannel WB: The natural history of congestive heart failure: The Framingham Study. *N Engl J Med* 1971; 285:1441–1445.

250. Kitzman DW, Higginbotham MB, Cobb FR, Sheikh KH, Sullivan MJ: Exercise intolerance in patients with heart failure and preserved left ventricular systolic function: Failure of the Frank–Starling mechanism. *J Am Coll Cardiol* 1991;17:1065–1072.

251. Kitzman DW, Higginbotham MB: Congestive heart failure with preserved left ventricular systolic function. *Primary Cardiol* 1992;18(4):55–61.

252. Cody RJ, Toree S, Clar M, Pnodolfina K: Age-related hemodynamic, renal, and hormonal differences among patients with congestive heart failure. *Arch Intern Med* 1989;149:1023–1028.

253. Packer M, Gheorghiade M, Young JB, et al: Withdrawal of digoxin from patients with chronic heart failure treated with angiotensin-converting-enzyme inhibitors. *N Engl J Med* 1993;329:1–7.

254. Kulick DL, Rahimtoola SH: Current role of digitalis therapy in patients with congestive heart failure. *JAMA* 1991;265:2995–2997.

255. Gaasch WH: Diagnosis and treatment of heart failure based on left ventricular systolic or diastolic dysfunction. *JAMA* 1994;271:1276–1280.

256. Woldow A, Wang RY, Rajagopal DE, Cohen JJ: The use of digoxin 0.125 mg versus 0.25 mg daily as maintenance dosage in patients older than 75 years of age. *Cardiol Elderly* 1993;1:3–7.

257. The CONSENSUS Trial Study Group: Effects of enalapril on mortality in severe congestive heart failure: Results of the Cooperative North Scandivavian Enalapril Survival Study (CONSENSUS). *N Engl J Med* 1987;316:1729–1735.

258. The SOLVD Investigators: Effect of enalapril on survival in patients with reduced left ventricular ejection fractions and congestive heart failure. *N Engl J Med* 1991;325:293–302.

26

Acute Myocardial Infarction in Women

Laura J. Collins, MD, and Pamela S. Douglas, MD

INTRODUCTION

Since 1908 the most frequent cause of death among U.S. women aged 40 and over has been coronary artery disease, with one-quarter of a million deaths annually (1). Cardiovascular disease actually accounts for a greater proportion of deaths in women (52%) than in men (46%) (2–4). Death rates from coronary artery disease have been declining since the 1950s; however, in women less than 65 years of age, deaths from coronary heart disease increased more than 50% (from 26% to 41%) from 1965 to 1985 (5,6). As of 1995, health care costs associated with cardiovascular disease in women are projected to exceed $68 billion annually, more than half of the cost for all cardiovascular disease (7).

Myocardial infarction in women differs from that of men on many levels including clinical presentation, in-hospital and late mortality, complications, eligibility and selection for treatment, response to treatment, and effect of risk factor modification. A fundamental dilemma is whether these discrepancies are primarily related to women's more advanced age and accordingly "older" cardiac status at the time of presentation and/or a greater burden of co-morbidities, or whether a distinct disadvantage due to gender-related differences exists. This discussion will focus on the sex-related differences apparent in acute myocardial infarction and highlight those areas lacking in information specific to gender-related issues.

CLINICAL PRESENTATION

Definitive data illustrating differences in the clinical presentation of acute myocardial infarction between men and women are lacking. For example, no data are available on whether gender-specific differences are present in the triggers of infarction, circadian variation of its occurrence, or risk of perioperative infarction during noncardiac surgery. However, the following observations have been made.

Compared with men, women present a decade later in age with their first symptoms of coronary disease or with their first myocardial infarction (8–11). A 26-year follow-up of the Framingham Heart Study revealed that angina pectoris was the most likely initial presentation of coronary artery disease in women, occurring in 47% of women, compared with 39% of men (11). Conversely, men were more likely to present with a myocardial infarction (43%) compared with women (29%) (11).

A significantly higher percentage of men presenting with angina subsequently had a myocardial infarction within 5 to 10 years of follow-up, which erroneously led many physicians to believe that anginal symptoms in women were less worrisome than in men (12,13). Two criticisms of this study are that no subjects over the age of 62 were included, and that the diagnosis of coronary artery disease was based on symptoms, which in women are unreliable indicators of angiographic coronary artery disease (14–17).

On average, women having a myocardial infarction are more likely to have a prior history of hypertension (8–10,18–22), congestive heart failure (8,18–20,23–25), unstable angina (11), diabetes (both type I and II) (18–20,22–24,26–28), a higher serum cholesterol (10,22,29) and less likely to have had a previous myocardial infarction (8,19,21,23, 27,30) or smoking history (9,19,21–23,27,29,31, 32). Women are also more likely to have concomitant obesity, valvular heart disease, cerebrovascular disease, and chronic dementia (22). Women typically present with a higher Killip class (22,23,27), and have a greater likelihood of rales and tachycardia on exam than men (23). Women seek medical attention for symptoms of an acute myocardial infarction 1 hour later than men on average (8,10), which may be partly accounted for by their more atypical symptoms including a greater incidence of abdominal pain, dyspnea, nausea, and fatigue (8,33) in addition to or in the absence of a chest pain syndrome. The Framingham Study revealed a higher incidence of silent (undetected) myocardial infarction in women (11).

In several studies from the thrombolytic era (8,18,22,34,35), women have been shown to have a higher incidence of non–Q wave (subendocardial) infarctions than men; however, a study by Marmor et al found no significant difference between the sexes (36). Two studies revealed higher myocardial enzyme levels for men (19,22); however, others report no significant difference between the sexes when adjusted for body mass index (29). One study reported a higher frequency of inferior infarctions for women (37). Anterior infarctions in women have been reported to cover a larger territory compared with those in men, more often involving both the anteroseptal and anterolateral walls of the left ventricle (29). Peri-infarct ventricular arrhythmias may be more common in men; however, they are independent of age and do not predict a worse prognosis in the setting of an acute myocardial infarction (29). Paradoxically, although women present at the time of their infarction with more co-morbid conditions and a higher likelihood of congestive heart failure, there is little conclusive evidence that this is due to a greater extent of myocardial damage, and women tend to have better left ventricular function after myocardial infarction than men (18,21,35). The mechanisms underlying this mismatch are unknown.

COMPLICATIONS OF MYOCARDIAL INFARCTION

Many studies have reported higher in-hospital and 1-year mortality rates for women (18,19,27–29,32, 38–43). These have been attributed in part to more advanced age, to more complications in the peri-infarct period, as well as to women being more critically ill upon initial presentation. Congestive heart failure, cardiogenic shock (8,19,23–25,27,29,32), recurrent chest pain or angina (8), and unrecognized myocardial infarction (44) have all been shown to occur more often in women, although these studies did not consistently adjust for age and other co-morbid conditions. Two large trials indicate a minimal, if any, increased risk of recurrent infarction in women compared with men in the thrombolytic era (28,45). One study revealed that mechanical complications and atrioventricular block in the peri-infarction period were more age than gender dependent (29).

The incidence of myocardial rupture is 1–3% after transmural myocardial infarction and whether this is more frequent in women is still controversial (see Ch. 16). There are an equal number of studies supporting both viewpoints; however, study numbers tend to be small and in most cases are not adjusted for baseline characteristics (46–50). MILIS (Multicenter Investigation of the Limitation of Infarct Study) (51) identified myocardial rupture in 1.7% of 845 patients and, in contrast to previous studies (48,49), there was not a higher incidence of rupture in women. Assessment of an unselected population of patients with acute myocardial infarction found that myocardial rupture was found in 3.2% and accounted for 17% of overall deaths from myocardial infarction. Women aged less than 70 years had the highest incidence of rupture, with nearly half of the deaths in this group due to rupture (48).

There are more complications seen post–myocardial infarction in diabetics than in nondiabetics. Both men and women diabetics have a higher incidence of cardiogenic shock, congestive heart failure, conduction disturbances, myocardial rupture, and recurrent myocardial infarction (52–55). However, female diabetics appear to fare worse than male diabetics, with higher rates of recurrent myocardial infarction (54), silent myocardial infarctions (56), and sudden death (54). Therefore, it appears that diabetes in women leads to a higher incidence of complications from myocardial infarction compared with both nondiabetics and diabetic men; however, the reasons are unclear.

EARLY MORTALITY

In the prethrombolytic era, most clinical trials presented assessments of early (in-hospital) and late mortality (unadjusted for age) that suggested that initial survival in men after myocardial infarction was almost two-fold greater than in women (18,38,39). The Framingham Heart Study reported a 30-day mortality rate of 28% for women vs 16% for men (38,39). A large multicenter study in Israel that included 1,524 women revealed a persistently higher in-hospital mortality for women despite adjustment for age (23.1% vs. 15.7%, $p < 0.0005$) and a 1-year age-adjusted cumulative mortality of 31.8% in women and 23% in men ($p < 0.0005$) (19).

The majority of mortality data from the large thrombolytic trials including ISIS-2 (The Second International Study of Infarct Survival) (40), ASSET (Anglo-Scandinavian Study of Early Thrombolysis) (56), GUSTO (Global Utilization of Streptokinase and Tissue Plasminogen Activator for Occluded Coronary Arteries) (41), and GISSI-1 (Gruppo Italiano per lo Studio della Streptochinasi nell' Infarto Miocardio) (42,43) supports a gender difference in mortality prior to adjustment for age or other clinical variables. These trials consistently reveal a higher early mortality (21–35 days) rate for women (≈2-fold) compared with men after thrombolysis (Table 26–1). However, ASSET revealed little difference between the sexes, with only a 1.2-fold increase in mortality for women compared with men (57).

Only three of the thrombolysis trials addressed whether women have a higher mortality than men after myocardial infarction after adjusting for critical baseline characteristics and age (Table 26–2). The International Tissue Plasminogen Activator/Streptokinase Mortality Study (n = 1,944 women, 6,317 men), which included 23% women, analyzed mortality with respect to gender, adjusting for age and covariables including body mass index, weight, hours to treatment, Killip class, previous history of hypertension, diabetes, previous infarction, angina, and smoking (27). Women typically had "worse" baseline characteristics and received thrombolytic therapy an average of 18 minutes later than men. Although women treated with thrombolysis had higher unadjusted in-hospital (12% vs. 7.2%, $p < 0.0001$) and 6-month (16.6% vs. 10.4%, $p < 0.0001$) mortality rates than men, these differences were eliminated after correction for the above variables with odds ratios of 1.11 and 1.02, respectively. The data from TAMI (Thrombolysis and Angioplasty in Myocardial Infarction) support the above findings (n = 348 women, 1,271 men) (28). When adjusted for clinical variables, with or without correcting for the extent of coronary artery disease, men and women had similar mortalities, with a relative risk of 1.31 for women, (95% CI 0.83–2.06, p = NS). In contrast, after 6 weeks of follow-up, TIMI-2 (Thrombolysis in Myocardial Infarction) found an increased mortality for women (RR = 1.54, 95% CI 0.98–2.43, $p = 0.01$) after controlling for age, clinical factors at time of presentation, and previous history of coronary risk factors (25). In the Minneapolis–St. Paul metropolitan area of the United States the community 28-day mortality after hospitalization for definite acute myocardial infarction declined from 13% to 10% between 1985 and 1990 in men and from 15 to 12% in women respectively (267).

Table 26–1. Unadjusted Mortality with Thrombolysis and Primary Angioplasty for Women and Men

Trial	% Women	Treatment	Follow-up	Mortality	Mortality
				W	M
GISSI-1 (42,43) $n = 11{,}806$	20%	SK	3 wk	18.5%	8.8%
			1 yr	28.3%	14.5%
ISIS-2 (40) $n = 17{,}187$	23%	SK	5 wk	13.3%	7.9%
		ASA		13.2%	8.2%
		Both		12.2%	6.7%
ASSET (56) $n = 5{,}011$	23%	rt-PA + heparin	4 wk	8.6%	6.8%
GUSTO (41,222) $n = 2{,}431$	25%	SK	4 wk	11.5%	5.9%
	25%	rt-PA		10.2%	5.0%
PAMI (63) $n = 395$	27%	PTCA	in hospital	4.0%*	2.1%

SK = intravenous streptokinase, ASA = aspirin, rt-PA = recombinant tissue plasminogen activator, PTCA = primary percutaneous transluminal angioplasty, W = women, M = men, *p = not significant for mortality difference between men and women. GISSI-1 = Gruppo Italiano per lo Studio della Streptochinasi nell' Infarto Miocardio, ASSET = Anglo-Scandinavian Study of Early Thrombolysis, GUSTO = Global Utilization of Streptokinase and Tissue Plasminogen Activator for Occluded Coronary Arteries, PAMI = Primary Angioplasty in Myocardial Infarction, ISIS-2 = The Second International Study of Infarct Survival.

Assessment of mortality data post–myocardial infarction is made difficult by the nonuniformity between studies in considering age and clinical variables, which may have a large effect on the final results, and the methods involved in controlling for these specifics. The relatively small number of women included in these studies poses yet another difficulty. Due to the rigorous entry criteria of clinical trials, these results may not be representative of actual myocardial infarction patients treated in the community.

Several studies in the prethrombolytic era have shown an almost 2.0-fold higher in hospital (58, 59) and late (60) mortality for women diabetics

Table 26–2. Gender Comparison of Thrombolytic Trials with Adjusted Mortality (Odds Ratio of Women:Men)

Trial	% Women	Treatment	Follow-up	Odds Ratio	p Value
TAMI (28)† $n = 1{,}619$	27%	rt-PA, UK, or both	in hospital	1.31	NS
TIMI-II (25)* $n = 3{,}339$	18%	rt-PA	6 wks	1.54	0.01
			1 yr	1.39	NS
International t-PA/SK (27)† $n = 8{,}261$	23%	rt-PA,SK, or both	in hospital	1.11	NS
			6 mos	1.02	NS

Mortality adjusted for age, baseline clinical, demographic, and angiographic factors for each study; see individual references for detail. UK = urokinase, rt-PA = recombinant tissue plasminogen activator, SK = streptokinase, TAMI = Thrombolysis and Angioplasty in Myocardial Infarction, TIMI = Thrombolysis in Myocardial Infarction, International t-PA/SK = International Tissue Plasminogen Activator/Streptokinase Mortality Study.

†Multivariable logistic regression—for age and other factors

*Using Cox proportional hazards model

after myocardial infarction. In GISSI-2, insulin-dependent diabetic women having an acute myocardial infarction treated with intravenous thrombolytic therapy had a 2-fold increase (RR = 2.2, 95% CI 1.4–3.5) in the risk of in-hospital mortality compared with nondiabetic women and 7-fold higher mortality at 6 months (Fig. 26–1) (52). There was a higher mortality for diabetic women than men even after adjustment for age and baseline clinical variables (52), which may be explained by gender differences in diabetic cardiovascular pathophysiology. Compared with diabetic men, diabetic women have been reported to have an altered fibrinolytic system with a lesser response to extrinsic thrombolysis (52), worsened left ventricular dysfunction in part due to diabetic cardiomyopathy (54,59,61), and a higher incidence of sudden death postinfarction (52).

A recent review of sex differences in mortality after myocardial infarction by Vaccarino et al attempted to address inconsistencies in mortality data (62). They reviewed all studies available on sex differences in mortality after myocardial infarction from 1966 through 1994 (pre- and postthrombolysis), and they included only those 27 studies which controlled at least for age and had 30 or more outcome events. In-hospital or early mortality was greater in women by an average of 40% prior to adjustment for age, with the exception of one study (30), which was limited to black patients. When the data were adjusted for age, the sex difference in mortality declined to less than 20% and was statistically significant only in two studies (19,26). The six studies that adjusted for additional covariables found that, although the relative risk of mortality remained >1 in all studies, less than half reached statistical significance (62). Vaccarino et al concluded that women may have a survival disadvantage early after myocardial infarction compared with men, but this can be partially explained by advanced age, worse clinical characteristics, and more co-morbid conditions (62). Therefore, intrinsic gender differences cannot be excluded as contributors to worsened early myocardial infarction mortality in women.

Primary angioplasty in the treatment of acute myocardial infarction has gained considerable favor over the past several years as an alternative to thrombolytic therapy, and it results in statistically

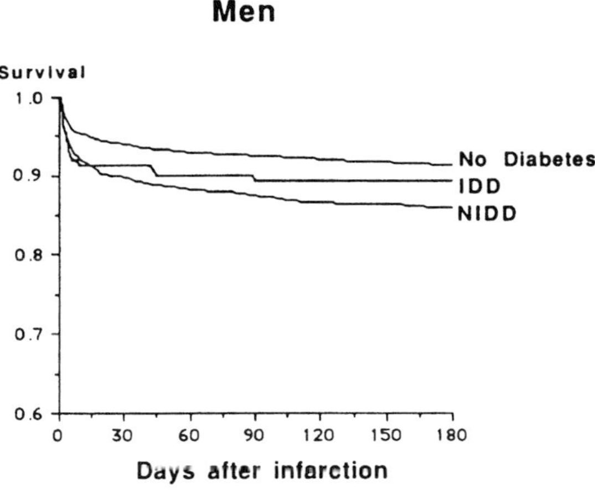

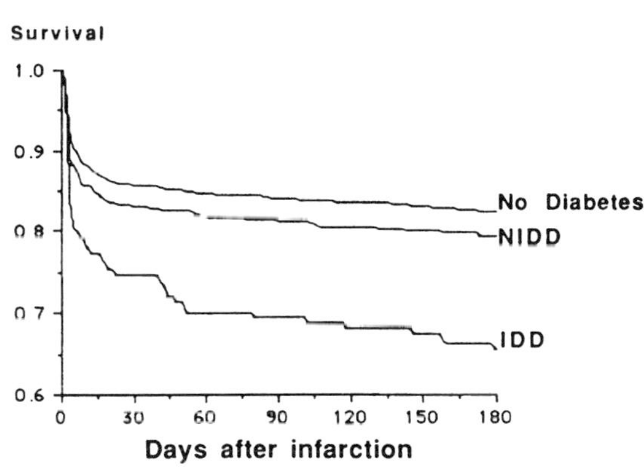

Figure 26–1. Survival curves demonstrating the gender difference after myocardial infarction at 6 months of follow-up for nondiabetics and insulin-dependent and non-insulin-dependent diabetics. Data are from GISSI-2 Study (52). *Reprinted with permission from the American College of Cardiology (Journal of the American College of Cardiology 1993;22:1788 1794).*

similar mortality in men and women (63,64). The PAMI (Primary Angioplasty in Myocardial Infarction) trial showed a trend toward higher early mortality in women than in men randomized to primary angioplasty (4.0% vs. 2.1%, p = 0.46), although these results were not adjusted for age or other covariables (63,64).

LATE MORTALITY

Vaccarino et al's (62) review of late mortality data following myocardial infarction showed similar variable results prior to age and other covariable adjustments, with four studies reporting a higher long-term mortality in women survivors (19,37,65, 66), one showing a higher mortality for men (34), and seven studies showing similar mortality between the sexes or a trend toward better survival in women (62). Over the five year period the improvement in hospital mortality was similar between men and women in the Minneapolis–St. Paul community where the risk of death within three years after hospitalization for definite myocardial infarction decreased by 26% among men and 17% among women, between 1985 and 1990 respectively. (267) Among patients surviving to day 28, the three year mortality declined in men from 16 to 12% and in women from 22 to 18%. When age adjustment was applied to mortality data, only one study (19,66a) reported a higher mortality in women, although Vaccarino et al thought this might be secondary to "incomplete age adjustment" (62). All other studies showed a similar mortality for men and women or a trend toward lower late (>1 year) mortality for women. When additional covariables were taken into consideration, women appeared to have a higher long-term survival rate than men.

PRIMARY AND SECONDARY PREVENTION OF MYOCARDIAL INFARCTION

The modification of risk factors in the primary and secondary prevention of myocardial infarctions has long been suspected to be of importance in women; however, most studies have included very few women or have not been specifically analyzed with respect to sex. Nevertheless, it is clear that gender differences exist in the evaluation and treatment of risk factors (66b,66c).

Determination of the relative contribution of each factor to the risk of a myocardial infarction is somewhat difficult to discern; however, it is widely accepted that cigarette smoking, diabetes, hypertension, and hyperlipidemia are among the more powerful risk factors for both men and women. Women with coronary disease also carry a greater burden of risk factors; women less than 55 years of age with symptomatic coronary artery disease have more risk factors (an average of 3.26/individual vs. 2.87, $p = 0.009$) than similarly aged men, and a more frequent incidence of diabetes, elevated cholesterol (>240 mg/dl) and physical inactivity (67).

Smoking

Discouragingly, one-quarter to one-third of the U.S. population continues to smoke tobacco, with more male smokers (32%) than female (26%), although the number of women beginning to smoke is higher (68). The Nurse's Health Study (69) and other studies (5,70,71) have demonstrated a dose response between tobacco use and the risk of fatal heart disease and nonfatal myocardial infarction in women. Smoking as few as 1 to 4 cigarettes per day is associated with a relative risk for myocardial infarction of 2.4, which progressively increases to 10.8 in those women smoking 45 or more cigarettes per day (69). Current Smoking has been identified as a stronger risk factor for women (relative risk 3.3) than for men (relative risk 1.9) (71a). Approximately 46–88% of all men and women presenting with their first myocardial infarction are smokers (72). Smokers account for 50% of all myocardial infarctions in women less than 55 years of age (69). The change to a low yield cigarette is not helpful in decreasing the risk of a first myocardial infarction (73). As in men, women who discontinue tobacco use decrease their risk of a first myocardial infarction to that of their nonsmoking peers within 2 to 3 years (74). Overall, patients who discontinue smoking after myocardial infarction have a 40–90% reduction in subsequent coronary heart disease events (75,76) (see Ch. 34).

Deleterious synergism between smoking and the use of some forms of oral contraceptives has been clearly established, with a 39-fold increase in the risk of myocardial infarction compared with women who use neither (77). Although this risk increases with age, young women do not escape this geometric increase (77).

Several studies (78) have demonstrated that smoking lowers HDL (high-density lipoprotein) cholesterol in a dose–response fashion in both sexes and may have a stronger effect in women. Taylor et al (79) found a 13% reduction in HDL cholesterol for women smokers compared with a 6% reduction in men smokers. One study (80) demonstrated a less pronounced difference between men and women, while yet another revealed a greater increase in LDL (low-density lipoprotein) cholesterol for young male smokers (40%) compared with females (17%) (81).

Lipoproteins

Primary Prevention

Cardiovascular risk in men has been clearly tied to total, LDL, and HDL cholesterol levels (82–88). In comparison, HDL cholesterol has been shown to be a stronger, negative predictor of cardiovascular death for women when compared with elevated LDL or total cholesterol (89–91). In women, an increase of HDL cholesterol by 10 mg/dl has been associated with a 42–50% reduction in the risk of a coronary event (85,89).

Elevated total cholesterol in women has also been associated with a higher risk of coronary heart disease (78). In the nine prospective studies that have addressed this issue, seven have reached statistical significance (78). Although men have higher rates of myocardial infarction (92) and other coronary events (93) than women with total cholesterols below 265 mg/dl, when women exceed cholesterol levels of 265 mg/dl they face a similar risk of coronary disease (92,93). This suggests that total cholesterol becomes a more important factor for women at higher levels compared with men, who have a significant increase in risk even with only a mild elevation.

The association or predictive value of LDL cholesterol with coronary heart disease in women is less clear. The Framingham Heart Study (11) found LDL cholesterol to be a significant, but less powerful, predictor of coronary heart disease in women than HDL cholesterol, while another study found no significant predictive value (90). It has been postulated that LDL cholesterol is less atherogenic in premenopausal women due to less dense particles (78) or the antioxidant effects of estrogen (94). If true, LDL cholesterol might be expected to be more atherogenic in postmenopausal women.

Triglyceride levels increase at a slower rate in women (95) and are now known to be an independent risk factor for coronary artery disease and myocardial infarction in women (95,96) with a 1.65 relative risk of cardiovascular mortality for mild to moderate elevation of triglyceride levels and a 3.44 relative risk for triglyceride levels greater than 400 mg/dl (97–99). Elevated triglyceride levels have not been shown to predict coronary heart disease risk in men (100).

Elevated Lp(a) levels have also been shown to be a strong predictor of myocardial infarction in women (101); however, a recent report suggests that this may only be true for premenopausal women (102).

Secondary Prevention

A recent prospective, randomized trial, the Scandinavian Simvastatin Survival Study (4S) (103) found a similar reduction in mortality for all subgroups analyzed including women and patients over age 60 years who were treated with simvastatin. The probability that a woman would escape any major coronary event over the 5.4-year follow-up period was 85% for the treated group versus 77.7% for the placebo group (RR = 0.65, p = 0.01). Overall, deaths from all causes and cardiovascular events were reduced by approximately one-third. There are also three older secondary prevention trials, separately analyzed with respect to gender, which revealed similar reductions in cardiovascular mortality based on similar degrees of cholesterol lowering (104–106) (see Ch. 34).

Thus both men and women gain significant benefit from cholesterol altering drug therapy with a reduction in cardiovascular events and mortality. It is impossible to discern which cholesterol fraction (LDL, HDL, or total) is responsible for the observed benefits or what optimal treatment for women might be. NCEP II guidelines (107) suggest that women aged 55 and older with one coronary risk factor and an LDL cholesterol of 160–190 mg/dl unresponsive to dietary modification be considered for drug therapy to reduce LDL cholesterol levels below 100 mg/dl. The effectiveness of such a strategy in women, in whom the importance of LDL cholesterol is equivocal, can be questioned. However, at least one study has demonstrated the validity of targeting LDL cholesterol reduction in women with coronary heart disease by revealing a resultant decrease in mortality (103). The choice of first-line therapy is unclear for women, although the NCEP II guidelines suggest that in selected postmenopausal women with elevated LDL cholesterol, estrogen should be considered as a first-line drug in lipid lowering therapy (107).

Hypertension

The Walnut Creek Study demonstrated a greater than 10-fold increase in the risk of premature death from coronary artery disease in hypertensive premenopausal women (108). In the elderly, hypertension appears to be a more significant risk factor for women than men (108). Overall, for men and women, the estimated risk reduction for first myocardial infarction is 2–3% for each 1 mm Hg drop in diastolic blood pressure (109). Following a myocardial infarction, poorly controlled hypertension is associated with a poor prognosis, with 40% higher reinfarction rates and 20% higher cardiovascular mortality (110) for both sexes. Evidence for the utility of antihypertensive therapy in secondary prevention is suggested by a 20% reduction in total mortality in those subjects with a history of myocardial infarction in the Hypertension Detection and Follow-up Program (HDFP) (111). Clearly, there is evidence that hypertension plays a significant role in the primary and secondary prevention of myocardial infarction; whether the benefit gained from modification of this risk factor is equivalent between the sexes is unknown.

Diabetes

For unclear reasons, diabetes poses a more than two-fold greater relative risk for the development of heart disease in women compared with men (54). GISSI-2 supports these Framingham data with a four-fold greater prevalence of insulin-dependent diabetes and a two-fold greater prevalence of non-insulin-dependent diabetics in its women subjects ($p < 0.01$) (52). Diabetes more commonly coexists with obesity, hypertension, and left ventricular hypertrophy in women, thus further increasing the risk for a myocardial infarction (54). The Diabetes Control and Complications Trial revealed that tight control of hyperglycemia in IDDM (insulin-dependent diabetes mellitus) is associated with a trend toward a decreased risk of macrovascular (cardiovascular and peripheral vascular) events (112). This trial was not subgroup analyzed with respect to sex, but approximately 50% of its participants were female. The benefit of tight hyperglycemic control in NIDDM (non-insulin-dependent diabetes mellitus) or in any form of diabetes after myocardial infarction is unknown.

Obesity

Obesity, including mild to moderate obesity, is associated with an increased risk of cardiovascular death in both men and women. Several studies (113–115) have demonstrated a weight-dependent increase in the risk of angina and myocardial infarction even after controlling for age and tobacco use. Distribution of body fat primarily to the abdominal area (apple-shape or central obesity) increases the risk of myocardial infarction in women (116–118) and is associated with increased androgens, insulin resistance, hypertension, and unfavorable lipid profiles. This particular body habitus is more closely associated with coronary risk in women than is body mass index (119). It is estimated that by maintaining ideal body weight and leading a physically active lifestyle, both men and women can reduce the risk of a first myocardial infarction by 35–55% (109).

Alcohol Consumption

Three prospective studies (120–122) have found a lower incidence of coronary heart disease but variable effects on mortality among women who consume alcohol compared with abstainers. The FHS (122) revealed a lowered risk of coronary heart disease, but not cardiovascular mortality, at all levels of alcohol consumption after controlling for other variables including lipids. Another study found a 36–39% reduction in the incidence of ischemic heart disease among women with light alcohol consumption (121). The NHS (Nurses Health Study) found a 40% reduction in the risk of coronary heart disease (120) with light to moderate alcohol consumption and a reduction in mortality (123) that was most significant among women 50 years of age or older with one or more coronary risk factors (RR = 0.81, 95% CI 0.74–0.91). In contrast, women 34–39 years of age had an elevated risk of mortality at any level of alcohol consumption (123). Because women are more likely to die of heart disease than of breast cancer or cirrhosis, the increased deaths from these diseases become important only at high levels of alcohol intake (124).

It is unclear if the reduction in incidence of ischemic heart disease and cardiovascular mortality is solely due to an ethanol-induced increase in HDL levels. The Lipid Research Clinics (LRC) Prevalence Study (90) revealed a dose-dependent relation between alcohol intake and HDL cholesterol levels, which was similar for men and women. In contrast, other studies have demonstrated a more pronounced increase in HDL levels with alcohol intake for men (125–127), suggesting that this mechanism of alcohol's benefit may be less important for women.

Aspirin

Primary Prevention

The benefit of aspirin use in the primary prevention of myocardial infarction has been well documented in men (128). Although for many physicians extension of these guidelines to women patients is routine practice, the actual benefit or detriment of this decision is unclear based on available data for women.

There have been four major studies addressing the issue of aspirin in the primary prevention of acute myocardial infarction in women. The Nurse's Health Study, a prospective nonrandomized observational study (n = 87,678), found that the use of 1 to 6 aspirin per week in women 34–59 years of age decreased the risk of first myocardial infarction by 25% with an age-adjusted relative risk of 0.68 (129). However, this benefit was not observed in women using higher doses of aspirin. The results of the Boston Collaborative Drug Surveillance Group, two large retrospective analyses that included both primary and secondary prevention cases, support the above findings with a similar but nonsignificant negative association between regular aspirin intake (daily aspirin, 4–7 days/week) and nonfatal myocardial infarction (130).

In contrast, two other studies have shown aspirin to be detrimental or neutral in the primary prevention of myocardial infarction. An observational cohort study of a California retirement community that included 8,881 women found that aspirin use was associated with a 70% increased risk of ischemic heart disease in women and a decrease in the risk of myocardial infarction in men only (131). Another prospective, but nonrandomized, study by the American Cancer Society ($n \geq 550{,}000$ women, over 35 years of age) found that aspirin use did not prevent death due to coronary disease for women, regardless of cardiovascular risk factors or prior cardiovascular disease (132).

Due to discrepancies in these data and the nonrandomized nature of all available studies, it may be best to individualize the use of aspirin in women for the primary prevention of myocardial infarction. The Women's Health Study, a large prospective, randomized trial addressing the use of aspirin for the primary prevention of acute myocardial infarction in women, is in progress.

Secondary Prevention

There are no conclusive data in women regarding the use of aspirin for the secondary prevention of acute myocardial infarction. The Acute Myocardial Infarction Study (AMIS) (133,134) demonstrated no clear effect of aspirin (1 gm/day) on survival of a small group of older women after myocardial infarction after 2 months to 5 years of follow-up. Other double blind randomized trials for secondary prevention have included even smaller numbers of women and have not demonstrated a significant survival benefit or have not been subgroup analyzed with respect to gender (135–138). There is no reason to believe that other antiplatelet agents (i.e. ticlid, persantine), which have not been recommended after myocardial infarction in men, should be more beneficial in women (see Ch. 32).

Hormone Replacement Therapy

Mechanisms

Over the past decade, much interest has centered on the use of estrogen replacement therapy for postmenopausal women for both the primary and secondary prevention of acute myocardial infarction. At least 25% (138–140) of estrogen's cardioprotective effect is believed to be secondary to favorable alteration of the circulating lipoprotein profile, particularly HDL elevation (90,139–142) and perhaps carbohydrate metabolism (143,144). Daily oral conjugated estrogen (0.625 mg) decreases LDL by 10–15% and increases HDL by 10–15% (145–155). The degree to which these effects are modulated by the addition of progestin is still unclear and likely depends on the type and dose of progestin replacement (152,154,156,157). Both estrogen and estrogen in combination with progestin have been shown to lower Lp(a), a recently described lipoprotein risk factor (158).

Several other areas have been implicated as contributing to the remainder of estrogen's cardioprotective effect. There is evidence that estrogen acts through its receptor on vascular smooth muscle cells to produce both vasodilatory and antiproliferative effects (159). Estrogen causes the upregulation of nitric oxide and prostacyclin synthesis, enhancing vasodilation (109,159,160,160a). Beneficial alteration of fibrinolytic parameters has also been demonstrated with estrogen replacement therapy (156,161,162). A recent analysis of 1,431 subjects in the Framingham Offspring Study found lower levels of plasminogen activator inhibitor (PAI-1) and t-PA (tissue-type plasminogen activator) antigen among premenopausal women and postmenopausal women on estrogen compared with age-matched men and postmenopausal women on no hormonal replacement (162). Previous studies have associated high levels of PAI-1 (163–168) and t-PA antigen (169,170) with an increased risk of coronary artery disease. Finally, estrogen replacement may improve cardiovascular biomechanics after menopause (170a).

Estrogen is also believed to possess intrinsic antioxidant properties (94) particularly important in relationship to the oxidation of LDL. Although some studies (171,172) have cited lower systemic blood pressure in women on estrogen replacement therapy, others have found no effect (145,173) or even an increase (174). A recent animal study (175) suggested that estradiol protects acutely ischemic myocardium in rabbits of both sexes. The estrogen-induced reduction in infarct size does not appear to be mediated through an increase in myocardial blood flow or alteration of hemodynamics (175).

Together, these studies suggest that estrogen contributes to the prevention of coronary disease through a variety of effects including modulation of coronary tone, enhancement of the fibrinolytic system, and reduction of important cardiovascular risk factors, such as hypercholesterolemia and hypertension, that predispose to atherosclerosis.

Primary Prevention

An overview of all prospective observational studies estimated that the reduction in relative risk of death from coronary artery disease is 0.50 (176) in both current and past users of estrogen replacement therapy compared with never users. Grady et al (155) estimated that overall cardiovascular mortality in current users of estrogen therapy is reduced by 35%. Data from the NHS suggest more than a 40% reduction in the risk of coronary heart disease and a 39–52% reduction in cardiovascular mortality in current users of estrogen replacement, while former users of hormone therapy enjoy a 16–21% reduction (177).

Data from the Framingham Study do not support these findings and suggest either no effect or an increase in the relative risk of death from coronary artery disease (178). Of importance is that the majority of women were using high-dose estrogen (1.25 mg or more). In support of this criticism, the NHS found that the use of higher doses of estrogen (≥1.25 mg per day) was associated with a higher relative risk (2.8) of coronary heart disease (177).

Further support for the use of hormonal therapy in the primary prevention of myocardial infarction comes from breast cancer trials with tamoxifen. A meta-analysis of 133 randomized trials shows a 25% reduction in deaths due to vascular causes associated with tamoxifen therapy (179). A Scottish trial revealed that 500 postmenopausal women treated with tamoxifen for breast cancer had a decreased incidence of fatal myocardial infarction compared with controls (180).

Several cross-sectional analyses have demonstrated a lower angiographic coronary atherosclerotic burden in estrogen users compared with nonusers (139,181,182). Sullivan et al reported that the relative risk of coronary artery disease (≥70% stenosis) in estrogen users compared with nonusers was 0.44 (95% CI 0.28–0.67) (181). Recent results from postmenopausal monkeys fed an atherogenic diet found that, although estrogen in combination with a progestin did not have a beneficial effect on lipoproteins, it protected against atherosclerosis (183,184).

Despite the lesser severity of coronary atherosclerosis, the rate of coronary artery bypass surgery among estrogen users is not reduced (RR = 1.21 for current users). The reason for this inconsistency is unclear; however, it has been suggested (177) that women on estrogen replacement therapy (ERT) may have better medical follow-up, and thus the diagnosis and treatment of coronary artery disease occurs at an earlier stage.

One study suggests that prolonged treatment may be necessary to achieve the beneficial reduction in coronary artery disease (RR = 0.5 with ≥15 years of usage, compared with a RR = 0.9 after less than 3 years of estrogen replacement) (185); however, another study suggests that there is no association between the degree of cardiovascular disease protection and the duration of use (177).

It appears that the benefit in risk reduction of coronary heart disease extends to even those women at the lowest level of risk. The NHS demonstrated an age-adjusted relative risk of 0.53 for the incidence of coronary heart disease in women without a history of smoking, hypertension, diabetes, hypercholesterolemia, or obesity (177). At this time it is unclear if the cardioprotective effect of estrogen replacement therapy declines with advancing age. The NHS (177) showed a nonsignificant trend toward a decreased benefit with increasing age, but Henderson et al (186) found a substantial benefit for women receiving estrogen in their seventies.

Three studies have assessed whether the combination therapy of estrogen and progestin alters the risk of coronary heart disease in women. The largest study (n = 23,174 women), from a cohort of women in Sweden aged 35 years and older, revealed a significant reduction in the risk of coronary heart disease among postmenopausal women taking estradiol and levonorgestrel (RR = 0.53, 95% CI 0.3–0.87) during the first year of follow-up (187). Two smaller studies did not support the above findings. A retrospective case-control study of 603 women aged 45–69 found a weak association (RR = 1.36, 95% CI 1.01–1.81) between "ever-use" of combination hormone replacement therapy in those women with a diagnosis of myocardial infarction or stroke (188). Another small study found no significant reduction in the risk of coronary heart disease in women taking estrogen and progestin replacement (189).

Many physicians and patients are reluctant to consider estrogen replacement therapy due to associated health risks including breast cancer, endometrial cancer, and other side effects such as vaginal bleeding and the need for monitoring, as well as an under-appreciation of the risk of cardiac death in women (189). To better understand the risks and benefits of hormone replacement therapy for a 50-year-old perimenopausal or recently postmenopausal woman, Grady et al used standard meta-analytical statistical methods and life-table methods to determine the relative risks of malignancies associated with hormone replacement therapy as well as its effect on the incidence of coronary heart disease, stroke, and hip fracture secondary to osteoporosis (155). This work suggests an 8.22 relative risk in the incidence of endometrial cancer and a 3.0 risk of death with long-term use of unopposed estrogen, which have been reported to persist even after the discontinuation of estrogen (190). The risk of endometrial cancer appears to be associated with both the dose and duration of estrogen therapy, although for unknown reasons (perhaps earlier diagnosis through better monitoring) estrogen replacement–induced malignancies have a lower case fatality rate compared to non–estrogen related cases (155,191). The incidence was estimated to decrease to 1.0 (190) with the addition of a progestin.

Data remain inconclusive as to how combination therapy of estrogen and progestin and duration of use will affect the risk of breast cancer. Based on Grady's model (155), the relative risks of developing and dying from breast cancer among long-term estrogen users are both 1.25. Due to inconsistencies between the available studies addressing the risk of breast cancer in users of estrogen and progestin, a "pooled" estimate of risk of combination therapy could not be performed; however, a "worst case" analysis of the data suggests an increase in relative risk from 1.25 to 2.00. It remains unclear if the risk of breast cancer increases with the duration of hormone usage; however, this is suggested by at least two studies (191,192), one of which showed an overall relative risk of 1.1, which increased to 1.7 ($p = 0.002$) after 9 years of estrogen use (192).

Estrogen decreases the relative risk of developing or dying from osteoporotic hip fractures to 0.75 (155) and possibly causes a minor reduction in the incidence of stroke (4%), neither of which is altered by progestins. One study, which showed a more significant reduction in the risk of stroke (185) had subjects with an average age of 73 years, suggesting that this benefit may be limited to older women. There is no association between thrombophlebitis or deep venous thrombosis in women (mean age 65 ± 9.5 years) taking low-dose conjugated estrogen preparations (193).

Recent studies have suggested that tamoxifen, an estrogen receptor antagonist, may favorably modify cardiovascular risk factors, including lipids, fibrinogen and body composition (193a,193b). Women receiving adjuvant tamoxifen for breast cancer have a reduced risk of myocardial infarction (193c).

Secondary Prevention

The use of estrogen replacement therapy in postmenopausal women for secondary prevention may afford an even greater reduction in cardiovascular mortality than in primary prevention, but few data are available. A retrospective observational analysis of 2,268 postmenopausal women found that women with a similar angiographic extent of coronary heart disease taking estrogen had an 84% lower rate of recurrent coronary events and prolonged survival compared with those not taking a hormone (194).

Antioxidant Therapy

The NHS, a prospective, observational study, suggested that in women aged 34–59 years, free of cardiovascular disease, the risk of coronary heart disease is decreased among users of dietary and supplemental vitamin E (195). There was a 22% reduced risk of nonfatal myocardial infarction or coronary disease in those women in the highest quintile of beta-carotene intake and a 44% reduction in risk for coronary disease in those with the highest level of vitamin E intake (195). The lack of adequate data from randomized trials, especially in older women, precludes the strong support of antioxidant vitamins as an effective modality for the prevention of myocardial infarction. Randomized trials addressing primary and secondary prevention of myocardial infarction with antioxidant therapy are under way.

Racial Issues

In general, the death rate from cardiovascular disease among black women has been reported to be 33% greater than white women, and the death rate from myocardial infarction is twice as high for black women (196). In contrast, the Charleston Heart Study found that there was no statistically significant difference between black and white mortality ratios after 30 years of follow-up (197). Black women are more likely to have preexisting hypertension, left ventricular hypertrophy, diabetes, decreased HDL, and end-stage renal disease (196). Whether black women have higher mortality after myocardial infarction than white women after adjustment for preexisting conditions is unclear.

Physical Activity/ Cardiac Rehabilitation

Although physical activity has long been viewed as reducing the risk of cardiovascular disease, only recent evidence has confirmed this suspicion (see Ch. 33). An observational study performed at the Cooper Clinic in Dallas, Texas, assessed physical fitness by treadmill testing as a predictor of overall and cause-specific mortality in 3,120 women (198). After 8 years of follow-up, women in the lowest fitness group had greater than a fourfold increase in overall mortality compared with those women in the highest fitness group. Further support of physical activity as a primary prevention strategy is found in a recent analysis from the Nurse's Health Study (199). Manson et al found that 1 hour of brisk exercise 4 to 5 times per week lowered a women's relative risk of myocardial infarction to 0.44 (95% CI 0.27–0.72) (199).

Secondary Prevention

Cardiac rehabilitation programs that include exercise lower overall and cardiovascular mortality (200) and the risk of recurrent infarction by

20–25% (200–202). However, the numbers of women in these studies are too small to make any specific gender-based conclusions. The above studies were also performed in the prethrombolytic, preangioplasty era, and very few of the patients had undergone coronary artery bypass grafting (CABG). Thus it is difficult to extrapolate the available data to today's population of women patients needing secondary prevention (see Ch. 33).

Women tend to utilize cardiac rehabilitation programs less frequently and may have higher attrition rates than men (203–206). Older age cannot be the full explanation, as more older men attend cardiac rehabilitation than their women peers (207) Higher rates of absenteeism among women who do complete programs have been attributed to the higher priority of women's domestic responsibilities (208). Interestingly, women increase their physical activity levels more rapidly after myocardial infarction than men, through an earlier return to household chores rather than formal exercise (209). However, other studies report that women return to work outside the home less frequently or after a longer period of time (203,210) and resume sexual activity later than men (203).

If women do participate in cardiac rehabilitation programs, they receive comparable benefits in coronary risk factor modification, improvement in behavioral traits and quality of life, and increased functional capacity (211,212). A recent comparison (n = 225; 51 women) of the outcome of men and women in cardiac rehabilitation (211) demonstrated that more women were unmarried, unemployed, non-white, or had hypertension, diabetes, or a higher cholesterol level compared with men. This study and one other suggest that although women consistently had a lower baseline exercise capacity than men, they achieved greater relative increases in their exercise time and peak METs compared with men (211,212). These findings suggest that cardiac rehabilitation may be more beneficial for women than for men.

TREATMENT OF MYOCARDIAL INFARCTION

Thrombolysis

The introduction of thrombolytic therapy for the treatment of acute myocardial infarction was a major advance affording the greatest improvement in mortality since the introduction of cardiopulmonary resuscitation and coronary intensive care units (see Ch. 19). The original thrombolysis placebo-controlled trials showed an overall 17–45% reduction in mortality (40,42,57) for both men and women (Table 26–3). For example, ISIS-2 found

Table 26–3. Mortality Reduction by Gender for Thrombolysis or Primary Angioplasty Versus Control Treatment

Study	% Women	Treatment	Follow-up	Control	Mortality	Reduction
					W	M
ISIS-2 (40) n = 17,187	23%	SK + ASA	in hospital	placebo	31%	45%
GISSI-1 (42) n = 11,711	20%	SK	in hospital	stnd care	19%	17%
GISSI-1 (43) n = 11,696	20%	SK	1 yr	stnd care	10% p = NS	10% p = 0.02
ASSET (56) n – 5,011	23%	rt-PA + heparin	in hospital	placebo + heparin	21%	28%
PAMI (62) n = 395	27%	PTCA	in hospital	rt-PA	29% p = 10.07	6% p = 0.46

Stnd Care = Standard Care

For abbreviations see Tables 26–1 and 26–2.

that women treated with intravenous streptokinase and aspirin had a 31% reduction in mortality compared with placebo, while men had a 45% reduction (40). Other trials showed a more closely matched reduction in early mortality for men and women (42,57). The benefit for long-term mortality is less clear. GISSI-1 demonstrated a similar magnitude of mortality reduction with streptokinase for men and women, although this did not reach statistical significance in women (43).

To date there is no evidence for a difference in the pharmacokinetics of thrombolytic agents between men and women in the setting of an acute myocardial infarction (213). However, there does appear to be a gender difference in the amount of endogenous t-PA and PAI-1 (214) (see the section on hormonal replacement).

Gender Bias in the Selection of Patients for Thrombolysis

In most trials, women were deemed "eligible" or received thrombolysis less often than men (8, 215–222), but once women received thrombolysis they did well (10,28,221,223–225). However, this benefit may be less available to women, as many studies indicate that there is still a greater tendency not to proceed with thrombolysis in eligible women (217,220,226). This reluctance can be partially explained by older age, atypical presentation, more non–Q wave myocardial infarctions, more co-morbid medical conditions, and later time of presentation; however, there is evidence that some degree of selection bias may exist on the basis of sex (226). This must be more fully examined.

MITI (Myocardial Infarction Triage and Intervention Registry) revealed that men with an acute myocardial infarction were almost twice as likely to receive thrombolysis (14% vs. 26%, $p < 0.0001$) compared with women (8). However, it is uncertain if this discrepancy is due to less frequent eligibility or to gender bias. In comparison, the Western Washington Emergency Department r-tPA trial found women to be less likely to be eligible for thrombolysis, but also demonstrated a gender bias, as eligible men received thrombolytic therapy more often than eligible women (78% vs. 55%) (220). The U.S. Thrombolysis Study Investigators, in addressing those factors accounting for gender bias in the utilization of thrombolytic therapy, found that women who were "strong" candidates for thrombolysis (i.e., short time to presentation, obvious EKG criteria, and without contraindications) received this therapy with the same frequency as the "strong" male candidates (217). However, if the decision to use thrombolysis became less clear, men were significantly more likely to receive thrombolysis than women. Their study did not address whether this was overutilization in men or underuse in women.

Overall, thrombolysis and primary angioplasty studies suggest that given the best therapy in the current era, and after controlling for clinical variables and age, gender differences in late postinfarction mortality can be reduced or eliminated. However, since women in the community are less likely to receive thrombolytic treatment (216), gender comparisons based on data from clinical trials, in which all patients receive such therapy, may not reflect true mortality.

Thrombolysis: Efficacy and Complications

The subgroup analyses comparing reperfusion rates after thrombolysis between men and women report similar pharmacokinetics and response to lytic therapy between the sexes (10,32,221, 223–225). The TIMI Phase 1 trial, a double-blinded, randomized trial ($n = 290$ patients), revealed no gender difference in the rate of reperfusion (221). This was further supported by a review of all data from TAMI, which found no difference in infarct-related artery patency, with 72.2% patency for men and 74.3% for women (28). In addition, a smaller series by Becker (213) was in agreement with the TIMI and TAMI trials. An assessment of noninvasive markers of reperfusion in GISSI-2 found that a decrease in ST segment elevation was achieved less often in diabetics, particularly insulin-dependent diabetic women (52). This finding may suggest an altered physiologic response to thrombolysis in insulin-dependent diabetic women.

Hemorrhagic complications in the setting of thrombolytic therapy are a major source of morbidity and mortality and are more common in women. Most studies show a 2–3 fold increase in the risk of hemorrhagic stroke in women, which is reduced but not fully eliminated by adjustment for age, body surface area, or body weight less than 70 kg, and the use of anticoagulation before admission (27,28,52,66,227). The PAMI trial also found an increased risk of intracranial hemorrhage among women treated with t-PA, at 5.3% compared with 0.7% for men (63). Less life-threatening hemorrhagic complications appear to be more common in women (228,229) as well. Currently, the major thrombolytic trials support a gender difference in the risk of intracranial bleeding, which is not solely attributable to advanced age or an inappropriate dose for body size.

Poor left ventricular function after myocardial infarction portends a poor prognosis for both sexes (230–233). Review of the TAMI database found similar improvement in left ventricular function prior to discharge for both sexes (28). Preliminary animal data in rats (234) suggest that females remodel differently post–myocardial infarction than males, with less cavity dilation and less hypertrophy of the noninfarcted walls. Unfortunately, gender subgroup analysis on left ventricular function after thrombolysis is not available for the majority of the studies.

Primary Angioplasty Versus Thrombolysis

The largest trial to date to address the issue of thrombolysis versus primary angioplasty in the treatment of acute myocardial infarction is PAMI (64). This multicenter trial randomized 395 patients, 27% of whom were women (without a separate randomization for each sex), who presented within 12 hours of the onset of myocardial infarction to either primary angioplasty or systemic thrombolysis with t-PA (100 mg or 1.25mg/kg for patients weighing less than 65 kg). The results revealed a lower in-hospital mortality for the angioplasty group and less complications, including less early reinfarction and intracranial bleeding, with similar post–myocardial infarction left ventricular function.

A separate analysis of the gender-specific outcome of the PAMI trial found a univariate trend toward reduced mortality among women treated with primary angioplasty compared with thrombolysis (4.0% vs. 14.0%, $p = 0.07$) (63). The group of women responsible for the increased mortality in the t-PA treated patients were women aged 65 years or older, while women less than 65 years of age had similar in-hospital mortality as men, regardless of treatment modality. The incidence of intracranial bleeding was higher in women ≥65 years of age treated with t-PA versus primary angioplasty (9.4% vs. 0%, $p = 0.07$).

Cardiac Catheterization

The MIDAS (Myocardial Infarction Data Acquisitions System) trial (235), the MITI trial (8), and others (22,236) revealed that women were less likely to undergo cardiac catheterization after myocardial infarction. MITI found that 58% of men in their population were referred for coronary angiography, compared with 40% of women ($p < 0.0001$) (8). These differences, and those in MIDAS (235), were not eliminated by controlling for age or multiple patient characteristics.

In contrast, other studies have found no difference in the usage of cardiac catheterization between men and women in the postinfarction period, especially after controlling for age and extent of coronary disease (31,215,237). Funk and Griffey found that the characteristics of old age, black race, treatment by a woman physician, chronic dementia, cerebrovascular disease, and a neurologic complication accompanying a myocardial infarction were all associated with a decreased likelihood of cardiac catheterization in the immediate peri-infarction period (31).

Thus it remains controversial as to whether women are truly referred less frequently than men for coronary angiography in the postinfarction period or whether this current referral pattern is justified by patient characteristics. Several factors may account for the differences in study results, including regional differences in aggressiveness of care or patient acceptance of catheterization. If future data do confirm a gender bias in the referral of patients for coronary angiography in the post–myocardial infarction period, further study will be required to determine if this represents a pattern of overuse in men versus an underuse in women.

Coronary Revascularization

Most studies reveal lower overall use of percutaneous transluminal coronary angioplasty (PTCA) in women post–myocardial infarction (8,22,235,236), but others (237,238) have demonstrated no difference in PTCA rates. However, once a women undergoes a cardiac catheterization, data suggests that she has the same rate of having a PTCA as a man (8,31,235), which is in support of Healy's (239) frequently quoted contention that once women are shown to have coronary artery disease they are treated "as men would be."

Available data suggest that women who undergo PTCA for post–myocardial infarction ischemia have similar procedural success rates as men (240,241). After PTCA, the rates of coronary artery bypass grafting (CABG), repeat PTCA, recurrent infarction, and mortality are similar to those in men after adjustment for age, severity of disease, and other clinical factors (240,241).

Surgical revascularization in women has been traditionally associated with a higher early mortality compared with men (242–245), which is also true after myocardial infarction (8). This has been attributed to several factors, including smaller vessel size, smaller body surface area (246), more co-morbid conditions, advanced age, a more critical status at the time of surgery, and more advanced disease at the time of CABG, perhaps due to delayed referral (247–250). In contrast, late mortality appears similar with a 6-year follow-up of the CASS (Coronary Artery Surgery Study) Registry revealing no difference in survival between men and women after CABG (248). Longer follow-up (15 years) also reveals no gender differences in survival for surgical treatment of left main coronary disease (248a).

Similar to the referral pattern for PTCA post–myocardial infarction, several studies reveal equivalent rates of CABG for men and women once they have undergone coronary catheterization (8,232,235). However, others have show a persistent difference even after adjusting for age, severity of coronary artery disease, and other clinical variables (236,237). The majority of data suggest that no specific gender discrepancy exists post–myocardial infarction in referral of patients for catheter or surgical revascularization.

Adjunctive Medical Therapy

Although reperfusion therapy has afforded the greatest reduction in mortality from myocardial infarction, adjunctive medical therapy remains important (see Ch. 12). Several studies have shown a mortality reduction for both men and women who receive beta blockers after myocardial infarction (251–255). Although the data are inconclusive, several studies suggest that women might experience more benefit than men (251–254). ISIS-1 (251) revealed a larger mortality reduction for women treated with atenolol compared with men. The Timolol Myocardial Infarction Trial revealed a 41% reduction in mortality for women, which was greater than that for men (35%) (252). BHAT (Beta-Blocker Heart Attack Trial), which included 602 women, also showed a trend (nonsignificant) toward greater reduction in mortality for women (253,254).

Available data suggest that calcium channel blockers do not reduce the risk of recurrent infarction (256,257) or cardiovascular death, and in some studies they have been associated with an increase in mortality (200,257). There is no reason to expect that women would receive more of a benefit from this therapy; however, specific gender analyzed data is unavailable.

Although it is widely recommended that angiotensin converting enzyme (ACE) inhibitors be used post–myocardial infarction in those patients with a left ventricular ejection fraction of 40% or less, no convincing data exist to support this for women. The SAVE (Survival and Ventricular Enlargement) trial demonstrated only a 2% (95% CI − 53–37%) reduction in deaths for women from all causes compared with a 22% (95% CI 6–36%) risk reduction for men (258). Likewise, there was a large discrepancy in the risk reduction of cardiovascular death and morbidity, with a 28% (95% CI 16–38%) reduction in men compared with a 4% reduction (95% CI − 32–30%) in women. Although the authors of the SAVE trial addressed the more favorable results in men by using a proportional-hazards model to show that the benefits of captopril therapy were independent of sex (259), it is difficult to conclude that men and women receive equivalent benefit from this therapy based on available data. Why men should have more benefit from this treatment is unclear. These data accentuate the need for further clarification of gender differences in the use of angiotensin converting enzyme inhibitors post–myocardial infarction, and in their optimal use in the female patient.

Two large randomized trials, ISIS-2 (40) and ISIS-2 Pilot Study (260), have demonstrated the benefit of aspirin in the setting of an acute myocardial infarction. In ISIS-2, less than 25% of the patients were women and subgroup analyses were determined to be unreliable (40).

An overview of six trials found the use of intravenous nitrates given during the early period of an acute myocardial infarction to reduce mortality by 45%; however, this analysis did not achieve conventional statistical significance (261). Although these trials did not specifically gender analyze, there are currently no data to suggest that women would receive less benefit from intravenous nitrates in this setting.

Gender Differences in the Use of Adjunctive Medical Therapy

Based on the available data, it is clear that following an acute myocardial infarction both beta blockers and aspirin may be indicated in women, without obvious contraindications, as adjuncts to reperfusion. Despite this knowledge, women and the elderly (those greater than 70 years of age) are more frequently discharged after myocardial infarction without prescription of these medications (29,262–266). For example, a study by Wilkinson et al (263) revealed that 23.3% of women compared with 41.4% of men ($p < 0.001$) were discharged on beta blockers after their initial admission for myocardial infarction. Beta blockers are also less likely to be given to women than men during the initial presentation of an acute myocardial infarction (43% vs. 37%, $p < 0.005$) (216).

The Worcester Heart Attack Study reported that men were more likely to be treated with antiplatelet therapy (25%) than women (19%, $p = 0.005$) in the acute phase of a myocardial infarction (216). There is also evidence that women are less likely to be discharged on aspirin therapy after myocardial infarction for secondary prevention (75% vs. 80%, $p < 0.01$) (264).

Several studies have reported the overuse of calcium channel blockers in the setting of an acute myocardial infarction or in the peri-infarction period (200,266), and at least two studies showed a trend toward a higher usage in women compared with men (25,47).

Women were also more likely than men to receive digoxin or diuretic therapy in the setting of an acute myocardial infarction and less likely to receive antiarrhythmic agents (216). Men are more likely to receive intravenous nitrates (216), which have been associated with a reduction in mortality (201,261). No gender-specific information is available concerning the pattern of use of ACE inhibitors post–myocardial infarction.

Whether these differential usage patterns in adjunctive medical therapy have any effect on short- or long-term morbidity and mortality after myocardial infarction in women is unclear. Data from an observational follow-up study of myocardial infarction patients in London (263) implicated the underutilization of beta blockers in women's relatively higher risk of recurrent ischemia postinfarction. However, after adjustment for other clinical factors, this difference became nonsignificant.

SUMMARY

Acute myocardial infarction in women is associated with more atypical symptoms, which may lead to delays in presentation and treatment and less aggressive care. It is important for physicians to recognize these differences. Women appear to have an early survival disadvantage after myocardial infarction that can be largely explained by more advanced age and other co-morbid conditions. However, some population-based studies which account for these factors still suggest that women do worse. To determine whether gender is truly an independent risk factor in mortality from myocardial infarction, any difference in the aggressiveness of diagnosis and treatment of coronary heart disease in men versus women must be eliminated. There appears to be no significant difference in long-term mortality, and there is even a suggestion that women may fare better.

Early reperfusion is an important predictor of early and late outcomes, and thrombolysis reduces mortality in women as well as men. To the extent that women are judged less eligible for thrombolysis, based on older age and concomitant disease, women are less likely to receive such therapy. Some studies have suggested an actual gender bias in the allocation of thrombolysis. Recent data suggest that primary angioplasty may be the preferred method of reperfusion, especially in elderly women; however, the availability of this therapy is limited.

Of all postinfarction medical therapy, only β-blockade has been carefully evaluated in women. Data regarding aspirin and angiotensin converting enzyme inhibitors in women are not conclusive. The suggestion that women are still less likely to be prescribed proven therapy than men (i.e. β-blockers) needs further investigation.

In the presence of diabetes, the onset of coronary artery disease is not delayed in women. Diabetic women are more prone to complications and have the worst survival following an acute MI. The etiologic mechanisms responsible for diabetics' worse prognosis are uncertain and probably multifactorial. Why diabetic women should fare considerably worse than diabetic men is also unknown.

Finally, the primary and secondary prevention of coronary heart disease is also different in women and less well studied. Determination of which lipid subfractions are most instrumental in the atherogenic process in women, and why, will be crucial to gender-specific tailoring of cholesterol lowering therapy. Hormone replacement therapy in postmenopausal women appears to be a very promising treatment for lipid abnormalities and reducing cardiovascular risk.

Careful attention to women's clinical presentation, response to treatment, complications, and mortality of acute myocardial infarction will be necessary to understanding their underlying pathophysiology and devising optimal treatment strategies for them.

REFERENCES

1. *Heart and Stroke Facts.* Dallas, American Heart Association, 1992.
2. Thom TJ. Cardiovascular disease mortality in U.S. women, in Eaker E, Packard B, Wenger N, Clarkson T, Tyroler HA (eds). *Coronary Heart Disease in Women.* New York, Haymarket Doyma, 1987, 33–41. As referenced by: Bush TL, Fried LP, Barrett-Connor E: Cholesterol, lipoproteins, and coronary heart disease in women. *Clin Chem* 1988;34(8B):B60–B70.
3. *Vital Statistics of the United States 1976: II. Mortality Part B,* Pub. no. 79–1102. Washington, DC, U.S. Department of Health, Education and Welfare, 1979. As referenced by: Bush TL, Fried LP, Barrett-Connor E: Cholesterol, lipoproteins, and coronary heart disease in women. *Clin Chem* 1988;34(8B): B60–B70.
4. *Vital Statistics of the United States 1976: II. Mortality Part A,* Pub. no. 80–1101. Washington, DC, U.S. Department of Health, Education and Welfare, 1980. As referenced by: Bush TL, Fried LP, Barrett-Connor E: Cholesterol, lipoproteins, and coronary heart disease in women. *Clin Chem* 1988;34(8B): B60–B70.
5. Department of Health and Human Services: *Reducing the Health Consequences of Smoking: 25 years of Progress: A report of the Surgeon General.* Washington, DC, Government Printing Office, 1989. (DHHS publication no. (CDC) 89–8411.)
6. National Center for Health Statistics: Advance report of final mortality statistics, 1986. *Monthly Vital Statistics Report* 1988;37(Suppl. 6):1–56.
7. Hodgson TA: American Heart Association extrapolation. *Health Care Financing Rev* 1984;5(4).
8. Maynard CM, Litwin PE, Martin JS, et al: Gender differences in the treatment and outcome of acute myocardial infarction: Results from the Myocardial Infarction Triage and Intervention Registry. *Arch Intern Med* 1992;152;972–976.
9. McCabe CH, Prior MJ, Fraulini T, et al: Gender differences between patients with acute myocardial infarction, non-Q-wave myocardial infarction, and unstable angina—results from TIMI II and T3B (abstract). *J Am Coll Cardiol* 1993;21:271A.
10. Jenkins JS, Flaker GS, Nolte B, et al: Causes of higher in-hospital mortality in women than in men after acute myocardial infarction. *Am J Cardiol* 1994;73:319–322.
11. Lerner DJ, Kannel WB: Patterns of coronary heart disease morbidity and mortality in the sexes: A 26-year follow-up of the Framingham population. *Am Heart J* 1986;111:383–390.
12. Kannel WB, Feinlib M: Natural history of angina pectoris in the Framingham Heart Study. *Am J Cardiol* 1972;29:154–163.

13. Murabito JM, Evans JC, Larson MG, et al: Prognosis after the onset of coronary heart disease. *Circulation* 1993;88:2548–2555.
14. Chaitman BR, Bourassa MG, Davis K, et al: Angiographic prevalence of high-risk CAD in patient subsets (CASS). *Circulation* 1993;88:2548–2555.
15. Weiner DA, Ryan TJ, McCabe CH, et al: Correlations among history of angina, ST-segment response and prevalence of coronary artery disease in the Coronary Artery Surgery Study (CASS). *N Engl J Med* 1979;301:230–235.
16. Welch PC, Proudfit WL, Sheldon WC: Coronary arteriographic findings in 1,000 women under age 50. *Am J Cardiol* 1975;35:211–215.
17. Waters DD, Halphen C, Theroux P, et al: Coronary artery disease in young women: Clinical and angiographic features an correlation with risk factors. *Am J Cardiol* 1978;42:41–47.
18. Tofler GH, Stone PH, Muller JE, et al: Effects of gender and race on prognosis after myocardial infarction: Adverse prognosis for women, particularly black women. *J Am Coll Cardiol* 1987;9:473–482.
19. Greenland P, Reicher-Reiss H, Goldbourt U et al: In hospital and 1-year mortality in 1,524 women after myocardial infarction: comparison with 4,315 men. *Circulation* 1991;83:484–491.
20. Henning R, Lundman T: The Swedish Cooperative Study, Part I: A description of the early stage. *Acta Med Scand* 1975;586(Suppl):27–29.
21. Dittrich H, Gilpin E, Nicod P, et al: Acute myocardial infarction in women: Influence of gender on mortality and prognostic variables. *Am J Cardiol* 1988;62:1–7.
22. Funk M, Griffey KA: Relation of gender to the use of cardiac procedures in acute myocardial infarction. *Am J Cardiol* 1994;74:1170–1173.
23. Fiebach NH, Viscoli CM, Horwitz RI: Differences between women and men in survival after myocardial infarction: Biology or methodology? *JAMA* 1990;263:1092–1096.
24. Goldberg RJ, Gorak EJ, Yarzebski J, et al: A communitywide perspective of sex differences and temporal trends in the incidence and survival rates after acute myocardial infarction and out of-hospital deaths caused by coronary heart disease. *Circulation* 1993;87:1947–1953.
25. Becker RC, Terrin M, Ross R, et al: Comparison of clinical outcomes for women and men after acute myocardial infarction. *Ann Intern Med* 1994;120: 638–645.
26. Puletti M, Sunseri L, Curione M, et al: Acute myocardial infarction: Sex-related differences in prognosis. *Am Heart J* 1984;108:63–66.
27. White HD, Barbash GI, Modan M, et al: After correcting for worse baseline characteristics, women treated with thrombolytic therapy for acute myocardial infarction have the same mortality and morbidity as men except for a higher incidence of hemorrhagic stroke. *Circulation* 1993;88(Pt 1):2097–2103.
28. Lincoff M, Califf RM, Ellis SG, et al: Thrombolytic therapy for women with myocardial infarction: Is there a gender gap? *J Am Coll Cardiol* 1993; 22(7):1780–1787.
29. Robinson K, Conroy RM, Mulchay R, et al: Risk factors and in-hospital course of first episode of myocardial infarction or acute coronary insufficiency in women. *J Am Coll Cardiol* 1988;11:932–936.
30. Liao Y, Cooper RS, Ghali JK, et al: Survival rates with coronary artery disease for black women compared with black men. *JAMA* 1992;268:1867–1871.
31. Murabito JM, Evans JC, Larson MG, et al. Prognosis after the onset of coronary heart disease: An investigation of differences in outcome between the sexes according to initial coronary disease presentation. *Circulation* 1993;88:2548–2555.
32. Jenkins JS, Flaker GC, Nolte B, et al: Causes of higher in-hospital mortality in women than in men after acute myocardial infarction. *Am J Cardiol* 1944;73:319–322.
33. Willich SN, Löwel H, Lewis M, et al: Unexplained gender differences in clinical symptoms of acute myocardial infarction (abstract). *J Am Coll Cardiol* 1993;21:238A.
34. Pohjola S, Siltanen P, Romo M: Five-year survival of 728 patients after myocardial infarction: A community study. *Br Heart J* 1980;43:176–183.
35. Johansson S, Bergstrand R, Schlossman D, et al: Sex differences in cardioangiographic findings after myocardial infarction. *Eur Heart J* 1984;5:374–381.
36. Marmor A, Geltman EM, Schechtman K, et al: Recurrent myocardial infarction: Clinical predictors and prognostic implications. *Circulation* 1982; 66:415–421.
37. Peter T, Harper R, Luxton M, et al: Acute myocardial infarction in women. The influence of age on complications and mortality. *Med J Aust* 1978;1: 189–191.
38. Kannel WB, Sorlie P, McNanamara AM: Prognosis after myocardial infarction. The Framingham Study. *Am J Cardiol* 1979;44:53–59.

39. Kannel WB, Thomas JT: Incidence, prevalence and mortality of cardiovascular diseases in the heart, arteries and veins, in Hurst JW (ed): *The Heart.* New York, McGraw Hill, 1986, pp 557–565.
40. ISIS-2 (Second International Study of Infarct Survival) Collaborative Group: Randomised trial of intravenous streptokinase, oral aspirin, both or neither among 17,187 cases of suspected acute myocardial infarction: ISIS-2. *Lancet* 1988;2:349–360.
41. The GUSTO Angiographic Investigators: The effects of tissue plasminogen activator, streptokinase or both on coronary-artery patency, ventricular function, and survival after myocardial infarction. *N Engl J Med* 1993;329:1615–1622.
42. Grupo Italiano per lo Studio della Streptochinasi nell' Infarto Miocardio (GISSI): Effectiveness of intravenous thrombolytic treatment in acute myocardial infarction. *Lancet* 1986;1:397–401.
43. Gruppo Italiano per lo Studio della Streptochinasi nell' Infarto Miocardio (GISSI): Long-term effects of intravenous thrombolysis in acute myocardial infarction: final report of the GISSI study. *Lancet* 1987;2:871–874.
44. Kannel WB, Abbot RD: Incidence and prognosis of unrecognized myocardial infarction: An update on the Framingham Study. *N Engl J Med* 1984;311: 1144–1147.
45. GISSI-2 Investigators, ANMCO and M Negri Institute, Italy: Predictors of nonfatal reinfarction in survivors of myocardial infarction after thrombolysis. Results from the GISSI-2 data base. *Circulation* 1993;88(Pt 2):I-490.
46. Held AC, Cole PL, Lipton B, et al: Rupture of the interventricular septum complicating acute myocardial infarction: A multicenter analysis of the clinical findings and outcome. *Am Heart J* 1988; 116:1330–1336.
47. Naeim F, de la Maza LM, Robbins SL: Cardiac rupture during myocardial infarction. A review of 44 cases. *Circulation* 1972;45:1231–1239.
48. Delborg M, Held P, Swedberg K, et al: Rupture of the myocardium. Occurrence and risk factors. *Br Heart J* 1985;54:11–16.
49. Rasmussen S, Leth A, Kjoller, et al: Cardiac rupture in acute myocardial infarction. A review of 72 consecutive cases. *Acta Med Scand* 1979;205:11–16.
50. Radford MJ, Johnson RA, Daggett WM Jr, et al: Ventricular septal rupture: A review of clinical and physiologic features and an analysis of survival. *Circulation* 1981;64:545–553.
51. Pohjola-Sintonen S, Mueller JE, Stone PH, et al, and the MILIS Study Group: Ventricular septal and free wall rupture complicating acute myocardial infarction: Experience of the Multicenter Investigation of Limitation of Infarct Size. *Am Heart J* 1989;117:809–818.
52. Zuanetti G, Latini R, Maggioni MD, et al, on behalf of GISSI-2 Investigators: Influence of diabetes on mortality in acute myocardial infarction: Data from the GISSI-2 study. *J Am Coll Cardiol* 1993;22:1788–1794.
53. Umachandran V, Ranjadayalan K, Kopelman PG, et al: Morbidity and mortality benefits in diabetics and the elderly (abstract). *Eur Heart J* 1991;12 (Suppl A): 321.
54. Abbott RD, Donahue RP, Kannel WB, et al: The impact of diabetes on survival following myocardial infarction in men versus women: The Framingham Study. *JAMA* 1988;260:3456–3460.
55. Singer DE, Moulton AW, Nathan DM: Diabetic myocardial infarction: Interaction of diabetes with other preinfarction risk factors. *Diabetes* 1989;38: 350–357.
56. Margolis JR, Kannel WB, Feinlib M, et al: Clinical features of unrecognized myocardial infarction: Silent and asymptomatic. *Am J Cardiol* 1973;32:1–7.
57. Wilcox RG, von der Lippe G, Olsson CG, et al: Trial of tissue plasminogen activator for mortality reduction in acute myocardial infarction. Anglo-Scandinavian Study of Early Thrombolysis (ASSET). *Lancet* 1988;2:525–530.
58. Stone PH, Muller JE, Hartwell T, et al: The effect of diabetes mellitus on prognosis and serial left ventricular function after acute myocardial infarction: Contribution of both coronary disease and diastolic left ventricular dysfunction to the adverse prognosis. *J Am Coll Cardiol* 1989;14: 49–57.
59. Savage MP, Krowlewski AS, Kenien GG, et al: Acute myocardial infarction in diabetes and significance of congestive heart failure as a prognostic factor. *Am J Cardiol* 1988;62:665–669.
60. Smith JW, Marcus FI, Serokman R, and the Multicenter Postinfarction Research Group: Prognosis of patients with diabetes mellitus after acute myocardial infarction. *Am J Cardiol* 1984;54:718–721.
61. Jacoby RM, Nesto RW: Acute myocardial infarction in the diabetic patient: Pathophysiology, clinical course and prognosis. *J Am Coll Cardiol* 1992; 20:736–744.

62. Vaccarino V, Krumholz HM, Berkman LF, et al: Sex differences in mortality after myocardial infarction: Is there evidence for an increased risk for women? *Circulation* 1995;91:1861–1871.
63. Stone GW, Grines CL, Browne KF, et al: Comparison of in-hospital outcome in men-versus-women treated by either thrombolytic therapy or primary coronary angioplasty for acute myocardial infarction. *Am J Cardiol* 1995;75:987–993.
64. Grines CL, Browne KF, Marco J, et al, for the Primary Angioplasty in Myocardial Infarction Study Group: A comparison of immediate angioplasty with thrombolytic therapy for acute myocardial infarction. *N Engl J Med* 1993;328:673–679.
65. Pardaens J, Lesaffre E, Willems JL, et al: Multivariate survival analysis for the assessment of prognostic factors and risk categories after recovery from acute myocardial infarction: The Belgian Situation. *Am J Epidemiol* 1985;122:805–819.
66. Maggioni AP, Franzosi MG, Santoro E, et al: The risk of stroke in patients with acute myocardial in farction after thrombolytic and antithrombotic treatment. *N Engl J Med* 1992;327:1–6.
66a. Goldbourt U, Greenland P: Sex differences in men and women after myocardial infarction. *Circulation* 1996;93:1260.
66b. Douglas PS, Ginsburg GS: Evaluation of chest pain in women. *New Engl J Med,* 1996, 334:1311–1315.
66c. Fetters JK, Peterson ED, Shaw LJ, Newby LK, Califf RM: Sex-specific differences in coronary artery disease risk factors, evaluation, and treatment: Have they been adequately evaluated? *Am Heart J* 1996, 131:796–813.
67. Bullemer F, Graham KJ, Pankow J, et al: Gender-related differences in risk factors of young patients with symptomatic coronary artery disease (abstract). *J Am Coll Cardiol* 1995; February/Special Issue: 267A.
68. Centers for Disease Control: Cigarette smoking in the United States, 1986. *Morb Mort Wkly Rep* 1987; 36:581–585.
69. Willett WC, Green A, Stampfer MJ, et al: Relative and absolute excess risks of coronary heart disease among women who smoke cigarettes. *N Engl J Med* 1987;317:1303–1309.
70. Doyle JT, Dawber TR, Kannel WB, et al: The relationship of cigarette smoking to coronary heart disease: The Second Report of the Combined Experience of the Albany, NY and Framingham, Mass. Studies. *JAMA* 1964;190:886–890.
71. Fiore M, Novotny T, Lynn W, et al: Smoking cessation data from the 1986 adult use of tobacco survey, in Aoki M, Hisamichi S, Tominaga S (eds): *Smoking and Health,* Tokyo, November 9–12, 1987. Amsterdam, Excerpta Medica, 1988, pp 189–194.
71a. Njolstad I, Arnesen E, Lung-Larsen PG: Smoking, serum lipids, blood pressure, and sex differences in myocardial infarction. A 12-year follow-up of the Finnmark Study. *Circulation* 1996;93:450–456.
72. Robinson JG, Leon AS: The prevention of cardiovascular disease. Emphasis on secondary prevention. *Med Clin North Am* 1994;78:69–98.
73. Palmer JR, Rosenberg L, Shapiro SS: "Low yield" cigarettes and the risk of nonfatal myocardial infarction in women. *N Engl J Med* 1989;320: 1569–1573.
74. Rosenberg L, Palmer JR, Shapiro, SS: Decline in the risk of myocardial infarction among women who stop smoking. *N Engl J Med* 1990;322:213–217.
75. Mulcahy R: Influence of cigarette smoking on morbidity and mortality after myocardial infarction. *Br Heart J* 1983;49:410–415.
76. Aberg A, Bergstrand R, Johansson S, et al: Cessation of smoking after myocardial infarction. Effects on mortality after ten years. *Br Heart J* 1983;49: 416–422.
77. Shapiro S, Sloane D, Rosenberg L, et al: Oral contraceptive use in relation to myocardial infarction. *Lancet* 1979;1:743–746.
78. Bush TL, Fried LP, Barrett-Connor E: Cholesterol, lipoproteins, and coronary heart disease in women. *Clin Chem* 1988;34(8B):B60–B70.
79. Taylor KG, Carter TJ, Valente AJ, et al: Sex differences in the relationships between obesity, alcohol consumption and cigarette smoking and serum lipid and apolipoprotein concentrations in a normal population. *Atherosclerosis* 1981;38:11–18.
80. Criqui MH, Wallace RB, Hess G, et al: Cigarette smoking and plasma high-density lipoprotein cholesterol. The Lipids Research Clinics Program Prevalence Study. *Circulation* 1980;62(Suppl IV): IV-70–IV-76.
81. Freedman DS, Srinivasan SR, Shear CL, et al: Cigarette smoking initiation and longitudinal changes in serum lipids and lipoproteins in early adulthood: The Bogalusa Heart Study. *Am J Epidemiol* 1977, 105:75–86.
82. Frost PH, Verter J, Miller D: Serum lipids and lipoproteins after myocardial infarction: Associations with cardiovascular mortality and experience

in the aspirin myocardial infarction study. *Am Heart J* 1987;113:1356–1364.

83. Bainton D, Burns-Cox CJ, Elwood PC, et al: Prevalence of ischemic heart disease and associations with serum lipoproteins in subjects aged 45 to 64 years. The Speedwell Study. *Br Heart J* 1982;47: 483–489.

84. Reardon MF, Nestel PJ, Craig IH, et al: Lipoprotein predictors of the severity of coronary artery disease in men and women. *Circulation* 1985;71: 881–888.

85. Gordon T, Castelli WP, Hjortland MC, et al: High density lipoprotein as a protective factor against coronary heart disease. *Am J Med* 1977;62:707–714.

86. The Pooling Project Research Group: Relationship of blood pressure, serum cholesterol, smoking habit, relative weight and ECG abnormalities to incidence of major coronary events: Final report of the Pooling Project. *Am Heart Assoc Monogr* 1978;60.

87. Keys A: Coronary heart disease in seven countries (abstract). *Circulation* 1970;41(Suppl I):I-211.

88. Shekelle RB, Shyrock AM, Paul O, et al: Diet, serum cholesterol and death from coronary heart disease. The Western Electric Study. *N Engl J Med* 1981;304:65–70.

89. Brunner D, Weisbort J, Meshulam N, et al: Relation of serum total cholesterol and high density lipoprotein cholesterol percentage to the incidence of definite coronary events: Twenty-year follow-up of the Donolo–Tel Aviv Prospective Coronary Artery Disease Study. *Am J Cardiol* 1987;59:1271–1276.

90. Bush TL, Barrett-Connor E, Criqui MH, et al: Cardiovascular mortality and non contraceptive use of estrogen in women: Results from the Lipid Research Clinics' Follow-up Study. *Circulation* 1987; 75:1102–1109.

91. Gordon DJ, Probstfield JL, Garrison RJ, et al: High-density lipoprotein cholesterol and cardiovascular disease: Four prospective studies. *Circulation* 1989;79:8–15.

92. AIMS Trial Study Group: Effect of intravenous APSAC on mortality after acute myocardial infarction: Preliminary report of a placebo-controlled clinical trial. *Lancet* 1985;1:545–549.

93. Collen D, Topol E, Teifanbrunn AJ, et al: Coronary thrombolysis with recombinant human tissue type plasminogen activator: A prospective, randomized, placebo controlled trial. *Circulation* 1984; 70:1012–1017.

94. Rifici VA, Khachadurian AK: The inhibition of low-density lipoprotein oxidation by 17-β estradiol. *Metabolism* 1992;41:1100–1104.

95. Castelli WP: The triglyceride issue: A view from Framingham. *Am Heart J* 1986;112:432–437.

96. Lapidus L, Bengtsson C, Lindquist O, et al: Triglycerides: Main risk for cardiovascular disease in women. *Acta Med Scand* 1985;217:481–489.

97. Castelli WP, Anderson K: A population as risk: Prevalence of high cholesterol levels in hypertensive patients in the Framingham Study. *Am J Med* 1986;80(2A):23–32.

98. Hypertension Detection and Follow-up Program Cooperative Group: Five-year findings of the hypertension detection and follow-up program. II. Mortality by race, sex and age. *JAMA* 1979;242: 2572–2577.

99. Kannel WB: Lipids, diabetes, and coronary heart disease: Insights from the Framingham Study. *Am Heart J* 1985;110:1100–1107.

100. Higgins M: Women and coronary heart disease: Then and now, in *Women's Health Issues,* pp 5–11. Presented at the 159th meeting of the National Heart, Lung and Blood Advisory Council, Sept. 6, 1990. U.S. Department of Health & Human Services, NIH, 1991.

101. Boston AG, Gagnon DR, Cupples A, et al: A prospective investigation of elevated lipoprotein (a) detected by electrophoresis and cardiovascular disease in women: The Framingham Heart Study. *Circulation* 1994;90:1688–1695.

102. Sunayama S, Mokuno H, Miyano H, et al: Lp(a) is a predictor of coronary artery disease in premenopausal but not in postmenopausal women (abstract). *J Am Coll Cardiol* 1995; February/Special Issue:25A.

103. Scandinavian Simvastatin Survival Study Group (4S): Randomized trial of cholesterol lowering in 4444 patients with coronary heart disease: The Scandinavian Simvastatin Survival Study. *Lancet* 1994;344:1383–1389.

104. Trial of clofibrate in the treatment of ischemic heart disease. Five-year study by a group of Physicians of the Newcastle upon Tyne region. *Br Med J* 1971;4:767–775.

105. Miettinen M, Turpeinen O, Karvonen MJ, et al: Effect of cholesterol-lowering diet on mortality from coronary heart disease and other causes. A 12-year clinical trial in men and women. *Lancet* 1972;2:835–883.

106. Ischaemic heart disease: A secondary prevention trial using clofibrate. Report by a Research Committee of the Scottish Society of Physicians. *Br Med J* 1971;4:775–784.

107. Expert panel in detection, evaluation, and treatment of high blood cholesterol in adults: Summary of the second report of National Cholesterol Education Program (NCEP) expert panel on detection, evaluation and treatment of high blood cholesterol in adults. *JAMA* 1993;269:3015–3023.

108. Perlman JA, Wolf PH, Ray R, Lieberknecht G: Cardiovascular risk factors, premature heart disease, and all cause mortality in a cohort of Northern California women. *Am J Obstet Gynecol* 1988; 158:1568–1574.

109. Manson JE, Tosteson H, Ridker PM, et al: The primary prevention of myocardial infarction. *N Engl J Med* 1992;326:1406–1416.

110. Kannel WB, Sorlie P, Castelli WP, et al: Blood pressure and survival after myocardial infarction: The Framingham Study. *Am J Cardiol* 1980;45: 326–330.

111. Langford HG, Stamler J, Wasserthiel-Smoller S, et al. All cause mortality in the Hypertension, Detection and Follow-up Program: Findings for the whole cohort and for persons with less severe hypertension with and without other traits related to the risk of mortality. *Prog Cardiovasc Dis* 1986;29 (Suppl 1):29–54.

112. Diabetes Control and Complications Trial Research Group: The effect of intensive treatment of diabetes on the development and progression of long-term complications in insulin-dependent diabetes mellitus. *N Engl J Med* 1993;329:977.

113. Manson JE, Colditz GA, Stampfer MJ, et al: A prospective study of obesity and risk of coronary heart disease in women. *N Engl J Med* 1990;322: 882–889.

114. Lew EA, Garfinkel L: Variations in mortality by weight among 750,000 men and women *J Chronic Dis* 1979;32:563–576.

115. Hubert HB, Feinleib M, McNamara PM, et al: Obesity as an independent risk factor for cardiovascular disease: A 26-year follow-up of participants in the Framingham Heart Study. *Circulation* 1983;67:968–977.

116. Kissebah AH, Vydelingum N, Murray R, et al: Relations of body fat distribution to metabolic complications of obesity. *J Clin Endocrinol Metab* 1982;54:254–260.

117. Krotkiewski M, Björntorp P, Sjöström L, et al: Impact of obesity on metabolism in men and women: Importance of regional adipose tissue distribution. *J Clin Invest* 1983;72:1150–1162.

118. Björntorp P: Regional patterns of fat distribution. *Ann Intern Med* 1985;103:994–995.

119. Folsom AR, Kaye SA, Sellers TA, et al: Body fat distribution and 5-year risk of sudden death in older women. *JAMA* 1993;269:483–487.

120. Stampfer MJ, Colditz GA, Willett WC, et al: A prospective study of moderate alcohol consumption and the risk of coronary disease and stroke in women. *N Engl J Med* 1988;319:267–273.

121. Garg R, Wagener DK, Madans JH: Alcohol consumption and the risk of ischemic heart disease in women. *Arch Intern Med* 1993;153:1211–1216.

122. Gordon T, Kannel WB. Drinking habits and cardiovascular disease: The Framingham Study. *Am Heart J* 1983;4:669–673.

123. Fuchs SC, Stampfer MJ, Colditz GA: Alcohol consumption and mortality among women. *N Engl J Med* 1995;332:1245–1250.

124. Silverberg E, Lubera J. Cancer statistics, 1987. *CA, Cancer J Clin* 1987;37:2–19.

125. Taylor KG, Carter TJ, Valente AJ, et al: Sex differences in the relationships between obesity, alcohol consumption and cigarette smoking and serum lipid and apolipoprotein concentrations in a normal population. *Atherosclerosis* 1981;38:11–18.

126. Haffner SM, Stern MP, Hazuda HP, et al: The role of behavioral variables and fat patterning in explaining ethnic differences in serum lipids and lipoproteins. *Am J Epidemiol* 1986;123:830–839.

127. Castelli WP, Gordon T, Hjortland MC, et al: Alcohol and blood lipids. The Cooperative Lipoprotein Phenotyping Study. *Lancet* 1977;2:153–155.

128. Steering Committee of the Physicians' Health Study Research Group: Final report on the aspirin component of the ongoing Physicians' Health Study. *N Engl J Med* 1989;321:129–135.

129. Manson JE, Stampfer MJ, Colditz GA, et al: A prospective study of aspirin use and primary prevention of cardiovascular disease in women. *JAMA* 1991;226:521–527.

130. Boston Collaborative Drug Surveillance Group: Regular aspirin intake and acute myocardial infarction. *Br Med J* 1974;1:440–443.

131. Paganini-Hill A, Chao A, Ross RK, et al: Aspirin use and chronic diseases: A cohort study of the elderly. *Br Med J* 1989;299:1247–1250.

132. Hammond EC, Garfinkel L: Aspirin and coronary heart disease: Findings of a prospective study. *Br Med J* 1975;2:269–271.
133. Aspirin Myocardial Infarction Study Research Group: A randomized, controlled trial of aspirin in persons recovered from myocardial infarction. *JAMA* 1980;243:661–669.
134. The Aspirin Myocardial Infarction Study Research Group: The Aspirin Myocardial Infarction Study: Final result. *Circulation* 1980;62(Suppl V): V-79–V-84.
135. Elwood PC, Sweetnam PM: Aspirin and secondary mortality after myocardial infarction. *Lancet* 1979;2:1313–1315.
136. Breddin K, Loew D, Lechner K, et al: Secondary prevention of acute myocardial infarction. Comparison of acetylsalicylic acid, phenprocoumon and placebo. A multicenter two-year prospective study. *Thromb Haemost* 1979;41:225–236.
137. Persantine–Aspirin Reinfarction Study Research Group: Persantine and aspirin in coronary heart disease. *Circulation* 1980;62:449–461.
138. Antiplatelet Trialists' Collaboration: Secondary prevention of vascular disease by prolonged antiplatelet treatment. *Br Med J* 1988;296: 320–331.
139. Gruchow HW, Anderson AJ, Barboriak JJ: Postmenopausal use of estrogen and occlusion of coronary arteries. *Am Heart J* 1988;115:954–963.
140. Walsh BW, Schiff I, Rosner B, et al: Effects of postmenopausal estrogen replacement on the concentrations and metabolism of plasma lipoproteins. *N Engl J Med* 1991;325:1196–1204.
141. Colvin PL, Auerbach BJ, Case LD, et al: A dose–response relationship between sex hormone–induced change in hepatic triglyceride lipase and high-density lipoprotein cholesterol in postmenopausal women. *Metabolism* 1991;40: 1052–1056.
142. Vaziri SM, Evans JC, Larson MG, et al: The impact of female hormone usage on the lipid profile: The Framingham Offspring Study. *Arch Intern Med* 1993;153:2200–2206.
143. Barrett-Connor E, Laakso M: Ischemic heart disease risk in postmenopausal women: Effects of estrogen use on glucose and insulin levels. *Arteriosclerosis* 1990;10:531–534.
144. Busby MJ, Bellantoni MF, Tobin JD, et al: Glucose tolerance in women: The effects of age, body composition, and sex hormones. *J Am Geriatr Soc* 1992;40:497–502.
145. Nabulsi A, Folsom A, White A, et al, for the Atherosclerosis Risk in Communities Study Investigators: Increased association of hormone-replacement therapy with various cardiovascular risk factors in postmenopausal women. *N Engl J Med* 1993;328:1069–1075.
146. Haarbo J, Hassager C, Jensen SB, et al: Serum lipids, lipoproteins, and apolipoproteins during postmenopausal estrogen replacement therapy combined with either 19-nortestosterone derivatives or 17-hydroxyprogesterone derivatives. *Am J Med* 1991;90:584–589.
147. Kable WT, Gallagher JC, Nachtigall L: Lipid changes after hormone replacement therapy for menopause. *J Reprod Med* 1990;35:512–518.
148. Cano A, Fernandes H, Serrano S, et al: Effect of continuous oestradiol-medroxyprogesterone administration on plasma lipids and lipoproteins. *Maturitas* 1991;13:35–42.
149. Yancey MK, Hannan CJ Jr, Plymate SR, et al: Serum lipids and lipoproteins in continuous or cyclic medroxyprogesterone acetate treatment in postmenopausal women treated with conjugated estrogens. *Fertil Steril* 1990;54:778–782.
150. Ottosson UB, Johansson BG, von Schoultz B: Subfractions of high-density lipoprotein cholesterol during estrogen replacement therapy: A comparison between progestogens and natural progesterone. *Am J Obstet Gynecol* 1985;151:746–750.
151. Christiansen C, Christensen MS, Grande P, et al: Low-risk lipoprotein pattern in postmenopausal women on sequential oestrogen/progestogen treatment. *Maturitas* 1984;5:193–199.
152. Wahl P, Walden C, Knopp R, et al: Effect of estrogen/progestin potency on lipid/lipoprotein cholesterol. *N Engl J Med* 1983;308:862–867.
153. Tikkanen MJ, Nikkila EA, Kuusi T, et al: High density lipoprotein-2 and hepatic lipase: Reciprocal changes produced by estrogen and norgestrel. *J Clin Endocrinol Metab* 1982;54:1113–1117.
154. Silfverstolpe G, Gustafson A, Samsioe G, et al: Lipid metabolic studies in oophorectomised women: Effects on serum lipids and lipoproteins of three synthetic progestogens. *Maturitas* 1982;4: 103–111.
155. Grady D, Rubin SM, Petitti DB, et al: Hormone therapy to prevent disease and prolong life in

postmenopausal women. *Ann Intern Med* 1992;117: 1016–1037.

156. The Writing Group for the PEPI Trial: Effects of estrogen–progestin regimens on heart disease risk factors in postmenopausal women: The Postmenopausal Estrogen–Progestin Intervention (PEPI) Trial. *JAMA* 1995;273:199–208.

157. Cauley JA, La Porte RE, Kuller KH, et al: Menopausal estrogen use, high density lipoprotein cholesterol subfractions and liver function. *Atherosclerosis* 1983;49:31–39.

158. Kim CJ, Jang HC, Min YK: Hormone replacement therapy lowers the plasma concentration of lipoprotein (a) in postmenopausal women (abstract). *Circulation* 1992;86(Suppl I):I-866.

159. Mendelsohn ME, Karas RH: Estrogen and the blood vessel wall. *Curr Opin Cardiol* 1994;9: 619–626.

160. Ylikorkala O, Kuusi T, Tikkanen MJ, et al: Desogestrel- and levonorgestel-containing oral contraceptives have different effects on urinary excretion of prostacyclin metabolites and serum high density lipoproteins. *J Clin Endocrin Metab* 1987;65: 1238–1242.

160a. Gerhard M, Ganz P: How do we explain the clinical benefits of estrogen? *Circulation* 1995;92:5–8.

161. Gebara OCE, Walsh B, Mittleman MA, et al: Fibrinolytic potential is increased by estrogen therapy in postmenopausal women (abstract). *J Am Coll Cardiol* 1995; February/Special Issue:328A.

162. Gebara OCE, Mittleman MA, Sutherland P, et al: Association between increased estrogen status and increased fibrinolytic potential in the Framingham Offspring Study. *Circulation* 1995;91: 1952–1958.

163. Kruithof EKO: Plasminogen activator inhibitor type 1: Biochemical, biological and clinical aspects. *Fibrinolysis* 1988;2:59–70.

164. Juhan-Vague I, Alessi MC, Joly P, et al: Plasma plasminogen activator inhibitor-1 in angina pectoris: Influence of plasma insulin and acute phase response. *Arteriosclerosis* 1989;9:362–367.

165. Hamsten A, Wiman B, deFaire U, et al: Increased plasma levels of a rapid inhibitor of tissue plasminogen activator in young survivors of myocardial infarction. *N Engl J Med* 1985;313: 1557–1563.

166. Keber I, Keber D: Increased plasminogen activator inhibitor activity in survivors of myocardial infarction is associated with metabolic risk factors of atherosclerosis. *Haemostasis* 1992;22:187–194.

167. Hamsten A, Walldius G, Szamosi A, et al: Plasminogen activator inhibitor in plasma: Risk factor for recurrent myocardial infarction. *Lancet* 1987;2: 3–9.

168. Gram J, Jespersen J: A selective depression of tissue plasminogen activator (t-PA) activity in euglobulins characterizes a risk group among survivors of acute myocardial infarction. *Thromb Haemost* 1987;57:137–139.

169. Ridker PM, Vaughan DE, Stampfer MJ, et al: Endogenous tissue-type plasminogen activator and risk of myocardial infarction. *Lancet* 1993;341: 1165–1168.

170. Jansson JH, Olofsson BO, Nilsson TK: Predictive value of tissue plasminogen activator mass concentration on long-term mortality in patients with coronary artery disease: A 7-year follow-up. *Circulation* 1993;88:2030–2034.

170a. Samaan SA, Crawford MH: Estrogen and cardiovascular function after menopause. *J Am Coll Cardiol* 1995;26:1403–1410.

171. Lobo RA: Estrogen replacement therapy and hypertension. *Postgrad Med* 1987;14:48–54.

172. Barret-Connor E, Wingard DL, Criqui MH: Postmenopausal estrogen use and heart disease risk factors in the 1980s: Rancho Bernardo, Calif., revisited. *JAMA* 1989;261:2095–2100.

173. Pettiti DB, Perlman JA, Sidney S: Noncontraceptive estrogens and mortality: Long-term follow-up of women in the Walnut Creek Study. *Obstet Gynecol* 1987;70:289–293.

174. Wren BG, Routledge PA: Blood pressure changes: Oestrogens in climateric women. *Med J Austr* 1981;2:528–531.

175. Hale SL, Kloner RA: Estradiol administered acutely, protects ischemic myocardium in both female and male rabbits (abstract). *J Am Coll Cardiol* 1995;February Special Issue:189A.

176. Stampfer MJ, Colditz GA: Estrogen replacement therapy and coronary heart disease: A quantitative assessment of the epidemiologic evidence. *Prev Med* 1991;20:47–63.

177. Stampfer MJ, Colditz GA, Willett WC, et al: Postmenopausal estrogen therapy and cardiovascular disease. Ten-year follow-up from the Nurse's Health Study. *N Engl J Med* 1991;325: 756–762.

178. Lufken EG, Carpenter PC, Ory SJ, et al: Estrogen replacement therapy: Current recommendations. *Mayo Clin Proc* 1988;63:453–460.

179. Early Breast Cancer Trialists' Collaborative Group: Systemic treatment of early breast cancer by hormonal, cytotoxic or immune therapy: 133 randomised trials involving 31,000 recurrences and 24,000 deaths among 75,000 women. *Lancet* 1992;339;1–15,71–85.

180. McDonald CC, Stewart HJ: Fatal myocardial infarction in the Scottish adjuvant tamoxifen trial. *Br Med J* 1991;303:435–437.

181. Sullivan JM, Zwaag RV, Lemp GF, et al: Postmenopausal estrogen use and coronary atherosclerosis. *Ann Intern Med* 1988;108:358–363.

182. McFarland KF, Boniface ME, Hornung CA, et al: Risk factors and noncontraceptive estrogen use in women with and without coronary disease. *Am Heart J* 1989;117:1209–1214.

183. Clarkson TB, Shivley CA, Morgan TM, et al: Oral contraceptives and coronary artery atherosclerosis of cynomoglus monkeys. *Obstet Gynecol* 1990;75:217–222.

184. Adams MR, Kaplan JR, Manuch SB, et al: Inhibition of coronary artery atherosclerosis by 17-beta estradiol in ovariectomized monkeys. Lack of an effect of added progesterone. *Arteriosclerosis* 1990;10:151–157.

185. Paganini-Hill A, Ross RK, Henderson BE: Postmenopausal oestrogen treatment and stroke: A prospective study. *Br Med J* 1988;297:519–522.

186. Henderson BE, Paganini-Hill A, Ross RK: Decreased mortality in users of estrogen replacement therapy. *Arch Intern Med* 1991;151:75–78.

187. Falkeborn M, Persson I, Adami HO, et al: The risk of acute myocardial infarction after oestrogen and oestrogen-progestogen replacement. *Br J Obst Gyn* 1992;99:821–828.

188. Thompson SG, Meade TW, Greenberg G: The use of hormonal replacement therapy and the risk of stroke and myocardial infarction in women. *J Epidemiol Community Health* 1989;43:173–178.

189. Nachtigall LE, Nachtigall RH, Nachtigall RD, et al: Estrogen replacement therapy II; a prospective study in the relationship to carcinoma and cardiovascular and metabolic problems. *Obstet Gynecol* 1979;54:74–79.

189a. Pilote L, Hlatky MA: Attitudes of women toward hormone therapy and prevention of heart disease. *Am Heart J* 1995;129:1237–1238.

190. Mack TM, Ake MC, Henderson BE, et al: Estrogens and endometrial cancer in a retirement community. *N Engl J Med* 1976;294:1262–1267.

191. Henderson BE, Ross RK, Lobo RA, et al: Re-evaluating the role of progestogen therapy after the menopause. *Fertil Steril* 1988;49(Suppl):9S–15S.

192. Bergkvist L, Adami HO, Persson I, et al: The risk of breast cancer after estrogen and estrogen-progestin replacement. *N Engl J Med* 1989;321:293–297.

193. Devor M, Barrett-Connor E, Renvall M et al: Estrogen replacement therapy and the risk of venous thrombosis. *Am J Med* 1992;92:275–282.

193a. Grey AB, Stapleton JP, Evans MC, et al: The effect of the anti-estrogen tamoxifen on cardiovascular risk factors in normal postmenopausal women. *J Clin Endocrinol Metab* 1995;80:3191–3195.

193b. Guetta V, Lush RM, Figg WD, et al: Effects of the antiestrogen tamoxifen on low-density lipoprotein concentrations and oxidation in postmenopausal women. *Am J Cardiol* 1995;76:1072–1073.

193c. McDonald CC, Alexander FE, Whyte BW, et al: Cardiac and vascular morbidity in women receiving adjuvant tamoxifen for breast cancer in a randomised trial. *British Med J* 1995;311:977–980.

194. Sullivan JM, Vander Zwaag R, Hughes JP, et al: Estrogen replacement and coronary artery disease. Effect of survival in postmenopausal women. *Arch Intern Med* 1990;150:2557–2562.

195. Stampfer MJ, Hennekens CH, Manson JE, et al: Vitamin E consumption and the risk of coronary disease in women. *N Engl J Med* 1993;328:1444–1449.

196. Eastman P. Coping with heart disease in African-American women. *Cardiology World News* 1995;Dec 15–Jan 15:6–7.

197. Keil JE, Sutherland SE, Knapp RG, et al: Mortality rates and risk factors for coronary disease in black as compared with white men and women. *N Engl J Med* 1993;329:73–78.

198. Blair SN, Kohl HW, Paffenbarger RS, et al: Physical fitness and all-cause mortality: A prospective study of healthy men and women. *JAMA* 1989;262:2395–2401.

199. Manson JE, Stampfer MJ, Willet WC, et al: Physical activity and incidence of coronary heart disease and stroke in women. *Circulation* 1995;91:927.

200. O'Connor GT, Buring JE, Yusuf S, et al: An overview of randomized trials of rehabilitation with exercise after myocardial infarction. *Circulation* 1989;80:234–244.

201. Lau J, Antman EM, Jiminez-Silva, et al: Cumulative meta-analysis of therapeutic trials for myocardial infarction. *N Engl J Med* 1992;327: 248–254.
202. Oldridge NB, Guyatt GH, Fischer ME, et al: Cardiac rehabilitation after myocardial infarction: Combined experience of randomized clinical trials. *JAMA* 1988;26:945–950.
203. Hamilton GA: Recovery from acute myocardial infarction in women. *Cardiology* 1990;77(Suppl 2): 58–70.
204. O'Callaghan WG, Teo KK, O'Riordan J, et al: Comparative response of male and female patients with coronary artery disease to exercise rehabilitation. *Eur Heart J* 1984;5:649–651.
205. Murdaugh C: Coronary artery disease in women. *J Cardiovasc Nurs* 1990;4:35–50.
206. Oldridge NB, LASalle D, Jones NL: Exercise rehabilitation of female patients with coronary heart disease. *Am Heart J* 1980;100:755–757.
207. Ades PA, Waldmann ML, Polk DM, et al: Referral pattern and exercise response in the rehabilitation of female coronary patients aged ≥62 years. *Am J Cardiol* 1992;69:1422–1425.
208. O'Callaghan WG, Teo KK, O'Riordan J, et al: Comparative response of male and female patients with coronary heart disease to exercise rehabilitation. *Eur Heart J* 1984;5:649–651.
209. Boogaard MAK, Briody ME: Comparison of the rehabilitation of men and women post myocardial infarction. *J Cardiopulmon Rehabil* 1985;5: 379–384.
210. Chirikos TN, Nickel JL: Work disability from coronary heart disease in women. *Women Health* 1984;9:55–74.
211. Cannistra LB, Balady GJ, O'Malley CJ, et al: Comparison of the clinical profile and outcome of women and men in cardiac rehabilitation. *Am J Cardiol* 1992;69:1274–1279.
212. Lavie CJ, Milani RV: Effects of cardiac rehabilitation and exercise training on exercise capacity, coronary risk factors, behavioral characteristics and quality of life in women. *Am J Cardiol* 1995; 75:340–343.
213. Becker RC: Coronary thrombolysis in women. *Cardiovasc Dis Women* 1990;77(Suppl 2):110–123.
214. Koh SC, Yuen R, Viegas OA, et al: Plasminogen activators t-PA, u-PA and its inhibitor (PAI) in normal males and females (abstract). *Thromb Haemost* 1991;66:581–585.
215. Ridolfo B, Jamrozik KD, Hobbs MST, et al: Gender bias in management of myocardial infarction: Prevalence and relevance to outcome (abstract). *J Am Coll Cardiol* 1993;21:238A.
216. Goldberg RJ, Gorak EJ, Yarzebski J, et al: A community wide perspective of sex differences and temporal trends in the incidence and survival rates after acute myocardial infarction and out of hospital deaths caused by coronary heart disease. *Circulation* 1993;87:1947–1953.
217. Caro JJ, O'Brien JA, Holden-Wiltse J, et al: Why do women receive thrombolysis less often for acute myocardial infarction? (abstract). *Circulation* 1993;88(Suppl I):I-508.
218. Pfeffer MA, Myoe LA, Braunwald E, et al: Selection bias in the use of thrombolytic therapy in acute myocardial infarction. The SAVE Investigators. *JAMA* 1991;266:528–532.
219. Varma VK, Murphy PL, Hood WP, et al: Are women with acute myocardial infarction managed differently from men? (abstract). *J Am Coll Cardiol* 1992;19:20A.
220. Maynard C, Althouse R, Cerqueira M, et al: Underutilization of thrombolytic therapy in eligible women with acute myocardial infarction. *Am J Cardiol* 1991;68:529–530.
221. Chesebro JH, Knatterud G, Roberts R, et al: Thrombolysis in Myocardial Infarction (TIMI) Trial, Phase I: A comparison between intravenous tissue plasminogen activator and intravenous streptokinase. *Circulation* 1987;76:142–154.
222. Weaver WD, Wilcox RG, Morris D, et al: Women in GUSTO: Baseline characteristics and effects of treatment regimen on mortality and complication rates (abstract). *Circulation* 1993;88(Suppl I): I-508.
223. Kasper W, Erbel R, Meinertz T, et al: Intracoronary thrombolysis with an acylated streptokinase–plasminogen activator (BRL 26921) in patients with acute myocardial infarction. *J Am Coll Cardiol* 1984;4:357–363.
224. Merx W, Dorr R, Rentrop P, et al: Evaluation of effectiveness of intracoronary streptokinase infusion in acute myocardial infarction: Post-procedure management and hospital course in 204 patients. *Am Heart J* 1981;102:1181–1817.
225. Been M, Debono DP, Muir AL: Coronary thrombolysis with intravenous anisoylated plasminogen–streptokinase complex BRL26921. *Br Heart J* 1985;53:253–259.

226. Kennedy JW, Martin GV, Davis KB, et al: The Western Washington intravenous streptokinase in acute myocardial infarction. *Circulation* 1988;77: 345–352.

227. DeJaegere PP, Arnold AA, Balk AH, et al: Intracranial hemorrhage in association with thrombolytic therapy: Incidence and clinical predictive factors. *J Am Coll Cardiol* 1992;19:289–294.

228. Califf RM, Topol EJ, George BS, et al: Hemorrhagic complications associated with the use of intravenous tissue plasminogen activator in treatment of acute myocardial infarction. *Am J Med* 1988;895:353–359.

229. Bovill EG, Terin ML, Stump DC, et al: Hemorrhagic events during therapy with recombinant tissue-type plasminogen activator, heparin, and aspirin for acute myocardial infarction. *Ann Intern Med* 1991;115:256–265.

230. Kannel WB, Abbott RD: Incidence and prognosis of myocardial infarction in women: The Framingham study, in Eaker ED, Packard B, Wenger NK, et al (eds): *Coronary Heart Disease in Women:* Proc NIH Workshop, New York, Haymarket Doymma, 1987, pp 208–214.

231. Hendel RC: Myocardial infarction in women. Cardiovascular disease in women. *Cardiology* 1990; 77:41–57.

232. Murdaugh CK, O'Rourke RA: Coronary heart disease in women: Special considerations. *Curr Prob Cardiol* 1988;13:73–156.

233. Kindwall KE: Therapy for coronary heart disease in women, in Douglas PS (ed): *Heart Disease in Women. Cardiovascular Clinics.* Philadelphia, Davis, 1989, pp 195–202.

234. Litwin SE, Katz SE, Forman DE, et al: Gender differences in post-infarction left ventricular remodeling and function (abstract). *J Am Coll Cardiol* 1994;February 1995;130A.

235. Kostis JB, Wilson AC, O'Dowd K, et al: Sex differences in the management and long-term outcome of acute myocardial infarction: A statewide study. *Circulation* 1994;90:1715–1730.

236. Ayanian JZ, Epstein AM: Differences in the use of procedures between women and men hospitalized for coronary heart disease. *N Engl J Med* 1991;325: 221–225.

237. Krumholz HM, Douglas PS, Lauer MS, et al: Selection of patients for coronary angiography and coronary revascularization early after myocardial infarction: Is there evidence for a gender bias? *Ann Intern Med* 1992;116:785–790.

238. Behar S, Gottlieb S, Hod H, et al, for the Israeli Thrombolytic Survey Group: Influence of gender in the therapeutic management of patients with acute myocardial infarction in Israel. *Am J Cardiol* 1994;73:438–443.

239. Healy B: The Yentl syndrome (editorial). *N Engl J Med* 1991;325:274–276.

240. Welty FK, Mittleman MA, Healy RW, et al: Similar results of percutaneous transluminal coronary angioplasty for women and men with post myocardial infarction ischemia. *J Am Coll Cardiol* 1994; 23:35–39.

241. Khan JK, Rutherford BD, McConahay DR, et al: Why is the mortal risk of balloon coronary angioplasty increased in women? (abstract). *J Am Coll Cardiol* 1991;17:266A.

242. Tyras DH, Barner HB, Kaiser GC, et al: Myocardial revascularization in women. *Ann Thorac Surg* 1978;25:449–453.

243. Douglas JS, King SB, Jones EL, et al: Reduced efficacy of coronary artery bypass in women. *Circulation* 1981;64(Suppl II):II-11–II-16.

244. Bolooki H, Vargas A, Green R, et al: Results of direct coronary artery surgery in women. *J Thorac Cardiovasc Surg* 1975;69:271–277.

245. Loop FS, Golding LR, MacMillan JP, et al: Coronary artery surgery in women compared with men: Analysis of risks and long-term results. *J Am Coll Cardiol* 1983;4:383–390.

246. James TN: Anatomy of the coronary arteries in health and disease. *Circulation* 1965;32:1020–1029.

247. Khan SS, Nessim S, Gray R, et al: Increased mortality of women in coronary artery bypass surgery: Evidence for referral bias. *Ann Intern Med* 1990;112:561–567.

248. Eaker ED, Kronmal R, Kennedy JW, et al: Comparison of the long-term, postsurgical survival of women and men in the Coronary Artery Surgery Study (CASS). *Am Heart J* 1989;117:71–81.

248a. Caracciolo EA, Davis KB, Sopko G, et al: Comparison of surgical and medical group survival in patients with left main coronary artery disease. Long-term CASS experience. *Circulation* 1995;91: 2325–2334.

249. King KB, Clark PC, Hicks GL, et al: Patterns of referral and recovery in women and men under-

going coronary artery bypass grafting. *Am J Cardiol* 1992;69:179–182.

250. Rankin SH: Differences in recovery from cardiac surgery: A profile of male and female patients. *Heart Lung* 1990:19:481–485.

251. ISIS-1 Collaborative Group: Randomised trial of intravenous atenolol among 16,027 cases of suspected acute myocardial infarction. *Lancet* 1986;2:57–67.

252. Rodda BE: The Timolol Myocardial Infarction Study: An evaluation of selected variables. *Circulation* 1983;67(6 Pt 2):I-101–I-106.

253. β-Blocker Heart Trial Research Group: A randomized trial of propranolol in patients with acute myocardial infarction. I. Mortality results. *JAMA* 1982;247:1707–1714.

254. β-Blocker Heart Trial Research Group: A randomized trial of propranolol in patients with acute myocardial infarction. II. Morbidity results. *JAMA* 1983;250:2814–2819.

255. Yusuf S, Pet R, Lewis J, et al: Beta-blockade during and after myocardial infarction: An overview of the randomized trials. *Progr Cardiovasc Dis* 1985;27:335–371.

256. Multicenter Diltiazem Post-infarction Research Group: The effect of diltiazem on mortality and reinfarction after acute myocardial infarction. *N Engl J Med* 1988;319:385–392.

257. Held PH, Yusuf S, Furberg CD: Calcium channel blockers in acute myocardial infarction and unstable angina: An overview. *Br Med J* 1989;299:1187–1192.

258. Pfeffer MA, Braunwald E, Moyè. LA, et al, on behalf of the SAVE Investigators: Effect of captopril on mortality and morbidity in patients with left ventricular dysfunction after myocardial infarction: Results of the Survival and Ventricular Enlargement Trial. *N Engl J Med* 1992;327:669–677.

259. Pfeffer MA, Braunwald E, Moye LA: ACE inhibitors after myocardial infarction: Letter to the editor. *N Engl J Med* 1993;328:968.

260. ISIS Pilot Study Investigators: Randomized factorial trial of high dose intravenous streptokinase, of oral aspirin and of intravenous aspirin in acute myocardial infarction. *Eur Heart J* 1987;8:634–642.

261. Yusuf S, Collins R, MacMahon S, et al: Effect of intravenous nitrates on mortality in acute myocardial infarction: An overview of the randomised trials. *Lancet* 1988;2:1088–1092.

262. Tsuyuki RT, Teo KK, Ikuta RM: Mortality risk and patterns of practice in 2,070 patients with acute myocardial infarction, 1987–1992: Relative importance of age, sex and medical therapy. *Chest* 1994;105:1687–1692.

263. Wilkinson P, Laji K, Ranjadayalan K, et al: Acute myocardial infarction in women: survival analysis in first six months. *Br Med J* 1994;309:566–569.

264. Clarke KW, Gray D, Keating NA, et al: Do women with acute myocardial infarction receive the same treatment as men? *Br Med J* 1994;309:563–566.

265. Hannaford PC, Clifton RK, Ferry S: Agism as explanation for sexism in provision of thrombolysis. *Br Med J* 1994;309:573.

266. Antman EM, Lau, J, Kupelnick B, et al: A comparison of results of meta-analyses of randomized control trials and recommendations of clinical experts: Treatments for myocardial infarction. *JAMA* 1992;268:240–248.

267. McGovern PG, Pankow JS, Shahar E, et al. Recent trends in acute coronary heart disease. Mortality, morbidity, medical care and risk factors. *NEJM* 1996;334:884–890.

PART IV

Management and Evaluation of the Post-Infarct Survivor

27

Invasive Electrophysiologic Testing and Holter Monitoring in Infarct Survivors

Anil K. Bhandari, MBBS, and Shahbudin H. Rahimtoola, MB, FRCP, MACP

Survivors of acute myocardial infarction are at an increased risk of sudden death after discharge from the hospital. The incidence of sudden death ranges from 3% to 8% in the first year and 2% to 4% per year thereafter (1–5). There is a need to reliably identify a high-risk subset who could be treated with antiarrhythmic prophylaxis; this area has been the focus of extensive investigation in the past two decades. Several investigators (6–24) have used predischarge Holter monitoring in these patients to predict the likelihood of subsequent arrhythmic events. More recently, electrophysiologic testing has also been used to identify the high-risk subset (25–37).

This chapter critically evaluates the clinical value of Holter monitoring and electrophysiologic testing in predicting the risk of subsequent arrhythmic events in survivors of acute myocardial infarction. The significance and management of sustained ventricular tachycardia or fibrillation during the in-hospital phase of acute myocardial infarction is discussed in Chapter 14. The value of signal-averaged electrocardiography is covered in Chapter 28.

ROLE OF HOLTER MONITORING

The use of Holter monitoring in risk stratification is based on two important assumptions: (i) spontaneous ventricular arrhythmia indicates the presence of an underlying myocardial electrical instability; (ii) the severity of electrical instability varies directly with the increasing frequency and complexity of the ventricular arrhythmias.

Prevalence of Ventricular Arrhythmias After Myocardial Infarction

In the reported studies (6–12), the prevalence of ventricular arrhythmias has ranged from 50% to 84% during the prehospital discharge phase of acute myocardial infarction (Table 27–1). The varying incidence probably reflects differences in the duration of Holter monitoring, in the time elapsed between the onset of myocardial infarction and the date of Holter application, in the number of patients studied, and in the proportion of patients with complicated myocardial infarctions. The prevalence of arrhythmias increased with longer duration of Holter monitoring. Although earlier studies used 1 to 8 hours, Holter recording has ranged from 24 to 48 hours in more recent studies. There is also an important temporal evolution of the ventricular arrhythmias after acute myocardial infarction. Ventricular arrhythmias are ubiquitous in the first 48 hours after infarction and are proba-

Table 27–1. Prevalence of Ventricular Arrhythmias During Predischarge Holter Monitoring in Survivors of Acute Myocardial Infarction

Study	Number of Patients	Duration of Holter (h)	Ventricular Arrhythmias (%)			
			None	PVC > 10/h	Multiform	Repetitive
Ruberman et al (8)	1,739	1	49	26	32	20
Moss et al (9)	940	6	50	—	13	3
Mukharji et al (10)	533	24	16	15	66	26
Bigger et al (11)	819	24	14	15	64	26
Kostis et al (12)	1640	24	16	13	32	20

PVC = premature ventricular complexes.

bly related to the pathophysiologic processes that characterize acute ischemic injury. The frequency and complexity of the arrhythmias, however, decline over the next 3 to 4 days and then begin to increase, reaching their peaks probably around 6 to 8 weeks after the infarction (16). In most previous studies (6–12), the incidence of ventricular arrhythmias has been studied between 1 and 3 weeks after infarction, because the risk of sudden death is highest in the first several months after discharge from the hospital (1–5).

Table 27–1 summarizes the results of several studies on the prevalence of ventricular arrhythmias during the late in-hospital phase of the myocardial infarction. Approximately 20% to 30% of the patients have no ventricular arrhythmias and another 30% to 40% have infrequent (<10 per hour) premature ventricular complexes (PVCs). Thus ventricular arrhythmias are absent or infrequent in about 50% to 70% of the survivors of acute myocardial infarction. In 15% to 25% of the patients, PVCs occur frequently (≥10 per hour), and 20% to 25% of the patients may have ventricular couplets. Nonsustained ventricular tachycardia (VT) occurs in about 3% to 11% of the patients, depending on the duration and the timing of Holter monitoring after the index infarction (Table 27–2) (6,7,9,17,18,20). The incidence was as low as 1% in a 6-hour recording performed just before hospital discharge in 940 infarct survivors. Kleiger et al (20) performed serial 10-hour Holter monitoring on 238 survivors of acute myocardial infarction at 2 weeks and then at monthly intervals for 6 months. The prevalence of VT was 3.4% at the 2-week recording, rose to a peak of 11.5% at 1 month, and then decreased to an average of 5% to 7% in the months thereafter. A similar time dependence in the frequency and complexity of PVCs was also reported by the Beta-Blocker Heart Attack Trial (BHAT) investigators (16).

The duration of ventricular tachycardia is generally brief, with the vast majority of runs consisting of

Table 27–2. Prevalence of Nonsustained Ventricular Tachycardia During Holter Monitoring in Survivors of Acute Myocardial Infarction

Study	Number of Patients	Duration of Holter (h)	Time After Acute MI	Prevalence of VT (%)
Moss et al (6)	100	6	21 d	4
Vismara et al (7)	64	10	11 d	6
Moss et al (9)	940	6	Predischarge	1
Anderson et al (17)	915	6	4–48 m	7
Bigger et al (18)	819	24	—	11
Kleiger et al (20)	238	10	2 w	3.4
	209	10	4 w	11.5
	207	10	12 w	7

h = hours, d = day, w = week, VT = ventricular tachycardia.

three to five beats. Most patients do not experience more than one to two runs of VT a day, and the majority are asymptomatic. The risk of development of ventricular arrhythmias is related to the size of the myocardial infarction (as measured by the serum enzymes) and to the severity of left ventricular dysfunction.

Prognostic Significance of Ventricular Arrhythmias

In the past two decades, several investigators have examined the relationship between spontaneous ventricular arrhythmias in the first few weeks after infarction and the occurrence of major arrhythmic events (that is, sudden cardiac death, or spontaneous sustained VT in the first years after discharge from the hospital. Table 27–3 summarizes the findings of five large studies involving a total of 5,671 patients who were followed up an average of 29 months. High-risk ventricular arrhythmias were defined as the presence of bigeminal, multiform, repetitive, or R-on-T phenomenon extrasystoles in the studies by Ruberman et al (8) and Moss et al (9); by the presence of frequent PVCs (≥10 per hour) in the study by Mukharji et al (10); and by the presence of frequent (≥10 per hour), repetitive, or multiform PVCs in the study by Kostis et al (12). The incidence of sudden cardiac death ranged from 3% to 6% in patients who had no or low-risk ventricular arrhythmias. In contrast, the presence of high-risk ventricular arrhythmias was associated with a significantly higher incidence of sudden cardiac death, ranging from 8% to 15%. In all of these studies, complex ventricular arrhythmias were an independent predictor of sudden and total cardiac mortality, and their presence was associated with twofold to threefold higher risk of cardiac mortality, depending on the frequency and complexity of the ventricular arrhythmia.

Despite the findings discussed, several problems are associated with the use of asymptomatic ventricular arrhythmias as a risk factor in infarct survivors. First, the sensitivity and specificity for predicting an untoward event are too low to be of clinical utility in a given patient. In the study of Kostis et al (12), the sensitivity for the prediction of subsequent sudden death was 25% for frequent PVCs, 34% for repetitive PVCs, and 43% if the presence of either was considered an abnormal finding (Table 27–4). The sensitivity increased to 92% if the presence of any PVC on a 24-hour Holter was considered a positive finding; however, one or more PVCs were present in 84% of the study population, and hence the specificity was low, at 16%.

Table 27–3. Relationship Between Ventricular Arrhythmias and Mortality in Survivors of Acute Myocardial Infarction

			High-Risk Ventricular Arrhythmias			No or Low-Risk Ventricular Arrhythmias		
Study	Number of Patients	Follow-up (mo)	Number of Patients	SCD	TCD	Number of Patients	SCD	TCD
Ruberman et al (8)	1,739	42	462[a]	68(15)[b]	139(30)	1,277	71(6)	178(14)
Moss et al (9)	940	36	216[a]	23(11)	46(21)	724	32(4)	69(10)
Mukharji et al (10)	533	18	78[c]	10(13)	23(29)	455	19(4)	43(9)
Bigger et al (11)	819	24	245[d]	30(12)	47(19)	574	24(4)	65(11)
Kostis et al (12)	1,640	25	665[e]	51(8)	101(15)	975	25(3)	62(6)
Total	5,671	29	1,666	182(11)	356(21)	4,005	171(4)	417(10)

SCD = sudden cardiac death, TCD = total cardiac death.

[a]Bigeminal, multiform, R-on-T phenomenon, or repetitive.

[b]Numbers in parentheses are percentage values.

[c]≥10 per hour mean frequency.

[d]≥3 per hour.

[e]≥10 per hour, repetitive, or multiform.

Table 27–4. Sensitivity and Specificity of Different Categorical Definitions of Premature Ventricular Complexes in Predicting Mortality

Definition	Prevalence (%)	Sudden Death (%)		Total Deaths (%)	
		Sensitivity	Specificity	Sensitivity	Specificity
Any PVC	84	92	16	92	17
>10 per hour	13	25	88	26	89
Repetitive PVC	20	34	81	33	82
>10 per hour or repetitive	26	43	75	44	77
Multiform	33	62	69	50	69
>10 per hour, pair, and multiform	7	16	93	14	94
>10 per hour, pair or multiform	41	67	60	62	61

PVC = premature ventricular complexes
Data from Kostis et al (12).

Some have favored the use of nonsustained VT as a prognostic marker. Nonsustained VT may be detected in 6% to 11% of the infarct survivors, and its presence appears to increase twofold the risk of total and sudden cardiac mortality. However, its sensitivity and positive predictive accuracy for sudden death are not significantly better than those of frequent PVCs. Moreover, nonsustained VT has not been shown to be an independent predictor of sudden cardiac mortality, and its day-to-day variability is too high to justify using it as a prognostic marker.

A second problem is that the ideal time for performance of Holter monitoring after acute myocardial infarction is also controversial. In reported studies, Holter monitoring was, in general, performed 10 to 21 days after infarction. As noted previously, the frequency of ventricular arrhythmias does not peak until 6 to 8 weeks after the infarction (16); thus, the sensitivity and predictive accuracy of ventricular arrhythmias may depend significantly on the timing of Holter recording relative to the onset of the initial infarct.

Third, it appears that the prognosis of ventricular arrhythmias may be different in patients with Q wave and non–Q wave infarcts. Maisel et al (19) performed 24-hour Holter monitoring in 777 survivors of acute myocardial infarction and followed them for 1 year, without any antiarrhythmic therapy. Multiform or repetitive PVCs occurred more frequently in nonsurvivors than in survivors of the non–Q wave infarcts, but their prevalence did not significantly differ between nonsurvivors and survivors of Q wave infarcts. This finding, however, needs to be confirmed, and its clinical implications are unclear.

Finally, the relationship between ventricular arrhythmias and left ventricular dysfunction in predicting prognosis after myocardial infarction has been controversial (13–15). Much of the controversy has arisen because the prevalence of ventricular arrhythmias bears a strong relationship to the presence of left ventricular dysfunction, and therefore, it has been argued that the ventricular arrhythmias do not contribute to increased risk of cardiac mortality after an adjustment is made for the presence of underlying left ventricular dysfunction. Schulze et al (13) examined the prognostic value of ventricular arrhythmias and left ventricular dysfunction (as defined by left ventricular radionuclide ejection fraction <0.40) in 81 patients 2 weeks after the infarction. As expected, complex ventricular arrhythmias (Lown grade 3 or higher) occurred more frequently in 26 to 45 patients (58%) with left ventricular dysfunction than in 3 of 36 patients (8%) with normal left ventricular function ($p < 0.01$). During a short follow-up of 7 months, all 8 sudden deaths occurred in the subset of 26 patients who manifested *both* complex ventricular arrhythmias and left ventricular dysfunction. In a study of 295 medically treated patients with coronary artery disease, Califf et al (14) failed to find a significant association between ventricular arrhythmias and cardiac mortality once an adjustment was made for left ventricular dysfunction. In the majority of the patients, however, the index infarction was not recent, and 47% had no history of previous myocardial infarction.

More recently, five large prospective studies (8–12) have examined the relationship between ventricular arrhythmias, left ventricular dysfunction, and subsequent cardiac mortality. All concluded that both left ventricular dysfunction and ventricular arrhythmias are *independent* predictors of both sudden cardiac and total cardiac mortality, and that the risk is synergistically increased when the high-risk ventricular arrhythmias coexist with left ventricular dysfunction. The incidence of sudden death was low and ranged from 0% to 2% in patients with no or low-risk arrhythmias and normal left ventricular function. In contrast, the incidence of sudden death ranged from 18% to 31% in patients who had both high-risk ventricular arrhythmias and left ventricular dysfunction (Table 27–5).

Thrombolysis and Ventricular Arrhythmias

Thrombolytic therapy, when administered within 12 hours of acute myocardial infarction, has been demonstrated to reduce 1-year cardiac mortality (21) (see Ch. 19). This beneficial effect on mortality may be related to the infarct size reduction, preservation of left ventricular function, better left ventricular remodeling, and patency of the infarct-related vessel. An improved electrical stability may be another potential mechanism of benefit of heart, but the available data are conflicting.

Table 27–6. Prevalence and Prognostic Significance of Ventricular Arrhythmias in 8,676 Patients in the GISSI-2 Trial

		6-Month Cardiac Mortality	
Category	Prevalence	Total	Sudden
No PVCs	36%	2%	0.6%
Infrequent PVCs	44%	2.7%	0.8%
Frequent PVCs*	20%	5.5%	2.1%

*Independent predictor of total and sudden cardiac mortality.

Nonsustained VT was seen in 6.7% of the patients, but it was not an independent predictor.

In GISSI-2 trial, 8,676 infarct survivors underwent Holter monitoring at a mean of 17 days after the infarction (22). As summarized in Table 27–6, the overall frequency and complexity of ventricular arrhythmias did not appear to be much different from that reported in the prethrombolytic era. The PVCs were absent in 36%, infrequent (1–10 per hour) in 44%, and frequent (>10 per hour) in 20% of the infarct survivors; nonsustained VT was seen in 7%. The presence of frequent PVCs was an independent predictor of the total- and sudden-cardiac mortality with odds ratio of 2.98 (95% confidence interval, 2.13–4.17) and 4.07 (95% confidence interval, 2.30–7.20), respectively. Other studies (23,24), albeit smaller in size, have reported similar findings. McClements and Adgey (23) performed Holter an average of 6 days after the infarct in 301 patients (68% of whom had received thrombolytic therapy) and reported the frequency of high-grade PVCs to be 26%. In a multivariate analysis, the occurrence

Table 27–5. Sudden Cardiac Death in Relation to Left Ventricular Dysfunction in Survivors of Acute Myocardial Infarction

	Ruberman et al (8)		Schulze et al (13)		Mukharji et al (10)	
Category	Number of Patients	SCD[a] (%)	Number of Patients	SCD (%)	Number of Patients	SCD (%)
Low-risk VA[b], no LV dys	883(51)	2	33(41)	0	314(59)	2
Low-risk VA, LV dys	393(23)	7	19(23)	0	141(26)	10
High-risk VA, no LV dys	267(15)	12	3(4)	0	38(7)	8
High-risk VA, LV dys	195(11)	20	26(32)	31	40(8)	18

LV dys = left ventricular dysfunction, SCD = sudden cardiac death, VA = ventricular arrhythmias.

[a]Cumulative probability.

[b]Low-risk VA = low or no VA.

of arrhythmic events during follow-up was independently predicted by the late potentials and impaired left ventricular ejection fraction, but not by the Holter findings.

Recently, Rouleau et al (23a) reported their findings regarding survival and risk factor analysis in 3178 patients with acute myocardial infarction enrolled between July 1990 and June 1992 at nine Canadian hospitals [Canadian Assessment of Myocardial Infarction (CAMI) Study]. The in-hospital mortality was 8.4% and a predischarge Holter was performed in 74% of the survivors. Frequent PVCs (≥10/h) were seen in 16% of the patients and the frequency of PVCs correlated with the 1-year post discharge mortality. However, in a multivariate model, the PVCs did not predict the arrhythmic or total mortality and the left ventricular ejection fraction was the most powerful predictor. Also, the 1-year incidence of sudden death was relatively low at 1.9%.

Holter-Guided Long-Term Antiarrhythmic Drug Trials

Although the presence of ventricular arrhythmia is an established risk factor for sudden death in survivors of acute myocardial infarction, an important question is whether arrhythmia suppression will be accompanied by a reduction in the incidence of sudden death (see also Ch. 28). Until recently, there were relatively few trials in such patients, and none were large enough to answer this question. The recent findings of the Cardiac Arrhythmia Suppression Trial have significantly influenced the management approach of asymptomatic ventricular arrhythmias in patients with recent myocardial infarction.

Table 27–7 summarizes the findings of 11 large studies in which infarct survivors were randomly assigned to either placebo or antiarrhythmic drugs(s) and followed up for at least 3 months and in which total mortality was reported. Before the Cardiac Arrhythmia Pilot Study and the Cardiac Arrhythmia Suppression Trial, there were eight trials involving a total of 2,171 patients; the antiarrhythmic drugs under evaluation included procainamide in one (38), phenytoin in two (39,40), tocainide in two (41,42), mexiletine in two (43,44), and aprinidine in one study (45). In none of these studies did the difference in total mortality between the treated group and the placebo group reach statistical significance. Indeed, the mortality tended to be higher in five studies, unchanged in one study, and lower in two studies.

Table 27–7. Long-Term Antiarrhythmic Drug Trials in the Survivors of Acute Myocardial Infarction

Study	Number of Patients		Antiarrhythmic Agent	Follow-up (mo)	Mortality (%)		*p* Value
	C	Rx			C	Rx	
Kosowsky et al (38)	39	39	Procainamide	36	2.6	10.3	NS
Collaborative Group (39)	285	283	Phenytoin	12	9.1	8.1	0.75
Peter et al (40)	76	74	Phenytoin	24	18.4	24.3	0.49
Bastian et al (41)	74	72	Tocainide	6	4.1	5.6	0.97
Ryden et al (42)	56	56	Tocainide	6	8.9	8.9	1.0
Chamberlain et al (43)	163	181	Mexiletine	4	11.7	13.3	0.78
IMPACT (44)	313	317	Mexiletine	9	4.8	7.6	NS
Gottlieb et al (45)	72	71	Aprindine	12	22	17	0.31
CAPS (46)	100	402	Encainide Flecainide Moricizine Imipramine	12	2	1.2	NS
CAST-I (47)	725	730	Flecainide	10	3	7.7	0.0003
CAST-II:							
(titration) (48)	665	660	Moricizine	0.5	0.5	1.4	0.02
(long-term) (48)	574	581	Moricizine	18	12.4	14.9	0.40

C = control, Rx = treated, NS = not significant.

All of these studies were subject to limitations that detracted from the significance of the findings. None were large enough to detect a significant drug-related reduction in mortality. Only a single antiarrhythmic agent was used at a fixed dose, and in most studies, the presence of ventricular arrhythmia was not a specific criterion for enrollment. Few studies documented an effective suppression of arrhythmias by drug therapy. It is of interest that in the International Mexiletine and Placebo Antiarrhythmic Coronary Trial (IMPACT) (44), mexiletine treated patients had a lower prevalence of ventricular arrhythmias at 1 and 4 months, even though the total and sudden cardiac mortality tended to be higher in the treated than in the placebo group (7.6% and 2.5% versus 4.8% and 1.3%).

Cardiac Arrhythmia Pilot Study

Because of the significant problems in the design of these studies, the National Heart, Lung and Blood Institute (NHLBI) sponsored a 10-center Cardiac Arrhythmia Pilot Study (CAPS) in 1983 (46). CAPS was designed to determine the feasibility of conducting a larger trial that would test the hypothesis whether PVC suppression results in reduction in mortality in infarct survivors. CAPS enrolled 502 patients who were less than 75 years of age and had an average of 10 or more PVCs per hour or 5 or more runs of nonsustained ventricular tachycardia ranging from three to nine beats in duration. Enrolled patients were randomized to placebo (100 patients) or one of the four active treatment tracks with encainide, flecainide, moricizine, or imipramine. The study design permitted administration of up to three doses of the first drug to be tested before the patient was enrolled in a trial of a second drug. Patients were followed for 12 months, during which 24-hour Holter electrocardiograms were recorded 3, 6, 9, and 12 months after the infarction. Except for imipramine, which had a low efficacy (52%) and was associated with a high incidence (20%) of intolerable noncardiac adverse effects, the other three drugs had high efficacy rates (66% to 83%) in achieving 70% or greater suppression of PVCs and a low incidence (<6%) of intolerable noncardiac side effects. The incidence of documented or suspected proarrhythmia was also relatively low (2% to 7%).

Cardiac Arrhythmia Suppression Trial

Encouraged by the CAPS results, the full-scale Cardiac Arrhythmia Suppression Trial (CAST) was begun in 1987 (47) (see Ch. 28). Eligibility criteria included the presence of both an average of 6 or more PVCs per hour on a screening Holter and a left ventricular ejection fraction <0.55 (if the Holter was performed within 6 to 90 days) or <0.40 (if the Holter was performed more than 90 days after the infarction). A total of 2,309 patients met the eligibility criteria and underwent open-label titration with encainide, flecainide, or moricizine. One hundred and thirty-five (6%) patients were excluded because they did not show greater than 80% suppression of PVCs, and 447 patients (19%) were excluded because they developed proarrhythmia, had intolerable side effects, or died. Two hundred and seventy-two patients were assigned to moricizine or placebo. The remaining 1,455 patients were assigned to placebo (725 patients) or to treatment with flecainide or encainide (730 patients). Although the study was due to be completed in 1992, a scheduled survey by the Data and Safety Monitoring Board found an unexpectedly high mortality in the patients treated with flecainide and encainide. During an average of 10 months of follow-up, compared with placebo, the encainide and flecainide groups had a 2.5-fold higher total mortality (3.0% versus 7.7%, $p < 0.0003$) and a 3.6-fold higher arrhythmic mortality (1.2% versus 4.5%, $p < 0.0006$). An analysis of the baseline characteristics of patients assigned to the flecainide and encainide groups and the placebo group did not reveal any significant differences to explain the increased mortality in the treated groups (Table 27–8). As a result, the flecainide and encainide treatment arms were discontinued, but in the moricizine arm, the patients were continued to be enrolled (CAST-II) (48). The moricizine therapy was associated with almost a threefold higher cardiac mortality in the first 2 weeks (0.5% vs. 1.4%, $p = 0.02$) but not in the subsequent long-term therapy (12.4% vs. 14.9%, $p = 0.4$).

CAST has several important clinical implications in the management of survivors of acute myocardial infarction (see Ch. 28). First, the results have conclusively shown that flecainide, encainide, and

Table 27–8. Characteristics and Mortality Results of Patients Participating in the Cardiac Arrhythmia Suppression Trial

	Encainide/ Flecainide (n = 730)	Placebo (n = 725)
Age	61 ± 10	61 ± 10
LVEF	0.40 ± 0.10	0.39 ± 0.09
CHF history	13.7%	11.5%
Anterior myocardial infarction	20%	18%
Thrombolysis	28.2%	24.3%
CABG and/or PTCA	53.6%	54.1%
PVCs per hour	127 ± 254	128 ± 249
Proportion of patients with ventricular tachycardia	21.2%	20.1%
Beta blockers	30.4%	33.1%
Digitalis	21.2%	18.5%
Total mortality	7.7%*	3.0%
Sudden death mortality	4.5%**	1.2%

CABG = coronary artery bypass graft surgery, CHF = congestive heart failure, LVEF = left ventricular ejection fraction, PTCA = percutaneous transluminal coronary angioplasty, PVCs = premature ventricular complexes, VT = ventricular tachycardia.

*$p < 0.0003$.

**$p < 0.0006$.

Data from the CAST Investigators Preliminary Report (47).

moricizine ought not to be used in those survivors of acute myocardial infarction who meet the CAST eligibility criteria. Whether other class Ic drugs (such as propafenone and recainam) will have similar detrimental effects in these patients remains to be determined. It should also be emphasized that a tendency toward increased cardiac mortality was also apparent in many of the previous trials that used class Ia (procainamide) or Ib (mexiletene, tocainamide, phenytoin) drugs. At present, there appears to be no justification for empiric use of currently available antiarrhythmic drugs in treating *asymptomatic* ventricular arrhythmia in survivors of acute myocardial infarction. CAST has also shown a relatively low risk of recurrent arrhythmic events in the untreated infarct survivors with asymptomatic ventricular arrhythmias. The mortality was especially low in patients who were enrolled more than 90 days after the infarct; however, it should be appreciated that CAST required the eligible patients to respond to antiarrhythmic therapy during the open-label phase, and the nonresponders were excluded. Also, there were 62 deaths during the open-label phase. Undoubtedly, many of the high-risk patients were excluded or died prior to randomization. Finally, CAST highlights the need for developing alternative risk stratification and treatment strategies for survivors of acute myocardial infarction. In this regard, the preliminary experience with signal-averaged electrocardiograms and electrophysiologic testing is promising and needs to be further explored (see also Ch. 28). Also, the failure of a class I antiarrhythmic agent needs to be contrasted against the consistently beneficial effect of the prophylactic use of beta-adrenergic blockers in reducing the incidence of sudden and total cardiac mortality (49,50). The benefit of beta-adrenergic blockers appears to be greatest in subsets of patients who have experienced an electrical or mechanical complication early after the acute myocardial infarction (see Ch. 12) (50). Many of these patients, however, do not tolerate the beta blocker therapy, and the beta blockers may worsen heart failure in 15% to 20% of such patients (49,50).

In recent years, there has been a resurgence of interest in the prophylactic role of amiodarone to the infarct survivors. In the Basal Antiarrhythmic Study of Infarct Survival (BASIS) (51), 312 infarct survivors with Lown class III or IVb ventricular arrhythmias on Holter were randomized to receive low-dose amiodarone (200 mg/day), individualized antiarrhythmic agents (other than amiodarone), or placebo. During 1-year follow-up, there were 2 cardiac deaths in the amiodarone group and 15 cardiac deaths in those on placebo ($p < 0.05$). Ten cardiac deaths occurred in the individualized therapy group, but the difference from the placebo group was not significant. The BASIS investigators demonstrated the persistence of mortality benefit in long-term follow-up even after amiodarone was discontinued (52). However, in a subset analysis, the beneficial effect of amiodarone was limited only to patients with left ventricular ejection fraction of 40% or greater (53). Ceremuzynski et al (54) also reported a beneficial effect of prophylactic therapy with amiodarone (up to 400 mg daily dose) in a double-blind, placebo-controlled trial ($p = 0.048$).

The beneficial effects of amiodarone have also been recently reported (presented at American College of Cardiology meeting Orlando, 1996) in two large placebo-controlled double-blind primary prevention trials in the infarct survivors. In the Canadian Myocardial Infarction Amiodarone Trial (CAMIAT), a total of 1202 patients were randomized to receive amiodarone or placebo. This study enrolled patients with frequent PVCs or runs of nonsustained VT, and the presence of impaired left ventricular ejection fraction was not required. Amiodarone reduced significantly the occurrence of sudden death or resuscitated VF by 40% but the total cardiac mortality was not reduced significantly (18% reduction). The European Myocardial Infarction Amiodarone Trial (EMIAT) enrolled patients with left ventricular ejection fraction ≤0.40 and did not require the presence of PVCs or VT. As compared to the placebo arm, there was no significant difference in total mortality in the amiodarone treated patients. However, there appeared to be a trend towards decreased mortality in the patients with clinical heart failure and lower left ventricular ejection fraction. In both EMIAT and CAMIAT studies, about two-thirds of the patients were receiving beta-blockers in both the placebo- and treatment-arms. Thus, the available data do not justify a routine use of prophylactic therapy with amiodarone in the high-risk survivors of acute myocardial infarction.

ROLE OF ELECTROPHYSIOLOGIC TESTING

In recent years, electrophysiologic study (EPS) has been shown to be useful in the diagnosis and management of patients with sustained ventricular tachycardia and patients with out-of-hospital cardiac arrest (56,57). More recently, this technique has been used in identifying patients at increased risk for sudden death after acute myocardial infarction (25–37).

Rationale for Electrophysiologic Testing

In post–myocardial infarction patients, the predominant mechanism of ventricular arrhythmias appears to be reentry (58,59). Histologic studies of surgically resected specimens of the recently infarcted myocardium have revealed the presence of scattered and surviving myocardial and Purkinje fibers trapped within the infarct region or at its margins (see Ch. 28) (60,61). On ultrastructural studies, these surviving cells show evidence of ischemic damage as manifested by decreased intracellular glycogen, increased lipid droplets, and relaxed sarcomeres with widened I-bands (60). Microcellular electrophysiologic studies have demonstrated significant abnormalities in the resting membrane potential, the action potential duration, and the rate of upstroke rise (V_{max}) (61–63), and the extent of these abnormalities shows a significant regional dispersion in the infarcted myocardium (see Ch. 14). These abnormalities would be expected to produce areas of slow conduction, dispersion of refractoriness, and unidirectional functional block to the conduction, especially when a ventricular stimulus is delivered prematurely; this is an appropriate substrate for reentrant arrhythmias. They are also in accord with observations in the experimental canine infarction model (59,63,64), in which detailed electrophysiologic mapping studies (with multielectrode arrays) have conclusively proven reentry to be the mechanism of inducible ventricular arrhythmias. In these experimental models, programmed ventricular stimulation has been shown to induce sustained VT or fibrillation in up to 50% of the animals, and inducibility is higher in animals with a large infarct size and a low left ventricular ejection fraction (64).

In survivors of acute myocardial infarction who present with clinical sustained VT or ventricular fibrillation, EPS has been reported to induce clinical arrhythmias in 70% to 95% of the patients (56,57). Furthermore, in patients with stable coronary artery disease and without history of documented ventricular arrhythmias, EPS only rarely induces sustained ventricular tachycardia or fibrillation (65). Thus it is reasonable to postulate that EPS may also be useful in predicting patients at risk of sudden death after a recent myocardial infarction. Inducibility of ventricular arrhythmias would be expected in infarct survivors who have the necessary anatomic and electrophysiologic substrate for the development of clinical sustained ventricular tachyarrhythmias and, hence, the risk for sudden death. Conversely, noninducibility may identify patients at low risk for the development of subsequent arrhythmic events.

Frequency of Inducibility of Ventricular Arrhythmias

Table 27–9 summarizes the results of several studies of the frequency of inducibility of ventricular arrhythmias in survivors of acute myocardial infarction. The wide variability in the reported incidence is probably related to the vigor of the stimulation protocol and the nature of the patient population under study. In general, ventricular arrhythmias are not inducible in about 70% of the patients when the protocol for EPS uses a maximum of two extrastimuli; however, the incidence of noninducibility declines to about 50% when three or more extrastimuli are used. Nonsustained VT is inducible in about 10% to 20% of the patients. The frequency of inducible sustained ventricular tachycardia or fibrillation is about 10% to 20% with two extrastimuli, but increases to 30% to 45% with the use of three extrastimuli. Inducibility of sustained ventricular tachycardia or fibrillation increases to 50% or higher when the stimulation protocol employs up to five extrastimuli. In addition to the number of extrastimuli, the frequency of inducibility is also influenced by the current strength of the delivered extrastimuli and by the number of stimulated ventricular sites. Left ventricular stimulation has not been routinely performed in these patients, but it appears to increase the yield of inducible sustained ventricular arrhythmias by 10% (32).

In most reported studies, the inducibility of sustained ventricular tachycardia (but not ventricular fibrillation, which accounts for about half of all inducible sustained arrhythmias) has correlated with

Table 27–9. Response to Electrophysiologic Stimulation in Survivors of Acute Myocardial Infarction

			PVS Protocol			Induced Response		
Study	Number of Patients	Days After Acute MI	Number of ES	Number of Sites	Stimulus Strength	Nonind (%)	NSVT (%)	Sus VT/VF (%)
Hamer et al (25)	70	11	2	1–2[a]	2–10 V[a]	72	17	11
Richards et al (26)	165	10	2	1	20 mA	77[b]		23[c]
Marchlinski et al (27)	46	22	2	1	2 × DT	78	11	11
Roy et al (28)	150	12	2	2	2 × DT	77	11	12
Santarelli et al (29)	50	25	2	1	10 mA	40	40	20
Breithardt et al (30)	132	22	2	1	2 × DT	54	25	21
Denniss et al (31)	403	7–28	2	1	20 mA	66[b]		34[c]
Bhandari et al (32)	75	14	3	3	2 × DT	48	8	44
Waspe et al (33)	50	16	3	2	4 × DT	66	12	22
Cripps et al (34)	75	21	3	1	2 × DT	38	32	30
Bhandari et al (35)	86	14	3	2	2 × DT	64	7	29
Richards et al (36)	361	6–28	5*	2	2 × DT, 20 mA	50	—	50[d]
Bourke et al (37)	1,209	11	5*	2	2 × DT, 20 mA	94[f]	—	6[e]

*Variable stimulation protocols.

ES = extrastimuli, Nonind = noninducible, NSVT = nonsustained ventricular tachycardia, PVS = programmed ventricular stimulation, Sus VT/VF = sustained ventricular tachycardia or fibrillation, 2 × DT = twice the diastolic threshold, 4 × DT = four times the diastolic threshold.

[a]Variable in different patients.

[b]Included patients with induced NSVT.

[c]Sus VT > 10 seconds in duration.

[d]Sus VT > 230 ms in 7%, VF, rapid VT in 43%.

[e]Only for sus VT > 230 ms; no values given for VF or rapid VT inducibility.

[f]Noninducibles included those with induced VF, nonsustained VT, and sustained polymorphic VT.

a higher prevalence of congestive heart failure, left ventricular aneurysm, severe left ventricular wall motion abnormalities, and depressed left ventricular ejection fraction. These findings are in accord with the experimental canine infarction model, in which the larger infarct size predisposes the animals to develop inducible ventricular tachycardia (64). Interestingly, the inducibility of ventricular arrhythmia has not shown a consistent relationship with the frequency or complexity of the spontaneous ventricular arrhythmia on Holter monitoring (25–37).

Prognostic Significance of Inducible Ventricular Arrhythmia

The prognostic significance of inducible ventricular arrhythmias after myocardial infarction remains controversial. Some investigators have reported favorable results; other have failed to confirm the prognostic value of inducibility. A meaningful interpretation of these studies is hampered further by the small numbers of patients in individual series and by the presence of major differences in the patient populations, in stimulation protocols, in the use of concomitant antiarrhythmic therapy, and in definitions of abnormal responses to electrophysiologic stimulation. Moreover, only few studies have compared the prognostic significance of the inducible ventricular arrhythmias with that of other simple clinical variables.

Although most of the reported studies included clinically stable survivors of acute myocardial infarction and excluded patients with unstable angina or severe congestive heart failure, the 1-year mortality ranged from 2% to 17%; therefore, it is clear that the patient populations differed significantly in their risk for subsequent arrhythmic events. This is so even though most studies did not systemically attempt to exclude either low- or high-risk survivors of acute myocardial infarction. As the predictive value of a given test depends on the prevalence of the disease and the endpoints, it is important that the prognostic value of EPS be judged separately in low- and high-risk survivors of acute myocardial infarction.

Table 27–10 summarizes the results of seven studies that included relatively low-risk survivors of acute myocardial infarction. In two studies (28,32), high-risk patients were specifically excluded; the other five studies (29–31,34,37) are included in the table because of their overall low 1-year total cardiac mortality. The incidence of sudden death was low (0% to 2.9%) in patients who did not have inducible sustained ventricular arrhythmias. In all studies, patients with inducible sustained arrhythmias fared worse than noninducible patients, but the difference did not reach statistical significance

Table 27–10. Prognostic Significance of Induced Ventricular Arrhythmias in Stable "Low-Risk" Survivors of Acute Myocardial Infarction

Study	Follow-up (mo)	Sudden Death (%) in Patients with: Nonind Sus VT/VF	Sudden Death (%) in Patients with: Ind Sus VT/VF	Spontaneous Sus VT (%) in Patients with: Nonind Sus VT/VF	Spontaneous Sus VT (%) in Patients with: Ind Sus VT/VF	Total Cardiac Mortality (%)
Roy et al (28)	10	0.8	5.6	0.8	5.6	3.3
Santarelli et al (29)	11	0	0	0	0	2
Breithardt et al (30)	15	2.9	3.6	1.9	25*	6.1
Bhandari et al (32)	18	2.3	9.1	2.3	6.1	6.7
Cripps et al (34)	16	0	0	0	27*	1.3
Denniss et al (31)[a]	12	1.5	5.9	—	—	5.5
Bourke et al (37)	12	1	7**	2	13**	5.5

Sus VT/VF = sustained ventricular tachycardia or fibrillation, Nonind = noninducible, Ind = inducible.

[a]Fifteen patients developed spontaneous sustained ventricular tachycardia, but the relationship to inducibility was not described.

*$p < 0.05$.

**$p < 0.0005$.

except in the study by Denniss et al (31) and Bourke et al (37). The largest reported study has been by Bourke et al (Westmead Group), who performed predischarge EPS in 1209 (37%) of the 3,286 postinfarction patients over a 4-year period. EPS induced sustained ventricular tachycardia of cycle length >235 msec in 75 (6%) patients. In a 1-year follow-up, sudden death occurred in 7% of the inducible patients and in 1% of the remainder ($p < 0.005$). However, the overall incidence of sudden death was low at 1.7%; the sensitivity and positive predictive accuracy of inducible sustained ventricular tachycardia for sudden death were 24% and 7%, respectively. Moreover, Bourke et al (37) used up to five extrastimuli with stimulus current strength of up to 20 mA. With such a protocol, rapid sustained VT of cycle length <230 msec and ventricular fibrillation (the prognostically nonspecific arrhythmias) are inducible in about 40% of the patients.

With regard to the development of spontaneous sustained VT during follow-up, three studies (28,29,32) did not show significant differences in the development of this complication between patients with and those without inducible sustained ventricular arrhythmias. In the studies by Breithardt et al (30) and Cripps et al (34), however, spontaneous sustained VT developed in about 25% of the patients with inducible sustained arrhythmias compared with less than 2% of the patients with noninducible sustained arrhythmias ($p < 0.05$). In these studies, the overall incidence of sustained ventricular tachycardia was relatively high at 7% and 8%, and it is possible that the study populations were biased toward inclusion of patients who were more likely to have developed this complication. It should be emphasized that sustained ventricular tachycardia develops in not more than 1% to 3% of the infarct survivors. In the study by Bourke et al (37), sustained ventricular tachycardia occurred in 2.5% of the patients, and its occurrence was higher in the inducible patients (13% vs. 2%, $p < 0.0005$). Neither of these studies specified the time course of development of this arrhythmia during follow-up.

Table 27–11 summarizes the results of five electrophysiologic studies of patients considered to be at high risk after myocardial infarction. Three of the studies (25,33,35) specifically included high-risk patients whose postinfarction course was complicated by congestive heart failure, angina, bundle branch block, or nonsustained VT. The other two (26,27) are included because of a high 1-year cardiac mortality. In two studies in which the stimulation protocol included a maximum of two extrastimuli at twice diastolic threshold (25,27), the inducibility of sustained ventricular arrhythmias did not correlate with subsequent sudden cardiac mortality; however, in the other three studies (26,33,35), where three extrastimuli were used or

Table 27–11. Prognostic Significance of Induced Ventricular Arrhythmias in High-Risk Survivors of Acute Myocardial Infarction

Study	Follow-up (mo)	Sudden Death (%) in Patients With: Nonind Sus VT/VF	Sudden Death (%) in Patients With: Ind Sus VT/VF	Spontaneous Sus VT (%) in Patients With: Nonind Sus VT/VF	Spontaneous Sus VT (%) in Patients With: Ind Sus VT/VF	Cardiac Mortality (%)
Marchlinski et al (27)	18	14.6	0	—	—	21.7
Hamer et al (25)	12	4	33[a]	—	—	17
Richards et al (26)	12	10.0	21.1[b]	1.5	10.5	10
Waspe et al (33)	23	7.7	27[c]	0	9.1	24
Bhandari et al (35)	11	4	16[d]	3.3	8.0	13

Sus VT/VF = sustained ventricular tachycardia or fibrillation, Nonind = noninducible, Ind = inducible.

[a] $p < 0.05$ (data for 37 of the 70 study patients; the stimulation protocol was incomplete in the remaining 33 patients).

[b] $p < 0.05$.

[c] $p < 0.001$.

[d] $p < 0.05$.

two extrastimuli were delivered at high current strength (20 mA), patients with inducible sustained ventricular tachycardia had a significantly higher incidence of subsequent sudden death and spontaneous sustained VT than those without inducible sustained ventricular arrhythmias.

Bhandari et al (35) performed EPS in 86 (21%) high-risk survivors of the 416 patients with acute myocardial infarction. These patients had one or more of the following: Killip class II or III heart failure, moderate angina, or nonsustained VT. During EPS performed a mean of 14 days after the infarct, sustained monomorphic VT was inducible in 19 patients (22%), polymorphic VT or ventricular fibrillation (VF) in 6 patients (7%), and no inducible sustained arrhythmia in 61% patients (71%). During follow-up of 11 months, sudden death occurred in 7 patients (8%) and spontaneous sustained VT in 4 patients (5%) (total arrhythmic events, 11). The arrhythmic events occurred in 6 (32%) of 19 patients with inducible sustained VT, in none of the 6 patients with inducible VF, and in 5 (8%) of the 61 patients without inducible sustained arrhythmias ($p < 0.003$). Thus, for patients surviving a complicated myocardial infarct, the sensitivity and positive predictive accuracy of the inducible sustained VT for major arrhythmic events were 55% and 32%, respectively; the inducible VF, however, appeared to be of no clinical significance. Other studies have also confirmed the lack of prognostic utility of the inducible polymorphic VT and VF (Table 27–12).

Clinical Implications

In evaluating the clinical value of EPS for risk stratification, several issues need to be considered (66). First, although EPS can be safely performed in post–myocardial infarction patients, it is an invasive and expensive test associated with a small but definite morbidity; thus, its routine use may not be recommended unless it has a high sensitivity and positive predictive accuracy for subsequent arrhythmic events. It should also provide prognostic information *independent* of the routine clinical evaluation. Finally, there must be an evidence of improved survival by antiarrhythmic therapy based on the results of EPS.

In patients who are clinically stable and whose postinfarction course is not complicated by congestive heart failure, angina, or nonsustained ventricular tachycardia, the risk of subsequent arrhythmic events is relatively low and ranges from 2% to 5% a year (4). About half of the survivors of acute myocardial infarction belong in this low-risk group. Yet the inducibility of sustained VT is 10% to 15% and of VF 8% to 20%, depending on the stimulation protocol. Even if the inducibility of VF is ignored and the study endpoints include both sudden death and nonfatal sustained ventricular arrhythmias, inducible sustained VT has a relatively low sensitivity of 50% and positive predictive accuracy of 25%. Thus at least half of the arrhythmic events would be missed even if antiarrhythmic therapy were to be administered to all patients with inducible sus-

Table 27–12. Comparison of Prognostic Significance of Inducible Sustained Ventricular Tachycardia Versus Ventricular Fibrillation

	No. Pts with Induced Arrhythmia		Major Arrhythmic Events in Patients with Inducible		
Study Value	Sus VT	VF	Sus VT	VF	Nonind Sus VT/VF
Cripps et al (34)	8(11)[a]	14(19)	6(75)	0	0
Bhandari et al (32)	19(25)	14(19)	4(21)	1(7)	2(4.6)
Denniss et al (31)	80(20)	56(14)	6[b](7.5)	2[b](3.4)	4[b](1.5)
Bhandari et al (35)	19(22)	6(7)	6(32)	0(0)	5(8.2)

Sus = sustained, VT = ventricular tachycardia, VF = ventricular fibrillation, Nonind = noninducible.

[a]Number in parentheses indicate percentage values.

[b]These values refer to the frequency of sudden death and do not include those who developed nonfatal spontaneous sustained ventricular tachycardia.

tained VT. Also, there are no available data that demonstrate a beneficial effect on mortality of the prophylactic antiarrhythmic therapy based on the EPS findings. Denniss et al (67) could not demonstrate any beneficial effect of empiric or EPS-based antiarrhythmic therapy during 3 years of follow-up in 96 survivors of acute myocardial infarction. Thus, at present, there is no clinical justification for performing routine predischarge EPSs in such patients.

On the other hand, the initial experience with EPS appears to be somewhat encouraging in patients whose postinfarction course is complicated by heart failure, bundle branch block, angina pectoris, or nonsustained ventricular tachycardia. In this setting, EPS may provide valuable information regarding the severity of conduction system disease and the potential of antiarrhythmic drugs to exacerbate preexisting conduction disturbances. Also, the inducibility of sustained ventricular tachycardia (but not ventricular fibrillation) has a relatively high sensitivity of 60%, and positive predictive accuracy of 35% for subsequent arrhythmic events. Others have recommended the use of an impaired left ventricular ejection fraction (37) and abnormal signal-averaged electrocardiogram in defining the high-risk subset in whom the predischarge EPS may be beneficial (37,67a). The recently presented findings of the Multicenter Automatic Defibrillation Implantation Trial (MADIT) at NASPE meeting Seattle, 1996 appear to provide substantial support for this approach. In this study, the post myocardial patients were enrolled if they had documented nonsustained ventricular tachycardia, left ventricular ejection fraction $\leq$0.35 and inducible sustained ventricular tachycardia during EPS but not suppressed by intravenous procainamide. The enrolled patients were randomized to conventional antiarrhythmic agents or ICD implant. The study enrollment was stopped after 196 patients in March 1996 because of an almost 50% reduction in total mortality in patients randomized to ICDs. Of note is that approximately 80% of the patients randomized to the medical treatment were receiving amiodarone.

Other Unresolved Issues

There are two other issues for which more data are needed in regard to the use of EPS after myocardial infarction. The first relates to the day-to-day variability in the inducibility of ventricular arrhythmias after myocardial infarction. In studies (68,69) where EPS was performed within a week of the myocardial infarction, there was a significant variability in the response to programmed ventricular stimulation; however, the variability improved when the EPS was performed a minimum of 1 week or later after the infarction (64,70). In a recent study (70), we reported 100% reproducibility in the induction of sustained ventricular tachycardia with cycle length $\geq$240 msec, compared with a 44% reproducibility in the induction of rapid polymorphic ventricular tachycardia or fibrillation ($p < 0.009$). These findings are in accord with those on the prognostic significance of inducible arrhythmias in postinfarction patients, which show a correlation between the inducibility of sustained ventricular tachycardia (and not of ventricular fibrillation) and the occurrence of subsequent arrhythmic events. It should also be emphasized that the inducibility of ventricular arrhythmia declines significantly over a more extended period in all patients. In one study (71), there was a 50% decline in the inducibility of sustained ventricular tachycardia or fibrillation from 2 to 20 weeks after the myocardial infarction.

The second issue relates to the effects of coronary thrombolysis on inducibility of ventricular arrhythmias (see Ch. 19). Thrombolytic therapy may improve the myocardial electric stability by reducing the overall infarct size, improving the regional and global left ventricular function, promoting a better left ventricular remodeling, and increasing the frequency of patent infarct-related artery (72). Several recent studies have compared the inducibility of ventricular arrhythmias in patients receiving or not receiving thrombolytic therapy. Sager et al (73) performed EPS in 21 patients with recent anterior myocardial infarction and left ventricular aneurysm. Twelve had received thrombolytic therapy and nine did not. During EPS, sustained ventricular tachycardia was inducible in only 1 (8%) of the 12 patients who had received thrombolytic therapy, compared with 7 (88%) of the 9 patients without such therapy. During follow-up of 11 $\pm$ 8 months, 4 of the 9 nonthrombolysed patients had major arrhythmic events, while none of the thrombolysed patients had such an event. Similarly,

Kersschot et al (74) reported a significantly lower incidence of inducible sustained monomorphic ventricular tachycardia in 21 patients who had received thrombolytic therapy at the time of acute infarction than in 15 patients not receiving such therapy (29% vs. 67%, $p < 0.05$). However, when the definition of sustained arrhythmias was expanded to include polymorphic ventricular tachycardia as well as ventricular fibrillation, such arrhythmias were inducible in as high as 48% of the thrombolysed patients and in 100% of the nonthrombolysed patients. Interestingly, none of the patients developed arrhythmic events during follow-up of 14 ± 4 months without any antiarrhythmic therapy.

Bourke et al (75) performed predischarge EPS in 97 (61%) of the 159 post–myocardial infarction patients enrolled from Westmead Hospital into ISIS-2 trial. Forty-seven patients had received streptokinase and 50 did not. Sustained ventricular tachycardia was inducible in 8 (16%) of the 50 patients on placebo and in none of the 47 patients treated with streptokinase ($p = 0.005$). They did not report on the frequency of inducible rapid polymorphic sustained ventricular tachycardia or ventricular fibrillation. During 39 ± 9 months follow-up, 3 placebo patients had sudden death or nonfatal spontaneous sustained ventricular arrhythmias, while no such event occurred in the streptokinase treated patients. Of interest is that none of the 8 patients with inducible sustained ventricular tachycardia in the placebo group had an arrhythmic event during follow-up.

In contrast to these studies, McComb et al (76) reported a high incidence of inducible ventricular tachycardia in 92 consecutive patients with acute myocardial infarction who had received thrombolytic therapy. Using a stimulation protocol of three extrastimuli, they could induce sustained ventricular tachycardia in 22% (20 patients) and nonsustained ventricular tachycardia in 13% (12 patients). Despite this high inducibility, there was only 1 sudden death and 1 spontaneous sustained ventricular tachycardia during follow-up of 30 ± 16 months. In this study, the morphology of inducible sustained arrhythmias was polymorphic in 11 of the 20 patients. If such patients were excluded (as was done in the Westmead Study) (75), the incidence of sustained monomorphic ventricular tachycardia would had been relatively low at 10% (9 patients).

Thus, at present, the available data are contradictory regarding the effects of thrombolysis on the inducibility of ventricular arrhythmias. Only a relatively small number of patients have been studied and the stimulation protocols have been variable. The available data do not support any potential concern regarding the arrhythmogenic effects of thrombolytic therapy, but it remains to be proven whether thrombolysis will decrease the development of late arrhythmic events in the postinfarction patients.

Heart Rate Variability

Heart rate variability (HRV) is a measure of the spontaneous variations and fluctuations in the R–R intervals (77–79). It may be measured in time or frequency domains. The time-domain measures are easier to determine and comprehend and, thus, are more frequently used. The most common measure is SDNN, which refers to the standard deviation (in msec) of all the normal R–R intervals in the entire 24-hour recording. The SDANN index refers to the standard deviation of the mean normal RR intervals for all 5 minute segments of a 24-hour recording. The SDNN index refers to the mean of the standard deviations of all normal RR intervals for 5 minute segments in a 24-hour recording. r-MSSD refers to the square root of the mean of the squared differences between adjacent normal R–R intervals in a 24 hour-recording, and pNN50 refers to the percentage of differences between adjacent normal R–R intervals that are greater than 50 msec in the entire 24-hour recording.

The frequency-domain measures are less frequently used and are based on a power spectral analysis using fast Fourier waveform (FFT) techniques. The *total global power* is measured in the range of frequencies between 0.01 and 0.40 Hz. More frequently, the spectral power is determined for different frequency bands and may be expressed as ultralow frequency power (<0.0033 Hz), very low frequency power (0.0033 to 0.04

Hz), low-frequency power (between 0.04 and 0.15 Hz), and high-frequency power (between 0.15 and 0.40 Hz).

Prognostic Significance of HRV

Heart rate variability reflects modulations of the autonomic nervous system (80,81). The parasympathetic system modulations are a major mechanism of respiratory sinus arrhythmia and contribute to HRV in the high-frequency zone. The sympathetic system modulations influence HRV in the low and very low frequency zones. Other, less appreciated contributors to the HRV include the renin–angiotensin system, the thermoregulation system, and other biocircadian rhythms.

The postinfarction state is associated with significant autonomic nervous system abnormalities that may lead to a loss of protective vagal reflexes, inappropriate sympathetic discharges, and local supersensitivity to the circulating catecholamines (80,81). These abnormalities are likely to be arrhythmogenic and may contribute to the development of sustained VT or VF in patients with recent myocardial infarctions. Being an index of automatic system modulations, the HRV would also be expected to be abnormal in such patients.

Kleiger et al (82) examined the prevalence and prognostic significance of the HRV in 808 survivors of acute myocardial infarction. The HRV was measured in the time domain, and a value of SDNN < 50 msec was defined as abnormal. The abnormal HRV was present in 16% of the patients. During mean follow-up of 31 months, the total mortality was 34% in patients with HRV < 50 msec, 14% in patients with HRV 50–100 msec, and 9% in patients with HRV > 100 msec. The presence of an abnormal HRV was an independent predictor of the total mortality. In the same cohort of patients, when HRV was determined using frequency-domain analysis, the presence of abnormal HRV continued to be an independent predictor of total mortality. In particular, the spectral powers in the ultralow frequency band and in the very low frequency band provided the best measures of total cardiac mortality and arrhythmic deaths (83,84).

More recently, Farrell et al (85) examined the prognostic utility of an abnormal HRV (<20 msec) against signal-averaged electrocardiogram, left ventricular ejection fraction, and Holter-detected PVCs in a consecutive series of 416 infarct survivors. In these patients, the mean HRV was 27 ± 11 msec (range 3–81 msec) and its value was abnormal (<20 msec) in 23% of the patients. Abnormal HRV correlated with the presence of impaired left ventricular ejection fraction, late potentials, and frequent PVCs, but it had no relation with anatomical location of the infarct, number of diseased coronary arteries, or patency of the infarct-related artery. During a 24-month mean follow-up, 47 patients died of cardiac causes and there were 24 major arrhythmic events (sudden death or spontaneous sustained ventricular tachycardia). By stepwise Cox regression analysis, abnormal HRV was the best predictor of both major arrhythmic events and total cardiac mortality. Other predictors of arrhythmic events included the presence of late potentials and repetitive PVCs. When the high risk subset was defined by the presence of all three abnormal variables (i.e., HRV, repetitive PVCs, and late potentials), the positive predictive accuracy for major arrhythmic events was as high as 58%, but the sensitivity was relatively low at 24% (Fig. 27–1).

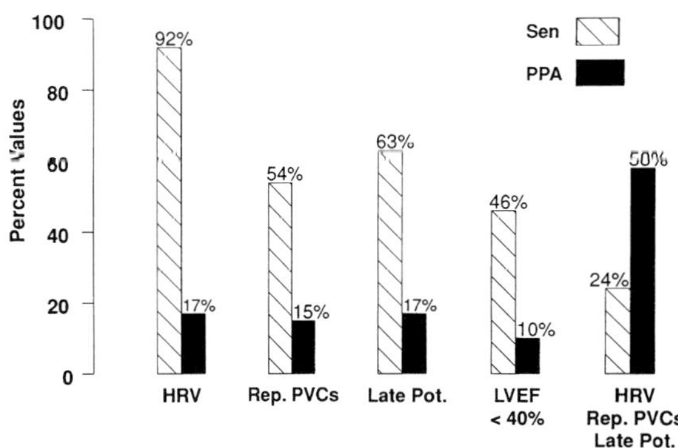

Figure 27–1. Comparative prognostic utility in predicting major arrhythmic events of abnormal heart rate variability (HRV), repetitive PVCs (rep PVCs), late potentials (late pot), and impaired left ventricular ejection fraction (LVEF) in 416 survivors of acute myocardial infarction. Sen = sensitivity; PPA = positive predictive accuracy. *Data from Farrell et al (85).*

Clinical Implications

At present, the HRV is a promising but investigational technique in the risk stratification of the infarct survivors (86). Although the range of the HRV is well defined in the normal subjects, there is a need to define its range for different age groups, gender, and types of heart disease. Significant variability exists in the methodology for determining HRV, and the definitions of abnormal HRV have varied from one study to another. Also, little or no data exist regarding the short- or long-term reproducibility of the HRV measurements. Finally, the available data on HRV are still based on less than 2,000 survivors of acute myocardial infarction. Many of the reported studies were retrospective in nature and did not take into account the effects of thrombolysis and aggressive anti-ischemic interventions. Therefore, there is a need for a large prospective trial to further assess the prognostic utility of abnormal HRV in the thrombolytic era.

CONCLUSIONS

A reliable identification of patients who are at increased risk for the development of arrhythmic events after acute myocardial infarction represents a difficult challenge for the clinical cardiologist. Although the presence of frequent and repetitive PVCs on Holter monitoring identifies a high-risk group, the sensitivity and positive predictive accuracy of this technique are too low to be of clinical utility in a given patient. Moreover, Holter-guided antiarrhythmic drug therapy has not been shown to be beneficial in infarct survivors with asymptomatic ventricular arrhythmias. To the contrary, the use of several antiarrhythmic drugs appears to be harmful in such patients. Electrophysiologic testing may be of prognostic value in patients who are clinically judged to be at high risk for the development of subsequent arrhythmic events; however, a larger cohort of patients needs to be studied to confirm this finding, and it remains to be shown whether EPS-guided antiarrhythmic therapy will improve survival in these patients. Until the answers to these questions are available, the routine use of Holter monitoring and EPS is not recommended in all infarct survivors.

REFERENCES

1. Moss AJ, DeCamilla J, Davis M: Cardiac death in the first 6 months after myocardial infarction: Potential for mortality reduction in the early post hospital period. *Am J Cardiol* 1977;39:816–820.
2. Kannel WB, Sorlie P, McNamara PM: Prognosis after initial myocardial infarction: The Framingham study. *Am J Cardiol* 1988;61:8–15.
3. Helmers C, Lundman T: Early and sudden death after myocardial infarction. *Acta Med Scand* 1979; 205:3–9.
4. Sang G, Costaner A, Betri U, et al: Determinants of prognosis in survivors of acute myocardial infarction. *N Engl J Med* 1981;306:1065–1070.
5. Gilpin EA, Koziol JA, Madsen EP, et al: Periods of differing mortality distribution during the first year after acute myocardial infarction. *Am J Cardiol* 1983;52:240–244.
6. Moss A, Schnitzler R, Green R, et al: Ventricular arrhythmias 3 weeks after acute myocardial infarction *Ann Intern Med* 1975;75:837–841.
7. Vismara LA, Anderson EA, Mason DT: Relation of ventricular arrhythmias in the late hospital phase of acute myocardial infarction to sudden death after hospital discharge. *Am J Med* 1975; 59:6–12.
8. Ruberman W, Weinblatt E, Goldberg JD, et al: Ventricular premature beats and mortality after acute myocardial infarction. *N Engl J Med* 1977; 297:750–757.
9. Moss AJ, Davis HT, DeCamilla J, Bayer LW: Ventricular ectopic beats and their relation to sudden and nonsudden cardiac death after myocardial infarction. *Circulation* 1979;60:998–1003.
10. Mukharji J, Rude RE, Poole WK, et al: The MILIS study group. Risk factors for sudden death after acute myocardial infarction: Two year follow-up. *Am J Cardiol* 1984;54:31–36.
11. Bigger JT, Fleiss JL, Kleiger K, et al: The multicenter post-infarction research group. The relationship between ventricular arrhythmias, left ventricular dysfunction and mortality in the two years after myocardial infarction. *Circulation* 1984;69:250–258.
12. Kostis JB, Byington R, Friedman LM, et al: Prognostic significance of ventricular ectopic activity in survivors of acute myocardial infarction. *J Am Coll Cardiol* 1987;10:231–242.
13. Schulze RA Jr, Strauss HW, Pitt B: Sudden death in the year following myocardial infarction: Relation

to ventricular premature contractions in the late hospital phase and left ventricular ejection fraction. *Am J Med* 1977;62:192–199.

14. Califf RM, McKinnis RA, Barks J, et al: Prognostic implications of ventricular arrhythmias during 24 hour ambulatory monitoring in patients undergoing cardiac catheterization for coronary artery disease. *Am J Cardiol* 1982;50:23–31.
15. Calbert A, Lown B, Gorlin R: Ventricular premature beats and anatomically defined coronary artery disease. *Am J Cardiol* 1977;39:627.
16. Lichstein E, Morganroth J, Harris R, et al: Effect of propranolol on ventricular arrhythmias: The beta-blocker heart attack trial experience. *Circulation* 1983;67(Suppl I):I-5–I-9.
17. Anderson KP, DeCamilla J, Moss AJ: Clinical significance of ventricular tachycardia (3 beats or longer) detected during ambulatory monitoring after myocardial infarction. *Circulation* 1978;57:890–896.
18. Bigger JT, Weld FM, Rolnitzky LM: Prevalance, characteristics and significance of ventricular tachycardia (three or more complexes) detected with ambulatory electrocardiographic recording in the late hospital phase of acute myocardial infarction. *Am J Cardiol* 1981;48:815.
19. Maisel AS, Scott N, Gilpin E, et al: Complex ventricular arrhythmias in patients with Q wave versus non–Q wave myocardial infarction. *Circulation* 1985;72:963–970.
20. Kleiger RE, Miller JP, Thanovaro S, et al: Relationship between clinical features of acute myocardial infarction and ventricular runs 2 weeks to 1 year after infarction. *Circulation* 1981;63:64–70.
21. Fibrinolytic Therapy Trialists Collaborative Group: Indications for fibrinolytic therapy in suspected acute myocardial infarction: Collaborative overview of early mortality and major morbidity results from all randomized trials of more than 1000 patients. *Lancet* 1994;343:311–322.
22. Maggioni AP, Zuanetti G, Franzosi MG, et al: Prevalence and prognostic significance of ventricular arrhythmias after acute myocardial infarction in the fibrinolytic era. GISSI-2 results. *Circulation* 1993;87:312–322.
23. McClements BM, Adgey AAJ: Value of signal averaged electrocardiography, radionuclide ventriculography, Holter monitoring and clinical variables for prediction of arrhythmic events in survivors of acute myocardial infarction in the thrombolytic era. *J Am Coll Cardiol* 1993;21:1419–1427.

23a. Rouleau JL, Talajic M, Sussex B et al: Myocardial infarction patients in the 1990s—their risk factors, stratification and survival in Canada: The Canadian Assessment of Myocardial Infarction (CAMI) Study. *J Am Coll Cardiol* 1996;27:1119–1127.

24. Odemuyiwa O, Farrell TG, Malik M, et al: Influence of age on the relation between heart rate variability, left ventricular ejection fraction, frequency of ventricular extrasystole and sudden death after myocardial infarction. *Br Heart J* 1992; 67:387–391.
25. Hamer A, Vohra J, Hunt D, Sloman G: Prediction of sudden death by electrophysiologic studies in high risk patients surviving acute myocardial infarction. *Am J Cardiol* 1982;50:223–229.
26. Richards DA, Cody DV, Denniss AR, et al: Ventricular electrical instability: A predictor of death after myocardial infarction. *Am J Cardiol* 1982;50: 223–229.
27. Marchlinski FE, Buxton AE, Waxman HL, Josephson ME: Identifying patients at risk of sudden death after myocardial infarction: Value of the response to programmed stimulation, degree of ventricular ectopic activity and severity of left ventricular dysfunction. *Am J Cardiol* 1983;52: 1190–1196.
28. Roy D, Marchand E, Theroux P, et al: Programmed ventricular stimulation in survivors of an acute myocardial infarction. *Circulation* 1985;72:487–494.
29. Santarelli P, Bellocci F, Loperfido F, et al: Ventricular arrhythmia induced by programmed ventricular stimulation after acute myocardial infarction. *Am J Cardiol* 1985;55:391–394.
30. Breithardt G, Borggrefe M, Haerten K: Role of programmed ventricular stimulation and noninvasive recording of ventricular late potentials for the identification of patients at risk of ventricular tachyarrhythmias after acute myocardial infarction, in Zipes DP, Jalife J (eds): *Cardiac Electrophysiology and Arrhythmias.* New York, Grune & Stratton, 1985, pp 553–561.
31. Denniss AR, Richards DA, Cody DV, et al: Prognostic significance of ventricular tachycardia and fibrillation induced at programmed stimulation and delayed potentials detected on the signal-averaged electrocardiograms of survivors of acute myocardial infarction. *Circulation* 1986;74:731–745.
32. Bhandari AK, Hong R, Kotlewski A, et al: Prognostic significance of programmed ventricular stimulation in survivors of acute myocardial infarction. *Br Heart J* 1989;61:410–416.

33. Waspe LE, Seinfeld D, Ferrick A, et al: Prediction of sudden death and spontaneous ventricular tachycardia in survivors of complicated myocardial infarction: Value of the response to programmed stimulation using a maximum of three ventricular extra stimuli. *J Am Coll Cardiol* 1985;5:1292–1301.
34. Cripps T, Bennett ED, Camm AJ, Ward DE: Inducibility of sustained monomorphic ventricular tachycardia as a prognostic variable. *J Am Coll Cardiol* 1989;14:289–296.
35. Bhandari AK, Widerhorn J, Sager PT, et al: Prognostic significance of programmed ventricular stimulation in patients surviving complicated acute myocardial infarction: A prospective study. *Am Heart J* 1992;124:87–96.
36. Richards D, Byth K, Ross D, Uther J: What is the best predictor of spontaneous sustained ventricular tachycardia and sudden death of the myocardial infarction? *Circulation* 1991;83:756–763.
37. Bourke JP, Richards DA, Ross DL, et al: Routine programmed electrical stimulation in survivors of acute myocardial infarction for prediction of spontaneous ventricular tachyarrhythmias during follow up: Results optimal stimulation protocol and cost effective screening. *J Am Coll Cardiol* 1991;18:780–789.
38. Kosowsky BD, Taylor J, Lown B, et al: Long-term use of procainamide following acute myocardial infarction. *Circulation* 1973;47:1204–1210.
39. Collaborative Group: Phenytoin after recovery from myocardial infarction controlled trial in 568 patients. *Lancet* 1971;2:1055–1057.
40. Peter T, Ross D, Duffield A, et al: Effect on survival after myocardial infarction of long-term treatment with phenytoin. *Br Heart J* 1978;40:1356–1360.
41. Bastian BC, Macfarlane PW, McLauchlan JH, et al: A prospective randomized trial of tocainide in patients following myocardial infarction. *Am Heart J* 1980;100:1017–1022.
42. Ryden L, Arnman K, Conradson TB, et al: Prophylaxis of ventricular tachyarrhythmias with intravenous and oral tocainide in patients with and recovering from acute myocardial infarction. *Am Heart J* 1980;100:1006–1012.
43. Chamberlain DA, Jewitt DE, Julian DG, et al: Oral mexiletine in high-risk patients after myocardial infarction. *Lancet* 1980;2:1324–1327.
44. IMPACT Research Group: International mexiletine and placebo antiarrhythmic coronary trial: Report on arrhythmia and other findings. *J Am Coll Cardiol* 1984;6:1148–1163.
45. Gottlieb SM, Achuff SC, Mellits ED, et al: Prophylactic antiarrhythmic therapy of high risk survivors of myocardial infarction: Lower mortality at 1 month but not at 1 year. *Circulation* 1987;75:792–799.
46. The Cardiac Arrhythmia Pilot Study (CAPS) investigators: Effects of encainide, flecainide, imipramine and moricizine on ventricular arrhythmias during the year after acute myocardial infarction: The CAPS. *Am J Cardiol* 1988;61:501–509.
47. The Cardiac Arrhythmia Suppression Trial (CAST) Investigators Preliminary Report: Effect of encainide and flecainide on mortality in a randomized trial of arrhythmia suppression after myocardial infarction. *N Engl J Med* 1989;321:406–412.
48. The Cardiac Arrhythmia Suppression Trial II Investigators: Effect of the antiarrhythmic agent moricizine on survival after acute myocardial infarction. *N Engl J Med* 1992;327:227–233.
49. Frishman WH, Furberg CD, Friedewald WT: Beta-adrenergic blockade for survivors of acute myocardial infarction. *N Eng J Med* 1984;321:406–412.
50. Furberg CD, Hawkins M, Lichstin E, et al: Effect of propranolol in postinfarction patients with mechanical or electrical complications. *Circulation* 1984;69:761–765.
51. Bukart F, Pfisterer M, Klowski W, Follath F, Burkhardt D: Effect of antiarrhythmic therapy on mortality in survivors of myocardial infarction with asymptomatic complex ventricular arrhythmias: Basal Antiarrhythmic Study of Infarct Survival (BASIS). *J Am Coll Cardiol* 1990;16:1711–1718.
52. Pfisterer M, Klowski W, Burkhardt D, Follath F, Burkart F: Longterm benefit of a 1 year amiodarone treatment for persistent complex ventricular arrhythmias after myocardial infarction. *Circulation* 1993;87:309–311.
53. Pfisterer ME, Klowski W, Burkhardt D, et al: Beneficial effect of amiodarone on cardiac mortality in patients with asymptomatic complex ventricular arrhythmias after acute myocardial infarction and preserved but not impaired left ventricular function. *Am J Cardiol* 1992;69:1399–1402.
54. Ceremuzynski L, Kleczar E, Krzeminskapalzula M, et al: Effects of amiodarone on mortality after myocardial infarction: A double-blind, placebo-controlled, pilot study. *J Am Coll Cardiol* 1992;20:1056–1062.
55. Cairns JA, Connolly SJ, Gent M, Roberts R: Post-myocardial infarction mortality in patients with ventricular premature depolarization: Canadian

Amiodarone Myocardial Infarction Arrhythmia Trial Pilot Study. *Circulation* 1991;84:550–557.

56. Marchlinski FE, Waxman HL, Buxton AE, et al: Sustained ventricular tachyarrhythmias during the early post-infarction period: Electrophysiologic findings and prognosis for survival. *J Am Coll Cardiol* 1983;2:240–250.

57. DiMarco JP, Lerman BBB, Kron IL, Sellers TD: Sustained ventricular tachyarrhythmias within 2 months of acute myocardial infarction: Results of medical and surgical therapy in patients resuscitated from the initial episode. *J Am Coll Cardiol* 1985;6:759–768.

58. Karagueuzian HS, Fenoglio JJ, Weiss MB, Wit AL: Protracted ventricular tachycardia induced by premature stimulation of the canine heart after coronary artery occlusion and reperfusion. *Circ Res* 1979;44:833–846.

59. El-Sherif M, Scherlag B, Lazzarra R, Hope RR: Reentrant ventricular arrhythmias in the late myocardial infarction period: I, Conduction characteristics in the infarction zone. *Circulation* 1977;55:686–702.

60. Fenoglio JJ, Phan TD, Harken AH, et al: Recurrent sustained ventricular tachycardia: Structure and ultrastructure of subendocardial regions in which tachycardia originates. *Circulation* 1983;68:518–533.

61. Spear JF, Horowitz LN, Hodess AB, et al: Cellular electrophysiology of human myocardial infarction: Abnormalities of cellular activation. *Circulation* 1979;59:247–256.

62. Ursell PC, Gardner PI, Albala A, et al: Structural and electrophysiological changes in the epicardial border zone of canine myocardial infarcts during infarct healing. *Circ Res* 1985;56:436–451.

63. Freidman PL, Fenoglio JJ, Wit AL: Time course for reversal of electrophysiological and ultrastructural abnormalities in subendocardial. Purkinje fibers surviving extensive myocardial infarction in dogs. *Circ Res* 1975;36:127–144.

64. Garan H, Ruskin J, McGovern B, Grant B: Serial analysis of electrically induced ventricular arrhythmias in a canine model of myocardial infarction. *J Am Coll Cardiol* 1985;5:1095–1106.

65. Bigger JT, Reiffel JA, Livelli FD, Wang PJ: Sensitivity, specificity and reproducibility of programmed ventricular stimulation. *Circulation* 1986;73(Suppl II): II-73–II-78.

66. Bhandari AK, Rahimtoola SH: Indications for intracardiac electrophysiologic testing in survivors of acute myocardial infarction. *Circulation* 1987;75 (Suppl III):III-166–III-168.

67. Denniss AR, Ross DL, Cody DV, et al: Randomized controlled trial of prophylactic antiarrhythmic therapy in patients with inducible ventricular tachyarrhythmias after recent myocardial infarction. *European Heart J* 1988;9:746–757.

67a. Gomes JA, Winters SL, Steward D, et al: A new non-invasive index to predict sustained ventricular tachycardia and sudden death in the first year after myocardial infarction: Based on signal averaged electrocardiogram, radionuclide ejection fraction and Holter monitoring. *J Am Coll Cardiol* 1987; 10:349–357.

68. Cobbe SM, Hoffman E, Ritzenhoff A, et al: Day to-day variations in inducibility of ventricular tachycardia during the late post myocardial infarction phase in conscious dogs. *Circulation* 1985;72: 200–204.

69. Kuck KH, Costard A, Schliiter M, Kunze KP: Significance of timing programmed ventricular stimulation after acute myocardial infarction. *J Am Coll Cardiol* 1986;8:1279–1288.

70. Bhandari A, Hong R, Kulick D, et al: Day-to-day reproducibility of response to programmed ventricular stimulation in patients with recent myocardial infarction. *J Am Coll Cardiol* 1990;15: 1075–1081.

71. Bhandari AK, Au PK, Rose JS, et al: Decline in inducibility of sustained ventricular tachycardia from two to twenty weeks after acute myocardial infarction. *Am J Cardiol* 1987;59:284–290.

72. Martin G, Kennedy JW: Thrombolytic therapy in the management of acute myocardial infarction: 2, Influence on mortality. *Mod Concepts Cardiovasc Dis* 1990;59:13–18.

73. Sager PT, Perlmutter RA, Rosenfeld LE, et al: The electrophysiologic effects of thrombolytic therapy in patients with a transmural anterior wall myocardial infarction complicated by left ventricular aneurysm formation. *J Am Coll Cardiol* 1988;12: 19–24.

74. Kersschot IE, Brugada P, Ramentol M, et al: Effects of early reperfusion in acute myocardial infarction on arrhythmias induced by programmed stimulation: A prospective randomized study. *J Am Coll Cardiol* 1986;7:1234–1242.

75. Bourke J, Young A, Richards D, Uther J: Reduction in incidence of inducible ventricular tachycardia of the myocardial infarction by treatment with

streptokinase during infarct evolution. *J Am Coll Cardiol* 1990;16:1703–1710.

76. McComb JM, Gold HK, Leinbach RC, et al: Electrically induced ventricular arrhythmias in acute myocardial infarction treated with thrombolytic agents. *Am J Cardiol* 1988;62:186–191.
77. Malik M, Camm AJ: Components of heart variability: What they really mean and what we really measure. *Am J Cardiol* 1993;72:821–822.
78. Ewing DJ, Neilson JMM, Travis P: New method for assessing cardiac parasympathetic activity using 24 hour electrocardiograms. *Br Heart J* 1984;52:396.
79. Costa O, Lago P, Rocha AP, et al: Heart rate variability in 24-hour Holter recordings. Comparative study between short- and long-term time and frequency domain analyses. *J Electrocardiol* 1994;27: 251–254.
80. Moser M, Lehofer M, Sedminek A, et al: Heart rate variability as a prognostic tool in cardiology. A contribution to the problem from a theoretical point of view. *Circulation* 1994;90:1078–82.
81. Schwartz PJ, Billman GE, Stone HL: Autonomic mechanisms in ventricular fibrillation induced by myocardial ischemia during exercise in dogs with healed myocardial infarction: An experimental preparation for sudden cardiac death. *Circulation* 1984;69:790.
82. Kleiger RE, Miller JP, Bigger JT, et al: Decreased heart rate variability and its association with increased mortality after acute myocardial infarction. *Am J Cardiol* 1987;59:256–262.
83. Bigger JT, Fleiss JL, Steinman RC, et al: Frequency domain measures of heart rate variability and mortality after acute myocardial infarction. *Circulation* 1992;85:164–171.
84. Bigger JT, Fleiss JL, Rolnitzky LM, Steinman RC: Frequency-domain measures of heart period variability to assess risk late after myocardial infarction. *J Am Coll Cardiol* 1993;21:729–736.
85. Farrell TG, Bashir Y, Cripps T, et al: Risk-stratification of arrhythmic events in post infarction patients based on heart rate variability ambulatory electrocardiographic variables and the signal-averaged electrocardiogram. *J Am Coll Cardiol* 1991;18:687–697.
86. ACC Position Statement by Cardiovascular Technology Assessment Committee: Heart rate variability for risk stratification of life threatening arrhythmias. *J Am Coll Cardiol* 1993;33:948–950.

28

The Prognostic Significance of the Signal Averaged Electrocardiogram in the Infarct Survivor

J. Anthony Gomes, MD

The mortality of patients with myocardial infarction (MI) after discharge from the hospital can be attributed to reinfarction with subsequent heart failure or arrhythmia, cardiac rupture, or primary ventricular tachyarrhythmia. Although sustained ventricular tachycardia degenerating into ventricular fibrillation has been shown to be the major cause of sudden cardiac death post–myocardial infarction, the exact mechanism that precipitates the arrhythmia has not been defined. Ischemia, the presence of an arrhythmic substrate (characterized by inhomogeneous and slow propagation of conduction) in scarred myocardium, and triggers such ventricular premature depolarizations preceded by a short–long cycle, have been implicated (1).

The natural history and prognosis of acute myocardial infarction has been substantially altered in recent years (2–13) (see Ch. 6). The use of thrombolytic therapy and beta-adrenergic blocking agents has resulted in a decline in the cardiac mortality post–myocardial infarction to 3–5% per annum (14) (see Ch. 31). However, mortality will continue to be high in certain subsets of patients—namely, those patients who do not undergo thrombolysis, those with large and multiple infarcts, those with a closed coronary artery, and those with late potentials, ventricular arrhythmias, and left ventricular dysfunction (15). Thus it is of clinical relevance to identify the patients at high risk, since appropriate preventive therapeutic modalities can be applied in this group of patients.

Risk stratification has been attempted with the use of a variety of clinical tests, noninvasive and invasive (16–23) (see Chs. 30–31). These have included 24-hour Holter monitoring to assess the frequency and characteristics of ventricular premature depolarizations (VPDs); heart rate variability, a measure of autonomic tone; exercise testing to assess the presence of ischemia; radionuclide angiography to determine the ejection fraction; coronary angiography to assess coronary anatomy; and programmed electrical stimulation for induction of ventricular tachyarrhythmias. Recently, the technique of signal averaging with high-gain application and filtering has been used to detect "late potentials" (24–33) in the terminal QRS complex or the ST segment, as a noninvasive test for risk stratification of patients post–myocardial infarction. This is an attractive noninvasive test for risk stratifying patients post–myocardial infarction, since the presence of late potentials on the signal-averaged electrocardiogram (ECG) is considered a noninvasive marker of the arrhythmic substrate. The purpose of this chapter is to discuss the technique of signal averaging to detect the presence of late potentials and its role as a predictor of a malignant arrhythmic event post–myocardial infarction.

TECHNIQUE OF SIGNAL AVERAGING

The QRS complex on the surface electrocardiogram is a reflection of the sum of the electrical activity due to depolarization of Purkinje elements and the ventricular myocardium. However, slow and inhomogeneous propagation of conduction in scarred myocardium is usually undetectable on the surface ECG because the voltage generated is of an amplitude too low to be detected there. These concealed low-amplitude electrical waveforms are clinically important, since slow and inhomogeneous conduction propagation is an important criterion for the occurrence of reentry. Furthermore, most clinically significant ventricular arrhythmias in the setting of a previous myocardial infarction are reentrant in origin. In humans, late potentials occurring in the terminal QRS complex or the ST segment of the ECG have been conventionally recorded by the use of intracardiac electrodes during cardiac catheterization or during intraoperative mapping. Over the last several years, their presence has been detected noninvasively by signal processing techniques (24–33).

The purpose of signal processing is to decrease random noise in the amplified ECG so as to enhance the detection of low-amplitude signals measuring a few microvolts. The primary source of noise is skeletal muscle activity, which measures 5 to 25 μV and cannot be eliminated by filtering because its frequency content is more than 25 Hz and similar to cardiac potentials. In ensemble averaging, sequential beats are averaged if they satisfy a template. A QRS detector provides a fiducial point to select a window that serves as a template. To reduce noise effectively, several conditions need to be met. These include the following. (i) The waveform of interest must be repetitive, such that multiple samples can be stacked to form an averaged waveform. Ventricular premature beats are excluded by comparing a new beat against a template of previous beats before averaging. (ii) The waveform of interest must have a fixed temporal relationship with a reference time that is the QRS complex, or the averaged waveform will be smoothed and high-frequency details will be lost. (iii) The noise has to be random in relationship to the signal of interest. To minimize contamination of the amplified ECG in this average, noise from skeletal muscle, electrodes, amplifiers, and power line interference is reduced to the square root of the number of beats averaged, improving the signal-to-noise (S/N) ratio. Averaging 100 to 400 beats will reduce noise by a factor of 10 to 20. Usually, averages of approximately 200 beats will yield noise levels of less than 1 μV. Signal averaging can be performed for a specific number of beats or a specific noise level. In our laboratory, signal averaging is performed for a noise level of less than or equal to 0.3 μV. After averaging, the signal-averaged QRS complex is filtered at corner frequencies of 25 to 80 Hz (high pass) and 250 Hz (low pass). Most laboratories use corner frequencies of 25 and/or 40 to 250 Hz. In our laboratory, high-pass filtering of 25 Hz as well as 40 Hz is used.

Various lead systems have been used for signal averaging, including precordial leads, orthogonal X, Y, Z leads, and the Frank leads. Although the best lead system with the highest sensitivity remains undefined, most laboratories use the orthogonal X, Y, Z lead systems. The signal-averaged QRS complex can be analyzed in the time-domain mode (i.e., voltage changes with time over a window of frequencies defined by filtering) or the frequency-domain mode performed by the Fourier transform (that is, amplitude versus frequencies). In the frequency domain the signal is mathematically decomposed into fundamental and harmonic frequencies. It remains unclear which of these two methods of analysis is optimal for analyzing the signal-averaged ECG. Because most studies in patients with myocardial infarction have used time-domain analysis, only this method of analysis will be discussed henceforth.

QUANTITATIVE ANALYSIS OF THE SIGNAL-AVERAGED ELECTROCARDIOGRAM IN THE TIME-DOMAIN MODE

The vector magnitude (Fig. 28–1) of the X, Y, and Z is used for quantitative analysis of the signal-

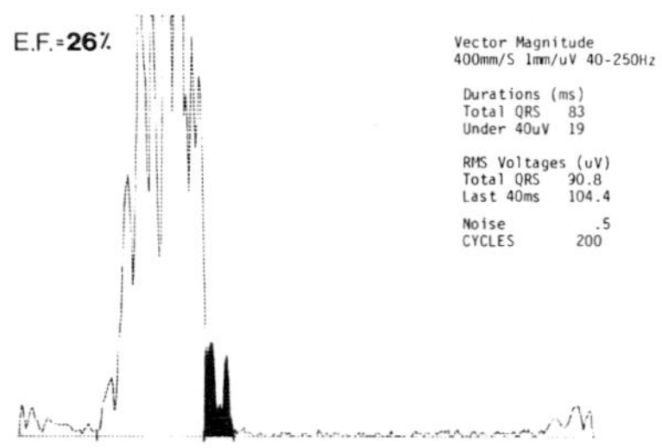

Figure 28–1. Normal vector magnitude in a patient with a previous myocardial infarction and depressed ejection fraction. The vector magnitude is filtered at 40–250 Hz. The dark area shows the duration of low-amplitude signals of <40 μV. The quantitative, SA variables are all normal. The SA-QRS duration is 83 msec, the duration of low amplitude signals of <40 μV is 19 msec, and the RMS-40 is 104.4 μV.

averaged (SA) ECG utilizing the method of Simson (27). In this method, the end of the QRS complex is determined by a computer algorithm that measures the level of noise in the ST segment. The ST segment is then scanned retrogradely for a point where consecutive 5-msec segments yields a root mean square (RMS) voltage of greater than 2.5 times the noise level. This point defines the end of the QRS complex. The quantitative signal-averaged parameters measured on the vector magnitude include (i) the entire duration of the SA-QRS complex (SA-QRS); (ii) the RMS voltage of the terminal 40 msec (RMS-40); and (iii) the duration of the low-amplitude signals of <40 μV (LAS). These quantitative parameters depend on the high-pass filter selected for analysis. As the high-pass filter is increased in order from 25 to 80 Hz, there is a marked decrease in the RMS 40 values and an increase in duration of the LAS, whereas the duration of the SA-QRS is less filter dependent (34). Thus normal values for quantitative SA parameters will depend on the high-pass filter selected for analysis.

DEFINITION OF LATE POTENTIALS

The definition of what constitutes late potentials or what consitutes an abnormal SA-ECG is shown in Table 28–1 (27,29,34,35). At 40-Hz high-pass filtering, an abnormal SA-ECG or the presence of late potentials is considered if one or more of the following three quantitative criteria are met: (i) the filtered QRS complex is greater than 114 to 120 msec (34,35); (ii) the duration of LAS is >38 msec (34); (iii) the RMS-40 is <20 μV (34,35). However, the predictive value of these variables depends on how they are used to define an abnormal SA-ECG. Whereas the RMS-40 is the most sensitive parameter, it is the less specific for predicting an arrhythmic event. In contrast, the duration of the SA-QRS complex has a lower sensitivity but the best specificity. Studies in our laboratory using Cox analysis have shown that the duration of the SA-QRS is the most significant independent variable in predicting an arrhythmic event in post–MI patients when a total of 27 clinical and noninvasive variables were compared (36). Additionally, our studies have also indicated that the combination of the SA-QRS and RMS-40 provides the highest positive predictive value when compared with the three variables used singly or in combination (36). We therefore believe that a late potential should be defined as a filtered QRS ≥ 114 msec and RMS-40 of <20 μV in the absence of bundle branch block. No criterion has yet been established in the presence of bundle branch block. In addition to quantitative assessment of the SA-ECG, a qualitative assessment needs to be done, since late potentials of very low amplitude (i.e., <2.5 times the noise level) are identified often as noise, giving a false reading of the end of the QRS complex and of the quantitative parameters (37).

Table 28–1. Abnormal Signal-Averaged Parameters at 25 and 40 Hz

Author	High-Pass Filtering	SA-QRS	LAS	RMS_{40}
Simson et al (27)	25 Hz	>110	—	<25 μV
Gomes et al (30)	25 Hz	>114	32 msec	<25 μV
Gomes et al (30)	40 Hz	>114	38 msec	<20 μV
Kuchar et al (35)	40 Hz	>120	—	<20 μV

ELECTROPHYSIOLOGIC BASIS OF LATE POTENTIALS

Studies in experimental myocardial infarction have shown that fragmented electrograms can be recorded from infarcted myocardium outlasting the QRS complex, and that the onset and the maintenance of ventricular tachycardia (VT) depends on continuous electrical activity in diastole (38,39). Fragmented electrograms occur in areas of chronic infarcts with surviving Purkinje muscle elements interspersed with connective tissue (40). Fragmentation of electrograms recorded from chronic infarcts are thought to represent asynchronous electrical activation of surviving muscle bundles. Microelectrode studies have revealed that fragmentation of electrograms is due to increased coupling resistance between surviving myocardial fibers (40). These changes would occur when muscle bundles do not have electrically tight connections. Late potentials recorded from the body surface by signal averaging originate from scarred myocardium with delayed, inhomogeneous propagation of conduction.

Berbari and coworkers (24) were the first to record delayed epicardial activation in the canine heart on the body surface with signal processing. Subsequently, Simson et al (42) found that late potentials detected on the body surface correlated with delayed, fragmented electrical activity recorded from endocardial sites. They also demonstrated that for late potentials to be detected on the body surface, fragmented activity needs to outlast normal ventricular activation. Removal of the arrhythmic substrate by endocardial resection abolishes late potentials, and this usually correlates with noninducibility of ventricular tachycardia in man. Thus the concept that the presence of late potentials is a noninvasive marker of the arrhythmic substrate has been rather well established. However, one must understand that the presence of an arrhythmic substrate should not be automatically equated with the occurrence of a sustained tachyarrhythmia, since other electrophysiologic characteristics such as differential refractoriness are equally important in maintaining a tachycardia. Furthermore, ischemia, autonomic factors, electrolyte disturbances, and other triggers, some of which are still undefined, may play a role in the final arrhythmic event that precipitates ventricular fibrillation (see Ch. 14). Additionally, it is important to keep in perspective that an arrhythmic substrate may indeed remain dormant, protected by entrance or exit block.

MORPHOLOGICAL CHARACTERISTICS OF LATE POTENTIALS

Late potentials usually occur in the terminal part of the QRS complex. Atypically, however, late potentials are seen late in the ST segment. These have been referred to as "late" late potentials (37). We have qualitatively analyzed signal-averaged ECGs in 48 patients with spontaneous and inducible ventricular tachycardia post—myocardial infarction. In this study, late potentials could be categorized into three morphological subtypes. Type 1 late potentials were usually seen in the setting of a broad QRS complex of more than 110 msec, were of higher amplitude, were confined to the terminal QRS complex, and occurred in 40% of patients. Type 2 late potentials (Fig. 28–2) were detected prior to the end of the QRS complex, similar to type 1, but extended into the ST segment and occurred in 33% of patients. Type 3 late potentials (Fig. 28–3) were noted to begin after the end of the surface QRS complex, were of extremely low amplitude, usually of a peak amplitude of less than 2 μV, and extended substantially beyond the QRS complex for as much as 61 ± 27 msec (Fig. 28–3).

Computer algorithms to assess quantitative variables underestimated the duration of low-amplitude signals by 20 to 72.5 msec and often missed type 3 late potentials. We found no significant correlation between the three types of late potentials and clinical features such as site of myocardial infarction, the rate of induced ventricular tachycardia, and so forth. Thus our findings suggest that the anatomic and geometric characteristics of the arrhythmic substrate probably define the three types of late potentials. Since type 3 late potentials are often missed by computer algorithm based on noise, they may be misclassified as normal and therefore are more suited for qualitative analysis.

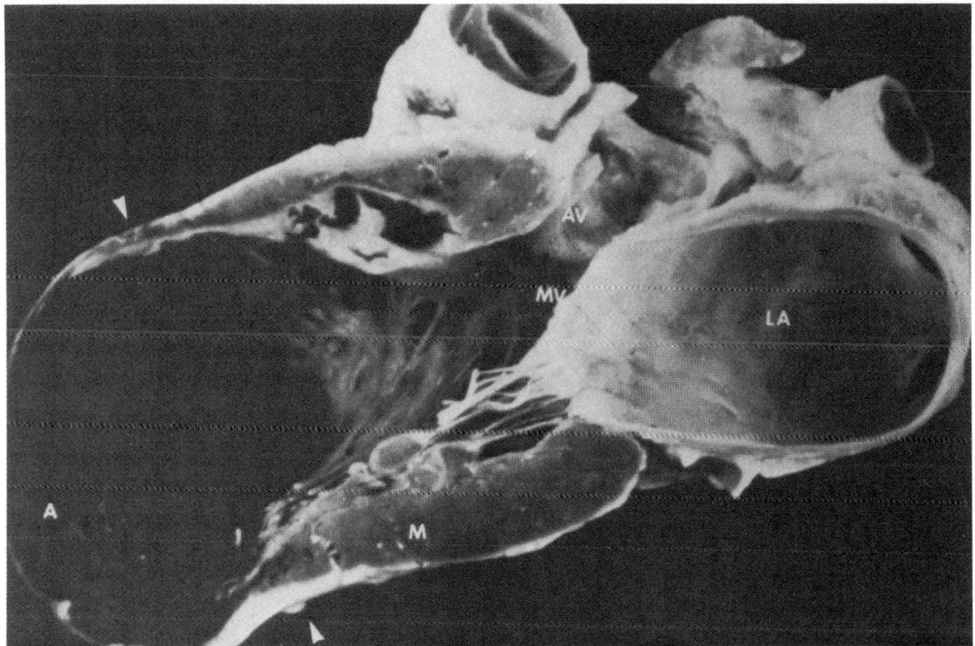

Figure 28–2. Vector magnitude showing type 2 late potentials in a patient with out-of-hospital sudden death following an inferoposterior infarct. The dark area shows the duration of low-amplitude signals of <40 μV. Note that all three quantitative variables are abnormal. The duration of the SA-QRS is 164 msec, the duration of low-amplitude signals of <40 μV is 82 msec, and the RMS-40 is 8.8 μV. The late potentials started before the end of the QRS complex and extended into the ST segment (type 2).

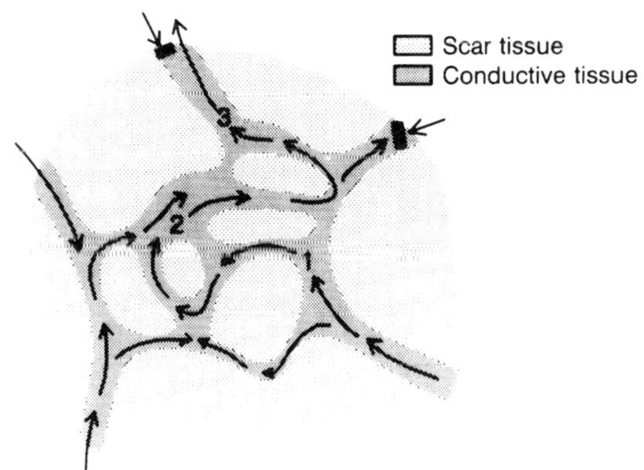

Figure 28–3. Vector magnitude showing the presence of type 3 late potentials. The open area shows the end of the QRS complex as determined by the computer algorithm. The dark arrow shows the end of the QRS complex determined qualitatively. The slanted arrows show the late potentials in the ST segment. At both 25 and 40 Hz, the late potentials commence after the end of the QRS complex (not shown) on the amplified, unfiltered ECG-QRS complex. Note that the quantitative variables assessed by computer significantly underestimate the quantitative variables assessed qualitatively.

PREVALENCE OF LATE POTENTIALS FOLLOWING MYOCARDIAL INFARCTION

The prevalence of late potentials following a myocardial infarction has ranged from 24% to 52%. This variability is related to substantial interstudy differences such as time of recording following an acute myocardial infarction, recording technique, and definition of late potentials. McGuire and coworkers (43) reported the incidence of late potentials in the first 10 days of myocardial infarction. In this study, late potentials were defined by the SA-QRS complex being >120 msec in duration or the RMS-40 being <20 μV at 40-Hz high-pass filtering. They found late potentials in 32% of patients on day 1 and in 52% of patients 7–10 days postinfarction. The incidence of late potentials will strongly depend on the definition used. In a study of 115 patients (36) who had signal averaging performed 10 ± 6 days post–myocardial infarction, the

RMS-40 was found to be abnormal in 35% of patients, the SA-QRS complex was abnormal in 23% of patients, and the duration of LAS was abnormal in 30% of patients at 40-Hz high-pass filtering. If late potentials were defined as one or more abnormal quantitative parameters, then 42% of patients had late potentials; if by two or more abnormal parameters, 27% had late potentials. If the duration of the SA-QRS complex and an abnormal RMS-40 were used jointly to define late potentials, only 14% had late potentials. It is clear from this study that the predictive value of late potentials will depend on the variables used to define the abnormality.

Several studies (43,44) have also observed time-dependent changes in the SA-ECG following acute myocardial infarction. Whereas an initial normal SA-ECG rarely becomes abnormal, approximately 16% of abnormal recordings became normal at 6 weeks and 30% at 1 year when compared with recordings obtained just prior to discharge. These changes are likely related to healing and remodeling of the myocardial infarct.

The prevalence of late potentials also depends on the site of myocardial infarction (36). The incidence of late potentials defined as at least one quantitative variable being abnormal was 56% in patients with inferior or inferior-posterior infarcts, as compared with 27% in patients with anterior or anteroseptal infarcts. These observations are likely related to differences in activation timing of the inferior-posterior segments of the left ventricle, which have a paucity of Purkinje fibers relative to the anteroseptal and anterior segments of the left ventricle.

RELATIONSHIP BETWEEN THE SIGNAL-AVERAGED ECG, WALL MOTION ABNORMALITIES, LEFT VENTRICULAR EJECTION FRACTION, AND 24-HOUR HOLTER MONITORING

Some previous studies have noted a good correlation between the presence of late potentials and wall motion abnormalities in patients with coronary artery disease. Observations in 50 patients post–acute myocardial infarction have found no significant correlation between the presence of late potentials and wall motion abnormalities. In this study (45), signal averaging of the surface QRS complex and radionuclide ventriculography was performed in 50 patients within 8 ± 5 days of the index infarction. A wall motion score was constructed according to the method of Hecht and Hopkins (46) and Currie et al (47). Both the right and left ventricles were divided into a total of 21 segments in the anterior, left anterior-oblique, and lateral views. Wall motion was subsequently scored as normal segment = 4, hypokinesis = 3, akinesis = 2, and dyskinesis = 1. Consequently, a normal segment had the highest score, and a dyskinetic segment had the lowest score. A patient with normal right and left ventricles would have a total score of 84. The incidence of dyskinesis, akinesis, hypokinesis, and normal wall motion was also assessed. No significant differences in distribution of wall motion abnormalities in patients with and without late potentials were found (Table 28–2). The total wall motion scores for the left ventricle and the right ventricle and the combined wall motion scores were not significantly different in patients with and in those without late potentials. These findings suggest that the type and degree of wall motion abnormality is not the source of late potentials in patients post–MI. Rather, it is possible that the likely source of late potentials in these patients is the amount of viable myocardium in the infarct area or the peri-infarct area, thus resulting in regional slow ventricular activation.

A lack of correlation between late potentials and left ventricular ejection fraction has also been shown. In a study (36) of 110 patients post–myocardial infarction in whom a signal-averaged ECG and radionuclide ventriculography were obtained within

Table 28–2. Left Ventricular Wall Motion Abnormalities in Patients With and Without Late Potentials

	Dyskinesis	Akinesis	N/H
LP(+)	57%	29%	14%
LP(−)	62%	10%	14%
p value	n.s.	n.s.	n.s.

N/H = normal or hypokinetic

Modified from Gomes et al (45), with permission of the American Journal of Cardiology.

10 ± 6 days of the MI, patients with late potentials had similar ejection fractions compared with patients with a normal SA-ECG. Furthermore, no significant correlation was found between any of the signal-averaged quantitative parameters and the ejection fraction.

Of substantial prognostic value is the observation that ejection fraction and the SA-ECG reveal opposing information in relation to the site of myocardial infarction (36). A significantly higher proportion of patients with an inferior wall MI have late potentials compared with patients with an anterior wall MI (56% vs. 27%). On the other hand, a significantly higher number of patients with an anterior wall MI have an abnormal ejection fraction dichotomized as less than 40% compared with patients with an inferior or inferior-posterior wall MI (66% vs. 32%). Thus the predictive value of these two tests will depend on the site of myocardial infarction.

A lack of correlation has been noted between the signal averaged ECG and the presence or absence of high-grade ventricular ectopy following myocardial infarction. In a prospective study (36) of 94 patients post–MI, an SA-ECG as well as 24-hour Holter was done within 10 ± 6 days of the infarction. No relationship was noted between the presence or absence of late potentials, and the frequency or the characteristics of ventricular premature depolarizations. Similar observations have also been reported by Kuchar and coworkers (35). In a more recent study by El Sherif and coworkers (48), serial recordings of the SA-ECG and 24-hour Holter monitoring were done in 156 patients with acute MI at ≤5 days (phase 1), 6–30 days (phase 2), and 31–60 days (phase 3) after the infarction. They found that the incidence of complex ventricular arrhythmias on the Holter monitor was 35% in the first 5 days after infarction, was 29% 6–30 days after infarction, and substantially increased in the second month postinfarction to 43%. In contrast, the incidence of an abnormal SA-ECG was 17% in phase 1, 25% in phase 2, and then decreased in phase 3 to 18%. Thus time-dependent changes in the SA-ECG were discordant with those noted on a 24-hour Holter monitor. The findings discussed here suggest that late potentials, ejection fraction, and the frequency and characteristics of VPDs on a Holter monitor following a myocardial infarction are independent of each other.

PROGNOSTIC SIGNIFICANCE OF LATE POTENTIALS IN PATIENTS POST–MYOCARDIAL INFARCTION

In recent years several prospective follow-up studies (Table 28–3) have assessed the prognostic significance of the signal-averaged ECG following myocardial infarction (see Ch. 31). A total of seven large prospective studies (35,36,48–52) comprised a total of 1,750 patients, who were studied anywhere from 6 days to as much as 6 weeks post–MI. Although the methods of defining late potentials and the recording techniques varied among studies, all reported significant differences in event rates defined as sustained ventricular tachycardia or the occurrence of sudden cardiac death in patients with,

Table 28–3. Prospective Studies of the Significance of Late Potentials Post–Myocardial Infarction

Authors	# of pts	LP+	LP−	Method of Analysis	Follow-up	Event Rate LP+	Event Rate LP−	*p* value
Breithardt et al (49)	511	193(38%)	315(62%)	Qualitative	18 ± 13 mos	41(21.2%)	11(4%)	<0.02
Deniss et al (50)	306	80(26%)	226(74%)	Qualitative	12 mos	15(19%)	8(4%)	<0.001
Kuchar et al (35)	200	78(39%)	122(61%)	Quantitative	14 mos	13(17%)	1(1%)	<0.001
Gomes et al (36)	115	48(42%)	67(58%)	Quantitative	14 ± 8 mos	13(27%)	3(4%)	<0.001
Cripps et al (51)	159	38(24%)	121(76%)	Quantitative	12 ± 6 mos	10(26%)	1(1%)	<0.001
El Sherif et al (48)	156	39(25%)	117(75%)	Quantitative	12 mos	9(23%)	3(3%)	<0.001
Pedretti et al (52)	303	77(27%)	226(67%)	Quantitative	15 ± 7 mos	12(16%)	7(2%)	<0.001
Total	1,750	553(32%)	1,197(68%)	—	14 mos	113(21%)	34(3%)	

LP = late potentials.

as compared with patients without, late potentials. Of the 1,750 patients, 32% had late potentials and 68% did not. For a mean follow-up period of 14 months, 21% of patients with late potentials had an arrhythmic event, in contrast to 4% of patients without late potentials. For details of the individual studies, see Table 28–3.

The predictive value of the signal-averaged ECG has been found to depend on the quantitative variable used to define late potentials, on high-pass filtering, and on the site of myocardial infarction. In a study of 115 patients in whom the SA-ECG was obtained within 10 ± 6 days post–MI, 16 patients had an arrhythmic event during a follow-up period of 14 ± 8 months. In this study, the sensitivity of late potentials for predicting an arrhythmic event was better at 40-Hz high-pass filtering in comparison with 25-Hz high-pass filtering (Table 28–4) (45). Also, it was noted that the sensitivity and specificity of the SA-ECG depended on the quantitative variable. When an abnormal SA-ECG was defined as at least one abnormal quantitative variable, the sensitivity for predicting an arrhythmic event was 81% and the specificity was 65% at 40-Hz high-pass filtering. When it was defined as at least two variables, the sensitivity was 69% and the specificity was 80%. If the presence of late potentials was defined as the occurrence of a prolonged QRS duration as well as an abnormal voltage in the terminal 40 msec (SA-QRS & RMS_{40}) then the specificity increased markedly to 95% but the sensitivity declined to 56%. However, this combination provided the highest positive predictive value of 58%.

The independent prognostic value of late potentials following a myocardial infarction has been reported in several large prospective studies. In a study by Kuchar et al (35), an abnormal signal-averaged ECG (defined as the presence of RMS-40 of less than 20 μV or a filtered QRS duration greater than 120 msec at 40-Hz high-pass filtering) and ejection fraction were related to the occurrence of an arrhythmic event on multivariate regression analysis. In this study, the frequency and characteristics of VPDs on a 24-hour Holter were not independently related to an event. Another study (53) done in 102 patients following myocardial infarction showed that ejection fraction, the presence of late potentials on the SA-ECG (defined as any one abnormal quantitative parameter), and the presence of nonsustained ventricular tachycardia on a 24-hour Holter monitor were independently related to an arrhythmic event when assessed in the Cox survivorship analysis. Subsequently, the prognostic value of 27 clinical and noninvasive variables, including quantitative signal-averaged vari-

Table 28–4. Relationship Between Quantitative SA Variables and Arrhythmic Event Rates Post–Myocardial Infarction

Event Rate (%)				
SA Variables (25 Hz)	Abnormal	Normal	Sn	Sp
SA-QRS duration	10/26	6/89	63	84
LAS	12/33	4/82	75	78
RMS-40	9/31	7/84	56	78
≥1 variable	12/51	4/64	75	61
≥2 variables	10/26	6/89	62	84
SA-QRS & RMS-40	8/16	8/99	50	92
SA Variables (40 Hz)				
SA-QRS duration	10/26	6/89	63	84
LAS	11/34	5/81	69	77
RMS-40	13/40	3/75	81	73
≥1 variable	13/48	3/67	81	65
≥2 variables	11/31	5/84	69	80
SA-QRS & RMS-40	9/16	7/99	56	95

LP = late potentials, SA-QRS = signal-averaged QRS complex, LAS = low-amplitude signals (<40 μV), RMS-40 = root mean square voltage of the terminal 40 msec. Sn = sensitivity, Sp = specificity.

Modified from Gomes et al (36), with permission of the American College of Cardiology.

ables determined at 25-Hz and at 40-Hz high-pass filtering, were assessed by the Cox hazards model in a total of 115 patients (36). This study showed that the total duration of the signal-averaged QRS complex at 40-Hz high-pass filtering, followed by couplets and ejection fraction, had the most significant relationship to the development of an arrhythmic event following MI. This study concluded that the duration of the signal-averaged QRS complex is the most important single variable relative to other clinical variables, findings of a 24-hour Holter monitor, and ejection fraction. Whereas the reason for this remains unclear, it is possible that an abnormal duration of the signal-averaged QRS complex reflects a greater mass of ventricular myocardium with inhomogeneous propagation of conduction. This subsequently could favor the occurrence of reentrant ventricular tachyarrhythmias and ventricular fibrillation. El-Sherif et al (54), writing for the Cardiac Arrhythmia Suppression Trial (CAST) Investigators, have reported similar findings. In CAST, a total of 1,958 patients without bundle branch block were followed for a total of 10.3 ± 3.2 months; 45 patients had a serious arrhythmic event. A Cox regression analysis including the six signal-averaged parameters at 25 and 40 Hz indicated that filtered QRS duration, at 40 Hz, ≥120 msec was the most predictive for arrhythmic events. The QRS duration, 40 Hz, ≥120 msec was the most significant predictor ($p < 0.0001$) in a regression analysis that included clinical, Holter, and ejection fraction variables. The positive, negative, total predictive accuracy, and odds ratio for QRS, 40 Hz, ≥120 msec were 17%, 98%, 88%, and 8.4, respectively.

PREDICTIVE VALUE OF LATE POTENTIALS AND EJECTION FRACTION RELATIVE TO THE SITE OF MYOCARDIAL INFARCTION

Since the incidence of late potentials and abnormal ejection fraction depends on the site of myocardial infarction, as previously discussed, clearly the predictive value of these two noninvasive variables will depend on the site of myocardial infarction (55) (see Ch. 31). To assess this, a total of 99 patients were studied, of which 50 had anterior wall MI and 49 had inferior wall MI. Of the 99 patients, 35 patients (group I) had an arrhythmic event, that is, documented sustained ventricular tachycardia and/or sudden cardiac death, ≥8 days and ≤24 months following the myocardial infarction. The remaining 62 patients (group II) had no arrhythmic events for ≤24 months post–MI. These patients were used as controls. In this study, the presence of late potentials was defined as one or more abnormal signal-averaged parameters being present (late potential 1 [LP1]), or as an abnormal signal-averaged QRS duration in combination with an abnormal RMS-40 (late potential Z [LP2]). An abnormal ejection fraction was dichotomized as less than 40% (LVEF1) or as less than or equal to 30% (LVEF2). The ejection fractions were obtained by radionuclide ventriculography.

The presence of late potentials in patients with and without sustained ventricular tachycardia in relation to site of myocardial infarction is shown in Fig. 28–4. As can be seen, there is a significant difference between the incidence of LP1 or LP2 in patients with sustained ventricular tachycardia in the setting of an anterior wall MI, in contrast to patients without sustained ventricular tachycardia. Similarly, there is a significantly higher incidence of the presence of LP1 as well as LP2 in patients with an inferior wall MI in the presence of sustained ventricular tachycardia in contrast to those without ventricular tachycardia. However, the incidence of LP1 is about 58% in patients with anterior wall MI, whereas it is about 95% in patients with inferior

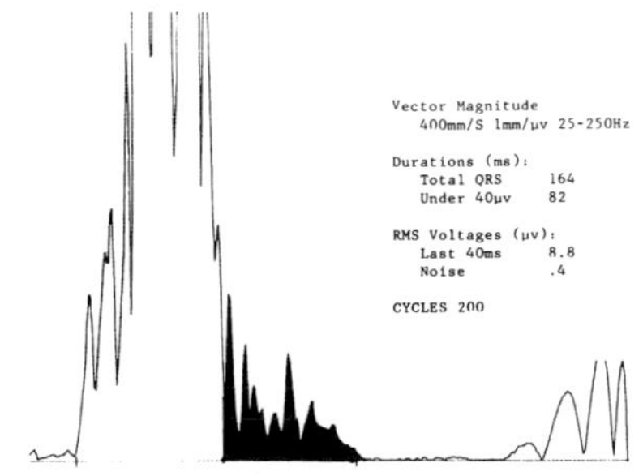

Figure 28–4. Bar graphs showing the prevalence of late potentials in patients with and without VTs relative to the site of myocardial infarction. For further explanation, see text.

wall MI. The incidence of LP1 in patients with anterior wall MI but without sustained ventricular tachycardia is only 18%, whereas it is 45% in patients without ventricular tachycardia but with an inferior wall MI. When looking at LP2, again the incidence of late potentials in anterior wall MI in the setting of sustained ventricular tachycardia was only about 44%. In contrast, the incidence of LP2 in patients without ventricular tachycardia in the setting of an anterior wall MI was only about 8%. In patients with an inferior wall MI and sustained ventricular tachycardia, LP2 occurred in about 85% of patients. In contrast, LP2 was present in only 20% of patients without sustained ventricular tachycardia and inferior wall MI.

A significant difference was noted between the presence of LVEF1 in patients with anterior wall myocardial infarction and sustained ventricular tachycardia, in contrast to those without sustained ventricular tachycardia (Fig. 28–5). Whereas 100% of patients with an anterior wall MI and sustained ventricular tachycardia had LVEF1, 60% of patients without ventricular tachycardia but an anterior wall MI also had LVEF1. Approximately 70% of patients with an inferior wall MI with ventricular tachycardia had LVEF1, whereas only about 30% of patients with an inferior wall MI but without ventricular tachycardia had LVEF1 (Fig. 28–5). LVEF2 was seen in about 85% of patients with anterior wall MI and sustained ventricular tachycardia, in contrast to about 30% of patients without ventricular tachycardia. No significant difference was found in LVEF2 in patients with and without sustained ventricular tachycardia in the setting of an inferior wall MI (Fig. 28–5).

Thus the sensitivity and specificity and predictive values of LP1 and LP2 and an abnormal LVEF depended strongly on the site of myocardial infarction, as shown in Table 28–5. Whereas LVEF1 and LVEF2 has a very high sensitivity in patients with anterior wall MI for predicting an arrhythmic event, their specificities are both lower than those of late potentials. Thus the positive predictive value of late potentials, both LP1 and LP2, is higher than that of the ejection fraction, whereas the negative predictive value of the ejection fraction is much higher than that of LP1 and LP2. Thus, in patients with anterior and anteroseptal wall MI, an abnormal ejection fraction should carry a higher weight than the absence of late potentials. On the other hand, the presence of late potentials should be given a higher weight when ejection fraction is normal. In inferior wall MI, the sensitivity of late potentials is extremely high, 94% for LP1; however, the specificity of LP1 is very low, namely 47%. LP2 has both a relatively good sensitivity of 82% and twice the specificity of LP1 at 84%. Thus, in infe-

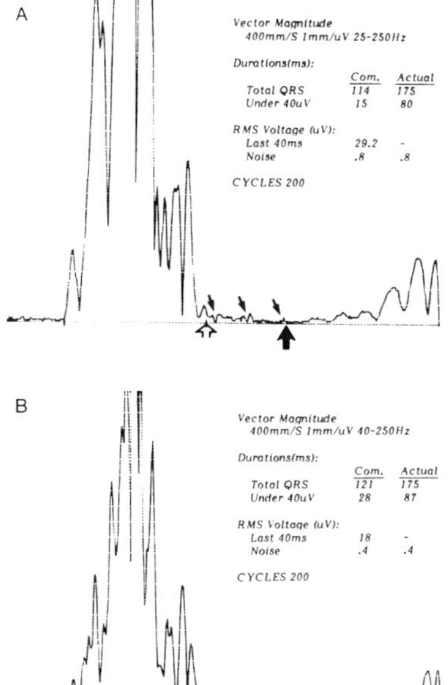

Figure 28–5. Bar graphs showing the presence of an abnormal ejection fraction relative to the site of myocardial infarction. For further explanation, see text.

Table 28–5. The Sensitivity, Specificity, and Predictive Value of LP1, LP2, and LVEF

	AWMI		IWMI	
	LP1	LP2	LP1	LP2
Sn	56%	39%	94%	82%
Sp	84%	94%	47%	84%
+Pv	67%	78%	48%	74%
−Pv	77%	73%	94%	90%

LP = late potentials, LVEF = left ventricular ejection fraction, Sn = sensitivity, Sp = specificity, Pv = predictive value, AWMI = anterior wall myocardial infarction, IWMI = inferior wall myocardial infarction.

rior wall MI, LP2 is superior for predicting an arrhythmic event than LP1. It is clear from this study that in patients post–anterior wall MI, LP2 has a higher positive predictive value than LP1, LVEF1, and LVEF2. However, both LVEF1 and LVEF2 have the best negative predictive values. In patients post–inferior wall MI, LP2 has a higher positive predictive value than LP1, LVEF1, LVEF2, and as good a negative predictive value as LP1. Thus the significance of late potentials and left ventricular ejection fraction in predicting malignant arrhythmic events and recommending electrophysiologic studies should be appraised in the context of the site of the myocardial infarction.

NONINVASIVE INDEX FOR PREDICTING VENTRICULAR ARRHYTHMIAS

The signal-averaged ECG, ejection fraction, results of 24-hour Holter monitoring, and heart rate variability have been assessed in combination to risk stratify patients post–myocardial infarction in several recent prospective studies (44, 48, 52–54). These invasive algorithms, which combine tests, assume importance because individual tests have a low positive predictive value for arrhythmic mortality. The results of six large studies comprising a total of 1,859 patients followed for a 10 to 16 months post–MI are listed in Table 28–6. In most of these studies, the SA-ECG was considered as abnormal if at least one variable was abnormal. A 24 hour Holter monitor was considered as abnormal if there were more than 10 VPDs per hour and or couplets and/or triplets. An ejection fraction was considered as abnormal if it was <40%. Multivariate analysis found that the SA-ECG, the duration of the filtered QRS couplex, complex ventricular arrhythmias on 24-hour Holter monitoring, ejection fraction, and an abnormal heart rate variability were independent predictors of arrhythmic events. These studies found that the combination of two or more abnormal variable was associated with a higher arrhythmic event rate than a single abnormal variable. Thus the combination of late potential (LP) and ejection fraction (EF) provided a positive predicted value of 34%. Patients' who had LP, abnormal EF, and abnormal Holter had event rate of 28–57%; in contrast, only 2% of patients without this abnormality had an event. Farrell and coworkers (56) used a combination of abnormal heart rate variability, LPs, and repetitive forms on the Holter. This combination provided a positive predictive value of 58% and a negative predictive value of 95%. Pedretti and coworkers (52) combined an abnormal EF with two or more runs of nonsustained VT and a filtered SA-QRS duration of ≥106 msec. They obtained a positive predictive value of 44% and a negative predictive value of 99%.

These noninvasive algorithms have more recently been used to select patients for invasive stimulation studies. Pedretti et al (52) used the algorithm that combined LP, Holter, and LVEF as originally proposed by Gomes et al (53) to select patients for programmed ventricular stimulation post–myocardial infarction. Of 303 patients studied, 67 (22%) of which were classified as high risk by Pedretti et al's aforementioned noninvasive algorithm, 47 consented to undergo programmed electrical stimulation. Inducible sustained normophormic VT (rate <270 beats/min) was found to be the strongest independent predictor of an arrhythmic event in these patients. The continued use of the noninvasive algorithm and programmed electrical stimulation had a 65% positive predictive accuracy for a future arrhythmic event. Needless to say, these approaches could have clinical relevance in the highest-risk patient population, where interventions such as the implantable cardioverter–defibrillator can be tested prospectively. What impact thrombolytic therapy would have on such approaches remains undefined.

IMPACT OF THROMBOLYSIS ON LATE POTENTIALS

Reperfusion of the infarct-related coronary artery (IRA) following thrombolytic therapy has contributed to the improvement in survival of post–MI patients (see Ch. 31). The mechanism by which this occurs is not fully understood but is likely related to an improvement in electrical stability and less propensity for inhomogeneous propagation of

Table 28–6. Noninvasive Index

Test Variables	Gomes et al (53)		Kuchar et al (44)		El Sherif et al (48)		Farrell et al (56)		Pedretti et al (52)		El Sherif et al (CAST) (54)	
	PPV	NPV	PPV	NPL	PPV	NPV	PPV	NPV	PPV	NPV	PPV	NPV
LP + EF	36	100	34	100	27	98	19	94				
LP + Holter	35	100	31	100	27	99	19	94				
LP + EF + Holter	50	100	—	—	57	98	28	97	—	—	32	97
LP + HRV + Holter	—	—	—	—	—	—	58	95				
EF + Holter + (QRS d > 106 msec)	—	—	—	—	—	—	—	—	44	99		

PPV = positive predictor value, NPV = negative predictor value, LP = late potentials, EF = ejection fraction, HRV = heart rate variability conduction and consequent reentrant malignant ventricular arrhythmias as well as improvement in LV EF. Following restoration of patency of the infarct-related artery, factors such as intramyocardial hemorrhage, influx of inflammatory cells, cellular edema, and calcium-induced contraction band necrosis may accelerate scar formation and stiffening of infarct tissue, reducing infarct expansion (57–59). Aneurysm formation following acute myocardial infarction in an unusual finding in patients with an open IRA (60). Thus prevention of ventricular dilation and aneurysm formation following reperfusion may decrease the incidence of VT/VF, resulting in a more favorable outcome.

In recent years several studies (61–67) have reported on the impact of the patent IRA on LPs and subsequent arrhythmic events. Gang and coworkers (61) obtained SA-ECGs in 106 patients within 48 hours of the index infarction. Of the 106 patients, 62 were treated conventionally and 46 received thrombolysis with t-PA. LPs were seen in 6% of patients with an open IRA and in 32% of patients with a closed IRA ($p < 0.02$). In this study, abnormalities of all three SA parameters were used as the definition of LPs. Turitto et al (62) studied 118 patients with acute MI with signal averaging. Of these patients, 46 received urokinase and 72 conventional treatment. LPs were observed in 8% of patients with an open IRA and in 15% of patients with a closed IRA. This difference, however, was not statistically significant.

Zimmerman et al (64) studied a total of 223 patients, of which 59 received t-PA and 164 were treated conventionally. LPs were present in 13% of patients with a patent IRA and in 26% of patients with a closed IRA ($p < 0.05$).

Vatterot et al (65) assessed 126 patients with acute acute MI with coronary angiography, SA-ECG, and measurement of LV function following thrombolytic therapy, or acute percutaneous transluminal coronary angioplasty, or standard care. Patients with a patent IRA had a 20% incidence of LPs, whereas patients with a closed IRA had a 71% incidence of LPs ($p = 0.001$). This study elegantly showed that the best prediction of LPs was a closed coronary artery, a prior MI, and age whereas EF was not a predictor of LPs. Of the SA parameters, the duration of the filtered QRS complex was the most significant independent predictor of an open IRA.

Pedretti et al (66) also reported that patients who did not receive thrombolytic therapy had a higher prevalence of LPs in contrast to patients who did (34% vs. 17%, $p < 0.001$). Likewise, when the patency of the IRA was assessed in relation to LPs, 9% of patients with a patent IRA had LPs, whereas 39% of patients with a closed IRA had LPs ($p < 0.001$). In their study, LPs were present in 75% of patients with arrhythmic events and in 18% of those without arrhythmic events ($p < 0.001$) for a follow-up period of 14 ± 8 months.

Steinberg et al (67), in a recently published multicenter study, reported on the effect of late thrombolytic therapy administered 6–24 hours after myocardial infarction on the SA-ECG parameters in 310 patients, of which 160 received placebo and 150 received t-PA. They noted that rt-PA was associated with fewer abnormalities on SA parameters compared with placebo; however, the effects of rt-PA were more dramatic in patients with ST elevation. In these patients rt-PA resulted in a 52% reduction in abnormal SA-ECG parameters and a significantly shorter filtered QRS duration (105.7 ± 10.9 msec versus 110.7 ± 15.9 msec, $p = 0.01$). In their study, however, the relationship of LPs to the IRA was not addressed.

The results of these studies clearly indicate that early thrombolysis, and perhaps even late thrombolysis (≤24 hours), results in a significant reduction of LPs and that this is independent of the effect of LVEF and is related to the presence of an open IRA. Thus it can be concluded that the reduction in mortality following thrombolytic therapy in patients with acute MI is partly related to the modulating effect of reperfusion on the arrhythmic substrate, which is more prevalent in patients with large infarcts.

IMPACT OF THROMBOLYTIC THERAPY ON THE PREDICTIVE VALUE OF LATE POTENTIALS

There has been a substantial decline of sustained ventricular tachycardias as well as in arrhythmic and total cardiac mortality in the thrombolytic era. Thus the predictive values of LPs, LV function, and asymptomatic VPDs in the risk stratification of ischemia need to be reassessed. The long-term predictive value of LPs following thrombolysis has been assessed in two independent studies.

Malik and associates (68) studied 331 patients with acute MI, of which 130 received thrombolytic therapy at <24 hours. During a follow-up period of ≥10 months, 17 patients (8.5%) who did not receive thrombolysis had arrhythmic events, whereas arrhythmic events occurred in 8 patients (6.2%) who had received thrombolysis. Significant differences in SA variables were noted in patients who did not receive thrombolysis and had arrhythmic events, whereas only RMS-40 was significant for those who had received thrombolysis. Receiver operator curves, retrospectively adjusted, showed that for a sensitivity of 30%, the maximal achievable positive predictive accuracy of LP was 100% in patients who did not undergo thrombolysis but only 27% in patient who underwent thrombolysis. Unfortunately, in this study, the data of groups that did and did not receive thrombolysis were not collected contemporaneously and no assessment was made of the success of thrombolytic therapy on the IRA. The latter would be important since patients who received streptokinase within 24 hours of the index infarction were included in the study.

Kawalsky et al (69) and Hammill and Vatterot (70) followed 121 patients with acute MI for 3–5 years (mean = 3.6 ± 1 year) who had SA-ECG and thrombolytic therapy or coronary angioplasty. They reported a death rate of 14.8% over the course of follow-up. Multivariate analysis showed that a prior MI, a closed coronary artery, and ejection fraction were the most powerful determinants of mortality. Survival at 4 years was 77% for patients with LPs and 88% for patients without LPs; however, this difference was not statistically significant. In contrast, the survival was 92% in patients with an open IRA versus 69% in patients with a closed IRA ($p < 0.05$). This study concluded that patency of the IRA and not the presence or absence of LPs was predictive of long-term survival. In this study, however, no separation was made of those dying from an arrhythmic event versus those dying from a nonarrhythmic event.

Although the value of LPs and other noninvasive tests, such as assessment of LV function and Holter monitoring, in risk stratification is somewhat controversial, it is likely that these tests will not provide a sufficiently high predictive accuracy in patients undergoing thrombolysis. Thus, in the era of thrombolytic therapy, risk stratification utilizing SA-ECG and other noninvasive tests is more appropriate in patients not undergoing thrombolysis and in those patients with a prior myocardial infarction.

REFERENCES

1. Gomes JA, Alexopoulos D, Winters SL, et al: The role of silent ischemia, the arrhythmic substrate and the short-long sequence in the genesis of sudden cardiac death. *J Am Coll Cardiol* 1989;14:1618–1625.
2. Norris RM: The changing natural history and Prognosis of Acute myocardial infarction, in Gersh BJ, Rahimtoola SH (eds): *Acute Myocardial Infarction,* New York, Elsevier, 1991, pp 87–97.
3. Norwegian Multicenter Study Group: Timolol-induced reduction in mortality and reinfarction in patients surviving acute myocardial infarction. *N Engl J Med* 1981;304:801–807.
4. Beta-Blocker Heart Attack Research Group: A randomized trial of propranolol in patients with acute myocardial infarction. *JAMA* 1982;247: 1717–1724.
5. Beta-Blocker Pooling Project Research Group: Subgroup findings from randomized trials in post infarction patients. *Eur Heart J* 1988;9:8–16.
6. ISIS-2 (Second International Study of Infarct Survival) Collaborative Group: Randomized trial of intravenous streptokinase, oral aspirin, both, or neither among 17,187 cases of suspected acute myocardial infarction: ISIS 2. *Lancet* 1988;2:349–369.
7. Muller DW, Topol EJ, George BS, et al: Long-term follow-up in the Thrombolysis and Angioplasty in Acute Myocardial Infarction (TAMI) trials: Comparison of trials with thrombolysis alone. *Circulation* 1989;80(Suppl II):II–520.
8. GISSI Trial Group: Long-term effects of intravenous thrombolysis in acute myocardial infarction: Final report of the GISSI study. *Lancet* 1987;2: 871–874.
9. Williams DO, Braunwald E, Knatterud G, et al: The Thrombolysis in Myocardial Infarction (TIMI) trial:

Outcome at one year of patients randomized to either invasive or conservative management. *Circulation* 1989;80(Suppl II):II-519.

10. Schroder R, Neuhaus KL, Leizorovicz A, et al: A prospective placebo-controlled double blind multicenter trial of streptokinase in acute myocardial infarction (ISAM): Long term mortality and morbidity. *J Am Coll Cardiol* 1987;9:197–203.
11. Simoons ML, Arnold A: One year follow-up of rt-PA without and with immediate PTCA (abstract). *Circulation* 1980;80(Suppl II):II-520.
12. Van de Werf F, Arnold AE: The European Cooperative rt-PA vs Placebo trial: 1 year follow-up (abstract). *Circulation* 1989;80(Suppl II):II-520.
13. Dalen JE, Gore GM, Braunwald F, et al: Six and twelve month follow-up of the phase I Thrombolysis in Myocardial Infarction (TIMI) trial. *Am J Cardiol* 1988;62:179–185.
14. Taylor GJ, Moses HW, Katholi RE, et al: Six-year survival after coronary thrombolysis and early revascularization for acute myocardial infarction. *Am J Cardiol* 1992;70:26–30.
15. Gomes JA, Winters SL, Ip J. Post infarction high risk of sudden death, in Akhtar M, Meyerburg RJ, Ruskin JN (eds): *Sudden Cardiac Death: Prevalence, Mechanism and Approaches to Diagnosis.* Baltimore, Williams & Wilkins, 1994, pp 531–538.
16. Fioretti P, Brower RW, Simonson ML, et al: Relative value of clinical variables, bicycle ergometry, rest radionuclide ventriculography, 24-hour ambulatory electrocardiographic monitoring at discharge to predict 1 year survival after myocardial infarction. *J Am Coll Cardiol* 1986;8:40–49.
17. Schultze RA, Strauss HW, Pitt B: Sudden death in the year following myocardial infarction. *Am J Med* 1977;62:192–199.
18. Bigger JT, Fleiss JF, Kliger R, Miller JP, Rolnitzky LM, and the Multicenter Post-Infarction Research Group: The relationship among ventricular arrhythmias, left ventricular dysfunction and mortality in the 2 years after myocardial infarction. *Circulation* 1984;69:250–258.
19. Mukarji J, Rude RE, Poole WK, et al, and the MILIS Study Group: Risk factors for sudden death after acute myocardial infarction: Two year follow-up. *Am J Cardiol* 198;54:31–36.
20. Hamer A, Vohra J, Hunt D, Slomen G: Prediction of sudden death by electrophysiologic studies in high-risk patients surviving acute myocardial infarction. *Am J Cardiol* 1982;50:223–229.
21. Richards DA, Cody DV, Denniss AR, Russell PA, Young AA, Uther JB: Ventricular electrical instability: A predictor of death after myocardial infarction. *Am J Cardiol* 1983;51:75–80.
22. Gomes JAC, Hariman RI, Kang PS, El-Sherif N, Chowdhry I, Lyons J: Programmed electrical stimulation in patients with high-grade ventricular ectopy: Electrophysiologic findings and prognosis for survival. *Circulation* 1984;70:43–51.
23. Waspe LE, Seinfeld D, Feerick A, Kim SG, Matos JA, Fisher JD: Prediction of sudden death and spontaneous ventricular tachycardia in survivors of complicated myocardial infarction: Value of the response to programmed stimulation using a maximum of three ventricular extrastimuli. *J Am Coll Cardiol* 1985;5:1292–1301.
24. Berbari BJ, Scherlag RJ, Hope RR, Lazzara R: Recording from the body surface of arrhythmogenic ventricular activity during the ST segment. *Am J Cardiol* 1978;41:697–702.
25. Fontaine G, Frank R, Gallais Hammono F, et al: Electrocardiographic des potentiels tardifs du syndrome de postexcitation. *Arch Mal Coeur* 1978;78: 851–861.
26. Rozanski JJ, Mortara D, Myerburg RJ, Castellanos A: Body surface detection of delayed depolarizations in patients with recurrent ventricular tachycardia and left ventricular aneurysm. *Circulation* 1981;63:1172–1178.
27. Simson MB: Use of signals in the terminal QRS complex to identify patients with ventricular tachycardia after myocardial infarction. *Circulation* 1981; 64:235–242.
28. Breithardt G, Becker R, Seipel L, Abendroth RR, Ostermeyer J: Non-invasive detection of late potentials in man: A new marker for ventricular tachycardia. *Eur Heart J* 1981;2:1–2.
29. Denes P, Santarelli P, Hauser RG, Uretz EF: Quantitative analysis of the high-frequency components of the terminal portion of the body surface QRS in normal subjects and in patients with ventricular tachycardia. *Circulation* 1983;67:1129–1138.
30. Gomes JAC, Mehra R, Barreca P, El-Sherif N, Hariman R, Holtzman R: Quantitative analysis of the high frequency components of the signal-averaged QRS complex in acute myocardial infarction. *Circulation* 1985;72:102–111.
31. El-Sherif N, Gomes JAC, Restivo M, Mehra R: Late potentials and arrhythmogenesis. *PACE* 1985; 8:440–462.

32. Kanovsky MS, Falcone RA, Dresden CA, Josephson ME, Simson MB: Identification of patients with ventricular tachycardia after myocardial infarction: Signal-averaged electrocardiogram, Holter monitoring and cardiac catheterization. *Circulation* 1984;79:264–270.

33. Gomes JAC, Mehra R, Barreca P, et al: A comparative analysis of signal averaging of the surface QRS complex and intracardiac electrode recordings in patients with ventricular tachycardia. *PACE* 1988;11:271–282.

34. Gomes JA, Winters SL, Stewart D, et al: Optimal band pass filters for time domain analysis of the signal-averaged electrocardiogram. *Am J Cardiol* 1987;60:1290–1298.

35. Kuchar DL, Thorburn CW, Sammel L: Prediction of serious arrhythmic events after myocardial infarction: Signal-averaged electrocardiogram, Holter monitoring and radionuclide ventriculography. *J Am Coll Cardiol* 1987;9:531–538.

36. Gomes JA, Winters SL, Martinson M, Machac J, Stewart D, Targonsky A: The prognostic significance of quantitative signal-averaged variables relative to clinical variables, site of myocardial infarction, ejection fraction and ventricular premature beats: A prospective study. *J Am Coll Cardiol* 1988; 13:377–384.

37. Gomes JA, Winters SL, Stewart D: "Late" late potentials on the signal-averaged ECG: Incidence, characteristics and significance (abstract). *Circulation* 1988;78(Suppl. II):II-52.

38. Scherlag BJ, El-Sherif N, Hope R, Lazzara R: Characterization and localization of ventricular arrhythmias resulting from myocardial ischemia and infarction. *Circ Res* 1974;35:372–383.

39. Josephson ME, Horowitz LN, Farshidi A: Continuous local electrical activity. A mechanism of recurrent ventricular tachycardia. *Circulation* 1978;57: 659–665.

40. Fenoglio JJ Jr, Pham TD, Harken AH, Horowitz LN, Josephson ME, Wit AL: Recurrent sustained ventricular tachycardia: Structure and ultrastructure of subendocardial regions where tachycardia originates. *Circulation* 1983;68:518.

41. Spear JF, Michelson EL, Moore EN: Reduced pace constant in slowly conducting regions of chronically infarcted canine myocardium. *Circ Res* 1983; 53:176–185.

42. Simson MB, Untereker WJ, Spelman SR, et al: Relations between late potentials on the body surface and directly recorded fragmented electrograms in patients with ventricular tachycardia. *Am J Cardiol* 1983;57:105–112.

43. McGuire M, Kuchar D, Ganes J, Sammel N, Thorburn C: Natural history of late potentials in the first ten days after acute myocardial infarction and relation to early ventricular arrhythmias. *Am J Cardiol* 1988;61:1187–1190.

44. Kuchar DL, Thorburn CW, Sammel NL: Late potentials detected after myocardial infarction: Natural history and prognostic significance. *Circulation* 1986;74:1280–1289.

45. Gomes JAC, Horowitz S, Milner M, Machac J, Winters SL, Barreca P: Signal averaging of the QRS complex in myocardial infarction: Relationship between ejection fraction and wall motion abnormalities. *Am J Cardiol* 1989;59:1071–1074.

46. Hecht HS, Hopkins JM: Exercise induced regional wall motion abnormalities on radionuclide angiography: Index of reliability for detection of coronary artery disease in the presence of coronary heart disease. *Am J Cardiol* 1981;47:861–865.

47. Currie PJ, Kelly MU, Harper RW, et al: Incremental value of clinical assessment, supine exercise electrocardiography, and biplane exercise radionuclide ventriculography in the prediction of coronary artery disease in men with chest pain. *Am J Cardiol* 1983;52:927–935.

48. El-Sherif N, Ursell SN, Bekheit S, et al: Prognostic significance of the signal-averaged electrocardiogram depends on the time of recording in the postinfarction period. *Am Heart J* 1989;118:256–264.

49. Breithardt G, Borggrefe M, Haarten K: Role of programmed ventricular stimulation and non-invasive recording of ventricular late potentials for the identification of patients at risk of ventricular arrhythmias after acute myocardial infarction in Zipes DP, Jalife J (eds): *Cardiac Electrophysiology and Arrhythmias.* Orlando, FL, Grune & Straton, 1984, pp 553–561.

50. Deniss AR, Richard DA, Cody DV, et al: Prognostic significance of ventricular tachycardia and fibrillation induced at programmed stimulation and delayed potentials detected on the signal-averaged electrocardiograms of survivors of acute myocardial infarction. *Circulation* 1986;74:731–745.

51. Cripps T, Bennett ED, Camm AJ, Ward DE: High-gain signal-averaged electrocardiogram combined with 24-hour monitoring in patients early after myocardial infarction for beside prediction of arrhythmic events. *Br Heart J* 1989;60:181.

52. Pedretti R, Etro MD, Laporta A, et al: Prediction of late arrhythmic events after acute myocardial infarction from combined use of non-invasive prognostic variables and inducibility of sustained monomorphic ventricular tachycardia. *Am J Caridol* 1993;71:1131–1141.
53. Gomes JA, Winters SL, Stewart D, Horowitz S, Milner M, Barreca P: A new noninvasive index to predict sustained ventricular tachycardia and sudden death in the first year after myocardial infarction: Based on signal-averaged electrocardiogram, radionuclide ejection fraction and Holter monitoring. *J Am Coll Cardiol* 1987;10:349–357.
54. El-Sherif N, Denes P, Katz R, et al, and the CAST/SA-ECG Substudy Investigators: Definition of the best prediction critria of the time domain signal-averaged electrocardiogram for serious arrhythmic events in the postinfarction period. *J Am Coll Cardiol* 1995;25:908–914.
55. Gomes JA, Winters SL, Deshmukh P, Pe E: The significance of late potentials and ejection fraction is dependent on the site of myocardial infarction (abstract). *Circulation* 1989;80:(Suppl II):II-635.
56. Farrell TG, Bashiz Y, Cripps E, et al: Risk stratification for arrhythmic events in post–myocardial infarction patients based on heart rate variability, ambulatory electrocardiographic variales and the signal averaged ECG. *J Am Coll Cardiol* 1991;18: 687–697.
57. Pirzada FA, Weiner JM, Hood WB Jr: Experimental myocardial infarction: Accelerated myocardial stiffening related to coronary reperfusion following ischemia. *Chest* 1978;74:190–195.
58. Braunwald E: Myocardial reperfusion, limitation of infarct size, reduction or left ventricular dysfunction and improved survival. Should the paradigm be expanded? *Circulation* 1989;14:779:441–444.
59. Kim CB, Braunwald E: Potential benefits of late reperfusion of infarcted myocardium the open artery hypothesis. *Circulation* 1993;88:2426–2436.
60. Forman MB, Collins HW, Kopelman HA, et al: Determinants of left ventricular aneurysm formation after acute myocardial infarction: A clinical and angiographic study. *J Am Coll Cardiol* 1986;8: 1256–1262.
61. Gang ES, Lew AS, Hong M, Wang FZ, Siebst CA, Peter T: Decreased incidence of late potentials after successful thrombolytic therapy of myocardial infarction. *N Engl J Med* 1989;321:712–716.
62. Turitto G, Risa AL, Zanchi E, Prate L: The signal-averaged electrocardiogram and ventricular arrhythmias after thrombolysis for acute myocardial infarction. *J Am Coll Cardiol* 1990;15:1270–1376.
63. Winters SL, Gomes JA: Thrombolytic therapy, infarct vessel patency and late potentials: Can the arrhythmic substrate be altered? *J Am Coll Cardiol* 1990;15:1277–8.
64. Zimmerman M, Adamee R, Ciaroni S, Malbois F, Tieche R: Reduction in the frequency of ventricular late potentials after cute myocardial infarction by early thrombolytic therapy. *Am J Cardiol* 1991; 67:697–703.
65. Vatterot PJ, Hammill SC, Bailey WR, Wiltgen CM, Gersh BJ: Late potentials on signal-averaged electrocardiograms and patency of the infarct-related artery in survivors of acute myocardial infarction. *J Am Coll Cardiol* 1991;17:330.
66. Pedretti R, Laporta A, Etro MD, et al: Influence of thrombolysis on signal averaged electrocardiography and late arrhythmic events after acute myocardial infarction. *Am J Cardiol* 1992;69:866–872.
67. Steinberg JS, Hachman JS, Morgan CD, et al: Effects of thrombolytic therapy administration 6 to 24 hours after myocardial infarction on the signal-averaged ECG. Results of a Multicenter Randomized Trial. *Circulation* 1994;90:746–752.
68. Malik M, Kulokowski P, Odemuyiloa O, et al: Effect of thrombolytic therapy on the predictive value of signal averaged electrocardiography after acute myocardial infarction. *Am J Cardiol* 1992;70: 21–25.
69. Kawalsky DL, Garratt KN, Hammill SC, et al: Infarct artery patency and late potentials after myocardial infarction. Long term follow-up (abstract). *Circulation* 1991;84(Suppl II):II-366.
70. Hammill SC, Vatterot PJ: The effect of reperfusion on the signal averaged ECG, in Gomes JA (ed): *Signal Averaged Electrocardiography: Concepts, Methods and Applications.* Dordrecht, Boston, London, Kluwer Academic Publishers, 1993, pp 469–476.

29

Angiotensin Converting Enzyme Inhibition Following Myocardial Infarction: From Left Ventricular Remodeling to Improved Survival

Scott D. Solomon, MD, and Marc A. Pfeffer, MD, PhD

INTRODUCTION

In the days, weeks, and months following a myocardial infarction (MI), a number of structural changes in the heart can occur that result in alterations in left ventricular size and shape, a phenomenon generally referred to as ventricular remodeling post–MI. The subsequent risk of congestive heart failure or death is related to the extent of this remodeling or enlargement. The finding that angiotensin converting enzyme (ACE) inhibitors could attenuate this process in animal models of myocardial infarction provided the initial rationale for this new clinical use. The initial patient experiences were small mechanistic trials, which demonstrated that the use of ACE inhibitors could attenuate these structural changes that follow myocardial infarction. Recent major clinical trials have demonstrated reduced mortality and incidence of congestive heart failure in survivors of myocardial infarction treated with ACE inhibitors. Thus ACE inhibitors join a select group of agents that have been proven to improve survival and reduce morbidity in patients with myocardial infarction. This chapter will review the process of ventricular remodeling that occurs following myocardial infarction and will focus on evidence that this process can be attenuated with ACE inhibitors. The recent clinical outcome trials experience of ACE inhibition in patients with myocardial infarction will be reviewed, and our perspective on an appropriate clinical use of these agents in MI will be offered.

LEFT VENTRICULAR REMODELING

Ventricular remodeling refers to the ability of the ventricle to respond to chronic alterations in its loading conditions by changing its size, configuration, and mass without increasing the number of myocytes. The inherent plasticity of the mammalian heart is best exemplified by the normal changes that occur throughout the development process, a profound example of which occurs when the left ventricle assumes the function of the systemic ventricle shortly after birth. Yet in addition to normal morphologic changes that occur throughout growth, pathologic changes in ventricular morphology and mass occur in a variety of disease states in which chronic abnormalities of ventricular loading are imposed.

Linzbach indicated that the increase in chamber mass that occurs during the remodeling process exhibits characteristic patterns that are particularly well suited to the type of pathophysiologic workload imposed (1). The left ventricular hypertrophy that occurs secondary to pressure overload due to systemic hypertension or aortic valve stenosis differs from the volume overload imposed by valvular insufficiency. Grossman et al have suggested that these different hypertrophic responses to increased workload are adaptive mechanisms to restore left ventricular wall stress toward normal (2). From the Laplace relationship, wall stress is proportional to the product of the chamber pressure and radius divided by the wall thickness. This relationship holds only qualitatively in the human heart, which under normal conditions more closely resembles a prolate ellipsoid than a sphere, and can demonstrate marked distortions in geometry in diseased states.

At a cellular level, the heart responds to an increased workload by myocyte hypertrophy. In conditions of increased ventricular pressure, such as aortic stenosis, this cellular hypertrophy results in increased wall thickness and, thus, helps normalize overall left ventricular wall stress, which is increased due to elevated cavity pressures. In a pressure-overload hypertrophied ventricle, increased wall thickness is the physiologic adaptation to increased wall stress that allows the ventricle to eject a stroke volume against a markedly increased load. In contrast to pressure-overload conditions in which cellular hypertrophy usually results in increased wall thickness, volume overload conditions such as aortic or mitral regurgitation produce *eccentric* hypertrophy, in which ventricular mass increases as the ventricular chamber dilates. Yet in the dilated ventricle, wall thickness is usually unchanged or thin, resulting in a greater overall wall stress. The increased wall stress predicted by the increased dilation is not offset by an increase in wall thickness, and thus, overall wall stress, by the Laplace relationship, increases. In these conditions, the adaptive response is dilatation, which serves to accommodate a greater volumetric load, maintaining, or even elevating, stroke volume.

REMODELING IN MYOCARDIAL INFARCTION

Early Phase of Myocardial Infarction—Expansion of the Infarcted Region

The ventricular enlargement that occurs following a myocardial infarction is distinct from global ventricular remodeling seen in other pathologic states. In MI, the ventricle is not responding to an extrinsic imposed load but to the intrinsic loss of myocytes and contractile tissue of a regional nature. Following large myocardial infarctions, marked changes in ventricular shape occur rapidly as a result of passive forces on infarcted tissue that can no longer generate tension (3–5). Myocardial infarction, by definition, involves necrosis of a region of the myocardium, which interfaces with normal viable contracting tissue. Fishbein et al described the histologic evolution of the infarction process from myocyte death, inflammatory response, and eventual replacement with fibrous connective tissue (6). In transmural infarctions, the change from contractile to fibrous connective tissue results in thinning of the infarcted region with a reduction in the number of myocytes across the wall. Hutchins and Bulkley observed that the infarcted region not only thins but in some instances also elongates (7). They termed the segmental elongation of the noncontractile region "infarct expansion," defined as "acute dilatation and thinning of the area of infarction not explained by additional myocardial necrosis." Histologically, infarct expansion is characterized by myocyte slippage and a decrease in the number of cells throughout the cardiac wall (8). Infarct extension, by contrast, is defined as an increase in the size of the noncontractile region in the setting of a continuing ischemic insult.

Thinning and elongation of an infarcted myocardial region in certain survivors of myocardial infarction results in distortion of ventricular topography and contributes to the early enlargement of the overall ventricular cavity (9). In patients demonstrating infarct expansion, the process can be detected by echocardiography within hours of an acute MI, and it may continue for several weeks. During this period, scar healing is characterized by fibroblast proliferation, collagen deposition, and connective tissue repair processes, all of which tend to increase the tensile strength of the infarcted region and help resist further distortion (10,11).

During the period of scar formation, the infarcted region is particularly vulnerable to further alterations in shape. Indeed, agents that interfere with the inflammatory response, such as glucocorticoids and nonsteroidal anti-inflammatory agents, have been shown in clinical and experimental infarct models to exacerbate the process of infarct expansion, resulting in thinner scars with greater segment elongation (12–15). Since these therapies have not been shown to actually lower the collagen content of the scar (16,17), it appears that their detrimental effect on scar formation may be related to prolonging the vulnerable period and delaying the point at which the infarcted region can resist further deformation. Although placebo-controlled clinical trial experience with anti-inflammatory agents is extremely limited, observational studies support the mechanistic concern for a potential harmful effect following MI (18).

The clinical diagnosis of infarct expansion is generally made with echocardiographic determinations of infarct lengthening without enzyme evidence of further myocardial necrosis (9,19). Patients with large transmural infarctions have a greater likelihood of developing infarct expansion than those with nontransmural infarctions (7,20). As a result of the reduced radius of curvature and wall thickness of the anterior apical region, infarcts involving this region of the left ventricle are more likely to manifest expansion than those involving other regions (21). Patients exhibiting infarct expansion have a greater likelihood of both early and late clinical complications, including death, myocardial rupture, aneurysm formation, and the development of clinical congestive heart failure, than do infarct patients without expansion (9,22,23). Animal experiments demonstrating that thinning in infarct expansion is the result of a reduction in the number of myocytes across the ventricular wall support the clinical view that myocardial rupture represents a tragic consequence of infarct expansion (4). In chronic survivors of infarction, eventual fibroblast proliferation and connective tissue repair of the infarcted region greatly reduce the risk of rupture, which renders this region more resistant to further stretch and distortion (24).

Later Phase of Myocardial Infarction—Remodeling of the Noninfarcted Region

In the acute phase of myocardial infarction, distortion of the ventricle occurs primarily during systolic contraction due to the effect of passive forces on a thinning, necrotic region of noncontracting myocardium. While the acute phase of myocardial infarction is dominated by changes in the infarct segment itself, elongation of the noninfarcted region can also be demonstrated even within the first week after infarction (22). In animal models, altered gene expression in the remote, noninfarcted region following MI is consistent with the pattern of the genetic response observed in other hyperfunctional conditions producing cardiac hypertrophy. Expression of angiotensin II and the proto-oncogenes c-myc and c-jun have been shown to be enhanced in noninfarcted left ventricular regions following MI (25). In addition, increased angiotensinogen gene expression in noninfarcted regions has been demonstrated in the setting of experimental myocardial infarction in the rat (26). The shift from the dominant VI myosin isoenzyme to the V3 isoenzyme in the noninfarcted myocardium is also seen in this as in other animal models of myocardial hypertrophy (27).

Morphologic changes that occur following infarction can thus be viewed as an overall process of global ventricular enlargement, and remodeling therefore involves both the infarcted and noninfarcted regions. In addition to an actual increase in ventricular circumference, the distortion of the ventricular topography following infarction results in a more spherical contour (28). Thus the global process of ventricular remodeling after myocardial infarction should be viewed as an overall change in the ventricular contour and size with contributions

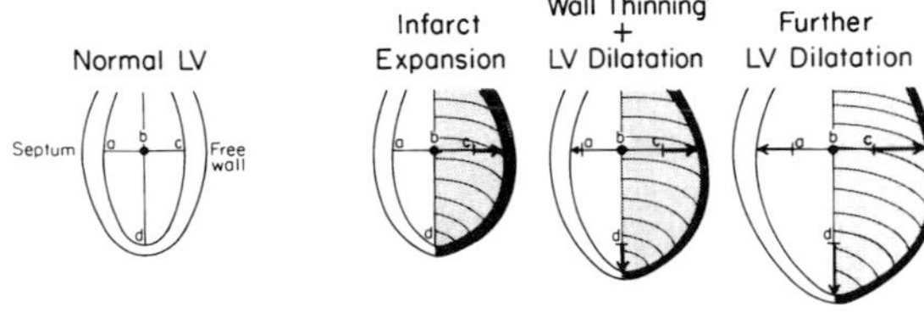

Figure 29–1. Morphologic changes occurring in the left ventricle (LV) during the early and late postinfarction periods. In the normal left ventricle, the lengths ba and bc represent the distance (minor radius) from the midpoint of the left ventricle to the septum and free wall, respectively; the length bd represents the distance (major radius) from the midpoint to the apex. These distances are also presented in the infarcted left ventricles, and they demonstrate the effect of infarct expansion, initial wall thinning and dilatation, and further ventricular dilatation. The shaded area represents an infarction comprising approximately 50% of the ventricle. *Reprinted with permission from Pfeffer: Progressive ventricular dilation in experimental myocardial infarction and its attenuation by angiotensin-converting-enzyme inhibition. Am J Cardiol Supplement 1991;68:17D–25D.*

from both the infarcted and noninfarcted regions (Fig. 29–1). Prior to fibrous tissue proliferation, the infarcted region makes a relatively larger contribution to the process of enlargement; however, dilatation of the noninfarcted region continues for a more protracted period and is more likely to be the major contributor to the late phase of ventricular enlargement (29).

REMODELING AS AN ADAPTATION

While infarct expansion results from passive mechanical forces, it is probable that the early remodeling process that affects noninfarcted myocardium is initially an active adaptive process. As stated previously, the principal adaptive advantage of ventricular enlargement is that it allows an impaired left ventricle to eject a greater stroke volume with less muscle shortening (30). As an adaptation, an enlarged cavity requires a smaller change in radius to eject the same stroke volume. McKay et al demonstrated that stroke volume returns to normal within 2 weeks following MI, despite a persistent reduction in ejection fraction (31). This improvement in stroke volume was associated with ventricular enlargement and a decline in left ventricular filling pressures, indicative that this cavity enlargement was dilatation, a true structural change rather than distention or enlargement due to higher filling pressure. Other studies have confirmed the association between ventricular enlargement and early restoration of stroke volume following large infarctions (32).

Although some ventricular enlargement is necessary to restore stroke volume in patients with infarcts involving 20% or greater of the left ventricular circumference (33), this adaptation does not come without a price. Patients whose ventricles remodel to restore global pump function following MI are at increased risk for progressive ventricular enlargement. In the long term, rather than conferring additional benefit in the form of improved pump function, this type of remodeling has a distinct mechanical disadvantage, as overall wall stress is higher in these ventricles. If the ratio between ventricular mass to volume is offset toward greater volume per unit mass, ventricular wall stress would be increased at any given pressure level throughout the cardiac cycle. The poorly contracting enlarged ventricle of any etiology may be viewed as an internally loaded ventricle, since wall stress is increased throughout the entire cardiac cycle. As opposed to the normal ventricle, in which the increase in pressure during systole is offset by wall thickening and a major reduction in the chamber radius, the impaired ventricle operates from a higher initial radius and exhibits less shortening. While cellular hypertrophy does occur as a response to the increased wall stress, this response appears to be limited and does not compensate fully for the increased stress (34). By Laplace's law, in a patient with ventricular enlargement, wall stress is increased during the ejection phase, in contrast to the decline in wall stress during ejection in the normal ventricle (35).

Thus, despite the adaptive nature of ventricular enlargement following myocardial infarction, these structural changes may have adverse long-term consequences, even in the setting of early restoration of global pump function. The loss of myocardium from MI may initiate a process whereby the infarcted and noninfarcted regions elongate, the cavity enlarges, shape is distorted, and as a consequence, wall stress remains chronically elevated.

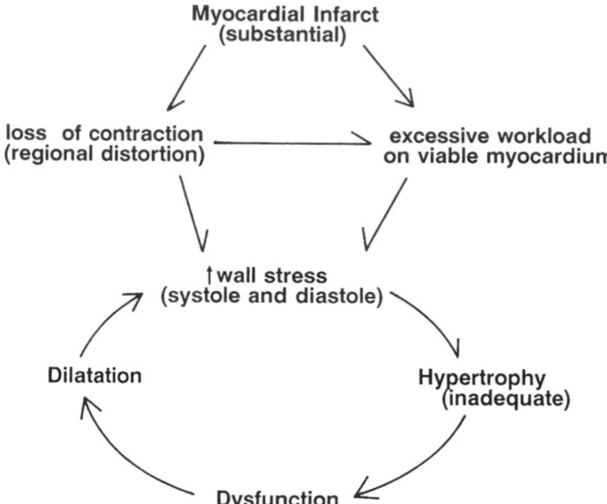

Figure 29–2. Pathologic scheme whereby the loss of substantial myocardium from an acute myocardial infarction can lead to a progressive process of enlargement and dysfunction.

This altered loading state may lead to further ventricular enlargement and perpetuate a vicious cycle producing a chronic augmentation in the workload of the viable myocardium (5). (Fig. 29–2).

REMODELING AND PROGNOSIS

Clinical studies have demonstrated that ventricular enlargement following myocardial infarction is associated with higher morbidity and mortality. Although an inverse relationship between the extent of cardiac enlargement and survival is common for all forms of systolic dysfunction, in survivors of acute myocardial infarction the impact of cardiac enlargement on mortality is particularly striking. Field et al demonstrated a markedly impaired prognosis in postinfarct patients not sustaining a normal left ventricular mass to volume ratio (36). X-ray studies relating clinical outcomes to cardiac dimensions following infarction have been consistent in demonstrating that adverse clinical events are much more frequent in patients with cardiac enlargement (37,38). Quantitative left ventriculography has shown that the relative risk of death is directly related to the actual magnitude of ventricular volume (39,40). Indeed, in a detailed study of survivors of MI, White and coworkers demonstrated that end-systolic and end-diastolic ventricular volumes were particularly powerful predictors of death in this patient population (39). In these studies, quantitative determinations of left ventricular volume were the most important predictors of reduced survival, providing major independent prognostic information above that provided by the extent of the coronary disease and left ventricular ejection fraction.

MODIFIERS OF INFARCT REMODELING

The extent of left ventricular remodeling after myocardial infarction is directly related to the extent of myocardial necrosis. By far, the interventions that will be most effective in preventing ventricular remodeling are those that prevent infarction in the first place (primary prevention). In the midst of a myocardial infarction, hyperacute therapies aimed at aborting or reducing the extent of myocardial necrosis by restoring coronary flow are the next most effective therapy in reducing long-term changes in ventricular morphology (see Ch. 19, 22). The initial rationale for ACE inhibition post–MI represented a strategy aimed at attenuating secondary damage from progressive left ventricular remodeling after myocardial infarction. As such, ACE inhibition therapy is intended to complement rather than replace other proven effective therapies.

Modification of Remodeling with ACE Inhibitors

That ventricular remodeling, both adaptive and pathologic, results from abnormal augmentations in regional left ventricular wall stress following infarction provides a compelling rationale for the use of pharmacologic agents that alter the most alterable determinant of wall stress, cavity pressure. Angiotensin converting enzyme (ACE) inhibitors represent a unique class of agents that have been used extensively in the treatment of hypertension and congestive heart failure. Their use following myocardial infarction has emerged over the past decade from both animal models and human studies that have shown them to be an effective therapy in attenuating the time-dependent changes in ventricular size and shape following myocardial infarction.

The initial rationale for administering ACE inhibitors to modify postinfarction ventricular enlargement was based on the concept that the progressive left ventricular enlargement and deterioration in function following MI was a consequence of increased wall stress. This concept developed out of the observation that ACE inhibitors could prevent both ventricular dilatation and transition to heart failure in spontaneously hypertensive rats (41). The extension of this concept to myocardial infarction was natural given observational studies of progressive ventricular enlargement after MI. In a direct study of experimental myocardial infarction in rats, administration of the ACE inhibitor captopril post–MI reduced left ventricular filling pressures and attenuated the normally progressive ventricular enlargement seen in that model (42). In the animal studies it was possible to dissociate the ACE inhibitor effects on distention (filling pressure) and dilatation (structural changes), as both components contribute to the lower operating volume in treated animals with MI. That improved survival was evident following a year of ACE inhibitor treatment for experimental myocardial infarction bolstered the importance of the functional studies (43). Studies with other ACE inhibitors in the experimental MI model have also demonstrated functional and survival benefits. These studies generally compared animals grouped by histologic infarct size and thereby underscore the fact that ACE inhibitor therapy exerts its benefit by reducing secondary damage after infarction rather than by limiting infarct size (44).

Initial Human Trials with ACE Inhibition

Based on animal studies demonstrating attenuation of remodeling and congestive heart failure with ACE inhibitors following moderate and large myocardial infarction, the initial human studies with ACE inhibitors following myocardial infarction focused on a group of patients that the animal studies had predicted would most benefit from the therapy: those with some degree of left ventricular (LV) dysfunction. In a small mechanistic study of patients with a first anterior myocardial infarction and left ventricular ejection fraction (LVEF) less than 45%, progressive left ventricular enlargement was observed in the group assigned to placebo. In contrast, in the ACE inhibitor treated group, end-diastolic volumes did not increase from 3 weeks to 1 year following the MI (45). In another early study of ACE inhibitor treatment of patients with asymptomatic LV dysfunction after myocardial infarction, significant reduction in left ventricular size was observed by serial echocardiography (46). In both of these early studies of ACE inhibition in MI, the therapy was found to be safe and effective in reducing left ventricular enlargement. Other studies of LV volumes following MI generated consistent information, solidifying the concept that ACE inhibition therapy could attenuate the progressive enlargement that occurred in selected survivors of MI (47,48).

ACE Inhibitors Prolong Survival After Myocardial Infarction

Selective Long-Term Studies

While these initial clinical trials demonstrated that ACE inhibitors could favorably alter ventricular remodeling following myocardial infarction, the clinical significance of these mechanistic remodeling trials remained to be determined. The Survival and Ventricular Enlargement (SAVE) trial (49) was a direct attempt to demonstrate the clinical utility of ACE inhibition post–myocardial infarction. The SAVE study randomized 2,231 patients with ejection fractions of 40% or less without symptomatic heart failure to receive either placebo or captopril within 3–16 days following myocardial infarction. Patients were followed for an average of 42 months. Mortality was significantly reduced in the captopril group (228 deaths, or 20%) versus the conventional therapy group (275 deaths, or 25%, $p = 0.019$). This reduction in all cause mortality was a consequence of reduced cardiovascular deaths and nonfatal events such as development of heart failure and recurrent myocardial infarction. An important observation was that similar efficacy was found for captopril therapy whether or not concomitant therapy with thrombolytics, aspirin, or beta blockers was utilized. These observations underscored that this new use of ACE inhibitors was to supplement rather than replace other proven beneficial therapies. Moreover, within the SAVE study population, the benefits of ACE inhibitor therapy were observed across most subgroups (50).

When interpreting the results of the SAVE study, it is important to appreciate the unique characteristics of the patient population and the study design. Patients enrolled in this trial, while asymptomatic, all had evidence of left ventricular dysfunction, as defined by radionuclide ejection fraction less than 40%, and therefore constituted a high-risk group for ventricular enlargement and progression to congestive heart failure (CHF). Second, because of a concern for a potential hazard associated with early ACE inhibitor administration in a precarious patient population, captopril was administered between 3 and 16 days following MI with a mean of 11 days. Thus, while providing compelling evidence that ACE inhibition was beneficial after MI in a select group of patients, this study left open questions regarding optimal patient population and timing of initiation of this therapy.

The international research community focused a great deal of effort on the role of ACE inhibition following MI in the early 1990s. With eight major clinical outcomes trials randomizing more than 100,000 patients, this area quickly became one of the best studied in cardiology. Trials of ACE inhibition following MI can be broadly grouped into trials that employed selective entry criteria and those that used this therapy on a broader patient population (Fig. 29–3). The AIRE (51) and TRACE (52) trials, like SAVE, enrolled selected high-risk patients and avoided administration of this potentially hypotensive agent on the initial day of the acute MI. In contrast, the CONSENSUS II (53), GISSI-3 (54), ISIS-4 (55), and Chinese Cardiac (56) trials tested ACE inhibition in a broad range of patients and initiated therapy in the early phase.

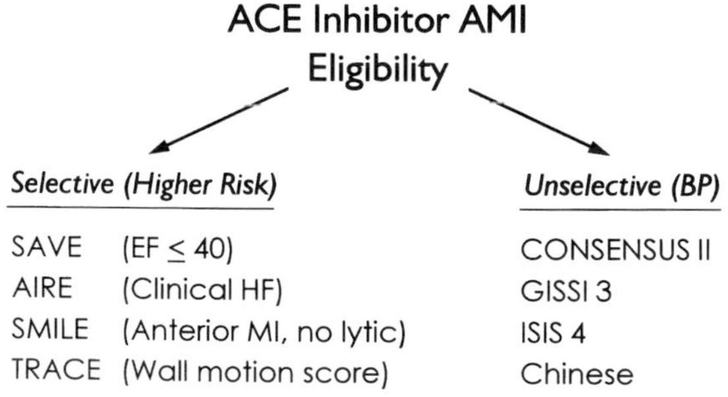

Figure 29–3. ACE inhibitor in MI trials categorized by eligibility.

The AIRE trial randomized 2,006 patients with clinical evidence of heart failure following MI to receive either ramipril or placebo within 3–10 days following MI. In enrolling patients with clinical evidence of transient CHF and not requiring an objective measure of left ventricular function, the AIRE trial complemented the SAVE study, which enrolled patients who were asymptomatic and had a left ventricular ejection fraction ≤40%. Follow-up was continued for a minimum of 6 months, with a mean follow-up time of 15 months. There were 170 deaths (17%) in the treatment group in contrast to 222 deaths (23%) in the placebo group, with an observed risk reduction of 27% ($p = 0.002$). The benefit was apparent within 30 days and did not differ significantly across subgroups. In addition, there was no interaction with either thrombolytic therapy, aspirin, or beta blocker usage.

The Trandolapril Cardiac Evaluation (TRACE) trial was an ACE inhibitor MI trial that also enrolled selected high-risk patients. To be eligible for TRACE, patients had to have echocardiographic evidence of left ventricular dysfunction within 3–7 days following MI. Eligible patients were randomized to receive either trandolapril or placebo. Of the 1,749 patients randomized, 304 (34.7%) died in the trandolapril group compared with 369 patients (42.3%) in the placebo group. This difference resulted in a relative risk reduction of 22% ($p = 0.001$). An important caveat to the TRACE trial was that the patient population was particularly high risk, as the number of placebo group deaths was higher than in both the SAVE and AIRE trials. In addition, the TRACE trial provided an important perspective on the incidence of left ventricular dysfunction in acute MI, since as part of the study design, echocardiographic screening was conducted on more than 7,000 consecutive enzyme-confirmed MI patients, with severe wall motion abnormalities or left ventricular dysfunction found in up to one-third of acute infarct patients.

The SAVE, AIRE, and TRACE trials thus selectively enrolled relatively high-risk patients and treated these patients long-term with ACE inhibitors commencing only after the initial day of myocardial infarction. Together, these trials with three different ACE inhibitors provided consistent evidence for the additional beneficial effect of this therapy in patients with symptoms of failure or asymptomatic LV dysfunction following MI.

Broader Inclusion, Shorter-Term Studies

Whether patients should receive ACE inhibitors early following MI had been the subject of intensive debate. The strongest argument for not administering ACE inhibitors early in the course of an MI was the potential risk, especially of hypotension, during this early extremely vulnerabel period. However, a justifiable rationale for early use was to favorably influence early infarct expansion. The CONSENSUS II trial attempted to answer this question by randomizing patients to receive intravenous enalaprilat or placebo within 24 hours of an MI. The ACE inhibitor was then planned to be continued orally for 6 months. CONSENSUS II was stopped prematurely, with 6,090 of the planned 9,000 patients enrolled, because of failure to show any benefit in mortality at 180 days. With an increased incidence of hypotension and a worrisome trend for excess mortality, the CONSENSUS II trial sent an important cautionary message regarding early broad use of ACE inhibitors, especially intravenous formulations.

Fortunately, at the time the CONSENSUS II trial was stopped, several even larger studies of broad early ACE inhibition therapy in MI were ongoing, which were permitted to go to completion by their respective data safety monitoring committees. GISSI-3 utilized a factorial design to randomize 19,394 patients to receive lisinopril or placebo and either transdermal nitrates or placebo. The ACE inhibitor lisinopril was started within 24 hours of acute MI and continued for 6 weeks. Lisinopril resulted in significant reductions in both overall mortality (12% reduced risk) and in combined mortality and CHF (10% reduced risk).

ISIS-4 randomized 58,050 patients in a 2 × 2 × 2 factorial design to receive either captopril or placebo, controlled release mononitrate or placebo, and IV magnesium versus open control within the first day of MI. Twenty-eight days of captopril therapy resulted in a 7% reduction in 35-day mortality. The survival advantage appeared to be greater in patients with heart failure, a history of previous MI, or anterior MI location.

Another large ACE inhibitor MI trial, the Chinese Cardiac Study (CCS-1) randomized 13,634 patients to receive either oral captopril or placebo within 36 hours of acute MI. Although not reaching statistical significance, there was a reduction in 4-week mortality in the captopril treated group versus the placebo group (9.05% vs. 9.59%, $p = 0.3$), which is equivalent to 5 lives saved per 1,000 treated patients, a risk reduction that was similar in magnitude to that seen in the ISIS-4 trial.

The ISIS-4, GISSI 3, and Chinese Cardiac trials resulted in from 5 to 8 saved lives per 1,000 patients treated with ACE inhibitor. Although more lives were saved per patient treated in the more selective trials, such as SAVE, AIRE, and TRACE, which resulted in 42, 57, and 76 lives saved per 1,000 treated patients respectively, in the less selective trials—ISIS-4, GISSI-3, and CCS-1, the time to ACE inhibitor administration and the follow-up periods were shorter. Moreover, these differences are likely also attributable to the much broader patient population enrolled in the GISSI and ISIS trials, yet underscore the fact that the patients who would most benefit from ACE inhibitors are those with the poorest left ventricular function.

The SMILE study (57), in which the ACE inhibitor zofenopril was administered early to a selective group of patients following anterior MI, represented a hybrid between nonselective early ACE inhibition trials (GISSI-3, ISIS-4, CCS-1) and selective later ACE inhibition trials (SAVE, AIRE, TRACE). In SMILE, 1,556 patients with acute anterior myocardial infarction not receiving thrombolytic therapy were randomized within 24 hours to receive either placebo or zofenopril for 6 weeks. The incidence of death at 6 weeks, although not significant, was 6.5% in the placebo group compared with 4.9% in the zofenopril group, equivalent to a 25% reduction in risk. After 1 year, however, the mortality rate was significantly lower in the group that had initially received zofenopril (10.0% versus 14.1%, $p = 0.011$). Together, the early ACE inhibition trials (GISSI-3, ISIS-4, CCS-1, SMILE) indicated that despite an increased incidence of symptomatic hypotension, oral ACE inhibitor

Table 29–1. Trials of ACE Inhibition After Acute Myocardial Infarction

	n	Duration	Placebo Mortality %	Risk Reduction %	Lives Saved per 1,000 pts
(Selective)					
SAVE	2,231	42	25	19	42
AIRE	2,006	15	23	27	57
SMILE	1,556	1	8	(22)	18
		12	14	33	41
TRACE	1,749	24	42	22	76
(Broad Inclusion)					
CONSENSUS II	6,090	5	9.4	null	—
GISSI-3	19,394	1.5	7.1	12	8
ISIS=4	58,043	1	7.6	7	5
Chinese CCS-1	13,634	1	9.6	9.1	5

therapy within the first day of myocardial infarction improves survival (Table 29–1).

Early Benefit of ACE Inhibition

Both the SAVE and AIRE trials demonstrated clearly that patients with left ventricular dysfunction post–MI benefit from ACE inhibition. In SAVE, the reduction in mortality was associated with echocardiographic evidence of attenuation of left ventricular remodeling. Taken together with animal work demonstrating that ACE inhibitors result in associated reductions in mortality and ventricular enlargement following myocardial infarction, it may be reasonable to conclude that the reduction in mortality associated with the long-term selective use of ACE inhibitors is, to a large extent, related to attenuation of ventricular remodeling. Yet results from the shorter-term studies that utilized early ACE inhibition post–MI suggest another potential mechanism for the reduction in mortality. In both the ISIS-4 and GISSI-3 studies, a major proportion of the mortality benefit occurred in the first day of the infarct. Specifically, in GISSI-3, of the 76 fewer fatal events in the lisinopril treated group, there were 21 fewer deaths by day 1 and 64, or 84% of the total, lives saved within the first week of the MI (58). Similarly, in ISIS-4, 31% of the lives saved with the ACE inhibitor, captopril, occurred by the end of the first day of therapy and 57% of the 143 lives saved attributed to the ACE inhibitor were within the first week.

One interpretation of these data would be that *early* ACE inhibition post–MI attenuates *early* infarct expansion during an extremely vulnerable period, and reduces the incidence of complications related to this process, such as ventricular rupture. This mechanism may be independent of the later effect of ACE inhibition on global left ventricular remodeling. Moreover, the observation in both the SAVE study (59) and the SOLVD studies (60) that ACE inhibitor treated patients actually had fewer subsequent myocardial infarctions suggests an additional completely novel mechanism of action, and a possible role for ACE inhibitors in primary or secondary prevention of MI.

New analysis indicates that the mortality benefit of ACE inhibition in the GISSI-3 and ISIS-4 trials was present by the first few days following MI, providing a compelling argument that most patients should receive the benefit of early ACE inhibition following MI. Indeed, these findings were felt to be so compelling that the Executive Committee of an ongoing multicenter trial, the HEART study, assessing early versus delayed use of the ACE inhibitor ramipril following anterior MI, terminated enrollment prematurely so as not to deny patients the potential benefit of early ACE inhibition (61) (Fig. 29–4).

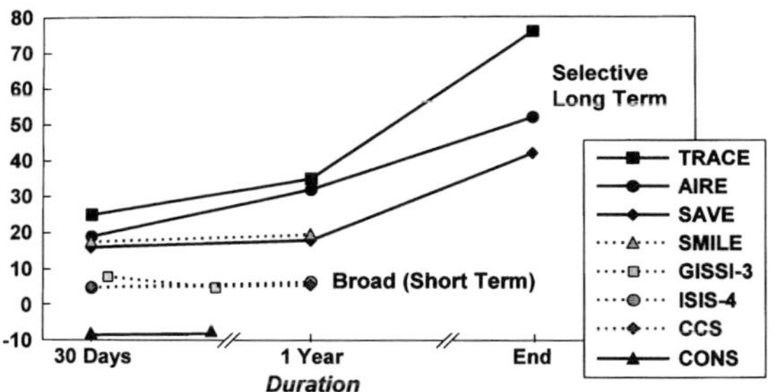

Figure 29–4. Lives saved per 1,000 treated patients in all of the major randomized clinical trials of ACE inhibition following MI. Lives saved per 1,000 patients are presented at the initial endpoint (usually 30 days), at 1 year, and at the end of the respective trials. The dark symbols represent the selective long-term trials (SAVE, AIRE, and TRACE), and the light symbols represent the broad inclusion short-term trials (GISSI-3, ISIS-4, CCS, and CONSENSUS II). The SMILE study represents a hybrid trial.

Recommendations for ACE Inhibition Following Myocardial Infarction

How do we translate the results of these clinical trials into the care of patients experiencing an MI? The results from the SAVE, AIRE, and TRACE trials clearly demonstrate that patients who are at greatest risk following MI, those with left ventricular dysfunction (asymptomatic or symptomatic), are those who will most benefit from long-term ACE inhibition therapy. Because these trials administered the ACE inhibitors beyond the first day following MI, they did not address the important question of whether this therapy was of benefit in the more hyperacute phase. Despite a potential hazard associated with early IV ACE inhibition uncovered in the CONSENSUS II trial, the two subsequent mega-trials, GISSI-3 and ISIS-4, did demonstrate a small survival advantage in a broad range of acute MI patients who received oral ACE inhibition starting in the first 24 hours.

The sum of these early broad inclusion trials suggests that ACE inhibition is, on average, of benefit to patients following MI. Moreover, there appears to be no excess hazard related to acute oral ACE administration following MI, and recent data demonstrate that a large proportion of the lives saved in the GISSI-3 and ISIS-4 trials occurred early. These new observations provide a compelling rationale for early administration of oral ACE inhibitors.

Thus, in light of mechanistic research and the growing number of clinical trials, we recommend early use (within 24 hours) of oral ACE inhibitors during acute myocardial infarction to patients without overt contraindications (clinical instability, systolic blood pressure less than 100 mm Hg, prior problem with ACE inhibition, or pregnancy). This therapy should be sustained long term in the higher-risk patients such as those developing congestive heart failure, exhibiting left ventricular dysfunction, having a prior MI, or with anterior electrocardiographic location. In lower-risk patients, ACE inhibition could be discontinued after preserved left ventricular function is documented.

As a result of intensive international investigative effort, the role of ACE inhibition in MI has been established and has earned a position as one of the few therapies that has been shown to decrease cardiovascular events and prolong survival after myocardial infarction. While individual treatment decisions are always best made at the bedside, the ACE inhibitor trials provide substantial support for the clinician in deciding who and when to treat with ACE inhibitors during and following MI.

REFERENCES

1. Linzbach AJ: Heart failure from the point of view of quantitative anatomy. *Am J Cardiol* 1960;5:370–382.
2. Grossman W, Jones D, McLaurin LD: Wall stress and patterns of hypertrophy in the human left ventricle. *J Clin Invest* 1975;56:56–64.
3. Erlebacher JA, Richter RC, Alonso DR, Devereux RB, Gay WA: Early infarct expansion. Structural or functional? *J Am Coll Cardiol* 1985;6:839–844.
4. Weisman HF, Bush DE, Mannisi JA, Weisfeldt ML, Healy B: Cellular mechanisms of myocardial infarct expansion. *Circulation* 1988;78:186–201.
5. Pfeffer MA, Braunwald E: Ventricular remodeling after myocardial infarction: Experimental observations and clinical implications. *Circulation* 1990;81:1161–1172.
6. Fishbein MC, MacLean D, Maroko PR: The histologic evolution of myocardial infarction. *Chest* 1978;73:843–849

7. Hutchins GM, Bulkley BH: Infarct expansion versus extension: Two different complications of acute myocardial infarction. *Am J Cardiol* 1978;41: 1127–1132.
8. Weisman H, Bush D, Mannisi J, Weisfeldt M, Healy B: Cellular mechanisms of myocardial infarct expansion. *Circulation* 1988;78:186–201.
9. Eaton LW, Weiss JL, Bulkley BH, Garrison JB, Weisfeldt ML: Regional cardiac dilatation after acute myocardial infarction. Recognition by two-dimensional echocardiography. *N Engl J Med* 1979;300:57–62.
10. Vracko R, Thorning D, Frederickson RG: Connective tissue cells in healing rat myocardium. *Am J Pathol* 1989;134:993–1006.
11. Parmley WW, Chuck L, Kivowitz C, Matloff JM, Swan HJC: In vitro length–tension relations of human ventricular aneurysms. *Am J Cardiol* 1973; 32:889–894.
12. Bulkley BJ, Roberts WC: Steroid therapy during acute myocardial infarction: A cause of delayed healing and of ventricular aneurysm. *Am J Med* 1974;56:244–250.
13. Jugdutt BI, Basualdo CA: Myocardial infarct expansion during indomethacin or ibuprofen therapy for symptomatic post infarction pericarditis. Influence of other pharmacologic agents during remodeling. *Can J Cardiol* 1989;5:211–221.
14. Brown EJ, Kloner RA, Schoen FJ, Hammerman H, Hale S, Braunwald E: Scar thinning due to ibuprofen administration after experimental myocardial infarction. *Am J Cardiol* 1983;51: 877–883.
15. Hammerman H, Kloner RA, Schoen FJ, Brown EJ, Hale S, Braunwald E: Indomethacin-induced scar thinning after experimental myocardial infarction. *Circulation* 1983;67:1290–1295
16. Hammerman H, Schoen FJ, Braunwald E, Kloner RA: Drug-induced expansion of infarct: Morphologic and functional correlations. *Circulation* 1984; 69:611–617.
17. Jugdutt BI: Delayed effects of early infarct-limiting therapies on healing after myocardial infarction. *Circulation* 1985;72:907–914.
18. Jugdutt BI, Michorowski BL: Role of infarct expansion in rupture of the ventricular septum after acute myocardial infarction: A two-dimensional echocardiographic study. *Clin Cardiol* 1987;10: 641–652.
19. Weiss JL, Bulkley BH, Hutchins GR, Mason SJ: Two-dimensional echocardiographic recognition of myocardial injury in man: Comparison with postmortem studies. *Circulation* 1981;63:402–408.
20. Weisman HF, Healy B: Myocardial infarct expansion, infarct extension, and reinfarction: Pathophysiologic concepts. *Prog Cardiovasc Dis* 1987;30: 73–110.
21. Pirolo JS, Hutchins GM, Moore GW: Infarct expansion: Pathologic analysis of 204 patients with a single myocardial infarct. *J Am Coll Cardiol* 1986;7: 349–354.
22. Erlebacher JA, Weiss JL, Eaton LW, Kallman C, Weisfeldt ML, Bulkley BH: Late effects of acute infarct dilation on heart size: A two dimensional echocardiographic study. *Am J Cardiol* 1982;49: 1120–1126.
23. Schuster EH, Bulkley BH: Expansion of transmural myocardial infarction: A pathophysiologic factor in cardiac rupture. *Circulation* 1979;60:1532–1538.
24. Vracko R, Thorning D, Frederickson RG: Connective tissue cells in healing rat myocardium. *Am J Pathol* 1989; 134:993–1006.
25. Reiss K, Capasso JM, Huang HE, Meggs LG, Li P, Anversa P: ANG II receptors, c-myc, and c-jun in myocytes after myocardial infarction and ventricular failure. *Am J Physiol* 1993;264:H760–769.
26. Lindpaintner K, Lu W, Neidermaier N, et al: Selective activation of cardiac angiotensinogen gene expression in post-infarction ventricular remodeling in the rat. *J Mol Cell Cardiol* 1993;25:133–143.
27. Michel JB, Lattion AL, Salzmann JL, et al: Hormonal and cardiac effects of converting enzyme inhibition in rat myocardial infarction. *Circ Res* 1988; 62:641–650.
28. Mitchell GF, Lamas GA, Vaughan DE, Pfeffer MA: Left ventricular remodeling in the year after first anterior myocardial infarction: A quantitative analysis of contractile segment lengths and ventricular shape. *J Am Coll Cardiol.* 1992;19(6):1136–1144.
29. Mitchell GF, Lamas GA, Vaughan De, Pfeffer MA: Infarct expansion does not contribute to late left ventricular enlargement (abstract). *Circulation* 1989; 80(Suppl II):II-589.
30. Gulch RW, Jacob R: Geometric and muscle physiological determinants of cardiac stroke volume as evaluated on the basis of model calculations. *Basic Res Cardiol* 1988;83:476–485.
31. McKay RG, Pfeffer MA, Pasternak RC, et al: Left ventricular remodeling following myocardial infarction: A corollary to infarct expansion. *Circulation* 1986;74:693–702.

32. Gaudron PJ, Eilles C, Strotmann J, Jarausch T, Ertl G, Kochsiek K: Time course of left ventricular dilatation and hemodynamics in patients after acute myocardial infarction. Dependence on infarct size abstract. *Circulation* 1989;80(Suppl II):II-253.

33. Klein MD, Herman MV, Gorlin R: A hemodynamic study of left ventricular aneurysm. *Circulation* 1967;35:614–630.

34. Anversa P, Loud AV, Levicky V, Guideri G: Left ventricular failure induced by myocardial infarction. I. Myocyte hypertrophy. *Am J Physiol* 1985; 248:H876–H882.

35. Weber KT, Janicki JS: The heart as a muscle-pump system and the concept of heart failure. *Am Heart J* 1979;98:371–384.

36. Feild BJ, Baxley WA, Russell RO Jr, et al: Left ventricular function and hypertrophy in cardiomyopathy with depressed ejection fraction. *Circulation* 1973;47:1022–1031.

37. Shanoff HM, Little JA, Csima A, Yano R: Heart size and ten-year survival after uncomplicated myocardial infarction. *Am Heart J* 1969;78:608–614.

38. Kostuk WJ, Kazamias TM, Gander MP, Simon AL, Ross J: Left ventricular size after acute myocardial infarction: Serial changes and their prognostic significance. *Circulation* 1973;47:1174–1179.

39. White HD, Norris RM, Brown MA, Brandt PWT, Whitlock RML, Wild CJ: Left ventricular end-systolic volume as the major determinant of survival after recovery from myocardial infarction. *Circulation* 1987;76:44–51.

40. Hammermeister KE, DeRouen TA, Dodge HT: Variables predictive of survival in patients with coronary disease: Selection by univariate and multivariate analyses from the clinical, electrocardiographic, exercise, arteriographic, and quantitative angiographic evaluations. *Circulation* 1979;59: 421–430.

41. Pfeffer JM, Pfeffer MA, Mirsky I, Braunwald E: Regression of left ventricular hypertrophy and prevention of ventricular dysfunction by captopril in the spontaneously hypertensive rat. *Proc Natl Acad Sci USA* 1982;79:3310–3314.

42. Pfeffer JM, Pfeffer MA, Braunwald E: Influence of chronic captopril therapy on the infarcted left ventricle of the rat. *Circ Res* 1985;57:84–95.

43. Pfeffer MA, Pfeffer JM, Steinberg C, Finn P: Survival following experimental myocardial infarction: Beneficial effects of chronic captopril therapy. *Circulation* 1985;72:406–412.

44. Richer C, Mulder P, Fornes P, Domergue V, Heudes D, Giudicelli JF: Long-term treatment with trandolapril opposes cardiac remodeling and prolongs survival after myocardial infarction in rats. *J Cardiovasc Pharmacol* 1992;20:147–156.

45. Pfeffer MA, Lamas GA, Vaughan DE, Parisi AF, Braunwald E: Effect of captopril on progressive ventricular dilatation after anterior myocardial infarction. *N Engl J Med* 1988;319:80–86.

46. Sharpe N, Murphy J, Smith H, Hannan S: Treatment of patients with symptomless left ventricular dysfunction after myocardial infarction. *Lancet* 1988; 1:255–259.

47. Sharpe N, Smith H, Murphy J, Greaves S, Hart H, Gamble G: Early prevention of left ventricular dysfunction after myocardial infarction with angiotensin-converting-enzyme inhibition. *Lancet* 1991;337:872–876.

48. Foy SG, Crozier IG, Turner JG, et al: Comparison of enalapril versus captopril on left ventricular function and survival three months after acute myocardial infarction (the "PRACTICAL" study). *Am J Cardiol* 1994;73:1180–1186.

49. Pfeffer MA, Braunwald E, Moye LA, et al: Effect of captopril on mortality and morbidity in patients with left ventricular dysfunction after myocardial infarction. Results of the Survival and Ventricular Enlargement trial. *N Engl J Med* 1992;327: 669–677.

50. Moye LA, Pfeffer MA, Wun CC et al: Uniformity of captopril benefit in the SAVE study: Subgroup analysis. *Eur Heart J* 1994;15:2–8.

51. The Acute Infarction Ramipril Efficacy (AIRE) Study Investigators: Effect of ramipril on mortality and morbidity of survivors of acute myocardial infarction with clinical evidence of heart failure. *Lancet* 1993;342:821–828.

52. The TRACE Study Group: The Trandolapril Cardiac Evaluation (TRACE) study: Rationale, design and baseline characteristics of the screened population. *Am J Cardiol* 1994;73(Suppl):44C–50C.

53. Swedberg K, Held P, Kjekshus J, Rasmussen K, Ryden L, Wedel H: Effects of the early administration of enalapril on mortality in patients with acute myocardial infarction—results of the Cooperative New Scandinavian Enalapril Survival Study II (CONSENSUS II). *N Engl J Med* 1992;327: 678–684.

54. Gruppo Italiano per lo Studio della Sopravvivenza nell' Infarto Miocardico: GISSI-3. Effects of lisinopril

and transdermal glyceryl trinitrate singly and together on 6-week mortality and ventricular function after acute myocardial infarction. *Lancet* 1994; 343:1115–1122.

55. ISIS-4 Collaborative Group: ISIS-4: A randomized factorial trial assessing early oral captopril, oral mononitrate, and intravenous magnesium sulphate in 58,050 patents with suspected acute myocardial infarction. *Lancet* 1995;345:669–685.

56. Chinese Cardiac Study Collaborative Group: Oral captopril versus placebo among 13,634 patients with suspected acute myocardial infarction: Interim report from the Chinese cardiac study (CCS-1). *Lancet* 1995;345:686–687.

57. Ambrosioni E, Borghi C, Magnani B, et al: The effect of the angiotensin-converting-enzyme inhibitor zofenopril on mortality and morbidity after anterior myocardial infarction. *N Engl J Med* 1995;332: 80–85.

58. Latini R, Maggioni AP, Flather M, Sleight P, Tognoni G: ACE inhibitor use in patients with myocardial infarction. *Circulation* 1995;92:3132–3137.

59. Rutherford JD, Pfeffer MA, Moye LA, et al: Effects of captopril on ischemic events after myocardial infarction. Results of the SAVE trial. *Circulation* 1994; 90:1731–1738.

60. The SOLVD Investigators: Effect of enalapril on survival in patients with reduced left ventricular ejection fractions and congestive heart failure. *N Engl J Med* 1991;325:293–302.

61. Pfeffer MA, Hennekens CH: When a question has an answer: Rationale for our early termination of the HEART trial. *Am J Cardiol* 1995;75(16): 1173–1175.

30

Assessment of the Survivors of Acute Myocardial Infarction: The Case for Coronary Angiography

Daniel L. Kulick, MD, and Shahbudin H. Rahimtoola, MB, FRCP, MACP

More than 600,000 patients are admitted annually to the hospital with acute myocardial infarction (MI) in the United States (1,2), and more than 80% survive to hospital discharge (2); with newer aggressive strategies, including reperfusion therapy, the percentage of patients surviving the hospital phase of acute MI may be substantially higher (3–5). For hospital survivors of acute MI, mortality in the first year approximates 10%, and it is 3% to 5% per year thereafter (1,2,6–10). Of patients who die in the first year after acute MI, approximately 50% to 75% do so in the first 3 to 6 months (2,8,9,11–13); importantly, the majority of deaths and morbid cardiac events are often observed in the first several weeks after acute MI (12,14,15). More recent data, most of which emanates from the era of acute reperfusion, suggest that mortality rates, both short-term and long-term, have declined (see Chs. 6 and 19). Nonetheless, identification of patients at increased risk of subsequent cardiac morbidity and mortality after acute MI is an issue of major clinical importance.

Before hospital discharge, survivors of acute MI may be subdivided into those at very high risk (with a 1-year cardiac mortality of up to 50%), those at low risk (with a 1-year mortality well below 5%), and those at intermediate risk (2,16,17). A history of prior myocardial infarction, before the index infarction, is clearly associated with an increased late cardiac mortality (2,8,9,18–20). Recurrent myocardial ischemia more than 24 to 48 hours after hospital admission is observed in up to 18% of patients with acute MI (21–23), and it is associated with a high incidence of cardiac mortality (21,24,25), recurrent MI (26,27), and multivessel coronary artery disease (21,23,28). Congestive heart failure occurring during hospitalization is associated with increased late cardiac mortality (2,9,17,20,25), as is severe left ventricular systolic dysfunction (2,16–18,29); residual left ventricular ejection fraction and in particular left ventricular end-systolic volume after acute MI may in fact be the most potent predictors of late survival (30,31). The occurrence of complex and/or frequent ventricular arrhythmias in the late hospital phase of acute MI is similarly associated with an increased risk of late cardiac mortality (9,17,32,33). Overall, the incidence of acute MI complicated by one or more of the preceding factors is 30% to 48% (23,34,35).

For these high-risk patients with complicated acute MI, the poor prognosis associated with conservative management mandates a more intensive approach; the majority of such patients may benefit from early cardiac catheterization and coronary angiography, and potentially from coronary artery revascularization, as well as aggressive management of left ventricular dysfunction and ventricular arrhythmias. The *critical management decision* is with the majority of patients who have an uncomplicated acute MI; some may have a relatively poor late prognosis, and others are at very low risk (<1% 1-year mortality). The *clinical challenge* is to correctly and nearly completely identify patients with uncomplicated acute MI who are at increased risk so that the appropriate interventions may be instituted before the occurrence of further adverse cardiac events.

Two approaches may be applied to patients surviving an uncomplicated acute MI in assessing cardiac risk before hospital discharge. One method is the initial use of noninvasive tests, including measures to detect myocardial ischemia and left ventricular dysfunction (see Ch. 11); invasive testing (that is, cardiac catheterization and angiography) is reserved for patients with abnormal or equivocal results of noninvasive testing, or for those patients in whom noninvasive testing cannot be performed for any reason. The second approach to risk assessment after acute MI comprises early cardiac catheterization and angiography in virtually all survivors; catheterization data may be integrated with selected, appropriate noninvasive test data to determine the prognosis for the patient. These two approaches are discussed separately and then compared and contrasted.

CARDIAC CATHETERIZATION AND ANGIOGRAPHY AFTER ACUTE MYOCARDIAL INFARCTION

Much valuable information may be learned from cardiac catheterization and angiography after MI, including anatomic and physiologic data on cardiac function and the coronary circulation; this information is summarized in Table 30–1. Cardiac catheterization is a relatively safe procedure, with a procedure-related mortality of 0.1% to 0.3% (36–39) and is similarly safe after acute MI (18,23,40–43), so that procedural risk is not a major factor in decision analysis. The exception may be in the performance of catheterization immediately after the administration of thrombolytic therapy, when procedural risk may be increased (44,45); catheterization immediately after thrombolytic therapy should generally be reserved for unstable patients who may be in need of emergent mechanical or surgical revascularization.

Table 30–1. Information Learned from Cardiac Catheterization and Angiography After Acute Myocardial Infarction

Cardiac hemodynamics
Left ventricular function (systolic and diastolic)
Coronary artery anatomy
Extent of disease
Severity of disease
Lesion morphology and location
Presence of residual thrombus
Coronary artery physiologic function
Estimation of "vulnerable," hibernating, and stunned myocardium
Concomitant valvular and pulmonary vascular disease

Patients sustaining an acute MI often have extensive coronary artery disease. Table 30–2 depicts the incidence of severe coronary artery disease in series reporting coronary arteriographic findings soon after acute MI. The severity of coronary artery disease increases with advancing age of the population studied, with an average incidence of significant multivessel coronary artery disease after acute MI of 62%; most series report an incidence of 50% to 75% (18,19,23,28,29,41,42,46–57). Importantly, most series report an incidence of severe three-vessel coronary artery disease of 25% to 50%, with a small percentage of patients having left main coronary artery disease. It is therefore clear that a large percentage, if not the majority, of survivors of acute MI have coronary artery disease severe enough to warrant consideration for coronary artery revascularization.

Severe Extensive Coronary Artery Disease

The common finding of severe extensive coronary disease after acute MI has important prognostic implications. In patients with stable coronary artery disease, survival is directly related to the number of vessels involved with significant disease

Table 30–2. Incidence of Severe Coronary Artery Disease After Acute Myocardial Infarction

Study		Maximum age	Incidence (%)		
			MVD	3VD	LMCAD
Savran et al,	1976 (46)	39	45	24	0
Veenbrink et al,	1985 (47)	59	25	5	NS
Sanz et al,	1982 (29)	60	59	26	1
Roubin et al,	1983 (41)	60	35	9	1
Abraham et al,	1986 (48)	60	43	13	0
Patterson et al,	1983 (49)	64	63	43	8
Tubau et al,	1980 (50)	65	64	28	6
DeFeyter et al,	1982 (28)	65	55	14	1
Gibson et al,	1983 (51)	65	61	22	2
Griffith et al,	1988 (52)	65	68	45	NS
Taylor et al,	1980 (18)	66	74	53	NS
Schulman et al,	1988 (19)	66	73	50	8
Bertrand et al,	1979 (42)	68	75	32	NS
Schwartz et al,	1981 (53)	68	71	NS	NS
Starling et al,	1981 (54)	68	72	40	2
Akhras et al,	1984 (55)	68	73	49	NS
Turner et al,	1980 (23)	69	67	35	8.5
Morris et al,	1984 (56)	83	88	47	12
Williams et al,	1973 (57)	NS	72	36	3
Pooled			62	32	4
Range			25–88	5–53	0–12

MVD = multivessel coronary disease, 3VD = three-vessel coronary artery disease, LMCAD = left main coronary artery disease, NS = not stated.
Modified from Kulick and Rahimtoola (136), with permission.

(58–64). Similarly, in patients with acute MI, the presence of significant multivessel coronary artery disease is closely associated with an increased mortality risk (18,29,48,51). Schulman et al (19) reported a 5-year event-free survival (freedom from death, coronary artery bypass surgery) of only 38% after acute MI in patients with three-vessel coronary artery disease. The finding of severe disease in the proximal segment of the left anterior descending coronary artery also confers an adverse prognosis after acute MI (19,28,65). Several series have demonstrated the presence or absence of multivessel disease after acute MI to be a better predictor of survival than clinical or noninvasive testing parameters (28,29,51,66).

Specific Coronary Angiographic Patterns

In addition to providing information regarding a potentially adverse prognosis, certain coronary angiographic patterns may be used to define a group of patients with a favorable prognosis after acute MI. The finding of single-vessel coronary artery disease after acute MI is associated with an excellent prognosis in most patients (19,67). Angiographic patency of the infarct-related coronary artery confers powerful prognostic information as well; long-term cardiac morbidity and mortality are favorably influenced by patency of the infarct related artery, as opposed to a persistently occluded artery (14,68–70).

In assessment of coronary angiograms, the finding of angiographically entirely normal coronary arteries has different implications than the observance of minimal luminal irregularities (no stenosis ≥50% diameter reduction). In patients with truly normal coronary arteries, the 5- to 7-year cardiac mortality is only 0% to 0.9%, whereas mortality increases to 2.0% to 5.1% in the presence of minimal coronary artery disease (71–74). In series of patients in whom coronary angiography was performed 18 to 23 months before the acute MI, 48% to 90% of patients were demonstrated to have had a stenosis of <50% diameter reduction in the future infarct-related coronary artery (75–77). The presence of luminal irregularities or ulcerations is related to an increased likelihood of development of acute MI (77–79). Such subtle abnormalities in coronary anatomy, although prognostically important, are not detectable by currently available noninvasive techniques. Although no specific therapy may be available when such findings are detected, such information may be very useful to both the physician and to the patient for long-term management and planning (aggressive risk factor control and lifestyle modification, and possible initiation of pharmacologic prophylactic measures).

Residual Left Ventricular Function

In addition to coronary artery anatomy, residual left ventricular function after acute MI, which may also be assessed with cardiac catheterization, is a potent predictor of late prognosis (2,16–19,28–30,80). The importance of left ventricular end-systolic volume as the major determinant of late outcome has been emphasized by White and associates (81) (see also Ch. 29). Importantly, the presence of viable, contracting myocardial segments subtended by a high-grade coronary artery stenosis ("vulnerable myocardium") is associated with a high incidence of adverse cardiac events after acute MI (19). Areas of hypocontractile myocardium that are still perfused after acute MI may still be viable, as a result of myocardial stunning or hibernation, and may improve function after myocardial revascularization (82–86); this subject is discussed later in the chapter. It is therefore clear that in addition to the independent prognostic information learned from coronary and left ventricular angiography after acute MI, an integrated analysis of the two provides further valuable information.

Coronary Flow Reserve

The introduction of methods to assess coronary flow reserve in the cardiac catheterization laboratory has allowed use of this excellent measure of coronary artery flow dynamics in the assessment of the functional significance of coronary artery stenoses of apparently moderate angiographic severity (87,88). This physiologic information may be a valuable adjunct to evaluation of coronary anatomy.

Application to Therapy

In addition to providing important prognostic information, cardiac catheterization and angiography findings after acute MI may be used to implement therapy designed to improve long-term survival. Clinical trials comparing coronary artery bypass surgery with conventional medical therapy have demonstrated survival benefit after bypass surgery in patients with left main coronary artery disease, as well as in those with three-vessel and two-vessel coronary artery disease (particularly in those patients with proximal left anterior descending coronary artery disease and/or left ventricular dysfunction) (83,89–92). After acute MI, myocardial revascularization likely provides survival benefit in patients with recurrent ischemia (93), severe multivessel coronary artery disease (55,94), and "vulnerable" myocardial segments (as described earlier) (94). Early cardiac catheterization and angiography thus provide important diagnostic, prognostic, and therapeutic information for the survivor of acute MI, and they are valuable aids in long-term patient management.

NONINVASIVE TESTING AFTER ACUTE MYOCARDIAL INFARCTION

Risk assessment using noninvasive testing is a widely advocated approach in patients surviving an uncomplicated acute MI (6,16,95–97) (see Ch. 11). The goal of this approach is to identify patients with residual myocardial ischemia, extensive coronary artery disease, left ventricular dysfunction, and/or complex ventricular arrhythmias, and then to apply invasive tests to this group of patients. Identification and management of patients with complex ventricular arrhythmias after acute MI are discussed in Chapter 27 and are not further addressed here. In analysis of a noninvasive risk assessment strategy for post–MI patients, it is important to evaluate not only the comparative incidences of cardiac events in patients with or without abnormal test results, but also the sensitivity of the test for detecting cardiac events (that is, how many patients who develop a late event are correctly identified) and the predictive accuracy of the test (that is, how likely are patients with a normal or abnormal test to have a late cardiac event).

The foundation of noninvasive risk assessment after acute MI is the predischarge exercise test, generally performed at a low to moderate workload, and limited either by the development of symptoms or by attainment of a predetermined workload. The safety of such testing is well established, and expected findings are the subject of detailed review (95,98–100). Selected aspects of predischarge exercise testing after acute MI are discussed here.

Numerous exercise variables have been evaluated for the ability to predict cardiac mortality in the months and years after uncomplicated acute MI. Although exercise-induced ST segment depression has been the most commonly studied variable and has been predictive of cardiac prognosis in most series, several series have found this variable to be of little or no predictive value (34,53,101–103). The magnitude of ST segment depression required to constitute an "abnormal" test has direct bearing on the utility of the test. Weld et al (101) found a criterion of 2 mm of ST segment depression to result in enhanced specificity for cardiac mortality after acute MI, as compared with 1 mm of depression, although this criterion reduced the sensitivity of the test for predicting cardiac mortality to only 19% (Table 30–3); when predischarge exercise testing is used for screening purposes, such levels of sensitivity are unacceptable. Exercise-induced ST segment elevation may also be predictive of an adverse late prognosis after acute MI (24). Other exercise variables demonstrated in some series to be predictive of an adverse late prognosis include development of angina pectoris during exercise (53,54,104); failure to attain an adequate workload (24,28,34,101–103,105), heart rate (24,49,66), or blood pressure response during exercise (24,34, 54,102); and development of ventricular arrhythmias during exercise (24,66,101,102). Rather than focusing on a single test variable, the predischarge exercise test is of maximal value if all data from the study are integrated and interpreted as a composite result (54,66,106).

An analysis of some of the reported series of predischarge exercise testing after acute MI is presented in Table 30–3. Series are presented with the prognostic exercise variable(s) analyzed and the late event(s) measured (24,25,28,34,51,53,101–109). Although each of these series was able to separate groups at high and low risk for adverse cardiac events after acute MI, these findings must be carefully analyzed. These series report variable sensitivities and specificities. A test sensitivity of 80% may be statistically attractive; however, clinically it implies that 20% of patients destined for an adverse event will be "missed" with noninvasive screening. More importantly, the predictive value of normal tests has major implications for individual patients; if a normal test is 95% predictive of absence of late cardiac events, the patient with a normal test has a 1 in 20 chance of sustaining a major adverse event in the year after acute MI. From Table 30–3, it is clear that certain variables may have greater prognostic value than others on careful analysis; in series comparing multiple variables, exercise duration and attained workload appear to confer much more predictive value that ST segment depression/elevation (28,101,109).

In addition to prognostic value, predischarge exercise testing after acute MI has other important uses, including provision of patient reassurance before hospital discharge, assessment of functional capacity and development of an exercise prescription, and assessment of physiologic significance of known coronary artery disease of moderate angiographic severity.

To improve the prognostic utility of simple exercise testing, other supplemental noninvasive modalities have been examined in survivors of acute MI. Addition of immediate and delayed thallium-201 scintigraphy to exercise testing has been observed to improve sensitivity and predictive value for late cardiac events in several series (51,66,110). Gibson et al (51) observed a sensitivity of 94% for late cardiac events with exercise thallium-201 scintigraphy, as opposed to a sensitivity of only 71% with exercise testing alone; in this series, however, a normal

Table 30–3. Prognostic Value of Exercise Testing After Acute Myocardial Infarction

Study		% of Patients with Abnormal Test*	Prognostic Variable Analyzed	Late Event Monitored	Incidence (%) of Late Events in Patients with		Ability of Test To predict events		
					Abnormal Test	Normal Test	Sens (%)	Spec (%)	Pred NL† (%)
Markiewicz et al,	1977 (107)	40	ST	DEATH, MI	41	0	100	71	100
Theroux et al,	1979 (104)	38	ST	DEATH	27	2	85	75	98
Starling et al,	1980 (106)	60	ST, AP, BP, and/or ARR	DEATH	13	0	100	43	100
Schwartz et al,	1981 (53)	44	AP	DEATH	27	3	75	82	97
Weld et al,	1981 (101)	51	ST-1	DEATH	13	8	33	79	92
			ST-2	DEATH	15	8	19	90	92
			DUR	DEATH	17	1	95	53	99
DeFeyter et al,	1982 (28)	68	ST and/or AP	DEATH	8	5	64	50	95
			DUR	DEATH	9	0	100	35	100
DeBusk et al,	1983 (108)	9	ST	DEATH, MI	10	4	20	91	96
Gibson et al,	1983 (51)	41	ST and/or AP	DEATH	9	2	71	61	98
Hung et al,	1984 (105)	27	ST	DEATH, MI	9	6	38	73	94
Williams et al,	1984 (103)	46	DUR	DEATH	17	5	42	84	95
Madsen et al,	1985 (109)	55	ST	DEATH, MI	9	4	74	47	96
			WORK	DEATH, MI	18	2	79	75	98
Waters et al,	1985 (24)	43	ST	DEATH	22	3	84	62	97
Deckers et al,	1987 (34)	44	BP	DEATH	13	1	75	79	99
Krone et al,	1985 (102)	40	BP	DEATH	18	3	32	93	97
Ross et al,	1989 (25)	37	ST and/or WORK	DEATH	6	1	83	65	99
Range		9–68			6–41	0–8	19–100	35–93	92–100

SENS = sensitivity of exercise test for predicting late cardiac events; SPEC = specificity of exercise test for predicting late cardiac events; PRED NL = predictive accuracy of normal exercise test for predicting freedom from late cardiac events; ST = ST segment depression during exercise (ST-1 = 1 mm depression, ST-2 = 2 mm depression); AP = angina pectoris during exercise; BP = abnormal blood pressure response during exercise; ARR = ventricular arrhythmias during exercise; DUR = duration of exercise; WORK = workload achieved during exercise; MI = myocardial infarction.

* Patient with a major test abnormality suggestive of possible myocardial ischemia; not necessarily the prognostic variable analyzed in next column.

† Predictive accuracy of abnormal test for predicting occurrence of late cardiac events is identical to column labeled "Incidence (%) of Late Events in Patients with Abnormal Test."

thallium scintigraphic study was less predictive of freedom from late events (94%) than was a normal exercise test (98%). Other investigators have failed to observe a major advantage from the addition of thallium-201 imaging to simple exercise testing (48, 105,111). At the time of this writing, no consensus is apparent regarding the additive value of exercise thallium-201 scintigraphy after an uncomplicated acute MI (see Ch. 11). In patients unable to exercise after acute MI, immediate and delayed thallium imaging after administration of dipyridamole has been evaluated; preliminary studies have been conflicting regarding the prognostic utility of this test (15,112), and further studies are necessary before recommendations may be made.

The occurrence of painless myocardial ischemia at rest, as detected by ambulatory monitoring, has recently been demonstrated to be predictive of an adverse late outcome after MI (113,114). The additional value of seeking painless myocardial ischemia at rest in patients already undergoing an extensive risk assessment evaluation after acute MI remains uncertain at present.

As mentioned earlier, resting left ventricular systolic function is a potent predictor of survival after acute MI (2,16–18,29). Left ventricular systolic function may be assessed noninvasively with either echocardiography or radionuclide angiography, and one of these tests is essential if a noninvasive approach to risk assessment is employed. Measurement of the exercise response of left ventricular ejection fraction, as assessed by exercise radionuclide angiography, has been found to add prognostic information after acute MI in some series (105,115,116), but not in others (117,118). Exercise two-dimensional echocardiography may similarly supply prognostic information after acute MI (119,120) (see Ch. 10).

The preceding noninvasive test modalities add a degree of complexity to the noninvasive evaluation of the survivor of acute MI. Many of these tests may not be widely available, and where available, the complex equipment and expert performance and interpretation required to attain the accurate results reported in the literature may not be present. Finally, the cost of complex noninvasive testing is not insignificant, particularly if multiple tests are often repeated.

LIMITATIONS OF NONINVASIVE TESTING AFTER ACUTE MYOCARDIAL INFARCTION

Several limitations of a noninvasive approach to risk assessment after acute MI merit discussion. Most reported series of noninvasive testing after acute MI have not included three important subgroups of patients: (i) those receiving thrombolytic therapy; (ii) the "elderly" (greater than 65 to 70 years of age); and (iii) those unable to perform an exercise test. The first two groups of patients are examined separately later in this chapter. Patients may be unable to exercise after acute MI not only because of severe cardiac disease, but also because of severe peripheral vascular disease, musculoskeletal disorders, or noncardiac medical illness; approximately 10% to 22% of patients are unable to perform an exercise test after acute MI (Table 30–4) (34,35,51,102,121–125). Inability to perform an exercise test after acute MI is a potent marker of an adverse late prognosis; such patients demonstrate a 10% to 14% mortality 12 to 22 months after acute MI (see Table 30–4) (25,34,102,122,125) and have a high incidence of recurrent myocardial infarction (9). The subgroup of patients unable to exercise after acute MI thus represents a high-risk subset that may benefit from early, aggressive intervention.

Submaximal predischarge exercise testing after acute MI, because of failure to attain a maximal workload, may be insufficient to reliably exclude potential sources of myocardial ischemia. As many as 35% of patients with a negative predischarge submaximal exercise test may demonstrate myocardial ischemia on a more strenuous test performed 6 to 12 weeks after acute MI (35,126); patients with a normal predischarge submaximal exercise test should, therefore, undergo a second, more rigorous test after hospital discharge. As the majority of cardiac deaths in the first year after hospital discharge for acute MI occur in the early weeks and months (9,12,14,15,127), a small but finite risk of mortality exists for the patient with a normal predischarge submaximal exercise test who may have potentially severe myocardial ischemia not yet detected by a full exercise test (128). Similarly, the day-to-day reproducibility of submaximal exercise testing after

Table 30–4. Inability to Perform Exercise Testing After Acute Myocardial Infarction

Study		% of Patients Unable to Perform Exercise Test	Late Mortality (%) in Patients Unable to Perform Exercise Test
Ibsen et al,	1975 (121)	15	NA
Chaitman et al,	1978 (123)	15	NA
Fuller et al,	1981 (35)	10	NA
Gibson et al,	1981 (124)	19	NA
Gibson et al,	1983 (51)	15	NA
Krone et al,	1985 (102)	22	14 (12 mo)
Gibson et al,	1986 (122)	12	13 (22 mo)
Deckers et al,	1987 (34)	16	10 (12 mo)
Krone et al,	1989 (125)	20	13 (12 mo)
Ross et al,	1989 (25)	*	11 (12 mo) *
RANGE		10–22	10–14

NA = not available from published report.

* % of patients unable to perform exercise test not separated from patients with indeterminate test results; late mortality includes those unable to perform test and those with indeterminate tests.

acute MI may be less that optimal; Handler and Sowton (129) observed only a 71% day-to-day reproducibility for demonstrable myocardial ischemia on consecutive predischarge submaximal exercise tests after acute MI.

As demonstrated in Table 30–3, a number of patients with normal results on predischarge exercise testing may still die or suffer a recurrent myocardial infarction in the first year after acute MI. Such noninvasive "false negatives" are a particular problem in managing individual patients. If a normal exercise test has a 97% predictive accuracy for the absence of late cardiac mortality, a 3% mortality in the first year may not be a satisfactory prognosis for a 40- or 50-year-old patient, particularly one with a young family. As also illustrated in Table 30–3, the wide range of sensitivities of exercise testing for detecting cardiac events after acute MI suggests that a significant number of patients who will sustain an adverse cardiac event may be missed with exercise testing.

Why might patients with a normal noninvasive evaluation after acute MI still be at risk of cardiac mortality? One possible explanation might be the inability of the test to detect significant multivessel coronary artery disease. The adverse prognostic implication of multivessel disease after acute MI has already been discussed in detail; the ability of noninvasive testing to reliably detect multivessel coronary artery disease might, therefore, be strongly related to its prognostic utility. Table 30–5 lists reported series evaluating the ability of exercise testing after acute MI to detect the presence of multivessel coronary artery disease. In 10 of the 14 series listed, the sensitivity of exercise testing for the presence of multivessel disease is <75%, suggesting that >25% of patients with significant multivessel disease may fail to be detected with exercise testing; similarly, in 10 of these 14 series, the predictive accuracy of a normal exercise test for the absence of multivessel coronary artery disease after acute MI is below 75%, implying that a patient with a normal exercise test will have a >25% chance of having multivessel coronary artery disease (35,47,48,50, 52–56,110,124,130–132). Gibson et al (124) found that addition of thallium-201 scintigraphy to exercise testing enhances the ability to detect multivessel coronary artery disease after acute MI; other investigators, however, have not demonstrated increased benefit from the addition of radionuclide imaging (48,110,111,133). In addition to possible failure to detect severe multivessel coronary artery disease in many patients after acute MI, noninvasive testing is unable to detect luminal ulcerations, thrombi, and other irregularities in noncritically stenosed coronary arteries; the prognostic importance of such findings has already been addressed.

A final consideration in review of noninvasive risk assessment after acute MI is the duration of clinical follow-up in reported series. Most series report follow-up of only 1 or 2 years; however, the patient and physician may benefit from a longer prognostic perspective. Although Waters et al (24) were able to identify a subset of patients with only a 3%

Table 30–5. Ability of Noninvasive Testing to Predict Multivessel Coronary Artery Disease After Acute Myocardial Infarction

		Exercise Testing				Exercise + Thallium-201 Scintigraphy			
Study		SENS (%)	SPEC (%)	PRED ABNL (%)	PRED NL (%)	SENS (%)	SPEC (%)	PRED ABNL (%)	PRED NL (%)
Paine et al,	1978 (130)	83	54	78	62				
Weiner et al,	1978 (131)	96	41	70	87				
Tubau et al,	1980 (50)	72	52	73	51				
Turner et al,	1980 (110)	50	83	93	28	46	83	92	26
Fuller et al,	1981 (35)	65	90	87	72				
Gibson et al,	1981 (121)	42	74	57	61	74	91	88	81
Schwartz et al,	1981 (53)	56	86	90	44				
Starling et al,	1981 (54)	88	69	88	69				
DeFeyter et al,	1983 (132)	67	67	71	63				
Akhras et al,	1984 (55)	94	94	98	86				
Morris et al,	1984 (56)	43	85	95	17				
Veenbrink et al,	1985 (47)	63	89	67	88				
Abraham et al,	1986 (48)	64	77	64	77	64	88	80	76
Griffith et al,	1988 (52)	46	85	87	42				
Range		42–96	41–94	57–98	17–88	46–74	83–91	80–92	26–81

SENS = sensitivity; SPEC = specificity; PRED ABNL = predicted accuracy of abnormal test for presence of multivessel coronary artery disease, PRED NL = predictive accuracy of normal test for absence of multivessel coronary artery disease.

1-year mortality with exercise testing after uncomplicated acute MI, the 5-year mortality in this "low-risk subset" was 12%; in this series, the results of predischarge exercise testing were far less predictive of survival beyond the first year after acute MI.

In conclusion, although noninvasive testing after acute MI may be able to identify groups of patients with differing prognosis, many patients will ultimately require invasive (see later), and certain limitations of this approach are apparent. These limitations, discussed in detail earlier, are summarized in Table 30–6.

Table 30–6. Potential Limitations of Noninvasive Risk Assessment After Acute MI

- Many clinically important subgroups are excluded from reported series (elderly, those who have received thrombolytic treatment, those unable to exercise).
- Submaximal exercise testing may not attain a sufficient workload to reliably exclude myocardial ischemia.
- Patients destined for adverse cardiac events may be "missed."
- Value is limited in the detection of multivessel coronary artery disease.
- Reported follow-up is of relatively short duration.
- High-quality, state-of-the-art testing may not be available in many centers.
- Many patients still ultimately require cardiac catheterization and angiography.

EXPECTED RESULTS FROM NONINVASIVE RISK ASSESSMENT AFTER UNCOMPLICATED ACUTE MYOCARDIAL INFARCTION

A scheme illustrating the results expected from a noninvasive risk assessment strategy for survivors of uncomplicated acute MI, based on a compilation of reported clinical series, is presented in Fig. 30–1. This scheme excludes the following groups of patients: patients failing to survive to hospital discharge; patients with acute MI complicated by recurrent ischemia, congestive heart failure, or late (>24 to 48 hours) complex ventricular arrhythmias; and patients excluded in most clinical series of exercise testing after acute MI (age >65 to 70 years; treatment with thrombolytic therapy). Approximately 10% to 22% of patients are unable to perform an exercise test before hospital discharge (34,35,51,102, 121–125); this number may be averaged to 15%. As patients unable to perform an exercise test after acute MI are at increased risk for late cardiac events, these 15 patients (15% of 100 patients) should undergo early cardiac catheterization and angiography.

Table 30–3 demonstrates that of patients able to perform an exercise test after acute MI, 9% to 68%

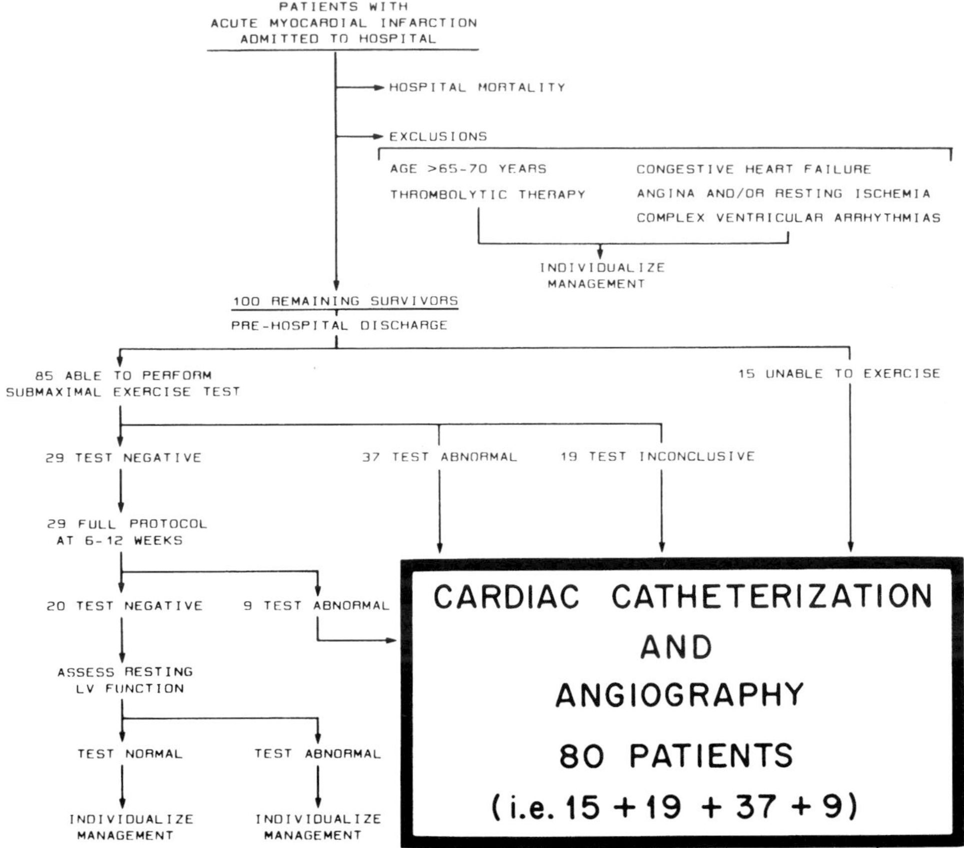

Figure 30–1. Projected scheme for expectations of noninvasive risk assessment in survivors of uncomplicated acute myocardial infarction. Details are given in text. *Modified from Kulick and Rahimtoola (135), with permission.*

demonstrate an abnormality on testing suggesting myocardial ischemia or left ventricular dysfunction; the average incidence of abnormal tests in these 15 series is 43%. Of the 85 remaining patients thus able to perform an exercise test, 43%, or 37 patients, have an abnormal test and require early cardiac catheterization and angiography. Inconclusive or indeterminate exercise test results are observed in 16% to 29% of patients, for an average of 22% (47,130); as patients with inconclusive test results may have a high incidence of multivessel coronary disease (130), such patients should also undergo cardiac catheterization (85 × 22% = 19 patients).

The remaining 29 patients with a normal predischarge submaximal exercise test after acute MI require maximal exercise testing at a later date; 25% to 35% of such tests may be expected to be abnormal (average, 30%) (35,126), resulting in an additional 9 patients who require cardiac catheterization. Of the remaining 20 patients with no exercise test abnormality, independent assessment of resting left ventricular systolic function will disclose some patients with occult left ventricular dysfunction, some of whom may require invasive evaluation. Overall, therefore, employment of a noninvasive risk assessment strategy after uncomplicated acute MI indicates that approximately 80% of patients will ultimately require cardiac catheterization and angiography.

Analysis of the data from the prospective study of Ross et al (25) reveals somewhat similar findings. Among 402 patients 75 years of age or younger surviving to hospital discharge after uncomplicated acute MI, 66% either had abnormal or indeterminate exercise test results or did not perform an exercise test; these patients had a 6% to 11% 1-year cardiac mortality, suggesting potential benefit of early cardiac catheterization and angiography in this high-risk group.

The addition of exercise thallium-201 scintigraphy to noninvasive risk assessment after acute MI yields similar results. Gibson et al (51) observed 70% of patients to either be unable to exercise or to demonstrate evidence of reversible ischemia with radionuclide imaging, suggesting a 70% requirement for cardiac catheterization and angiography.

In a multicenter registry (from Sweden, Canada, and the United States) (134), after evaluation by history, clinical and noninvasive, 70% of the patients were considered to be in the medium- and high-risk subgroups, suggesting a 70% requirement for cardiac catheterization and angiography.

It is evident, therefore, that although noninvasive risk assessment after acute MI may be able to identify subsets of patients with differing late prognosis, a significant majority of such patients ultimately require cardiac catheterization and angiography.

COST CONSIDERATIONS IN RISK ASSESSMENT AFTER ACUTE MYOCARDIAL INFARCTION

The performance of early cardiac catheterization and angiography in all survivors of acute MI is perceived as resulting in a significantly increased cost, but this may not be entirely correct. An aggressive approach to patients with acute MI, including early cardiac catheterization, need not be significantly more costly (135,136). The cost of noninvasive testing is not insignificant, particularly if complex, multiple, and often repetitive tests are employed; as discussed earlier, the majority of patients ultimately require cardiac catheterization after noninvasive risk assessment.

Also discussed earlier, cardiac catheterization and angiography as a single test provide powerful prognostic information after acute MI. Some patients may still require exercise testing after cardiac catheterization to help assess the functional significance of moderate coronary artery disease; a combination of selected invasive and noninvasive variables may provide the most complete prognostic profile (51,66). Early cardiac catheterization and angiography in virtually all survivors of acute MI need not be more expensive than an initial noninvasive approach, if all tests are carefully and judiciously selected.

SPECIAL PATIENT SUBSETS

Patients with Non-Q Wave Myocardial Infarction

Approximately 25% of acute MIs are of the non-Q wave variety (137–139); this percentage is likely to increase with the more widespread use of thrombolytic therapy to limit myocardial infarct size. Although the in-hospital mortality after non-Q wave MI is lower than that associated with Q wave MI, the late (1- to 3-year) mortality is similar, suggesting that hospital survivors of non-Q wave MI have a higher late mortality than survivors of Q wave MI (137–141); the late mortality after non-Q wave MI is particularly high in the presence of persistent ST segment depression (142) or anterior location (143) (see Ch. 18).

Patients with non-Q wave MI do not have a greater incidence of severe multivessel coronary artery disease than patients with Q wave MI, suggesting that the extent of coronary artery disease is an unlikely cause of the increased late risk in these patients (23,122,137,144,145). The likely cause of increased late cardiac morbidity and mortality in survivors of non-Q wave MI is the high incidence of recurrent myocardial ischemia observed in such patients. As illustrated in Table 30–7, recurrent myocardial ischemia is observed in 35% to 66% of patients during the first year after non-Q wave MI (22,122,140,146–148), and recurrent MI in 6% to 21% of patients (26,122,140,141,143,146). Gibson et al (122) demonstrated abnormal exercise thallium-201 scintigraphic patterns suggestive of myocardial ischemia in 75% of survivors of non-Q wave MI and a high incidence of need for early coronary revascularization. Demonstration of recurrent ischemia after non-Q wave MI is clearly

Table 30–7. Myocardial Ischemia in the First Year After Non-Q Wave Myocardial Infarction

Study		Incidence (%)	
		Recurrent Ischemia	Recurrent Myocardial Infarction
Madigan et al,	1976 (146)	64	21
Hutter et al,	1981 (141)	—	21
Nicholson et al,	1983 (148)	64	—
Gibson et al,	1986 (122)	54	18
Gibson et al,	1986 (147)	43	—
Bosch et al,	1987 (22)	35	—
Kao et al,	1989 (143)	—	19
Nicod et al,	1989 (140)	66	6
Range		35–66	6–21

related to an increased morbid cardiac rate (26,122,149).

In patients with uncomplicated non-Q wave MI, Krone, Roger and their workers (125,150) demonstrated noninvasive test variables to be of limited value for predicting subsequent cardiac morbidity and mortality. As such patients are clearly in a high-risk group for late cardiac events, early cardiac catheterization and angiography are appropriate for most, if not all, survivors of non-Q wave MI, particularly those with a non-Q wave anterior MI. This remains an area of controversy (see Ch. 18).

Recent data analyses from the TIMI-II Study indicated that of 2,634 patients who were eligible for a selected analysis, 767 (29.1%) had a non-Q wave infarct (151). Patients with non-Q wave infarcts, when compared with those with Q wave infarcts, were less commonly men (75.6% versus 85.3%, $p < 0.001$) and had an anterior wall infarct less frequently (43.7% versus 53.8%, $p < 0.001$). With recombinant tissue-type plasminogen activator (r-tPA) infusion, TIMI grade 3 flow was achieved in a higher percentage of patients with non-Q wave MI (72.2% versus 62.2%, $p < 0.001$); they also had a higher resting left ventricular ejection fraction (54.6% versus 48.6%) and more often had a left ventricular ejection >55% (43.4% versus 24.1%, $p = 0.001$). In the patients assigned to the conservative strategy, 47.5% of those with non-Q wave infarction had cardiac catheterization and 27.6% had percutaneous transluminal coronary angioplasty (PTCA) or coronary bypass surgery. Of patients with non-Q infarction, death occurred in 2.2% in 42 days and reinfarction in 5.4%. However, of patients with non-Q wave infarction, 11% had no coronary vessels with ≥60% stenosis and 61.4% had one-vessel disease; only 7.4% had three-vessel disease. Thus this group of patients with non-Q wave infarction were in general a low-risk group of patients; nevertheless, many had cardiac catheterization and revascularization.

Young Patients

Cardiac catheterization and angiography have been recommended in all "young" survivors of acute MI (6,96); which age constitutes "young" remains uncertain. In fact, as demonstrated in Table 30–2, younger patients have a lower incidence of extensive coronary artery disease than the overall cohort of post–MI patients; series restricted to patients 60 years of age or younger have demonstrated an incidence of multivessel coronary artery disease in 25% to 59% of patients, and of three-vessel coronary artery disease in 5% to 26% (29,41,46–48). Nonetheless, given the limitations of noninvasive screening after acute MI already discussed and the ultimately longer life expectancy of younger patients, it is appropriate to perform early cardiac catheterization and angiography on these younger survivors.

The Elderly

The proportion of elderly patients in the United States is increasing; three-fourths of all deaths from coronary artery disease occur in patients older than 65 years (152) (see Ch. 25). In the MITI study (153), the in-hospital mortality was 2% in those aged <55 years, 4.6% in patients aged 55–64 years, 12.3% in those aged 65–74 years, and 17.8% in those aged ≥75 years. In the GUSTO-I trial (154), age was the most significant factor influencing 30-day mortality, with rates of 1.1% in the patients <45 years and 20.5% in patients >75 years.

Patients older than 60 to 70 years have a threefold or greater late mortality after acute MI than younger patients (11,20,80,138,140,142,155–157). Such older patients also have a much higher incidence of multivessel coronary artery disease than younger survivors of acute MI (55,152).

More recently, the EPESE program (158) documented that the 6-month mortality after acute myocardial infarction of patients aged 65–74 years was 26%, of those aged 75–84 years was 47%, and of those aged ≥85 years was 50%. Thus the older patients also have a high mortality in the first 6 months after myocardial infarction.

Few data are available on noninvasive risk assessment of elderly patients after acute MI, as most reported series have excluded patients older than 65 to 70 years of age. Morris et al (56), in a series evaluating patients up to 83 years of age, observed an 88% incidence of multivessel coronary artery disease, and exercise testing failed to correctly identify 57% of such patients. Similarly, radionuclide left ventricular ejection fraction may not be predictive of late mortality in elderly patients after acute MI (157). Moreover, it is likely that a higher percentage of elderly patients, as compared with those <65 years of age, will not be able to perform or satisfactorily complete an exercise test.

As older patients generally do well after coronary artery revascularization, either by coronary artery bypass surgery (159) or by PTCA (160,161), appropriate older patients in otherwise good medical condition should undergo cardiac catheterization and angiography after acute MI.

Patients with Inferior Myocardial Infarction

Several series have demonstrated a particularly high incidence of multivessel coronary artery disease in survivors of inferior MI (28,42,48,50, 57,162); severe left anterior descending or left main coronary artery disease has been observed in 31% to 52% of such patients (23,28,123,162). The presence or absence of anterior ST segment depression associated with inferior MI does not reliably predict the presence or absence of multivessel coronary artery disease (163). Chaitman et al (123) observed 33% of patients with significant multivessel coronary artery disease after inferior MI to have negative exercise tests. For these reasons, cardiac catheterization and angiography are appropriate in survivors of inferior MI.

Patients with Hibernating and/or Stunned Myocardium

After acute MI, areas of partially infarcted but reperfused myocardium may be overtly hypocontractile but still viable; such "stunned" myocardium may exhibit delayed recovery of function (82) (see Chs. 3, 21). Similarly, areas of chronically hypoperfused myocardium may be hypofunctional, or "hibernating," with the ability to recover contractility after coronary artery revascularization (83–86).

At present, with currently available diagnostic tests, no single method will reliably diagnose hibernating myocardium in all patients (85,164). In a retrospective review from UCLA of 20 patients with old Q wave infarction, 20% of left ventricular regions in the area of infarction were shown to have hibernating myocardium by positron emission tomography (PET) (165). More recently, the group from Scotland (166) showed that $^{32}/_{41}$ (78%) patients had evidence of hibernating myocardium in the area of infarction identified electrocardiographically, and in one-third of the patients this was a single large area of hibernating tissue.

In one study of 84 patients who had a myocardial infarction ≥1 month previously, 17 (20%) had a cardiac event on follow-up (167). On stepwise multivariate regression analysis, presence of viable but hypocontractile myocardium by PET and the number of stenosed vessels on angiography were independent predictors of an untoward event. At 3 years, almost 60% of those with viable but hypocontractile myocardium by PET had an untoward event as opposed to less than 10% of those without viable myocardium. Performance of cardiac catheterization and angiography, with subsequent coronary artery revascularization, may result in marked improvement of left ventricular function in many such patients after acute MI. Improvement in left ventricular function after PTCA in a patient with acute MI who had received thrombolytic therapy is illustrated in Fig. 30–2. In a prospective randomized trial of PTCA in a small number of patients (168), those assigned to PTCA had a higher coronary blood flow, greater reduction in abnormal thallium-201 images, and greater improvement of left ventricular segmental wall motion and global ejection fraction.

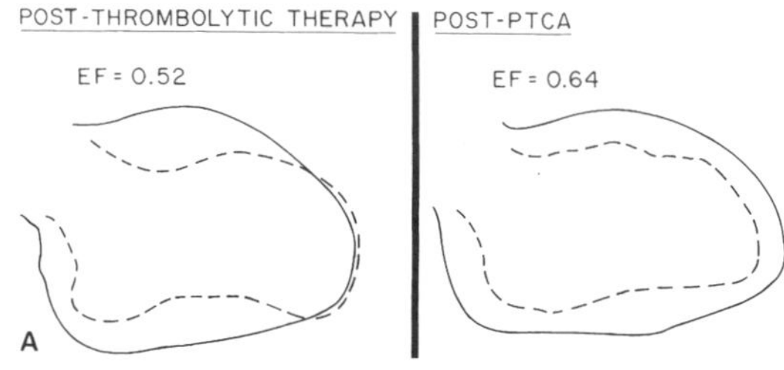

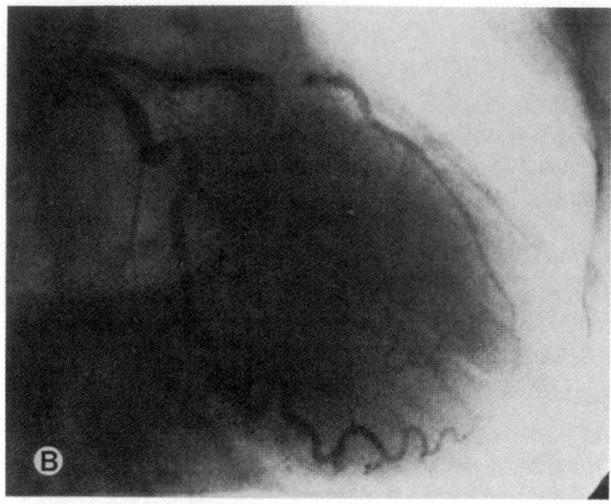

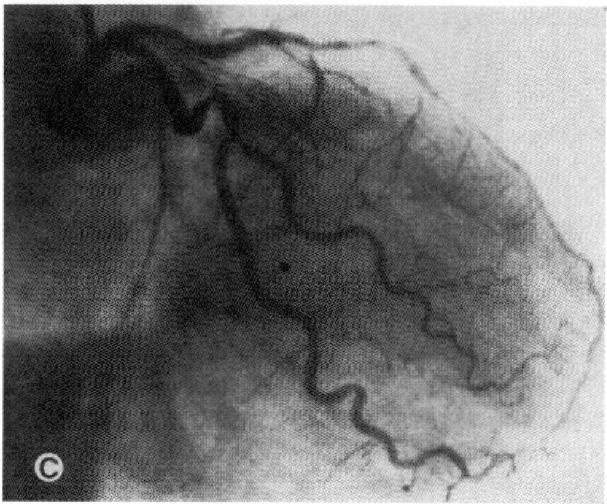

Figure 30–2. Forty-eight-year-old female sustaining an acute anterior wall myocardial infarction was treated with tissue-type plasminogen activator 2 hours after the onset of chest pain. Twenty-four hours later, the patient had recurrent angina and underwent emergency cardiac catheterization and coronary angiography. **A.** Tracings of the right anterior oblique ventriculograms. On the left, anterior akinesis is demonstrated (with a small area of dyskinesis) after thrombolytic therapy. After percutaneous transluminal coronary angioplasty (PTCA) of a high-grade left anterior descending (LAD) coronary artery stenosis, repeat ventriculography performed 1 week later, shown on the right, demonstrated dramatic recovery of wall motion; this reversible wall motion abnormality likely represents a combination of stunned and hibernating myocardium. **B.** High-grade, eccentric proximal LAD lesion before PTCA. **C.** Marked reduction of the stenosis immediately after PTCA. EF = left ventricular ejection fraction.

Patients Treated with Thrombolytic Therapy

According to the reported criteria (<76 years of age, chest pain of no more than 4 hours duration, presence of ST segment elevation, and absence of standard exclusion criteria), only 9% to 15% of patients with acute MI are eligible to receive thrombolytic therapy (see Chs. 11, 19, and 22) (169,170). Given the dramatic reduction in mortality observed with this therapeutic modality (4,5,171), these patients represent a critically important subset, and the number of patients managed with thrombolytic therapy is likely to increase. The subject of thrombolytic therapy for acute MI is addressed in detail elsewhere in this book (see Chs. 19 and 20). The assessment of patients after thrombolytic therapy is briefly discussed here.

Thrombolytic therapy fails to achieve patency of the infarct-related coronary artery in at least 20% of patients (172,173), and coronary artery reocclusion and recurrent ischemia may occur in as many as 20% of patients after initially successful thrombolysis (172–174). In the GUSTO-I trial (175), with accelerated t-PA, TIMI grade 3 flow was established in 54% of the patients, TIMI grade 2 flow was present in 27%, and TIMI grade 1 or 0 in 19%; reocclusion had occurred in 5.9%. In the GUSTO-I trial (175), the 30-day mortality of patients with TIMI grade 0 or 1 flow was 8.9%, with grade 2 flow 7.4%, and with grade 3 flow 4.4%. After successful thrombolysis, severe residual coronary artery stenoses are often present (176). Patency of the infarct-related coronary artery after successful thrombolysis is a potent prognostic variable; a patent coronary artery after thrombolytic therapy, as opposed to a persistently occluded artery, is associated with markedly improved late survival (14,69,70) and recovery of left ventricular function (69,177). Noninvasive markers of reperfusion after thrombolysis are unreliable; coronary angiography remains the only proven reliable method to establish coronary artery patency after administration of thrombolytic therapy (178).

Very limited data are available on noninvasive testing of patients after thrombolytic therapy. Exercise testing with thallium-201 scintigraphy does not reliably predict infarct vessel patency after thrombolytic therapy, although reversible thallium defects in the infarct zone may suggest viability of myocardium (179). Noninvasive testing appears to be a poor predictor of multivessel coronary artery disease after thrombolytic therapy, with reported sensitivities of only 35% to 44% (179,180). Recent data of Haber and coworkers (181) showed that for the detection of multivessel coronary artery disease postthrombolysis the sensitivity and specificity of ST segment depression on the exercise ECG were 29% and 96%, respectively; those of thallium-201 redistribution were 35% and 82%, respectively; and those of either test jointly as a single variable were 58% and 78%, respectively. Tilkemeier et al (182) determined that low-level exercise thallium-201 testing was useful in identifying patients at high risk for cardiac events at a mean follow-up of 374 days. The sensitivity and specificity of ST segment depression on the ECG in those not treated with thrombolysis were 48% and 72%, respectively; and in those treated with thrombolytics, these were 11% and 83%, respectively. The sensitivity and specificity of thallium-201 redistribution in those not treated with thrombolysis were 77% and 37%, respectively; and in those treated with thrombolytics, these were 55% and 63%, respectively. Topol et al (183) demonstrated that a combination of exercise testing and early cardiac catheterization and angiography facilitates early discharge from the hospital after thrombolytic therapy.

In the Thrombolysis in Myocardial Infarction Phase II Trial (TIMI-IIB) (3,184,185), an invasive approach, consisting of early (18 to 48 hours) cardiac catheterization and PTCA in suitable patients, was compared with a conservative approach after administration of intravenous tissue-type plasminogen activator. In the conservative limb of this study, cardiac catheterization was reserved for patients with recurrent clinical ischemia or demonstrable ischemia on exercise testing. Even in the conservative limb of this trial, at the end of 1 year, cardiac catheterization and angiography had been performed in 45% of the patients; 20.5% had undergone PTCA, and 17.3% had undergone bypass surgery (186). In this trial, equivalent cardiac mortality and recurrent myocardial infarction incidences were observed in the two treatment limbs, both at 42 days and at 1 year after acute MI. Before the findings of this trial may be widely applied to all patients managed with thrombolytic therapy, however, several key issues must be addressed.

As noted earlier, criteria for entry into the TIMI-IIB trial were quite specific and similar to those used in many other trials of acute reperfusion therapy (see Ch. 19). They included age <76 years, ability to initiate therapy within 4 hours of onset of symptoms, diagnostic ST segment elevation, no history of PTCA in the preceding 6 months, no history of coronary artery bypass surgery, no history of cerebrovascular disease, and blood pressure <180 mm Hg systolic and <110 mm Hg diastolic. The results of this trial may *not* be applicable to patients not fulfilling these criteria, but they probably do apply to the majority of patients receiving thrombolytic therapy in the current environment; in particular, ST segment elevation on the electrocardiogram remains one of the most important selection criteria for such therapy. No exclusion registry for the trial had been published at the time of this writing; thus, the number of potentially eligible patients actually enrolled remains unknown. In this regard, it should be noted that the data of Cragg et al from Michigan (187) indicated that of 1,374 consecutive patients seen at that medical center from April 1986 through June 1988, only 230 (17%) were included in randomized trials of thrombolysis. The mortality of the 230 patients included in these trials was 4% and that of 1,144 patients not included was 19%. The mortality in the total group was 16%. As the TIMI-IIB trial was carried out over approximately 2 years and involved 50 hospitals that were largely active, high-volume centers, the 3,262 patients in the study represent an enrollment of only slightly more than 30 patients per year at each center; the possibility of selection bias cannot be excluded until details about patients excluded from this trial are available. Similarly, no subgroup analysis is available at the time of this writing; it remains very possible that selected subgroups may have demonstrated benefit from one of the treatment limbs. As the incidence of multivessel coronary artery disease in reported trials of thrombolytic therapy after acute MI has been lower than that observed in unselected groups of patients with acute MI (as outlined in Table 30–2), it is possible that patients included in these trials represent a lower-risk cohort; data from several reported trials of thrombolytic therapy that include coronary arteriographic findings are presented in Table 30–8 (44, 45,188–193). Data from GUSTO-I (175) also show a low incidence of one-vessel disease and a higher mortality in those with multivessel disease (Table 30–9). In general, the incidence of multivessel disease in patients presenting with ST segment elevation is far lower than that encountered among historic controls, including infarct patients with ST segment depression (194).

Patients failing thrombolytic therapy in the TIMI-IIB trial (that is, those with an occluded coronary artery at the time of diagnostic catheterization) were not offered salvage angioplasty; many of these patients may have derived long-term benefit from attainment of delayed patency of the infarct-related coronary artery (68). Importantly, 35% of the deaths in the invasive limb of the TIMI-IIB trial occurred in the first 24 hours after hospital admission, before the invasive study. If early deaths in this trial are excluded, a possible benefit in the invasive limb becomes apparent; between 1 week and 1 year, the cardiac mortality in the conservative limb of the trial was 4.5%, as opposed to only 3.1% in the invasive limb (184). Evaluation of these patients beyond the first year after treatment remains to be defined; availability of long-term follow-up data is important. In the series of Simoons et al (193), 5-year event-free survival (freedom from death, recurrent myocardial infarction, or need for revascularization therapy) was only 40% after thrombolytic therapy for acute MI. Predictors of survival in this series are outlined in Table 30–10; as is clear from the table, 5-year outcome was best predicted by

Table 30–8. Incidence of Multivessel Coronary Artery Disease in Trials of Patients Treated with Thrombolytic Therapy for Acute Myocardial Infarction

		Incidence (%)	
Study		MVD	3VD
Kennedy et al,	1983 (188)	46	16
Topol et al (TAMI-I),	1987 (45)	42	10
TIMI-IIA,	1988 (44)	33	10
Bassand et al (APSIM),	1989 (189)	40	14
Erbel et al,	1989 (190)	55	21
Magnani (PAIMS),	1989 (191)	62	24
Rentrop et al,	1989 (192)	52	16
Simoons et al,	1989 (193)	51	NA
Pooled		48	16
Range		33–62	10–24

MVD and 3VD = multivessel and three-vessel coronary artery disease, respectively; NA = not addressed specifically in published data.

Table 30–9. Extent of Coronary Artery Disease and 30-Day Mortality in the GUSTO-I Trial

	Incidence	30-Day Mortality*
One-vessel disease	62%	3.5%
Two-vessel disease	24%	6.5%
Three-vessel disease	14%	11.2%

* 1-VD vs. 2-VD $p = 0.003$
2-VD vs. 3-VD $p = 0.02$
1-VD vs. 3-VD $p < 0.001$

Data from the GUSTO Investigators (175).

Table 30–10. Predictors of 5-Year Outcome After Acute Myocardial Infarction: ICI Netherlands Trial (533 Patients)

5-Year event-free survival (death, MI, CBS, PTCA) = 40%
Multivariate Predictors
- Death
  - Left ventricular ejection fraction
  - Stenosis severity of infarct-related coronary artery
  - Extent of coronary artery disease
  - Age
  - History of prior MI
- Reinfarction
  - Initial thrombolytic therapy
  - Inferior MI
  - Residual stenosis >90% in infarct-related coronary artery
- Death or Reinfarction
  - Left ventricular ejection fraction
  - Residual stenosis ≥90% in infarct-related coronary artery
  - History of prior MI

CBS = coronary bypass surgery; MI = myocardial infarction; PTCA = percutaneous transluminal coronary angioplasty.

Reproduced from Simoons et al (193), with permission.

clinical parameters, as well as left ventricular function and the extent and severity of coronary artery disease. Five-year survival in this series was 95% if left ventricular ejection fraction was 0.40 or greater and there was no remaining coronary stenosis >50%; in contrast, 5-year survival was only 55% if ejection fraction was <0.40 *and* there was a residual severe stenosis (>90%) in the infarct-related coronary artery or multivessel coronary artery disease was present. Of critical importance, results of predischarge exercise testing were *not* predictive of 5-year survival or reinfarction after acute MI in this series.

Invasive therapy in the TIMI-IIB trial was performed 18 to 48 hours after administration of thrombolytic therapy; the increased risk of invasive procedures performed this soon after thrombolysis is well documented (44,45) and may be less if cardiac catheterization is electively performed in stable patients before hospital discharge. Finally, the TIMI-IIB trial was an evaluation of cardiac catheterization *and* PTCA versus conservative management, the issue of sole cardiac catheterization, without a predetermined requirement for angioplasty, was not addressed. Nonetheless, recent additional information tends to support the trial's original conclusions, if applied to patients with similar characteristics (31,185,195). As summarized next, cardiac catheterization after administration of thrombolytic therapy provides valuable information and is not merely part and parcel of mechanical revascularization.

In summary, the role of diagnostic cardiac catheterization and angiography after thrombolytic therapy has not been independently prospectively evaluated to date. In addition to the important information learned from cardiac catheterization in survivors of acute MI presented in Table 30–1, specific valuable information is learned from this procedure after thrombolytic therapy; this information is presented in Table 30–11. After diagnostic cardiac catheterization and angiography, it is important to apply coronary revascularization procedures judiciously, only to selected patients most likely to benefit from such therapy. Diagnostic catheterization should not lead to "automatic," perhaps premature, intervention. At present, diagnostic cardiac catheterization and angiography may be advised in

Table 30–11. Value of Cardiac Catheterization after Thrombolytic Therapy

Aids establishment of prognosis; provides reassurance to patient
Establishes patency of infarct-related coronary artery
(Noninvasive variables unable to reliably predict Patency)
Limitations of exercise testing after Thrombolytic Therapy
Limited prognostic data available
Poor ability to detect multivessel coronary artery disease
Enables coronary artery revascularization to be offered to appropriate patients
Facilitates early hospital discharge

patients receiving thrombolytic therapy for acute MI. In the relatively lower-risk cohort of patients suitable for entry into randomized trials, a policy of conservative management may well be appropriate (31,185,195); further data in such patients, as well as in higher-risk patients such as the elderly or those with ST segment depression, are clearly needed.

In the aforementioned trial of Simoons et al (193), 5-year survival after acute MI depended most on residual left ventricular function and the extent of coronary artery disease, irrespective of whether patients received thrombolytic therapy. If late prognosis is thus predicted by coronary anatomy and left ventricular function, patients receiving thrombolytic therapy may not require special consideration apart from the overall cohort of patients with acute MI.

Five-year follow-up data from 1,088 patients randomized in two trials of thrombolytics performed by the European Cooperative Study Group is now available. It shows that the five-year survival in those with TIMI grade 3 flow was significantly better than that of those with TIMI grade 2 or TIMI grade 1-0 flow (91% versus 84%, p=0.01) (195a). In the GUSTO-I trial (175) TIMI grade 3 flow was established in 54% of the patients. Thus, thrombolytic therapy alone may not be satisfactory in approximately 46% of patients.

CONCLUSION

Ideally, the best and most complete information in survivors of acute MI is obtained by knowledge of the extent and severity of coronary artery disease, the state of left ventricular function, the inducibility or spontaneous occurrence of myocardial ischemia, and the presence and extent of reversible resting left ventricular dysfunction. The value of additional information that can be obtained by assessment of propensity for ventricular tachyarrhythmias is not fully known at present. The relative predictive value of obtaining only two of these variables noninvasively (left ventricular function and myocardial ischemia), without knowledge of coronary anatomy, remains unknown in the individual patient.

A noninvasive approach to risk assessment in survivors of acute MI can effectively subdivide patients into groups with differing risk profiles after hospital discharge, but some patients at risk of adverse cardiac events may be incorrectly identified; data derived from early cardiac catheterization and angiography provide complementary and generally more powerful prognostic information. Many patient subgroups may gain particular benefit from early cardiac catheterization and angiography, including patients with acute MI complicated by recurrent myocardial ischemia, congestive heart failure, and/or complex ventricular arrhythmias; patients with abnormal or inconclusive results from noninvasive testing or those patients unable to perform an exercise test; "young" patients (below 50 years of age?); older patients (above 60 to 70 years of age?); patients with non-Q wave myocardial infarction; and patients receiving thrombolytic therapy. For these reasons, early cardiac catheterization and angiography in all survivors of acute MI, with *selective* use of appropriate noninvasive tests, may provide a more efficacious means of risk assessment after acute MI; if all tests are performed judiciously, the cost of such an approach need not be excessive. While reducing costs is important, this should be a secondary consideration to optimal or better patient care.

The potential risks of performing coronary arteriography in all survivors of acute MI include the following: (i) Adequate care and attention may not be paid to the proper performance of the procedure(s). Detailed and proper analyses of the data may not be performed. (ii) The need for additional noninvasive test(s) in selected patients may be ignored. (iii) The decision to perform revascularization may be premature or even unnecessary (196). (iv) The decision to perform revascularization may be correct, but the improper revascularization procedure may be selected.

For optimal patient care, the clinician must obtain all necessary data, avoid unnecessary and repetitive tests, know the accuracy of individual tests at his or her own facility, interpret all data in the proper context, and then counsel patients objectively about available management strategies. With this approach, all patients who might *appropriately* benefit from coronary artery revascularization will be correctly identified, and truly low-risk patients (minimal residual coronary artery disease and preserved left ventricular function) may be similarly identified. Comprehensive patient care must not be neglected, including lifestyle modification, risk factor control, and other aspects of post–MI care, which are addressed elsewhere (see Chs. 33, 34).

REFERENCES

1. Dwyer EM: After the myocardial infarction: A review and approach to risk stratification. *Cardiol Clin* 1988;6(1):153–163.
2. Moss AJ: Prognosis after myocardial infarction. *Am J Cardiol* 1983;52:667–669.
3. The TIMI Study Group: Comparison of invasive and conservative strategies after treatment with intravenous tissue plasminogen activator in acute myocardial infarction: Results of the thrombolysis in myocardial infarction (TIMI) phase II trial. *N Engl J Med* 1989;320:618–627.
4. Gruppo Italiano per lo Studio della Streptochinasi nell' Infarto Miocardico (GISSI): Effectiveness of intravenous thrombolytic treatment in acute myocardial infarction. *Lancet* 1986;1:397–401.
5. ISIS-2 Collaborative Group: Randomized trial of intravenous streptokinase, oral aspirin, both, or neither among 17,187 cases of suspected acute myocardial infarction: ISIS-2. *Lancet* 1988;2:349–360.
6. Kelly DT: Clinical decisions in patients following myocardial infarction. *Curr Prob Cardiol* 1985;10(1):1–45.
7. Gomez-Marin I, Folsom AR, Kottke TE, et al: Improvement in long-term survival among patients hospitalized with acute myocardial infarction, 1970–1980. *N Engl J Med* 1987;316:1353–1359.

8. Madsen EB, Gilpin E, Henning H, et al: Prediction of late mortality after myocardial infarction from variables measured at different times during hospitalization. *Am J Cardiol* 1984;53:47–54.
9. Dwyer EM, McMaster P, Greenberg H, and the Multicenter Post-Infarction Research Group: Nonfatal cardiac events and recurrent infarction in the year after acute myocardial infarction. *J Am Coll Cardiol* 1984;4:695–702.
10. Kannel WB, Sorlie P, McNamara PM: Prognosis after initial myocardial infarction: The Framingham study. *Am J Cardiol* 1979;44:53–59.
11. Davis HT, DeCamilla J, Bayer LW, Moss AJ: Survivorship patterns in the post-hospital phase of myocardial infarction. *Circulation* 1979;60:1252–1258.
12. Moss AJ, DeCamilla JJ, Davis H: Cardiac death in the first six months after myocardial infarction: Potential for mortality reduction in the early post-hospital period. *Am J Cardiol* 1977;39:816–820.
13. Mulcahy R, Hickey N, Graham I, McKenzie G: Factors influencing long-term prognosis in male patients surviving a first coronary attack. *Br Heart J* 1975;37:158–165.
14. Dalen JE, Gore JM, Braunwald E, et al, and the TIMI Investigators: Six- and twelve-month follow-up of the phase I thrombolysis in myocardial infarction (TIMI) trial. *Am J Cardiol* 1988;62: 179–185.
15. Gimple LW, Hutter AM, Guiney TE, Boucher CA: Prognostic utility of predischarge dipyridamole–thallium imaging compared to predischarge submaximal exercise electrocardiography and maximal exercise thallium imaging after uncomplicated acute myocardial infarction. *Am J Cardiol* 1989;64: 1243–1248.
16. Epstein SE, Palmeri ST, Patterson RE: Evaluation of patients after myocardial infarction: Indications for cardiac catheterization and surgical intervention. *N Engl J Med* 1982;307:1487–1492.
17. The Multicenter Post-Infarction Research Group: Risk stratification and survival after myocardial infarction. *N Engl J Med* 1983;309:331–336.
18. Taylor GJ, Humphries JO, Mellits ED, et al: Predictors of clinical course, coronary anatomy, and left ventricular function after recovery from acute myocardial infarction. *Circulation* 1980;62: 960–970.
19. Schulman SP, Achuff SC, Griffith LSC, et al: Prognostic cardiac catheterization variables in survivors of acute myocardial infarction: A five year prospective study. *J Am Coll Cardiol* 1988;11: 1164–1172.
20. Henning H, Gilpin E, Covell JW, et al: Prognosis after acute myocardial infarction: A multivariate analysis of mortality and survival. *Circulation* 1979; 59:1124–1136.
21. Schuster EH, Bulkley BH: Early post-infarction angina: Ischemia at a distance and ischemia in the infarct zone. *N Engl J Med* 1981;305:1101–1105.
22. Bosch X, Theroux P, Waters DD, et al: Early post-infarction ischemia: Clinical, angiographic, and prognostic significance. *Circulation* 1987;75: 988–995.
23. Turner JD, Rogers WJ, Mantle JA, et al: Coronary angiography soon after myocardial infarction. *Chest* 1980;77:58–64.
24. Waters DD, Bosch X, Bouchard A, et al: Comparison of clinical variables and variables derived from a limited predischarge exercise test as predictors of early and late mortality after myocardial infarction. *J Am Coll Cardiol* 1985;5:1–8.
25. Ross J, Gilpin EA, Madsen EB, et al: A decision scheme for coronary angiography after acute myocardial infarction. *Circulation* 1989;79:292–303.
26. Marmor A, Geltman EM, Schechtman K, et al: Recurrent myocardial infarction: Clinical predictors and prognostic implications. *Circulation* 1982; 66:415–421.
27. Figueras J, Cinca J, Valle V, et al: Prognostic implications of early spontaneous angina after acute transmural myocardial infarction. *Int J Cardiol* 1983;4:261–272.
28. DeFeyter PJ, Van Eenice MJ, Dighton DH, et al: Prognostic value of exercise testing, coronary angiography, and left ventriculography six to eight weeks after myocardial infarction. *Circulation* 1982; 66:527–536.
29. Sanz G, Castaner A, Betriu A, et al: Determinants of prognosis in survivors of myocardial infarction: A prospective clinical angiographic study. *N Engl J Med* 1982;306:1065–1070.
30. Norris RM, Barnaby PF, Brandt PWT, et al: Prognosis after recovery from first acute myocardial infarction: Determinants of reinfarction and sudden death. *Am J Cardiol* 1984;53:408–413.
31. Barbash GI, Hod H, Roth A, et al: Randomized controlled trial of late in-hospital angiography and angioplasty vs. conservative management after RT-PA treatment in acute myocardial infarction (abstract). *J Am Coll Cardiol* 1990;15:76A.

32. Moss AJ, DeCamilla JJ, Davis HT, Bayer I: Clinical significance of ventricular ectopic beats in the early post-hospital phase of myocardial infarction. *Am J Cardiol* 1977;39:635–640.
33. Bigger JT, Fleiss JL, Kleiger R, et al, and the Multicenter Post-Infarction Research Group: The relationships among ventricular arrhythmias, left ventricular dysfunction, and mortality in the two years after myocardial infarction. *Circulation* 1984; 69:250–258.
34. Deckers JW, Fioretti P, Brower RW, et al: Prediction of one year outcome after complicated and uncomplicated myocardial infarction: Bayesian analysis of predischarge exercise test results in 300 patients. *Am Heart J* 1987;113:90–95.
35. Fuller CM, Raizner AE, Verani MS, et al: Early post–myocardial infarction treadmill stress testing: An accurate predictor of multivessel coronary disease and subsequent cardiac events. *Ann Intern Med* 1981;94:734–739.
36. Braunwald E: Deaths related to cardiac catheterization. *Circulation* 1968;37(Suppl III):III-17–III-26.
37. Davis K, Kennedy JW, Kemp HG, et al: Complications of coronary arteriography from the collaborative study of coronary artery surgery (CASS). *Circulation* 1979;59:1105–1112.
38. Bourassa MG, Noble J: Complication rate of coronary arteriography: A review of 5250 cases studied by a percutaneous femoral technique. *Circulation* 1976;53:106–114.
39. Wyman RM, Safian RD, Portway V, et al: Current complications of diagnostic and therapeutic cardiac catheterization. *J Am Coll Cardiol* 1988;12: 1400–1406.
40. Betriu A, Castaner A, Sanz GA, et al: Angiographic findings one month after myocardial infarction: A prospective study of 259 survivors. *Circulation* 1982;65:1099–1105.
41. Roubin GS, Harris PJ, Bernstein L, Kelly DT: Coronary anatomy and prognosis after myocardial infarction in patients 60 years of age and younger. *Circulation* 1983;67:743–749.
42. Bertrand ME, Lefebvre JM, Laisne CL, et al: Coronary arteriography in acute transmural myocardial infarction. *Am Heart J* 1979;97:61–69.
43. DeWood MA, Spores J, Notske R, et al: Prevalence of total coronary occlusion during the early hours of transmural myocardial infarction. *N Engl J Med* 1980;303:897–902.
44. The TIMI Research Group: Immediate vs. delayed catheterization and angioplasty following thrombolytic therapy for acute myocardial infarction: TIMI II-A results. *JAMA* 1988;260:2849–2858.
45. Topol EJ, Califf RM, George BS, et al, and the Thrombolysis and Angioplasty in Myocardial Infarction Study Group: A randomized trial of immediate versus delayed elective angioplasty after intravenous tissue plasminogen activator in acute myocardial infarction. *N Engl J Med* 1987;317:581–588.
46. Savran SV, Bryson AL, Welch TG, et al: Clinical correlates of coronary cineangiography in young males with myocardial infarction. *Am Heart J* 1976;91:551–555.
47. Veenbrink TWG, Van Der Werf T, Westerhof PW, et al: Is there an indication for coronary angiography in patients under 60 years of age with no or minimal angina pectoris after a first myocardial infarction? *Br Heart J* 1985;53:30–35.
48. Abraham RD, Freedman SB, Dunn RF, et al: Prediction of multivessel coronary artery disease and prognosis early after acute myocardial infarction by exercise electrocardiography and thallium-201 myocardial perfusion scintigraphy. *Am J Cardiol* 1986;58:423–427.
49. Patterson RE, Horowitz SF, Eng C, et al: Can noninvasive exercise test criteria identify patients with left main or three vessel coronary artery disease after a first myocardial infarction? *Am J Cardiol* 1983;51:361–372.
50. Tubau JF, Chaitman BR, Bourassa MG, Waters DD: Detection of multivessel coronary disease after myocardial infarction using exercise stress testing and multiple ECG lead systems. *Circulation* 1980;61:44–52.
51. Gibson RS, Watson DD, Craddock GB, et al: Prediction of cardiac events after uncomplicated myocardial infarction: A prospective study comparing predischarge exercise thallium-201 scintigraphy and coronary angiography. *Circulation* 1983;68:321–336.
52. Griffith LSC, Varnauskas E, Wallin J, et al: Correlation of coronary arteriography after acute myocardial infarction with predischarge limited exercise test response. *Am J Cardiol* 1988;61:201–207.
53. Schwartz KM, Turner JD, Sheffield LT, et al: Limited exercise testing soon after myocardial infarction: Correlation with early coronary and left ventricular angiography. *Ann Intern Med* 1981;94: 727–734.

54. Starling MR, Crawford MH, Richards KL, et al: Predictive value of early post–myocardial infarction modified treadmill exercise testing in multivessel coronary artery disease detection. *Am Heart J* 1981; 102:169–175.
55. Akhras F, Upward J, Keates J, Jackson G: Early exercise testing and elective coronary artery bypass surgery after uncomplicated myocardial infarction: Effect on morbidity and mortality. *Br Heart J* 1984; 52:413–417.
56. Morris DD, Rozanski A, Berman DS, et al: Noninvasive prediction of the angiographic extent of coronary artery disease after myocardial infarction: Comparison of clinical, bicycle exercise electrocardiographic, and ventriculographic parameters. *Circulation* 1984;70:192–201.
57. Williams RA, Cohn PF, Vokonas PS, et al: Electrocardiographic, arteriographic, and ventriculographic correlations in transmural myocardial infarction. *Am J Cardiol* 1973;31:595–599.
58. Mock MB, Ringqvist I, Fisher LD, et al, and the Coronary Artery Surgery Study: Survival of medically treated patients in the coronary artery surgery study (CASS) registry. *Circulation* 1982;66: 562–568.
59. Humphries JO, Kuller L, Ross RS, et al: Natural history of ischemic heart disease in relation to arteriographic findings. *Circulation* 1974;49:489–497.
60. Platia EV, Grunwald L, Mellits ED, et al: Clinical and arteriographic variables predictive of survival in coronary artery disease. *Am J Cardiol* 1980;46: 543–552.
61. Bruschke AVG, Proudfit WL, Sones FM: Progress study of 590 consecutive nonsurgical cases of coronary disease followed 5–9 years: Arteriographic correlations. *Circulation* 1973;47:1147–1153.
62. Reeves TJ, Oberman A, Jones WB, Sheffield LT: Natural history of angina pectoris. *Am J Cardiol* 1974;33:423–430.
63. Burggraf GW, Parker JO: Progress in coronary artery disease: Angiographic, hemodynamic, and clinical factors. *Circulation* 1975;51:146–156.
64. Harris PJ, Harrell FE, Lee KL, et al: Survival in medically treated coronary artery disease. *Circulation* 1979;60:1259–1269.
65. Rahimtoola SH: Left main equivalence is still an unproved hypothesis but proximal left anterior descending coronary artery disease is a "high risk" lesion. *Am J Cardiol* 1984;53:1719–1721.
66. Kaul S, Lilly DR, Gascho JA, et al: Prognostic utility of the exercise thallium-201 test in ambulatory patients with chest pain: Comparison with cardiac catheterization. *Circulation* 1988;77:745–758.
67. Wilson WW, Gibson RS, Nygaard TW, et al: Acute myocardial infarction associated with single vessel coronary artery disease: An analysis of clinical outcome and the prognostic importance of vessel patency and residual ischemic myocardium. *J Am Coll Cardiol* 1988;11:223–234.
68. Cigarroa RG, Lange RA, Hillis LD: Prognosis after acute myocardial infarction in patients with and without residual antegrade coronary blood flow. *Am J Cardiol* 1989;64:155–160.
69. Sheehan FH, Doerr R, Schmidt WG, et al: Early recovery of left ventricular function after thrombolytic therapy for acute myocardial infarction: An important determinant of survival. *J Am Coll Cardiol* 1988;12:289–300.
70. Kennedy JW, Ritchie JL, Davis KB, et al: The Western Washington randomized trial of intracoronary streptokinase in acute myocardial infarction. *N Engl J Med* 1985;312:1073–1078.
71. Bruschke AVG, Proudfit WL, Sones FM: Clinical course of patients with normal, and slightly or moderately abnormal coronary arteriograms: A follow-up study on 500 patients. *Circulation* 1973; 47:936–945.
72. Proudfit WL, Welch CC, Siqueira C, et al: Prognosis of 1000 young women studied by coronary angiography. *Circulation* 1981;64:1185–1190.
73. Kemp HG, Kronmal RA, Vlietstra RE, et al, and participants in the Coronary Artery Surgery Study: Seven year survival of patients with normal or near normal coronary arteriograms: A CASS Registry Study. *J Am Coll Cardiol* 1986;7:479–483.
74. Ljungberg S, Forsberg SA, Paulin S, Werko L: Coronary arteriography in 486 patients: Arteriographic pathology and prognosis. *Acta Med Scand* 1979;206:145–151.
75. Hackett D, Verwilghen J, Davies G, Maseri A: Coronary stenoses before and after acute myocardial infarction. *Am J Cardiol* 1989;63:1517–1518.
76. Ambrose JA, Tannenbaum MA, Alexopoulos D, et al: Angiographic progression of coronary artery disease and the development of myocardial infarction. *J Am Coll Cardiol* 1988;12:56–62.
77. Little WC, Constantinescu M, Applegate RJ, et al: Can coronary angiography predict the site of a

subsequent myocardial infarction in patients with mild-to-moderate coronary artery disease? *Circulation* 1988;78:1157–1166.

78. Ellis S, Alderman EL, Cain K, et al, and the participants of the Coronary Artery Surgery Study (CASS): Morphology of left anterior descending coronary territory lesions as a predictor of anterior myocardial infarction: A CASS Registry study. *J Am Coll Cardiol* 1989;13:1481–1491.
79. Wilson RJ, Hilida MD, White CW: Quantitative angiographic morphology of coronary stenoses leading to myocardial infarction or unstable angina. *Circulation* 1986;73:286–293.
80. Ahnve S, Gilpin E, Dittrich H, et al: First myocardial infarction: Age and ejection fraction identify a low-risk group. *Am Heart J* 1988;116:925–932.
81. White HO, Norris RM, Brown MA, et al: Left ventricular end-systolic volume as the major determinant of survival after recovery from myocardial infarction. *Circulation* 1987;76:44–51.
82. Braunwald E, Kloner RA: The stunned myocardium: Prolonged, postischemic ventricular dysfunction. *Circulation* 1982;66:1146–1149.
83. Rahimtoola SH: A perspective on the three large multicenter randomized clinical trials of coronary bypass surgery for chronic stable angina. Circulation 1985;72(Suppl V):V-123–V-135.
84. Braunwald E, Rutherford JD: Reversible ischemic left ventricular dysfunction: Evidence for the hibernating myocardium. *J Am Coll Cardiol* 1986;8:1467–1470.
85. Rahimtoola SH: The hibernating myocardium. *Am Heart J* 1989;117:211–221.
86. Cohen M, Charney R, Hershman R, et al: Reversal of chronic ischemic myocardial dysfunction after transluminal coronary angioplasty. *J Am Coll Cardiol* 1988;12:1193–1198.
87. Wilson RF, Laughlin DE, Ackell PH, et al: Transluminal, subselective measurement of coronary artery blood flow velocity and vasodilator reserve in man. *Circulation* 1985;72:82–92.
88. Gould KL, Lipscomb K, Hamilton GW: Physiologic basis for assessing critical coronary stenosis: Instantaneous flow response and regional distribution during coronary hyperemia as measures of coronary flow reserve. *Am J Cardiol* 1974;33:87–94.
89. Chaitman BR, Fisher LD, Bourassa MG, et al: Effect of coronary bypass surgery on survival patterns in subsets of patients with left main coronary artery disease: Report of the collaborative study in coronary artery surgery (CASS). *Am J Cardiol* 1981;48:766–777.
90. Varnauskas E, and the European Coronary Surgery Study Group: Survival, myocardial infarction, and employment status in a prospective randomized study of coronary bypass surgery. *Circulation* 1985;72(Suppl V):V-90–V-101.
91. Bounous EP, Mark DB, Pollock BG, et al: Surgical survival benefits for coronary disease patients with left ventricular dysfunction. *Circulation* 1988;78 (Suppl I):I-151–I-157.
92. Pigott JD, Kouchouskos NT, Oberman A, Cutter GR: Late results of surgical and medical therapy for patients with coronary artery disease and depressed left ventricular function. *J Am Coll Cardiol* 1985;5:1036–1045.
93. Rahimtoola SH: Coronary bypass surgery for unstable angina. *Circulation* 1984;69:842–848.
94. Rogers WJ, Smith LR, Oberman A, et al: Surgical vs. nonsurgical management of patients after myocardial infarction. *Circulation* 1980;62(Suppl I): I-67–I-74.
95. Froelicher VF, Perdue ST, Atwood JE, et al: Exercise testing of patients recovering from myocardial infarction. *Curr Probl Cardiol* 1986;11(7):369–444.
96. Crawford MH, O'Rourke RA: The role of cardiac catheterization in patients after myocardial infarction. *Cardiol Clin* 1984;2(1):105–111.
97. DeBusk RF, Blomqvist CG, Kouchoukos NT, et al: Identification and treatment of low-risk patients after acute myocardial infarction and coronary artery bypass graft surgery. *N Engl J Med* 1986;314:161–166.
98. Baron DB, Licht JR, Ellestad MH: Status of exercise stress testing after myocardial infarction. *Arch Intern Med* 1984;144:595–601.
99. Theroux P, Marpole DGF, Bourassa MG: Exercise stress testing in the post–myocardial infarction patient. *Am J Cardiol* 1983;52:664–667.
100. Cohn PF: The role of noninvasive cardiac testing after an uncomplicated myocardial infarction. *N Engl J Med* 1983;309:90–93.
101. Weld FM, Cho KL, Bigger JT, Rolnitzky LM: Risk stratification with low-level exercise testing two weeks after acute myocardial infarction. *Circulation* 1981;64:306–314.
102. Krone RJ, Gillespie JA, Weld FM, et al, and the Multicenter Post-Infarction Research Group: Low-level exercise testing after myocardial infarc-

tion: Usefulness in enhancing clinical risk stratification. *Circulation* 1985;71:80–89.

103. Williams WL, Nair RC, Higginson LAJ, et al: Comparison of clinical and treadmill variables for the prediction of outcome after myocardial infarction. *J Am Coll Cardiol* 1984;4:477–486.

104. Theroux P, Waters DD, Halphen C, et al: Prognostic value of exercise testing soon after myocardial infarction. *N Engl J Med* 1979;301:341–345.

105. Hung J, Goris ML, Nash E, et al: Comparative value of maximal treadmill testing, exercise thallium myocardial perfusion scintigraphy and exercise radionuclide ventriculography for distinguishing high- and low-risk patients soon after myocardial infarction. *Am J Cardiol* 1984;53: 1221–1227.

106. Starling MR, Crawford MH, Kennedy GT, O'Rourke RA: Exercise testing early after myocardial infarction: Predictive value for subsequent unstable angina and death. *Am J Cardiol* 1980;46: 909–914.

107. Markiewicz W, Houston N, DeBusk RF: Exercise testing soon after myocardial infarction. *Circulation* 1977;56:26–31.

108. DeBusk RF, Kraemer HC, Nash E: Stepwise risk stratification soon after myocardial infarction. *Am J Cardiol* 1983;52:1161–1166.

109. Madsen EB, Gilpin E, Ahnve S, et al: Prediction of functional capacity and use of exercise testing for predicting risk after acute myocardial infarction. *Am J Cardiol* 1985;56:839–845.

110. Turner JD, Schwartz KM, Logic JR, et al: Detection of residual jeopardized myocardium three weeks after myocardial infarction by exercise testing with thallium-201. *Circulation* 1980;61:729–737.

111. Van Der Wall EE, Eenige Van MJ, Visser FC, et al: Thallium-201 exercise testing in patients 6–8 weeks after myocardial infarction: Limited value for the detection of multivessel disease. *Eur Heart J* 1985;6:29–36.

112. Younis LT, Byers S, Shaw L, et al: Prognostic value of intravenous dipyridamole thallium scintigraphy after an acute myocardial ischemic event. *Am J Cardiol* 1989;64:161–166.

113. Gottlieb SO, Gottlieb SH, Achuff SC, et al: Silent ischemia on Holter monitoring predicts mortality in high-risk post-infarction patients. *JAMA* 1988; 259:1030–1035.

114. Tzivoni D, Gavish A, Zin D, et al: Prognostic significance of ischemic episodes in patients with previous myocardial infarction. *Am J Cardiol* 1988; 62:661–664.

115. Nicod P, Corbett JR, Firth BG, et al: Prognostic value of resting and submaximal exercise radionuclide ventriculography after acute myocardial infarction in high-risk patients with single and multivessel disease. *Am J Cardiol* 1983;52:30–36.

116. Corbett JR, Dehmer GJ, Lewis SE, et al: The prognostic value of submaximal exercise testing with radionuclide ventriculography before hospital discharge in patients with recent myocardial infarction. *Circulation* 1981;64:535–544.

117. Morris KG, Palmeri ST, Califf RM, et al: Value of radionuclide angiography for predicting specific cardiac events after myocardial infarction. *Am J Cardiol* 1985;55:318–324.

118. Borer JS, Rosing DR, Miller RH, et al: Natural history of left ventricular function during one year after acute myocardial infarction: Comparison with clinical, electrocardiographic, and biochemical determinations. *Am J Cardiol* 1980;46:1–12.

119. Ryan T, Armstrong WF, O'Donnell JA, Feigenbaum H: Risk stratification after acute myocardial infarction by means of exercise two dimensional echocardiography. *Am Heart J* 1987;114: 1305–1316.

120. Armstrong WF, O'Donnell J, Ryan T, Feigenbaum H: Effect of prior myocardial infarction and extent and location of coronary disease on accuracy of exercise echocardiography. *J Am Coll Cardiol* 1987;10:531–538.

121. Ibsen H, Kjoller E, Styperek J, Pedersen A: Routine exercise ECG three weeks after acute myocardial infarction. *Acta Med Scand* 1975;198:463–469.

122. Gibson RS, Beller GA, Gheorghiade M, et al: The prevalence and clinical significance of residual myocardial ischemia two weeks after uncomplicated non-Q wave infarction: A prospective natural history study. *Circulation* 1986;73:1186–1198.

123. Chaitman BR, Waters DD, Corbara F, Bourassa MG: Prediction of multivessel disease after inferior myocardial infarction. *Circulation* 1978;57: 1085–1090.

124. Gibson RS, Taylor GT, Watson DD, et al: Predicting the extent and location of coronary artery disease during the early post-infarction period by quantitative thallium-201 scintigraphy. *Am J Cardiol* 1981;47:1010–1019.

125. Krone RJ, Dwyer EM, Greenberg H, et al, and the Multicenter Post-Infarction Research Group:

Risk stratification in patients with first non-Q wave myocardial infarction: Limited value of the early low level exercise test after uncomplicated infarcts. *J Am Coll Cardiol* 1989;14:31–37.

126. Starling MR, Crawford MH, Kennedy GT, O'Rourke RA: Treadmill exercise tests predischarge and six weeks post-myocardial infarction to detect abnormalities of known prognostic value. *Ann Intern Med* 1981;94:721–727.

127. Gilpin EA, Koziol JA, Madsen EB, et al: Periods of differing mortality distribution during the first year after acute myocardial infarction. *Am J Cardiol* 1983;52:240–244.

128. Senaratne MPJ, Hsu L, Rossall RE, Kappagoda CT: Exercise testing after myocardial infarction: Relative values of the low level predischarge and the post-discharge exercise test. *J Am Coll Cardiol* 1988;12:1416–1422.

129. Handler CE, Sowton E: Diurnal variation and reproducibility of predischarge submaximal exercise testing after myocardial infarction. *Br Heart J* 1984;52:299–303.

130. Paine TD, Dye LE, Roitman DI, et al: Relation of graded exercise test findings after myocardial infarction to extent of coronary artery disease and left ventricular dysfunction. *Am J Cardiol* 1978;42: 716–723.

131. Weiner DA, McCabe C, Klein MD, Ryan TJ: ST segment changes post-infarction: Predictive value for multivessel coronary disease and left ventricular aneurysm. *Circulation* 1978;58:887–891.

132. DeFeyter PJ, Van Eenige MJ, Dighton DH, Roos JP: Exercise testing early after myocardial infarction: Detection of multivessel coronary artery disease and extent of left ventricular dysfunction six to eight weeks after infarction using a 12-lead exercise electrocardiogram. *Chest* 1983;83: 853–859.

133. Rigo P, Bailey IK, Griffith LSC, et al: Stress thallium-201 myocardial scintigraphy for the detection of individual coronary arterial lesions in patients with and without previous myocardial infarction. *Am J Cardiol* 1981;48:209–216.

134. Nicod P, Gilpin EA, Dittrich H, et al: Trends in use of coronary angiography in subacute phase of myocardial infarction. *Circulation* 1991;84: 1004–1015.

135. Chapekis AT, Burek K, Topol EJ: The cost:benefit ratio of acute intervention for myocardial infarction: Results of a prospective, matched pair analysis. *Am Heart J* 1989;118:878–882.

136. Kulick DL, Rahimtoola SH: Is noninvasive risk stratification sufficient, or should all patients undergo cardiac catheterization and angiography after a myocardial infarction? in Cheitlin MD (ed): *Dilemmas in Clinical Cardiology,* Vol. 21. Philadelphia, FA Davis Co., 1990, pp 3–25.

137. Gibson RS: non-Q wave myocardial infarction: Diagnosis, prognosis, and management. *Curr Prob Cardiol* 1988;13:1–72.

138. Krone RJ, Friedman E, Thanavaros S, et al: Long-term prognosis after first Q wave (transmural) or non-Q wave (non-transmural) myocardial infarction: Analysis of 593 patients. *Am J Cardiol* 1983;52:234–239.

139. Connolly DC, Elveback LR: Coronary heart disease in residents of Rochester, Minnesota: VI, Hospital and post-hospital course of patients with transmural and subendocardial myocardial infarction. *Mayo Clin Proc* 1985;60:375–381.

140. Nicod P, Gilpin E, Dittrich H, et al: Short- and long-term clinical outcome after Q wave and non-Q wave myocardial infarction in a large patient population. *Circulation* 1989;79:528–536.

141. Hutter AM, DeSanctis RW, Flynn T, Yeatman LA: Nontransmural myocardial infarction: A comparison of hospital and late clinical course of patients with that of matched patients with transmural anterior and transmural inferior myocardial infarction. *Am J Cardiol* 1981;48:595–602.

142. Schechtman KB, Capone RJ, Kleiger RE, et al, and the Diltiazem Reinfarction Study Research Group: Risk stratification of patients with non-Q wave myocardial infarction: The critical role of ST segment depression. *Circulation* 1989;80: 1148–1158.

143. Kao W, Khaja F, Goldstein S, Gheorghiade M: Cardiac event rate after non-Q wave acute myocardial infarction and the significance of its anterior location. *Am J Cardiol* 1989;64:1236–1242.

144. Abraham RD, Roubin GS, Harris PJ, et al: Coronary and left ventricular angiographic anatomy and prognosis of survivors of first acute myocardial infarction. *Am J Cardiol* 1983;52:257–260.

145. Schulze RA, Pitt B, Griffith LSC, et al: Coronary angiography and left ventriculography in survivors of transmural and nontransmural myocardial infarction. *Am J Med* 1978;64:108–113.

146. Madigan NP, Rutherford BD, Frye RL: The clinical course, early prognosis, and coronary anatomy of subendocardial infarction. *Am J Med* 1976; 60:634–641.

147. Gibson RS, Boden WE, Theroux P, et al, and the Diltiazem Reinfarction Study Group: Diltiazem and reinfarction in patients with non-Q wave myocardial infarction: Results of a double-blind, randomized multicenter trial. *N Engl J Med* 1986;315:423–429.

148. Nicholson MR, Roubin GS, Bernstein L, et al: Prognosis after an initial non-Q wave myocardial infarction related to coronary anatomy. *Am J Cardiol* 1983;52:462–465.

149. Boden WE, Gibson RS, Kleiger RE, et al, and the Diltiazem Reinfarction Study Research Group: Importance of early recurrent ischemia on one-year survival after non-Q wave acute myocardial infarction. *Am J Cardiol* 1989;64:799–801.

150. Roger VL, Kopecky SL, Gibbons RJ, et al: Exercise radionuclide angiography after non-Q wave myocardial infarction (abstract). *J Am Coll Cardiol* 1988;11(Suppl A):216A.

151. Aguirre FV, Younis LT, Chaitman BR, et al: Early and 1-year clinical outcome of patients evolving non-Q wave versus Q wave myocardial infarction after thrombolysis. Results from the TIMI II study. *Circulation* 1995;91:2541–2548.

152. *Report of the Working Group on Arteriosclerosis of the National Heart, Lung and Blood Institute.* US Dept of Health and Human Services, Public Health Service publication No. (NIH) 81-2034, 1981, p 39.

153. Weaver WD, Litwin PE, Martin JS, et al: Effect of age on use of thrombolytic therapy and mortality in acute myocardial infarction. *J Am Coll Cardiol* 1991;18:657–662.

154. Lee KL, Woodlief LH, Topol EJ, et al: Predictors of 30-day mortality in the era of reperfusion after acute myocardial infarction. Results from an international trial of 41,021 patients. *Circulation* 1995;91:1659–1668.

155. Norris RM, Caughey DE, Mercer CJ, Scott PJ: Prognosis after myocardial infarction: Six-year follow-up. *Br Heart J* 1974;36:786–790.

156. Henning H, Gilpin EA, Covell JW, et al: Prognosis after acute myocardial infarction: A multivariate analysis of mortality and survival. *Circulation* 1979;59:1124–1136.

157. Tofler GH, Muller JE, Stone PH, et al, and the MILIS Study Group: Factors leading to shorter survival after acute myocardial infarction in patients ages 65 to 75 years compared with younger patients. *Am J Cardiol* 1988;62:860–867.

158. Berkman LF, Leo-Summers L, Horwitz RI: Emotional support and survival after myocardial infarction. A prospective population-based study of the elderly. *Ann Intern Med* 1992;117:1003–1009.

159. Rahimtoola SH, Grunkemeier GL, Starr A: Ten year survival after coronary artery bypass surgery for angina in patients aged 65 years and older. *Circulation* 1986;74:509–517.

160. Simpfendorfer C, Raymond R, Schraider J, et al: Early and long-term results of percutaneous transluminal coronary angioplasty in patients 70 years of age and older with angina pectoris. *Am J Cardiol* 1988;62:959–961.

161. Holt GW, Sugrue DD, Bresnahan JF, et al: Results of percutaneous transluminal coronary angioplasty for unstable angina pectoris in patients 70 years of age and older. *Am J Cardiol* 1988;61: 994–997.

162. Miller RR, DeMaria AN, Vismara LA, et al: Chronic stable inferior myocardial infarction: Unsuspected harbinger of high-risk proximal left coronary arterial obstruction amenable to surgical revascularization. *Am J Cardiol* 1977;39:954–960.

163. Mirvis DM: Physiologic basis for anterior ST segment depression in patients with acute inferior wall myocardial infarction. *Am Heart J* 1988;116: 1308–1322.

164. Stadius M, McAnulty JH, Culter J, et al: Specificity, sensitivity and accuracy of the nitroglycerine ventriculogram as a predictor of surgically reversible wall motion abnormalities (abstract). *Am J Cardiol* 1980;45:399.

165. Brunken R, Tillisch J, Schwaiger M, et al: Regional perfusion, glucose metabolism, and wall motion in patients with chronic electrocardiographic Q wave infarctions: Evidence for persistence of viable tissue in some infarct regions by positron emission tomography. *Circulation* 1986; 73:951–963.

166. Adams JN, Norton M, Trent R, et al: Hibernating myocardium after acute myocardial infarction treated with thrombolysis (abstract). *Eur Heart J* (August) 1995. 16 (Abstract Suppl.). p 36

167. Tamaki N, Kawamoto M, Takahashi N, et al: Prognostic value of an increase in fluorine-18 deoxyglucose uptake in patients with myocardial

infarction: Comparison with stress thallium imaging. *J Am Coll Cardiol* 1993;22:1621–1627.

168. Montalscot G, Faraggi M, Drobinski G, et al: Myocardial viability in patients with Q wave myocardial infarction and no residual ischemia. *Circulation* 1992;86:47–55.

169. Lee TH, Weisberg MC, Brand DA, et al: Candidates for thrombolysis among emergency room patients with acute chest pain: Potential true- and false-positive rates. *Ann Intern Med* 1989;110: 957–967.

170. Doorey AJ, Michelson EL, Weber FJ, Dreifus LS: Thrombolytic therapy of acute myocardial infarction: Emerging challenges of implementation. *J Am Coll Cardiol* 1987;10:1357–1360.

171. Gruppo Italiano per lo Studio della Streptochinasi nell' Infarto Miocardico (GISSI): Long-term effects of intravenous thrombolysis in acute myocardial infarction: Final report of the GISSI study. *Lancet* 1987;2:871–874.

172. Mardor VJ, Sherry S: Thrombolytic therapy: Current status. *N Engl J Med* 1988;318:1512–1520, 1585–1595.

173. Bang NU, Wilhelm OG, Clayman MD: After coronary thrombolysis and reperfusion, what next? *J Am Coll Cardiol* 1989;14:837–849.

174. Ellis SG, Topol EJ, George BS, et al: Recurrent ischemia without warning: Analysis of risk factors for in-hospital ischemic events following successful thrombolysis with intravenous tissue plasminogen activator. *Circulation* 1989;80:1159–1165.

175. The GUSTO Investigators: The effects of tissue plasminogen activator, streptokinase, or both on coronary artery patency, ventricular function, and survival after acute myocardial infarction. *N Engl J Med* 1993;329:1615–1622.

176. Satler LF, Pallas RS, Bond OB, et al: Assessment of residual coronary arterial stenosis after thrombolytic therapy during acute myocardial infarction. *Am J Cardiol* 1987;59:1231–1233.

177. Schroder R, Neuhaus KL, Linderer T, et al: Impact of late coronary artery reperfusion on left ventricular function one month after acute myocardial infarction (results from the ISAM study). *Am J Cardiol* 1989;64:878–884.

178. Califf RM, O'Neill W, Stack RS, et al, and the TIMI Study Group: Failure of simple clinical measurements to predict perfusion status after intravenous thrombolysis. *Ann Intern Med* 1988;108: 658–662.

179. Touchstone DA, Beller GA, Nygaard TW, et al: Functional significance of predischarge exercise thallium-201 findings following intravenous streptokinase therapy during acute myocardial infarction. *Am Heart J* 1988;116:1500–1507.

180. Burns RJ, Freeman MR, Liu P, et al, and the TPAT Study Group: Limitations of exercise thallium single photon tomography early after myocardial infarction (abstract). *J Am Coll Cardiol* 1989;13:125A.

181. Haber HL, Beller GA, Watson DD, et al: Exercise thallium-201 scintigraphy after thrombolytic therapy with or without angioplasty for acute myocardial infarction. *Am J Cardiol* 1993;71:1257–1261.

182. Tilkemeier PL, Guiney TE, LaRaia PJ, et al: Prognostic value of predischarge low-level exercise thallium testing after thrombolytic treatment of acute myocardial infarction. *Am J Cardiol* 1990;66:1203–1207.

183. Topol EJ, Burek K, O'Neill WW, et al: A randomized controlled trial of hospital discharge three days after myocardial infarction in the era of reperfusion. *N Engl J Med* 1988;318:1083–1088.

184. Williams DO, Braunwald E, Knatterud G, et al, and TIMI investigators: The Thrombolysis in Myocardial Infarction (TIMI) trial: Outcome at one year of patients randomized to either invasive or conservative management (abstract). *Circulation* 1989;89(Suppl II):II-519.

185. Baim DS, Braunwald E, Feit F, et al: The Thrombolysis in Myocardial Infarction (TIMI) Trial Phase II: Additional information and perspectives. *J Am Coll Cardiol* 1990;15:1188–1192.

186. Williams DO, Braunwald E, Knatterud, et al: One-year results of the Thrombolysis in Myocardial Infarction Investigation (TIMI) Phase II trial. *Circulation* 1992;85:533–542.

187. Cragg DR, Friedman HZ, Bonema JD: Outcome of patients with acute myocardial infarction who are ineligible for thrombolytic therapy. *Ann Intern Med* 1991;115:173–177.

188. Kennedy JW, Ritchie JL, Davis KB, et al: Western Washington randomized trial of intracoronary streptokinase in acute myocardial infarction. *N Engl J Med* 1983;309:1477–1482.

189. Bassand JP, Machecourt J, Cassagnes J, et al, for the APSIM study Investigators: Multicenter trial of intravenous anisoylated plasminogen streptokinase activator complex (APSAC) in acute myocardial infarction: Effects on infract size and left

ventricular function. *J Am Coll Cardiol* 1989;13: 988–997.

190. Erbel R, Pop T, Diefenbach C, Meyer J: Long-term results of thrombolytic therapy with and without percutaneous transluminal coronary angioplasty. *J Am Coll Cardiol* 1989;14:276–285.

191. Magnani B, for the PAIMS investigators: Plasminogen Activator Italian Multicenter Study (PAIMS): Comparison of intravenous recombinant single-chain human tissue-type plasminogen activator (rt-PA) with intravenous streptokinase in acute myocardial infarction. *J Am Coll Cardiol* 1989;13:19–26.

192. Rentrop KP, Feit F, Sherman W, et al: Late thrombolytic therapy preserves left ventricular function in patients with collateralized total coronary occlusion: Primary endpoint findings of the second Mount Sinai–New York University reperfusion trial. *J Am Coll Cardiol* 1989;14:58–64.

193. Simoons ML, Vos J, Tijssen JGP, et al: Long-term benefit of early thrombolytic therapy in patients with acute myocardial infarction: 5 year follow-up of a trial conducted by the Interuniversity Cardiology Institute of the Netherlands. *J Am Coll Cardiol* 1989;14:1609–1615.

194. Califf R, Topol E, Gersh BJ: From myocardial salvage to patient salvage in acute myocardial infarction: The role of reperfusion therapy. *J Am Coll Cardiol* 1989;14:1382–1388.

195. Rogers WJ, Babb JD, Baim DS, et al, for the TIMI investigators: Is predischarge coronary arteriography beneficial in patients with myocardial infarction treated with thrombolytic therapy? (abstract). *J Am Coll Cardiol* 1990;15:64A.

195a. Lenderink T, Simoons ML, Van Es G-A, Van de Werf F, Verstraete M, Arnold AER. Benefit of Thrombolytic Therapy is Sustained Throughout Five Years and is Related to TIMI Perfusion Grade 3 but Not Grade 2 Flow at Discharge. *Circulation* 1995;92:1110–1116.

196. Rahimtoola SH: Coronary arteriography in asymptomatic patients after myocardial infarction: The need to distinguish between clinical investigation and clinical care. *Chest* 1980;77:53–57.

31

A Systematic Approach to Patients After Myocardial Infarction

Robert A. O'Rourke, MD

INTRODUCTION

There has been an impressive reduction in the early and 1- to 5-year mortality rates after acute myocardial infarction (MI) during the past 30 years (1,2). Improved early management, more effective therapeutic options, better noninvasive techniques for risk stratification, and more widely applied secondary prevention are all contributing factors to this improved survival (1,3,3a,4,4a). The common use of thrombolytic therapy to institute early myocardial reperfusion in patients treated within 6 hours of the onset of symptoms has had a tremendous positive effect on patient survival (1–6) (see Ch. 19). Also, early reperfusion by primary percutaneous transluminal coronary angioplasty (PTCA) has improved mortality rates in many patients with acute myocardial infarction, for example, patients not eligible for thrombolytic therapy and patients at high risk, including those with cardiogenic shock (3,7) (see Ch. 22).

There are considerable differences between myocardial infarction patients studied comprehensively before the widespread use of thrombolytic therapy and those evaluated after the onset of the thrombolytic era. Patients undergoing thrombolytic therapy have a lower early mortality rate, a markedly reduced cardiac event rate during late follow-up, better left ventricular systolic function, and a lower incidence of multivessel coronary artery disease (8,8a). Interestingly, postthrombolytic patients have a better survival for any extent of depressed left ventricular ejection fraction (9,10), and the prevalence of life-threatening arrhythmias is less in those who have undergone successful thrombolysis (11–14).

In the 70% of patients with acute myocardial infarction who do not receive thrombolytic therapy, risk stratification based on the patient's preinfarction history, in-hospital clinical characteristics, and often noninvasive testing has resulted in a more aggressive diagnostic and therapeutic approach for those at high risk. Secondary prevention by risk factor reduction and drug therapy is recommended for both high- and low-risk patients after infarction.

There is considerable controversy concerning the indications for and the timing of coronary arteriography for patients with myocardial infarction who have been treated without thrombolytic agents or PTCA, and even more so for those after thrombolytic therapy (15,16). Several multicenter trials have assessed routine coronary arteriography with PTCA of the infarct-related coronary artery when feasible in patients with thrombolytic therapy as compared with a more conservative approach with coronary arteriography and PTCA reserved for patients who have spontaneous or stress-induced myocardial ischemia after thrombolytic therapy (17–22). In general, these studies have shown no advantage of *routine* cardiac catheterization with coronary angioplasty prior to hospital discharge after thrombolytic therapy and a poorer prognosis and greater complication rate when immediate catheterization and angioplasty are performed within the first 2 hours after treatment with thrombolytic agents (23–25).

The accuracy of noninvasive tests for separating patients at high versus low risk after thrombolytic therapy is still being defined. Several studies using one or more noninvasive tests for determining the risk of subsequent major cardiac events in postthrombolytic patients have had disappointing results (22,22a,22b). Other studies using myocardial perfusion imaging or dobutamine echocardiography have identified most patients at high risk (26,27).

In this chapter, the methods used to determine the need for and the timing of cardiac catheterization and coronary arteriography in patients with myocardial infarction not undergoing thrombolytic therapy are delineated, and the factors affecting patient treatment decisions after thrombolytic therapy are discussed.

INDICATORS OF HIGH RISK BEFORE MYOCARDIAL INFARCTION

Certain patient characteristics present before the onset of myocardial infarction indicate an unfavorable prognosis (4,15). The mortality due to infarction increases with age, reaching 50% in patients >80 years of age. The mortality rate in the first 2 years after myocardial infarction is twice as great in patients with a history of previous MI or chronic angina (14,15). The presence of diabetes mellitus increases the mortality rate by three- to fourfold (28). A history of hypertension increases the late mortality rate, as does cigarette smoking in patients who continue to smoke. Also, the mortality rate is higher in women than in men, which is only partially explained by a later age at onset (4).

Table 31–1. High-Risk Factors Before Institution of Thrombolytic Therapy

Age of 70 years or older
Female gender
History of diabetes mellitus
History of prior myocardial infarction
ECG evidence of evolving anterior infarction
ECG showing atrial fibrillation
Pulmonary congestion by physical examination
Systemic arterial hypotension and sinus tachycardia

Data compiled from Hillis L, Forman S, Braunwald E, et al: Risk stratification before thrombolytic therapy in patients with acute myocardial infarction. J Am Coll Cardiol 1990;16:313–315 (with permission).

Data from Hillis et al (29), with permission.

In 3,339 patients enrolled in phase II of the Thrombolysis in Myocardial Infarction (TIMI) trial, the presence or absence of each of eight risk factors (Table 31–I) before the initiation of thrombolytic therapy was recorded (29). The factors included the following: age 70 years or older, female gender, a history of diabetes mellitus or previous MI, electrocardiographic (ECG) evidence of an evolving anterior infarction or atrial fibrillation, and findings on physical examination of mild pulmonary congestion or hypotension and tachycardia. Of the 26% of patients who had none of these risk factors, the mortality rate at 6 weeks was only 1.5%. In contrast, 5.3% of those with one or more risk factors died in 6 weeks (>0.001). Among those with one or more risk factors, the death rate at 6 weeks was related to the number of risk factors on admission; those with four or more factors had a 6-week mortality rate of 17.2%.

INDICATORS OF HIGH RISK DURING CORONARY CARE UNIT MONITORING

As many as 50% of the patients who are at high risk after myocardial infarction can be identified on the basis of certain clinical characteristics observed during their first 4 days of hospitalization in a coronary care unit (15). Continuing myocardial ischemia, moderate to severe depression of left ventricular systolic function, and electrical instability >24 hours after admission identify patients at high risk of dying within the first year. Continuing myocardial ischemia or necrosis may be manifested by chest pain after the first 24 hours, new or recurrent ST or T wave changes on the ECG, or new cardiac enzyme elevations.

The severity of left ventricular dysfunction depends on the preinfarction left ventricular function and the extent of the current myocardial infarction. The severity of left ventricular systolic dysfunction as quantitated by the ejection fraction correlates with the subsequent survival both in patients undergoing usual therapy and in those undergoing early thrombolytic therapy (10,30). An ejection fraction below 30% is particularly associated with a marked increase in the early and late postinfarction mortality. Persistent tachycardia or hypotension, a continuing third heart sound on auscultation, cardiomegaly, and pulmonary venous congestion are all usually indicators of left ventricular dysfunction.

Death after myocardial infarction is sudden in about one-half of cases and is not necessarily related to further MI or heart failure. The primary cause of death appears to be ventricular fibrillation in most instances (see Chs. 14, 27, 28). Frequent premature ventricular beats reflecting electrical instability may identify patients at increased risk for ventricular tachyarrhythmias. Several studies have shown that frequent and/or complex ventricular premature beats occurring >24 hours after hospitalization are an independent risk factor for increased first-year mortality. Specifically, more than 10 premature ventricular beats per hour is associated with increased risk after infarction. The risk is even greater in patients with depressed left ventricular function or recurrent myocardial ischemia. Patients with new bundle branch block, typically occurring in association with an anterior myocardial infarction, are also at higher risk for ventricular tachyarrhythmias. Atrial arrhythmias, especially atrial fibrillation, often occur in patients with large infarctions and left ventricular dysfunction and are associated with a higher mortality. Asystole and second- or third-degree block are also indicators of a poor prognosis.

Patients with a complicated hospital course involving recurrent ischemia, complex ventricular arrhythmias, hypotension, and significant heart failure (Killip class III or IV) are typically referred for cardiac catheterization without additional noninvasive testing. Patients who do not appear to be at high risk based on their clinical characteristics often can be risk stratified by noninvasive testing. A management algorithm for survivors of acute myocardial infarction is illustrated in Figs. 31–1 and 31–2 (31). This approach is effective for patients managed without thrombolytic therapy for myocardial infarction; however, its utility for patients receiving thrombolytic therapy is less clear.

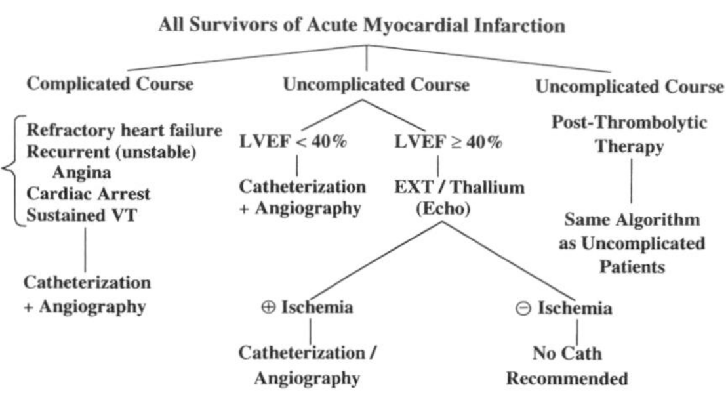

Figure 31–1. Management strategy for survivors of acute myocardial infarction based on the patient's clinical characteristics, the left ventricular ejection fraction (LVEF), and the presence or absence of inducible myocardial ischemia and ventricular tachycardia (VT). *Modified from Roberts et al (31), with permission.*

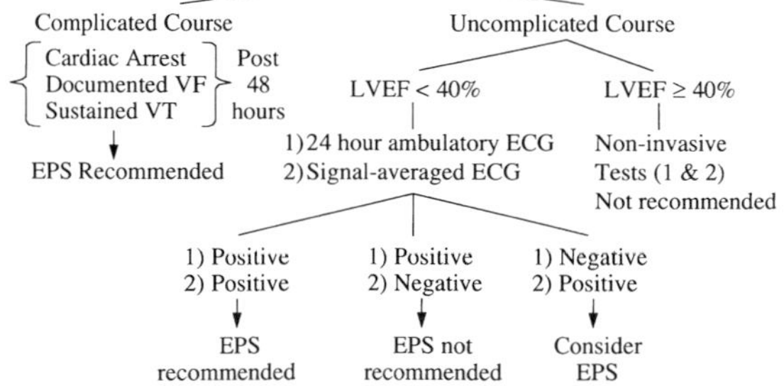

Figure 31–2. Management strategy for survivors of acute myocardial infarction to determine risk of ventricular tachyarrhythmias and sudden death during post–hospital discharge follow-up. VF-ventricular fibrillation; VT-ventricular tachycardia; EPS-electrophysiological study; LVEF-left ventricular ejection fraction. *Modified from Roberts et al (31), with permission.*

THE ARGUMENT AGAINST ROUTINE CORONARY ARTERIOGRAPHY

Some physicians recommend coronary arteriography routinely for almost all patients who have had a recent myocardial infarction (see Ch. 30). The presence of severe three-vessel disease, left main coronary artery disease, and multivessel disease with severe stenosis of the proximal left anterior descending coronary artery indicates a high risk, which is even greater when there is associated moderate to severe left ventricular dysfunction. However, the majority of such patients also have clinical characteristics or noninvasive test results indicating the likelihood of high risk (15,16). In addition, coronary arteriography does not accurately predict subsequent coronary events (32,33). In several studies performed using serial coronary arteriography, the infarct-related coronary artery was less than 50% stenosed at the original study. Also, in many patients the artery with the most severe stenosis was not the site where plaque rupture and thrombosis subsequently resulted in coronary artery occlusion. In comparison studies performed in patients not receiving thrombolytic therapy, coronary arteriography did not supersede noninvasive testing for risk stratification (34). In addition, routine coronary arteriography frequently results in coronary angioplasty or other interventional techniques that are not necessarily indicated on the basis of clinical signs and symptoms; such procedures are not entirely free of complications. Moreover, in a report by Dittus and associates (35), ECG exercise testing accompanied by myocardial perfusion imaging as necessary was superior to coronary arteriography for the cost-effective management of patients after infarction.

Guidelines for Coronary Arteriography

Guidelines for the use of coronary arteriography in patients with acute myocardial infarction were published in 1990 by the American College of Cardiology/American Heart Association Task Force on the Assessment of Diagnostic and Therapeutic Procedures (4). These guidelines have recently been revised (4a). Coronary arteriography in the early hours of MI is usually recommended for patients who develop pump failure or cardiogenic shock, for patients suspected of having an acute ventricular septal defect, and for those patients with persistent or recurrent ischemia (4) (see Chs. 13, 16). Often-recommended indications for early coronary arteriography include its use during the first 6 hours for patients who are candidates for primary coronary angioplasty or coronary artery bypass surgery and for patients who have had one or more previous aortocoronary vein grafts if a graft is the suspected infarct-related vessel.

The Task Force Report recommends coronary arteriography after the initial 6 hours and up to but not including predischarge evaluation in patients with myocardial infarction who have recurrent episodes of ischemic chest pain, particularly if accompanied by ECG changes (4). Cardiac catheterization also is recommended for patients suspected of having acute mitral regurgitation, ruptured ventricular septum, or a ventricular pseudoaneurysm. Cardiac catheterization in this time interval is also indicated when cardiogenic shock or severe pump failure develops.

Cardiac catheterization with coronary arteriography is acceptable and often beneficial in patients with congestive heart failure despite optimal medical therapy, and in patients with recurrent ventricular tachycardia or ventricular fibrillation on antiarrhythmic therapy (4). Cardiac catheterization after 6 hours generally is not indicated for patients with an uncomplicated completed myocardial infarction in whom no early mechanical or surgical intervention is contemplated.

Cardiac catheterization with coronary arteriography immediately before hospital discharge or up to 8 weeks thereafter is recommended for patients with postinfarction angina pectoris and for patients with evidence of myocardial ischemia on noninvasive testing (4). Predischarge or early postdischarge cardiac catheterization and coronary arteriography may provide important information about patients who need to return to unusually active and vigorous physical employment and for patients with a left ventricular ejection fraction of <40%.

Although not established by hard evidence, predischarge cardiac catheterization and arteriography is recommended by some as a routine approach during convalescence for patients without symptoms and with uncomplicated infarction who are <45 years of age and for patients with uncomplicated non-Q wave infarction despite lack of evidence of myocardial ischemia (4) (see Ch. 18). The results of the TIMI-IIIB trial indicate that routine cardiac catheterization with coronary angioplasty when feasible is no better than a conservative approach in the absence of recurrent or provocable ischemia for predicting 6-week mortality and reinfarction rates in patients with non-Q wave myocardial infarction (22) (Fig. 31–3). Cardiac catheterization and arteriography are not indicated for patients with debilitating diseases that preclude their being considered for invasive intervention, for patients with coexisting disease likely to be primarily responsible for a shortened life expectancy, or for patients with advanced left ventricular dysfunction (ejection fraction <20%) in the absence of angina pectoris or evidence of myocardia ischemia (4). Candidates for aneurysmectomy or cardiac transplantation are possible exceptions. Catheterization and coronary arteriography are also generally not indicated in this time period for patients with ventricular arrhythmias who have no clinical evidence of ischemia, a well-preserved exercise tolerance, and no suggestion of aneurysm formation. The patient with inducible sustained ventricular tachycardia may be an exception.

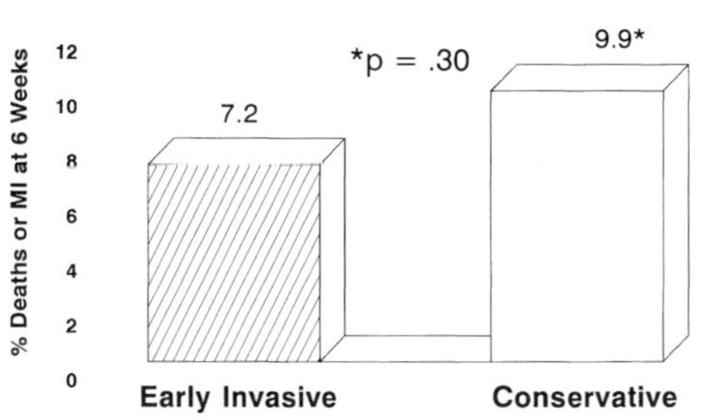

Figure 31–3. Six-week mortality or reinfarction rate in 476 patients with non-Q wave myocardial infarction (MI) randomized to early invasive or conservative management. *Data from Table 4 of TIMI IIIB Investigators (22).*

Coronary Arteriography After Thrombolytic Therapy

The effects on morbidity and mortality of early coronary angioplasty (PTCA) performed in the immediate period *after thrombolytic therapy* has been evaluated in three studies (23–25) (see Chs. 19, 22). The TIMI-IIA study assessed whether immediate cardiac catheterization with PTCA, when technically feasible, would confer an advantage compared with the same procedures performed 18 to 48 hours later (23). All patients were treated with intravenous tissue-type plasminogen activator (t-PA) within 4 hours of the onset of acute myocardial infarction. No difference between the two PTCA groups was observed in the predischarge left ventricular ejection fraction as measured by contrast ventriculography before discharge. Immediate catheterization/angioplasty was associated with more frequent bleeding and more often with the need for coronary artery bypass surgery. Twenty percent of patients undergoing PTCA within 2 hours after thrombolysis required blood transfusions, compared with 7.2% when PTCA was delayed ($p < 0.001$). Coronary artery bypass graft surgery was necessary for 16.4% of the immediate PTCA group, compared with 7.7% of those undergoing later PTCA ($p < 0.01$).

In the Thrombolysis and Angioplasty in Myocardial Infarction (TAMI)-1 trial, patients randomized to an immediate angioplasty approach had a higher mortality rate (4% versus 1%) compared with patients assigned to a deferred catheterization and angioplasty strategy (24). Also, a higher requirement for urgent coronary bypass surgery existed (7% versus 2%), as did an increase in transfusion requirement (21% versus 14%) in those undergoing immediate angioplasty after intravenous thrombolysis.

In the European Cooperative Study (25), patients randomized to immediate coronary arteriography and angioplasty of the infarct-related artery had a high rate of immediate reocclusion and early recurrent ischemia. A higher mortality rate was observed at 1 year (9.3% versus 5.4%) in the group undergoing immediate angioplasty compared with a control group. All three of these studies indicate that *routine immediate coronary angioplasty* early after thrombolysis confers no additional benefit and may be deleterious.

Several clinical studies have evaluated the potential benefit of deferred, pre–hospital discharge coronary arteriography and angioplasty compared with a conservative approach with coronary arteriography and PTCA reserved for patients with spontaneous myocardial ischemia or myocardial ischemia during stress (17–20). In the TIMI-IIB trial, patients receiving t-PA were randomly assigned to treatment according to either an invasive strategy consisting of coronary arteriography 18 to 48 hours after the administration of t-PA followed by prophylactic coronary angioplasty when technically feasible, or to conservative management with arteriography and PTCA performed only in patients with spontaneous or exercise-induced myocardial ischemia (17).

In the group assigned to the invasive strategy, PTCA was attempted in 56.7% of cases; the procedure was anatomically successful in 93.3%. In the group assigned to the conservative strategy, 13.3% of the patients underwent clinically indicated PTCA within 2 weeks of the onset of symptoms. Reinfarction or death within 42 days occurred in 10.9% of the group assigned to the invasive strategy and in 9.7% of those assigned to the conservative strategy (p = NS) (Fig. 31–4). At 2-year follow-up, cumulative death or reinfarction rates were 17.6% for the invasive strategy group and 17.9% for the conservative strategy group (p = NS), with mortality rates of 8.9% and 8.7% (p = NS), respectively (2). The 3-year mortality rate was 11.5% for the invasive strategy group and 11.0% for the conservative strategy group (p = NS). The invasive and conservative strategies in TIMI-IIB had similar favorable outcomes, and death occurred infrequently in the second and third years after study entry. No significant difference was observed between the two groups in the left ventricular ejection fraction at rest or during exercise either at hospital discharge or 6 weeks after randomization. An invasive strategy of coronary arteriography and PTCA when feasible 18 to 48 hours after the onset of symptoms did not reduce the mortality or reinfarction rates.

In the Should We Intervene Following Thrombolysis (SWIFT) trial, 397 patients after infarction were randomized to receive arteriography plus appropriate intervention at 18–48 hour postinfarction, and 403 were randomized to receive conservative care (18). The mortality rate at 12 months (Fig. 31–4) was no different (5.8% versus 5.0%) in the invasive strategy group compared with the conservative treatment group. The reinfarction rate at 12 months (15.1% versus 12.9%) was also similar in the two groups.

Two additional studies compared patients undergoing cardiac catheterization with prophylactic coronary angioplasty at 4 or more days after intravenous thrombolysis with a group undergoing a conservative strategy after thrombolytic therapy. In a study by Barbash et al (19), 97 patients were randomized to an invasive group who underwent routine coronary arteriography and angioplasty 5 ± 2 days after thrombolytic therapy, and 104 patients to a conservative group who underwent arteriography only for recurrent postinfarction angina or exercise-induced ischemia. In the invasive group, the total mortality after a mean follow-up of 10 months was 8 of 97, compared with only 4 of 104 in the conservative group (p = NS). However, a higher rate of rehospitalization was observed among patients assigned to the conservative group.

In the TOPS (Treatment of Post-thrombolytic Stenoses) study, 87 patients treated within 6 hours of chest pain with thrombolytic therapy and with negative functional tests for inducible ischemia

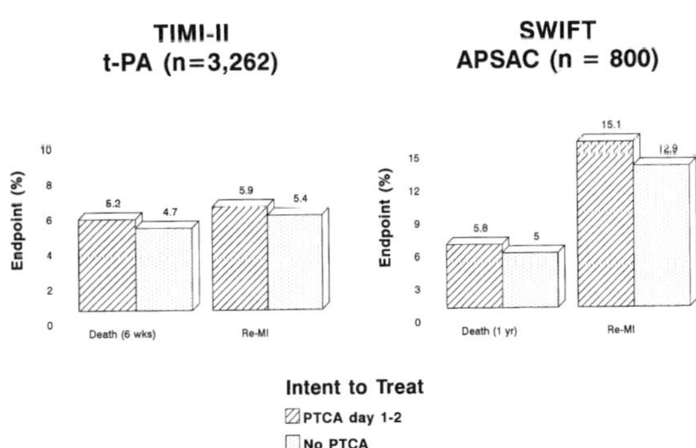

Figure 31–4. Incidence of death and recurrent myocardial infarction at 6 weeks or 1 year after thrombolytic therapy in patients undergoing coronary angioplasty (PTCA) at 18 to 48 hours versus those undergoing no catheterization/angioplasty unless spontaneous or provocable myocardial ischemia had occurred. *Data from the TIMI Study Group (17) and SWIFT Trial Study Group (18).*

were randomized to a strategy of PTCA 4 to 14 days after myocardial infarction or a no PTCA strategy (20). PTCA was successful in 38 of 42 patients (88%) but was complicated by a non-Q wave myocardial infarction because of early closure of the angioplasty site in 3 of 42 (9.5%). No difference was observed between the two groups in the 6-week resting ejection fraction or increase in ejection fraction with exercise; no deaths occurred in either group. There was no functional or clinical benefit from routine late PTCA after thrombolytic therapy for MI in this relatively low-risk group of patients.

To determine whether predischarge arteriography is beneficial in patients with acute myocardial infarction treated with t-PA, heparin, and aspirin, Rogers et al (21) compared outcomes in 197 patients in the TIMI-IIA study assigned to conservative management with routine predischarge coronary arteriography and in 1,461 patients in the TIMI-IIB study who were assigned to a conservative strategy with no coronary arteriography unless ischemia occurred spontaneously or on predischarge exercise testing (Fig. 31–5). During the initial hospital study, coronary arteriography was performed in 93.9% of the patients in the routine catheterization group and 34.7% of the patients in the selective catheterization group ($p < 0.001$), but the frequency of coronary revascularization was no different in the two groups (24.4% versus 20.7%, p = NS). Interestingly, coronary arteriograms showed a predominance of either no or only one-vessel disease (stenosis ≥60%) in both groups.

At the end of 1 year, coronary arteriography had been performed one or more times in 98.9% of patients in the routine catheterization group and in 59.4% of the patients in the selective catheterization group ($p < 0.001$), and death and nonfatal reinfarction had occurred in 10.2% versus 7.0% (p = 0.10) and 8.6% versus 9.0%, respectively (Fig. 31–5). The selective coronary arteriography strategy reduced the number of patients exposed to the small but definite risks and inconvenience of the procedure by about 40% without increasing the 1-year mortality or reinfarction rates. Thus it would appear to be an appropriate management strategy for postthrombolytic therapy.

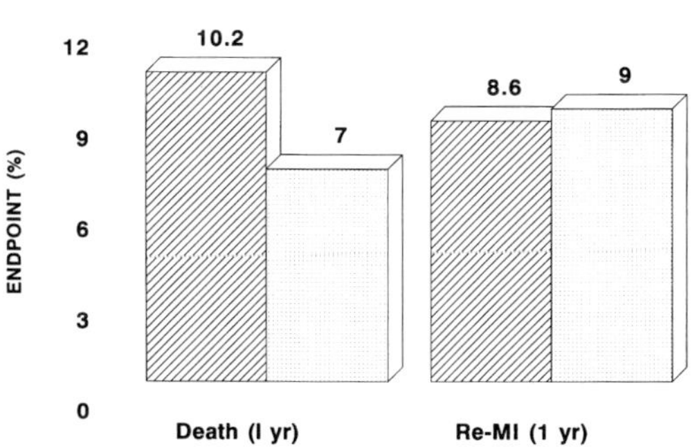

Figure 31–5. A nonrandomized comparison of patients from the TIMI-II trial treated with routine coronary arteriography versus those treated with selective coronary arteriography, with death and recurrent myocardial infarction used as endpoints. *Data from Rogers et al (21).*

NONINVASIVE TESTING AFTER NONTHROMBOLYTIC THERAPY

The use of noninvasive testing for risk stratification is most pertinent to postinfarction patients who by their clinical characteristics do not appear to be at high risk. Such individuals often undergo noninvasive testing during exercise or during pharmacologic stress testing to detect evidence of provocable myocardial ischemia (see Chs. 10, 11, 27, 28). The commonly used noninvasive methods for identifying ischemia and the types of stress most often used are listed in Table 31–2.

Table 31–2. Detection of Myocardial Ischemia

Methods
Electrocardiography
Myocardial perfusion imaging (thallium-201, technetium sestamibi)
Wall motion assessment (echocardiography, radionuclide ventriculography)
Stress testing
Exercise
Coronary vasodilators (dipyridamole, adenosine)
Positive inotropes (dobutamine)
Pacing

O'Rourke (16), with permission.

Several studies of postinfarction patients after nonthrombolytic therapy who were able to complete adequate exercise (5 METs or greater) and who had ECGs interpretable for exercise-induced ischemia indicate a higher incidence of reinfarction and cardiac death in the first year after infarction in those with ST segment depression or angina during low-level ECG exercise testing performed either at hospital discharge or 3 weeks after infarction (4,15). Other studies, with myocardial revascularization often prescribed as an intervention for patients with positive exercise tests, have shown no difference in cardiac events between those with positive and negative ECG stress tests (36).

Exercise stress-redistribution scintigraphy with thallium-201 commonly is used 4–10 days after infarction for predischarge risk stratification and the detection of residual myocardial ischemia (see Ch. 11). Dipyridamole or adenosine pharmacologic stress often is used in patients unable or unlikely to exercise sufficiently (37). Thallium imaging is more sensitive and specific for detecting ischemia than exercise ECG testing alone in postinfarction patients who have undergone nonthrombolytic therapy. Similar information can be obtained with myocardial perfusion imaging using intravenous technetium sestamibi injections during stress and at rest.

Regional wall motion abnormalities usually develop during exercise-induced myocardial ischemia and commonly before abnormalities in global left ventricular systolic function, often in the absence of diagnostic ECG changes or angina. Therefore, the detection of exercise induced left ventricular wall motion abnormalities by two-dimensional echocardiography or radionuclide ventriculography has been used after infarction to determine which patients are at increased risk for subsequent events (see Ch. 10). Recently, the intravenous administration of incremental doses of dobutamine during echocardiographic examination of multiple wall motion segments has been shown to be a useful method for detecting myocardial ischemia with a sensitivity and specificity similar to myocardial perfusion imaging during stress (38).

An assessment of left ventricular systolic function for risk stratifying patients undergoing nonthrombolytic ("standard") therapy for infarction is well accepted. A radionuclide ventriculogram showing a left ventricular ejection fraction of <40% or a two-dimensional echocardiogram indicating moderate to severe left ventricular dysfunction identifies patients who are likely to benefit from a more aggressive diagnostic therapeutic approach (31). The mortality rate in postinfarction patients with a left ventricular ejection fraction of <40% in the prethrombolytic area was five times that occurring in patients with a normal left ventricular ejection fraction (30).

An aggressive management approach also is recommended for patients who have episodes of recurrent ventricular tachycardia or ventricular fibrillation 24 hours or later after myocardial infarction. In such patients the presence of >10 premature depolarizations per hour, a positive signal-averaged ECG for late potentials (see Chs. 27, 28), the presence of exercise-induced ventricular arrhythmias, or diminished heart rate variability increases the likelihood of subsequent monomorphic sustained ventricular tachycardia or sudden death during follow-up (30,39). Such patients usually undergo cardiac catheterization, coronary arteriography, and often electrophysiologic testing.

AN INTEGRATED APPROACH AFTER NONTHROMBOLYTIC THERAPY

On the basis of the considerations just discussed, a management strategy has been outlined that leads to cardiac catheterization and coronary arteriography for high-risk patients after infarction who have undergone nonthrombolytic therapy (Figs. 31–1 and 31–2). Further noninvasive testing is most useful in patients who are not at high risk on the basis of their medical history or prior postinfarction clinical characteristics. This approach emphasizes the increased morbidity and mortality associated with recurrent myocardial ischemia, persistent left ventricular systolic dysfunction, late in-hospital ventricular tachyarrhythmias, and combinations thereof. Cardiac catheterization and coronary arteriography is recommended for those at high risk by their clinical characteristics or after noninvasive testing. Electrophysiologic testing should be considered for those at increased risk for recurrent ventricular tachycardia. The applicability of this strategy to patients with acute MI who received thrombolytic therapy is the subject of the subsequent discussion.

MANAGEMENT DECISIONS AFTER THROMBOLYTIC THERAPY

The plan for managing patients who have received thrombolytic therapy for acute myocardial infarctions is influenced by several factors. These include the presence or absence of high-risk characteristics before the index MI or the development of high-risk clinical features during or after thrombolytic therapy (15,29). Also pertinent are the results of studies comparing *routine* coronary arteriography/angioplasty and late *routine* coronary arteriography/angioplasty with selective coronary arteriography and revascularization for those with spontaneous or stress-induced myocardial ischemia (17–25). The availability and reliability of noninvasive tests for the further risk stratification of patients who appear clinically to be at low or moderate risk for recurrent cardiac events after thrombolytic therapy is another important consideration (8,16). A fourth factor is the probability of an open infarct-related coronary artery and whether or not its patency 48 hours postinfarction or later will alter the prognosis in patients with normal or depressed left ventricular function (9, 11,12).

Noninvasive Testings

Because of the lack of proven efficacy of routine cardiac catheterization after myocardial infarction, the noninvasive assessment assumes great importance in identifying high-risk patients who may benefit from invasive procedures. However, the usefulness of noninvasive testing for separating patients at low and high risk after successful thrombolysis has not been completely defined.

In the prethrombolytic era, an inverse relationship between *left ventricular ejection fraction* and 1-year mortality rate was observed. This relationship also exists for patients treated with thrombolytic therapy. In the European Cooperative Group Study, the 1-year mortality rate in patients with a left ventricular ejection fraction of <40% was 8.2% versus 1.8% for those with an ejection fraction of >40% (40). At 5-year follow-up after treatment for acute myocardial infarction with thrombolytic therapy, the same relationship between low ejection fraction and increased risk for cardiac events was evident (41).

In a recent report from the TIMI-II study, radionuclide measurements of left ventricular ejection fraction were related to all cause mortality and cardiac mortality at 1 year (10). In addition, the relationship between the ejection fraction and the 1-year mortality in this study was compared with the relationship between low ejection fraction and increased risk as established previously in the prethrombolytic era by the Multicenter Post-Infarction Research Group (30). A distinct inverse relationship was noted between left ventricular ejection fraction at rest and all cause mortality. The highest mortality rate (9.9%) was noted in patients with an ejection fraction of <30% (Fig. 31–6). Those post-thrombolytic patients unable to undergo this rest and exercise evaluation had a 1-year mortality rate of 6.2%. When compared with the Multicenter Post-Infarction Research Group data, there was strong evidence of difference in survival in the two studies. At any level of ejection fraction, the 1-year mortality was lower in TIMI-II patients than in patients in the prethrombolytic era (Fig. 31–7).

In some patients an improvement in left ventricular dysfunction occurs during the first 2 weeks

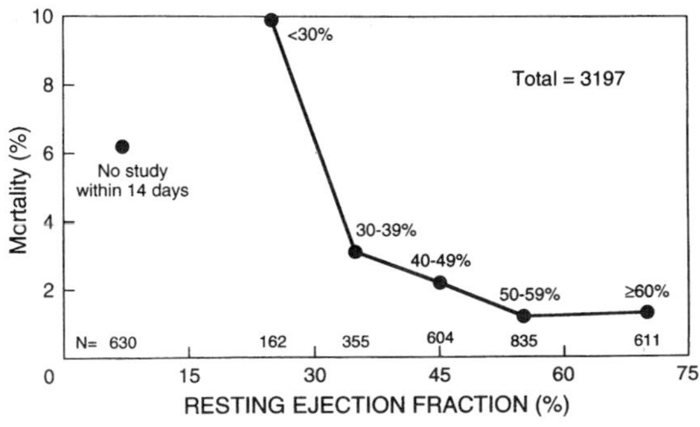

Figure 31–6. Relation of rest ejection fraction to all cause mortality in the TIMI-II study. Note the hyperbolic shape of the curve and the mortality rate for patients who did not undergo radionuclide ventriculography within 14 days. *From Zaret et al (10).*

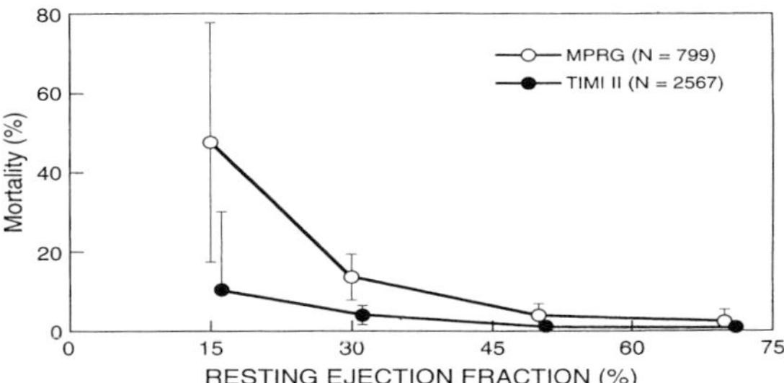

Figure 31–7. Comparison of cardiovascular mortality rate curves in relation to rest ejection fraction. Note the increased mortality in the Multicenter Post-Infarction Research Group (MPRG) studies at the lower levels of ejection fraction. The data from the Thrombolysis in Myocardial Infarction Phase II trial (TIMI II) have been regrouped according to specifications outlined in the MPRG study (1). Vertical bars represent confidence intervals. *From Zaret et al (10).*

postinfarction, with the early reduction in ejection fraction presumably related to stunned myocardium. Nevertheless, a predischarge ejection fraction of <40%, whether obtained by invasive or noninvasive testing, is associated with a higher mortality. An ejection fraction of <30% indicates an extremely high risk of early mortality during follow-up and frequently is used as an indication for aggressive management.

Several studies suggests that the positive and negative predictive accuracy of *exercise ECG testing* and *myocardial perfusion imaging* for detecting myocardial ischemia, determining the presence of multivessel disease, or predicting future cardiac events are less useful in patients undergoing successful thrombolytic therapy than in patients undergoing nonthrombolytic therapy (see Ch. 11). Importantly, the risk for subsequent cardiac events, in general, is significantly reduced in those patients who receive thrombolytic therapy.

Haber and associates (42) studied the ability of exercise thallium scintigraphy to identify multivessel coronary artery disease in 88 consecutive patients who received thrombolytic therapy and subsequently underwent both predischarge noninvasive testing and coronary arteriography. The sensitivity and specificity of ST segment depression alone for detecting multivessel disease were 29% and 96%, respectively. The sensitivity and specificity of a redistribution thallium-201 defect outside the area of infarction (remote) for indicating multivessel disease were 35% and 87%, respectively, and were not significantly different from ST segment depression alone. When taken as a single variable, the presence of either ST depression or a remote thallium defect had a sensitivity of 58%, but specificity was reduced to 78%.

In a study by Tilkemeier et al (43), the usefulness of low-level exercise thallium testing for identifying high-risk patients after thrombolytic therapy for acute myocardial infarction was evaluated. Sixty-four patients who received early thrombolytic therapy and 107 patients without thrombolytic treatment were studied. The accuracy of exercise ECG and of thallium imaging for predicting future cardiac events were compared. After a mean follow-up of 374 days, cardiac events including death, recurrent infarction, coronary bypass graft surgery, and coronary angioplasty occurred in 25% of patients with thrombolytic therapy and 32% of those without. Seventy-five percent of the events occurred within the first 3 months after the index MI. The sensitivity of exercise thallium testing was 55% in the thrombolytic therapy group and 81% in the group not receiving thrombolytic therapy. In patients receiving thrombolytic therapy for acute MI, approximately half of the cardiac events after discharge were not predicted by exercise thallium testing.

In a very recent study, Dakik and associates (44) performed exercise thallium-201 tomography and coronary arteriography prior to hospital discharge in 71 patients who received thrombolytic therapy for acute myocardial infarction. Eleven of seventy-one patients (15%) had ischemic ST segment depression during exercise, whereas 27 patients (38%) had scintigraphic evidence of ischemia. Twenty-five of sixty-eight patients (37%) had a cardiac event consisting of either death, recurrent myocardial infarction, congestive heart failure, or unstable angina over a follow-up averaging 26 months. By multivariate analysis, the significant two predictors of risk were ejection fraction ($p < 0.0005$) and ischemic perfusion defect size ($p = 0.005$). Thus exercise thallium-201 SPECT imaging may provide important prognostic information in patients receiving thrombolytic therapy, particularly when imaging results are combined with measurement of the left ventricular ejection fraction.

Also, in the TIMI-II trial 1,658 patients treated with t-PA were assigned to the conservative strategy, with cardiac catheterization and revascularization recommended only if the exercise test was abnormal (45). Of these, 1,594 patients survived >14 days. Of this group, 1,261 performed a predischarge submaximal bicycle ergometry test; 333 were unable to exercise. The 1-year mortality in patients with ST segment depression or chest pain and therefore treated aggressively was only 1.4%. The 1-year mortality was 9.3% in those unable to exercise. Thus, the recommendation of performing cardiac catheterization and revascularization only when the predischarge test was abnormal resulted in a low 1-year mortality for those with exercise-induced angina or ST segment depression, comparable with the mortality for patients without these test findings. Those unable to perform the submaximal exercise test, as in previous studies, had the worst prognosis.

Pharmacologic stress testing, including dobutamine echocardiography, is being used to risk stratify patients after thrombolytic therapy for myocardial infarction (26,46) (see Ch. 10). The usefulness of this method for identifying high-risk postthrombolytic therapy patients has not been definitively proven in prospective studies with long-term follow-up as of this writing.

Risk factors for recurrent sustained *ventricular tachycardia* and *sudden death* in post–myocardial infarction patients studied in the prethrombolytic era included depressed left ventricular function (ejection fraction <40%), the presence of frequent premature ventricular depolarizations or nonsustained ventricular tachycardia on ambulatory ECG monitoring, a positive signal-averaged ECG, a lack of normal heart rate variability, and exercised-induced ventricular tachycardia (see Chs. 4, 28). Several of these markers also pertain to patients treated with thrombolytic therapy. McClements and Adgy (13) reported a series of 300 consecutive survivors of myocardial infarction, of whom 205 received thrombolytic therapy. Patients had signal-averaged ECG (SA-ECG), ambulatory ECG recordings, and radionuclide ventriculography prior to discharge in an effort to predict arrhythmic events defined as sudden death or sustained ventricular tachycardia. During the mean follow-up of 1 year, 13 patients (4.3%) had an arrhythmic event. An ejection fraction of <40% was the best predictor of arrhythmic events, with a sensitivity of 74% and a specificity of 81% (Fig. 31–8). The SA-ECG was 64% sensitive and 82% specific for predicting events. High-grade ventricular ectopy on ambulatory ECG recordings was only 38% sensitive and 74% specific. Although the positive predictive accuracy of the SA-ECG and of left ventricular ejection fraction of <40% were 11 and 14%, respectively, the negative predictive value was high at 98% for the SA-ECG and 99% for left ventricular ejection fraction. These results indicate that the SA-ECG and left ventricular ejection fraction are useful for predicting the absence of subsequent arrhythmic events in patients treated with thrombolytic therapy and that the ambulatory ECG recording is less reliable.

As indicated earlier, the 1-year mortality after myocardial infarction decreased with the advent of thrombolytic therapy. Patients receiving thrombolytic therapy are less likely to have depressed left ventricular function and multivessel coronary artery disease. The incidence of signal-averaged ECGs that are positive for late potentials is also significantly reduced when thrombolytic therapy is successful. This reduction in positive SA-ECGs appears independent of left ventricular function and

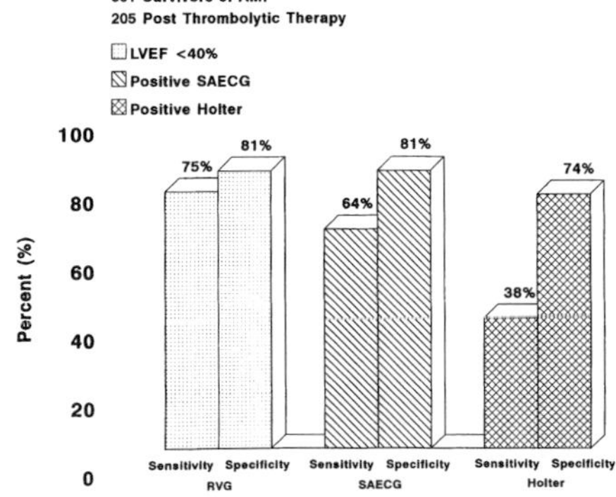

Figure 31–8. Sensitivity and specificity of three noninvasive techniques for detecting subsequent sudden death or sustained ventricular tachycardia (VT) in patients who survived acute myocardial infarction (AMI). LVEF-left ventricular ejection fraction; SAECG-signal-averaged electrocardiogram; Holter-ambulatory ECG recordings. *Data from McClements and Adgey (13).*

implies "an electrical stability" after myocardial reperfusion (12).

Of 2,546 patients in the TIMI-II trial without congestive heart failure or hypotension during the first 24 hours after study entry, sustained ventricular tachycardia or ventricular fibrillation developed in 49 patients (1.9%; group I) within 24 hours of admission, whereas neither developed in 2,497 patients (98%; group II) (14). In patients undergoing protocol arteriography 18–48 hours after t-PA therapy, infarct artery patency was more common in patients in group II (87% of 1,169) than in patients in group I (15% of 22 patients, $p = 0.001$). More patients in group I than in group II died within 21 days (20.4% versus 1.6%, $p < 0.001$). Thus ventricular tachyarrhythmias should not be considered as markers for reperfusion after thrombolytic therapy; such arrhythmias are associated with occlusion rather than patency of the infarct-related artery. Early mortality is increased when ventricular tachycardia and fibrillation develop in patients with infarction treated with thrombolytic agents, even in the absence of congestive heart failure and hypotension.

The "Open Artery" Hypothesis

The clinical importance of a patent as opposed to an occluded infarct-related coronary artery for patients with acute myocardial infarction is widely recognized (9,11,12). The "open artery" hypothesis is founded on the principle that early reperfusion of the infarct-related coronary artery causes myocardial salvage, thus preserving ventricular function and improving patient survival. In the GUSTO trial, the better 30-day survival in patients treated with t-PA compared with that of patients treated with streptokinase appears to be related primarily to the attainment of early reperfusion (6). Earlier reperfusion resulted in a higher left ventricular ejection fraction.

Since there is a higher mortality rate among patients with an occluded infarct-related artery or only partial perfusion at 90 minutes, it is important to utilize accurate noninvasive methods for defining the early success or failure of thrombolytic therapy so that patients who may benefit from immediate retreatment with thrombolytic agents or urgent revascularization can be identified at the earliest time (11,12). Routine immediate coronary arteriography after thrombolytic therapy is not the most cost-effective strategy, for reasons previously enumerated. Several noninvasive methods (Table 31–3) are being reevaluated or are undergoing new clinical assessments for this purpose (16,47–52). A rapid and progressive decrease in chest pain when present results in a presumptive identification of myocardial reperfusion (47,48). Frequent or continuous ECG ST segment monitoring may be used as an accurate indicator of successful thrombolysis and a patent infarct-related coronary artery (47–49). ST segment monitoring may also detect reocclusion early in the post–myocardial infarction period. In the TAMI-7 study (49), continuous 12-lead ST segment recovery analysis was used as a noninvasive method for the detection of failed myocardial reperfusion. All patients had 12-lead continuous ST segment monitoring and early coronary arteriography with each analyzed in an independent blinded core laboratory. ST segment recovery and reelevation were analyzed up to the moment of arteriography, at which time patency was predicted (Fig. 31–9). Infarct-artery occlusion was seen on first injection in 27% of patients. The positive predictive value of incomplete ST recovery or ST elevation by this technique was 71%, and the negative predictive value was 87%, with 90% specificity and 64% sensitivity for coronary occlusion. ST recovery analysis predicted patency in 94% of patients with TIMI grade 3 flow versus 81% of patients with TIMI grade 2 flow and predicted occlusion in 57% of patients with collateralized occlusion versus 72% of patients with noncollateralized occlusion (49).

Table 31–3. Noninvasive Methods for Determining the Patency of the Infarct-Related Coronary Artery

Rapid and progressive decrease in chest pain
Frequent or continuous electrocardiographic ST segment monitoring
The use of creatine kinase MM and MB isoforms
Prethrombolytic and postthrombolytic therapy imaging with ^{99m}Tc-labeled sestamibi
Multiple indicators currently in early development, such as magnetic resonance imaging of the coronary arteries

O'Rourke (16), with permission.

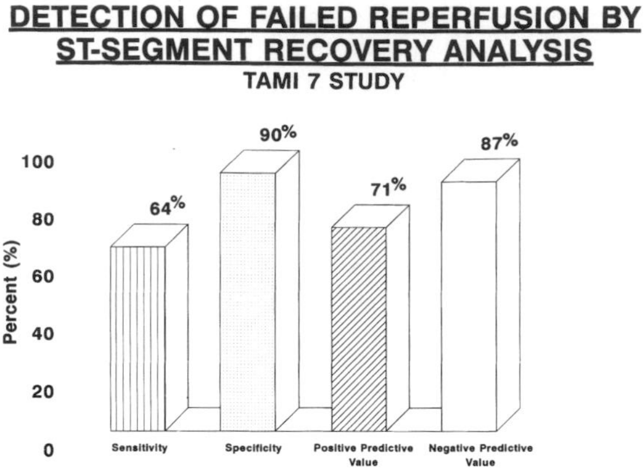

DETECTION OF FAILED REPERFUSION BY ST-SEGMENT RECOVERY ANALYSIS

TAMI 7 STUDY

Figure 31–9. Sensitivity, specificity, and positive and negative predictive value of continuous ST segment monitoring for detecting failed reperfusion with thrombolytic therapy. *Adapted from Krucoff et al (49), with permission.*

A recently described noninvasive method for detecting myocardial reperfusion utilizes measurements of the serum creatine kinase MM and MB isoforms, which have been identified and separated electrophoretically into the two types found in cardiac muscle, $MB_2$and MM_3 (50) (see Ch. 8). After these isoforms are released into the serum, they are converted by the enzyme carboxypeptidase N to the serum isoforms MB_1 and MM_1. Creatine kinase MB_2 and creatine kinase MM_3 are released more rapidly when reperfusion occurs than if the artery remains occluded. Both an elevated ratio of MB_2/MB_1 and the rapid rate of rise in the concentration of MM_3 appear to correlate with vessel patency on coronary arteriography (12,50).

Imaging with ^{99}mTc-labeled sestamibi may also be useful for assessing postthrombolytic infarct-related coronary artery patency noninvasively after thrombolytic therapy (51,52) (See Ch. 11). Sestamibi, like thallium-201, rapidly accumulates in viable myocardial cells in proportion to the myocardial perfusion; however, unlike thallium, it does not redistribute significantly as a function of time (see Ch. 11). Therefore, sestamibi imaging has been used to define myocardium at risk during the pretreatment phase of acute myocardial infarction and subsequently to determine myocardial perfusion and salvage after thrombolytic therapy (51,52). Importantly, the use of these noninvasive techniques for determining successful thrombolysis or of others now being developed or refined (e.g., magnetic resonance imaging) should identify most patients with acute MI who do not undergo successful thrombolysis.

A better survival rate has been observed in patients with acute myocardial infarction when reperfusion was achieved after substantial myocardial salvage was no longer possible, that is, the "time-independent" effect of reperfusing the infarct-related artery (12). In the SAVE trial (53,53) patency of the infarct-related artery was identified as an independent indicator of a lower incidence (36% versus 51%) of a combined clinical endpoint (cardiovascular death, severe heart failure, recurrent infarction, or marked deterioration in ejection fraction) at an average follow-up of 42 months.

Possible mechanisms responsible for the potential benefits of an open infarct-related artery include improved healing of infarcted tissue, prevention of infarct expansion and ventricular remodeling, and perfusion of "hibernating" myocardium (12). Patency of an infarct-related artery appears to be associated with greater electrical stability and thus fewer instances of ventricular tachyarrhythmias (12,14). Probably, a diminished ventricular remodeling accounts for this salutary effect; dilated hearts have greater arrhythmogenicity and more dispersion of refractory periods than do normal hearts (12).

SA-ECGs, which detect late potentials generated by asynchronous conduction through ischemic or fibrotic myocardium, are useful in identifying patients after infarction who are at increased risk for future ventricular arrhythmias (54,55) (see Ch. 28). Late potentials can be detected during the first 10 days in at least 30% of patients with acute myocardial infarction who do not receive thrombolytic therapy (54,55). Lang et al (56) reported late potentials in 8% and 40% of patients with open and closed infarct-related arteries, respectively. Although the presence of late potentials in patients receiving thrombolytic agents appears to correlate with persistent occlusion of the infarct-related artery, considerable overlap exists, with many patients having occluded arteries but no positive signal-averaged ECG and vice versa (16).

While a patent coronary artery is important particularly early and probably late after myocardial infarction, it must be emphasized that both spontaneous recanalization and reocclusion of the infarct-related coronary artery occur both during acute and long-term follow-up (see the next section).

SELECTIVE CORONARY ARTERIOGRAPHY AFTER THROMBOLYSIS

Coronary arteriography defines the severity of coronary artery stenoses and the extent of coronary artery disease, thus providing information concerning the risk for future cardiac events. However, coronary arteriography early after myocardial infarction often fails to discriminate between the severity of the underlying coronary artery stenosis and the presence of partial thrombosis (8). Coronary artery remodeling occurs for several days after the acute cardiac event. Moreover, patients treated with thrombolytic agents often have no significant residual stenosis or only single-vessel coronary artery disease (8,17–25). Serial coronary arteriographic studies indicate that the arteriographic measurement of coronary artery stenoses usually does not predict subsequent acute coronary events or which artery is likely to become the infarct-related coronary vessel (32,33). Also, pathologic studies using intravascular ultrasonography and coronary angioscopy have shown that coronary arteriography does not always accurately delineate the severity of coronary atherosclerosis (8,12).

Clinical studies assessing routine catheterization in patients after thrombolytic therapy show no advantage of this strategy versus a conservative approach where patients undergo cardiac catheterization only if spontaneous or stress-provoked myocardial ischemia is present. The major benefit of routine coronary arteriography is the detection of the 20% to 25% of patients whose infarct-related coronary artery is occluded despite thrombolytic therapy. Clinically used noninvasive techniques are not completely reliable for separating a patent infarct-related artery from an occluded vessel (8,12,16). As has been discussed, a patent infarct-related coronary artery is associated with an improved long-term prognosis, particularly in patients with a left ventricular ejection fraction of <40%.

Better methods for identifying patients with an occluded infarct-related artery who will benefit from predischarge opening of the vessel at the time of coronary arteriography remain to be defined. The number of such patients is likely to vary depending on the site of infarction, the affected coronary artery, the collateral circulation, the status of left ventricular function, and the amount of viable myocardium distal to significant coronary artery stenoses. In the TAMI-6 study, patients undergoing PTCA of occluded infarct-related arteries 48 hours after the onset of symptoms had improved left ventricular ejection fraction compared with that in patients who did not receive this procedure; however, the global systolic function was no different at the 6-month follow-up (57). Also, 38% of totally occluded coronary arteries at 48 hours had spontaneously opened at 6 months, and the percentage of patients with open coronary arteries after PTCA had declined from 81% to 60% (Fig. 31–10). Spontaneous reocclusion also occurs; in the APRICOT trial (58), the reocclusion rate at 3 months in those with initially patent infarct-related coronary arteries after thrombolysis averaged 30% (Fig. 31–11).

If cardiac catheterization and coronary arteriography are recommended as routine procedures in

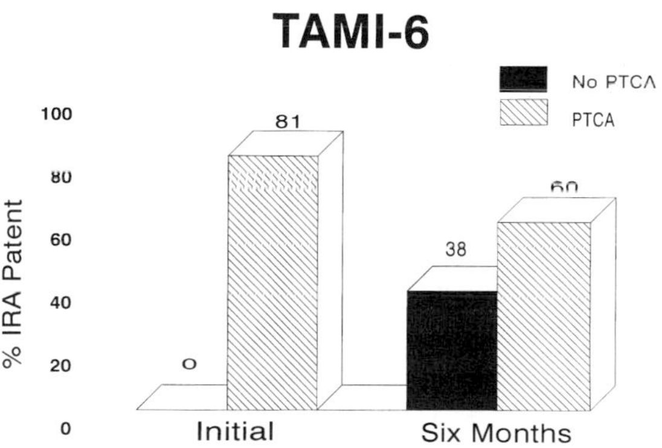

Figure 31–10. A comparison of patients treated in the TAMI-6 trial randomized to either PTCA or no PTCA of an initially occluded infarct-related artery. Bar graph shows percentage of patent infarct-related arteries after initial treatment strategy (PTCA vs. no PTCA) and at 6-month follow-up. Thirty-eight percent of patients randomized to no PTCA had spontaneous reperfusion by 6 months. *Data from Topol, et al (57).*

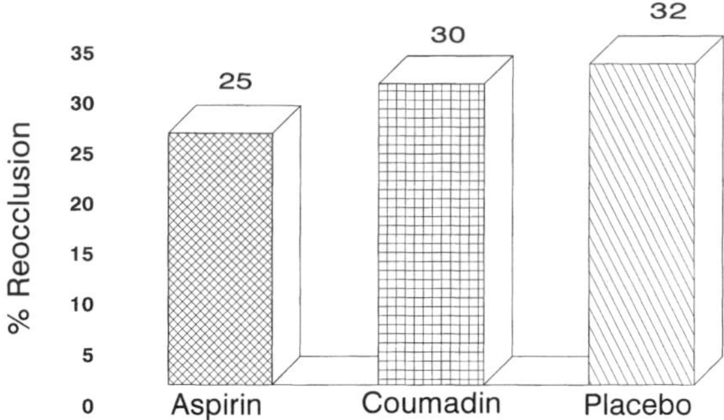

Figure 31–11. Coronary artery reocclusion rates at 3 months after successful thrombolysis in patients treated with aspirin, coumadin, or placebo in the APRICOT study. *Data from Meijer et al (58).*

patients after thrombolytic therapy, then coronary angioplasty or coronary artery bypass graft surgery should be reserved only for those with clinical indications such as provocable ischemia during noninvasive testing. Mortality rates are as high as 30% to 40% in patients after *failed* attempts at either direct or salvage PTCA, and thus a cautious approach is recommended in the use of *routine* coronary angioplasty in patients with acute infarction (59).

The European Cooperative Study Group evaluated the role of coronary arteriography before hospital discharge in 1,043 hospital survivors of two clinical thrombolytic trials (60). Forty-two of these patients (4.0%) died between 1 and 489 days after predischarge coronary arteriography. In a stepwise multivariate regression model, the use of diuretics or digitalis, a history of previous infarction, and age greater than 60 years were retained in the model using clinical data only. Also, inability to perform exercise testing and an exercised-induced systolic blood pressure rise of less than 30 mm Hg were markers of a poor prognosis. Large enzymatic infarct size, radionuclide left ventricular ejection fraction below 40%, and multivessel disease were also important determinants of mortality after hospital discharge.

The risk function that included coronary arteriography was no better for predicting late mortality than the risk function based on clinical data and noninvasive testing. Patients without a history of previous infarction, not treated with diuretics or digitalis, and with a systolic blood pressure increase of 30 mm Hg or more during exercise had an excellent survival rate (98.6%) in the first year after hospital discharge, irrespective of whether symptoms of recurrent ischemia occurred. This low-risk group, 47% of the total patient population, did not benefit from coronary arteriography. A diagnostic strategy approach recommended by the European Cooperative Study Group (60) is illustrated in Fig. 31–12. Using echocardiography or radionuclide ventriculography, patients with severe left ventricular dysfunction can be identified. Myocardial perfusion imaging can be used to verify whether exercised-induced ST segment changes without angina represent a significant area of ischemia.

Recommending cardiac catheterization and coronary arteriography only for selected patients after thrombolysis is consistent with the data from multicenter trials discussed earlier in this chapter. A conservative approach, with catherization reserved for selected patients at increased risk, has been shown to be as effective in reducing subsequent acute cardiac events as routine cardiac catheterization. The cost savings of avoiding 40% or more of the cardiac catheterizations and related myocardial revascularization procedures of questionable necessity after thrombolytic therapy are considerable (61). Noninvasive testing with a measurement of

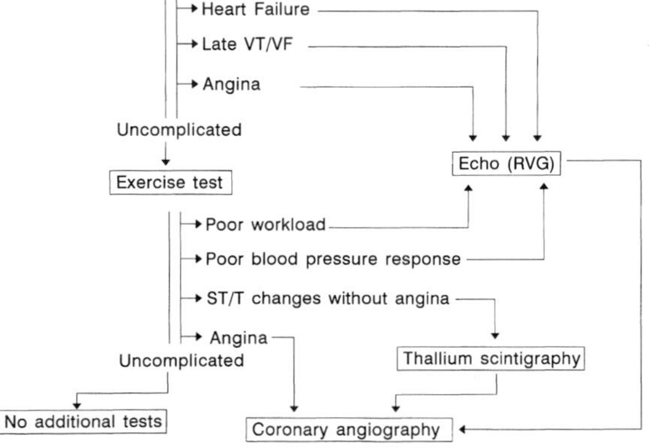

Figure 31–12. Management approach to patients with postthrombolytic myocardial infarction based on a multivariate analysis in 1,043 patients. VT = ventricular tachycardia; VF = ventricular fibrillation; RVG = radionuclide ventriculography. *Modified from Arnold et al (60), with permission.*

left ventricular systolic function and stress testing to evoke myocardial ischemia (Fig. 31–1) is considerably less expensive than coronary arteriography, which provides only anatomic information and often results in unnecessary revascularization procedures for residual stenosis in the infarct-related coronary artery even though the long-term outcome is likely to be favorable without the procedure.

As mentioned, Rogers et al (21) used the TIMI-II data to compare selective and routine angiography after thrombolysis and found that routine angiography offered no benefit. Although the 1-year mortality rate between the two groups did not differ, the in-hospital mortality rate of 8% for patients undergoing routine predischarge catheterization was high compared with 4% for patients undergoing selective catheterization ($p = 0.001$).

The selective use of postthrombolytic catheterization enhances the continuity of care in local community centers and decreases the need for interhospital transfer for the purpose of performing predischarge arteriography (8). In the TIMI-II trial, a conservative strategy after thrombolytic therapy was equally effective in community hospitals despite the greater use of coronary arteriography and angioplasty at tertiary hospitals (62). Therefore, a selective arteriography approach is highly practical because the frequency of unnecessary procedures, transfers, and PTCA is diminished, with a reduction in cost and risk (8).

Specific indications for coronary arteriography after thrombolytic therapy are listed in Table 31–4. Early coronary arteriography often is recommended for patients in whom persistent pain, continuing ST segment elevation, or a slow rise in serum creatine kinase enzyme levels suggests that thrombolysis has been unsuccessful. After the first 6 hours but before predischarge evaluation, coronary arteriography is commonly recommended for patients with recurrent episodes of ischemic chest pain, for those with congestive heart failure that persists despite intensive medical therapy, and for patients with recurrent ventricular tachycardia or ventricular fibrillation during intensive antiarrhythmic therapy (4).

Concerning patients with an uncomplicated myocardial infarction who have received thrombolytic therapy, predischarge cardiac catheterization and coronary arteriography are usually recommended for those with episodes of postinfarction angina pectoris, for those with stress-provoked ischemia during noninvasive testing, and for patients with a left ventricular ejection fraction of less than 40% (4). In the last group, an open infarct-related coronary artery likely is important for favorably affecting long-term prognosis; also, many of these patients will have severe multivessel disease and thus be candidates for coronary artery bypass surgery.

Table 31–4. Catheterization and Coronary Arteriography After Thrombolytic Therapy

Early
Pump failure/shock syndrome
Mechanical complications (VSD, severe MR)
Persistent or recurrent ischemia
Late
Recurrent episodes of ischemic chest pain
CHF during intensive medical therapy
Recurrent VT or VF during intensive antiarrhythmic therapy
Predischarge
Postinfarction angina pectoris
Provocable ischemia (noninvasive testing)
LVEF <40%

VSD = ventricular septal defect; MR = mitral regurgitation; CHF = congestive heart failure; VT = ventricular tachycardia; VF = ventricular fibrillation; LVEF = left ventricular ejection fraction.

O'Rourke (16), with permission.

SECONDARY PREVENTION AFTER THROMBOLYSIS

Risk factor modification after myocardial infarction is important both for patients receiving nonthrombolytic treatment and for those undergoing thrombolysis (see Chs. 32, 33, 34). Major risk factors for recurrent acute coronary events that can be altered include hypertension, smoking, increased serum cholesterol levels, sedentary lifestyle, and obesity. Definite evidence indicates that the treatment of hypertension, the cessation of smoking, and the reduction of hypercholesterolemia decrease major recurrent cardiac events in patients who have recovered from an MI (63–74). The direct beneficial effects of exercise, weight reduction, and modification of type A behavior for the secondary prevention of coronary disease need further confirmation (63,75).

Patients with persistent hypertension after myocardial infarction have a greater risk of subsequent cardiac death compared with normotensive patients if those who had a substantial decline in diastolic blood pressures are excluded from analysis. Treatment of hypertension benefits survivors of MI. Patients with a history of MI who were randomly assigned to the treatment group in a hypertension detection follow-up program had a 20% reduction in total mortality, which was statistically significant (65).

Observational studies comparing patients who continue to smoke postinfarction with those who quit smoking indicate that continuing to smoke is associated with a relative increase of 1.6% to 1.9% in the subsequent mortality rate (67–69). Reduced death rates have also been observed in several clinical trials of treatments to lower serum cholesterol levels in patients after myocardial infarction (66,71–74). While specific prospective studies have not compared the salutary effects of modifying these three important risk factors on the subsequent numbers of cardiac events in patients receiving thrombolytic therapy as compared with those receiving nonthrombolytic treatment, there is no reason to believe that risk factor modification is not beneficial for the postthrombolytic patient group.

Postinfarction pharmacologic therapies with beta blockers, aspirin, coumadin, and angiotensin converting enzyme (ACE) inhibitors (particularly in patients with a left ventricular ejection fraction of less than 40%) have been shown to reduce mortality reinfarction mortality rates in patients who receive these drugs for secondary prevention (58,70, 76–82) (scc Chs. 29 and 32).

The long-term beneficial effects of beta blocker therapy that particularly pertain to patients at high risk after infarction also appear relevant to patients who have received thrombolytic therapy (16). While prospective long-term data to prove this premise are lacking, the results of the TIMI-IIB trial indicate that the early initiation of beta blocker therapy reduces the incidence of ischemic events at least short term compared with their frequency during the initial hospitalization in patients who did not receive beta blocker therapy until the sixth day after thrombolytic therapy (17) (see Chs. 12, 32).

The salutary effects of aspirin early during the treatment of patients with acute myocardial infarction were well documented in the ISIS-2 study (80). The continuation of long-term aspirin therapy for secondary prevention appears applicable to patients who did or did not receive thrombolytic agents, considering the pathogenesis of acute coronary artery syndromes (16). In the APRICOT study (58), the effects of three antithrombotic regimens on the arteriographic and clinical courses after successful thrombolysis were assessed. Coronary artery patency and left ventricular function were reevaluated in 248 patients after 3 months of therapy with aspirin, coumadin, or placebo (Fig. 31–11). Reocclusion rates were not significantly different: 25% with aspirin, 30% with warfarin, and 32% with placebo. Reinfarction occurred in 3% of patients on aspirin, 8% of those on coumadin, and 11% of patients on placebo (aspirin versus placebo, $p < 0.025$). An event-free clinical course was observed in 93% of patients with aspirin, 82% of patients with warfarin, and 76% of patients with placebo; the difference between aspirin and the other two regimens was statistically significant. At 3 months after thrombolytic therapy, aspirin as compared with placebo significantly reduced the reinfarction rate, improved event-free survival, and better preserved left ventricular function (see Ch. 20).

In the Warfarin Re-infarction Study (81), daily treatment of warfarin for an average of 37 months caused a 24% reduction in the number of total deaths and a 34% reduction in the incidence of recurrent myocardial infarction as compared with placebo therapy. Several ongoing clinical trials are comparing the usefulness of warfarin anticoagulation versus aspirin therapy or their combination in lower doses for the secondary prevention of cardiac events in postinfarction patients, including those treated with thrombolytic therapy.

In the Survival and Ventricular Enlargement (SAVE) trial (82), all cause mortality during an average of 42 months follow-up was reduced by 19% in patients post–myocardial infarction with a left ventricular ejection fraction (LVEF) of less than

40% who were treated daily with the ACE captopril compared with those randomized to placebo therapy (see Ch. 29). In these patients with an impaired left ventricular systolic function, daily therapy with an ACE inhibitor reduced the occurrence of both fatal and nonfatal major cardiovascular events. Approximately 30% of the patients in both the captopril and placebo treated groups received thrombolytic therapy before randomization (83). Accordingly, it is highly likely that the ACE inhibitor therapy reduction in the incidence of major cardiovascular events for postinfarction patients with LVEF < 40% occurs both in patients receiving and those not receiving thrombolytic therapy (see Ch. 29).

SUMMARY

On the basis of the available data concerning the indications for and the timing of coronary arteriography after treatment of myocardial infarction, the inevitable conclusion is that conservative instead of aggressive management is indicated for the 40% to 50% of patients who are characterized as at low risk by clinical characteristics and after noninvasive testing for depressed left ventricular systolic function, stress-induced myocardial ischemia, and indicators of recurrent ventricular tachyarrhythmias. This applies both to patients who receive thrombolytic therapy and to those who do not. Factors to be considered in treatment decisions for individual patients after thrombolytic therapy include risk factors before and after thrombolytic therapy, the results of studies assessing conservative versus aggressive postthrombolytic management, the accuracy of risk stratification by noninvasive testing, and the relevance of the "open artery" hypothesis. The low-risk patient with a left ventricular ejection fraction above 40% and no ischemia during adequate stress testing has a low 3- to 5-year mortality rate.

While routine coronary arteriography usually determines the severity and extent of coronary artery disease and whether the infarct-related artery is patent, selective coronary arteriography is a more feasible and less expensive approach for appropriate patients. The low annual mortality rate with this approach is equal to that obtained when patients undergo routine coronary arteriography with myocardial revascularization based on the coronary arteriographic results.

The modification of various coronary risk factors appears as valuable for patients who have undergone thrombolytic therapy as for those who did not. Specifically, the cessation of smoking, the control of hypertension, and the treatment of hypercholesterolemia are indicated for patients after thrombolysis when any of these modifiable risk factors is present.

Secondary prevention with pharmacologic agents appears to be similar for those who have undergone nonthrombolytic or thrombolytic therapy. Long-term aspirin therapy is routine for secondary prevention, long-term beta blocker therapy is useful for high-risk patients; and long-term treatment with angiotensin converting enzyme inhibitors is indicated for patients who have a low left ventricular ejection fraction after thrombolysis.

REFERENCES

1. O'Rourke RA: Overview of trends in heart disease: Changing prognoses after acute myocardial infarction. *Am J Epidemiol* 1993;3:541–546.
2. Terrin ML, William DO, Kleinman NS, et al: Two and three year results of the Thrombolysis in Myocardial Infarction (TIMI) phase II clinical trial. *J Am Coll Cardiol* 1993;22:1763–1772.
3. Reeder GS, Gersh BJ: Modern management of acute myocardial infarction. *Curr Prob Cardiol* 1993;2: 81–156.

3a. Reeder GS, Gersh BJ: Modern management of acute myocardial infarction. *Current Problems in Cardiology* 1996 (Sept) (In press).

4. Gunnar RM, Bourdillon PDV, Dixon DW, et al: ACC/AHA Task Force report. Guidelines for the early management of patients with acute myocardial infarction. *J Am Coll Cardiol* 1990;16:249–292.

4a. Ryan TJ, Anderson JL, Antman EM et al: ACC/AHA Guidelines for the management of the patients with acute myocardial infarction. *J Amer Col Cardiol* and *Circulation* 1966 (In press).

5. The GUSTO Investigators: An international randomized trial comparing four thrombolytic strategies for acute myocardial infarction. *N Engl J Med* 1993;329:673–682.

6. The GUSTO Angiographic Investigators: The effects of tissue plasminogen activator, streptokinase or both on coronary-artery patency, ventricular function and survival after acute myocardial infarction. *N Engl J Med* 1993;329:1615–1622.
7. Grines CL, for the Primary Angioplasty in Myocardial Infarction Group: A comparison of immediate angioplasty with thrombolytic therapy for acute myocardial infarction. *N Engl J Med* 1993;328: 673–679.
8. Topol EJ, Holmes DR, Rogers WJ: Coronary angiography after thrombolytic therapy for acute myocardial infarction. *Ann Intern Med* 1991;114; 877–885.

8a. Newby LK, Califf RM, Guerci A: Early discharge in the thrombolytic era: an analysis of criteria for uncomplicated infarction from the global utilization of streptokinase and t-PA for occluded coronary arteries (GUSTO) trial. *J Amer Col Cardiol* 1996;27:625–632.

9. Fortin D, Califf R: Long-term survival from acute myocardial infarction: Salutary effect of an open coronary vessel. *Am J Med* 1990;88(Suppl I): 1N–9N.
10. Zaret BL, Wackers FJT, Terrin ML, et al, for the TIMI Study Group: Value of radionuclide rest and exercise left ventricular ejection fraction in assessing survival of patients after thrombolytic therapy for acute myocardial infarction: Results of Thrombolysis in Myocardial Infarction (TIMI) Phase II Study. *J Am Coll Cardiol* 1995;26:73–79.
11. Braunwald E: The open-artery theory is alive and well again. *N Engl J Med* 1993;329:1650–1652.
12. Kim CB, Braunwald E: Potential benefits of late reperfusion of infarcted myocardium. The open artery hypothesis. *Circulation* 1993;88:2426–2436.
13. McClements BM, Adgey AAJ: Value of signal-averaged electrocardiography, radionuclide ventriculography, Holter monitoring and clinical variables for the prediction of arrhythmic events in survivors of acute myocardial infarction in the thrombolytic era. *J Am Coll Cardiol* 1993;21: 1419–1427.
14. Berger PB, Ruocco NA, Ryan TJ, et al: Incidence and significance of ventricular tachycardia and fibrillation in the absence of hypotension or heart failure in acute myocardial infarction treated with recombinant tissue type plasminogen activator: Results from the TIMI phase II trial. *J Am Coll Cardiol* 1993;22:1773–1779.
15. O'Rourke RA: Non-invasive and invasive testing after myocardial infarction. *Curr Prob Cardiol* 1991; 11:727–763.
16. O'Rourke RA: Management of patients after myocardial infarction and thrombolytic therapy. *Curr Prob Cardiol* 1994;19:177–228.
17. The TIMI Study Group: Comparison of invasive and conservative strategies after treatment with intravenous tissue plasminogen activator in acute myocardial infarction. Results of the Thrombolysis in Myocardial Infarction (TIMI) phase II trial. *N Engl J Med* 1989;320:618–627.
18. SWIFT Trial Study Group: SWIFT trial of delayed elective intervention versus conservative treatment after thrombolysis with anistreplase in acute myocardial infarction. *Br Med J* 1991;302: 555–560.
19. Barbash GI, Roth A, Hod H, et al: Randomized controlled trial of late in-hospital angiography and angioplasty versus conservative management after treatment with recombinant tissue-type plasminogen activator in acute myocardial infarction. *Am J Cardiol* 1990;66:538–545.
20. Ellis SG, Mooney MR, George BS, et al: Randomized trial of late elective angioplasty versus conservative management for patients with residual stenoses after thrombolytic treatment of myocardial infarction. *Circulation* 1992;86:1400–1406.
21. Rogers WJ, Babb JD, Baim DS, et al: Selective versus routine predischarge coronary arteriography after therapy with recombinant tissue-type plasminogen activator, heparin and aspirin for acute myocardial infarction. *J Am Coll Cardiol* 1991;17: 1007–1016.
22. TIMI IIIB Investigators: Management of unstable angina and non-Q-wave myocardial infarction. *Circulation* 1994;89:1545–1560.

22a. Reeder GS, Gibbons RJ. Commentary: Acute myocardial infarction: Risk stratification in the thrombolytic era. *Mayo Clin Proc* 1995;70:87–94.

22b. Pitt B. Evaluation of the postinfarction patient. *Circulation* 1995;91:1855–1860.

23. The TIMI Research Group: Immediate vs delayed catheterization and angioplasty thrombolytic therapy for acute myocardial infarction. TIMI IIA results. JAMA 1988;260:2849–2858.
24. Topol EJ, Califf RM, George BS, et al: A randomized trial of immediate versus delayed elective angioplasty after intravenous tissue plasminogen acti-

vator in acute myocardial infarction. *N Engl J Med* 1987;317:581–588.

25. Simoons ML, Arnold A, Betriu A, et al: Thrombolysis with rt-PA in acute myocardial infarction: No beneficial effects of immediate PTCA. *Lancet* 1988; 1:197–203.

26. Mahmarian JJ, Mahmarian AC, Marks GF, Pratt CM, Verani MS: Role of adenosine thallium-201 tomography for defining long-term risk in patients after acute myocardial infarction. *J Am Coll Cardiol* 1995;25:1333–1340.

27. Jaarsma W, Cramer MJM, Suttorp MJ, et al: Risk stratification thrombolysis in acute myocardial infarction with dobutamine stress echocardiography (abstract). *Circulation* 1993;88:(Suppl I):I-120.

28. Smith J, Marcus FI, Serkoman R, with the Multicenter Post-Infarction Research Group: Prognosis of patients with diabetes mellitus after acute myocardial infarction. *Am J Cardiol* 1984;54:718–721.

29. Hillis LD, Forman S, Braunwald E, et al: Risk stratification before thrombolytic therapy in patients with acute myocardial infarction. *J Am Coll Cardiol* 1990;16:313–315.

30. The Multicenter Post-Infarction Research Group: Risk stratification and survival after myocardial infarction. *N Engl J Med* 1983;209:331–336.

31. Roberts R, Morris D, Pratt GM, et al: Pathophysiology, recognition and treatment of acute myocardial infarction and its complications, in Schlant RC, Alexander RW (eds): *The Heart*, 8th ed. New York, McGraw-Hill, 1994, pp 1107–1184.

32. Little WC, Downes T, Applegate R: The underlying coronary lesion in myocardial infarction: Implications for coronary angiography. *Clin Cardiol* 1991; 14:868–874.

33. Little WC, Constantinescu M, Applegate RJ, et al: Can coronary angiography predict the site of a subsequent myocardial infarction in patients with mild to moderate coronary artery disease? *Circulation* 1988;78:1157–1166.

34. Gibson R, Watson D, Craddock G, et al: Prediction of cardiac events after uncomplicated myocardial infarction: A prospective study comparing predischarge exercise thallium-201 scintigraphy and coronary angiography. *Circulation* 1983;68:321–326.

35. Dittus RS, Roberts SD, Adolph RJ: Cost-effective analysis of patient management alternatives after uncomplicated myocardial infarction: A model. *J Am Coll Cardiol* 1987;10:868–878.

36. O'Rourke, RA: Risk stratification after myocardial infarction. Clinical overview. *Circulation* 1991;84 (Suppl I):I-177-I-181.

37. Verani MS: Pharmacologic stress myocardial perfusion imaging. *Curr Prob Cardiol* 1993;8:481–528.

38. Hoffmann R, Lethen H, Kleinhans E, et al: Comparative evaluation of bicycle and dobutamine stress echocardiography with perfusion scintigraphy and bicycle electrocardiogram for identification of coronary artery disease. *Am J Cardiol* 1993; 72:55–559.

39. Gomes JA, Winters SL, Stewart D, et al: A new noninvasive index to predict sustained ventricular tachycardia and sudden death in the first year after myocardial infarction: Based on signal-averaged electrocardiogram, radionuclide ejection fraction and Holter monitoring. *J Am Coll Cardiol* 1987;10: 349–357.

40. Arnold AER, Simoons ML, Van de Werf F, et al: Recombinant tissue-type plasminogen activator and immediate angioplasty in acute myocardial infarction. One-year follow-up. *Circulation* 1992;86: 111–120.

41. Simoons ML, Vos J, Tijssen JG, et al: Long-term benefit of early thrombolytic therapy in patients with acute myocardial infarction: 5 year follow-up of a trial conducted by the Interuniversity Cardiology Institute of the Netherlands. *J Am Coll Cardiol* 1989;14:1609–1615.

42. Haber HL, Beller GA, Watson DD, et al: Exercise thallium-201 scintigraphy after thrombolytic therapy with or without angioplasty for acute myocardial infarction. *Am J Cardiol* 1993;71:1257–1261.

43. Tilkemeier PL, Guiney TE, LaRaia PJ, et al: Prognostic value of predischarge low-level exercise thallium testing after thrombolytic treatment of acute myocardial infarction. *Am J Cardiol* 1990;66: 1203–1207.

44. Verani M: Personal communication & Dakik HB, Mahmarian JJ, Kimball KY et al. Prognostic value of exercise thallium-201 tomography in patients treated with thromobolytic therapy during acute myocardial infarction. *Circulation* 1996 (In press).

45. Chaitman BR, McMahon RP, Terrin M, et al: Impact of treatment strategy on predischarge exercise test in the Thrombolysis in Myocardial Infarction (TIMI) II trial. *Am J Cardiol* 1993;71:131–138.

46. Takuchi M, Araki M, Nakashima Y, et al: The detection of residual ischemia and stenosis in patients

with acute myocardial infarction with dobutamine stress echocardiography. *J Am Soc Echocardiogr* 1994; 7:252–252.

47. Hohnloser SH, Zabel M, Kasper W, et al: Assessment of coronary artery patency after thrombolytic therapy: Acute prediction using the combined analysis of three non-invasive markers. *J Am Coll Cardiol* 1991;18:44–49.
48. Shah PK, Cercek B, Lew AS, et al: Angiographic validation of bedside markers of reperfusion. *J Am Coll Cardiol* 1993;21:55–61.
49. Krucoff MW, Croll MA, Pope JF, et al: Continuous 12-lead ST-segment recovery analysis in the TAMI 7 study. Performance of a non-invasive method for real-time detection of failed reperfusion. *Circulation* 1993;88:436–446.
50. Roberts R, Kleiman NS: Earlier diagnosis and treatment of acute myocardial infarction necessitates the need for a "New Diagnostic Mind-set." *Circulation* 1994;89:872–881.
51. Christian TF, Behrenbeck T, Pellikka PA, et al: Mismatch of left ventricular function and infarct size demonstrated by technetium-^{99}m isonitrile imaging after reperfusion therapy for acute myocardial infarction: Identification of myocardial stunning and hyperkinesia. *J Am Coll Cardiol* 1990; 16:1632–1638.
52. Wackers FJ, Gibbons RJ, Verani MS, et al: Serial quantitative planar technetium-^{99}m isonitrile imaging in acute myocardial infarction: Efficacy for noninvasive assessment of thrombolytic therapy. *J Am Coll Cardiol* 1989;14:186–173.
53. Lamas GA, Flaker GC, Mitchell G, et al: Effect of captopril therapy on post-MI outcome in patients with and without a patent infarct-related artery (abstract). *J Am Coll Cardiol* 1993;21:44A.

53a. Lamas GA, Flaker GC, Mitchell G et al: Effect of infarct artery patency on prognosis after acute myocardial infarction. *Circulation* 1995;92:1101–1109.

54. Kjellgren O, Gomes JA: Current usefulness of the signal-averaged electrocardiogram. *Curr Prob Cardiol* 1993;6:361–420.
55. Graceffo M, O'Rourke RA, Hibner C, Boulet AJ: The time course and relationship of positive signal-averaged electrocardiograms by time domain and spectral temporal mapping analyses in post-infarction patients. *Am Heart J* 1995;129:238–251.
56. Lang R, Cigarroa R, Wells P, et al: Influence of anterograde flow in the infarct artery on the incidence of late potentials after acute myocardial infarction. *Am J Cardiol* 1990;65:554–558.
57. Topol EJ, Califf RM, Vandormael M, et al: A randomized trial of late reperfusion for acute myocardial infarction. *Circulation* 1992;85:2090–2099.
58. Meijer A, Verheugt FWA, Christ JPJ, et al: Aspirin versus coumadin in the prevention of reocclusion and recurrent ischemia after successful thrombolysis: Prospective placebo-controlled angiographic study: Results of the APRICOT study. *Circulation* 1993;87:1524–1530.
59. Ryan TJ, Bauman WB, Kennedy JW, et al: ACC/AHA Task Force report: Guidelines for percutaneous transluminal coronary angioplasty. *J Am Coll Cardiol* 1993;22:2033–2054.
60. Arnold AER, Simoons ML, Detry JMR, et al: Prediction of mortality hospital discharge after thrombolysis for acute myocardial infarction: Is there a need for coronary arteriography? *Eur Heart J* 1993;14:306–315.
61. Charles ED, Rogers WJ, Reeder GS, et al: Economic advantages of a conservative strategy for AMI management: rt-PA without obligatory PTCA (abstract). *J Am Coll Cardiol* 1989;13:152A.
62. Felt F, Mueller HS, Braunwald E, et al: Thrombolysis in Myocardial Infarction (TIMI) phase II trial: Outcome comparison of a "conservative strategy" in community versus tertiary hospitals. *J Am Coll Cardiol* 1990;16:1529–1534.
63. Siegel D, Grady D, Browner W, et al: Risk factor modification after myocardial infarction. *Ann Intern Med* 1988;109:213–218.
64. Kannel WB, Sorlie P, Castelli W, et al: Blood pressure and survival after myocardial infarction: The Framingham study. *Am J Cardiol* 1980;45:326–330.
65. Langforg H, Stamler J, Wassertheil-Smoller S, et al: All cause mortality in the Hypertension Detection and Follow-up Program: Findings for the whole cohort and for persons with less severe hypertension, with and without other traits related to the risk of mortality. *Prog Cardiovasc Dis* 1986;29(Suppl 1): 29–54.
66. The Coronary Drug Project Research Group: Natural history of myocardial infarction in the Coronary Drug Project: Long-term prognostic importance of serum lipid levels. *Am J Cardiol* 1978;42: 489–498.
67. Wilhelmsson C, Vedin J, Elmfeldt D, et al: Smoking and myocardial infarction. *Lancet* 1975;1:415–420.

68. Mulcahy R, Hickey N, Graham I, et al: Factors affecting the 5-year survival rate of men with acute coronary heart disease. *Am Heart J* 1977;93: 556–559.

69. Sparrow D, Dawber T: The influence of cigarette smoking on prognosis after a first myocardial infarction: A report from the Framingham Study. *J Chronic Dis* 1978;31:425–432.

70. Smith SC, Blair SN, Criqui et al: Preventing heart attack and death in patients with coronary disease. *Circulation* 1995;92:2–4.

71. Scandinavian Simvastatin Survival Study Group: Baseline serum cholesterol and treatment effect in the Scandinavian Survival Study (4S). *Lancet* 1995; 1274–1280.

72. Pederson TR, Kjekshus J, Berg K, et al: Randomised trial of cholesterol lowering in 4444 patients with coronary heart disease: The Scandinavian Simvastatin Survival Study (4S). *Lancet* 1994; 344:1383–1389.

73. Levine GN, Keaney JF Jr, Vita JA: Cholesterol reduction in cardiovascular disease: Clinical benefits and possible mechanisms. *N Engl J Med* 1995;332: 512–521.

74. Quinn TG, Alderman EL, McMillan A, Haskell W: Development of new coronary atherosclerotic lesions during a 4-year multifactor risk reduction program: The Stanford Coronary Risk Intervention Project (SCRIP). *J Am Coll Cardiol* 1994;24: 900–908.

75. Hambrecht R, Niebauer J, Marburger C, et al: Various intensities of leisure time physical activity in patients with coronary artery disease: Effects on cardiorespiratory fitness and progression of coronary atherosclerotic lesions. *J Am Coll Cardiol* 1993; 22:468–477.

76. Beta Blocker Heart Attack Trial Research Group: A randomized trial of propranolol in patients with acute myocardial infarction. 1. Mortality results. *JAMA* 1982;247:1701–1714.

77. The Norwegian Multicenter Study Group: Timolol-induced reduction in mortality and reinfarction in patients surviving acute myocardial infarction. *N Engl J Med* 1981;304:801–807.

78. Hjalmarson A, Herlitz J, Malek I, et al: Effect on mortality of metoprolol in acute myocardial infarction: ISIS-1. *Lancet* 1986;2:57–65.

79. Furberg C, Hawkins C, Lichstein E, et al. Effect of propranolol in post-infarction patients with mechanical or electrical complications. *Circulation* 1984;69:761–765.

80. ISIS-2 Collaborative Group: Randomized trial of IV streptokinase, oral aspirin both or neither group among 17,187 cases of suspected acute myocardial infarction. *Lancet* 1988;2:349–360.

81. Smith P, Arnesen H, Holme I: The effect of warfarin on mortality and reinfarction after myocardial infarction. *N Engl J Med* 1990;323:147–152.

82. Pfeffer MA, Braunwald E, Moye L, et al: Effect of captopril on morbidity in patients with left ventricular dysfunction after myocardial infarction: Results of the Survival and Ventricular Enlargement Trial. *N Engl J Med* 1992;327:669–676.

83. Rouleau JL, Moye LA, Pfeffer MA, et al: A comparison of management patterns after acute myocardial infarction in Canada and the United States. *N Engl J Med* 1993;328:779–784.

32

Secondary Prevention Postinfarction: The Role of β-Adrenergic Blockers, Calcium Channel Blockers, and Aspirin

William H. Frishman, MD, and Alan E. Skolnick, MD

Despite a decline in the incidence of coronary heart disease in the United States, more than 600,000 patients are admitted to hospitals annually with a diagnosis of acute myocardial infarction (MI) (1). For patients having their first infarction, there is a 10% in-hospital mortality; the figure is higher for patients with recurrent infarctions (2). On discharge from the hospital, patients continue to have an increased risk of cardiovascular morbidity and mortality. Patients under 70 years of age who survive the in-hospital phase of MI have a 10% mortality rate in the first year postdischarge, with the highest proportion of deaths occurring in the first 3 months (2). Subsequently, there is a 5% annual mortality rate, six times higher than the expected rate in an age-matched population without coronary disease (2). Approximately 85% of deaths that occur after hospital discharge are related to coronary artery disease, and almost half are sudden deaths. Ventricular fibrillation appears to be the primary cause of sudden death.

Prospective epidemiologic studies have identified subsets of infarct patients with a high, intermediate, or low risk of mortality (3,4). Prolonging life in this heterogeneous group of patients is a major goal of preventive therapy. To reach this goal, a variety of therapeutic approaches have been evaluated, including lifestyle measures (dietary modification, cessation of smoking, physical exercise) and coronary artery reconstructive procedures (5). Specific pharmacologic agents have included anticoagulants, cholesterol lowering drugs, thrombolytic drugs, drugs that inhibit platelet aggregation, antiarrhythmic drugs, angiotensin converting enzyme (ACE) inhibitors, calcium entry blockers, and β-adrenergic blockers (5) (see Ch. 12). The calcium entry blockers and β-adrenergic blockers always have appeared attractive preventive measures in patients because of their anti-ischemic, antiarrhythmic, and antihypertensive actions (6); aspirin because of its antithrombotic activity (7). In this chapter the clinical use of β-adrenergic blockers, calcium channel blockers, and aspirin for patients with MI will be discussed.

β-ADRENERGIC BLOCKADE

β-Adrenergic blockers have been proven safe and effective for the treatment of patients with various cardiovascular disorders (8). Since 1965 they have been considered as possible therapies for extending life in patients surviving MI (5) (see Ch. 12). On the basis of multiple long-term clinical studies, the efficacy of beta blockers in reducing the risk of mortality and nonfatal reinfarction in survivors of an acute MI has been proven (5,9). They also have been shown to reduce the extent of myocardial injury and mortality during the acute phase of MI (5). Finally, beta blockers have been suggested for the primary prevention of MI and death in patients with hypertension, stable angina, and unstable angina; their protective effects in these conditions, however, are less well defined (10,10a).

Long-Term Reduction of Cardiovascular Mortality Risk in Survivors of Acute Myocardial Infarction

The presumed major mechanisms for increased risk of cardiovascular mortality during the postinfarction period include persistent myocardial ischemia, cardiac arrhythmias, and left ventricular (LV) dysfunction (1–5,10). Elevations in plasma cat echolamine levels or enhanced sympathetic drive can increase both the severity of myocardial ischemia and the frequency of ventricular arrhythmias. After the clinical introduction of propranolol for therapy of angina pectoris and arrhythmias, it was proposed that a beta blocker might favorably influence the natural history of patients with MI by attenuating the undesirable consequences resulting from increased sympathetic nervous system activity (5,10,11). Depression of LV function, the other major risk factor contributing to mortality after infarction, can be caused by beta-blockade (8,11). For this reason, beta blockers were initially avoided or used in small doses in patients with MI. Only in the past 15 years have the results of long-term studies demonstrated the benefit of beta-blockade in reducing total mortality and nonfatal reinfarction (5,9,10).

Long-Term Beta Blocker Prevention Trials

Since 1974, 15 major randomized controlled trials with beta blockers after acute MI have been reported, with treatment and mean follow-up extending from 9 months to 6 years (12–32). More than 18,000 survivors of acute MI were studied in an attempt to document reductions in total mortality, cardiovascular mortality, coronary mortality, sudden death, and nonfatal reinfarction. Ten different beta blockers have been evaluated in these studies: acebutolol, atenolol, alprenolol, metoprolol, oxprenolol, pindolol, practolol, propranolol, sotalol, and timolol (Table 32–1) (12–32). The 15 trials met the following criteria for study design: a trial endpoint of total mortality or a clearly defined cause-specific mortality, a total sample size of at least 200, and random assignment of patients to either the beta blocker group or a concurrently followed control group. The study populations contained from 230 to 3,837 patients (12–32). Fourteen of the fifteen trials used a placebo treated control group and had a double-blind phase. The time between the infarction and the start of beta blocker or placebo treatment ranged from under 24 hours to 7.5 years. In 12 trials, patients in the low- and intermediate-risk groups were studied predominately (12–14, 16–19,24–31), and in 3 trials only high-risk patients were evaluated (15,23,32).

The results from 12 of the 15 long-term trials showed a lower mortality rate in the beta blocker group than in the placebo group (Table 32–2)

Table 32–1. Pharmacologic Properties of the β-Adrenoceptor Blocking Drugs Tested in Long-Term Trials

Drug	Relative β_1-Selectivity	Intrinsic Sympatho-mimetic Activity	Membrane Stabilizing Activity
Acebutolol	+	+	0
Alprenolol*	0	+	+
Atenolol	+	0	0
Metoprolol	+	0	0
Oxprenolol*	0	+	+
Pindolol	0	++	0
Practolol*	+	+	0
Propranolol	0	0	++
Sotalol*	0	0	0
Timolol	0	0	0

*Not available for clinical use in the United States

Reproduced from Frishman et al (5), with permission.

Table 32–2. Results of Long-Term (More than 9 Months) Beta Blocker Trials

	Number of Patients (Randomized)		Mortality		
Trial	Control	Intervention	Control (%)	Intervention (%)	P^a
Wilhelmsson et al (31)	116	114	12.1	6.1	0.18
Ahlmark and Saetre (12)[b]	93	69	11.8	7.2	0.48
Barber et al(17)[c]	147	151	31.3	27.2	0.51
Multicenter International Study (28)	1,520	1,533	8.2	6.3	0.051
Andersen et al (14)[c]	242	238	26.2	25.2	0.92
Baber et al (16)	365	355	7.4	7.9	0.91
Norwegian Multicenter Study (27)	939	945	16.2	10.4	0.0003
BHAT (18)	1,921	1,916	9.8	7.2	0.005
Hansteen et al (23)	282	278	13.1	9.0	0.16
Julian et al (25)	583	873	8.9	7.3	0.32
Taylor et al (29)	471	632	10.2	9.5	0.78
Pindolol Study Group (15)	266	263	17.7	17.1	0.36
European Infarction Study (19)	880	861	5.1	6.6	0.14
Lopressor Intervention Trial (26)	1,200	1,195	5.2	5.5	0.90
Boissel et al (32)	309	298	11.0	5.7	0.013

[a]*p* values computed for chi-square test comparing the proportion of deaths in each group.

[b]Incomplete reporting.

[c]Mortality includes all in-hospital deaths.

Adapted from Frishman WH: Clinical Pharmacology of the β-Adrenoceptor Blocking Drugs, 2nd ed. New York, Appleton-Century-Crofts, 1984, p 319, with permission.

(12–15,17,18,23–25,27–32). In the 3 large studies, the reduction in mortality with beta-blockade was statistically significant (18,24,27,28). In the remaining 9 trials, the results were not always conclusive with regard to overall mortality.

Combining the results of all 15 beta blocker trials, mortality was reduced by approximately 21%. Caution is advised in interpreting such results from pooled data due to the inherent differences among the studies in the patient population, type and dosage of beta blocker, and time of initiation and duration of treatment (5,9,10,21).

Preliminary data from the APSI trial, in which acebutolol, a beta blocker with mild intrinsic sympathomimetic activity, was compared with a placebo, documented a 48% reduction in overall mortality and a 58% reduction in vascular mortality (32).

Ten of the eleven trials reporting on the incidence of nonfatal reinfarction showed lower rates in the actively treated groups (5,10,32). In only one of the trials was this lower incidence statistically significant. A comparison of the effect of treatment on the incidence of nonfatal reinfarction is complicated for many reasons. The diagnostic criteria for infarction differed among the trials, for example, resulting in large differences in incidence. A statistical test for homogeneity, however, indicated that the result of each trial was consistent with those of the other. When all the findings from the 10 placebo-controlled, double-blind trials are pooled, the reduction in nonfatal reinfarction is 22%, a benefit almost identical to that for overall mortality.

It has been suggested that beta blocker treatment should be started on admission to the hospital to reduce the high rate of mortality among inpatients. In general, short-term intravenous treatment trials were designed to provide information about infarct size, arrhythmias, and pain relief, not mortality (9,10,33). In three large studies where intravenous beta blocker treatment was followed by oral treatment, a true reduction of about 15% was observed in the in-hospital mortality compared with placebo or control (34–36).

Possible Mechanisms of Benefit

Antiarrhythmic Effects

An analysis of cause-specific mortality in the beta blocker trials indicates that the reductions in total mortality were caused by a reduction in cardiovascular deaths (5,10). Although different definitions of sudden death were reported in the trials, a large part of the benefit from beta blocker therapy appears to have stemmed from the prevention of these deaths (5,10,20). Eight trials reported on sudden death; the rates of sudden cardiac death were lower in the beta blocker group for all eight trials (Table 32–3) (20,32). Beta blocker treatment appears to manifest a trend toward a greater overall reduction in sudden cardiac death than in all cause mortality. The weighted risk ratios for sudden cardiac death vary between 0.15 to 0.84 (mean 0.67), indicating an overall reduction of 33% in sudden cardiac death. Indeed, if sudden cardiac deaths are subtracted from all cause mortality, the remaining death rate is 3.5% in the intervention group and 4.4% in the control group, which represents an intervention/control risk ratio of nonsudden death of 0.8. Thus, although nonsudden deaths are reduced by 20% in these trials, the sudden cardiac death rate is reduced to a greater extent.

In the five largest trials, the intervention/control risk ratio for nonsudden death ranged from 0.75 to 1.02 (18,23,25,28). The two smallest trials had the most favorable risk ratios of intervention to control, that is, 0.51 and 0.61 for all cause mortality and 0.25 and 0.15 for sudden cardiac death (12,31); these same studies, however, had intervention/control risk ratios of 1.4 and 2.8 for nonsudden death. Moreover, it may be argued that this unfavorable difference in nonsudden cardiac death may relate to the specific beta blocker used; however, a more probable explanation is the potential for chance associated with small patient numbers.

For witnessed instantaneous deaths, an even larger relative benefit from beta blocker therapy was recorded. The reduction was 59% in one study (27), 46% in the second (23), and 37% in the third (17), corresponding to an average reduction in instantaneous death of 46%. For these three trials, the pooled reduction in all cause mortality was 31%, indicating that the relative reduction in instantaneous deaths is about 50% higher than that in all cause mortality. When the instantaneous deaths are removed from the all-cause mortality, the pooled reduction in death in the remaining patients becomes 23%, and the relative reduction in instantaneous deaths is twice as great.

Three of the seven trials obtained 24-hour ambulatory electrocardiographic (ECG) records on a subset of their participants, both at trial entry and at a subsequent follow-up visit (18,25,27). The findings of these three trials are similar. In the subgroup of survivors who entered the trial with frequent ventricular premature beats, fewer patients demonstrated this type of arrhythmia at a later follow-up visit than in the placebo groups (25,37,38). Among patients with frequent ventricular premature beats at entry, many continued to have this type of arrhythmia at follow-up, although fewer patients on beta blockers did than those on placebo (25,37,38). Although the recorded episodes of ventricular tachycardia were few in all trials at follow-up, this arrhythmia was less common in patients receiving beta blockers than in those on placebo (38a).

In the trials, a higher serum potassium and a shorter corrected ECG QT interval were noted in patients receiving beta blockers compared with those receiving placebo (22,25,39). Beta blockers have been observed to attenuate transmembrane potassium fluxes in response to high catecholamine levels (40). Perhaps part of the protective effect of beta-blockade comes from its ability to preserve normal serum potassium levels, especially in those patients receiving concurrent diuretic therapy (39).

Anti-ischemic Effects

Given that the incidence of nonsudden cardiac deaths and nonfatal reinfarction were reduced by beta-blockade in the long-term trials, the anti-ischemic actions of the drugs also may have contributed to their beneficial effects in the postinfarction period (38a).

Stimulation of cardiac β-adrenergic receptors by endogenous catecholamines increases myocardial oxygen consumption and can thereby aggravate the ischemic process. Drugs that block the β-adrenergic receptor reduce the effects of catecholamines and

Table 32–3. Selected Results From Some Long-Term Beta Blocker Trials

Trial	Number of Patients (Randomized)		All Cause Mortality			Sudden Cardiac Death			
	Intervention	Control	Intervention (%)	Control (%)	RR (%)	D (hr)	Intervention (%)	Control (%)	RR (%)
Wilhelmsson et al (31)	114	116	6.1	12.1	0.51	≤24	2.6	9.5	0.28
Ahlmark and Saetre (12)	69[a]	93[a]	7.2	11.8	0.61	≤24	1.4	9.7	0.15
Multicenter International Study (28)	1,533	1,520	6.7	8.4	0.80	≤1	2.9[b]	4.2[b]	0.70
Norwegian Multicenter Study (27)	945	939	10.4	16.2	0.64	≤24	7.0	11.7	0.60
BHAT (18)	1,916	1,921	7.2	9.8	0.74	≤1	3.3	4.6	0.72
Hansteen et al (23)	278	282	9.0	13.1	0.69	≤1	4.0	8.2	0.49
Julian et al (25)	873	583	7.3	8.9	0.82	≤24	5.5	6.5	0.84
Total	5,728	5,454	7.7	10.7	0.72		4.2	6.3	0.67

RR = risk ratio (intervention/control), D = time of sudden death.

[a]Incomplete reporting.

[b]Sudden cardiac death rates underestimated due to missing information.

Adapted from Frishman et al (20), with permission.

decrease myocardial oxygen requirements by reducing systemic arterial pressure, heart rate, and myocardial contractility at rest and during exercise (5,8). The effects of these drugs on coronary blood flow are less well defined. Beta blockers may decrease coronary blood flow by allowing the unopposed influence of coronary vasoconstrictor impulses to prevail. Furthermore, these drugs may also augment or maintain overall coronary blood flow by slowing the heart rate and increasing diastolic perfusion time (5,8,41). More controversial are those studies reporting favorable effects of beta blockers on myocardial metabolism, the coronary microvasculature, collateral blood flow, the dis tribution of myocardial blood flow, and oxygen–hemoglobin affinity. One or several of these anti-ischemic mechanisms may underlie the beneficial effects of beta blocker therapy in survivors of MI.

Prevention of Atherosclerotic Plaque Tears

Coronary thrombi, large enough to be detected by angiography, are often associated with tears (fissures) in the caps of atherosclerotic plaques (42,43) (see Chs. 2, 4). These tears allow blood to penetrate into the arterial wall, leading to thrombus formation within the intima; this may be followed by propagation of thrombosis into the vessel lumen. This process was described more than 60 years ago (44–46); however, its clinical importance has been realized more recently after the microanatomy of coronary thrombi was established by serial histological sectioning (47–50). Plaque tears have been recognized in the angiograms of living patients with unstable angina (51,52), acute MI (53,54), and in patients resuscitated from sudden cardiac death (55). Angioscopy in living patients with unstable angina has also confirmed the presence of mural thrombi on torn atherosclerotic plaques in the coronary arteries (56,57).

Why a plaque becomes susceptible to rupture is not known. It is presumed to be a dynamic, reversible disorder caused by changes in the constituents in the plaque, its blood supply through the vasa vasorum, or the functional integrity of the overlying endothelium (58). Computer modeling of different forms of plaque have shown that the distribution of circumferential tensile stress across the intima can be radically influenced by atherosclerotic plaques. Regions of high circumferential stress correlated closely with the sites of intimal tears found on autopsy.

It has been proposed that sudden increases in blood pressure precipitated by physical or mental stress and surges in sympathetic tone could produce hemodynamic changes leading to plaque rupture (see Ch. 5). These surges in sympathetic nervous activity could also increase platelet aggregability and possibly coronary vascular tone. β-Adrenergic blockade may modulate or attenuate the consequences of these sympathetic nervous system surges by inhibiting the effects of catecholamines on blood pressure, heart rate, and myocardial contractility (59).

Beta blockers are known to protect the aorta from acute dissection, as well as reducing the incidence of recurrent dissection (8). This is accomplished, in part, by the ability of beta blockers to reduce blood pressure and myocardial contractility. Comparing propranolol with hydralazine, using Doppler ultrasonography, Spence found that propranolol was more likely to reduce the velocity of blood flow and the likelihood of nonlaminar blood flow in the aorta (60), thereby reducing turbulance and vortex formation (as heart rate–blood velocity product is a determinant of arterial blood flow disturbance). It is postulated that this effect of beta blockers could also reduce the risk of endothelial damage and plaque rupture; subsequent coronary thrombosis would be less likely to occur. In addition, some beta blockers also have weak antiplatelet effects that might additionally prevent the development and/or propagation of clots (7,61).

β-Adrenoceptor Blockade in the Early Phase of Myocardial Infarction

β-Adrenergic blockers have been considered for use as standard therapy in patients with acute MI in order to prevent the undesirable consequences of increased sympathoadrenal discharge: arrhythmogenesis and extension of myocardial injury (9,18,35) (see Ch. 12). The drugs can alter those factors that determine increases in myocardial oxygen consumption, and they may augment coronary blood flow by increasing diastolic perfusion time

(41). They also may reduce the incidence of ventricular fibrillation. On the other hand, β-adrenergic blockade can have unfavorable consequences in some cases of acute infarction. Cardiac impulse formation may be impaired greatly, and conduction diminished to a degree that causes cardiac arrest (41). Furthermore, exacerbation of congestive heart failure in those patients dependent on the positive inotropic effect of catecholamines is a well-recognized sequela of beta-blockade (41).

Clinical Trials

Intravenous (IV) administration of a beta blocker within a few hours after the onset of chest pain markedly reduces pain and the need for narcotic analgesia in patients with MI (33) (see Ch. 12). Pain relief is associated closely with a reduction in the systolic blood pressure–heart rate product. Beta-blockade also reduces the number of episodes of ventricular fibrillation compared with placebo treatment in patients with MI (33). With the use of crude measures of infarct size, such as cumulative creatine phosphokinase (CPK) release and development of Q waves on the ECG, it is clear that beta-blockade is associated with less CPK release and better preservation of the R wave on the ECG than placebo (9,10,33,62–70). β_1-Adrenergic blockade appears to be necessary. Compared with placebo, the pyrexial response that accompanies MI is diminished by beta-blockade (33), serum potassium is preserved at a more normal level (39,71), and the number of patients with threatened infarction going on to frank infarction is often reduced (33,70).

The MIAMI (Metoprolol in Acute Myocardial Infarction) study set out to evaluate the effect of metoprolol on mortality in patients entering the hospital within 24 hours of the onset of chest pain (36). Included in the study were 5,778 patients considered to be in a low-risk category, in that patients with bradycardia, hypotension, and LV failure were excluded. Patients received either placebo or IV metoprolol (15 mg) followed by oral metoprolol for 15 days. A nonsignificant reduction in mortality of 13% was observed (36). Retrospective subgroup analysis suggested that an older population of patients with associated risks (previous angina, previous infarction, diabetes) experienced a 29% reduction in mortality (36).

The First International Study of Infarct Survival (ISIS-1) study was a large, simple, open, randomized investigation designed to establish the effect of short-term atenolol treatment on total mortality and cardiovascular mortality at 1 week and 1 year after the onset of chest pain (35). IV atenolol (5–10 mg) was administered, followed by oral atenolol, 100 mg daily for 1 week. As in the MIAMI trial, a low-risk population was studied (4.5% mortality at 1 week in the control group) (35). More than 16,000 patients were randomized; 80% were admitted to the study within 8 hours of chest pain. A significant reduction in cardiovascular mortality of 15% was observed with atenolol therapy. The benefit of atenolol was confined to the first 36 hours. The reduction in mortality on day 0 to day 1 was 32% (similar to that observed in the MIAMI study). Nonfatal cardiac arrests were not reduced by atenolol treatment, suggesting a reduction in infarct size as a cause for the mortality reduction (33,35), but a subsequent analysis implied a major benefit from atenolol on the frequency of cardiac rupture (72).

Patients in ISIS were followed for 1 year. The cardiovascular mortality was 10.1% in the atenolol group and 11.3% in the control group, representing a 10.6% reduction in mortality (35). The extra lives saved during days 8 to 365 most likely were related to IV beta-blockade because, at hospital discharge, more patients in the atenolol group remained on beta blocker than in the control group (35% vs. 26%) (35). An early intervention study in 1,395 MI patients randomized to receive metoprolol IV followed by 200 mg per day orally or placebo for 3 months (34) showed that the significant early benefit in mortality reduction at 90 days was still present 2 years later. The benefit, however, was not present 5 years later (73).

Clinical Use

It has been demonstrated conclusively that beta blockers can prolong life in patients who have had infarction (10). Should all patients receive beta blockers after an MI? There are obvious contraindications to the use of beta blockers, such as advanced congestive heart failure, Raynaud's phenomenon, bronchospastic conditions, significant disorders of atrioventricular and sinus node function, and possibly vasospastic angina. These conditions restrict the postinfarction population in whom beta blocker therapy can be administered. Moreover, in the major postinfarction beta blocker studies, approximately 50% of the eligible patients (including many high-risk individuals) were excluded (10).

Similar patient selection should be utilized if comparable mortality reduction is to be achieved in standard clinical practice. It is estimated that up to 80% of infarction patients could receive long-term β-adrenergic blockade. However, in a recent study of physician practices, it was found that cardiologists were more likely to be prescribing beta blockers than internists and family practitioners (74). Investigators have concluded that practicing physicians need to be more aware of the results of published clinical trials (75–78,78a,78b).

It appears from the findings of recent studies that the greatest benefit from beta blocker therapy is achieved in patients who are more than 60 years of age, and in the medium- or high-risk postinfarction groups (patients with LV dysfunction and/or arrhythmias) (9,10,32,79). There is a serious question whether low-risk postinfarction patients (first infarct, no LV dysfunction, normal predischarge exercise test results, and absence of complex ventricular arrhythmias) who have a 1-year post–hospital discharge mortality of 2%, require prophylactic treatment with beta blockers (79). It also is not known whether beta blockers should be used as long-term prophylactic therapy in those patients who have undergone successful coronary bypass surgery or angioplasty (10). Certain postinfarction patients with angina pectoris, hypertension, supraventricular arrhythmias, or strongly positive graded exercise tests should be considered for treatment with beta blockers as soon as these indications arise (10).

Is one β-adrenergic blocker superior to another in survivors of acute MI, or is there a common protective effect seen with all the drugs in this class? Trials investigating 10 different beta blockers found favorable mortality trends, suggesting that the benefit is conferred by the drug class rather than by a specific beta blocker.

When should treatment be initiated with beta blockers, by what route, at which dose, and for how long? It appears from multiple studies that β-adrenergic blockade can be initiated early and safely to hemodynamically stable patients with and without thrombolysis (approximately 50% of patients with MIs) (9). Caution should be exercised in administering beta blockers to patients with transmural inferior wall MI, where hemodynamic complications of a right ventricular infarction might be unmasked.

IV metoprolol and atenolol are currently approved for use in MI. Timolol was the first orally active beta blocker to be approved by the FDA as a long-term prophylactic agent in survivors of an acute MI at a fixed daily dose of 20 mg in 2 divided doses. Propranolol was also approved for this use at a range of 180–240 mg daily in 2 to 3 divided doses to be started 5 to 21 days after the onset of infarction. Oral metoprolol in doses of 100 mg twice daily and oral atenolol are approved for long-term use. Whether or not the sustained-release form of propranolol or metoprolol will be effective as a postinfarction treatment needs to be determined. It also is not clear whether a fixed-dose regimen of these drugs is preferable to a titration until clinical β-adrenergic blockade is achieved.

No conclusive data are available regarding the effect of beta blocker therapy on mortality if the drugs are started months to years after acute infarction. Nevertheless, it is reasonable to assume that mortality and morbidity would be reduced if treatment were initiated within a few months after hospitalization. Support of this view arose from retrospective subgroup analyses of a long-term prevention study with oxprenolol in coronary heart disease (CPRG). A beneficial effect on survival was noted if treatment was started within 4 months of an acute MI, but no benefit was noted when therapy was started 4 months or more after the event (29).

Some studies suggest that the major beneficial effects of beta blockers accrue during the first 12–18 months following infarction, and that the incremental benefit thereafter is small (80). Limited information from one trial shows more deaths in the placebo treatment group than in the beta blocker group as far out as 72 months (80), which suggests a sustained benefit from continued therapy.

If concern exists over the extended use of these drugs in the general postinfarction population, patients in the intermediate- and high-risk subsets, who benefit the most from beta blocker therapy, might be candidates for longer courses of therapy. An argument for stopping beta blocker treatment after a fixed time period stems from the recent observation that some beta blockers can lower plasma high-density lipoprotein (HDL) cholesterol levels and triglyceride levels, potentially increasing the risk of atherogenesis (81). Whether this should be a concern in patients who already have advanced heart disease is debatable.

Finally, in the long-term postinfarction trials, there was no evidence of a beta blocker "withdrawal reaction" in patients who discontinued active treatment (82). Patients who require continued beta blocker treatment for other reasons (angina pectoris, hypertension, migraine, and arrhythmias) should be maintained on this treatment regimen as needed.

How will postinfarction beta blocker therapy affect utilization of coronary reconstructive procedures in this population? Myocardial revascularization surgery appears to be of benefit in patients with significant angina and angiographically documented severe left main or three-vessel coronary artery disease. Therapy with beta blockers should reduce the frequency and severity of angina and, therefore, may diminish clinical indications for coronary angiography and bypass surgery. In addition, because there is a documented reduction in 1-year postinfarction mortality with beta blockers, risk–benefit considerations may now favor continued medical therapy, rather than surgical intervention, in many patients (10,79).

Is there a difference in the postinfarction safety profiles of the different beta blockers? Severe side effects from β-adrenergic blocking drugs were infrequent in the postinfarction trials. Compared with placebo, there appeared to be a higher incidence of symptomatic congestive heart failure, sinus bradycardia, hypotension, bronchial obstruction, fatigue, and mental depression with the beta blockers (83,84). Caution still should be exercised, however, when using beta blockers in high-risk patients whose myocardial function may depend on stimulation from the sympathetic nervous system. The different beta blockers used in these trials appeared to demonstrate comparable safety profiles, except for practolol, which caused a unique series of side effects leading to its withdrawal from the world market (10).

How do beta blockers protect certain patients with previous MI from death and reinfarction? By virtue of their basic pharmacologic actions, the drugs, as a group, can attenuate sympathetic cardiac stimulation and perhaps the potential for plaque rupture, coronary thrombosis, reentrant ventricular arrhythmia, and sudden death (38,59,84a). The drugs inhibit lipolysis and can reduce stress-induced increases in free fatty acids that can induce arrhythmia. All beta blockers have been found to exert a powerful suppressive effect on plasma renin levels (8). Owing to the concomitant aldosterone lowering effect and inhibitory actions on transmembrane potassium fluxes, beta blockers also might protect patients from the dangers of hypokalemia (8,40). The drugs may prevent formation of free radicals (85). The platelet inhibiting actions of some beta blockers probably do not contribute to their benefit in infarct survivors, given that this effect is related to nonspecific membrane stabilization and not to β-adrenergic blockade (timolol lacks this membrane stabilizing property) (10). Other less probable mechanisms for benefit include favorable effects on the oxygen dissociation curve (10) and reduction in transmembrane myocardial calcium fluxes (10).

Conclusion

Independent of mechanism, appropriate use of beta blockers in postinfarction patients should improve the outcome of many patients with MI. The addition of beta blockers to acute thrombolysis may improve patient outcome to a greater extent than either drug alone. This was suggested by the results of the Thrombolysis in Myocardial Infarction (TIMI-II) trial, where metoprolol was combined with recombinant tissue-type plasminogen activator (t-PA) in patients with MI (86). The benefit of combining beta blockers with antiplatelet agents, angiotensin converting enzyme inhibitors, cholesterol lowering drugs, and calcium entry blockers to further improve long-term patient outcome also needs to be examined.

CALCIUM CHANNEL BLOCKADE

The calcium channel blockers (diltiazem, nifedipine, and verapamil) are a heterogeneous groups of compounds that share the common ability to reduce transmembrane calcium ion fluxes from the extracellular to the intracellular compartments of both cardiac and vascular smooth muscle (87) (see Ch. 12). Despite this common basic action, the effects of these drugs on regional circulatory beds, sinus and atrioventricular node function, and myocardial contractility vary considerably (88). These drugs do, however, share antianginal, antiarrhythmic, and antihypertensive properties, which suggest their potential benefit during the acute phase of MI, as well as for reducing the risk of mortality and nonfatal reinfarction in survivors of an acute MI.

Calcium channel blockers exert a number of theoretical benefits in the setting of acute MI (Table 32–4). Pharmacologically, they produce a favorable reduction in myocardial oxygen demand by causing reductions in heart rate, ventricular afterload, and myocardial contractility (87). In addition, they enhance coronary blood flow to ischemic zones by relieving coronary spasm and constriction, and by vasodilatation of collateral beds (87). On a cellular level, calcium overload has been implicated as the final common pathway in ischemia-induced myocardial necrosis. Calcium channel blockers can prevent intracellular calcium overload in ischemia, thereby preserving mitochondrial structure and function, while decreasing the availability of intracellular calcium for stimulating ATPase, lipase, and protease, which can magnify cellular damage (89). Finally, some calcium channel blockers have been shown to inhibit epinephrine-induced platelet aggregation (90).

On the basis of these theoretical benefits, the calcium channel blockers have been examined both in experimental models and in patients in order to evaluate their effects on myocardial infarct size and the incidence of arrhythmias. Long-term placebo-controlled mortality studies also have been conducted using each drug in survivors of acute MI.

Table 32–4. Possible Benefits of Calcium Channel Blockers in Acute Myocardial Infarction

1. Reduction of blood pressure, heart rate (verapamil, diltiazem), and myocardial contractility.
2. Coronary vasodilatation, reversal of coronary artery spasm, and coronary constriction.
3. Enhancing coronary collateral flow.
4. Reducing intracellular calcium accumulation in ischemia, preserving mitochondrial structure and function, decreasing availability of calcium to stimulate proteolytic enzymes and ATPase.
5. Antiarrhythmic activity.
6. Inhibition of platelet aggregation (verapamil, nifedepine).

Reprinted from Frishman et al (6), with permission.

Experimental Studies in Acute Myocardial Infarction

Multiple experimental studies in various animal models have been performed to examine the effects of calcium channel blockers on MI size, the incidence of arrhythmias, and their ability to augment coronary collateral flow to the ischemic zone. The results of these studies have revealed conflicting results, with some investigators reporting reductions in predicted MI size utilizing diltiazem (91), nifedipine (92), and verapamil (93); augmentation of coronary collateral blood flow into ischemic myocardium with nifedipine (94) and verapamil (93); and reduction in the incidence of arrhythmias using either diltiazem (91) or verapamil (95). In contrast, other investigators have reported no effect on infarct size with nifedipine or verapamil (96). Moreover, increases of coronary collateral flow only to the nonischemic myocardium were demonstrated with verapamil (97), whereas treatment with nifedipine (98) was shown to have no effect on collateral flow at all. Finally, a greater benefit on infarct size was reported when calcium entry blockade was combined with thrombolytic therapy (99).

These differences in study findings may relate to the various animal models used, the length and intensity of ischemic injury, the time to drug intervention, and the histologic techniques used to assess necrosis. The results of these studies are confounded by too many experimental design variables to extrapolate the findings to human beings. There are vast differences in the pathophysiology and natural history of acute MI in humans versus animals. In addition, many of the experimental protocols involved short coronary artery occlusion periods, as well as very early, often prophylactic, administration of the study drug, two factors unlikely to be replicated in clinical studies. In addition, the coronary circulation of humans, similar to that of other primates, contains a less developed collateral circulation than in dogs. Despite these shortcomings and the varied findings of experimental studies, trials examining the effects of calcium channel blockers in patients with acute MI have been conducted over the past decade.

Clinical Trials

Verapamil

In 1984 the Danish Multicenter Group on Verapamil and Myocardial Infarction (100–103) reported the results of a study in which 1,436 patients with acute MI were randomized within 48 hours of the onset of chest pain. One group received verapamil 0.1 mg/kg IV followed by 120 mg orally 3 times daily for 6 months, and a second group received placebo in a comparable manner. The patients were followed up for 1 year, and none of them receive concomitant therapy with beta blockers. The study's major findings revealed no overall difference in mortality at 6 months or 1 year, and no difference in the rate of reinfarction was seen at 6 months. Subgroup analysis yielded additional interesting results. Mortality was greatest during the first week in patients treated with verapamil, but was greatest on days 22 to 180 in the placebo group. In those patients aged 65 or older who were treated with verapamil, mortality was decreased at 6 months. Six-month mortality was also decreased in patients treated with verapamil who had symptoms lasting 6 to 24 hours. The incidence of second- and third-degree heart block and sinoatrial block was greater in the verapamil group, but the incidence of ventricular fibrillation and premature ventricular contractions was decreased in the group of patients taking verapamil (102). Heart failure was more frequent in the verapamil group, while the incidence of angina was greater in the placebo group. Finally, it must be noted that treatment was stopped more frequently in the verapamil group after 6 months due to side effects (100–103).

A subgroup of the Danish Multicenter Study (104) included 100 patients who were randomized within 4 hours after the onset of symptoms of acute MI and who were treated with either verapamil, as just described, or with placebo. For the members of this subgroup, infarct size was assessed by MBCK release, and no significant differences were found between the two treatments.

A second subgroup of 472 patients was examined 2 to 3 weeks after stopping 6 months of treatment. The patients who had been given verapamil experienced worsening or reappearance of angina more frequently than did those given placebo (105). In addition, a subgroup of 48 patients who were followed up at 3 months of treatment showed no alteration of platelet function following therapeutic doses of verapamil after acute MI (106).

The Danish Multicenter Study Group on Verapamil and Acute Myocardial Infarction (DAVIT-II) has completed a new clinical trial that was begun in February 1985. In the trial, 1,775 patients were randomized in a double-blind placebo-controlled fashion to receive either placebo or verapamil 120 mg orally 3 times daily, starting in the second week after admission and continued for 18 months. Preliminary results reported the incidence of death or reinfarction at 18 months was 18% in the verapamil treated patients compared with 21.6% in placebo controls, $p < 0.03$. Apparently the major benefit was noted in patients without heart failure (72). Future analysis of the data is awaited with interest. The results of a study which used sustained-release verapamil in patients with acute myocardial infarction were recently reported. Patients received verapamil retard 360 mg/day (n = 531) or placebo (n = 542) 7–21 days after myocardial infarction. After 2 mean follow-up of 2305 months there were no differences in total mortality seen when comparing verapamil to placebo with a nonsignificant lower reinfarction ratio with verapamil (106).

The only clinical trial reporting any benefit from verapamil in the setting of early acute MI was conducted by Bussman et al (107) in Germany. Fifty-four patients were treated with verapamil 5 or 10 mg/hour IV for at least 48 hours beginning 8 ± 5 hours after the onset of symptoms. With this protocol, a 30% reduction in MBCK release was demonstrated. In the verapamil group, the enzyme activity curves increased less sharply, and their peaks were lower than those in the control group.

The group treated with verapamil required less lidocaine and diuretic therapy than the control group, and it had lower mean arterial pressures as well as decreased coronary perfusion pressures. These positive results can be interpreted only with the following caveats: the study was not double blind and was of small size, and the MBCK values were calculated assuming that no BBCK fraction was present.

Crea et al (108) reported the results of a single-blind, placebo-controlled study involving 17 patients with acute MI. The patients were randomized to receive either verapamil 10 mg IV every 30 minutes up to 10 mg, followed by 80 mg orally 3 times daily until discharge from the hospital, or placebo given in a similar manner. Treatment was started 6.5 ± 3 hours after the onset of symptoms. The study was terminated early because verapamil clearly failed to prevent angina and reinfarction after acute MI.

In 1978 Hagemeijer (109) studied 16 patients with acute MI who had experienced more than 20 minutes of sustained supraventricular tachycardia. Patients were given IV verapamil in 1 mg increments every minute for up to 20 minutes. Verapamil effectively converted 7 of 8 patients having atrial flutter with 2:1 block in sinus rhythm. However, only 1 of 8 patients with atrial fibrillation converted to sinus rhythm, while the other patients slowed their ventricular rate below 100 and subsequently required the administration of digitalis.

The results of the clinical trials indicate that verapamil given in the setting of acute MI is not as effective as beta blockers in reducing both mortality (100,108,109) and the incidence of reinfarction (100). It is, however, able to convert atrial flutter to sinus rhythm (109), reduce myocardial oxygen consumption, and improve the contractile functioning of ischemic LV segments (110).

Nifedipine

In 1984 the Nifedipine Angina Myocardial Infarction Study (111), a multicenter trial, reported the assessment of two groups: 105 patients with threatened MI and 66 patients with acute MI. The patients in both groups had greater than 45 minutes of chest pain and new ECG changes that were consistent with acute MI. The groups were distinguished by early MBCK values at the time of randomization, and patients in each group were randomly assigned to receive nifedipine 20 mg orally every 4 hours for 14 days, beginning 4.6 ± 0.1 hours after the onset of chest pain, or placebo. The primary endpoints of the study were the occurrence of acute MI in the threatened MI patients, and mortality in the patients of both groups. In addition, the study measured infarct size by MBCK values. It was found that nifedipine did not reduce the likelihood of progression from threatened acute MI to acute MI, since 75% of each group developed acute MI. Infarct size was also similar in the nifedipine and placebo groups. Two-week mortality in the nifedipine and placebo groups was 7.9 and 0% respectively, but the 6 month mortality rates were similar, 10.8% in the nifedipine group and 11.4% in the placebo group. The finding of increased early mortality in the nifedipine group raises the possibility that nifedipine exacerbated the consequences of acute MI. The timing of peak MBCK values with respect to onset of chest pain was not significantly different between the two groups, which indicates that reperfusion did not occur in the nifedipine group.

The authors of the Nifedipine Angina Myocardial Infarction Study (111) concluded that the lack of benefit seen in the nifedipine group may be due to delay in treatment, or the lack of coronary collateral flow in the human, and not due to reduced coronary perfusion pressure secondary to decreased afterload. However, in the subset of patients in whom therapy began within 4 hours following the onset of chest pain, there were no significant differences in progression from threatened to acute MI between the two groups. One possible reason that the study failed to realize a potential benefit with nifedipine is that the study had only an 80% probability of detecting even a 36% reduction in infarct size. Thus small changes may have been missed.

The Norwegian Nifedipine Multicenter Trial (112) was a double-blind, placebo-controlled study that enrolled 227 patients with suspected acute MI. The patients were randomized to receive either oral nifedipine 10 mg 5 times daily for 2 days followed by 10 mg 4 times daily for the next 6 weeks, or placebo during the same period. The mean time to treatment was 5.5 ± 2.9 hours from the onset of chest pain. Of the patients who were proven to have an acute MI, 13% of the nifedipine group and 21% of the placebo group were currently taking beta blockers. The primary endpoint of the study was mortality at 6 weeks, and infarct size was estimated by MBCK values. There were no significant differences in infarct size between the two groups. Indeed, the nature of the MBCK peaks was similar in both groups, indicating that reperfusion did not occur in the nifedipine group. At 6 weeks, there were 10 deaths in each group, all in patients who had suffered an acute MI. Although the number of patients in the nifedipine group concomitantly receiving beta blockers was small, the combination did not cause any significant reductions in infarct size. In the nifedipine group there were significant decreases in systolic blood pressure and increases in heart rate after the first dose. The placebo group, however, required significantly more furosemide than the nifedipine group. The authors concluded that the lack of benefit with nifedipine may have been due to delay in treatment, the lack of coronary collateral flow in humans, or unfavorable changes in the myocardial oxygen supply and demand equation.

In 1986 the results of the trial of Early Nifedipine in Acute Myocardial Infarction (113) were reported. In this large trial involving 4,491 patients with suspected acute MI, patients were randomized to receive either two doses of nifedipine (10 mg sublingually followed by 10 mg orally 4 times daily) until follow-up after 28 days, or the same regimen of placebo. Treatment began within 24 hours following onset of symptoms, with 68% of the patients receiving treatment within 8 hours. Similar numbers of patients in each group were receiving beta blockers at the start of the study. The primary endpoint of the study was 1-month mortality in the patients who had suffered an acute MI. After 1 month, the mortality rate in patients with proven MI was 10.2% in the nifedipine group and 9.3% in the placebo group. The proportion of patients diagnosed as suffering an acute MI was lower among those who had been taking beta blockers, irrespective of taking nifedipine or placebo. However, mortality was greater in those patients taking beta blockers who had suffered an acute MI, regardless of which group they were in. Mortality in those patients treated before 4 hours had elapsed from the onset of symptoms was similar in both groups. Those patients who were treated with nifedipine after 8 hours had elapsed did slightly worse than those receiving placebo. Compared with the placebo group, the nifedipine treated patients were found to have significant decreases in both systolic and diastolic blood pressures and increases in heart rate. Both groups experienced similar incidences of ventricular fibrillation and asystole.

Gottlieb et al (114) reported a trial of nifedipine in the setting of acute MI. The study included 132 patients (Killip class I or II, LV ejection fraction <35%), who were randomized to receive either nifedipine 120 mg orally for 6 weeks, or placebo. Treatment began at a mean of 8 ± 2.5 hours after the onset of symptoms of acute MI. The primary endpoints of the study were mortality at 6 weeks, incidence of angina after MI, and the need for coronary artery bypass graft (CABG). The study assessed infarct size calculated by MBCK levels, and LV ejection fraction at 10 days and 8 weeks. There was an insignificant trend toward lower peak CK values in the nifedipine group. There were no significant differences between the two groups with regard to the 6-week mortality, recurrent MI, the need for CABG, or the incidence of postinfarction angina. Global LV ejection fraction remained stable, and there were no significant differences between the groups at the time of randomization, at 10 days, or after 8 weeks.

Branagan et al (115) reported the results of a trial involving 98 patients with suspected acute MI. Patients were randomized to receive either nifedipine 10 mg sublingually on admission to the coronary care unit (CCU), and again 4 hours later, followed by 10 mg orally 4 times daily for 2 days, or placebo. Therapy was begun an average of 3.3 hours from the onset of symptoms. There was a significant difference in the average age of patients who had suffered acute MI as opposed to the group with acute coronary insufficiency. The primary endpoints of the study were 1-month mortality in the acute MI group and morbidity in the acute coronary insufficiency group. The study also estimated infarct size by MBCK values, and the patients who sustained acute MI showed an insignificant trend toward higher MBCK values. There was no significant difference between the two groups in 1-month mortality of patients with acute MI, nor was there any significant difference at 1 month in the progression from acute coronary insufficiency to acute MI.

Walker et al (116) reported the results of a trial in Ireland on 434 patients with suspected acute MI. The patients were randomized to receive either nifedipine 10 mg sublingually every 4 hours for 24 hours, followed by 10 mg orally every 4 hours for 24 hours, or placebo. Therapy began an average 111 minutes after onset of symptoms for the nifedipine group, and 129 minutes afterward for the placebo group. There were no significant differences between the groups with respect to infarct size, the incidence of ventricular arrhythmias, or in-hospital mortality.

The Secondary Prevention Reinfarction Nifedipine Trial (117,118), which involved 2,279 patients with acute MI, reported its results in 1986. Patients were randomized to receive nifedipine 10 mg orally 3 times daily for 1 year, or the same regimen of placebo beginning 7–21 days after the onset of symptoms. The mortality in the placebo group was less than half of what was expected when the study was conceived. No significant difference in cardiac enzyme levels was detected between the groups. The trial was terminated early since low mortality in the placebo group precluded the demonstration of any beneficial effect of nifedipine in the setting of recent acute MI.

Erbel et al (119) reported the results of a trial including 149 patients with chest pain lasting longer than 30 minutes and ECG changes. Initially, patients were randomized to receive either nifedipine 20 mg sublingually or placebo. Treatment continued with intracoronary nifedipine 0.2 mg before reperfusion of the infarct-related vessel with streptokinase and 0.2 mg afterward, followed by nifedipine 20 mg orally 3 times daily for the duration of the hospital stay, or similar treatment with placebo. All patients received therapy within 2.5 hours of chest pain onset, and the mean time to reperfusion was 3.5 hours. In the group receiving nifedipine, peak MBCK values were larger and occurred significantly earlier than in the control group. During the hospital stay, the mortality rate was 13% in the nifedipine group and 8% in the placebo group. Patients treated with nifedipine had a 16% incidence of reinfarction, compared with 11% in the placebo group. Reocclusion of the infarct-related vessel occurred in 20% of the nifedipine group versus 13% of the placebo group. None of the reported differences is significant. During reperfusion in the patients receiving nifedipine, a decreased incidence of second- and third-degree heart block, ventricular tachycardia, and ventricular fibrillation was also found to be insignificant. Regional and global LV ejection fractions were similar following either treatment or control regimens. Thus early nifedipine administration, in conjunction with intracoronary administration, did not enhance the salvage of ischemic myocardium achieved with reperfuson by streptokinase. Compared with simple reperfusion, the regimen combining nifedipine with thrombolytic therapy revealed an insignificant but disturbing trend toward increased cardiovascular morbidity and mortality.

In 1986 the results of the Holland Interuniversity Nifedipine/Metoprolol Trial (120) were published. The study was a double-blind, placebo-controlled trial comparing nifedipine, metoprolol, and the combination of the two in 515 patients with unstable angina. Prior to randomization, 338 patients were not pretreated with a beta blocker, whereas 177 patients were pretreated with a beta blocker. Patients who were not previously given a beta blocker were randomized to receive either both nifedipine and metoprolol, nifedipine and metoprolol placebo, metoprolol and nifedipine placebo, or double placebo. Patients previously receiving beta blockers were randomized to receive either nifedipine or placebo. Patients previously given beta blockers were either continued on the same agent or given metoprolol, depending on when they entered the trial. Dosages given were metoprolol 100 mg twice daily and nifedipine 10 mg every 4 hours for at least 48 hours, and preferably for the duration of the hospital stay. The primary endpoints studied were incidence of acute MI and incidence of recurrent ischemia within 48 hours. The effects of the trial medications were expressed as ratios of event rates, comparing therapy with placebo. The study was terminated early because interim analysis revealed that the risk of developing an acute MI was higher in the group receiving nifedipine alone than in the other groups. In patients who had not received previous beta-blockade, metoprolol had a beneficial effect on unstable angina. The combination of metoprolol and nifedipine provided no further benefit, and nifedipine alone may be detrimental; however, addition of nifedipine to existing beta-blockade in the setting of acute MI may be beneficial.

Five studies (121–125) attempted to determine whether nifedipine in the setting of acute MI can confer beneficial changes in the myocardial oxygen supply and demand equation. Verma et al (123) reported the results of a study on the hemodynamic effects of nifedipine 20 mg given sublingually in 40 patients studied within 18 hours of the onset of symptoms of acute MI. To examine the effects of preload and afterload on the hemodynamic response, the patients were stratified into four groups on the basis of blood pressure and pulmonary capillary wedge pressure (PCWP). In all groups, nifedipine significantly reduced blood pressure and systemic vascular resistance, whereas it increased heart rate and cardiac index, although the greatest reduction in blood pressure was seen in the hypertensive groups. PCWP dropped only in those treated hypertensive patients in whom it was initially elevated; nifedipine also raised the stroke volume index in this group. In the hypertensive patients who presented with normal PCWP, the stroke work index was reduced. We suggest that the study identifies a particular subgroup of hypertensive patients, with or without elevated PCWP, where nifedipine treatment in the setting of acute MI may be of particular value.

The results of the clinical trials have shown that nifedipine therapy in the setting of acute MI is ineffective in reducing the mortality when given alone (110,114–118,125a), with thrombolytic therapy (119), or in conjunction with beta-blockade (111, 113,120). During acute MI, nifedipine had an insignificant effect on the progression of acute coronary insufficiency to acute MI (110,115), MBCK-estimated infarct size (110–120), the incidence of postinfarction angina (114), or the incidence of ventricular arrhythmias (116,119,124). Treatment with nifedipine decreased the PCWP when elevated (122,123,125) and decreased blood pressure (111, 113,121–125). Nifedipine, however, often caused reflex tachycardia (113,121,123–125), thereby increasing myocardial oxygen consumption.

Diltiazem

In 1986 the Multicenter Diltiazem Reinfarction Study (126) described a double-blind, placebo-controlled trial involving 576 patients with non-Q wave MI (see Ch. 18). Patients were randomized to receive either diltiazem 90 mg orally 4 times daily, or a similar regimen of placebo for 14 days, or until discharge. The mean treatment period was 10.5 days. Treatment began between 24–72 hours after onset of symptoms, with a mean time of 53 ± 13.8 hours in the diltiazem group and 53.5 ± 13.7 hours in the placebo group. Of 287 patients in the diltiazem group, 61.3% were being treated with beta blockers at the time of randomization compared with 64.3% in the placebo group, while more than 80% overall were taking nitrates. The reinfarction rate was significantly lower in the diltiazem group than in placebo group: 5.2% and 9.3%, respectively. Regarding patients who suffered reinfarction, 8 of 15 patients in the diltiazem group and 15 of 27 patients in the placebo groups were also taking beta blockers (127). As similar numbers of the patients were given beta-blockade in each group, the effect of diltiazem on the rate of reinfarction appears to be due to its own actions. The 14-day mortality rate was similar in the two groups, 3.8% in the diltiazem group and 3.1% in the placebo group (126), but diltiazem reduced the frequency of postinfarction angina by 49.7%. The patients in the diltiazem group were more likely to experience atrioventricular block, especially first-degree heart block, bradycardia, and sinus pauses greater than 3 seconds. Although there were significant numbers of drug withdrawals in the diltiazem group, the authors concluded that diltiazem was safe and effective in preventing early reinfarction and severe angina after non-Q wave MI (126).

In 1987 the results from this study were further analyzed (128) with particular attention to the prognostic significance of diltiazem and its beneficial effects on the incidence of early recurrent ischemia in the setting of non-Q wave MI. This analysis stratified the patients from the Diltiazem Reinfarction Study (126) into three categories: no angina, angina without ST–T wave abnormalities on ECG, and angina with ST–T wave abnormalities on ECG. The major differences in the baseline characteristics of these groups was that the last included significantly more diabetics and fewer smokers. Correction for this difference was achieved by using the Cox proportional-hazards model. Within the 2 weeks of randomization, reinfarction (12.2% vs. 3.6%) and death (6.1% vs. 1.5%) were more likely to occur in those patients with postinfarction angina than in those without angina. Patients with angina and ST–T wave abnormalities indicative of ischemia had significantly greater incidence of reinfarction (20% vs 5.3%), greater myocardial damage as assessed by MBCK levels, and higher mortality (11.3% vs. 1.5%) than those patients without postinfarction angina. Patients in the diltiazem group had significantly less angina with ECG changes than did patients in the placebo group. They (128) concluded that patients with postinfarction angina after non-Q wave MI are at an increased risk of reinfarction and death. Patients who experience angina with associated ECG abnormalities also appear to be at an increased risk of cardiovascular morbidity and mortality. This high-risk group of patients seemed to benefit from prophylactic treatment with diltiazem.

In the Multicenter Diltiazem Postinfarction Trial Research Group (MDPIT) (129), 2,466 patients with acute MI were randomized within 2–15 days to receive either diltiazem 60 mg orally 4 times daily, or placebo, and were followed up for 12–52 months, with a mean of 25 months. The primary endpoints of the study were total mortality and first cardiac event (cardiac death or nonfatal MI). In the placebo group, 167 patients died, in contrast to 166 in the diltiazem group. There were 226 cardiac events in the placebo group and 202 in the diltiazem group. While the incidence of cardiac events was 11% lower in the diltiazem group, this difference was not significant. Compared with patients given placebo, the patients receiving diltiazem had a slightly increased incidence of atrioventricular block, atrial bradycardia, and hypotension.

Subgroup analysis from the MDPIT study revealed interesting interactions between certain preselected covariates and treatment assignment (129–132). A significant bidirectional interaction was noted between the presence or absence of pulmonary congestion on chest roentgenogram and diltiazem treatment (129). In 1909 patients (80%) without pulmonary congestion on chest roentgenogram, diltiazem was associated with a significant reduction in the incidence of cardiac events (Cox hazard ratio [CHR] 0.77; 95% confidence interval, 0.61 to 0.98) (129). In 490 patients (20%) with pulmonary congestion on chest roentgenogram, diltiazem was associated with a significantly increased incidence of cardiac events (CHR 1.41; 95% confidence interval, 1.01 to 1.96) (129). An analogous bidirectional interaction was observed between pulmonary congestion and diltiazem treatment when death from cardiac causes was used as the endpoint (129). With respect to the interaction between the presence or absence of anterolateral Q wave infarction and treatment assignment, again a corresponding bidirectional trend was observed, although this was of borderline statistical significance (129).

Regarding the interaction of radionuclide LV ejection fraction and diltiazem treatment, a similar bidirectional interaction was observed (129,130). In the 68% to 80% of patients with an LV ejection fraction greater than 40%, diltiazem was associated with a decreased incidence of cardiac death (CHR ≤ 0.85) (130). Conversely, in those patients with an LV ejection fraction less than 40%, diltiazem was associated with a significant increase in cardiac death (CHR > 1.5) (130). Moreover, a dose–response effect in the hazard ratios for cardiac events, when diltiazem was compared with placebo treatment, was observed if severity of pulmonary congestion and the LV ejection fraction were taken into account (129).

The effectiveness of beta blockers in combination with diltiazem after MI during the MDPIT study was also analyzed (129). There was an insignificant interaction between treatment with diltiazem and pretreatment with beta blockers. Of 2,466 patients in the trial at 1 year, 53% of 996 patients still taking diltiazem were also given a beta blocker, while 56% of 965 patients assigned to the placebo group were also taking a beta blocker. Treatment with beta blockers had a negligible effect on the bidirectional interaction between radiologic evidence of pulmonary congestion and diltiazem treatment.

One of the drawbacks of the Multicenter Diltiazem Reinfarction Study (126) is that the beneficial effect of reinfarction can only be interpreted in the context of the 14-day study period. Subgroup analysis from the MDPIT study involving a cohort of 634 patients with non-Q wave MI regarding cardiac events (cardiac death and nonfatal reinfarction) has been reported (131). During a follow-up period of 1 year, there were 46 cardiac deaths and 62 nonfatal reinfarctions, with a cumulative 1-year cardiac event rate of 15% in the placebo group and 9% in the diltiazem group. Thus, in contrast to the placebo group, a 40% reduction (CHR 0.65; 95% confidence interval, 0.43 to 0.96) in the number of cardiac events could be detected among diltiazem treated patients. The results of this analysis show that long-term prophylactic diltiazem in patients with non-Q wave MI is associated with highly significant reduction in 1-year mortality and reinfarction.

Further subgroup analysis from the MDPIT study evaluated the effect of diltiazem on ventricular arrhythmias (132). This analysis was based on the premise that the difference in the reduction of mortality after MI seen with beta blockers and not with calcium channel blockers may be due to the differences in their antiarrhythmic properties. To evaluate the ability of diltiazem to control ventricular arrhythmias 3 months after MI, 24-hour ECG recordings were made in 797 patients of the placebo group and 806 patients from the diltiazem group. Both groups experienced similar incidences of ventricular arrhythmias, although there was a significant increase in the R–R interval among patients given diltiazem. Although its inability to reduce the frequency of ventricular arrhythmias may explain diltiazem's lack of effect on mortality after MI, the analysis fails to analyze whether or not the interaction of beta blockers and diltiazem on the incidence of ventricular arrhythmias is synergistic.

Zannad et al (133) reported on the results of a double-blind placebo-controlled study involving 34 patients admitted within 6 hours of the onset of symptoms of acute MI. The patients were randomized and either received a single 10 mg dose of diltiazem IV followed by 72 hours of a 15 mg/hour infusion before being given 60 mg orally 4 times daily for the remaining part of the 21-day study period, or placebo. The mean time to treatment was 4.6 ± 0.9 hours in the diltiazem group and 4.4 ± 1.0 hours in the placebo group. The study assessed MI size by measuring plasma CK and MBCK values, by analyzing perfusion defect scores from serial thallium-201 single-photon emission computer tomography, and by using LV ejection fractions measured by radionuclide angiography. All patients received anticoagulant doses of heparin and a constant IV infusion of lidocaine 600–800 mg/24 hours. There was an insignificant trend toward higher MBCK values in the placebo group, and one death occurred in each group. The group treated with diltiazem showed significant decreases in thallium-201 perfusion defect scores at 21 days and an increase in LV ejection fraction at 48 hours and at 21 days after randomization. A 24–48 hour Holter monitor test showed no significant differences in ventricular premature beats (Lown grades 0 to 4b) between the two groups. The authors (133) concluded that diltiazem may reduce ischemic injury in acute MI, but this conclusion must be considered in the context of the small study group. A study is in progress comparing long-acting diltiazem and aspirin alone in up to 920 patients with an uncomplicated first myocardial infarction within 36 to 96 hours of receiving thrombolysis (133a).

The results of the completed clinical trials have shown that diltiazem, given in the setting of Q wave acute MI, is ineffective in reducing mortality when given alone (126,129,133) or in conjunction with beta-blockade (126,129). Prophylactic diltiazem therapy in the setting of non-Q wave MI has, however, been shown both to reduce the incidence of reinfarction at 2 weeks (126) and at 1 year (131), and also to lower the 1-year mortality rate (131). In addition, diltiazem given during non-Q wave MI reduced the incidence of refractory angina (126) and angina associated with ST T wave abnormalities (128). Diltiazem administration was also shown to have a bidirectional interaction with the incidence of cardiac events (129,130). Thus those patients with either pulmonary congestion on chest roentgenogram, anterior Q wave infarction, or an LV ejection fraction less than 40% had significantly greater risk of sustaining cardiac death or reinfarction when treated with diltiazem. Diltiazem therapy in the setting of acute MI is associated with reductions in myocardial oxygen consumption (125, 134–136) both at rest and during exercise (137), but it is ineffective in reducing the incidence of ventricular arrhythmias (132,133).

Conclusion

Despite a promising theoretical rationale for the use of calcium channel blockers in acute MI, these agents have not been shown to be as effective as beta blockers in reducing mortality or infarct size (138,139). Table 32–5 summarizes the cumulative evidence against the ability of the calcium channel blockers to reduce mortality in the setting of acute MI. These findings reinforce a retrospective statistical analysis in which Held et al (140) reviewed the effects of the calcium antagonists on the development of acute MI, reinfarction, and mortality in 21 clinical trials. They found that calcium antagonists do not prevent initial infarction in patients with acute ischemia, nor do they reduce the incidence of reinfarction or mortality.

Indeed, the MDPIT study identifies a subgroup of patients where diltiazem may be detrimental in the setting of an acute MI. Patients with pulmonary congestion (129), anterior wall MI (129), and poor LV ejection fraction (129,130) appear to be at an increased risk of cardiovascular morbidity and mortality. On a more promising note, there is a subgroup of patients that may benefit from treatment with diltiazem. The results from the Diltiazem Reinfarction Study (126,128) and the MDPIT study (129,131) indicate that diltiazem is effective in reducing the incidence of cardiovascular morbidity and mortality in patients with non-Q wave MIs.

The possible mechanisms by which diltiazem benefits patients with non-Q wave MI may be related to the pathophysiology of their disease. DeWood et al (141) have shown that in non-Q wave MI, the infarct-related vessel is rarely occluded completely. Furthermore, they demonstrated collateral circulation in a significant portion of their subjects. Thus it is highly possible that diltiazem is beneficial in non-Q wave MI because it vasodilates both collateral vessels and partially occluded arteries. It is also important that diltiazem does not produce any unfavorable hemodynamic effects and is well tolerated by most patients.

The results with nifedipine, on the other hand, have been disappointing. In fact, several studies were terminated prematurely (113,117). The Nifedipine Angina Myocardial Infarction Study trial (111) showed that nifedipine was associated with an excess mortality at 2 weeks but not at 6 months. Even when administered in conjunction with thrombolysis by streptokinase (115), nifedipine has been ineffective and has resulted in an insignificant but distressing trend toward increased cardiovascular morbidity and mortality. The problems with nifedipine are most likely due to its unfavorable hemodynamic effects, which cause increased myocardial oxygen demand. In some circumstances,

Table 32–5. Mortality in the Clinical Trials Evaluating Calcium Channel Blockers in Acute Myocardial Infarction

		Deaths/Patients	
Agents	# Studies	Calcium Blockers	Controls
Acute, short-term			
Diltiazem (126)	1	11/287	9/289
Nifedipine (111–114,120)	5	198/2,594	175/2,600
Verapamil (108)	1	0/8	2/9
Subtotal		209/2,889	186/2,898
Long-term			
Diltiazem (129)	1	167/1,234	166/1,232
Nifedipine (117)	1	66/1,140	64/1,139
Lidoflazine (138)	1	177/896	168/896
Verapamil (72,100,133a)	3	204/1,595 234/2,126	237/1,614 266/2,156
Subtotal		614/4,865 644/5,396	635/4,883 664/5,425
TOTAL		823/7,754 853/8,285	821/7,781 850/8,323

Modified from Yusuf and Furberg (139), with permission.

nifedipine may even reduce coronary perfusion pressure and extend infarct size by causing significant reduction in blood pressure, which triggers reflex tachycardia.

Finally, the results with verapamil have also shown little benefit (100–106,108) in acute MI other than the preliminary data from DAVIT-II (see earlier text). Only one study (106) was able to show any reduction in infarct size, and its protocols were not ideal. Verapamil may, however, be effective in the treatment of supraventricular tachyarrhythmias during acute MI (109), although few studies have addressed this question.

From review of clinical trials, it becomes apparent that the calcium channel blockers function somewhat differently during impending acute MI or acute MI from the way they do in controlling stable and unstable angina. Calcium channel blockers seem to be ineffective in the former clinical setting, but they are effective in the latter.

ASPIRIN

Complex interactions among the components of blood and those of the vessel wall are involved in the pathogenesis of atherosclerotic vascular disease and associated thrombotic complications (142). Considerable evidence, both clinical and experimental, has suggested that blood platelets not only play an important role in atherogenesis, arteriothromboembolic disorders, and MI, but they also may contribute to unstable, stable, and variant angina syndromes (7,142–146). Thus there is a high level of interest in the use of platelet modifying drugs, such as aspirin, in ischemic heart disease.

Aspirin has been evaluated for use in virtually every facet of atherosclerotic coronary artery disease (7,146a) (see Ch. 20). We will review the use of aspirin in the secondary prevention of MI and mortality.

Mechanism of Action

Cyclooxygenase inhibitors include the nonsteroidal anti-inflammatory drugs, such as aspirin, ibuprofen, naproxen, and many others, as well as the uricosuric agent sulfinpyrazone. Aspirin irreversibly inactivates platelet cyclooxygenase by acetylating the enzyme at the active site (145,147,148). Because platelets are not capable of synthesizing proteins, including new enzymes, one dose of aspirin inhibits cyclooxygenase for the life span of the circulating platelets, about a week (147,149). Only after new platelets enter the circulation is platelet function fully restored.

As a result of cyclooxygenase inhibition, therefore, platelets from patients taking aspirin fail to synthesize thromboxane A_2, and thus they show reduced aggregation in response to many stimuli, such as collagen, epinephrine, ADP, or arachidonate (150,151). Second-phase aggregation in response to epinephrine and ADP is abolished altogether. Bleeding time roughly doubles from baseline values for at least 24 hours (150). Release of granule contents, such as ADP, serotonin, platelet factor 4, or platelet-derived growth factor, is impaired in aspirin treated platelets, except when the platelets are activated by thrombin (145). As we know, thrombin produces platelet aggregation and release independently of thromboxane A_2, so that normal aggregation and release occur when platelets are stimulated by thrombin. This produces a very mild hemostatic defect as long as thrombin generation remains normal. When it is deficient, during anticoagulation or in hemophilia, for example, aspirin treatment can lead to severe bleeding problems (145).

Because aspirin does not impair either the primary aggregation responses to epinephrine or ADP, or the full aggregation response to thrombin, the overall effect is to inhibit thromboxane A_2 synthesis and to diminish platelet aggregation. The action of aspirin on platelets, therefore, is to modify mechanical occlusion of small vessels by platelet aggregates, but not to abolish aggregation altogether. Similarly, aspirin only partially inhibits the release of atherogenic substances, for example, platelet-derived growth factor. When blood flow and hematocrit are within normal limits, aspirin does not affect platelet adhesion to subendothelial structures or to collagen (145).

The dose of aspirin required to produce antiplatelet effects is very small. Ingestion of a single aspirin (325 mg) produces almost total inhibition of thromboxane A_2 synthesis and inhibits platelet aggregation by arachidonate, epinephrine, and collagen (152). This inhibition lasts about 48 hours, followed by a slow return to normal over a week to 10 days. Even a daily 20 mg dose of aspirin has been shown to markedly inhibit platelet aggregation responses and to reduce thromboxane A_2 generation by greater than 90% (153).

Because aspirin acts very early in the arachidonate pathway, it will affect prostaglandin synthesis in other tissues, as well as platelets, notably the synthesis of prostacyclin in the vessel wall. It originally was thought that vascular synthesis of prostacyclin was inhibited only by high doses of aspirin. This proved untrue. Jaffe and Weksler (151), for example, showed that in human vascular cell cultures, endothelial and platelet cyclooxygenases are equally sensitive to the inhibitory effect of low-dose aspirin. The difference is that the effect of aspirin on cyclooxygenase in the vessel wall is temporary because these cells can resynthesize the enzyme. So in the study just mentioned, endothelial cells began to regain their ability to produce prostacyclin as soon as aspirin was removed, and it was recovered fully in 36 hours (154).

More recent in vivo studies, on the other hand, have suggested that the effects of low-dose aspirin on prostacyclin synthesis in blood vessels might be more prolonged. Preston and coworkers obtained vein segments by biopsy from healthy volunteers after a single low dose of aspirin (150–300 mg) and measured prostacyclin synthesis (using a radioimmunoassay) for its stable metabolite 6-keto-prostaglandin F_{1a} (152). They found that there was no recovery in prostacyclin production for up to 8 hours. Simultaneous platelet production of thromboxane A_2, measured as thromboxane B_2, remained absent for up to 48 hours (152). It was proposed by Clarke et al (155) that a controlled-release aspirin could affect the formation of thromboxane A_2 but not prostacyclin by reducing the aspirin concentration that reaches the posthepatic circulation. They used a controlled-release aspirin preparation designed to release 10 mg/hour of drug. It was proposed that this slow release of aspirin would inhibit cyclooxygenase of platelets in the prehepatic circulation while the extremely low levels of drug in the posthepatic circulation would have no effect on the inhibition of prostacyclin production by the vasculature. In comparing the sustained-release aspirin to the immediate-release form, a greater preservation of prostacyclin was seen with the former (155). However, no definitive patient outcome studies are available.

Inhibition of cyclooxygenase does not fully account for aspirin's antithrombotic activity. Possible additional mechanisms include the inhibition of vitamin K–dependent clotting factor synthesis, stimulation of fibrinolysis, and antagonism of the lipooxygenase pathway of arachidonic acid metabolism in platelets and leukocytes (156). Recently it was reported that aspirin could inhibit nuclear factor KB mobilization and monocyte adhesion in stimulated human endothelial cells (157,158). Aspirin appears to modify the way in which blood neutrophils and platelets interact, some of which is endothelin dependent (159). Aspirin also may possess antiarrhythmic properties (159,160) and may augment collateral blood flow to ischemic myocardium (161), both by mechanisms independent of platelet inhibition.

Clinical Trials

There have been seven prospective, randomized, placebo-controlled, double-blind clinical trials concerned with aspirin therapy in the post-MI patients (Table 32–6) (7,147,162–167). The trials differed widely in aspirin dosage, patient numbers, female patient enrollment, time from qualifying MI to entry, and duration of patient follow-up. In six of seven trials, mortality was reduced by aspirin therapy (147, 162,164,166,167); however, the Aspirin Myocardial Infarction Study Research Group reported increased mortality (165), though none of these differences were statistically significant. In all seven trials, reductions in nonfatal recurrent infarction were found, though only in the Persantine–Aspirin Reinfarction Study (PARIS-II) (166), in which dipyridamole was concurrently administered, was this reduction statistically significant. Because these were intent-to-treat trials in which data from all enrolled patients were used regardless of whether or not they continued the prescribed therapy, it is possible that a small benefit with aspirin therapy may have been "diluted" beyond statistical significance (168). Nevertheless, one is left with the general

Table 32–6. Results of Clinical Trials of Aspirin and Aspirin Plus Dipyridamole in Post–Myocardial Infarction Patients[a]

						Nonfatal MI (%)		Death (%)					
								All Causes		MI		Sudden	
Trial	Drug Dose (mg)	Sex	Entry Time After MI	Time Observed	Number of Patients	Drug	Placebo	Drug	Placebo	Drug	Placebo	Drug	Placebo
MRC-I, 1974 (162)	A 300 daily	M	1–6 mo	2.5 y	1,239	—	—	8.3	10.9	—	—	—	—
CDPAS, 1976 (163)	A 324 TID	M	75% ≥ 5 y	10–28 mo	1,529	3.7	4.2	5.8	8.3	—	—	2.6	3.2
MRC-II, 1979 (164)	A 300 TID	B	50% within 7d	1 y	1,682	7.1	10.9	12.3	14.8	—	—	—	—
GAMPCT, 1979 (147)	A 1,500 daily	B	30–42 d	1 y	620	3.5	4.9	8.5	10.6	1.6	3.2	2.5	3.9
AMIS, 1980 (165)	A 500 BID	B	2–60 mo	3 y	1,524	6.3	8.1	10.8	9.7	6.0	6.0	2.7	2.0
PARIS, 1980 (166)	A 324 TID	B	2–60 mo	3–4 y	1,216	6.9	9.9	10.5	12.8	2.5	5.7	5.6	4.4
	A 324 + D 75 TID	B	2–60 mo	3–4 y	1,216	7.9	9.9	10.7	12.8	4.0	5.7	3.7	4.4
PARIS-II, 1986 (167)	A 330 + D 75 TID	B	1–4 mo	1–2 y	3,128	4.5	7.1	7.1	7.3	—	—	2.4	2.0

M = males. B = both males and females, TID = three times daily, A = aspirin, D = dipyridamole.

[a]Values are for analyzable deaths of eligible patients. Sudden death is recorded for the total time of the study.

Adapted from Mustard et al (168), with permission.

impression that aspirin reduces mortality by about 20% and recurrent infarction by about 25%, with the reduction in death but not in reinfarction being most marked during the first 6 months (the high-risk "early" postrecovery period).

By using statistical methods able to compensate for protocol and cohort differences, Peto (169) pooled the results of six of these studies (excluding PARIS-II), which involved a total of 10,703 patients. He assumed that if aspirin did not reduce mortality, the sum of the differences between the number of observed and expected (if aspirin had no effect) deaths in each trial would differ only randomly from zero. By showing that this quantity was significantly different from zero, Peto claimed a significant difference in favor of aspirin in overall death (probability $p < 0.03$). This, in turn, was the sum of a nonsignificant difference ($p > 0.03$) against aspirin in noncardiovascular mortality plus a more significant ($p < 0.01$) 16% reduction in cardiovascular mortality with aspirin therapy. By these methods, the reduction in cardiovascular morbidity was found to be even more significant ($p < 0.0001$), with a 21 ± 5% reduction in recurrent infarction.

More recently the Antiplatelet Trialists' Collaboration described and summarized their findings of all unconfounded controlled randomized trials of therapy in patients with cardiovascular disease that were available for review by March 1990 (170). Their overview comprised 145 randomized trials and 29 randomized active-control comparison studies. The most widely used regimen was aspirin in a dose range of 75–325 mg/day. In their analysis, they found that among 20,000 subjects with hyperacute MI who participated in these randomized trials (1 month duration), there was a significant reduction in vascular events including mortality, nonfatal reinfarction, and stroke (10% antiplatelet therapy, 14% controls, a reduction of 40 events/1,000 patients treated with aspirin). Among 20,000 patients who received aspirin as a long-term post–MI treatment (the studies previously discussed are included), there was a significant reduction in vascular events (13% antiplatelet therapy, 17% controls, a reduction of 40 events/1,000 patients treated).

In the hyperacute phase of MI, there is now clear evidence of aspirin's utility in reducing reinfarction, as a monotherapy and in combination (171) with a thrombolytic agent. In the Second International Study of Infarct Survival (ISIS-2), aspirin used in a dose of 162.5 mg/day had an independent effect in reducing vascular deaths, strokes, and reinfarction both short term (1 month) and long term, an action that was augmented by thrombolysis with streptokinase (172). This action probably extends to all thrombolytic agents. The protective action of aspirin was again demonstrated in the ISIS-3 study, where an additional benefit was demonstrated when both heparin and aspirin (173) were administered together with thrombolysis during the hyperacute phase of MI.

Aspirin, with and without heparin, has also been shown to be a useful treatment in the management of unstable angina, a condition associated with platelet activation (174), reducing the incidence of both MI and mortality by 50–70% from controls (175–177). Similar benefit with aspirin has also been shown in patients with stable angina pectoris (178).

Conclusion

There is now definitive evidence showing a reduction in mortality and morbid cardiovascular events when aspirin is used in the hyperacute phase of MI as an adjunctive therapy to thrombolysis and as a long-term prophylactic agent for reducing mortality, reinfarction, and stroke in survivors of acute MI (179). The Food and Drug Administration has approved aspirin, in part, based on Peto's statistical analysis (169), as a once-daily therapy (325 mg daily). However, some investigators have suggested using lower doses (75–160 mg/daily) (146a,179). Some have even suggested using the new controlled-release aspirin (155) ticlopidine or specific thromboxane inhibitors now under development. Despite the favorable outcomes with aspirin, it is still underutilized in clinical practice (179).

Based on the available information, our recommendation regarding aspirin is to use one 325 mg aspirin tablet upon initiation of therapy and at least 75 mg daily (¼ tablet) as maintenance therapy. In those patients intolerant of aspirin, dipyridamole or ticlopidine could be used; however, there is no evidence for their benefit in MI patients.

CLINICAL RECOMMENDATIONS

Pharmacologic interventions are now available for prolonging life in survivors of MI and for treating patients immediately after an acute MI. These interventions are summarized in Table 32–7.

Immediately after acute MI, IV β-adrenergic blockade has been proven efficacious in reducing the extent of myocardial injury and prolonging life, although the benefit is modest and only a fraction of the patients are eligible for treatment. Beta blockers should be administered within 4 hours of symptom onset to achieve their maximum effect. Beta-blockade does not appear to improve survival as well as thrombolysis, and unlike beta-blockade (180), thrombolysis can be used in most patients early in the course of infarction. A 1989 study demonstrated that early in MI, thrombolysis and β-adrenergic blockade (metoprolol) resulted in fewer recurrent ischemic episodes (86). Complete studies of calcium channel blockade in early infarction, however, are unfavorable, although there appears to be some benefit in administering oral diltiazem to patients with non-Q wave MI. Nonetheless, this benefit is not clearly greater than that achieved with beta-blockade alone.

β-Adrenergic blockade has a clear advantage over calcium channel blockade when the long-term risk of mortality and reinfarction is considered in survivors of MI. Calcium channel blockade may even be contraindicated in such patients with LV dysfunction. In patients with non-Q wave MI, either diltiazem or beta blockers can be used for long-term treatment, but beta blockers are more beneficial in patients with LV dysfunction. Finally, adjunctive therapies, such as aspirin (7), angiotensin converting enzyme (ACE) inhibitors, and pharmacologic and nonpharmacologic approaches to hyperlipidemia hypertension, and cigarette smoking should be considered for the survivors of MI. These therapies may further decrease cardiovascular morbidity and mortality (181).

Table 32–7. Recommendations for Cardiovascular Drug Treatment in Patients with Acute Myocardial Infarction*

Hyperacute phase	Thrombolysis + heparin, β-adrenergic blockade, aspirin, or combination. ACE inhibitors may be used with caution.
Long-term treatment of survivors	
Q wave infarction (good LV function)	β-Adrenergic blockade, aspirin, or combination; calcium entry blockers (diltiazem or verapamil) in patients who cannot tolerate beta-blockade.
Q wave infarction (diminished LV function)	β-Adrenergic blockade (if tolerated), aspirin, ACE inhibition or combination; avoid calcium channel blockade.
Non-Q wave infarction (good LV function)	Calcium channel blockade (diltiazem), aspirin, β-adrenergic blockade, or combination.
Non-Q wave infarction (diminished LV function)	β-Adrenergic blockade (if tolerated), aspirin, ACE inhibition, or combination.

*In all situations, therapy should be given to reduce LDL cholesterol below 100 mg% and patients encouraged to stop smoking.

Adapted from Skolnick AE, Frishman WH: Calcium channel blockers in myocardial infarction. Arch Intern Med 1989;149:1675, with permission.

REFERENCES

1. May GS, Furberg CD, Eberlein KA, et al: Secondary prevention after myocardial infarction: A review of short-term acute phase trials. *Prog Cardiovas Dis* 1983;25:335–359.
2. May GS, Eberlein KA, Furberg CD, et al: Secondary prevention after myocardial infarction: A review of long-term trials. *Prog Cardiovasc Dis* 1982;24: 331–352.
3. Davis HT, DeCamilla J, Bayer LW, et al: Survivorship patterns in posthospital phase of myocardial infarction. *Circulation* 1979;60:1252–1258.
4. Multicenter Postinfarction Research Group: Risk stratification after myocardial infarction. *N Engl J Med* 1983;309:331–336.
5. Frishman WH, Furberg DC, Friedewald WT: β-Adrenergic blockade for survivors of acute myocardial infarction. *N Engl J Med* 1984;310:830–836.
6. Frishman WH, Skolnick AE, Lazar EJ, Fein S: β-Adrenergic blockade and calcium channel block-

ade in myocardial infarction. *Med Clin North Am* 1989;73(2):409–436.

7. Miller KP, Frishman WH: Platelets and antiplatelet therapy in ischemic heart disease. *Med Clin North Am* 1988;72(1):117–184.
8. Frishman WH, Sonnenblick EH: β-Adrenergic blocking drugs, in Schlant RC, Alexander RW (eds): *The Heart,* 8th ed. New York, McGraw-Hill, 1994, pp 1271–1290.
9. Yusuf S, Peto R, Lewis J, Collins R, Sleight P: β-Blockade during and after myocardial infarction: An overview of the randomized trials. *Prog Cardiovasc Dis* 1985;27:335–371.
10. Opie LH, Sonnenblick EH, Frishman WH, Thadani U: β-Blocking drugs, in Opie LH (ed): *Drugs for the Heart,* 4th ed. Philadelphia, Saunders, 1995, pp 1–30.
10a. Hoes AW, Grobbee DE, Lubsen J, et al: Diuretics, β-blockers, and the risk for sudden cardiac death in hypertensive patients. *Ann Intern Med* 1995;123: 481–487.
11. Frishman WH: β-Adrenoceptor antagonists. New drugs and new indications. *N Engl J Med* 1981;305: 500 506.
12. Ahlmark G, Saetre H: Long-term treatment with β-blockers after myocardial infarction. *Eur J Clin Pharmacol* 1976;10:77–83.
13. Ahlmark G, Saetre H, Korsgren M. Reduction of sudden deaths after myocardial infarction. *Lancet* 1974;2:1563.
14. Andersen MP, Bechsgaard P, Frederiksen J, et al: Effect of alprenolol on mortality among patients with definite or suspected acute myocardial infarction: Preliminary results. *Lancet* 1979;2: 865–868.
15. Australian and Swedish Pindolol Study Group: The effect of pindolol on the 2 year mortality after complicated myocardial infarction. *Eur Heart J* 1983;4:367–375.
16. Baber NS, Wainwright-Evans D, Howitt G, et al: Multicentre postinfarction trial of propranolol in 40 hospitals in the United Kingdom, Italy, and Yugoslavia. *Br Heart J* 1980;44:96–100.
17. Barber JM, Boyle DMcC, Chaturvedi NC, Singh N, Walsh MJ: Practolol in acute myocardial infarction. *Acta Med Scand* 1975;587(Suppl):213–219.
18. β-Blocker Heart Attack Trial Research Group: A randomized trial of propranolol in patients with acute myocardial infarction. I. Mortality results. *JAMA* 1981;247:1707–1714.
19. European Infarction Study Group: A secondary prevention study with slow-release oxprenolol after myocardial infarction: Morbidity and mortality. *Eur Heart J* 1984;5:189–202.
20. Frishman WH, Laifer LI, Furberg CD: β-Adrenergic blockers in the prevention of sudden death, in Josephson ME (ed): *Sudden Cardiac Death.* Philadelphia, FA Davis, 1985, pp. 249–264.
21. Furberg CD, Bell RL: Effect of β-blocker therapy on recurrent nonfatal myocardial infarction. *Circulation* 1983;67(6 Pt 2):I-83–I-85.
22. Furberg CD, Byington RP, Prineas RJ: Potassium, β-receptor blockade, and mortality, the BHAT experience (abstract). *Circulation* 1984;70(Suppl II): II-7.
23. Hansteen V, Moinichen E, Lorentsen E, et al: One year's treatment with propranolol after myocardial infarction: Preliminary report of Norwegian multicentre trial. *Br Med J* 1982;284:155–160.
24. Improvement in prognosis of myocardial infarction by long-term β-adrenoceptor blockade using protocol. A multicenter international study. *Br Med J* 1975;3:735–740.
25. Julian DG, Prescott RJ, Jackson FS, Szekely P: A controlled trial of sotalol for 1 year after myocardial infarction. *Lancet* 1982;1:1142–1147.
26. Lopressor Intervention Trial Research Group: The Lopressor Intervention Trials: Multicentre study of metoprolol in survivors of acute myocardial infarction. *Eur Heart J* 1987;8:1056–1064.
27. Norwegian Multicenter Study Group: Timolol-induced reduction in mortality and reinfarction in patients surviving acute myocardial infarction. *N Engl J Med* 1981;304:801–807.
28. Green KG, Chamberlain DA, Fulton RM, et al: Reduction in mortality after myocardial infarction with long-term β-adrenoceptor blockade; multicenter international study. Supplementary Report. *Br Med J* 1977;2:419–421.
29. Taylor SH, Silke B, Ebbutt A, Sutton GC, Prout BJ, Burley DM: A long-term prevention study with oxprenolol in coronary heart disease. *N Engl J Med* 1982;307:1293–1301.
30. Vedin A, Wilhelmsson C, Werko L: Chronic alprenolol treatment of patients with acute myocardial infarction after discharge from hospital: Effects on mortality and morbidity. *Acta Med Scand* 1975; 575(Suppl):1–40.
31. Wilhelmsson C, Vedin JA, Wilhelmsen L, et al: Reduction of sudden deaths after myocardial infarction

by treatment with alprenolol: Preliminary results. *Lancet* 1974;2:1157–1160.

32. Boissel J-P, Leizorovicz A, Picolet H, et al: Secondary prevention after high-risk acute myocardial infarction with low-dose acebutolol. *Am J Cardiol* 1990;66:251–260.
33. Cruickshank JM, Prichard BNC: β-Blockers in Clinical Practice. *Edinburg, Churchill Livingstone, 1994, pp. 569–630.*
34. Hjalmarson A, Elmfeldt D, Herlitz J, et al: Effect on mortality of metoprolol in acute myocardial infarction: A double-blind randomized trial. *Lancet* 1981; 2:823–827.
35. ISIS-1 (First International Study of Infarct Survival) Collaborative Group: Randomized trial of intravenous atenolol among 16,027 cases of suspected acute myocardial infarction. ISIS-1. *Lancet* 1986;2:57–66.
36. MIAMI Trial Research Group: Metoprolol in acute myocardial infarction (MIAMI). A randomized placebo-controlled international trial. *Eur Heart J* 1985;6:199–226.
37. Lichstein E, Morganroth J, Harrist R, Hubble E: Effect of propranolol on ventricular arrhythmias. The β-Blocker Heart Attack Trial. *Circulation* 1983; 67(Suppl I):I-5–I-10.
38. von der Lippe G, Lund-Johansen P: Effect of timolol on late ventricular arrhythmias after myocardial infarction. *Acta Med Scand* 1981;651(Suppl): 253–258.
38a. Kendall MJ, Lynch KP, Hjalmarson A, et al: β-blockers and sudden cardiac death. *Ann Intern Med* 1995;123:358–367.
39. Nordrehaug JE, Johannessen KA, von der Lippe G, Sederholm M, Grottum P, Kjekshus J: Effect of timolol on changes in serum potassium concentration during acute myocardial infarction. *Br Heart J* 1985;53:388–393.
40. Brown MJ, Brown DC, Murphy MB: Hypokalemia from β_2-receptor stimulation by circulating epinephrine. *N Engl J Med* 1983;309: 1414–1419.
41. Frishman WH: Multifactorial actions of β-adrenergic blocking drugs in ischemic heart disease. Current concepts. *Circulation* 1983;67(6 Pt 2):I-11–I-18.
42. Richardson PD, Davies MJ, Born GVR: Influence of plaque configuration and stress distribution on fissuring of coronary atherosclerotic plaques. *Lancet* 1989;2:941–944.
43. Davies MJ, Thomas AC: Thrombosis and acute coronary artery lesions in sudden cardiac ischemic death. *N Engl J Med* 1984;310:1137–1140.
44. Benson RL: The present status of coronary arterial disease. *Arch Pathol* 1926;2:870–916.
45. Contantinides P: Plaque fissuring in human coronary thrombosis. *J Atheroscl Res* 1966;6:1–17.
46. Chandler AB: Mechanisms and frequency of thrombosis in the coronary circulation. *Thromb Res* 1974;4:3–22.
47. Fulton WFM: *The Coronary Arteries: Arteriography, Microanatomy and Pathogenesis of Obliterative Coronary Disease.* Illinois, Charles C. Thomas, 1965, pp 230–296.
48. Davies MJ, Thomas AC: The pathological basis and microanatomy of occlusive thrombus formation in human coronary arteries. *Phil Trans R Soc Lon D* 1981;294:225–229.
49. Davies MJ, Thomas AC: Plaque fissuring—the cause of acute myocardial infarction, sudden ischaemic death and crescendo angina. *Br Heart J* 1985;53:363–373.
50. Levin DC, Fallon JT: Significance of the angiographic morphology of localised coronary stenosis: Histopathologic correlations. *Circulation* 1982;66: 316–320.
51. Ambrose JA, Winters SL, Aora RR: Angiographic evolution of coronary artery morphology in unstable angina. *J Am Coll Cardiol* 1986;7:472–478.
52. Ambrose JA, Winters SL, Stern A, et al: Angiographic morphology and the pathogenesis of unstable angina pectoris. *J Am Coll Cardiol* 1985;5: 609–616.
53. Ambrose JA, Winters SL, Aora RR: Coronary angiograph morphology in acute myocardial infarction: Link between the pathogenesis of unstable angina and myocardial infarction. *J Am Coll Cardiol* 1985;6:1233–1238.
54. Ambrose JA, Tannenbaum MA, Alexopoulos DA, et al: Angiographic progression of coronary artery disease and the development of myocardial infarction. *J Am Coll Cardiol* 1988;12:56–62.
55. Lo Y-SA, Cutler JE, Blake K, Wright AM, Kron J, Swerdlow CD: Angiographic coronary morphology in survivors of cardiac arrest. *Am Heart J* 1988; 115:781–785.
56. Sherman CT, Litvack F, Grundfest W, et al: Coronary angioscopy in patients with unstable angina pectoris. *N Engl J Med* 1986;315:913–919.

57. Forrester JS, Litvack F, Grundfest W, Hickey A: A perspective of coronary disease seen through the arteries of a living man. *Circulation* 1987;75:505–513.
58. Muller JE, Tofler GH, Stone PH: Circadian variation and triggers of onset of acute cardiovascular disease. *Circulation* 1989;79:733–743.
59. Frishman WH, Lazar EJ: Reduction of mortality, sudden death and non-fatal reinfarction with beta-adrenergic blockers in survivors of acute myocardial infarction: A new hypothesis regarding the cardioprotective action of beta-adrenergic blockade. *Am J Cardiol* 1990;66:66G 70G.
60. Spence JD: Effects of hydralazine versus propranolol on blood velocity in patients with carotid stenosis. *Clin Sci* 1983;65:91–93.
61. Weksler BB, Gillich M, Pink J: Effect of propranolol on platelet function. *Blood* 1977;49:185–196.
62. Hjalmarson A, Herlitz J: Limitation of infarct size by β-blockers and its potential role of prognosis. *Circulation* 1983;67(Suppl I):I-68–I-71.
63. International Collaborative Study Group: Reduction in infarct size with the early use of timolol in acute myocardial infarction. *N Engl J Med* 1984; 310:9–15.
64. Frishman WH: Saving lives post myocardial infarction: The role of beta-adrenergic blockers. *Mt Sinai Med J* 1990;57:75–84.
65. McIlmoyle EA, Evans A, McCBoyle D, et al: Early, intervention in myocardial ischemia (abstract). Proceedings of the British Cardiac Society. *Br Heart J* 1982;47:189.
66. The MIAMI Trial Research Group: Metoprolol in acute myocardial infarction. *Am J Cardiol* 1985;56: 27G–29G.
67. Muller J, Roberts R, Stone P: Failure of propranolol administration to limit infarct size in patients with acute myocardial infarction (abstract). *Circulation* 1983;68(Suppl III):III-394.
68. Peter T, Norris RM, Clarke ED, et al: Reduction of enzyme levels by propranolol after acute myocardial infarction. *Circulation* 1978;57:1091–1095.
69. Rogue F, Amuchastegui LM, Lopez-Morillos MA, et al: Beneficial effects of timolol on infarct size and late ventricular tachycardia in patients with acute myocardial infarction. *Circulation* 1987;76:610–617.
70. Yusuf S, Sleight P, Rossi P, et al: Reduction in infarct size, arrhythmias and chest pain by early intravenous β-blockade in suspected myocardial infarction. *Circulation* 1983;67(Suppl I):I-32–I-41.
71. Jardine RM, Obel IW, Smith AM: Intravenous acebutolol raises serum potassium in acute myocardial infarction. *Eur Heart J* 1986;7:140–145.
72. Hansen F, and the DAVIT II (Danish Verapamil Infarction Trial) Investigators: Presented at the 39th Annual Scientific Sessions of the American College of Cardiology, March 1990.
73. Herlitz J, Hjalmarson A, Swedberg K, et al: Effects on mortality during 5 years after early intervention with metoprolol in suspected acute myocardial infarction. *Acta Med Scand* 1988;223:227–231.
74. Ayanian JZ, Hauptman PJ, Guadagnoli E, et al: Knowledge and practices of generalist and specialist physicians regarding drug therapy for acute myocardial infarction. *N Engl J Med* 1994;331: 1136–1142.
75. Lamas GA, Pfeffer MA, Hamm P, et al: Do the results of randomized clinical trials of cardiovascular drugs influence medical practice? *N Engl J Med* 1992;327:241–247.
76. Gurwitz JH, Goldberg RJ, Chen Z, Gore JM, Alpert JS: Beta-blocker therapy in acute myocardial infarction: Evidence for underutilization in the elderly. *Am J Med* 1992;93:605–610.
77. Greco PJ, Eisenberg JM: Changing physicians' practices. *N Engl J Med* 1993;329:1271–1273.
78. Manolio TA, Cutler JA, Furberg CD, Psaty BM, Whelton PK, Applegate W: Trends in pharmacologic management of hypertension in the United States. *Arch Intern Med* 1995;155:829–837.
78a. Kennedy HL, Rosenson RS: Physician use of beta-adrenergic blocking therapy: A changing perspective. *J Am Coll Cardiol* 1995;26:547–552.
78b. Sial SH, Malone M, Freeman JL, et al: Beta blocker use in the treatment of community hospital patients discharged after myocardial infarction. *J Gen Intern Med* 1994;9:599–604.
79. Goldman L, Sia STB, Cook EF, et al: Costs and effectiveness of routine therapy with long-term β-adrenergic antagonists after myocardial infarction. *N Engl J Med* 1988;319:152–157.
80. Pedersen TR: Six year follow up of the Norwegian Multicenter Study on timolol after acute myocardial infarction. *N Engl J Med* 1985;313:1055–1058.
81. Frishman WH: β-Adrenergic blocker withdrawal. *Am J Cardiol* 1987;59:26F–32F.
82. Lardinois CK, Neuman SL: The effects of antihypertensive agents on serum lipids and lipoproteins. *Arch Intern Med* 1988;148:1280–1288.

83. Friedman LM: How do the various β-blockers compare in type, frequency and severity of their adverse effects? *Circulation* 1983;67(Suppl I):I-89–I-90.

84. Hjalmarson AC: Use of β-blockers in postinfarct prophylaxis. Aspects on quality of life. *Am Heart J* 1987;114(Pt 2):245–250.

84a. Szabo' BM, Crijns HJGM, Wiesfeld ACP, et al: Predictors of mortality in patients with sustained ventricular tachycardias or ventricular fibrillation and depressed left ventricular function: importance of β-blockade. *Am Heart J* 1995;130: 281–286.

85. Maza SR, Frishman WH: Therapeutic options to minimize free radical damage and thrombogenicity in ischemic/reperfused myocardium. *Med Clin North Am* 1988;72:227–242.

86. TIMI Study Group: Comparison of invasive and conservative strategies after treatment with intravenous tissue plasminogen activator in acute myocardial infarction: Results of the Thrombolysis in Myocardial Infarction (TIMI) trial phase II. *N Engl J Med* 1989;320:618–627.

87. Opie LH, Frishman WH, Thadani U: Calcium channel antagonists, in Opie LH, Chatterjee K, Frishman WH, et al (eds): *Drugs for the Heart,* 4th ed. Philadelphia, WB Saunders, 1995, pp 50–82.

88. Frishman WH, Sonnenblck LH: Calcium channel blockers, in Schlant RC, Alexander RW (eds): *The Heart,* 8th ed. New York, McGraw-Hill, 1994, pp 1291–1308.

89. Reimer KA, Jennings RB: Effects of calcium-channel blockers on myocardial preservation during experimental myocardial infarction. *Am J Cardiol* 1985;55:107B–115B.

90. Johnson GJ, Leis LA, Francis GS: Disparate effects of the calcium channel blockers nifedipine and verapamil on α_2-adrenergic receptors and thromboxane α_2-induced aggregation of human platelets. *Circulation* 1986;73:847–854.

91. Bush LR, Romson JL, Ash JL, et al: Effect of diltiazem on extent of ultimate myocardial injury resulting from temporary coronary occlusion in dogs. *J Cardiovasc Pharmacol* 1982;4:285–296.

92. Downey JM, Hearse DJ, Yoshida S, et al: Verapamil and nifedipine limit infarct size in the dog. *Adv Myocardiol* 1985;6:529–543.

93. Wende W, Bleifeld W, Meyer J, et al: Reduction of the size of acute, experimental myocardial infarction by verapamil. *Basic Res Cardiol* 1975;70:198–208.

94. Gross GJ, Warltier DC, Hardman HF: Comparative effects of nicorandil, a nicotinamide derivative, and nifedipine on myocardial reperfusion injury in dogs. *J Cardiovasc Pharmacol* 1987;10:535–542.

95. Temsey-Armos PN, Legenza M, Southworth SR, et al: Effects of verapamil and lidocaine in a canine model of sudden coronary death. *J Am Coll Cardiol* 1985;6:874.

96. Alps BJ, Calder C, Wilson A: The beneficial effect of nicardipine compared with nifedipine and verapamil in limiting myocardial infarct size in baboons. *Arzneim-Forsch/Drug Res* 1983;33:868–876.

97. Karlsberg RP, Henry PD, Ahmed SA, et al: Lack of protection of ischemic myocardium by verapamil in conscious dogs. *Eur J Pharmacol* 1977;42: 339–346.

98. Weintraub WS, Hattori S, Agarwal JB, et al: Effect of nifedipine on myocardial blood flow by layer in normal, ischemic, and lateral border zones (abstract). *Circulation* 1981;64(Suppl IV):IV-281.

99. Knabb RM, Rosamond TL, Fox KAA, et al: Enhancement of salvage of reperfused ischemic myocardium by diltiazem. *J Am Coll Cardiol* 1986; 8:861–871.

100. Danish Multicenter Study Group on Verapamil in Myocardial Infarction: Verapamil in acute myocardial infarction. *Am J Cardiol* 1984;54:24E–28E.

101. The Danish Study Group on Verapamil in Myocardial Infarction: The Danish studies on verapamil in acute myocardial infarction. *Br J Clin Pharmacol* 1986;21:197S–204S.

102. Hansen JF: Letter to the editor. *Eur Heart J* 1986; 6:910–911.

103. The Danish Study Group on Verapamil in Myocardial Infarction: Verapamil in acute myocardial infarction. *Eur Heart J* 1984;5:516–528.

104. The Danish Study Group on Verapamil in Myocardial Infarction: Effect of verapamil on enzyme release after early intravenous administration in acute myocardial infarction: Double-blind randomised trial (abstract). *Br Med J* 1983;286:1107–1108.

105. The Danish Study Group on Verapamil in Myocardial Infarction: Abrupt withdrawal of verapamil in ischaemic heart disease. *Eur Heart J* 1984; 5:529–532.

106. Kristensen SD, Schmidt EB, Dyerberg J: Verapamil does not alter platelet function in patients with recent myocardial infarction. *Thromb Res* 1983;32:437–442.

106a. Rengo F, Carbonin P, Pahor M, et al: A controlled trial of verapamil in patients after acute myocardial infarction: Results of the Calcium Antagonist Reinfarction Italian Study (CRIS). *Am J Cardiol* 1996;77:365–369.

107. Bussman WB, Seher W, Gruengras M: Reduction of creatinine kinase and creatinine kinase-MB indexes of infarct size by intravenous verapamil. *Am J Cardiol* 1984;54:1224–1230.

108. Crea F, Deanfield J, Crean P, Sharom M, Davies G, Maseri A: Effects of verapamil in preventing early postinfarction angina and reinfarction. *Am J Cardiol* 1985;55:900–904.

109. Hagemeijer F: Verapamil in the management of supraventricular tachyarrhythmias occurring after a recent myocardial infarction. *Circulation* 1978;57: 751–755.

109a. Yusuf S: Verapamil following uncomplicated myocardial infarction: promising, but not proven. *Am J Cardiol* 1996;77:421–422.

110. Heikkila J, Nieminen M: Effects of verapamil in patients with acute myocardial infarction: Hemodynamics and function of normal and ischemic left ventricular myocardium. *Am Heart J* 1984; 107:241–247.

111. Muller JE, Morrison J, Stone PH, et al: Nifedipine therapy for patients with threatened and acute myocardial infarction: A randomized double-blind, placebo-controlled comparison. *Circulation* 1984;69:740–747.

112. Sirnes PA, Overskeid K, Pedersen TR, et al: Evolution of infarct size during the early use of nifedipine in patients with acute myocardial infarction: The Norwegian Nifedipine Multicenter Trial. *Circulation* 1984;70:638–644.

113. Wilcox RG, Hampton JR, Banks DC, et al: Trial of early nifedipine in acute myocardial infarction: The TRENT study. *Br Med J* 1986;295:1204–1208.

114. Gottlieb SO, Weiss JL, Flaherty JT, et al: Effect of nifedipine on clinical course and left ventricular function in low risk acute myocardial infarction: A double-blind randomized trial (abstract). *Circulation* 1984;70(Suppl II):II-257.

115. Branagan JP, Walsh K, Kelly P, Collins WC, McCafferty D, Walsh MJ: Effect of early treatment with nifedipine in suspected acute myocardial infarction. *Eur Heart J* 1986;7:859–865.

116. Walker L, MacKenzie G, Adgey J: Effect of nifedipine in the early phase of acute myocardial infarction on enzymatically estimated infarct size and arrhythmias (abstract). *Br Heart J* 1987;57: 83–84.

117. Neufeld HN: Calcium antagonists in secondary prevention after acute myocardial infarction: The Secondary Prevention Reinfarction Nifedipine Trial (SPRINT). *Eur Heart J* 1986;7(Suppl B): 51–52.

118. Moss AJ: Secondary prevention with calcium channel blocking drugs in patients after myocardial infarction: A critical review. *Circulation* 1987; 75(Suppl V):V-148–V-152.

119. Erbel R, Pop T, Meinertz T, et al: Combination of calcium channel blocker and thrombolytic therapy in acute myocardial infarction. *Am Heart J* 1988;115:529–538.

120. Report of the Holland Interuniversity Nifedipine/Metoprolol Trial (HINT) Research Group: Early treatment of unstable angina in the coronary care unit: A randomised, double-blind, placebo-controlled comparison of recurrent ischaemia in patients treated with nifedipine or metoprolol or both. *Br Heart J* 1986;56:400–413.

121. Majid PA, Niznick J, Nishizaki S, Haq A: Hemodynamic effects of nifedipine in acute myocardial infarction with observations on infarct size. *J Cardiovasc Pharmacol* 1986;8:262–267.

122. Gordon GD, Mabin TA, Isaacs S, Lloyd EA, Eichler HG, Opie LH: Hemodynamic effects of sublingual nifedipine in acute myocardial infarction. *Am J Cardiol* 1984;53:1228–1232.

123. Verma SP, Silke B, Taylor SH, et al: Nifedipine following acute myocardial infarction: Dependence of response on baseline haemodynamic status. *J Cardiovasc Pharmacol* 1987;9:478–485.

124. Roberts R, Jaffe AS, Henry PD, Sobel BE: Nifedipine and acute myocardial infarction. *Herz* 1981;6:90–97.

125. Drexler H, Hummler S, Zeiher A, Kasper W, Meinertz T, Just H: Hemodynamic effect of intravenous diltiazem and nifedipine in acute myocardial infarction: A randomised study. *Dtsch Med Wochenschr* 1987;112:1412–1417.

125a. Furberg CD, Psaty BM, Meyer JV: Nifedipine. Dose-related increase in mortality in patients with coronary artery disease. *Circulation* 1995,92. 1326–1331.

126. Gibson RS, Boden WE, Theroux P, et al: Diltiazem and reinfarction in patients with non-Q wave

myocardial infarction: Results of a double-blind, randomized multicenter trial. *N Engl J Med* 1986;315:423–429.

127. Roberts S, Gibson RS, Schectman K: Reply to letters to the editor. *N Engl J Med* 1987;316:220–221.

128. Gibson RS, Young PM, Boden WE, et al: Prognostic significance and beneficial effect of diltiazem on the incidence of early recurrent ischemia after non-Q wave myocardial infarction: Results from the multicenter diltiazem reinfarction study. *Am J Cardiol* 1987;60:203–209.

129. The Multicenter Diltiazem Post-Infarction Trial Research Group: The effect of diltiazem on mortality and reinfarction after myocardial infarction. *N Engl J Med* 1988;319:385–392.

130. Moss AJ, Oakes D, Benhorin J, et al: Effect of diltiazem on outcome in post-infarction patients with and without left ventricular dysfunction (abstract). *Circulation* 1988;78(Suppl II):II-97.

131. Boden WE, Krone RJ, Kleiger RE, et al: Diltiazem reduces long-term cardiac event rate after non-Q wave infarction: Multicenter Diltiazem Post Infarction Trial (MDPIT) (abstract). *Circulation* 1988;78(Suppl II):II-96.

132. Bigger JT, Coromilas J, Kleiger RE, et al: Effect of diltiazem on ventricular arrhythmias after myocardial infarction (abstract). *Circulation* 1988;78 (Suppl II):II-97.

133. Zannad F, Amor M, Karcher G, et al: Effect of diltiazem on myocardial infarct size estimated by enzyme release, serial thallium 201 single-photon emission computed tomography and radionuclide angiography. *Am J Cardiol* 1988;61:1172–1177.

133a. Boden WE, Scheldewaert R, Walters EG, et al: Design of a placebo-controlled clinical trial of long-acting diltiazem and aspirin versus aspirin alone in patients receiving thrombolysis with first acute myocardial infarction. *Am J Cardiol* 1995; 75:1120–1123.

134. Ogawa H, Yasue H, Nakamura M, Obata K, Sonoda R: Hemodynamic effects of intravenous diltiazem in patients with acute myocardial infarction. *Clin Cardiol* 1987;10:323–328.

135. Renard M, Sterling I, Van Camp G, Coupez R, Bernard R: Comparison of the effects of intravenous diltiazem and a placebo on hemodynamics and blood gases in the acute phase of myocardial infarction. *Ann Cardiol Angiol* 1987;36: 509–512.

136. Gibelin P, Benoit P, Camous JP, Baudouy M, Morand P: Clinical and hemodynamic tolerance of intravenous diltiazem in the acute phase of myocardial infarction. *Ann Cardiol Angiol* 1985;34: 263–367.

137. Cobelli F, Opasich C, Riccardi G, Rossetti S, Guffanti E, Specchia G: Haemodynamic effects of diltiazem at rest and during exercise in patients with previous myocardial infarction. *Eur Heart J* 1987;8:710–716.

138. DeGeest, Kesteloot H, Piessens J: Secondary prevention of ischemic heart disease: A long term controlled lidoflazine study. *Acta Cardiol* 1979;24 (Suppl): 7–46.

139. Yusuf S, Furberg CD: Effects of calcium channel blockers on survival after myocardial infarction. *Cardiovasc Drug Ther* 1987;1:343–344.

140. Held PH, Yusuf S, Furberg CD: Calcium channel blockers in acute myocardial infarction and unstable angina. An overview. *Br Med J* 1989;299: 1187–1192.

141. De Wood MA, Stifter WF, Simpson CS, et al: Coronary arteriographic findings soon after non-Q-wave myorcardial infarction. *N Engl J Med* 1986;315:417–423.

142. Willard JE, Lange RA, Hillis LD: The use of aspirin in ischemic heart disease. *N Engl J Med* 1993; 327:175–181.

143. Del Zoppa GJ, Harker LA: Blood/vessel interaction in coronary disease. *Hosp Pract* 1984;19(5): 163–182.

144. Eichner ER: Platelets, carotids, and coronaries, critique on antithrombotic role of antiplatelet agents, exercise and certain diets. *Am J Med* 1984; 77:513–523.

145. Frishman WH: Antiplatelet therapy in coronary heart disease. *Hosp Pract* 1982;17(5):73–86.

146. Mehta J: Current understanding of the role of platelet function in coronary artery disease. *Pract Cardiol* 1985;11:166.

146a. Hirsh J, Dalen JE, Fuster V, Harker LB, Patrono C, Roth G: Aspirin and other platelet-active drugs. *Chest* 1995;108(Suppl):247s–257s.

147. Breddin K, Loew D, Lechner K, Uberla K, Walter E: Secondary prevention of myocardial infarction. Comparison of acetylsalicylic acid, phenprocoumon, and placebo. A multicenter two-year prospective study. *Thromb Haemost* 1979; 41:225–236.

148. Vane JR: Inhibition of prostaglandin synthesis as a mechanism of action for aspirin-like drugs. *Nature* 1971;231:232–235.

149. Roth GJ, Calverley DC: Aspirin platelets and thrombosis; theory and practice *Blood* 1994;83: 885–898.

150. Bishopric N, Mehta J, Mehta P: Platelet activation and platelet suppressive drugs, in Mehta J, Mehta P (eds): *Platelets and Prostaglandins in Cardiovascular Disease*. New York, Futura Publishing, 1981, p 71.

151. Zucker MB, Rothwell KG: Differential influences of salicylate compounds on platelet aggregation and serotonin release. *Curr Ther Res* 1978;23:194–199.

152. Preston FE, Whipps S, Jackson CA, French AJ, Wyld PJ, Stoddard CJ: Inhibition of prostacyclin and platelet thromboxane A_2 after low dose aspirin. *N Engl J Med* 1981;304:76–79.

153. Weksler BB, Tack Goldman K, Subramanian VA, Gay WA Jr: Cumulative inhibitor effect of low dose aspirin on vascular prostacyclin and platelet thromboxane production in patients with atherosclerosis. *Circulation* 1985;71:332–340.

154. Jaffe E, Weksler BB. Recovery of endothelial cell prostacyclin production after inhibition by low doses of aspirin. *J Clin Invest* 1979;63:532–535.

155. Clarke RJ, Mayo G, Price P, Fitzgerald GA: Suppression of thromboxane A2 but not of systemic prostacyclin by controlled-release aspirin. *N Engl J Med* 1991;325:1137–1141.

156. DeGaetano G, Cerletti C, Dejana E, Latini R: Pharmacology of platelet inhibition in humans. Implications of the salicylate–aspirin interaction. *Circulation* 1985;72:1185–1193.

157. Ware JA, Heistad DD: Platelet–endothelium interactions. *N Engl J Med* 1993;328:628–635.

158. Weber G, Erl W, Pletsch A, Weber PC: Aspirin inhibits nuclear factor KB mobilization and monocyte adhesion in stimulated human endothelial cells. *Circulation* 1995;91:1914–1917.

159. Lopez-Farre A, Caramelo C, Esteban A, et al: Effects of aspirin on platelet–neutrophil interactions: Role of nitric oxide and endothelin-1. *Circulation* 1995;91:2080–2088.

160. Moschos CB, Haider B, DelaCruz C, Lyons MM, Regan TJ: Antiarrhythmic effects of aspirin during nonthrombotic coronary occlusion. *Circulation* 1978;57:681–684.

161. Capurro NL, Marr KC, Aamodt R, Goldstein RE, Epstein SE: Aspirin-induced increase in collateral flow after acute coronary occlusion in dogs. *Circulation* 1979;59:744–747.

162. Elwood PC, Cochrane AL, Burr ML, et al: A randomized controlled trial of acetyl salicylic acid in the secondary prevention of mortality from myocardial infarction. *Br Med J* 1974;1:436–440.

163. The Coronary Drug Project Research Group: Aspirin in coronary heart disease. *J Chron Dis* 1976; 29:625–642.

164. Elwood PC, Sweetnam PM: Aspirin and secondary mortality after myocardial infarction. *Lancet* 1979;2:1313–1315.

165. The Aspirin Myocardial Infarction Study Research Group: A randomized controlled trial of aspirin in persons recovered from myocardial infarction. *JAMA* 1980;243:661–669.

166. The Persantine–Aspirin Reinfarction Study Research Group: Persantine and aspirin in coronary heart disease. *Circulation* 1980;62(Suppl IV/V): V-85–V-88.

167. Klimt CR, Knatterud GL, Stamler J, Meier P: Persantine–Aspirin Reinfarction Study. Part II. Secondary coronary prevention with persantine and aspirin. *J Am Coll Cardiol* 1986,7.251–269.

168. Mustard JF, Kinlough-Rathbone RL, Packham MA: Aspirin in the treatment of cardiovascular disease. A review. *Am J Med* 1983;74(6A):43–49.

169. Peto R: Aspirin after myocardial infarction (editorial). *Lancet* 1980;1:1172–1173.

170. Antiplatelet Trialists' Collaboration: Collaborative overview of randomised trials of antiplatelet therapy. I: Prevention of death, myocardial infarction and stroke by prolonged antiplatelet therapy in various categories of patients. *Br Med J* 1994; 308:81–106.

171. Popma JJ, Topol EJ: Adjuncts to thrombolysis for myocardial perfusion. *Ann Intern Med* 1991;115: 34–44.

172. ISIS-2 (Second International Study of Infarct Survival) Collaborative Group: Randomised trial of intravenous streptokinase, oral aspirin, both, or neither among 17,187 cases of suspected acute myocardial infarction: ISIS-2. *Lancet* 1988;332: 349–360.

173. ISIS-3 (Third International Study of Infarct Survival) Collaborative Group: ISIS-3: A randomized comparison of streptokinase vs tissue plasminogen activator vs anistreplase and of aspirin plus heparin vs aspirin alone among 41,299 cases

of suspected acute myocardial infarction. *Lancet* 1992;339:753–770.

174. Fitzgerald DJ, Roy L, Catella F, Fitzgerald GA: Platelet activation in unstable coronary disease. *N Engl J Med* 1986;315:983–989.

175. Lewis HD, Davis JW, Archibald DG, et al: Protective effects of aspirin against acute myocardial infarction and death in men with unstable angina. *N Engl J Med* 1983;309:396–403.

176. Theroux P, Ouimet H, McCans J, et al: Aspirin, heparin or both to treat unstable angina. *N Engl J Med* 1988;319:1105–1111.

177. RISC Group: Risk of myocardial infarction and death during treatment with low dose aspirin and intravenous heparin in men with unstable coronary artery disease. *Lancet* 1990;336:827–830.

178. Juul-Moller S, Edvardsson N, Jahnmatz B, et al: Double-blind trial of aspirin in primary prevention of myocardial infarction in patients with stable chronic angina pectoris. *Lancet* 1992;340:1421–1425.

179. Roth GJ, Calverley DC: Aspirin, platelets and thrombosis: Theory and practice. *Blood* 1994;83: 885–898.

179a. Shahar E, Folsom AR, Romm FJ, et al: Patterns of aspirin use in middle-aged adults: The Atherosclerosis Risk in Communities (ARIC) Study. *Am Heart J* 1996;131:915–922.

180. Yusuf S: Interventions that potentially limit myocardial infarct size: Overview of clinical trials. *Am J Cardiol* 1987;60:11A–17A.

181. Frishman WH (ed): *Current Cardiovascular Drugs,* 2nd ed. Philadelphia, Current Medicine, 1995.

33

Exercise Training in Cardiac Rehabilitation After Myocardial Infarction

Gerald F. Fletcher, MD

INTRODUCTION

Early in the 1900s, subjects remained at bed rest for a minimum of 6 to 8 weeks after myocardial infarction (MI); and because of the perceived risk of ventricular aneurysm formation or ventricular rupture, even minimal physical activity, such as bathing, dressing, and self-feeding, was restricted. In 1951, Levine and Lown (1) introduced the "chair treatment of acute coronary thrombosis." Activity remained restricted, but subjects were allowed to sit in a chair for 1 to 2 hours daily, beginning the first day after an acute MI. In the decade that followed, several studies further supported the concept of early activity after MI (2). These results led to several worldwide investigations of the benefits of exercise, including the National Exercise and Heart Disease Project (NEHDP) in the United States (3,4). In the 1980s, the concept of more rapid mobilization of the post-MI subject, early exercise testing, and risk stratification began to emerge with long-term exercise-based rehabilitation (5) (see Ch. 34). Position papers on outpatient cardiac rehabilitation were published by several clinical and scientific organizations (6–8). These reports cited many benefits of cardiac rehabilitation with exercise—an increase in functional capacity, favorable changes in ventricular function and perfusion, effective coronary risk factor modification, decreased morbidity and mortality, and improvement in psychosocial function (8a). In recent years, a series of controlled trials of survivors of MI have collectively shown lower mortality in subjects randomized to supervised endurance training. Training programs typically consisted of 2 to 4 exercise sessions per week, lasting 20 to 60 minutes each at 70% to 85% of maximal heart rate. Individual trials, however, have been too small and too short in duration to render unequivocal results; and because of the complexity and cost of such trials, it is unlikely that a single, well-designed mortality trial with a large enough sample size and of sufficient duration will be performed.

The only controlled trial in the United States, the NEHDP, was initiated as a 3-year collaborative pilot trial involving 651 men between 30 and 64 years of age who had survived an acute MI (3,4). Subjects were randomized 2 to 36 months after MI and observed for 3 years. During the first 8 weeks, the participants attended three 1-hour exercise sessions per week and trained at 85% of peak heart rate with continuous electrocardiographic (ECG) monitoring. Subsequent exercise sessions were supervised but unmonitored and consisted of 15 minutes of jogging, cycling, or swimming at target heart rate, followed by 25 minutes of recreational sports 3 times per week. Study results revealed that total mortality rate was reduced by 37% (4.6% versus 7.3% in the intervention and control [usual and customary care] groups, respectively), and deaths from cardiovascular causes were 29% lower in the exercise group (7% versus 5.3%). However, these results were not statistically significant, primarily because of the small sample size. (If these trends had continued, a sample size of 1,500 subjects would have produced statistically significant results.) When deaths due to MI alone were analyzed, only 1 (0.3%) occurred in the exercise group in comparison with 8 in the control group (2.4%), for a significant difference ($p < 0.05$). Nonfatal MIs were nonsignificantly increased in the intervention group (4.6% versus 3.4%).

In a significant Finnish study, Kallio and coworkers (9,10) randomized 301 men and 74 women into a multifactorial rehabilitation program that included exercise training. In the intervention group, the 3-year cumulative mortality rate was 18.6% in comparison with 29.4% in the control group ($p = 0.02$). This difference was largely attributed to a reduction in sudden deaths—5.8% versus 14.4% in the intervention and control groups, respectively ($p < 0.01$). The rates of nonfatal reinfarction in the two groups were similar. After 10 years of follow-up, the incidence of sudden death in the intervention group remained significantly lower than that in the control group (12.8% versus 23%, $p = 0.01$), whereas reinfarction rates remained similar in the two groups. Coronary heart disease (CHD) mortality was significantly lower ($p = 0.02$) in the intervention (35.1%) compared with the control group (47.1%).

Several studies *with exercise as the only intervention* have shown favorable trends in mortality and, less consistently, in morbidity. Carson et al (11) randomized 303 subjects to a 12-week exercise regimen and observed the subjects for a mean of 2.1 years. Total mortality rate was 14% in the control and 8% in the intervention group, whereas the incidence of nonfatal MI was insignificantly higher in the intervention group (7.3% versus 6.6%). Wilhelmsen et al (12) reported a mortality of 22.3% in a control group ($n = 157$) and a 17.7% mortality among subjects randomized to intervention ($n = 158$) 3 months after MI with a follow-up of 4 years. Reinfarction rates were also slightly reduced in the intervention group (15.8% versus 17.8%). Roman et al (13) randomized 193 subjects to 3 times weekly exercise training beginning 2 months after MI. During a mean follow-up period of 55 months, the annual mortality rate was 3.6% in the intervention group and 5.8% in the control group. Annual reinfarction rates were 3.6% and 4.9%, respectively. Vermeulen et al (14) randomized 98 middle-aged men to a 6- to 8-week exercise program beginning 4 to 6 weeks after MI. Both total mortality and reinfarction rates were lower in the intervention group (4.3% versus 9.8% and 4.3% versus 7.8%, respectively) after 5 years of follow-up. In contrast to these studies, Rechnitzer et al (15), reporting for the Ontario Exercise Heart Collaborative Study ($n = 733$), and Marra et al (16) ($n = 167$) revealed insignificant mortality trends slightly favoring the control group (4% versus 3.7% in the former study and 7.4% versus 6.3% in the latter). Compared with the controls, however, reinfarction rates were somewhat lower in the intervention group in Marra's study (6.1% versus 11.2%) but not in Rechnitzer's analysis (10.3% versus 9.3% in the intervention and control groups, respectively).

In a meta-analysis evaluation, O'Conner et al (17) reported an overview of 22 randomized trials of *exercise rehabilitation* after MI involving 4,554 subjects and evaluated effects on total and cardiovascular mortality, sudden death, and both fatal and nonfatal MI. Total and cardiovascular mortality rates after 3 years in the exercise rehabilitation group were 20% and 22% lower, respectively, than in the control group. Fatal reinfarction was also significantly reduced, by 25%. In the intervention group, sudden death was significantly reduced only at 1 year, but favorable trends were apparent at 2 and 3 years. There were, however, no differences between the two groups in nonfatal reinfarction rates. Most of the trials included in this analysis had comprehensive cardiac rehabilitation with coronary risk factor reduction in addition to exercise training. The odds ratios for cardiovascular-related mortality and sudden death were lower in these multifactorial trials than in the exercise-only studies, but the relatively small number of exercise-only interventions did not allow definitive conclusions about the independent effect of exercise on these endpoints.

The hemodynamic adaptations capable of improving the long-term prognosis in subjects with coronary disease after exercise training are well documented. Exercise training at the usual intensity, frequency, and duration (typically, 3 to 4 sessions weekly lasting 20–30 minutes each at target heart rates of 70% to 85% of capacity) yields an average of 10% to 30% improvement in maximal oxygen uptake and work capacity. The magnitude of improvement is generally inversely proportional to the exercise capacity before training (18). Routine submaximal activities after training are thus performed more easily, with less perceived exertion, fatigue, and dyspnea, and with delayed onset of angina (19). The documented changes involve predominately peripheral adaptations, although prolonged exercise at higher intensities over a period of months may also lead to improvement in myocardial performance and perfusion (20,21). Antiarrhythmic properties of the myocardium also may be evoked by exercise training (22), but this is less well documented.

Therefore, rather extensive data support that exercise-based cardiac rehabilitation programs in middle-aged men consistently decrease all cause and cardiovascular mortality after MI but do not usually protect against reinfarction. Reinfarction in trained individuals, however, is less likely to be fatal. It is possible that the improvement in mortality with cardiac rehabilitation programs is related at least in part to closer subject surveillance rather than by the hemodynamic and metabolic effects of exercise. Regardless of the exact mechanisms involved, based on one report, cardiac rehabilitation programs with exercise have the potential to save approximately 13,000 lives annually (23).

STRATIFICATION OF RISK FOR EXERCISE

Activity Classification

After appropriate medical clearance for the post-MI subject is complete, they can be classified by risk based on certain characteristics and may enter exercise training as early as 2 weeks post-MI. Such entry time is determined clinically based on the individual's activity classification as recommended in standards by the American Heart Association (AHA) as follows (8) (paraphrased directly from the standards):

AHA Class B

Known, stable coronary disease with low risk for vigorous exercise but slightly greater than that for apparently healthy individuals. Moderate activity is not believed to be associated with increased risk in this group.

Clinical characteristics: (i) New York Heart Association (NYHA) class 1 or 2; (2) exercise capacity over 6 METs (one MET or metabolic equivalent equals 3.5 ml/kg/min of oxygen consumed); (iii) no evidence of heart failure; (iv) no ischemia or angina at rest or on the exercise test at or below 6 METs; (v) appropriate increase in systolic blood pressure during exercise; (vi) no *sequential* ectopic ventricular contractions; and (vii) ability to satisfactorily self-monitor intensity of activity.

Activity guidelines: Activity should be individualized with exercise prescription (based on exercise testing) by qualified personnel trained in basic cardiopulmonary resuscitation (CPR) or with electronic ECG monitoring at home.

ECG and blood pressure monitoring: Only during the early phase of training—usually 6–12 sessions.

Supervision required: Medical supervision during prescriptive sessions and nonmedical for other exercise sessions until the individual understands how to self-monitor activity.

AHA Class C

Those at moderate to high risk for cardiac complications during exercise, and/or unable to self-regulate activity or to understand recommended activity level. This group includes post–MI subjects with clinical characteristics outlined as follows:

Clinical characteristics: (i) Two or more MIs; (ii) NYHA class 3 or greater; (iii) exercise capacity less than 6 METs; (iv) ischemic horizontal or downsloping ECG ST depression of 4.0 mm or more, or angina during exercise; (v) significant fall in systolic blood pressure with exercise; (vi) associated medical condition that the physician believes may be "life-threatening"; (vii) previous episode of primary cardiac arrest; and (viii) ventricular tachycardia at a workload of less than 6 METs.

Activity guidelines: Activity should be individualized with exercise prescription by qualified personnel.

ECG and blood pressure monitoring: Continuous during exercise sessions until safety is established, usually 6–12 sessions or more.

Supervision: Medical supervision during all exercise sessions until safety is established.

AHA Class D

Unstable cardiac disease with activity restriction. This group includes individuals with (i) unstable ischemia; (ii) uncompensated heart failure; (iii) uncontrolled arrhythmias; (iv) severe aortic stenosis; and (v) other medical conditions that could be aggravated by exercise.

Activity guidelines: No activity is recommended for exercise training purposes. Attention should be directed to appropriate management of the subject and restoration to class C or higher. Daily activities must be prescribed based on individual assessment by the subject's personal physician.

These classifications are presented as a means of beginning exercise post–MI with the lowest possible risk. Co-morbidities are not considered (e.g., insulin-dependent diabetes mellitus, morbid obesity, severe pulmonary disease, or debilitating neurologic or orthopedic conditions) that may necessitate closer supervision during training sessions. In most instances, as safety of exercise and improvement in working capacity are demonstrated, "graduation" of a subject to class B is appropriate.

Monitoring

Class B, low-risk, individuals, should be monitored and supervised until they understand desirable activity levels (usually 6–12 sessions). Those in class C (moderate–high risk) should be medically supervised with ECG monitoring until they understand the safe level of activity and the medical team determines that the exercise is safe and effective. Usually 6–12 sessions or more are needed.

Monitoring sessions should ideally be performed with continuous ECG by either "hardwired" apparatus or telemetry. Sessions should be conducted by personnel who understand the exercise principles involved and who have a basic knowledge of electrocardiography. The sessions should also be supervised by either a physician or a nurse trained in emergency CPR, preferably with previous experience in intensive cardiac care. Standing orders for management of complications should be immediately available.

Monitored sessions should also include symptom assessment by the staff, blood pressure recording, rating of perceived exertion, and instructions to subjects about selection and proper use of exercise equipment. The ECG-monitored sessions should include instruction in the different modes and progression of exercise.

ROLE OF EXERCISE TESTING IN DIAGNOSIS AND IN PRESCRIBING EXERCISE TRAINING

In designating an exercise prescription for exercise training after MI, the exercise test is of vast importance, both for diagnosis and for designation of the proper levels of intensity and duration for each subject. The test offers a mechanism by which to observe important subjective, physiologic, and hemodynamic responses to activity. Exercise testing should emphasize the electrocardiographic response but also other important components of the exercise response, such as symptoms, changes in the physical examination, heart rate response and variation, blood pressure changes, and the overall exercise capacity. Moreover, the interpretation should consider any alterations to the exercise response induced by ongoing pharmacologic therapy.

Symptoms during testing are a valuable extension of the history and physical examination. Therefore, the subject should be questioned carefully about exercise-induced symptoms and about whether the symptoms reproduce those experienced during usual daily activity.

Exercise-induced typical anginal chest pain can be a valuable indicator of the presence and degree of coronary artery disease. The presence of diagnostic

ECG ST depression in association with exercise-induced chest discomfort is highly predictive of significant coronary artery disease (24).

In the early post–MI period, predischarge exercise testing has been used as a tool for risk stratification. Theroux and coworkers (25) exercised subjects at a mean of 11 days post–MI and found that 65% of those in whom chest discomfort developed during testing reported subsequent angina pectoris during the following year, in comparison with 36% of those who had no chest discomfort at the time of testing. Starling et al (26) reported on a group of 123 subjects, 34 of whom experienced exercise-induced angina post–MI; 5 of these subjects died, and 4 had recurrent infarctions. Furthermore, when angina and ST depression were combined, there was a statistically significant increased incidence of cardiac death.

Dyspnea on exertion is a more difficult symptom to assess due to its resemblance to hyperventilation in response to near-maximal or maximal exertion. Furthermore, true dyspnea may have either a pulmonary or a cardiac component or may be a combination of both. Cardiopulmonary testing can help distinguish the etiology of dyspnea, which may, in some instances, represent true angina.

A limited *physical examination* should be done on all subjects prior to an exercise test. Immediately after testing, certain components of the examination should be repeated and compared with those before testing. The development of an abnormal precordial impulse, or "gallop sounds," could be a consequence of left ventricular dysfunction. A new systolic murmur of papillary muscle dysfunction may represent exercise-induced ischemia. After exercise, auscultation can be done with the subject supine or in a sitting position if orthopnea or severe angina is of concern. The pre- and postexercise physical examinations should be included in the test interpretation.

Heart rate increases linearly with an exercise stress. Subjects with cardiac failure have a similar relationship between heart rate and oxygen consumption (VO_2), but there is a limit to the maximum heart rate they can attain, and they have a decreased exercise capacity. An inappropriate heart rate response (chronotropic incompetence) to exercise may be detected with testing. This may be secondary to the cardiac disease or to beta blocker therapy. In addition, disturbances of heart rhythm may be detected.

Blood pressure is recorded at regular intervals (at least every 3 minutes) during the exercise test. Figure 33–1 reveals both normal and abnormal systolic responses. Of special concern is a poor systolic response (≤30 mm Hg over baseline) or a drop in systolic pressure with exercise. The latter may reflect left ventricular dysfunction, especially in association with significant ST segment depression.

The assessment of *functional* or *exercise capacity* has been often overlooked in the search for cardiac pathology. Moreover, in the 1995 *Exercise Standards,* the American Heart Association includes functional capacity among the various exercise responses that should be included (8). Standard functional classifications of daily activities are subjective and poorly reproducible. As subjects become symptomatic, they often significantly restrict their pace of normal living activities and may still report themselves as functionally unchanged. Maximum oxygen uptake ($VO_{2,max}$), as a measure of the functional limits of the cardiovascular system therefore is the best objective index of functional capacity.

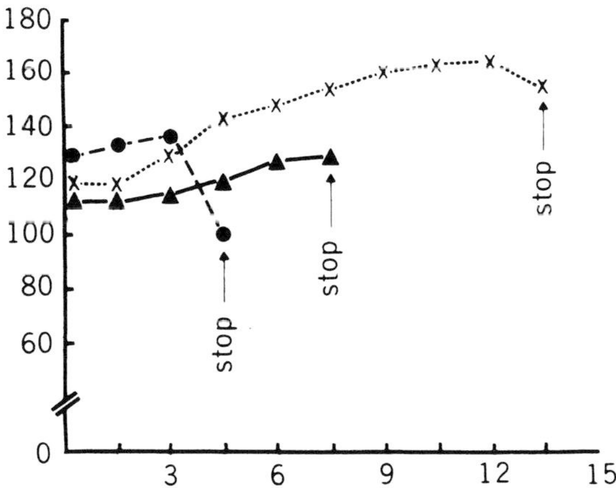

Figure 33–1. Normal and abnormal systolic blood pressure responses to exercise tests. x: Normal—blood pressure drops at peak of normal exercise capacity; •: Abnormal—blood pressure increases initially but drops early in exercise; ▲: Abnormal—blood pressure fails to increase to 130 mm Hg or higher. *Reproduced with permission* of Futura Publishers.

Maximum VO_2 depends on age, sex, physical conditioning, genetics, and the overall status of the cardiovascular system. In normal individuals, the $VO_{2,max}$ is approximately 30 ml O_2/min/kg and declines with age as cardiac output drops, which may be more manifest in presence of a previous MI.

The term *MET* (metabolic equivalent) is used to describe the metabolic unit of sitting at rest, representing an average VO_2 of 3.5 ml O_2/min/kg (27). The MET value is used to estimate the energy cost of various physical activities as well as to approximate the VO_2 during each stage of testing protocols. Such a measure is used both in normal and post–MI subjects.

The somewhat "cumbersome" methods of metabolic gas exchange instrumentation before the 1980s made the direct measurement of oxygen uptake impractical in the clinical testing laboratory. However, as computer technology has advanced and instrumentation has become more user friendly, the measurement of actual maximal oxygen uptake has become practical and convenient in the clinical setting. Such, therefore, should be done if possible to precisely measure functional capacity.

Scales of *perceived exertion* are useful in repeated testing and correlate well with the percent of maximal work or heart rate performed (28). The intensity of muscular exertion performed can also be designated in percentages of maximum VO_2, as shown in Table 33–1 (29). The perceived exertion is quite helpful in writing the exercise prescription.

Table 33–1. Classification of Intensity of Exercise Based on 20 to 60 Minutes of Endurance Training

Relative Intensity (%)		
HR_{max} (%)	$VO_{2,max}$ or HR_{max} Reserve (%)	Intensity
<35	<30	Very light
35–59	30–49	Light
60–79	50–74	Moderate
80–89	75–84	Heavy
≥90	≥85	Very heavy

HR_{max} = maximum heart rate (beats per minute); $VO_{2,max}$ = maximum oxygen uptake.

Revised with permission from Pollock and Wilmore: Exercise in Health and Disease: Evaluation and Prescription for Prevention and Rehabilitation, 2nd ed. Philadelphia PA, WB Saunders, 1990.

SPECIFIC GUIDELINES FOR EXERCISE—THE PRESCRIPTION

Exercise within the first 2 weeks after MI should focus on "offsetting" the effects of bed rest. When the subject is stable as determined by symptoms, vital signs, and ECG, he or she can begin walking. Although this activity is well tolerated and safe, certain precautions are recommended as outlined in Table 33–2. A symptom-limited exercise test should be performed after the individual is stable and is walking without difficulty (as early as 2–6 weeks after the cardiac event). If more studies such as nuclear studies or angiography are not indicated, a physical conditioning program can be initiated at that point.

General Principles of Conditioning Activity

For exercise training purposes, large-muscle group activities should be performed for at least 30 minutes (preceded by warm-up and followed by

Table 33–2. Guidelines for Helping Patients Resume Walking Soon After Myocardial Infarction

Before Exercise

Ask about chest discomfort, dyspnea, and faintness (if present, check with physician before proceeding).

Measure blood pressure and heart rate (if >160/100 or <90/60 mm Hg, or if heart rate is >110 or <60 bpm, check with physician before starting).

Check orthostatic blood pressure before beginning standing range of motion exercise or walking. If blood pressure falls more than 20 mm Hg or if fall is associated with symptoms of faintness, have patient lie down and notify physician.

During Exercise

Ask patient to report symptoms, particularly chest discomfort, dyspnea, or faintness. If symptoms occur, discontinue exercise until checking with physician.

Ask for rating of perceived exertion.

Immediately After Exercise

Ask patient about symptoms.

Measure heart rate, blood pressure, and rating of perceived exertion. If symptoms occur, blood pressure falls more than 20 mm Hg, or heart rate rises more than 20 bpm over resting rate, check with physician before continuing.

bpm = beats per minute

Reproduced from Fletcher et al (8), with permission.

cool-down) at least 3–4 times weekly. The intensity of exercise should be gauged by exercise prescription (described subsequently). Follow-up supervised group sessions are recommended to ensure that the participant is tolerating the program, to check that progress is occurring, and to provide medical supervision in high-risk situations.

General Principles of Exercise Prescription

In absence of ischemia or significant arrhythmias, exercise intensity should approximate 50% to 80% of $VO_{2,max}$, which can be ascertained by an exercise test and using the appropriate heart rate endpoint achieved within this range. (If a test is not done initially, the measurement of 20 beats/min above resting heart rate is adequate until testing is performed.) The steps in this process are as follows:

Table 33–3. Borg Scale for Rating Perceived Exertion

15-grade scale	10-grade scale	
6	0	Nothing
7 Very, very light	0.5	Very, very weak (just noticeable)
8	1	Very weak
9 Very light	2	Weak (light)
10	3	Moderate
11 Fairly light	4	Somewhat strong
12	5	Strong (heavy)
13 Somewhat hard	6	
14	7	Very strong
15 Hard	8	
16	9	
17 Very hard	10	Very, very strong (almost maximum)
18		
19 Very, very hard		* Maximum
20		

The rating of perceived exertion scales. The original scale (6–20) on the left and the newer 10-point scale with ratio properties on the right.

From Borg GA: Med Sci Sports Exerc 1982;14:377–387. Reproduced with permission.

1. The *target heart rate* may be considered as 50% to 75% of heart rate reserve ([maximal testing heart rate − resting heart rate] × 50% to 75% + resting heart rate. This rate endpoint can be used for dynamic leg exercise. Activities can be prescribed as the target work intensity that achieves the training heart rate after 5 to 10 minutes at that workload (steady state). Such may be expressed as watts on an ergometer, speed on a treadmill, or in METs. If an individual wishes to exercise but cannot assess intensity, then heart rate counting (manually or with a cardiotachometer) is useful. Heart rate counters are widely available and are generally quite accurate for low to moderate intensity exercise.
2. Individuals can also judge the intensity of exercise as the rating of *perceived exertion,* which can be equated to a desirable heart rate during exercise testing and to their activities. The original scale is a 15-grade category scale ranging from 6 to 20, with a verbal description at every odd number. (See Table 33–3.)
   The following rating of perceived exertion values should be followed:
   <12 light, 40% to 60% of maximal
   12–13 somewhat hard (moderate), 60% to 75% of maximal
   14–16 hard (heavy), 75% to 90% of maximal
3. Activities can progress as tolerance is demonstrated. The appropriate initial intensity of training is 50% to 60% of $VO_{2,max}$ or a rating of perceived exertion of 12 to 13 on a scale of 6 to 20. After safe activity levels have been established, duration is increased in 5-minute increments per week. Later, intensities can be increased as heart rate response to exercise decreases with conditioning.
   There is limited data to support that high intensity (75% to 90% of maximal) exercise improves left ventricular ejection (29a) over time and is also associated with more regression of atherosclerosis (30). These reports have reflected no increase in adverse events with the higher intensity.

An exercise test is most desirable for all post–MI subjects and, in the presence of ischemia or arrhythmias, is mandatory for this type of prescription. The manifestations of arrhythmias or ischemia that require such precautions can vary but usually include ventricular ectopic beats in sequence, an arrhythmia that is symptomatic or hemodynamically unstable, chest discomfort suggesting angina, ECG ST depression of 2 mm or more, or fall in systolic blood pressure of 20 mm Hg or more from baseline.

The exercise test is performed in the usual manner, but the conditioning *work intensity is derived from the heart rate associated with the abnormality.* If the exercise test continues to a high level of effort, the heart rate at 50% to 60% of heart rate maximum can be used if it falls at least 10 beats/min below the abnormal level. Otherwise, the recommended training heart rate is 10 beats/min less than that associated with the abnormality. More specifics with regard to risk stratification are addressed previously, and supervision will be addressed subsequently.

TYPES OF EXERCISE TRAINING

Exercise training for post–MI subjects should incorporate the components of intensity, frequency, and duration, as well as specific guidelines for the mode and progression of the exercise. Activities that cause the greatest increase in $VO_{2,max}$ qualify the exercise as endurance or cardiovascular. These characteristics include dynamic exercise, alternately contracting and relaxing the muscles (as opposed to isometric or resistive exercise), and large-muscle group activities such as walking or running.

With regard to intensity, frequency, and duration, exercise should be performed at least 3–4 times per week for a minimum of 30–60 minutes per session, at a minimum intensity of 50% to 60% $VO_{2,max}$. With regard to mode, in addition to walking and running, other endurance or cardiovascular activities include cycling and stair-stepping. Activities of higher intensity should be done with care in subjects with previous MI.

Exercising at a low intensity for 5–10 minutes before (warm-up) and after (cool-down) the training session is a routine recommendation. Such activities help stretch and "warm up" muscles and ligaments in preparation for the activity session. The cool-down period also prevents hypotension, which may occur with sudden cessation of exercise (31).

In addition to dynamic (endurance) exercise, properly selected resistive exercise (calisthenics and weights) are helpful in promoting muscle strength and flexibility. These are all important components of physical conditioning.

Resistive exercise involves activities that utilize low to moderate repetition movements against a resistance, generating an increase in muscle tension, such as is seen with weight lifting. The increased muscle tension during such exercise leads to a restriction in muscle blood flow during contraction due to compression of arterioles and capillaries that perfuse the muscle bed (32), as well as a centrally mediated pressor response. The blood pressure and heart rate responses during resistive exercise are proportional to the relative intensity of muscular contraction (i.e., the percent of maximal voluntary contraction), the size or mass of the muscle groups involved, and the duration of the contraction (33). Unlike dynamic (aerobic) exercise, which provokes changes in skeletal muscle aerobic capacity through changes in mitochondrial number and enzymes necessary for glycogen and fat metabolism (34), the effects of long-term resistive exercise on the skeletal muscle appear limited to muscle cell hypertrophy through synthesis of increased contractile protein and thickening of connective tissue (35). Subsequent increases in muscle strength (or maximal voluntary contraction) after training lead to a decreased heart rate and blood pressure response to a given load, because that load now represents a lower percentage of the maximal voluntary contraction (36). Of note, during maximal upper body resistive exercise, the heart rate–blood pressure product is lower than that observed during maximal dynamic effort (37), primarily due to a lower peak heart rate response.

Several reports document the improvements in muscle strength after a resistive training program in subjects with cardiac disease (38–42). Strength gains of 22% to 29% (38–42), as well as increases in the number of repetitions in a given submaximal load that can be performed (42), have been achieved in cardiac subjects. No adverse outcomes have been reported during supervised light to moderate intensity resistive training in cardiac rehabilitation.

As such, appropriate resistive training is encouraged as part of an overall exercise program for post-MI subjects. This can be performed using a wide variety of equipment including free weights, wall-mounted pulleys, or exercise machines equipped with weight stacks. Resistive exercise should be performed in a variety of body positions, both to isolate specific muscle groups and to ensure maximum orthopedic stability. To avoid the additive cardiovascular responses of the Valsalva maneuver, subjects should be trained to exhale during the contraction phase of the movement. Resistive training should include 8–10 exercises that involve the major muscle groups of the body, e.g., arms, shoulders, chest, abdominals, back/trunk, hips, and legs. The intensity of each weight training exercise can be adjusted by alterations in any of the following factors: weight load, number of repetitions per set, number of sets, and rest period between sets. Generally, for post–MI subjects, 2–3 days per week of resistive training using one set of 10–15 repetitions to moderate fatigue is recommended. Once 15 repetitions can be completed, the weight can be increased an additional 5% and more sets added. Initial weight training activities may be introduced during the first 2 weeks of an outpatient program, and these include the use of light calisthenics and 3- to 5-lb dumbbell weights. Later in the program, if subjects are medically stable, they can be cleared for regular weight training activities using barbells and weight machines. This sequence of range of motion exercise and strength training has been shown to be safe for use in subjects post–MI (43).

In summary, the types of exercise training should consist of "cardiovascular endurance," or dynamic, exercise preceded by a warm-up period and followed by a cool-down period. Calisthenics and resistive training are useful for promoting strength and flexibility. All training should follow the exercise prescription individually designated for the subject.

Program Types

For the implementation of exercise training in post-MI subjects, a number of "settings" may be considered.

Medically Supervised Group (Moderate- High-Risk Subjects)

These programs provide close medical supervision for subjects who are at high risk for a complication associated with physical activity. Such are largely from class C (as previously described).

These groups require careful medical supervision and surveillance to assure that the activity is well tolerated and safe. A physician should be readily available, although the presence of a properly trained nurse in the exercise room is sufficient if the physician is not available. The qualifications of the physician may vary, but experience in internal medicine and cardiovascular disease, and in treatment of subjects with heart disease, is recommended. Training programs should be medically supervised until low risk of activity has been established. All subjects entering these programs should be screened as described in Table 33–4. The program should also provide staff, space, equipment, and facilities (see Table 33–5).

Medically Supervised Group (Low-Risk Subjects)

Low-risk subjects (class B, as described previously) benefit from medically supervised programs because exercise can be conducted more safely, and the group dynamics and interchange often help subjects comply with good health behaviors. Immediate medical supervision of low-risk subjects can be provided by a well trained nurse working under a physician's orders. The person supervising subjects should have successfully completed an AHA-sponsored course in advanced cardiac life support and capable of providing emergency medications. All subjects entering these programs should be screened as outlined in Table 33–6. The program should provide the same basic requirements as for high-risk subjects as detailed in Table 33–5.

Home-Monitored Programs

The use of transtelephonic ECG monitoring at home has been utilized as a substitute for attending a group "clinic" program (44,45). Such programs

Table 33–4. Screening Process for Medically Supervised Programs for Moderate- to High-Risk Patients

Consent of attending physician
Stable clinical course
Exercise test with current medications (for prescription)
Patient's assurance of willingness to accept responsibility for higher risk and to follow instructions for modifying risk
Exercise prescription with ECG monitoring at beginning and for change in activity levels to ensure activity is well tolerated and to define desirable levels of exercise

Reproduced from Fletcher et al (8), with permission.

Table 33–5. Basic Requirements for Medically Supervised Programs for Moderate- to High-Risk Patients

Adequately ventilated and temperature-controlled space
Capability to assess patients with blood pressure and ECG analysis
ECG monitoring during initial sessions to ascertain desirable exercise levels
Supervision by either a nurse or physician in the exercise room. If a physician is not present, he or she must be readily available for consultation.
Medically qualified staff (completion of an AHA-sponsored advanced cardiac life support course [or the equivalent] and a minimum of two staff members present who are trained in cardiopulmonary resuscitation)
Appropriate drugs and equipment (emergency medications [as outlined in the AHA's *Textbook of Advanced Cardiac Life Support*] and cardioverter/defibrillator)
Standard orders for the nurse
Written procedures for the following:
- Identification of conditions needed to conduct session
- Management of problems that do not require hospitalization, such as acute, well-tolerated arrhythmias and neuromuscular injuries
- Ruling out myocardial infarction and management of problems requiring hospitalization, including postresuscitation problems
- Management of cardiac arrest, including procedure for immediate treatment and transportation to hospital

AHA = American Heart Association.
Reproduced from Fletcher et al (8), with permission.

have the disadvantage of lacking immediate emergency medical care, although local care in the community setting has been shown to be adequate through clinical experience. These programs may be particularly useful in following subjects in the event "clinics" are not readily available.

Table 33–6. Screening Process for Medically Supervised Programs for Low-Risk Patients

Permission of patient's personal physician, who judges patient to be either NYHA functional class 1 or 2
Exercise test without severe ischemic changes or high-grade ventricular ectopy
Willingness to accept responsibility for higher risk and to follow instructions for modifying risk
Exercise prescription with ECG monitoring at beginning and for change in activity levels to ensure activity is well tolerated and to define desirable levels of exercise heart rates

NYHA = New York Heart Association.
Reproduced from Fletcher et al (8), with permission.

Unmonitored Home Programs

In the first 1–2 weeks after discharge from the hospital after MI, subjects who are clinically stable may walk at a slow, regular pace with increasing duration, starting with 10-minute periods and working up to 1 hour. Such activity need not be supervised. Unmonitored exercise (46) can also be used for conditioning after the individual has recovered from the MI (2 weeks or more after hospital discharge) or in other cases of stable CHD. Medically supervised and monitored exercise, however, is preferred. If cardiac rehabilitation facilities are not available, physical activity guidelines can still be provided to cardiac subjects, and they should be encouraged to exercise. Activity should be restricted to *low–moderate intensity* walking (not race walking) or equivalent activities. If individuals carefully watch for symptoms and signs of intolerance and are attentive to heart rate and rating of perceived exertion, this activity level is considered safe. Walking is a safe, low-impact, exercise that usually generates an intensity level that is 50% to 70% of $VO_{2,max}$.

It is recommended that all activity be prescribed from the exercise test results. Although walking is most desirable, an activity other than walking (i.e., cycle ergometry) can be prescribed, provided the intensity is similar to walking and that it is dynamic (as opposed to static). Range of motion exercises and light calisthenics can also be performed in an unmonitored setting. Activities are considered safe and appropriate if they meet the criterion of moderate intensity.

It is permissible for subjects to participate in physical training classes (health clubs, YMCA, etc.) if they carefully follow the recommended guidelines for unmonitored exercise. In some cases, classes are desirable because of the "social interchange" and group dynamics.

SPECIAL CATEGORIES OF SUBJECTS

In exercise training for post–MI subjects, certain co-morbid conditions must be considered. For purposes of this discussion, the areas of concern will be confined to the elderly and those with heart failure, peripheral arterial disease, diabetes mellitus, or physical disabilities.

The Elderly

Special considerations must be addressed when prescribing exercise for the elderly population (46a,46b,46c) (see Ch. 25). In this group, (with time) maximal end-diastolic volume increases, while maximal heart rate, ejection fraction, and cardiac output all decrease. There is a decline in the heart rate response to isoproterenol with age (47,48). The elderly, however, have a similar stroke volume response to exercise as do the young (49); therefore, the decrease in cardiac output in the elderly primarily results from the heart rate decrease. Two factors contribute to the age-related reduction in cardiac ejection and the relative increase in end-systolic volume with exercise. Aortic impedance is increased, and there is reduced contractile reserve of the left ventricle (47). This reflects in large part the attenuated end-organ response to beta-adrenergic stimulation, such that beta-adrenergic modulation of contractility is reduced progressively with increasing age (47,48,50,51). Table 33–7 presents similarities between aging and beta-adrenergic blockade in response to exercise (52). However, the available data suggest that there is a dissociation between the inotropic responsiveness and lusitropic (diastolic) responsiveness in the aged heart, with maintenance of the responsiveness of left ventricular relaxation to beta-adrenergic stimuli (51). Thus, with the decrease in inotropic response to catecholamines, the lusitropic response is selectively well maintained. In the presence of disease, these factors may affect the cardiac response to a given exercise prescription. In addition, exercise-induced arrhythmias increase in frequency in older individuals and may be of concern in cardiac exercise programs (52).

Table 33–7. Similarities Between Aging and Beta-Adrenergic Blockade in Response to Exercise

	Aging	Beta-blockade
Maximal heart rate	Decreases	Decreases
Maximal ejection fraction	Decreases	Decreases
Maximal end-diastolic volume	Increases	Increases
Maximal cardiac output	Decreases	Decreases
Maximal plasma catecholamines	Increase	Increase

Reproduced with permission from Fleg JL: Effects of aging on the cardiovascular response to exercise, in Fletcher GF (ed): Cardiovascular Response to Exercise. Mount Kisco, NY, Futura Publishing, 1994, pp 387–404.

Reproduced from Fleg (52), with permission.

Heart Failure

Medically stable post MI subjects with compensated heart failure may participate in exercise training programs. Benefits are derived from conditioning of the musculoskeletal system. These specifically involve changes in ventilatory threshold, increased skeletal muscle vascular conductance and oxygen extraction, and decreased skeletal muscle lactate production (53). Figure 33–2 displays results of training in 12 subjects with heart failure. Subjects with persistent rales and uncontrolled edema on maximal medical therapy with diuretics, digoxin, and vasodilators have not been included. Subjects with active ischemia and severe left ventricular dysfunction should be considered for angiography and, if possible, myocardial revascularization before

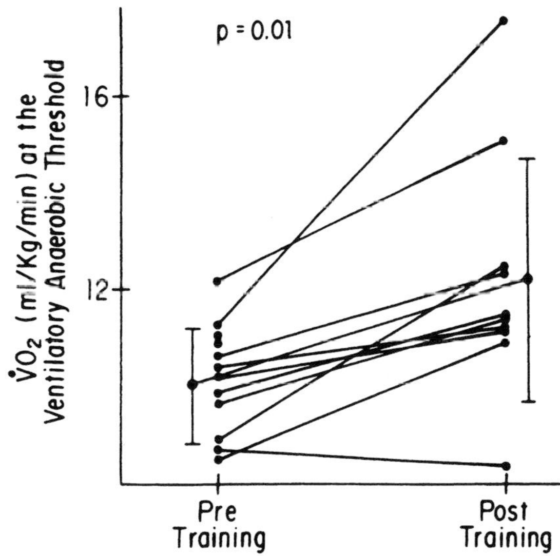

Figure 33–2. Graph showing individual changes in ventilatory threshold after exercise training in 12 subjects with heart failure. *Reproduced with permission from Sullivan MJ, et al: Exercise training in patients with chronic heart failure delays ventilatory anaerobic threshold and improves submaximal exercise performance. Circulation 1989;79:324–329.*

exercise training. Previous studies have indicated that this group may have the largest absolute mortality reduction from surgical (or possibly angioplasty) intervention (54,55) and may not achieve a marked training benefit if they undergo training with ongoing severe ischemia (56).

Studies examining the long-term effects of exercise training on morbidity and mortality in subjects with left ventricular dysfunction are currently unavailable. In lieu of recent studies (57–69a,69) appears that subjects with severe left ventricular dysfunction and stable class I–III heart failure controlled on medical therapy achieve a clinically important improvement in exercise performance and symptoms through exercise conditioning. Exercise conditioning therefore likely represents a valuable therapeutic adjunct to the pharmacological management of subjects with heart failure.

Peripheral Arterial Disease

In the post–MI subject, there is often associated peripheral arterial disease (PAD), especially in the lower extremities. Such is usually manifest by claudication. If there is no evidence of skin ulceration or other indications of impending tissue compromise secondary to poor circulation, these subjects can exercise.

Treadmill exercise is an effective mode of exercise therapy for those with claudication, and these subjects should have a similar exercise prescription to that of others. The beginning training workload, determined from a symptom-limited maximal treadmill test on entry, is at an intensity that precipitates claudication pain in 3 to 5 minutes. In subsequent visits, the speed or grade is increased if the subject can walk for 10 minutes or longer at the lower workload without reaching moderate claudication pain. Either speed or grade can be increased, but an increase in grade is recommended if the subject can walk at 2 mph. An additional goal of the program is to increase walking speed up to 3.0 mph from the average walking speed of 1.5 to 2.0 mph in subjects with PAD.

Subjects with PAD have improvements in muscle metabolism with exercise training. The primary evidence for this adaptation is that, after training, there is an increase in the extraction of oxygen across the leg during exercise despite no change in total blood flow (70). Another metabolic adaptation with exercise training in subjects with PAD involves changes in carnitine metabolism. Under both normal and abnormal conditions, the formation of acylcarnitine reflects the underlying metabolic state of the cellular acyl-CoA pool (71). Elevated muscle acylcarnitine concentrations at rest have been associated with functional impairment in subjects with PAD, such that those with the highest levels have the most impaired exercise performance (72). Exercise training reduces the plasma concentration of short chain acylcarnitines, and treated subjects who have the greatest response to training also have the greatest reduction in plasma short chain acylcarnitine concentration (73).

Other potential factors that may be associated with improved exercise performance are alterations in gait and perception of claudication pain, but further study is needed in these areas.

Diabetes Mellitus

Numerous studies have reported that regular exercise will improve glucose tolerance and enhance insulin sensitivity in diabetic as well as nondiabetic persons (75a,75b) (see Ch. 33). Benefits are most likely related to an increased tissue sensitivity to insulin due to regular exercise conditioning (76). In normal subjects, insulin binding to monocytes is increased by exercise conditioning (77), which may be regulated, in part, by an increase in muscle glucose transporters (78). In post–MI subjects with diabetes, the exercise prescription does not greatly differ from a prescription for a nondiabetic person in type, intensity, frequency, duration, and specificity of exercise required for conditioning (79). More frequent exercise, however, may be necessary to gain the expected benefits on "glucoregulation" in these diabetic individuals.

High-intensity aerobic exercise and true isometric exercise are contraindicated in the subject with proliferative retinopathy because of an increased risk for the development of retinal or vitreous hemorrhages and retinal detachment (80). However, the risk of moderate-intensity aerobic exercise is considered acceptable in these subjects (81). Subjects with peripheral neuropathy should not engage in exercise (such as jogging) that may traumatize an insensitive foot. In addition, properly fitted footwear and checking of the feet for injury after exercise are recommended precautions. Data evaluating the potential problem of exercise-induced hypoglycemia in subjects taking oral agents or insulin are lacking. However, in nondiabetic individuals taking oral hypoglycemic drugs, hypoglycemia may develop during prolonged exercise (82). Therefore, post–MI subjects with diabetes should be advised by their physicians regarding how to reduce their medication, either oral agent or insulin, before exercising and to not exercise alone.

Subjects with Physical Disabilities

There is a group of post–MI subjects who have physical (musculoskeletal) impairments. These include those after a stroke or amputation with resultant hemiplegia, paraplegia, or other limb impairments that render useless (or quite limited) any or most of the four extremities. Special modes of testing have evolved with this group of subjects (83), and this group is now more often considered for exercise post–MI.

These subjects can perform exercise training both at home and in group programs. One study (84) involved 83 men with documented coronary disease (including infarction) and a physical disability with functional use of ≥2 extremities, including one arm. They were randomized either to a 6-month exercise program at home using wheelchair ergometry or to usual and customary care at home. Using initial and follow-up echocardiographic studies, the home exercise group improved both peak exercise left ventricular ejection fraction (p = 0.0007) and fractional shortening (p = 0.01) from baseline to 6 months. Exercise training effects of decreased heart rate (p = 0.03) and decreased peak rate pressure product (p = 0.03) were also found in the treatment group. There were no exercise-related complications.

Therefore, exercise testing and training can be effectively and safely done in physically disabled subjects post–MI.

PSYCHOSOCIAL ISSUES

Psychosocial problems are common in post–MI subjects. Moderate to severe depression occurs in 10% to 20% of subjects after an MI, and anxiety disorders are manifest in approximately 5% to 10% (85,86). Recent data (87) have shown that depression that occurs in hospital post–MI is a significant predictor of post–MI cardiac mortality, and that this risk associated with depression is greater in subjects with ≥15 premature ventricular complexes (PVCs) per hour. About one-quarter of subjects do not resume sexual activity, and one-half decrease their sexual activity after an MI (88). Family and marital problems, as well as social isolation, are common. Health education and counseling, psychotherapy, and stress management show promising results in improving the quality of life and reducing psychosocial distress among such subjects, especially in the early phases of recovery (89,90).

Therefore, subjects entering cardiac rehabilitation exercise programs should be assessed for depressive or anxiety disorders, sexual dysfunction, excessive distress/stress and anger, work-related concerns, alcohol or drug abuse and dependence, and inadequate social support. Referral liaisons with psychiatrists, psychologists, social workers, or mental health workers should be established to assist with the continued evaluation and management of these problems as needed. Short-term stress management and/or group sessions focusing on psychosocial issues may be of additional benefit. The exercise program itself is often a means to alleviate depression. The group reinforcement component is effective, with the guidance of a sensitive and knowledgeable nurse or other professional.

COMPLIANCE

Compliance with exercise post–MI demonstrates a negatively accelerating curve, with approximately 20% to 25% of subjects dropping out of the intervention within the first 3 months, 40% to 50% between 6 and 12 months, and a relatively flat curve for the next 3 or 4 years (91). Although not confirmed, this trend for high early dropout rates may relate to the cost of the intervention, insurance reimbursement, inconvenience associated with program scheduling and facility location, family demands, or simply poor motivation. Although there is considerable knowledge regarding compliance enhancing strategies in some health behavior treatments for chronic conditions, there is little information on the effectiveness of such strategies for multidisciplinary cardiac exercise rehabilitation programs.

Two studies of multidisciplinary cardiac exercise rehabilitation have examined the impact of different compliance enhancing strategies on dropout rates. The first studied dropouts following an intervention used at entry to the study to enhance attendance during 3 months of multidisciplinary cardiac exercise rehabilitation intervention and to collect attendance data over the next 9 months (92). In this study, subjects randomized to both the intervention and comparison groups, as well as all spouses, received a mailed pamphlet describing the intervention, its benefits and drawbacks, and the need to attend regularly. In addition, all intervention subjects and their spouses received an educational intervention, consisting of telephone counseling about the items in the pamphlet and a request for an oral commitment to attend the program twice a week. The intervention resulted in a nonsignificant increase of 2% in attendance; adjustment for covariates suggested a 12% increase in attendance, with the strongest effect on subjects with high school education or less (92). The other study examined the impact of self-management strategies utilized throughout a 6-month multidisciplinary cardiac exercise rehabilitation intervention in subjects randomized to either an intervention or a control group (93). The strategies consisted of a signed agreement to comply with the intervention for 6 months and to record information in a diary about exercise responses, activity levels, and changes in weight and smoking habits. The increase in compliance in the intervention group was a nonsignificant 12% when compared with the control group; however, in those who initially consented to sign the agreement, compliance was significantly higher, 65%, compared with 42% in the control group and 20% in the intervention group who refused to sign the initial agreement (93).

The information on compliance enhancement strategies in supervised multidisciplinary cardiac exercise rehabilitation is thus limited, and the increase in compliance in the two noted studies of compliance enhancing strategies is small. Both experimental and observational studies are needed to better understand the impact of compliance on the "nonspecific" or indirect, as well as the direct, effects of an intervention (94). These nonspecific effects may be especially important in a multidisciplinary intervention such as cardiac exercise rehabilitation where the objectives include decreasing coronary risk factors, increasing exercise tolerance, and improving subject psychosocial status, including return to occupational and recreational activities.

Improving patient–provider communication with more information about cardiovascular disease, MI, and its treatments would likely result in more informed decision making by the subject, which may improve compliance. For example, increased involvement by the subject in clinical decision making has been shown to improve satisfaction (95), compliance (93,95), and outcome (96). Successful cooperation and frequently improved compliance is enhanced by (97–99)

1. Clear, open communication between subject and provider
2. Emotional support and alleviation of fears and anxieties
3. Understandable and sensible explanations about regimens that are compatible with the subject's values, preferences, and expressed needs and that acknowledge the individual's social and cultural norms
4. Integrating and coordinating care and providing continuity and transition

One recent study (29a), the Training Level Comparison study, is a randomized, multicenter clinical trial designed to compare the effects of two exercise training programs, low and high intensity, on left ventricular function in subjects with documented evidence of coronary heart disease (many of whom were postinfarction). The target heart rates for the low- and high-intensity programs corresponded to 50% and 85%, respectively, of the

$VO_{2,max}$ achieved on a baseline exercise test with a window of ±5 beats per minute. All subjects were to attend three 1-hour supervised exercise sessions per week for 2 years. Dropouts occurred more frequently in the high-intensity group than in the low-intensity group, and in smokers and those with a history of MI.

At 6 months, 55% of the low-intensity subjects maintained heart rates within their target ranges, in contrast to 31% of the high-intensity subjects. Similar results were observed at 1 year. In the low-intensity group, heart rates outside the range were typically above the target range, whereas those in the high-intensity group were more likely to fall short of the range. Nonetheless, there were statistically significant differences between the low- and high-intensity groups with respect to maintained heart rates at 6 months and 1 year.

The study achieved moderate success in implementing the treatment regimens. The greater dropout rate among the high-intensity subjects and the lower proportion who maintained heart rates within the target range suggest that this level of exercise training may be too demanding. Potential benefits of a high-intensity program may be compromised by a lack of attendance at exercise sessions and an inability to achieve the target heart rate. As the low-intensity target range was exceeded by a high proportion of subjects, this program may not have been sufficiently challenging. These results suggest that the optimal intensity level of exercise may be between the low and high intensity levels used in this study (100).

Overall compliance (long-term) is, therefore, an ongoing concern in exercise training for post–MI subjects. The lack of compliance and associated risk factor modification is likely a reason for recurrence of events in these subjects.

IMPACT ON EMPLOYMENT—RETURN TO WORK

Approximately 80% of subjects with uncomplicated MI who are under age 65 and employed at the time of infarction return to work within 2 to 3 months. Although the rate of early return to work is high, the subsequent dropout each year is also high. Subjects who have had coronary bypass surgery return to work and remain at work very inconsistently, despite substantial decrease in symptoms, improvement in functional capacity, and reported enhancement of quality of life (101).

Factors that determine return to work after a cardiac event include work status before the event, education level, employer attitude, psychological factors, and age. Certain other factors influence reemployment after a cardiac event in subjects nearing retirement. These include disability insurance, social security, early retirement incentives, early retirement benefits, and employer policy and attitude.

Almost half of controlled studies (8 of 19) (102) describe a favorable outcome regarding return to work in subjects who participated in cardiac rehabilitation exercise training. Exercise testing itself, as used for an exercise prescription, may enhance a subject's confidence in returning to work, particularly when the results of exercise testing are discussed relative to occupational work demands (103).

With regard to specific studies, DeBusk et al (104) studied male survivors of uncomplicated acute MI with a mean age of 54 years. They were randomly assigned to supervised gym training (n = 28), home training (n = 12), or control (n = 30) 3 weeks following the event. After follow-up of 11 weeks, more than half of the subjects in all groups had returned to work, with no significant differences among the three groups.

Mayou et al (105) conducted a study in an outpatient rehabilitation program in England, where health care providers included physicians, cardiac nurses, and physical therapists. Subjects were post–MI men with evaluation age of between 28 and 60 years (mean of 57). There were 15 who either died or were excluded, with 115 in the final sample, randomized and controlled. Randomization was to a control group (n = 37), an exercise group (n = 43) with 8 exercise sessions 2 times per week over 4 weeks within 4 weeks of event, or an advice group of 3 to 4 sessions given by a cardiac nurse to couples (n = 35). The length of follow-up was 18 months, and groups were well matched at baseline. The same proportion of all three groups eventually returned to work; however, the advice group showed greater hours of working than either of the other two groups ($p = 0.05$).

Lamm et al (106) studied 2,054 male MI survivors for 3 years in a European multicenter study. Return to work was higher in the rehabilitation group than in the control group in 15 of 17 centers, though significant differences were found in only 5 centers.

Hedback et al (107) studied post–MI survivors below the age of 65, with follow-up for 5 years. There were 147 rehabilitation subjects (124 male) and 158 in the control group (134 male), with a mean age of 57 years in both groups. After exclusion, 84 subjects (80 men) remained in the rehabilitation group as a final sample. Return to work was greater in the rehabilitation group versus controls at 2 years ($p < 0.001$). Among subjects under age 55 at baseline, 89% in the rehabilitation group versus 67% of the controls were working at 5 years ($p < 0.05$).

Hertzeanu et al (108) studied 41 post–MI subjects (2 to 19 years post–index event) with left ventricular ejection fractions less than 40%. The mean age was 61, and subjects were either NYHA functional class 2 or 3. The length of follow-up was between 36 and 60 months. Return to work was reported as 82% of each of two rehabilitation groups versus 40% of the controls (no p value given).

Therefore, modest evidence supports the benefit of cardiac rehabilitation in return-to-work status for post–MI subjects. Further observations in these subjects and specific subsets will likely delineate the type of rehabilitative effort that will be most beneficial.

FUTURE ISSUES AND CONSIDERATIONS WITH REGARD TO BASIC SCIENCE AND CLINICAL RESEARCH IN EXERCISE FOR THE POSTINFARCTION SUBJECT

As reflected in previous details of this chapter, progress has been made and guidelines established for exercise training for the post–MI subject (108a). Basic and clinical research have addressed areas of importance in basic science issues, as well as human anatomy and physiologic adaptations.

For the future, specific concerns will address practical matters such as more appropriate arm exercise testing for occupational adaptation and exercise training, and activity in the work setting. Home and worksite exercise activity interventions will be further explored. Use of improved metabolic studies with regard to oxygen consumption and ventilatory threshold endpoints resulting from exercise testing and training will be used appropriately to alleviate fatigue at the worksite.

As medical professionals deal more with the importance of being physically active after MI, both in the early phases of recovery and later, it will be important to consider the impact this will have on return-to-work status. It is believed that the physically active individuals post–MI will more likely return to work and stay at work more effectively after their cardiac event. These individuals will continue to have fewer recurrent events secondary to their physical activity and overall health enhancement.

Therefore, the future is quite important in both basic and clinical research with regard to exercise in subjects who have had compromise of their coronary circulation with resultant myocardial damage. Collaborative work with research experts at the "bench level" and appropriate clinical research will bring new insights in this area of continuing cardiovascular care.

REFERENCES

1. Levine SA, Lown B: The "chair" treatment of acute coronary thrombosis. *Trans Assoc Am Physicians* 1951; 64:316.
2. May GS, Eberlein KA, Furberg CD, et al: Secondary prevention after myocardial infarction: A review of long-term trials. *Prog Cardiovasc Dis* 1982;24:331.
3. Oberman A, Naughton J: The national exercise and heart disease project, in Pollock ML, Schmidt DH (eds): *Heart Disease and Rehabilitation,* 2nd ed. New York, John Wiley & Sons, 1986, pp 369–385.
4. Shaw LW: Effects of a prescribed supervised exercise program on mortality and cardiovascular morbidity in patients after a myocardial infarction. *Am J Cardiol* 1981;48:39.

5. DeBusk RF, Kraemer HC, Nash E, et al: Stepwise risk stratification soon after myocardial infarction. *Am J Cardiol* 1983;52:1161.
6. American Association of Cardiovascular and Pulmonary Rehabilitation: Scientific evidence of the value of cardiac rehabilitation services with emphasis on patients following myocardial infarction. Section I. Exercise conditioning component (position paper). *J Cardiopulm Rehab* 1990;10:79.
7. Cardiac Rehabilitation Services: Health and Public Policy Committee, American College of Physicians. *Ann Intern Med* 1988;109:671.
8. Fletcher GF, Balady G, Froehlicher VF, et al: Exercise standards: A statement for health professionals from the American Heart Association. *Circulation* 1995;91:580–615.

8a. Kavanagh T, Shephard RJ, Tuck JA: Depression following myocardial infarction: the effects of distance running. *Ann N Y Acad Sci* 1977;301:1029–38.

9. Hamalainen H, Luurila OJ, Kallio V, et al: Long-term reduction in sudden deaths after a multifactorial intervention programme in patients with myocardial infarction: 10-year results of a controlled investigation. *Eur Heart J* 1989;10:55.
10. Kallio V, Hamalainen H, Hakkila J, et al: Reduction in sudden deaths by a multifactorial intervention programme after acute myocardial infarction. *Lancet* 1979;2:1091.
11. Carson P, Phillips R, Lloyd M, et al: Exercise after myocardial infarction: Controlled trial. *J R Coll Physicians Lond* 1982;16:147.
12. Wilhelmsen L, Sanne H, Elmfeldt D, et al: A controlled trial of physical training after myocardial infarction: Effects of risk factors, nonfatal reinfarction and death. *Prev Med* 1975;4:491.
13. Roman O, Gutierrez M, Luksic I, et al: Cardiac rehabilitation after acute myocardial infarction: 9 year controlled follow-up study. *Cardiology* 1983;70:223.
14. Vermeulen A, Lie KI, Durrer D: Effects of cardiac rehabilitation after myocardial infarction: Changes in coronary risk factors and long-term prognosis. *Am Heart J* 1983;105:798.
15. Rechnitzer PA, Cunningham DA, Andrew GM, et al: Relation of exercise to the recurrence rate of myocardial infarction in men: Ontario Exercise Heart Collaborative Study. *Am J Cardiol* 1983;51:65.
16. Marra S, Paolillo V, Spadaccini F, et al: Long-term follow-up after a controlled randomized post-infarction rehabilitation programme: Effects on morbidity and mortality. *Eur Heart J* 1985;6:656.
17. O'Conner GT, Buring JE, Yusuf S, et al: An overview of randomized trials of rehabilitation with exercise after myocardial infarction. *Circulation* 1989;80:234.
18. Detry JMR, Rousseau M, Vandenbroucke G, et al: Increased arteriovenous oxygen difference after physical training in coronary heart patients. *Circulation* 1971;44:109.
19. Laslett L, Paumer L, Amsterdam EA: Exercise training in coronary artery disease. *Cardiol Clin* 1987;5:211.
20. Ehsani AA, Martin WH III, Heath GW, et al: Cardiac effects of prolonged and intense exercise training in patients with coronary artery disease. *Am J Cardiol* 1982;50:246.
21. Schuler G, Hambrecht R, Schlierf G, et al: Regular physical exercise and low-fat diet: Effects on progression of coronary artery disease. *Circulation* 1992;86:1.
22. Haskell WL, Leon AS, Caspersen CJ, et al: Cardiovascular benefits and assessment of physical activity and physical fitness in adults. *Med Sci Sports Exerc* 1992;24:S201.
23. Oberman A: Does cardiac rehabilitation increase long-term survival after myocardial infarction. *Circulation* 1989;80:416.
24. Weiner DA, McCabe C, Hueter DC, et al: The predictive value of anginal chest pain as an indicator of coronary disease during exercise testing. *Am Heart J* 1978;96:458–462.
25. Theroux P, Waters DD, Halphen C, et al: Prognostic value of exercise testing soon after myocardial infarction. *N Engl J Med* 1979;301:341–345.
26. Starling MK, Crawford MH, Kennedy GT, et al: Exercise test after myocardial infarction: Predictive value for subsequent unstable angina and death. *Am J Cardiol* 1980;46:909–914.
27. Wade OL, Bishop JM: *Cardiac Output and Regional Blood Flow.* Philadelphia, FA Davis, 1962.
28. Borg G: Perceived exertion as an indicator of somatic stress. *Scand J Rehabil Med* 1970;2-3:92–98.
29. Weber KT, Janicki JS: *Cardiopulmonary Exercise Testing: Physiologic Principles and Clinical Applications.* Philadelphia, WB Saunders, 1986.

29a. Oberman A, Fletcher GF, Lee J, et al. Efficacy of high-intensity exercise training on left ventricular ejection fraction in men with coronary artery disease (the Training Level Comparison Study). *Am J Cardiol* 1995;76:643–7.

30. Hambrecht R, Niebauer J, Marburger C, et al: Various intensities of leisure time physical activity in patients with coronary artery disease: Effects on cardiorespiratory fitness and progression of coronary atherosclerotic lesions. *J Am Coll Cardiol* 1993; 22(2):468–477.

31. Dimsdale JE, Hartley LH, Guiney T, Ruskin JN, Greenblatt D: Postexercise peril: Plasma catecholamines and exercise. *JAMA* 1984;251:630–632.

32. Asmussen E: Similarities and dissimilarities between static and dynamic effort. *Circ Res* 1981; Suppl I:I-3–I-10.

33 Seals DR, Washborn RH, Hanson PG, Painter PL, Nagle FJ: Increased cardiovascular response to static contraction of large muscle groups. *J Appl Physiol* 1983;58:434–437.

34. Holloszy JO, Coyle EF: Adaptations of skeletal muscle to endurance exercise and their metabolic consequences. *J Appl Physiol* 1984;56:831–838.

35. Sharkey B: Specificity of exercise, in American College of Sports Medicine (eds): *Resource Manual for Guidelines for Exercise Testing and Prescription.* Philadelphia, Lea and Febiger, 1988, p 5.

36. Franklin BA, Bonzheim K, Gordon S, Timmis GC: Resistance training in cardiac rehabilitation. *J Cardiopulmon Rehabil* 1991;11:99–106.

37. DeBusk RF, Valdez R, Houston N, Haskell N: Cardiovascular responses to dynamic and static effort soon after myocardial infarction. *Circulation* 1978; 58:368–375.

38. Kelemen M, Stewart KJ, Gillilan RE, et al: Circuit weight training in cardiac patients. *J Am Coll Cardiol* 1986;7:38–42.

39. Stewart KJ, Manson M, Kelemen MH: Three-year participation in circuit weight training improves muscular strength and self efficacy in cardiac patients. *J Cardiopulmon Rehabil* 1988;8:292–296.

40. Ghilarducci LEC, Holly RG, Amsterdam EA: Effects of high resistance training in coronary artery disease. *Am J Cardiol* 1989;64:866–870.

41. Sparling PB, Cantwell JD, Dolan CM, Neiderman RK: Strength training in a cardiac rehabilitation program: A six-month follow-up. *Arch Phys Med Rehabil* 1990;71:148–152.

42. McCartney N, McKelvie RS, Haslam DRS, Jones NL: Usefulness of weight lifting training and improving strength and maximal power output in coronary artery disease. *Am J Cardiol* 1991;67:939–945.

43. Sennett SM, Pollock ML, Pels AE III, et al: Medical problems of patients in an outpatient cardiac rehabilitation program. *J Cardiopulmon Rehabil* 1987;7:458–465.

44. Fletcher GF, Chiaramida AJ, LeMay MR, Johnston BL, Thiel JE, Spratlin MC: Telephonically-monitored home exercise early after coronary artery bypass surgery. *Chest* 1984;86:198–202.

45. DeBusk RF, Haskell WL, Miller N II, et al: Medically directed at-home rehabilitation soon after clinically uncomplicated acute myocardial infarction: A new model of patient care. *Am J Cardiol* 1985;55:251–257.

46. Fletcher BJ, Lloyd A, Fletcher GF: Outpatient rehabilitative training in patients with cardiovascular disease: Emphasis on training method. *Heart Lung* 1988;17:199–205.

46a. Ades PA, Hanson JS, Gunther PG, et al: Exercise conditioning in the elderly coronary patient. *J Am Geriatr Soc* 1987;35:121–4.

46b. Ades PA, Grunvald MH. Cardiopulmonary exercise testing before and after conditioning in older coronary patients. *Am Heart J* 1990;120:585–9.

46c. Ades PA, Waldmann ML, Gillespie C. A controlled trial of exercise training in older coronary patients. *J Gerontol A Biol Sci Med Sci* 1995;50A:M7–11.

47. Lakatta EG: Alterations in the cardiovascular system that occur in advanced age. *Fed Proc* 1979; 38:163–167.

48. Lakatta EG: Age-related alterations in the cardiovascular response to adrenergic mediated stress. *Fed Proc* 1980;39:3173–3177.

49. Rodeheffer RJ, Gerstenblith G, Becker LC, Fleg JL, Weisfeldt ML, Lakatta EG: Exercise cardiac output is maintained with advancing age in healthy human subjects: Cardiac dilatation and increased stroke volume compensate for a diminished heart rate. *Circulation* 1984;69:203–214.

50. Guarnieri T, Filburn CR, Zitnik G, Gerstenblith G, Weisfeldt ML, Lakatta EG: Contractile and biochemical correlates of beta-adrenergic stimulation of the aged heart. *Am J Physiol* 1980;239:H501.

51. Lakatta EG, Gerstenblith G, Angell CS, Weisfeldt ML: Diminished inotropic response of aged myocardium to catecholamines. *Circ Res* 1979;44:517–523.

52. Fleg JL: Effects of aging on the cardiovascular response to exercise, in Fletcher GF (ed): *Cardiovascular Response to Exercise.* Mount Kisco, NY, Futura Publishing, 1994, pp 387–404.

53. Sullivan MJ: Role of exercise conditioning in patients with severe left ventricular dysfunction, in Fletcher GF (ed): *Cardiovascular Response to Exercise.*

Mount Kisco, NY, Futura Publishing, 1994, pp 359–376.

54. Alderman EL, Fisher LD, Litwin P, et al: Results of coronary artery surgery in patients with poor left ventricular function (CASS). *Circulation* 1983;68:785.

55. Vigilante GJ, Weintraub WS, Klein LW, et al: Improved survival with coronary bypass surgery in patients with three-vessel coronary disease and abnormal left ventricular function. Matched case-control study in patient with potentially operable disease. *Am J Med* 1987;82:697.

56. Arvan S: Exercise performance of the high risk acute myocardial infarction patient after cardiac rehabilitation. *Am J Cardiol* 1988;62:197–201.

57. Letac B, Cribier A, Desplanches JF: A study of left ventricular function in coronary patients before and after physical training. *Circulation* 1977;56: 375–378.

58. Cobb FR, Williams RS, McEwan P, Jones RH, Coleman RE, Wallace AG: Effects of exercise training on ventricular function in patients with recent myocardial infarction. *Circulation* 1982;66: 100–108.

59. Lee AP, Ice R, Blessey R, Sanmarco ME: Long-term effects of physical training on coronary patients with impaired ventricular function. *Circulation* 1979;60:1519–1526.

60. Hagberg JM, Ehsani AA, Holloszy JO: Effect of 12 months of intense exercise training on stroke volume in patients with coronary artery disease. *Circulation* 1983;67:1194–1199.

61. Conn EH, Williams RS, Wallace AG: Exercise responses before and after physical conditioning in patients with severely depressed left ventricular function. *Am J Cardiol* 1982;49:296–300.

62. Coats AJS, Adamopoulos S, Meyer TE, Conway J, Sleight P: Effects of physical training in chronic heart failure. *Lancet* 1990;335:63–66.

63. Sullivan MJ, Higginbotham MB, Cobb FR: Exercise training in patients with severe left ventricular dysfunction: Hemodynamic and metabolic effects. *Circulation* 1988;78:506–515.

64. Sullivan MJ, Higginbotham MB, Cobb FR: Exercise training in patients with chronic heart failure delays ventilatory anaerobic threshold and improves submaximal exercise performance. *Circulation* 1989;79:324–329.

65. Coats AJS, Adamopoulos S, Radaelli A, et al: Controlled trial of physical training in chronic heart failure: Exercise performance, hemodynamics, ventilation, and autonomic function. *Circulation* 1992; 85:2119–2131.

66. Giannuzzi P, Temporelli PL, Tavazzi L, et al, and the EAMY Study Group: Cami-exercise training in anterior myocardial infarction: An ongoing multicenter randomized trial. *Chest* 1972;101(10): 3155–3225.

67. Kellermann JJ, Ben-Ari E, Fisman E, Hayet M, Drory Y, Haimovitz D: Physical training in patients with ventricular impairment. *Adv Cardiol* 1986;34: 131–147.

68. Hoffmann A, Duba J, Lengyel M, Majer K: The effect of training on the physical working capacity of MI patients with left ventricular dysfunction. *Eur Heart J* 1987;8:43–49.

69. Van Camp SP, Peterson RA: Cardiovascular complications of outpatient cardiac rehabilitation programs. *JAMA* 1986;256:1160–1163.

69a. Hambrecht R, Niebauer J, Fiehn E, et al: Physical training in patients with stable chronic heart failure: effects on cardiorespiratory fitness and ultrastructural abnormalities of leg muscles. *J Am Coll Cardiol* 1995;25:1239–49.

69b. Coats AJ, Adamopoulos S, Radaelli A, et al: Controlled trial of physical training in chronic heart failure. Exercise performance, hemodynamics, ventilation, and autonomic function. *Circulation* 1992; 85:2119–31.

70. Zetterquist S: The effect of active training on the nutritive blood flow in exercising ischemic legs. *Scand J Clin Lab Invest* 1970;25:101.

71. Brass EP, Hoppel CL: Relationship between acid-soluble carnitine and coenzyme A pools in vivo. *Biochem J* 1980;190:495.

72. Hiatt WR, Wolfel EE, Regensteiner JG, et al: Skeletal muscle carnitine metabolism in patients with unilateral peripheral arterial disease. *J Appl Physiol* 1992;73:346.

73. Hiatt WR, Regensteiner JG, Hargarten ME, et al: Benefit of exercise conditioning for patients with peripheral arterial disease. *Circulation* 1990;81: 602.

74. Holloszy JO, Schultz J, Kusnierkiewicz J, et al: Effects of exercise on glucose tolerance and insulin resistance: Brief review and some preliminary results. *Acta Med Scand Suppl* 1986;711:55.

75. Rogers MA, Yamamoto C, King DS, et al: Improvement in glucose tolerance after 1 week of exercise in patients with mild NIDDM. *Diabetes Care* 1988;11:613.

75a. Rosenthal M, Haskell WL, Solomon R, et al: Demonstration of a relationship between level of physical training and insulin-stimulated glucose utilization in normal humans. *Diabetes* 1983;32: 408–11.

75b. King DS, Dalsky GP, Clutter WE, et al: Effects of exercise and lack of exercise on insulin sensitivity and responsiveness. *J Appl Physiol* 1988;64: 1942–6.

76. King DS, Dalsky GP, Clutter WE, et al: Effects of exercise and lack of exercise on insulin sensitivity and responsiveness. *J Appl Physiol* 1988;64: 1942.

77. Soman VJ, Koivisto VA, Deibert D, et al: Increased insulin sensitivity and insulin binding to monocytes after physical training. *N Engl J Med* 1979;301: 1200.

78. Douen AG, Ramlal T,Cartee GD, et al: Exercise modulates the insulin-induced translocation of glucose transporters in rat skeletal muscle. *FEBS Lett* 1990;261:256.

79. Schneider S, Ruderman NB: Exercise and NIDDM. *Diabetes Care* 1991;14 (Suppl 2):52.

80. National Institutes of Health: Consensus development conference on diet and exercise in non-insulin-dependent diabetes mellitus. *Diabetes Care* 1987;10:639.

81. Bernbaum M, Albert SG, Cohen JD, et al: Cardiovascular conditioning in individuals with diabetic retinopathy. *Diabetes Care* 1989;12:740.

82. Kemmer FW, Tacken M, Berger M: Mechanism of exercise-induced hypoglycemia during sulfonylurea treatment. *Diabetes* 1987;36:1178.

83. Fletcher BJ, Lloyd A, Whaling JF, Fletcher GF: Exercise testing in the patient with musculoskeletal handicaps. *Arch Phys Med Rehabil* 1988;69:123–127.

84. Fletcher BJ, Dunbar SB, Felner JM, et al: Exercise testing and training in physically disabled men with clinical evidence of coronary artery disease. *Am J Cardiol* 1994;73:170–174.

85. Taylor CB, DeBusk RF, Davidson DM, Houston N, Burnett K: Optimal methods for identifying depression following hospitalization for myocardial infarction. *J Chronic Dis* 1981;34:127–133.

86. Shuster JK, Stern TA, Tesar GE: Psychological problems and their management, in Wenger NK, Hellerstein HK (eds): *Rehabilitation of the Coronary Patient.* New York, Churchill Livingstone, 1992, pp 483–510.

87. Frasure-Smith N, Lesperance F, Talajic M: Depression and 18-month prognosis after myocardial infarction. *Circulation* 1995;91:999–1005.

88. Papadoupoulos C: A survey of sexual activity after myocardial infarction. *Cardiovasc Med* 1978; 3:821.

89. Miller NH, Taylor CB, Davidson DM, Hill MN, Krantz DS: The efficacy of risk factor intervention and psychosocial aspects of cardiac rehabilitation. *J Cardiopulmon Rehabil* 1990;10:198–209.

90. Ott CR, Sivarajan ES, Newton KM, et al: A controlled randomized study of early cardiac rehabilitation: The Sickness Impact Profile as an assessment tool. *Heart Lung* 1983;12:162–170.

91. Oldridge NB: Cardiac rehabilitation exercise program: Compliance and compliance-enhancing strategies. *Sports Med* 1988;6:42–55.

92. Daltroy LH: Improving cardiac patient adherence to exercise programs: A clinical trial of health education. *J Cardiac Rehabil* 1985;5:40–49.

93. Oldridge NB, Jones NL: Improving patient compliance in cardiac exercise rehabilitation: Effects of written agreement and self-monitoring. *J Cardiac Rehabil* 1983;3:257–262.

94. Horwitz RI, Horwitz SM: Adherence to treatment and health outcomes. *Arch Intern Med* 1993; 153:1863–1868.

95. Roter BL: Patient's participation in patient–provider interaction: The effect of patient "question asking" in the quality of interaction, satisfaction, and compliance. *Health Ed Monograph* 1977;5: 281–315.

96. Kaplan FH: Assessing the effect of physician–patient interaction on the outcome of chronic disease. *Medical Care* 1989;27(Suppl 3):S110–S127.

97. Gorlin R: Must cardiology lose his heart? *J Am Coll Cardiol* 1992;19:1635–1640.

98. Friedman HS: Patient–physician interaction, in Shoemaker S (ed): *The Handbook of Health Behavior Changes.* New York, Springer Publishing, 1990, pp 85–101.

99. Delbanco TL: In reaching the doctor–patient relationship by inviting the patient's participation. *Ann Intern Med* 1992;116:414–418.

100. Lee IM. Physical activity, fitness, and cancer. In: Bouchard C, Shephard RJ, Stephens T, eds. Physical Activity, Fitness, and Health: International Proceedings and Consensus Statement. Champaign, IL: *Human Kinetics,* 1994:814–831.

101. Fletcher GF: Current status of cardiac rehabilitation, in *Current Problems in Cardiology.* St. Louis, Mosby Year Book, 1992.

102. Wenger NK, Froelicher ES, Smith LK, et al: Cardiac Rehabilitation. Clinical Practice Guideline No. 17. Rockville, MD: U.S. Department of Health and Human Services, Public Health Service, Agency for Health Care Policy and Research and the National Health, Lung, and Blood Institute. ACHCPR Publication No. 96-0672, October 1995.

103. Bar FW, Hoppener P, Diederiks J, et al: Cardiac rehabilitation contributes to the restoration of leisure and social activities after myocardial infarction. *J Cardiopulmon Rehabil* 1992;12:117–125.

104. DeBusk RF, Houston N, Haskell W, et al: Exercise training soon after myocardial infarction. *Am J Cardiol* 1979;44(7):1223–1229.

105. Mayou R, MacMahon D, Sleight P, Florencio MJ. Early rehabilitation after myocardial infarction. *Lancet* 1981;2:1399–1402.

106. Lamm G, Denolin H, Dorossiev D, Pisa Z. Rehabilitation and secondary prevention of patients after acute myocardial infarction. WHO collaborative study. *Adv Cardiol* 1982;31:107–111.

107. Hedback B, Perk J. Five-year results of a comprehensive rehabilitation programme after myocardial infarction. *Eur Heart J* 1987;8(3):234–242.

108. Hertzeanu HL, Shemesh J, Aron LA, et al: Ventricular arrhythmias in rehabilitated and nonrehabilitated post myocardial infarction patients with left ventricular dysfunction. *Am J Cardiol* 1993;71:24–27.

108a. Smith SC, Jr., Blair SN, Criqui MH, et al: Preventing heart attack and death in patients with coronary disease. *Circulation* 1995;92:2–4.

34

Cardiac Rehabilitation and Risk Factor Modification

Charles E. Rackley, MD, and Fred Kuhn, MD

INTRODUCTION

The goal of risk factor modification in the post–myocardial infarction patient is to reduce the incidence of future ischemic events (see also Ch. 33). The risk factors for coronary artery disease have been widely publicized by the National Cholesterol Education Program (NCEP) (1). Fixed risk factors include age, gender, and family history, and modifiable factors consist of elevated low-density lipoprotein (LDL) cholesterol, low high-density lipoprotein (HDL) cholesterol, smoking, hypertension, and diabetes (Table 34–1) (2). The angiographic regression trials with diet and lipid lowering drugs have shown not only improvement in coronary anatomy with regression and slowing of progression of the atherosclerotic process, but also a significant reduction in cardiovascular events (3,4). Based on these angiographic trials, the new NCEP guidelines emphasize further reduction of LDL cholesterol in patients with established atherosclerotic disease. This chapter will review the metabolic and molecular basis for risk factor reduction, which primarily recognizes the role of oxidized LDL in the pathogenesis of coronary atherosclerosis. Specific risk factor modification will focus on LDL and HDL cholesterol, smoking, hypertension, diabetes, and hormone replacement in females.

PATHOGENESIS OF CORONARY ATHEROSCLEROSIS AND INFLUENCE OF RISK FACTORS

The prevailing theory for atherosclerosis based on extensive laboratory studies implicates the oxidation of LDL as being an initial pathologic step in the process. Various substances and clinical conditions can enhance the oxidation of LDL, which can damage the endothelium, create foam cells, and induce production of growth factors and inflammation (Table 34–2) (5). Oxidized LDL impairs the function of the endothelium and inhibits the production of the endothelial-derived relaxing factor (EDRF) (6,7). Normal release of EDRF produces relaxation in response to stimulations of neurotransmitters, cold, and other forms of stress. The loss of the relaxing factor results in an abnormal response to acetylcholine, which then induces vasoconstriction of the vessel (8–11). Oxidized LDL promotes binding of monocytes to the endothelial surface, conversion to macrophages, and formation of foam cells with increased LDL uptake. Oxidized LDL also stimulates growth factors that influence the fibromuscular hyperplasia and migration with foam cells into the endothelial space. Proteoglycans, P-selectin, monocyte chemoattractant factor, and

Table 34–1. Risk Factors for Coronary Artery Disease

Fixed Risk Factors	Modifiable Risk Factors
• Age: Males ≥45 years Females ≥55 years or premature menopause without estrogen replacement	• Elevated LDL • Low HDL • Smoking • Hypertension • Diabetes
• Family history of premature coronary artery disease (definite MI or sudden death <55 in male first-degree relative or <65 in female first- degree relative)	
"Negative" Risk Factor	
• HDL ≥ 60 mg/dl	

vascular adhesion molecules are all influenced by oxidized LDL and thus promote development of a fatty streak and eventually a soft plaque (12). Mildly oxidized LDL can induce these inflammatory molecules by increasing the rate of gene transcription. Auto-antibodies to oxidatively modified LDL have been demonstrated in carotid and coronary atherosclerosis (13–16). The soft lipid core of the plaque, subjected to the influence of abnormal vasoconstriction and inflammatory mechanisms, can eventually rupture and cause thrombosis of the lumen (Fig. 34–1) (17). In this manner, mild atherosclerotic lesions that do not hemodynamically impair coronary blood flow can rupture, and the resulting thrombosis can partially or totally occlude the vessel.

Several recent studies indicate that abnormal endothelial responsiveness induced by elevated cholesterol can be normalized with cholesterol reduction. Treasure and colleagues (9) noted improved endothelial responsiveness to acetylcholine in patients treated with lovastatin. Interestingly this benefit was seen in approximately 6 months suggesting that entholelial function can improve

Table 34–2. Role of Oxidized LDL in Atherosclerosis

1. Endothelial damage
2. Alteration in vascular tone
3. Monocyte/macrophage recruitment
4. Increased uptake of LDL by foam cells
5. Induction of growth factors
6. Formation of auto-antibodies to oxidized LDL

Adapted from Steinberg et al (5).

Role of Risk Factors in Myocardial Infarction

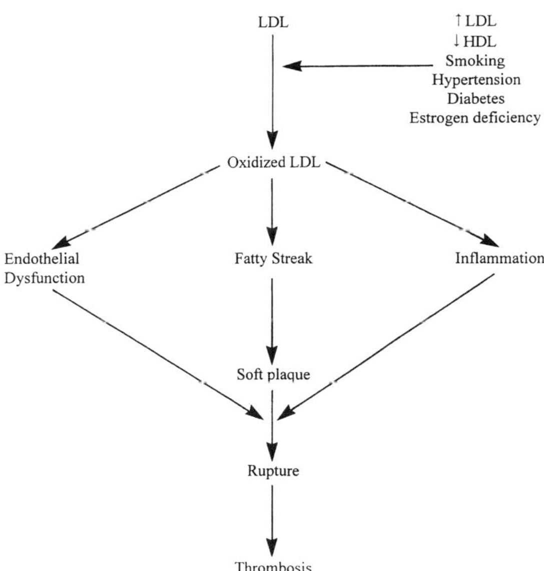

Figure 34–1. Role of risk factors in myocardial infarction.

rapidly. Similar results were seen by Anderson and colleagues in patients randomly assigned to lovastatin and the antioxidant probucol (10). Taken together these studies suggest that beneficial effects of lipid lowering noted in clinical trials may indeed be related to plague stabilization.

Evidence that cholesterol lowering can indeed reduce secondary events in patients following acute myocardial infarction was recently reported in the CARE trial (17b).

The results of clinical thrombolytic trials have revealed that after restoration of flow, the infarct-related vessel often has a residual stenosis of less than 60% (17). Such ischemic events provide a clinical basis for the role of oxidized LDL and rupture of soft plaques before hemodynamic embarrassment of blood flow through the vessel develops. Inflammatory cells have been identified at the margins of ruptured plaques in patients with acute myocardial infarction (18). Clinically, cytokines such as tumor necrosis factor and interferon along with elevations in C-reactive protein have been observed in patients with stable and unstable angina

(19). Angioscopic studies of human coronary arteries have reported an increased incidence of subsequent ischemic events in those individuals with yellowish plaques compared with those with whitish plaques, once again providing supporting evidence for the influence of lipid accumulation on plaque instability and tendency to rupture with subsequent ischemic events (20). Thus a large body of experimental data on isolated cells and vascular studies is now supported by clinical observations on the role of cholesterol, and in particular oxidized LDL cholesterol, in the atherosclerotic process in human coronary arteries.

Elevated levels of LDL, low levels of HDL, cigarette smoking, elevated blood pressure, high blood sugar, and reduced estrogen levels have all been shown to influence the oxidation of the LDL molecule (21–25). Therefore, modification of plasma lipids and the associated clinical interactions of smoking, hypertension, diabetes, and estrogen deficiency becomes a scientific approach for slowing the atherosclerotic process and reducing ischemia events in post–myocardial infarction patients. Clinical interventions to slow the rate of oxidation of LDL can stabilize the surface of the plaque by restoring endothelial function, decreasing lipid accumulation, and diminishing inflammation mechanisms.

LIPIDS

In 1993 the National Cholesterol Education Program revised its original 1987 guidelines with particular emphasis on goals for patients with established atherosclerosis. This would particularly apply to the post–myocardial infarction patient with clinical coronary artery disease. The original guidelines had targeted patients with two or more risk factors to achieve a total cholesterol of less than 200 and LDL below 130 mg/dl. Influenced by the results of the angiographic regression trials, which demonstrated both anatomic improvement and reduction in clinical events, the new goal for LDL in clinical atherosclerosis was recommended to be below 100 mg/dl. This would equate to a total cholesterol in the range of 160–180 mg/dl.

To apply the guidelines for lipid reduction goals to patients with acute myocardial infarction, physicians must be aware of the changes that occur in lipid values with acute myocardial infarction. These changes occur within the first 24–48 hours after an onset of chest pain (Table 34–3) (26). These new values generally reach their nadir at day 7 postinfarction, with LDL and HDL cholesterol fractions 48% and 32%, respectively, below baseline values, while the triglyceride levels may rise as high as 58% above baseline levels. These values may require 30–60 days before returning to preinfarction levels. Total cholesterol may remain stable during the first 24 hours after infarction, and the HDL fraction may be constant for 2–3 days after the acute event. However, the LDL decreases by an average of 31% on the day after myocardial infarction. In addition to the metabolic changes surrounding the acute event, beta blocking drugs, furosemide and other diuretic agents, and heparin can contribute to the alteration of lipid levels. An accurate baseline lipid profile probably cannot be obtained until 2 months after the acute myocardial infarction. Thus any prior information from the patient record on dyslipidemia for comparison with the infarction profile would be most helpful. Nevertheless, knowledge of

Table 34–3. Lipid Changes with Acute Myocardial Infarction

	Time After Symptom Onset			
Lipid	Day 1	Day 2	Day 7	Day 30
Cholesterol	−4% to −15%	−6% to −16%	−24% to −31%	−14%
LDL	−31%	−33%	−48%	−29%
HDL	−7%	−9%	−32%	Baseline
Triglyceride	+12%	+25%	+58%	+8%

Adapted from Rosenson (26).

the lipid changes after myocardial infarction would permit extrapolation to preinfarction values, which could serve as useful guides.

The angiographic regression trials provided an important clinical basis for aggressive lipid lowering in the treatment of coronary artery disease. The Familial Atherosclerotic Treatment Study (FATS) by Brown and colleagues in Seattle, Washington, provided the first objective evidence of angiographic regression and lack of progression after 2 1/2 years of combined treatment with lovastatin, colestipol, or niacin (27). Coronary events were more common in the control group and included myocardial infarction, angioplasty, bypass surgery, or death. This was the first major clinical study to document anatomic and clinical improvement with lipid lowering efforts in coronary artery disease. Additional regression trials included the Monitored Atherosclerosis Regression Study (MARS) and the Canadian Coronary Atherosclerosis Intervention Trial (CCAIT) (28,29). Both of these trials showed slowing of the progression of the disease, and the CCAIT trial demonstrated a 50% reduction in the development of new lesions. The Multicenter Anti-Atheroma Study (MAAS) was conducted in the Netherlands with simvastatin and again demonstrated significant slowing of progression of anatomic disease over a 4-year period (30). Trials employing pravastatin as the lipid lowering agent included the Pravastatin Limitation of Atherosclerosis in Coronary Arteries (PLAC I) and the Regression Growth Evaluation Statin Study (REGRESS), both of which use quantitative angiographic endpoints and demonstrated significantly less progression in the treated group compared with that in the placebo control groups (31,32). Several studies employed B-mode echocardiography to measure carotid intimal medial thickness with co-A reductase inhibitors. These trials included the Asymptomatic Carotid Artery Progression Study (ACAPS) employing lovastatin, and the Pravastatin, Lipids, and Atherosclerosis in Carotids (PLAC II) Study (33,34). Both of these studies demonstrated a significant reduction in cardiovascular events over a 3-year period of follow-up.

Two important studies on a single agent co-A reductase inhibitor and cardiovascular events were the Pravastatin Multinational Study and the Scandinavian Simvastatin Survival Study (4S) (35,36). The Pravastatin Multinational Study measured cholesterol reduction over a period of 26 weeks in controlled and treated patients who had a high incidence of cardiovascular risk factors. At the end of the study period there was a 92% reduction of cardiovascular events in the treated group compared with the placebo control group. In the 4S multicenter trial, patients were followed for 5.4 years, and this was a major study demonstrating not only a 42% reduction in cardiovascular mortality but a 30% reduction in overall mortality. Thus the angiographic, echocardiographic, and clinical trials using co-A reductase inhibitors have demonstrated not only the anatomic slowing or regression of coronary lesions but also a significant reduction in the development of unstable angina, acute myocardial infarction, the need for angioplasty or bypass surgery, and finally a reduction in cardiovascular and total mortality.

Diet and exercise remain a mainstay of initial treatment of lipid disorders in the postinfarction patient. The Lifestyle Heart Study by Ornish has demonstrated a reduction in symptoms and slowing of angiographic progression with the use of a vegetarian diet, exercise, and stress modification without lipid lowering drugs (37). Schuler and colleagues documented regression of anatomical coronary disease on a regimen of physical exercise and a low-fat diet along with a reduction in stress-induced myocardial ischemia (38). Thus dietary modification remains an important intervention in lipid modification and the impact on anatomical coronary disease and clinical events (39,40).

The goal for lipid values of the postinfarction patient should be an LDL less than 100 mg/dl. As discussed earlier, the lipid profile may not return to normal for 2 months, but any lipid profile obtained during the acute phase of the myocardial infarction can be related via Table 34–3 for extrapolation to a baseline value for LDL and other lipid components. Thus the postinfarction patient should be discharged not only with instructions on a standard American Heart Association low-fat diet and an exercise program, but also the use of a lipid lowering drug if the LDL is above 100 mg/dl. A co-A reductase inhibitor would be the drug of first choice to lower the LDL below 100. Two-month postinfarction lipid profiles should be measured, and if the LDL remains above 130 or the HDL remains below 35 mg/dl, a second agent might be considered. These agents would either be gemfibrozil or niacin. When either niacin or gemfibrozil is combined with a co-A reductase inhibitor, the baseline liver function studies, in particular the liver enzymes and creatine phosphokinase (CPK) should be obtained at baseline and after 6–8 weeks to monitor the compatibility of these drugs. Although warnings were initially published about the concern of rabdomyalysis with the combination of these agents, recent trials have reported a low incidence of enzyme abnormalities. Nevertheless, patients should be monitored every 2–3 months with lipid profiles and liver function studies. Brown and colleagues in Seattle has found that patients frequently require more than a single agent to achieve the optimal goal of an LDL below 100 (27).

In addition to goals for LDL cholesterol in the postinfarction patient, elevation of the HDL should also be considered. The Framingham Study was the first to recognize that low levels of HDL were associated with an increased risk for cardiovascular disease (41). Angiographic studies have reported that an abnormally low HDL value more frequently correlates with the presence of anatomic coronary disease than do elevated values for total cholesterol and LDL (42). In patients experiencing a myocardial infarction under the age of 60, the most commonly observed lipid abnormality is an abnormally low HDL value (43). Experimentally and clinically, HDL appears to antagonize the oxidation of LDL and facilitates removal of cholesterol from the vascular walls (44,45). Additional protective mechanisms of HDL include an increase in prostacyclin production, stabilization of serum prostacyclin, reduction in platelet aggregability, increase in antithrombotic activities, and promotion of regenerated endothelial proliferation (46–50). The angiographic regression trials have generally shown elevations of HDL and reductions of LDL in response to diet and drug treatment. The range for HDL elevation in males has been between 40 and 50 in the successful regression trials. Although the optimal range has not been established for women, studies have reported that females with HDLs under 50 are at greater risk for atherosclerotic disease, and reaching this level could be construed as a reasonable goal. Regular exercise, even when performed only modestly, is the best nontherapeutic intervention to raise HDL. Niacin and gemfibrozil are two pharmacologic agents with the potential for raising HDL (39,51). Niacin can raise the values as high as 30%, whereas gemfibrozil may raise them 15–20%. In postmenopausal females, estrogen has also been associated with a 20–30% elevation of HDL (51). Therefore, the goals for optimal lipid modification in the postinfarction patient could include an LDL value below 100 and an HDL value above 35.

SMOKING AND HEART DISEASE

Cigarette smoking is a major modifiable risk factor for coronary artery disease (see Ch. 33). The risk of coronary heart disease has been estimated to increase anywhere from 2-to 11-fold in smokers. Several studies suggest that the impact of smoking is dose related. In the Pooling Project, a 2-fold increase in risk was noted in individuals who smoked one-half pack of cigarettes per day (52). This risk increased to 3-fold with greater than 1 pack per day. In the Nurse's Health Study, women who smoked as little as 1–4 cigarettes daily increased their risk 2.5-fold, whereas those who smoked more than 45 cigarettes daily had an 11-fold increase in risk (53). The attributable risk in this study was particularly high in older individuals, in whom smoking is in fact a dominant risk factor contributing to coronary heart disease. The impact of smoking on coronary heart disease appears to be additive to other risk factors (54). In both men and women the absolute risk of smoking is highest in those at greatest risk, namely those with other risk factors for coronary heart disease (52,53). Although the data clearly indicate that a dose–response relationship exists, low nicotine cigarettes do not appear to be any less hazardous (55–57). Recent evidence from the MRFIT study suggests that even passive smoking may increase cardiovascular risk, as there was a significant increase in heart disease in men whose wives smoked (58).

Smoking may increase the risk of cardiovascular disease through several mechanisms. First, smoking acts indirectly by producing deleterious alterations in other risk factors. Compared with nonsmokers, smokers have higher LDL cholesterol and triglycerides and lower HDL values (59). Smoking may also increase the risk of hypertension and limit effectiveness of antihypertensive therapy (60). Recent evidence suggests that smoking may also have a more direct action on lipid metabolism by promoting oxidation of LDL, which is thought to enhance its atherogenic potential (61). In the MARS trial, a coronary regression study, smokers were more likely to have had progression of coronary artery disease and less likely to have undergone regression than nonsmokers (62). Smoking also alters endothelial function and promotes paradoxical vasoconstriction in response to endothelial-dependent vasodilators, suggesting that it may impair release of EDRF (63). Thus smokers may be more prone to abnormal vasoconstriction, which in turn could contribute to plaque rupture. Smoking is also procoagulant. Smokers have higher fibrinogen levels and enhanced platelet aggregation compared with nonsmokers (64,65). Thus smoking may contribute to coronary heart disease through its ability to enhance plaque formation via increased lipid accumulation and oxidation, as well as its effects on vasomotion, coagulation, and platelet function, which enhance plaque rupture and thrombosis.

The benefits of smoking cessation are clear and rapid. Rosenberg and colleagues have shown that the risk of myocardial infarction returns to baseline within 3 to 4 years of smoking cessation in women (66). Interestingly, this rapid benefit was independent of age, duration, and quantity of smoking. Similar results have been reported in men (67). There is also an important secondary preventive benefit to smoking cessation. Mortality rates following acute myocardial infarction are lower in those who quit compared with the rates in those who continue to smoke (68). In the CASS study, long-term survival was significantly higher in those who quit smoking following bypass surgery (69). Indeed, nonquitters who had undergone surgery had a similar overall mortality to the medically treated group.

It is estimated that interventions to promote smoking cessation are more cost-effective than almost any other health care intervention in terms of cost per year of life saved (70,71). Thus smoking cessation is a cost-effective approach, which can significantly lower cardiovascular risk in a relatively short period of time.

HYPERTENSION

Hypertension is among the most common modifiable risk factors for heart disease. It is estimated that more than 50 million adults in the United States—1 in 4—are hypertensive (72). The prevalence of hypertension increases with age and is higher in African Americans than in whites (73). Hypertension increases risk of coronary heart disease, stroke, congestive heart failure, and renal failure (74). Elevated systolic and diastolic blood pressure are both independently associated with increased risk of coronary heart disease and stroke (75,76). According to data from the MRFIT study, risk rises in a curvilinear fashion without evidence of a threshold effect (77). Moreover, hypertension interacts with other risk factors such as hypercholesterolemia, diabetes mellitus, and smoking in a synergistic fashion (75).

Hypertension may contribute to atherosclerotic coronary heart disease via a number of mechanisms. Hypertension increases shear stress, which promotes arterial injury especially at areas of turbulent blood flow such as branch points. Increased levels of Oxygen derived free radicals have been reported in essential hypertension, as well as enhanced LDL oxidation (23,24). These areas may be more prone to lipid accumulation and are often the initial sites of plaque development (78). Hypertension has been shown to impair endothelial function by reducing release of endothelial-derived relaxing factor (EDRF) (79). In this setting, abnormal vasoconstrictive responses to endothelial-dependent vasodilators can occur. Such abnormal vasoconstriction may contribute to plaque rupture and ultimately acute ischemic events and infarction. Hypertension is also associated with smooth muscle proliferation, which could therefore enhance atherosclerotic plaque formation and abnormal vasoconstriction (80). Neurohumoral abnormalities, which are thought to contribute to hypertension, may themselves contribute to the pathogenesis of atherosclerosis. Evidence that the renin–angiotensin system may have an intimate role in atherogenesis stems from the Survival and Ventricular Enlargement (SAVE) trial, in which an angiotensin converting enzyme (ACE) inhibitor was associated with a lower rate of reinfarction following myocardial infarction (81).

Recognition of the cardiovascular impact of hypertension along with increasing evidence of treatment benefit have led to an increasingly strict definition of hypertension. In the most recent report of the Joint National Committee on Detection, Evaluation and Treatment of High Blood Pressure (JNC V), normal blood pressure was defined as systolic and diastolic blood pressures below 130 and 85 mm Hg, respectively (82). Pressures between 130 and 139 mm Hg systolic and between 85 and 89 mm Hg diastolic are to be considered high normal. Blood pressures above these values are considered high and warrant further evaluation and treatment according to published guidelines.

Blood pressure control clearly reduces cardiovascular morbidity and mortality. Antihypertensive therapy has been associated with a significant reduction in stroke. In a recent meta-analysis of 14 clinical trials, a 5–6 mm Hg reduction in diastolic blood pressure was associated with a 42% reduction in stroke (83). Reductions in coronary heart disease (CHD) have been more difficult to prove. A modest 14% reduction for CHD events was noted in the same meta-analysis. Several reasons have been advanced for the discrepancy between stroke and cardiac benefits of antihypertensive therapy. Some of the benefits of blood pressure lowering in early trials may have been offset by adverse events related to diuretic therapy, but this is a matter of intense controversy. A much larger overall reduction in CHD events of 27% was noted in the Medical Research Council (MRC) trial (84). This greater benefit may have been related to differences in study population, as the MRC trial primarily involved older patients who might be expected to be at higher overall cardiovascular risk and therefore likely to derive the greatest benefit of antihypertensive therapy. Other trials, including the Systolic Hypertension in the Elderly Program (76), have confirmed that the elderly derive substantial cardiovascular benefit from treatment of systolic hypertension.

Guidelines for treatment of hypertension are published elsewhere (82). In general all patients should be instructed to perform lifestyle modifications including limiting salt intake, reducing weight, performing regular exercise, and limiting alcohol intake and stress. Pharmacologic therapy should be considered when these measures fail. According to the JNC, diuretics and beta blockers are recommended as first-line therapy unless contraindicated, because compared with other agents, they have been most extensively studied in long-term trials in which reductions in morbidity and mortality have been demonstrated. The use of beta blockers demonstrated reduction in post–myocardial infarction mortality and thus provided additional anti-ischemia benefits in the treatment of hypertension (85). Angiotensin converting enzyme inhibitors after myocardial infarction have shown long-term protective benefits, with reduction in both development of severe heart failure and mortality (86). Other agents may provide similar benefits, but results of large long-term trials are needed to evaluate the impact of other drugs on cardiovascular morbidity and mortality.

DIABETES

Insulin deficiency has long been associated with lipid abnormalities and accelerated atherosclerosis. Lipid abnormalities include elevated cholesterol, triglycerides, and LDL with depressed values of HDL. Glycosylated LDL is prone to oxidative modification. Lack of insulin can significantly raise triglycerides, which further lower HDL. High blood sugar levels enhance the oxidation of LDL.

The Multicenter Diabetes Control and Complication Trial demonstrated improvement in lipid values with tight glucose control (87). Standard diabetic control is 1 to 2 injections per day, but tight control was defined as 3 or more injections per day. Since the entry age in the study was 13 to 39 years, a significant reduction in cardiovascular events was not shown over the 6-year period. Tight glucose control can be supplemented with the reductase inhibitors gemfibrozil, niacin, and the bile salt resins. Lipid lowering agents favored for diabetes are the reductase inhibitors for elevated cholesterol and LDL, and gemfibrozil for high triglycerides and low HDL. If a reductase inhibitor is the initial drug to lower LDL, a persistently low HDL may require addition of gemfibrozil or niacin. A combination of agents should be monitored every 2 or 3 months with liver function studies and blood glucose values since niacin can elevate the blood sugar.

HORMONE REPLACEMENT IN FEMALES

Cardiovascular disease is now widely recognized as the major health factor in the postmenopausal female (88,89). Menopause is associated with a slight rise in cholesterol and LDL and stable or declining HDL values (90). Estrogen replacement in the postmenopausal female has been associated with a reduced incidence of anatomic coronary disease (51,91). This reduced incidence of anatomic coronary disease with hormone replacement has been associated with significant elevation of the HDL fraction. Estrogen deprivation both in experimental animals and clinical subjects has been attended by abnormal vasoconstriction of both the coronary and peripheral vessels when challenged by acetylcholine. This abnormal vasoconstriction can be reversed by the infusion of estradiol into the coronary arteries, and oral estrogen will restore endothelium-dependent flow in peripheral arteries (92,93). Furthermore, estrogen replacement in females slows the oxidation of LDL (94). Thus experimental and clinical evidence strongly support estrogen replacement in the postmenopausal female. Therefore, any female who has experienced a myocardial infarction should be a strong candidate for estrogen replacement (95).

Even though retrospective findings on lipid abnormalities and abnormal vasoactivity in the postmenopausal female are impressive, major prospective trials are under way to document the benefits of estrogen replacement and/or the combination with progesterone. Preliminary reports on the Postmenopausal Estrogen and Progesterone Interventional Trial have shown the highest elevation of HDL with estrogen replacement alone, but the withdrawal bleeding required interruption in a large number of study patients (96). Smaller doses of progesterone along with the estrogen still permit beneficial influence on the lipid components. While clinical trials will confirm the influence of estrogen and progesterone on coronary artery disease in women, retrospective data strongly support estrogen replacement in the postinfarction, postmenopausal female, along with other lipid lowering agents (97). In the hysterectomized individual, replacement estrogen on a daily basis with either premarin or estradiol would be the agent of choice. For the woman with an intact uterus, a combination of estrogen and progesterone with either monthly or quarterly interruptions with progesterone would seem appropriate. Mammograms and pap smears probably should be done on a yearly basis in these individuals.

ANTIOXIDANT THERAPY

Based on laboratory research and observational studies, antioxidants appear promising but unproved clinically to decrease risks of cardiovascular disease (5). Beta-carotene, vitamin C, or vitamin E can influence the effects of oxidized LDL. Beta-carotene does not inhibit oxidation of LDL in plasma but may prevent endothelial damage by decreasing uptake of oxidized LDL (98). The Nurse's Health Study indicated a reduced risk of coronary artery disease with intake of vitamin E supplements (99). Trends were observed with beta-carotene, but there was no relation to vitamin C intake. In contrast, data from the Iowa Women's health study 99a revealled on inverse relationship between dietary vitamin E intake and risk of cardiovascular disease. There was no benefit noted from vitamin E supplements and no association between vitamin A or C intake and cardiovascular disease. The Health Professionals Follow-up Study showed significant trend to lower coronary artery disease risk with increased vitamin E and beta-carotene (100). The National Health and Nutrition Examination Survey suggested lower cardiovascular mortality with high vitamin C intake (101). In a small subgroup of the Physicians Health Study, 50 mg beta-carotene on alternate days was reported to produce a 51% reduction in the combined endpoint of cardiovascular events (102). However, in a 12-year follow-up of the Health study, no relationship was noted between Beta carotene supplementation and cardiovascular disease (103).

SUMMARY RECOMMENDATIONS

The postinfarction patient should enter an exercise rehabilitation program as outlined by Fletcher in Chapter 33. A standard American Heart Association low-fat diet should be instructed and implemented (104). If the LDL cholesterol prior to discharge is greater than 100, a reductase inhibitor should be initiated (Table 34–4). Strong emphasis on smoking cessation with enrollment in a program and the use of patches should be advised. Blood pressure should be controlled and a beta blocker or an ACE inhibitor used, not only for the postinfarction benefits of reduced ischemic events and remodeling, but also for the optimization of systemic blood pressure. Diabetic control should be established with blood sugars in the normal range. In women, who generally will be postmenopausal with their infarctions, estrogen replacement should be strongly considered. Those with an intact uterus should be placed on a combination of estrogen and progesterone, whereas those with previous hysterectomies can take daily estrogen. At 2 months, a lipid profile should be obtained for measuring total cholesterol, HDL, triglyceride, and LDL cholesterol. If the LDL is still above 100, a second agent, either gemfibrozil or niacin, should be considered. Furthermore, these agents would also benefit the HDL value, which may be below 35. Patients should continue their lifestyle modification with the diet and daily exercise program. Lipids should be checked every 2–3 months until stable, and thereafter at least 3 times a year. Lifestyle modification for diet, exercise, stress modification, and medication compliance should be frequently reinforced. The goal of risk factor modification and treatment in the postinfarction patient is reduction of future ischemic events. With these measures, the natural history of coronary artery disease can be changed.

Table 34–4. Postinfarction Risk Factor Treatment

Factor	Goal	Therapy
1. LDL	<100 mg/dl	Reductase inhibitors, niacin, gemfibrozil, resins
2. HDL	>35 mg/dl	Exercise, niacin, gemfibrozil
3. Smoking	Cessation	Programs, patches
4. Hypertension	<140/90 mm Hg	Diuretics, β blockers, ACE inhibitors
5. Diabetes	Normal blood sugar	Diet, insulin
6. Estrogen	Replacement	Estrogen, progesterone

REFERENCES

1. Expert Panel on Detection, Evaluation and Treatment of High Blood Cholesterol in Adults: Summary of the second report of the National Cholesterol Education Program (NCEP) Expert Panel on Detection, Evaluation, and Treatment of High Blood Cholesterol in Adults (Adult Treatment Panel II). *JAMA* 1993;269:3015–3023.
2. Rackley CE: Analysis of cardiovascular risk factors, in Forker AD, Piepho RW (eds): *Clinical Pharmacology of Cardiovascular Risk Factors.* Norwalk, CT, GEM Communications, 1995, pp 4–7.
3. Superko HR, Krauss RM: Coronary artery disease regression: Convincing evidence for the benefit of aggressive lipoprotein management. *Circulation* 1994; 90:1056–1069.
4. Rackley CE: Monotherapy with HMG co-A reductase inhibitors and secondary prevention in coronary artery disease. *Clin Cardiol,* Sept. 1996.
5. Steinberg D, Parthasarathy S, Carew TE, Khoo JC, Witztum JL: Beyond cholesterol: Modifications of low-density lipoprotein that increases atherogenicity. *N Engl J Med* 1989;320:915–924.
6. Kuhn FE, Mohler ER, Rackley CE: Cholesterol and lipoproteins: Beyond atherogenesis. *Clin Cardiol* 1992;15:883–890.
7. Liao JK, Shin WS, Lee WY, Clark S: Oxidized low-density lipoprotein decreases the expression of endothelial nitric oxide synthase. *Circulation* 1994;90: I-407.

8. Kuhn FE, Mohler ER, Satler LF, Reagan K. Lu DY, Rackley CE: Effects of high-density lipoprotein and acetylcholine induced coronary vasoreactivity. *Am J Cardiol* 1991;68:1425–1430.
9. Treasure CB, Klein JL, Weintraub WS, et al: Beneficial effects of cholesterol-lowering therapy on the coronary endothelium in patients with coronary artery disease. *N Engl J Med* 1995;332: 481–487.
10. Anderson TJ, Meredith IT, Yeung HZ, Frei B, Selwyn AP, Ganz P: Cholesterol lowering therapy improves endothelial function in patients with coronary atherosclerosis. *N Engl J Med* 1995;332: 488–493.
11. Quyyumi AA, Dakak N, Andrews NP, et al: Nitric oxide activity in the human coronary circulation: Impact of risk factors for coronary atherosclerosis. *J Clin Invest* 1995;95:1749–1755.
12. Berliner JA, Navab M, Fogelman AM, et al: Atherosclerosis: Basic mechanisms, oxidation inflammation and genetics. *Circulation* 1995;91:2488–2496.
13. Salonen JT, Yea-Herttuala S, Yamamoto R, et al: Autoantibody against oxidized LDL and progression of carotid atherosclerosis. *Lancet* 1992;339: 883–887.
14. Bui MN, Sack MN, Moutsatsos G, et al: Autoantibody titers to oxidatively modified low-density lipoprotein in patients with coronary atherosclerosis. *Am Heart J;* 1996;131:663–667.
15. Maggi E, Chiesa R, Melissano G, et al: LDL oxidation in patients with severe carotid atherosclerosis: A study of in vitro and in vivo oxidation markers. *Arterioscler Thromb* 1994;14:1892–1899.
16. Holvoet P, Perez G, Zhian Z, Brouwers E, Bernar H, Collen D: Malondialdehyde-modified low-density lipoproteins in patients with atherosclerotic disease. *J Clin Invest* 1995;95:2611–2619.
17. Brown BG, Zhao X-Q, Sacco DE, Albers JJ: Lipid lowering and plaque regression: New insights in the prevention of plaque disruption and clinical events in coronary disease. *Circulation* 1993;87:1781–1791.

17a. Anderson TJ, Meredith IT, Yeung AC, et al: The effect of cholesterol-lowering and antioxidant therapy on endothelium-dependent coronary vasomotion. *N Engl J Med* 1995;332:488–490.

17b. Pfeffer MA, Sacks FM, Moye LA, et al: Cholesterol and recurrent events: a secondary prevention trial for normolipidemic patients. *Amer J Cardiol* 1995; 76:98C.

18. van der Wal AC, Becker AE, van der Loos CM, Das P: Site of intimal rupture or erosion of thrombose in coronary atherosclerotic plaques is characterized by an inflammatory process irrespective of the dominant plaque morphology. *Circulation* 1994;89:36–44.
19. Vaddi K, Nicolini FA, Mehta P, Mehta JL: Increased secretion of tumenecrosis factor/α and inerfuron/γ by mononuclear leukocytes in patients with ischemic heart disease: Relevance in superoxide anine generation. *Circulation* 1994;90: 694–699.
20. Miatke T, Arakawa K, Satomura K, et al: Efficacy of angioscopic findings for prediction of cardiac events in patients with chronic ischemic heart disease. *J Am Coll Cardiol* 1995;Feb:428A.
21. Lavy A, Brook GJ, Danker G, Amotz AB, Aviram M: Enhanced in vivo oxidation of plasma lipoproteins derived from hypercholesterolemic patients. *Metabolism* 1991;40:794–799.
22. Cominacini L, Pastorino AM, Garbia U, et al: Susceptibility to oxidation of LDL derived from hypercholesterolemic patients and its relation to preformed lipid hydroperoxides in native LDL, in Ursini F, Cadenas E. (eds): *Dietary Lipids, Antioxidants and the Prevention of Atherosclerosis.* Padova, Italy, CLUEP, 1993, pp 97–99.
23. Sagar S, Kallo JI, Kaul N, Grangaly NK, Sharma BK: Oxygen-free radicals in essential hypertension. *Mol Cell Biochem* 1992;111:103–108.
24. Maggi E, Marchesi E, Ravetta V, Falaschi F, Finardi G, Belloma G: Low-density lipoprotein oxidation in essential hypertension. *J Hyperten* 1993;11: 1103–1111.
25. Mohler ER, Fineberg NS, Hathaway DR: Breath pentane, a by-product of lipid peroxidation in elevated and antioxidant vitamins decreased in smokers. *Circulation* 1992;86(Suppl I):I-8.
26. Rosenson RS: Myocardial injury: The acute phase response in lipoprotein metabolism. *J Am Coll Cardiol* 1993;22:933–940.
27. Brown BG, Albers JJ, Fisher LD, et al: Regression of coronary artery disease as a result of intensive lipid lowering therapy in men with high levels of apolipoprotein B. *N Engl J Med* 1990;323: 1289–1298.
28. Blankenhorn DH, Azen SP, Kramsch DM, et al, and the MARS Research Group: Coronary angiographic changes with lovastatin therapy: The Monitored

Atherosclerosis Regression Study (MARS). *Ann Intern Med* 1993;119:969–976.

29. Waters W, Higginson L, Gladstone P, et al, and the CCAIT Study Group: Effects of monotherapy with an HMG co-A reductase inhibitor on the progression of coronary atherosclerosis as assessed by serial quantitative arteriography. The Canadian Coronary Atherosclerosis Intervention Trial. *Circulation* 1994;89:959–968.
30. MAAS Investigators: Effect of simvastatin on coronary atheroma: The Multicenter Anti-Atheroma Study (MAAS). *Lancet* 1994;344:633–638.
31. Pitt B, Macini GBJ, Ellis SG, Rosman HS, McGovern ME, for the PLAC I Investigators: Pravastatin limitation of atherosclerosis in the coronary arteries (PLAC I). *J Am Coll Cardiol* 1994;Feb:131A.
32. Jukema JW, Burschke AVG, van Boven AJ, et al, on behalf of the REGRESS Study Group: Effects of lipid lowering by pravastatin on progression and regression of coronary artery disease in symptomatic men with normal to moderately elevated serum cholesterol levels: The Regression Growth Evaluation Statin Study (REGRESS). *Circulation* 1995;91: 2528–2540.
33. Furberg CD, Adams HP Jr, Applegate WB, et al, for the Asymptomatic Carotid Artery Progression Study (ACAPS) Research Group: Effect of lovastatin on early carotid atherosclerosis in cardiovascular events. *Circulation* 1994;90:1679–1687.
34. Crouse JR III, Byington RP, Bond MG, et al: Pravastatin, lipids, and atherosclerosis in the carotid arteries (PLAC II). *Am J Cardiol* 1995;75: 455–459.
35. The Pravastatin Multinational Study Group of Cardiac Risk Patients: Effects of pravastatin in patients with serum total cholesterol levels from 5.2 to 7.8 mmol/L (200–300 mg/dl) plus two additional atherosclerotic risk factors. *Am J Cardiol* 1993;72: 1031–1037.
36. The Scandinavian Simvastatin Survival Study Group: Randomized trial of cholesterol lowering in 4,444 patients with coronary heart disease: The Scandinavian Simvastatin Survival Study (4S). *Lancet* 1994;344:1383–1389.
37. Ornish D, Brown SE, Scherwitz LW, et al: Can lifestyle changes reverse coronary heart disease? The Lifestyle Heart Trial. *Lancet* 1990;336:129–133.
38. Schuler G, Hambrecht R, Schlierf G, et al: Myocardial perfusion and regression of coronary artery disease in patients on a regimen of intensive physical exercise and low-fat diet. *J Am Coll Cardiol* 1992;19:34–42.
39. Rackley CE: Coronary artery disease hyperlipidemia, in Hurst JW (ed): *Current Therapy in Cardiovascular Disease,* 4th ed. St. Louis, Mosby, 1994, pp 143–145.
40. Gould KL: Reversal of coronary atherosclerosis: Clinical promise as the basis for noninvasive management of coronary artery disease. *Circulation* 1994;90:1558–1571.
41. Castelli WP, Garrison RJ, Wilson PWF, Abbott RD, Kalousidan S, Kannel WB: Incidence of coronary heart disease and lipoprotein cholesterol levels. The Framingham Study. *JAMA* 1986;256:2835–2838.
42. Hong MK, Romm PA, Reagan K, Green C, Rackley CE: Effects of estrogen replacement therapy on serum lipid values in angiographically defined coronary artery disease in post-menopausal women. *Am J Cardiol* 1992;68:176–178.
43. Genest JJ Jr, Martin-Munley SS, McNamara JR, et al: Familial lipoprotein disorders in patients with premature coronary artery disease. *Circulation* 1992;85:2025–2033.
44. Eisenberg S: High-density lipoprotein metabolism. *J Lipid Res* 1984;25:1017–1058.
45. Ohta T, Takata K, Horiuchi S, Morino Y, Matsuda I: Protective effects of lipoproteins containing apoprotein A-I on Cu^{2+} catalyzed oxidation of human low-density lipoprotein. *FEBS Lett* 1989; 257:435–438.
46. Tauber J, Cheng J, Gospodarowicz D: Effects of high- and low-density lipoproteins on proliferation of cultured bovine vascular endothelial cells. *J Clin Invest* 1980;66:696–708.
47. Fleisher LN, Tall AR, Witte LD, Miller RW, Cannon PI: Stimulation of arterial endothelial cell prostacyclin synthesis by high-density lipoproteins. *J Bio Chem* 1982;257:6653–6655.
48. Saku K, Ahmad M, Glas-Greenwalt P, Kashyap MI: Activation of fibrinolysis by apolipoproteins of high-density lipoproteins in man. *Thromb Res* 1985;39:1–8.
49. Yui Y, Aoyama T, Morishita H, Takahashi M, Takatsu Y, Kawai C: Serum prostacyclin stabilizing factor is identical to apolipoprotein A-1 (apo A-1): A novel function of Apo A-1. *J Clin Invest* 1988;82: 803–807.
50. Aoyama T, Yui Y, Morishita H, Kawai C: Prostaglandin I_2 halflife regulated by high-density lipoprotein is decreased in acute myocardial infarc-

tion and unstable angina pectoris. *Circulation* 1990; 81:1784–1791.

51. Frick MH, Elo O, Haapa K, Heinonen OP, Heinsalmi P: Helsinki Heart Study: Primary prevention trial with gemfibrozil in middle-aged men with dyslipidemia: The safety of treatment, changes in risk factors in incidence of coronary heart disease. *N Engl J Med* 1987;317:1237–1245.
52. The Pooling Project Research Project Group: Relationship of blood pressure, serum cholesterol, smoking habit, relative weight, and ECG abnormalities to incidence of major coronary events: Final report of the Pooling Project. *J Chron Dis* 1978;31:301–306.
53. Willet WC, Green A, Stampher MJ, et al: Relative and absolute excess risk of coronary heart disease among women who smoke cigarettes. *N Engl J Med* 1987;317:1303–1309.
54. Kannel WB: Hypertension, blood lipids, and cigarette smoking as co-risk factors for coronary heart disease. *Ann NY Acad Sci* 1978;304:128.
55. Palmer J, Rosenberg L, Shapiro S: "Low yield" cigarettes and the risk of nonfatal myocardial infarction in women. *N Engl J Med* 1989;320:1569–1573.
56. Kaufman DW, Helmrich SP, Rosenberg L, Miettinen OS, Shapiro S: Nicotine and carbon monoxide content of cigarette smoke and the risk of myocardial infarction in young men. *N Engl J Med* 1983, 308:409–413.
57. Borland C, Chamberlain A, Higenbottam T, Shipley M, Rose G: Carbon monoxide yield of cigarettes and its relation to cardiorespiratory disease. *Br Med J* 1983;287:1583–1586.
58. Svendsen KH, Kuller LH, Martin MJ, Ockene JK: Effects of passive smoking in the Multiple Risk Factor Intervention Trial. *Am J Epidemiol* 1987; 126:783.
59. Migas OD: The lipid effects of smoking. *Am Heart J* 1988;115:272.
60. Langford HG, Stamler J, Wassertheil-Smoller S, Prineas RJ: All cause mortality in the Hypertension Detection and Follow-up Program. Findings for the whole cohort and for persons with less severe hypertension with and without other traits related to risk of mortality. *Prog Cardiovasc Dis* 1986;29:29.
61. Morrow JD, Frei B, Longmire AW, et al: Increase in circulating products of lipid peroxidation (F_2-isoprostanes) in smokers: Smoking as a cause of oxidative damage. *N Engl J Med* 1995;332: 1198–1203.
62. Blankenhorn DH, Azen SP, Kramsch DM, and the MARS Research Group: Coronary angiographic changes with lovastatin therapy: The Monitored Antherosclerosis Regression Study (MARS). *Ann Intern Med* 1993;119:970–976.
63. Quyyumi AA, Dakak N, Andrews NP, et al: Nitric oxide activity in the human coronary circulation: Impact of risk factors for coronary atherosclerosis. *J Clin Invest* 1995;95:1747–1755.
64. Meade TW, Imeson J, Stirling Y: Effects of changes in smoking and other characteristics on clotting factors and the risk of ischemic heart disease. *Lancet* 1987;2:986.
65. Nowak J, Murray JJ, Oates JA, Fitzgerald GA: Biochemical evidence of a chronic abnormality in platelet and vascular function in healthy individuals who smoke cigarettes. *Circulation* 1987;76:6.
66. Rosenberg L, Palmer JR, Shapiro S: Decline in the risk of myocardial infarction among women who stop smoking. *N Engl J Med* 1990;322:213–217.
67. Salonen JT: Stopping smoking and long-term mortality after acute myocardial infarction. *Br Heart J* 1980;43:463–469.
68. Burr ML, Holliday RM, Fehily AM, Whitehead PJ: Haematological prognostic indices after myocardial infarction: Evidence from the diet and reinfarction trial (DART). *Eur Heart J* 1992;13: 166–170.
69. Cavender JB, Rogers WJ, Fisher LD, Gersh BJ, Coggin CJ, Myers WO: Effects of smoking on survival and morbidity in patients randomized to medical or surgical therapy in the Coronary Artery Surgery Study (CASS): 10 year follow-up. *J Am Coll Cardiol* 1992;20:287–294.
70. Tsevat J: Impact and cost-effectiveness of smoking interventions. *Am J Med* 1992;93:43S–47S.
71. Krumholtz HM, Cohne BJ, Tsevat J, Pastrenak RC, Weinstein MC: Cost-effectiveness of a smoking cessation program after myocardial infarction. *J Am Coll Cardiol* 1993;22:1697–1702.
72. Joint National Committee: The 1988 report of the Joint National Committee on Detection, Evaluation, and Treatment of High Blood Pressure. *Arch Intern Med* 1988;148:1023–1038.
73. Hypertension Detection and Follow-up Program Cooperative Group: Race, education, and prevalence of hypertension. *Am J Epidemiol* 1977;106: 351.
74. MacMahan S, Peto R, Cutler J, et al: Blood pressure, stroke, and coronary heart disease, Part 1:

Prolonged differences in blood pressure: Prospective observation studies corrected for the regression dilutional basis. *Lancet* 1990;335:765–774.

75. Levy D, Wilson PWF, Anderson KM, Castelli WP: Stratifying the patient at risk from coronary artery disease: New insights from the Framingham Heart Study.
76. SHEP Cooperative Research Group: Prevention of stroke by antihypertensive drug treatment in older patients with isolated systolic hypertension: Final results of the Systolic Hypertension in the Elderly Program (SHEP). *JAMA* 1991;265:3255–3264.
77. Neaton JW, Wentworth D, for the Multiple Risk Factor Intervention Trial Research Group: Serum cholesterol, blood pressure, cigarette smoking, and death from coronary heart disease: Overall findings and differences by age for 316,099 white men. *Arch Intern Med* 1992;152:56–64.
78. Chobanian AV: The influence of hypertension and other hemodynamic factors in atherogenesis. *Prog Cardiovasc Dis* 1983;26:177–196.
79. Luscher TF, Yang Z, Diedrich D, Buhle FR: Endothelium derived vasoactive substances: Potential role in hypertension, atherosclerosis, and vascular occlusion. *J Cardiovasc Pharmacol* 1989;14(Suppl 6): S63.
80. Aalkjaer C, Heagerty AM, Bailey I, et al: Evidence for increased media thickness, increases neuronal amine uptake, and depressed excitation–contraction coupling in isolated resistance vessels from essential hypertensives. *Circ Res* 1987;61:181.
81. Pfeffer MA, Braunwald E, Moye LA, et al: Effect of captopril on mortality and morbidity in patients with left ventricular dysfunction after myocardial infarction: Results of the Survival and Ventricular Enlargement Trial. *N Engl J Med* 1992;327: 669–677.
82. The Fifth Report of the Joint National Committee on Detection, Evaluation, and Treatment of High Blood Pressure (JNC V). *Arch Intern Med* 1993;153: 154–183.
83. Collins R, Peto R, MacMahon S, et al: Blood pressure, stroke and coronary heart disease, part 2: Short term reduction in blood pressure: Overview of randomized drug trials in their epidemiological context. *Lancet* 1990;335:827–838.
84. MRC Working Party: Medical Research Council trial of treatment of hypertension in older adults: Principal results. *Br Med J* 1992;304:405–412.
85. Fishman WH, Furberg CD, Friedewald WT: β-Adrenergic blockade for survivors of acute myocardial infarction. *N Engl J Med* 1984;310: 830–837.
86. Pfeffer MA, Braunwald E, Moye LA, et al: Effect of captopril on mortality and morbidity in patients with left ventricular dysfunction after myocardial infarction. *N Engl J Med* 1992;327:669–677.
87. The Diabetes Control and Complication Trial Research Group: Effect of intensive diabetes management on macrovascular events in risk factors in the diabetes control and complications trial. *Am J Cardiol* 1995;75:894–903.
88. Lerner DJ, Kannel WB: Patterns of coronary heart disease morbidity and mortality in the sexes: A 26 year follow-up of the Framingham population. *Am Heart J* 1986;111:383–390.
89. Kuhn FE, Rackley CE: Coronary artery disease in women: Risk factors, evaluation, treatment and prevention. *Arch Intern Med* 1993;153:2626–2636.
90. Bush TL, Barrett-Connor E, Cowen LD, et al: Cardiovascular mortality in non-contraceptive use of estrogen in women: Results from the Lipid Research Clinic Program Follow-up Study. *Circulation* 1987;75:1102–1109.
91. Sullivan JM, Vander, Zwaag R, et al: Post-menopausal estrogen use in coronary atherosclerosis. *Ann Intern Med* 1988;108:358–363.
92. Reis SE, Gloth ST, Blumenthal RS, et al: Ethinyl estradiol acutely attenuates abnormal coronary vasomotor responses to acetylcholine in post-menopausal women. *Circulation* 1994;89:52–60.
93. Lieberman EH, Gerhard MD, Uehata A, et al: Estrogen improved endothelium dependent flow mediated vasodilation in post-menopausal women. *Ann Intern Med* 1994;121:936–941.
94. Sack MN, Rader DJ, Cannon RO III: Oestrogen and inhibition of low-density lipoproteins in post-menopausal women. *Lancet* 1994;343:269.
95. Rackley CE: Estrogen and coronary artery disease in post-menopausal women. *Am J Med;* 1995;99: 117–118.
96. The Writing Group for the PEPI Trial: Effects of estrogen or estrogen/progestion regimens on heart disease risk factors in post-menopausal women. *JAMA* 1995;273:199–208.
97. The American College of Physicians: Guideline for counseling post-menopausal women about preventive hormone therapy. *Ann Intern Med* 1992;117:1038.

98. Keaney JF Jr, Gaziano JM, Xu A, et al: Dietary anti-oxidants preserve endothelium-dependent vessel relaxation in cholesterol-fed rabbits. *Proc Natl Acad Sci USA* 1993;90:11880–11884.

99. Stampfer MJ, Hennekens CH, Manson JE, Colditz GA, Rosner B, Willett WC: Vitamin E consumption and the risk of coronary disease in women. *N Engl J Med* 1993;328:1444–1449.

99a. Kushi LH, Folsom AR, Prineas RJ, et al: Dietary antioxidant vitamins and death from coronary heart disease in postmenopausal women. *N Engl J Med* 1996;334:1156.

100. Rimm EB, Stampfer MJ, Ascherio A, Giovannucci E, Colditz GA, Willett WC: Vitamin E consumption and the risk of coronary heart disease in men. *N Engl J Med* 1993;328:1450–1456.

101. Enstrom JE, Kanin LE, Klein MA: Vitamin C intake and mortality among a sample of the United States population. *Epidemiology* 1992;3:194–202.

102. Gaziano JM, Manson JE, Ridker PM, Buring JE, Hennekens CH: Beta-carotene therapy for chronic stable angina. *Circulation* 1991;82(Suppl III):III-202.

103. Hennekens CH, Buring JE, Manson JE, et al: Lack of effect of long-term supplementation with beta carotene on the incidence of malignant neoplasms and cardiovascular disease. *N Engl J Med* 1996;334.

104. Rackley CE, Schlant RC: Prevention of coronary artery disease, in Schlant RC, Alexander, RW (eds): *The Heart*, 8th ed. New York, McGraw-Hill, 1994, chapter 62, pp 1205–1222.

INDEX